ETHICAL ISSUES IN MODERN MEDICINE: CONTEMPORARY READINGS IN BIOETHICS

SEVENTH EDITION

Bonnie Steinbock

University at Albany/State University of New York
Alden March Bioethics Institute

Alex John London

Carnegie Mellon University

John D. Arras

University of Virginia

McGraw Hill

Boston   Burr Ridge, IL   Dubuque, IA   Madison, WI   New York   San Francisco   St. Louis
Bangkok   Bogotá   Caracas   Kuala Lumpur   Lisbon   London   Madrid   Mexico City
Milan   Montreal   New Delhi   Santiago   Seoul   Singapore   Sydney   Taipei   Toronto

The *McGraw·Hill* Companies

McGraw-Hill
Higher Education

Published by McGraw-Hill, an imprint of The McGraw-Hill Companies, Inc., 1221
Avenue of the Americas, New York, NY 10020. Copyright © 2009, 2003, 1999, 1995, 1989,
1983, 1977. All rights reserved. No part of this publication may be reproduced or
distributed in any form or by any means, or stored in a database or retrieval system,
without the prior written consent of The McGraw-Hill Companies, Inc., including, but
not limited to, in any network or other electronic storage or transmission, or broadcast
for distance learning.

This book is printed on acid-free paper.

1 2 3 4 5 6 7 8 9 0 DOC/DOC 0 9 8

ISBN: 978-0-07-340735-7
MHID: 0-07-340735-6

Editor in Chief: *Michael Ryan*
Publisher: *Lisa Moore*
Sponsoring Editor: *Mark Georgiev*
Marketing Manager: *Pam Cooper*
Project Manager: *Amanda Peabody*
Manuscript Editor: *Sharon O'Donnell*
Design Manager: *Laurie Entringer*
Cover Designer: *Pam Verros*
Production Supervisor: *Randy Hurst*
Composition: *International Typesetting & Composition*
Printing: *45# New Era Pub Matte, R. R. Donnelley & Sons*

Cover: Microscopic HIV virus—Geostock/Getty Images

Library of Congress Cataloging-in-Publication Data

Ethical issues in modern medicine: contemporary readings in bioethics / [edited by]
   Bonnie Steinbock, John Arras, Alex John London.—7th ed.
     p.; cm.
   Includes bibliographical references.
   ISBN-13: 978-0-07-340735-7 (alk. paper)
   ISBN-10: 0-07-340735-6 (alk. paper)
   1. Medical ethics. I. Steinbock, Bonnie. II. Arras, John. III. London, Alex John.
[DNLM: 1. Ethics, Medical—Collected Works. 2. Bioethical Issues—Collected Works.
3. Professional-Patient Relations—Collected Works. W 50 E826 2006]
R724.E788 2008
174'.2—dc22

                                    2007039863

The Internet addresses listed in the text were accurate at the time of publication. The inclusion
of a Web site does not indicate an endorsement by the authors or McGraw-Hill, and McGraw-
Hill does not guarantee the accuracy of the information presented at these sites.

www.mhhe.com

CONTENTS

Preface   xiv

The Contributors   xvii

INTRODUCTION: MORAL REASONING IN THE MEDICAL CONTEXT   1

Bioethics: Nature and Scope   1

Sources of Bioethical Problems and Concerns   2

Challenges to Ethical Theory   6

Moral Theories and Perspectives   8

Religious Ethics   20

"Rights-Based" Approaches   23

Communitarian Ethics   26

Feminist Ethics   29

Virtue Ethics   31

Nonmoral Considerations   35

Modes of Moral Reasoning   35

PART ONE

FOUNDATIONS OF THE HEALTH PROFESSIONAL–PATIENT RELATIONSHIP   43

SECTION 1   AUTONOMY, PATERNALISM, AND MEDICAL MODELS   61

The Hippocratic Oath   61

The Refutation of Medical Paternalism 62
Alan Goldman

Beneficence Today, or Autonomy (Maybe) Tomorrow? 70

Commentary 71
Bernice S. Elger

Commentary 72
Jean-Claude Chevrolet

Why Doctors Should Intervene 73
Terrence F. Ackerman

Four Models of the Physician-Patient Relationship 78
Ezekiel J. Emanuel and Linda L. Emanuel

SECTION 2 INFORMED CONSENT AND TRUTH-TELLING 87

Antihypertensives and the Risk of Temporary Impotence:
A Case Study in Informed Consent 87
John D. Arras

Informed Consent—Must It Remain a Fairy Tale? 89
Jay Katz

Errors in Medicine: Nurturing Truthfulness 97
Françoise Baylis

Bioethics in a Different Tongue: The Case of Truth-Telling 101
Leslie J. Blackhall, Gelya Frank, Sheila Murphy, and Vicki Michel

Offering Truth 110
Benjamin Freedman

SECTION 3 CONFLICTING PROFESSIONAL ROLES AND RESPONSIBILITIES 117

Vitaly Tarasoff et al. v. *The Regents of the University of California et al.,*
Defendants and Respondents 117

Please Don't Tell! 123

Commentary 123
Leonard Fleck

Commentary 124
Marcia Angell

Disclosing Misattributed Paternity 126
Lainie Friedman Ross

SARS Plague: Duty of Care or Medical Heroism? 134
Dessmon YH Tai

The Lessons of SARS 138
Ezekiel J. Emanuel

What Should the Dean Do?   141

Commentary   142
Gregory L. Eastwood

Commentary   143
Daniel Fu-Chang Tsai and Ding-Shinn Chen

Commentary   144
James Dwyer

**The Limits of Conscientious Objection—May Pharmacists Refuse
to Fill Prescriptions for Emergency Contraception?**   145
Julie Cantor and Ken Baum

When Law and Ethics Collide—Why Physicians Participate in Executions   150
Atul Gawande

"To Comfort Always": Physician Participation in Executions   158
Ken Baum

Dialysis for a Prisoner of War   166

Commentary   166
Daniel Zupan, Gary Solis, and Richard Schoonhoven

Commentary   168
George Annas

Recommended Supplementary Reading   169

PART TWO

ALLOCATION, SOCIAL JUSTICE, AND HEALTH POLICY   173

SECTION 1   JUSTICE, HEALTH, AND HEALTH CARE   191

An Ethical Framework for Access to Health Care   191
President's Commission for the Study of Ethical Problems
in Medicine and Biomedical and Behavioral Research

Equal Opportunity and Health Care   200
Norman Daniels

**Freedom and Moral Diversity: The Moral Failures
of Health Care in the Welfare State**   203
H. Tristram Engelhardt, Jr.

Social Determinants of Health: The Solid Facts   213

Why the United States Is Not Number One in Health   222
Ichiro Kawachi

Justice, Health, and Healthcare   231
Norman Daniels

Opportunity Is Not the Key   235
Gopal Sreenivasan

SECTION 2 ALLOCATING SCARCE RESOURCES   237

**Bone Marrow Transplants for Advanced Breast Cancer:
The Story of Christine deMeurers**   237
Alex John London

Justice and the High Cost of Health   244
Ronald Dworkin

Imposing Personal Responsibility for Health   251
Robert Steinbrook

Responsibility in Health Care: A Liberal Egalitarian Approach 255
Alexander W. Cappelen and Ole Frithjof Norheim

**Last-Chance Therapies and Managed Care: Pluralism,
Fair Procedures, and Legitimacy**   261
Norman Daniels and James Sabin

Illegal Immigrants, Health Care, and Social Responsibility   273
James Dwyer

**Rationing Vaccine During an Avian Influenza Pandemic:
Why It Won't Be Easy**   281
John D. Arras

Who Should Get Influenza Vaccine When Not All Can?   292
Ezekiel J. Emanuel and Alan Wertheimer

SECTION 3 ORGAN TRANSPLANTATION: GIFTS VERSUS MARKETS   297

The Case for Allowing Kidney Sales   297
Janet Radcliffe-Richards, Abdallah S. Daar, Ronald D. Guttmann,
Raymond Hoffenberg, Ian Kennedy, Margaret Lock, Robert A. Sells,
Nicholas L. Tilney, International Forum for Transplant Ethics

An Ethical Market in Human Organs   300
Charles A. Erin and John Harris

Body Values: The Case against Compensating for Transplant Organs 301
Donald Joralemon and Phil Cox

SECTION 4 POVERTY, HEALTH, AND JUSTICE BEYOND NATIONAL BORDERS 309

Responsibilities for Poverty-Related Illness   309
Thomas W. Pogge

Do We Owe the Global Poor Assistance or Rectification?   314
Mathias Risse

Recommended Supplementary Reading   319

PART THREE

DEFINING DEATH, FORGOING LIFE-SUSTAINING TREATMENT, AND EUTHANASIA   323

SECTION 1 **THE DEFINITION OF DEATH**   339

Defining Death   339
President's Commission for the Study of Ethical Problems
in Medicine and Biomedical and Behavioral Research

The Whole-Brain Concept of Death Remains Optimum Public Policy   348
James L. Bernat

An Alternative to Brain Death   356
Jeff McMahan

SECTION 2 **DECISIONAL CAPACITY AND THE RIGHT TO REFUSE TREATMENT**   361

State of Tennessee Department of Human Services v. *Mary C. Northern*   361

Transcript of Proceedings: Testimony of Mary C. Northern   365

Deciding for Others: Competency   368
Allen Buchanan and Dan W. Brock

A Chronicle: Dax's Case as It Happened   379
Keith Burton

Commentary   383
Robert B. White

Commentary   384
H. Tristram Engelhardt, Jr.

SECTION 3 **ADVANCE DIRECTIVES**   387

The Health Care Proxy and the Living Will   387
George J. Annas

Enough: The Failure of the Living Will   391
Angela Fagerlin and Carl E. Schneider

Testing the Limits of Prospective Autonomy: Five Scenarios   402

NORMAN L. CANTOR

SECTION 4 **CHOOSING FOR ONCE-COMPETENT PATIENTS**   405

**Erring on the Side of Theresa Schiavo: Reflections of the Special
Guardian ad Litem**   405
Jay Wolfson

"Human Non-Person": Terri Schiavo, Bioethics, and Our Future   409
Wesley J. Smith

In the Matter of Claire C. Conroy   411

The Severely Demented, Minimally Functional Patient: An Ethical Analysis   420
John D. Arras

Nutrition and Hydration: Moral and Pastoral Reflections   429
U.S. Bishops' Pro-Life Committee

**Quality of Life and Non-Treatment Decisions for Incompetent Patients:
A Critique of the Orthodox Approach**   436
Rebecca S. Dresser and John A. Robertson

The Limits of Legal Objectivity   447
Nancy K. Rhoden

SECTION 5   CHOOSING FOR NEVER-COMPETENT PATIENTS   455

**Termination of Life-Support for a Never-Competent Patient:
The Case of Sheila Pouliot**   455
Alicia R. Ouellette

Extreme Prematurity and Parental Rights After Baby Doe   459
John A. Robertson

Resuscitation of the Preterm Infant against Parental Wishes   467
John J. Paris, Michael D. Schreiber, and Alun C. Elias-Jones

SECTION 6   PHYSICIAN-ASSISTED DEATH   473

Death and Dignity: A Case of Individualized Decision Making   473
Timothy E. Quill

Physician-Assisted Suicide: A Tragic View   477
John D. Arras

Assisted Suicide: The Philosophers' Brief Introduction   484
Ronald Dworkin

The Philosophers' Brief   488
Ronald Dworkin, Thomas Nagel, Robert Nozick, John Rawls,
Thomas Scanlon, and Judith Jarvis Thomson

Euthanasia: The Way We Do It, the Way They Do It   496
Margaret P. Battin

Is There a Duty to Die?   511
John Hardwig

**"For Now Have I My Death": The "Duty to Die" versus the Duty
to Help the Ill Stay Alive**   521
Felicia Nimue Ackerman

Recommended Supplementary Reading   529

PART FOUR

REPRODUCTION   535

SECTION 1 **THE MORALITY OF ABORTION**   545

The Unspeakable Crime of Abortion   545
Pope John Paul II

Why Abortion Is Immoral   547
Don Marquis

Why Most Abortions Are Not Wrong   555
Bonnie Steinbock

A Defense of Abortion   567
Judith Jarvis Thomson

The Morality of Abortion   576
Margaret Olivia Little

SECTION 2 **OBLIGATIONS TO THE NOT-YET-BORN**   585

The Rights of "Unborn Children" and the Value of Pregnant Women 585
Howard Minkoff and Lynn M. Paltrow

**Reproductive Freedom and Prevention of Genetically
Transmitted Harmful Conditions**   588
Allen Buchanan, Dan W. Brock, Norman Daniels, and Daniel Wikler

Cheap Listening? Reflections on the Concept of Wrongful Disability 595
Richard J. Hull

SECTION 3 **ASSISTED REPRODUCTION**   599

The Presumptive Primacy of Procreative Liberty   599
John Robertson

**Instruction on Respect for Human Life in Its Origin
and on the Dignity of Procreation**   609
Vatican, Congregation for the Doctrine of the Faith

What Are Families For? Getting to an Ethics of Reproductive Technology 618
Thomas H. Murray

Grade A: The Market for a Yale Woman's Eggs   623
Jessica Cohen

Payment for Egg Donation   627
Bonnie Steinbock

SECTION 4 **REPRODUCTIVE CLONING**   637

The Case against Cloning-to-Produce-Children   637
The President's Council on Bioethics

Reproductive Cloning: Another Look
Bonnie Steinbock
651

Even If It Worked, Cloning Wouldn't Bring Her Back
Thomas H. Murray
661

Recommended Supplementary Reading
664

PART FIVE

GENETICS

669

SECTION 1 **PRENATAL GENETIC TESTING**
675

Prenatal Diagnosis and Selective Abortion: A Challenge to Practice and Policy
Adrienne Asch
675

Disability, Prenatal Testing, and Selective Abortion
Bonnie Steinbock
686

Ethical Issues and Practical Problems in Preimplantation Genetic Diagnosis
Jeffrey R. Botkin
694

**Using Preimplantation Genetic Diagnosis to Save a Sibling:
The Story of Molly and Adam Nash**
Bonnie Steinbock
704

SECTION 2 **THERAPEUTIC CLONING AND STEM CELL RESEARCH**
707

Embryo Ethics—The Moral Logic of Stem-Cell Research
Michael J. Sandel
707

Acorns and Embryos
Robert P. George and Patrick Lee
709

Surplus Embryos, Nonreproductive Cloning, and the Intend/Foresee Distinction
William FitzPatrick
716

Recommended Supplementary Reading
724

PART SIX

EXPERIMENTATION ON HUMAN SUBJECTS

727

SECTION 1 **BORN IN SCANDAL: THE ORIGINS OF U.S. RESEARCH ETHICS**
739

The Nuremberg Code
739

The Jewish Chronic Disease Hospital Case
John D. Arras
740

The Willowbrook Hepatitis Studies 749
David J. Rothman and Sheila M. Rothman

Racism and Research: The Case of the Tuskegee Syphilis Study 753
Allan M. Brandt

The Belmont Report: Ethical Principles and Guidelines
for the Protection of Human Subjects of Research 764
The National Commission for the Protection of Human Subjects of Biomedical
and Behavioral Research

SECTION 2 THE ETHICS OF RANDOMIZED CLINICAL TRIALS 771

Ethical Difficulties with Randomized Clinical Trials Involving
Cancer Patients: Examples from the Field of Gynecologic Oncology 771
Maurie Markman

Of Mice but Not Men: Problems of the Randomized Clinical Trial 774
Samuel Hellman and Deborah S. Hellman

A Response to a Purported Ethical Difficulty with Randomized Clinical
Trials Involving Cancer Patients 779
Benjamin Freedman

SECTION 3 ETHICAL ISSUES IN INTERNATIONAL RESEARCH 783

Unethical Trials of Interventions to Reduce Perinatal Transmission of the Human
Immunodeficiency Virus in Developing Countries 783
Peter Lurie and Sidney M. Wolfe

AZT Trials and Tribulations 788
Robert A. Crouch and John D. Arras

The Ambiguity and the Exigency: Clarifying "Standard of Care" Arguments
in International Research 793
Alex John London

Research in Developing Countries: Taking "Benefit" Seriously 803
Leonard H. Glantz, George J. Annas, Michael A. Grodin, and Wendy K. Mariner

Fair Benefits for Research in Developing Countries 808
Participants in the 2001 Conference on Ethical Aspects of Research
in Developing Countries

SECTION 4 RESEARCH ON CHILDREN 811

Children and "Minimal Risk" Research: The Kennedy-Krieger
Lead Paint Study 811
Alex John London

Research on Children and the Scope of Responsible Parenthood 815
Thomas H. Murray

In Loco Parentis: Minimal Risk as an Ethical Threshold for Research upon Children 829
Benjamin Freedman, Abraham Fuks, and Charles Weijer

Recommended Supplementary Reading 835

PART SEVEN

EMERGING TECHNOLOGIES AND PERENNIAL ISSUES   839

SECTION 1   EMERGING TECHNOLOGIES 845

The Designer Baby Myth 845
Steven Pinker

Applications of Behavioural Genetics: Outpacing the Science? 848
Mark A. Rothstein

Neuroethics 856
Walter Glannon

SECTION 2   ENHANCEMENT 871

Growth Hormone Therapy for the Disability of Short Stature 871
David B. Allen

The Genome Project, Individual Differences, and Just Health Care 874
Norman Daniels

Genetic Interventions and the Ethics of Enhancement of Human Beings 879
Julian Savulescu

The Case Against Perfection: What's Wrong with Designer Children, Bionic Athletes, and Genetic Engineering 890
Michael J. Sandel

Anyone for Tennis, at the Age of 150? 900
Ronald Bailey

SECTION 3   FREE WILL AND RESPONSIBILITY 903

Neurobiology, Neuroimaging, and Free Will 903
Walter Glannon

Recommended Supplementary Reading 913

PREFACE

In 1977 when John Arras published the first edition of *Ethical Issues in Modern Medicine (EIMM)* with his first coeditor Robert Hunt, he had a great deal of difficulty locating five decent articles for each of five chapters. The field was in its infancy in those days, consisting largely of assorted biomedical prophets and academic malcontents fed up with the insularity and irrelevance of their home disciplines. There were no professional associations, no yearly conventions, no degree-granting programs, no field of clinical ethics, certainly no Web sites, and only one journal, *The Hastings Center Report*, which could fit an exhaustive bibliography of all bioethics-related books and articles published during the preceding months onto a single back page of each issue.

Needless to say, although the coeditors of this volume have confronted many obstacles in bringing it to press, a dearth of good materials wasn't one of them. Even though our text has expanded from five to seven "parts" or chapters, each one subdivided into an average of four "sections," each of which in turn contains five or six articles of its own—in other words, even though the scope and bulk of the book have expanded easily five- or sixfold over the past thirty years—we now find it increasingly difficult to cull over 120 articles and case studies from a veritable sea of resources available in hundreds of books, scores of journals, and a dizzying array of Web sites and databases. Editing a book like this ain't what it used to be.

On the other hand, the editorial philosophy governing our collective effort has remained remarkably stable over the years. We consider the construction of a new edition a serious undertaking, requiring a lot more than adding a few new articles and slapping on a new cover with a higher price tag. Each new edition of *EIMM*, including the one you currently hold in your hands, has represented a near-total overhaul of the preceding version. Readers of a philosophical bent might well wonder if a book that undergoes such comprehensive revisions can plausibly qualify metaphysically as a new edition of the same book. This edition, for example, contains 55 new readings and cases out of a total of 120, and an entirely new part (for which Bonnie Steinbock claims responsibility) titled

"Emerging Technologies and Perennial Issues." The addition discusses topics such as behavioral genetics, neuroethics, and human genetic enhancement.

Moreover, each of the major parts has undergone substantial revision and updating. The section titled "Conflicting Professional Roles and Responsibilities" in Part 1, for example (for which Alex London had primary responsibility), has been updated to reflect current issues such as the boundary between obligation and heroism for medical professionals in the face of pandemics, emergency contraception and the limits of conscientious objection for pharmacists, the participation of physicians in capital punishment, and medical obligations toward prisoners of war.

Part 2 (which Alex London oversaw) now includes essays on the significance of the social determinants of health for theories of health care justice and entirely new material on justice-based obligations to meet the urgent health-related needs of the global poor. This crucially important part also features fresh reflections on the role of personal responsibility in rationing health care, on the exclusion of illegal immigrants from health benefits, and on the fair allocation of potentially life-saving vaccines in the face of a global pandemic of avian influenza. We have also included new developments in organ transplantation, including the pressing issue of whether organs should continue to be treated as gifts, as mandated by federal law, or sold on the free market in order to boost supply and possibly save many lives.

Finally, again just by way of example, Part 3 (for which Bonnie Steinbock had primary responsibility) includes new articles on the continuing debate among the partisans of whole-brain and neocortical conceptions of death, the failure of living wills to resolve end-of-life dilemmas, a discussion of the tragic case of Terri Schiavo, and dilemmas concerning the terminal care of never-competent patients, such as newborns and those with severe cognitive disabilities. Additional examples of new materials and fresh thinking could be drawn from any of the remaining subsequent parts of the book. In brief, this has been a comprehensive revision and updating. We are confident that the book before you represents the state of the art in contemporary bioethical scholarship and debate.

Continuing the precedent set by the previous edition, the seventh incarnation of *EIMM* has arisen from a rather uneven (some might even say unjust) division of labor. More simply and directly put, Bonnie Steinbock and Alex London have done the lion's share of the work, while John Arras has done a lot of kvetching from the sidelines. In keeping with his recently adopted role as the *éminence grise* behind this project—and we use the word *grise* advisedly—John has assisted Bonnie and Alex in combing the vast bioethics literature, selecting the choicest articles and cases, and working up these raw materials into pedagogically exciting and intellectually coherent parts. Once that enormous hurdle was successfully cleared, Bonnie and Alex undertook the hard slog of writing new part introductions, overseeing the compilation of useful bibliographies, and arguing with publishers over rights and fees. Through it all, incredibly, we have remained close colleagues and the best of friends. One might dream of having collegial relationships this enduring and fruitful, but one is rarely as fortunate as we have been in actually enjoying them in real life.

Each new edition of this text engenders scores of new debts to those who have helped make this book what it has become, and now is the time to express our profound gratitude to one and all. John Arras no longer presides over the actual construction of the book, so his debts are fewer than in previous editions. Still, he wishes to thank his indefatigable and indispensable administrative assistant, Carolyn Randolph, as well as his two most recent graduate assistants, Elizabeth Fenton and Amy Gilbert, for their stimulating philosophical companionship and generous willingness to read bluebooks.

Bonnie Steinbock owes a debt of gratitude to Juliette Stevens for her invaluable research assistance. The experience was so richly fulfilling for Juliette that she has vowed never to repeat the experience, for any amount of money. Bonnie also wishes to thank Glenn McGee, director of the Alden March Bioethics Institute, for helping fund Juliette's assistance. She also thanks Roopali Malhotra for assistance with the recommended readings, her undergraduate students over the years in her course Moral Problems in Medicine, her graduate students in her Bioethics course, and the minors in bioethics at the University at Albany for their insights and enthusiasm. Most of all, she thanks her coeditors, John and Alex, for their friendship, wit, and intelligence. She has learned more from them than she can express.

For Alex London, the preparation of the seventh edition overlapped with frenzied preparations for the arrival of Alexandra and Sophia who, with their older brother, Joshua, are an infinite joy. He could not have dedicated the full measure of time and energy necessary to complete the book without the unvarying support of his wife Tracy. He would also like to thank his parents, John and Elaine, for all the many ways in which their being the perfect grandparents makes it possible for him to hive off time to think and to write.

For Alex, planning for the seventh edition began in earnest with the publication of the sixth edition. He is grateful to the hundreds of talented and eager undergraduates from his Medical Ethics course who have offered their feedback about the book, both constructive and critical, over the past four years. He extends special thanks, however, to Emily Evans whose acumen, engagement, and sheer joy still stand out. Similarly, although he has been fortunate to have some truly excellent graduate students as teaching assistants, he bears a special debt to Erica Lucast, David Gray, and Peter Gildenhuys for their discerning reflections on the book and the course.

Finally, Alex extends his deep gratitude to his colleagues at Carnegie Mellon for their encouragement and support, especially Teddy Seidenfeld, Richard Scheines, Clark Glymour, Robert Cavalier, and Preston Covey, whose untimely death is a loss to us all.

Last, but certainly not least, the three of us wish to express our gratitude to our new editor, Mark Georgiev, who has been both patient and encouraging. We hope he finds the latest edition worth the wait.

THE CONTRIBUTORS

Felicia Nimue Ackerman, PhD,
is professor of philosophy at Brown University, Providence, Rhode Island.

Terrence F. Ackerman, PhD,
is professor and chair of the Department of Human Values and Ethics, and chair of the Institutional Review Board at the University of Tennessee Health Science Center.

David B. Allen, MD,
is professor of pediatrics at the University of Wisconsin School of Medicine and Public Health, and director of Endocrinology and Residency Training at the University of Wisconsin Children's Hospital, Madison, Wisconsin.

Marcia Angell, MD, FACP,
is a senior lecturer in social medicine at the Harvard Medical School, and former editor-in-chief of the New England Journal of Medicine.

George J. Annas, JD, MPH,
is professor and chair of the Health Law Department, Boston University School of Public Health, and professor at the Boston University School of Medicine and School of Law.

John D. Arras, PhD,
is the William and Linda Porterfield Professor of Bioethics, and professor of philosophy at the University of Virginia, Charlottesville.

Adrienne Asch, PhD,
is the Edward and Robin Milstein Professor of Bioethics, Wurzweiler School of Social Work, Yeshiva University, New York.

Ronald Bailey
is the science correspondent for the public policy magazine Reason, *and the author of* Liberation Biology: The Scientific and Moral Case for the Biotech Revolution.

Margaret P. Battin, MFA, PhD,
is Distinguished Professor of Philosophy and adjunct professor of internal medicine in the Division of Medical Ethics at the University of Utah.

Ken Baum, MD, JD,
is an attorney at Bartlit Beck Herman Palenchar & Scott LLP.

Françoise Baylis, PhD,
is professor and Canada research chair in bioethics and philosophy at Dalhousie University.

James L. Bernat, MD,
is a neurologist and professor of medicine (neurology) at Dartmouth Medical School, Lebanon, New Hampshire.

Leslie J. Blackhall, MD, MTS,
is associate professor of internal medicine and medical education, University of Virginia, Charlottesville.

Jeffrey R. Botkin, MD, MPH,
is a pediatrician and professor of pediatrics and medical ethics at the University of Utah.

Allan M. Brandt, PhD,
is the Amalie Moses Kass Professor of the History of Medicine at Harvard Medical School, Boston, Massachusetts.

Dan W. Brock, PhD,
is the Frances Glessner Lee Professor of Medical Ethics in the Department of Social Medicine, and director of the Division of Medical Ethics at the Harvard Medical School. He is also director of the Harvard Program in Ethics and Health.

Allen Buchanan, PhD,
is James B. Duke Professor of Philosophy and James B. Duke Professor of Public Policy Studies at Duke University, Durham, North Carolina.

Keith Burton
is managing director at Golin/Harris International in Chicago. He was a freelance journalist when he made the 1985 documentary Dax's Case.

Julie D. Cantor, MD, JD,
is an attorney with Munger, Tolles & Olson, and a lecturer at the UCLA School of Law.

Norman L. Cantor, JD,
is professor of law and justice Nathan Jacobs Scholar at the Rutgers University School of Law, Newark, New Jersey.

Alexander W. Cappelen, Dr. Oecon (PhD in economics),
is professor at the Norwegian School of Economics and Business Administration.

Ding-Shenn Chen, MD,
is dean and professor of medicine at the National Taiwan University College of Medicine, Taipei, Taiwan.

Jean-Claude Chevrolet, MD,
is professor of medicine and head of the Intensive Care Department, Faculty of Medicine, University Hospital of Geneva, Switzerland.

Jessica Cohen
was an undergraduate at Yale University when she wrote "Grade A: The Market for a Yale Woman's Eggs."

Phil Cox, PhD,
is associate professor of philosophy at the University of Massachusetts, Dartmouth.

Robert A. Crouch, MA,
is from the Center for the Study of Ethics and American Institutions at Indiana University, Bloomington, Indiana.

Abdallah S. Daar, DPhil (Oxon), FRCP (Lon), FRCS, FRCSC,
is senior scientist and codirector of the Program on Life Sciences, Ethics and Policy in the McLaughlin-Rotman Centre for Global Health;, director of Ethics and Policy, McLaughlin Centre for Molecular Medicine; Senior Fellow of Massey College at the University of Toronto; and health network professor of public health sciences and professor of surgery at the University of Toronto.

Norman Daniels, PhD,
is Mary B. Saltonstall Professor of Population Ethics in the Department of Population and International Health at the Harvard School of Public Health.

Rebecca S. Dresser, JD,
is professor of law and ethics in medicine at Washington University, St. Louis, Missouri.

Ronald Dworkin, LLB,
is Bentham Professor of Jurisprudence at University College London, and professor of law and philosophy at New York University.

James Dwyer, PhD,
is associate director of education at the Center for Bioethics and Humanities at the State University of New York Upstate Medical University.

Gregory L. Eastwood, MD,
is interim president at Case Western Reserve University, Cleveland, Ohio.

Bernice S. Elger, MD, PhD,
is MER (assistant professor) at the University of Geneva, Institute of Biomedical Ethics, and an internist at the University Hospital of Geneva, Switzerland.

Alun C. Elias-Jones, MD,
is consulting neonatologist at Leicester General Hospital, Leicester, United Kingdom.

Ezekiel J. Emanuel, MD, PhD,
is chair of the Department of Clinical Bioethics at the Warren G. Magnuson Clinical Center at the National Institutes of Health.

Linda L. Emanuel, MD, PhD,
is director of the Buehler Center on Aging, professor of health industry management at the Kellogg School, and professor of medicine at Northwestern University Medical School.

H. Tristram Engelhardt, Jr., PhD, MD,
is professor of medicine and community medicine at Baylor College of Medicine, Houston, Texas.

Charles A. Erin, PhD,
is senior lecturer in applied philosophy and a Fellow of the Institute of Medicine, Law and Bioethics at the University of Manchester, United Kingdom.

Angela Fagerlin, PhD,
is a research health science specialist at the Ann Arbor Veterans Administration, and a research assistant professor at the University of Michigan.

William FitzPatrick, PhD,
is associate professor of philosophy at Virginia Polytechnic Institute and State University (Virginia Tech).

Leonard M. Fleck, PhD,
is professor of philosophy and medical ethics in the Center for Ethics and Humanities in the Life Sciences at Michigan State University.

Gelya Frank, PhD,
is professor in the Division of Occupational Science & Occupational Therapy at the School of Dentistry, and professor of anthropology at the University of Southern California.

Benjamin Freedman, PhD,
was professor at the McGill Centre for Medicine, Ethics, and Law, Montreal, Canada, and clinical ethicist at the Sir Mortimer B. Davis-Jewish General Hospital, Montreal.

Abraham Fuks, BSc, MD, CM, FRCP(C),
is professor of medicine, pathology and oncology, Faculty of Medicine, McGill University.

Atul Gawande, MD, MPH,
is assistant professor of surgery at Brigham and Women's Hospital and the Harvard Medical School, assistant professor in the Department of Health Policy and Management in the Harvard School of Public Health, and assistant director of the Brigham and Women's Hospital Center for Surgery and Public Health.

Robert P. George, PhD,
is McCormick Professor of Jurisprudence and director of the James Madison Program in American Ideals and Institutions at Princeton University in New Jersey. He is a member of the President's Council on Bioethics.

Walter Glannon, PhD,
is associate professor of philosophy and Canada research chair in biomedical ethics and ethical theory at the University of Calgary, Canada.

Leonard H. Glantz, JD,
is professor of health law at Boston University School of Public Health.

Alan Goldman, PhD,
is professor of philosophy at the University of Miami, Florida.

Michael A. Grodin, MD,
is professor of health law, psychiatry, socio-medical sciences and community medicine, Boston University School of Public Health and Medicine.

Ronald D. Guttmann, MD, FRCPC,
is emeritus professor of medicine at McGill University, Montreal, Canada.

John Hardwig, PhD,
is professor of philosophy and department head at the University of Tennessee, Knoxville.

John Harris, DPhil (Oxon),
is the Sir David Alliance Professor of Bioethics at the University of Manchester; a member of the United Kingdom Human Genetics Commission and the Ethics Committee of the British Medical Association; and a Fellow of the Academy of Medical Sciences.

Deborah S. Hellman, MA, JD,
is associate professor of law at the University of Maryland, Baltimore.

Samuel Hellman, MD,
is the A.N. Pritzker Distinguished Service Professor in the Department of Radiology and Cellular Oncology at the Cancer Research Center, University of Chicago School of Medicine.

Sir Raymond Hoffenberg, MD, FRCP,
is the former president of Wolfson College, Oxford, and a past president of the Royal College of Physicians.

Richard J. Hull, PhD,
is lecturer in philosophy and director of the Centre of Bioethical Research and Analysis at the National University of Ireland, Galway.

Donald Joralemon, PhD,
is professor of anthropology at Smith College.

Jay Katz, MD,
is Elizabeth K. Dollard Professor Emeritus of Law, Medicine, and Psychiatry and Harvey L. Karp Professorial Lecturer in Law and Psychoanalysis at Yale Law School, New Haven, Connecticut.

Ichiro Kawachi, PhD,
*is professor of social epidemiology at the Harvard School of
Public Health, and a recipient of the Robert Wood Johnson
Investigator Award in Health Policy Research.*

Sir Ian Kennedy, LLD,
*is emeritus professor of health law, ethics and policy at
University College London; chair of the Healthcare
Commission in the UK; and former chair of the Nuffield
Council of Bioethics.*

Patrick Lee, PhD,
*is professor of bioethics and director of the Bioethics Institute at
the Franciscan University of Steubenville, Ohio.*

Margaret Olivia Little, PhD,
*is associate professor in the Philosophy Department, and a
senior research scholar in the Kennedy Institute of Ethics at
Georgetown University, Washington, DC.*

Margaret Lock, PhD,
*is the Marjorie Bronfman Professor in Social Studies in
Medicine, and is affiliated with the Department of Social
Studies of Medicine and the Department of Anthropology at
McGill University. She is a Fellow of the Royal Society of
Canada and an Officier de L'Ordre national du Québec.*

Alex John London, PhD,
*is associate professor of philosophy and director of the Center
for the Advancement of Applied Ethics and Political
Philosophy at Carnegie Mellon University, Pittsburgh,
Pennsylvania.*

Peter Lurie, MD, MPH,
*is deputy director of Public Citizens Health Research Group,
Washington, DC.*

Wendy K. Mariner, JD, LLM, MPH,
*is professor of health law, Boston University School of Public
Health.*

Maurie Markman, MD,
*is director of the Cleveland Clinic Taussig Cancer Center,
Cleveland, Ohio; and chair of the Department of
Hematology/Oncology at the Cleveland Clinic Foundation,
where he holds the Lee and Jerome Burkons Research Chair in
Oncology.*

Sir Michael Marmot, MBBS, MPH, PhD, FRCP,
   FFPHM,
*is director of the UCL International Institute for Society and
Health; professor of Epidemiology and Public Health at*

*University College London; and chair of the Commission on
Social Determinants of Health.*

Don Marquis, PhD,
*is professor of philosophy at the University of Kansas,
Lawrence.*

Jeff McMahan, PhD,
is professor of philosophy at Rutgers University, New Jersey.

Vicki Michel, JD,
*is coordinator of the Southern California Bioethics Committee
Consortium and adjunct professor at Loyola Law School.*

Howard Minkoff, MD,
*is Distinguished Professor, SUNY Downstate; and chair of
Obstetrics and Gynecology at Maimonides Medical Center,
New York.*

Sheila T. Murphy, PhD,
*is associate professor in the Annenberg School for
Communication at the University of Southern California.*

Thomas H. Murray, PhD,
*is president of The Hastings Center, a bioethics research
institute in Garrison, New York.*

Thomas Nagel, PhD,
*is professor of law and professor of philosophy at New York
University.*

Ole Frithjof Norheim, MD, PhD,
*is professor in the Division for Medical Ethics at the
University of Bergen.*

Robert Nozick, PhD,
*was the Arthur Kingsley Porter Professor of
Philosophy/Pellegrino University Professor at Harvard
University, Cambridge, Massachusetts.*

Alicia R. Ouellette, JD,
is associate professor at Albany Law School.

Lynn M. Paltrow, JD,
*is executive director of National Advocates for Pregnant
Women, New York City.*

John J. Paris, SJ, PhD,
*is the Walsh Professor of Bioethics at Boston College and
clinical professor of family medicine and community health,
Tufts University School of Medicine, Boston, Massachusetts.*

Steven Pinker, PhD,
*is the Johnstone Professor of Psychology at Harvard
University, Cambridge, Massachusetts.*

Thomas W. Pogge, PhD,
*is professor of political science at Columbia University,
New York.*

Pope John Paul II
*was pope of the Roman Catholic Church from October 16,
1978, until his death on April 2, 2005.*

Timothy E. Quill, MD,
*is associate chief of medicine at the Genesee Hospital, professor
of medicine and psychiatry at the University of Rochester
School of Medicine and Dentistry, and a primary care internist
in Rochester, New York.*

John Rawls, PhD,
*was professor emeritus of philosophy at Harvard University,
Cambridge, Massachusetts.*

Nancy K. Rhoden, JD,
*was professor of law at the University of North Carolina at
Chapel Hill, and a coeditor of the third edition of* Ethical
Issues in Modern Medicine.

Janet Radcliffe-Richards, BPhil (Oxon),
*is director of the Centre for Biomedical Ethics and Philosophy,
University College London.*

Mathias Risse, PhD, MS,
*is associate professor of philosophy and public policy at the
John F. Kennedy School of Government, Harvard University,
Cambridge, Massachusetts.*

John A. Robertson, JD,
*is the Vinson & Elkins Chair of Law at the University of
Texas School of Law, Austin, Texas, and is chair of the Ethics
Committee of the American Society of Reproductive
Medicine.*

Lainie Friedman Ross, MD, PhD,
*is the Carolyn and Matthew Bucksbaum Professor of Clinical
Medical Ethics; a professor in the Departments of Pediatrics
and Medicine; section chief of Community Health Sciences in
the Institute for Molecular Pediatric Sciences; and associate
director of the MacLean Center for Clinical Medical Ethics at
the University of Chicago.*

David J. Rothman, PhD,
*is Bernard Schoenberg Professor of Social Medicine and
director of the Center for the Study of Society and Medicine,
Columbia College of Physicians and Surgeons, Columbia
University, New York.*

Sheila M. Rothman, PhD,
*is professor of public health in the Sociomedical Sciences
Division of the Joseph L. Mailman School of Public Health, and
deputy director of the Center for the Study of Society and
Medicine, College of Physicians and Surgeons, Columbia
University, New York.*

Mark A. Rothstein, JD,
*is the Herbert F. Boehl Chair of Law and Medicine, and
director of the Institute for Bioethics, Health Policy
and Law at the University of Louisville, School of Medicine,
Kentucky.*

James E. Sabin, MD, PhD,
*is director of the Ethics Program at Harvard Pilgrim Health
Care, and clinical professor of psychiatry at Harvard Medical
School, Boston, Massachusetts.*

Michael J. Sandel, PhD,
*is the Anne T. and Robert M. Bass Professor of Government at
Harvard University, Cambridge, Massachusetts.*

Julian Savulescu, PhD,
*is the Uehiro Professor of Practical Ethics and director of the
Oxford Uehiro Centre for Practical Ethics at the University of
Oxford, and director of the Program on Ethics and the New
Biosciences in the 21st Century School at the University of
Oxford, United Kingdom.*

Thomas Scanlon, PhD,
*is professor of philosophy at Harvard University, Cambridge,
Massachusetts.*

Carl E. Schneider
*is the Chauncey Stillman Professor of Law and professor
of internal medicine at the University of Michigan,
Ann Arbor.*

Richard Schoonhoven, PhD,
*is associate professor in the Department of Philosophy and
English at the United States Military Academy.*

Michael D. Schreiber, MD,
*is vice-chair of pediatrics and professor of pediatrics at the
University of Chicago Pritzker School of Medicine.*

Robert A. Sells, MD,
*is past president of the British Transplantation Society and
recently retired from his position as consultant transplant
surgeon at the Royal Liverpool University Hospital, Liverpool,
United Kingdom.*

Wesley J. Smith, JD,
is a Senior Fellow at the Discovery Institute, an attorney for the International Task Force on Euthanasia and Assisted Suicide, and a special consultant to the Center for Bioethics and Culture.

Gary Solis, JD, LLM, PhD,
is a retired U.S. Marine with 26 years of active duty, a West Point retiree, a 2006–2007 scholar in residence at the Library of Congress, and an adjunct professor of law at Georgetown University Law Center.

Gopal Sreenivasan, PhD,
is a Canada research chair in the Department of Philosophy at the University of Toronto, Canada.

Bonnie Steinbock, PhD,
is professor of philosophy at the University at Albany, State University of New York, and a faculty member of the Alden March Bioethics Institute at Albany Medical College, and the Bioethics Program of Union Graduate College and the Mount Sinai School of Medicine.

Robert Steinbrook, MD,
is national correspondent for The New England Journal of Medicine.

Dessmon YH Tai, MBBS, MRCP (UK),
is clinical senior lecturer, Yong Loo Lin School of Medicine, National University of Singapore.

Judith Jarvis Thomson, PhD,
is professor of philosophy at the Massachusetts Institute of Technology, Cambridge, Massachusetts.

Nicholas L. Tilney, MD,
is the Francis D. Moore Professor of Surgery at Brigham and Women's Hospital and the Harvard Medical School.

Daniel Fu-Chang Tsai, MD, PhD,
is associate professor in the Department of Social Medicine and Department of Family Medicine, National Taiwan University College of Medicine; and attending physician in the Department of Medical Research, National Taiwan University Hospital.

Charles Weijer, MD, PhD, FRCPC,
is Tier I Canada research chair in bioethics and associate professor of philosophy and medicine at the University of Western Ontario.

Alan Wertheimer, PhD,
is professor emeritus of political science at the University of Vermont, and senior research scholar in the Department of Clinical Bioethics at the National Institutes of Health.

Robert B. White, MD,
is professor emeritus of psychiatry at the University of Texas Medical Branch, Galveston.

Daniel Wikler, PhD,
is Mary B. Saltonstall Professor of Population Ethics, Harvard School of Public Health, Cambridge, Massachusetts.

Richard G. Wilkinson, M Med Sci,
is professor of social epidemiology at the University of Nottingham Medical School, Nottingham, United Kingdom.

Sidney M. Wolfe, MD,
is director of the Public Citizen Research Group in Washington, DC.

Jay Wolfson, Dr PH, JD,
is Distinguished Professor of Public Health and Medicine and associate vice president of USF Health at the University of South Florida.

Daniel Zupan, PhD,
is a colonel in the United States Army and is currently deputy head of the Department of Philosophy and English at the United States Military Academy at West Point.

MORAL REASONING IN THE MEDICAL CONTEXT

BONNIE STEINBOCK / JOHN D. ARRAS / ALEX JOHN LONDON

BIOETHICS: NATURE AND SCOPE

Dr. Deborah Brody was not looking forward to Jim Lasken's next visit. Mr. Lasken, a Forty-year-old former postal carrier, devoted husband, and father of two teenagers, was at a critical juncture in his treatment for amyotrophic lateral sclerosis, a progressive and ultimately fatal degenerative disease of the nervous system, known to most people as Lou Gehrig's disease. Dr. Brody had been seeing Mr. Lasken for the past ten years, during which time his condition had been steadily deteriorating. Mr. Lasken was now in very bad shape. In the past three years he had lost the ability to walk, work, dress himself, and sit up without supports. He was now incontinent, and could speak only a few short words at a time, and only with agonizing difficulty. Mr. Lasken's psychological state had tracked his physical decline. Although he had kept up a brave front as many of his faculties declined over the first years of his illness, Mr. Lasken was becoming more and more despondent as his condition worsened.

Editors' note: Although this article represents a complete reworking and expansion of the introduction from previous editions of this book, the authors gratefully acknowledge the enduring contributions of Robert Hunt, coeditor of the first edition, to these pages.

Dr. Brody suspected that Mr. Lasken was in a deep depression, but, given his life prospects, she could not really blame him.

Dr. Brody dreaded Mr. Lasken's next visit not simply because he was seriously ill and getting progressively worse, but because Mr. Lasken had been asking her to help him "end it." As he and his wife, Jane, had explained, his life had become unbearable. He could no longer enjoy his former hobbies, he could no longer communicate with anyone without enduring monumental frustration and fatigue, he knew he was a tremendous burden to his family, and was well aware that things were just going to get worse. It had become clear, in fact, that Mr. Lasken would soon have to be hooked up to a mechanical ventilator to do his breathing for him, or else he would drown in his own secretions.

This was apparently the last straw. Mr. Lasken was now adamant: He saw no point in either going on the respirator or dying a slow, wasting death without it. He wanted to die now, and he wanted Dr. Brody to help him. "Give me a shot," he implored, "it's all you can do for me now. My life is over."

Dr. Brody now had a serious problem. Should she help her patient commit suicide? Indeed, since Mr. Lasken could no longer actively do anything to take his own life, the doctor would have to do it herself, engaging in what is called "active euthanasia." She knew that it was against the law in her state either to assist someone in a suicide or directly to kill another person, but could such an act be ethically permitted if the patient were sufficiently desperate and helpless? Supposing that *someone* might be justified in performing euthanasia, was this the sort of thing that a *doctor* could or should do? As a physician, she empathized with her patient's pain, isolation, and desperation, and would have done just about anything to alleviate his terrible suffering. "A big part of my job is to combat suffering, not just death," she thought. "If my patient's mental and physical suffering can only be ended by death, and if his life is no longer of any use to him, why should I not help him?" On the other hand, she recalled the Hippocratic oath, a version of which she took upon graduation from medical school, which condemned giving patients "deadly drugs." The message, transmitted from one generation of doctors to the next, was that physicians are supposed to be healers, not killers.

Dr. Brody's dilemma is also society's problem. More and more individuals are claiming that just as they have a right to control what happens to their own bodies during life, so they have a right to control the timing and manner of their deaths. Celebrated cases, like that of Dr. Kevorkian in Michigan, focus public attention on the question of whether the laws that currently constrain Dr. Brody should be changed. Given appropriate circumstances, checks, and balances, should doctors be given legal permission to prescribe deadly drugs for their suicidal patients? Should they be allowed to kill outright? What are the social implications of allowing individuals such a right to die? Should these practices become widespread, what would be the likelihood of abuse and the "slippery slope" toward killing those who are mentally infirm, elderly, and poor?

Problems of this sort lie at the heart of contemporary bioethics, the field introduced by this anthology. Like its parent disciplines, moral philosophy and religious ethics, bioethics is a study of moral conduct, of right and wrong. As such, it is inescapably *normative*. As opposed to some historical or social scientific approaches to moral conduct that emphasize description of the way the world is, or causal conjectures about why it is the way it is, bioethics inquires about the rightness or wrongness of various actions, character traits, and social policies. Thus, instead of fixing on such issues as

the history of physicians' participation in their patients' suicides, or the way in which their attitudes are shaped by age, gender, specialty, and so on, "bioethicists" typically ask whether assisted suicide or euthanasia can be morally justified, whether either practice would be good social policy, and whether these practices are compatible with the character traits of a good physician. (This is not to say, however, that good normative reasoning can or should take place without careful attention to empirical details, which often prove crucial to the careful resolution of practical moral problems.)

In addition to these straightforward normative concerns, bioethicists are also increasingly interested in what philosophers call "metaethical" themes. That is, they are concerned not just with the question, say, of whether assisted suicide is morally justified, but also with broader and more abstract questions bearing on the nature of moral justification and the kind of thinking that supports it. As we shall see near the end of this article, some bioethicists might claim, for example, that the justifiability of physician-assisted suicide must be sought in the articulation and application of various moral theories or principles, while others might claim that justification must proceed the other way around, beginning with concrete and unmistakable instances of good and bad behavior, and then gradually developing principles that capture and distill our most fundamental moral responses to cases. It is a question, in other words, of whether ethical thought should proceed from the "top down" or from the "bottom up."

SOURCES OF BIOETHICAL PROBLEMS AND CONCERNS

Since its birth in the early 1970s, the contemporary bioethics movement has grown from a mere blip on the radar of public consciousness to a major academic- and service-oriented profession with its own research centers, journals, conferences, and degree programs. Not a week goes by, it seems, without some controversial biomedical case or issue making its way into the nation's headlines and talk shows: "Gene for Homosexuality Discovered!" "Parents Insist on Treatment for Baby Without a Brain!" "Patients Subjected to Radiation Experiments

Without Their Consent!" "Dr. Kevorkian Strikes Again!" Why are we beset in this present age with so many fundamental and fascinating questions?

Technological Innovation

Obviously, much of the ferment in contemporary biomedical ethics is due to the unrelenting pace of technological advance. The story is by now familiar: Clever physicians, researchers, and technicians discover newer and better ways to do things, such as sustaining the lives of terminally ill patients, diagnosing fetal abnormalities in utero, and facilitating conception for infertile couples. Before we know it, however, these new techniques and services begin to take on lives of their own, expanding well beyond the problems and patients for whom they were originally intended.

Cardiopulmonary resuscitation, for example, originally intended for otherwise healthy victims of drowning or electrocution, has gradually and unceremoniously become a violent and final "rite of passage" for many aged, moribund patients in our nation's hospitals. The administration of artificial nutrition and hydration, originally intended as a temporary bridge to the restoration of patients' digestive functioning, now is routinely delivered to thousands of patients who have irretrievably lost all higher brain functions.

Prenatal diagnosis, originally intended for fetuses at high risk of a metabolic or genetic disorder, is now routinely offered to, and sought by, many women in their late twenties or early thirties who are at no special health risk. The availability of this technology has thus expanded choice, while simultaneously imposing new pressures on many women by altering their definition of an "acceptable risk" during pregnancy.

Finally, in vitro fertilization (IVF), originally developed to aid infertile married couples, is now offered to single women, to adult daughters volunteering to serve as surrogate mothers for their own mothers' children (i.e., to be the mothers of their own siblings), and to postmenopausal women in their late forties and fifties. In conjunction with the newly developed techniques of embryo freezing and "embryo splitting," a kind of cloning, IVF might soon make it possible for a woman grown from a split embryo to give birth to her own previously frozen identical twin.

Needless to say, problems such as these, as they spawn new possibilities for remaking ourselves, our families, and our society, call into question the adequacy of our traditional ways of thinking. In some instances, it is clear that scientific and technological developments have brought about a change in values and moral beliefs. As Emmanuel Mesthene has remarked, "By adding new options . . . technology can lead to changes in values in the same way that the appearance of new dishes on the heretofore standard menu of one's favorite restaurant can lead to changes in one's tastes and choices of food."[1] Often, what science and technology make possible soon becomes permissible and, eventually, normal and expected. For example, when the use of anesthesia during childbirth was introduced around 150 years ago, it was condemned as morally wrong. Women were "supposed" to suffer through labor: it was "unnatural" if they did not. But what *could* be done *was* done, and eventually those beliefs were revised.

In the more recent past, we have noted a change in attitude toward heart transplants; at first, many people had moral reservations about this procedure, not because it was new and risky, but because the heart was associated with the soul or personality. Today, although heart transplants continue to raise social policy problems, this particular moral reservation has completely vanished.

Most readers may feel comfortable about the attitudinal changes just mentioned, but in other areas the influence of technology on values and morals has had more controversial results. For example, developments in medical knowledge and techniques have played a major role in reshaping cultural and legal attitudes toward contraception and abortion, and more recent developments—for example, the "abortion pill," RU 486, and long-acting contraceptives such as Norplant—promise to erode traditional moral qualms even further. Yet not everyone believes that these developments constitute an unalloyed good; some regard them as a profound insult to their conception of the sanctity of life,

---

1. Emmanuel Mesthene, "The Role of Technology in Society," in *Technology and Man's Future,* edited by A. Teich (New York: St. Martin's Press, 1972), 137.

while others suspect that they will be coercively targeted at vulnerable minority groups. And what about the near future? Already there is widespread concern regarding the ethical implications of techniques and procedures that are still in their developmental stages. Will developments in genetic knowledge made possible by the human genome project and advances in reproductive technologies help usher in a "brave new world"? Is there, perhaps, some knowledge that we ought not try to seek? Or are our reservations about such matters as in vitro fertilization for women old enough to be grandmothers as time-bound and unwarranted as those of the people who opposed anesthesia and heart transplants?

As Nicholas Rescher has pointed out, the phenomenon of value change is a complex one, and technological developments may lead to "value restandardization."[2] The value of good health may not have changed position in our hierarchy of values, but as a result of technology the standard of what constitutes good health may have been revised considerably upward. As technology increases the possibilities in life, as values diversify and expectations rise, abnormalities—and common conditions—that were once taken for granted come to be viewed as pathological conditions requiring treatment and/or prevention. It is, after all, a comparatively recent assumption that medical relief can and should be sought for such conditions as acne, obesity, short stature, crooked teeth, small breasts, and the failure to achieve orgasm.

In addition to curing disease, medicine is now increasingly capable of *optimizing* more or less normal conditions that nevertheless can be improved upon. Drugs like Prozac, for example, promise a future in which individuals might not merely manage clinical depression better, but also alter their personalities in significantly positive ways. Having problems with self-esteem? Having trouble mustering the courage to ask for that promotion? "Cosmetic psychopharmacology" may be able to provide just what you need.[3]

Related to all these issues is, of course, the restandardization of what constitutes adequate health care. Today we expect not only to be cured of ills that were previously incurable, but also to be prevented from experiencing a variety of infirmities and misfortunes that were once the common lot of humankind. And we feel wronged if these expectations go unfulfilled. Driven by the pressure of consumer demand, treatments that many might regard today as "frills," such as in vitro fertilization and cosmetic personality-altering drugs, may well be regarded tomorrow as essential ingredients in the "pursuit of happiness."

The impact of technology on our value systems is also seen in the fact that the development of new knowledge and techniques may blur, rather than sharpen, the very concepts that are central to our norms and values. The advent of organ transplantation and critical-care technologies, for example, has forced physicians and society at large to rethink the very meanings of life and death. The traditional "definition" of life as the presence of respiration and heartbeat has been replaced in every U.S. state over the past twenty years by the notion of whole-brain death, yet few people, even today, can identify a noncontroversial philosophical rationale for the new law's insistence that the entire brain, both "higher" and "lower," must have ceased functioning irreversibly for a patient to be dead. As a result, the moral and legal status of patients with no higher brain functions, those in persistent vegetative states, poses an ongoing challenge to the current approach to brain death. If a patient has permanently lost the capacity for any kind of thought, feeling, and human interaction—if, to put it somewhat crudely, "no one is home"—why not consider him or her to be dead? (Issues such as this also raise methodological questions: e.g., Is the definition of death primarily a matter of discovery, death being some kind of brute fact with contours that merely need better tracing, or is it, rather, something that the citizens of a political community must *invent* for themselves?)

The definition of death is perhaps the most salient conceptual puzzle served up by the new medicine, but it is by no means the only one. Similar issues are posed by the advent of new reproductive technologies (Is a woman who donates an egg to another woman the "mother" of the child born?

---

2. Nicholas Rescher, "What Is Value Change? A Framework for Research," in *Values and the Future*, edited by K. Baier and N. Rescher (New York: Free Press, 1969).

3. Peter Kramer, *Listening to Prozac* (New York: Viking Press, 1993).

Is she a mother in any sense that matters?), the human genome project (Is the otherwise healthy twenty-year-old carrier of a gene associated with the development of coronary artery disease in later life "diseased" in some sense?), and, of course, abortion (Is the fetus a "person" or full-fledged human being deserving of our respect and protection, is it merely a clump of cells, or is it perhaps something in-between?).

Finally, technology drives the bioethical agenda by virtue of its phenomenal success in addressing medical needs and desires. Hundreds of years ago, when medicine could offer little more than bleeding, blistering, and purging—when the leech represented the cutting edge of biotechnology—there weren't many "tragic choices" to be made. With the advent of technological success, however, has come the need to pay for increasingly expensive curative, diagnostic, and palliative procedures, access to which is increasingly perceived as a matter of right. But as costs skyrocket and as the demand for access spreads, the inevitability of limits and priority-setting gradually comes into focus. Assuming that meeting every conceivable health care need would either break the bank or devour funds earmarked for other important societal needs—such as food, shelter, education, transportation, and the arts—the question of the explicit rationing of health care acquires real seriousness and urgency. Can we afford to pay for a patient's third organ transplant, for his or her experimental bone marrow transplant for advanced cancer, or for the short but otherwise normal child's synthetic growth hormone injections? Can we afford these things when millions of people lack basic health insurance and decent preventive and primary care? Conceived in their broadest framework, these questions ask how our health care system might be reformed to provide universal access to a good package of "basic" services, without either bankrupting society or destroying the doctor–patient relationship.

Other Sources of Bioethical Problems

Although the urgency and frequency of bioethical controversies owe much to the magnitude and pace of technological change, there are other factors at work driving the recent explosion of bioethical issues. Some long-standing moral problems in medicine, such as the limits of confidentiality, truth-telling, and euthanasia, have more to do with the ethics of human relationships—with what we owe to one another and may (or may not) do to one another—than with the advent of new technologies. More important than technology in reshaping the physician–patient relationship are such widespread social phenomena as the increasing demand, modeled on the civil rights movement, for patients' rights to information and health care; the growing distrust of professional privilege; women's critiques of male dominance within medicine; and the assimilation of medicine to our consumerist and entrepreneurial culture.

Even here, however, it remains true that advances in biology and medicine have often given a characteristically modern spin to some of these traditional problems. Truth-telling, for example, is perhaps now more important and more difficult an obligation than ever before, due in large measure to the vast proliferation of possible treatments and diagnostic interventions available to physicians and their patients. Likewise, our traditional norms governing the confidentiality of medical information are sorely tested when new genetic tests reveal serious abnormalities not only in patients coming for diagnosis and/or treatment, but also, of necessity, in some of their family members as well.

Still, many highly controversial practices require surprisingly little technological assistance in threatening our fundamental values and established customs. Artificial insemination with donated sperm, for example, allows infertile married couples to have children, but it also enables single women and lesbian partners to give birth without the presence of a male spouse; in addition, it makes possible the practice of so-called surrogate motherhood, in which, for example, a woman agrees to be inseminated with the sperm of the husband of a childless marriage. For some, these developments signal serious threats to the welfare of children and to the institution of marriage, the very bedrock of our society; for others, they merely represent the next logical step in the growth of reproductive rights for all individuals, whether they be married or single, straight or gay, fertile or infertile. Ironically, at the heart of this impassioned debate about rights, marriage, and society lies the most ordinary of technological means: the humble turkey baster.

CHALLENGES TO ETHICAL THEORY

The issues raised in the preceding section pose challenging factual, conceptual, and moral problems. People often have strong feelings about some of these issues (for example, abortion and euthanasia). On some issues, many of us do not know what to think (for example, IVF for older women, or using children born without a higher brain as sources of transplantable organs). The assumption in philosophical bioethics is that careful analysis can help us at least make progress on some of these issues, if not resolve all of them. However, some are skeptical about this assumption. They believe, for a variety of reasons, that ethical disputes are, in principle, unresolvable by rational means.

Moral Nihilism

Princeton philosopher Gilbert Harman defines "moral nihilism" as "the doctrine that there are no moral facts, no moral truths, and no moral knowledge."[4] Extreme nihilists think that nothing is right or wrong; that morality, like religion, is an illusion that should be abandoned. This implies that torturing, raping, and killing a young child is not wrong—something few people could accept. More moderate nihilists do not recommend abandoning morality, but, rather, offer a theory about the meaning of moral terms that explains why there are no moral facts, truths, or knowledge.

Ethics and Feelings

The theory of moral language that is offered by moderate moral nihilists is known as "emotivism." Emotivists believe that moral utterances do not express facts, or tell us anything about how the world is. Rather, they express our feelings. Therefore, such statements are not—indeed, cannot be—true or false, any more than "Go, Yankees!" is true or false. The statement "Abortion is wrong" does not say anything about abortion, but rather expresses someone's negative feelings about abortion.

How plausible is this thesis about moral language? Undoubtedly, moral claims often do express feelings, but it is debatable that that is all they do. Consider Dr. Brody's quandary. She might ask herself, "I wonder if euthanasia is wrong." In an emotivist analysis, this can only mean, "I wonder if I have negative feelings about euthanasia." Is this Dr. Brody's question? It seems rather that she wonders what she *thinks* about euthanasia. Should she be motivated by her empathy for her patient and her desire to alleviate his suffering? Or should she act according to that part of the Hippocratic oath that requires doctors to be healers, not killers? What would be the larger implications for society if doctors were to engage in terminating their patients' lives? Dr. Brody's internal debate is of a kind familiar to most of us. In other words, when we face a moral dilemma, instead of trying to resolve our puzzlement by an introspective attempt at ascertaining which of our feelings is really the strongest, we tend to look "outward" at various external or objective aspects and implications of the alternatives in order to determine which is right.

We do not deny a relationship between feelings and ethical decisions, for moral issues often, if not always, provoke deep emotional responses. But to assign feelings ultimate authority in these matters is, we think, to put the cart before the horse. Our feelings may provoke us to moral inquiry, but the inquiry does not terminate there.

Ethics and Culture

Another form of moderate moral nihilism denies the possibility of moral truth *independent of a particular culture*. This view, known as "ethical relativism," says that morality is relative to the society one lives in and the way one was brought up. The rightness or wrongness of an action or practice cannot be determined apart from the cultural or social context in which it occurs.

Support for ethical relativism comes from three sources. First, it stems from an observation that different cultures have different moral beliefs and practices. However, simply noting moral differences in various cultures does not establish ethical relativism. Ethical relativism goes beyond noting that cultures differ in their moral beliefs and practices;

---

4. Gilbert Harman, *The Nature of Morality: An Introduction to Ethics* (New York: Oxford University Press, 1977), 11.

it maintains that when there are moral differences, no one is right (or wrong). According to relativism, right and wrong are always relative to, and determined by, culture.

A reason for thinking that morality is always relative to culture is that there does not seem to be any way to prove that an ethical belief or practice is right (or wrong). Infanticide, for example, is treated as murder in our culture, but is accepted or tolerated in others. Who's to say who's right? The inability to prove an ethical belief is contrasted with the ability to prove factual claims. If we come across people who think that Earth is flat, we can (in principle) show them that it is round. Note that the difference between ethics and science is not that ethics has a monopoly on disagreement. There are plenty of heated disagreements among scientists. However, scientists agree (in principle) about what kinds of evidence would settle a dispute. There is no such agreement in ethics. In other words, we do not have a decision procedure for resolving ethical disputes. This is the second source of support for ethical relativism.

The previous two reasons offered in support of relativism make observations about the world, and then offer a theory about the nature of reality that is consistent with these observations. We might characterize these as intellectual reasons for relativism. The third reason for relativism is quite different. It offers a moral reason for adopting relativism: namely, that relativism promotes tolerance toward people who hold moral beliefs different from one's own. This apparently was the motivation of nineteenth-century anthropologists who wished to prevent Western imperialists from imposing their culture on indigenous peoples.

Assume that we accept the plausible claim that different cultures do in fact differ in their moral beliefs. (Even this statement can be questioned, but let us accept it for the sake of argument.) What about the second support for relativism, that there is no decision procedure in ethics? This claim seems most plausible when we think of controversial issues, such as abortion or euthanasia, about which intelligent people of good will can disagree. Suppose, however, we think instead of a practice that virtually everyone thinks is wrong: for example, slavery. In the eighteenth and nineteenth centuries, slavery was often justified on the grounds that the Africans

were inherently inferior to their European masters, incapable of learning or governing themselves. This is a "factual" claim, and it is clearly false. Indeed, had the slaves really been incapable of learning, laws prohibiting the teaching of reading to slaves would have been pointless—there were no laws outlawing the teaching of reading to cows, for example. These and other justifications of slavery are clearly false and self-serving.

Slavery can also be criticized as inconsistent with other fundamental values, such as the equality of all men (or as we would say today, all human beings), as proclaimed in the Declaration of Independence. It seems likely that the discrepancy between the value of equality and the practice of slavery was a motivation for the abolition of slavery, along with its recognition as cruel, exploitative, and unjust. These terms also have considerable factual content, so that it is not "just a matter of opinion" whether a practice is cruel, exploitative, or unjust.

A further point against relativism (parallel to the argument we presented against emotivism) is that it gives an inaccurate account of the meaning of certain moral claims, notably those of moral reformers. According to relativism, right and wrong are always relative to culture. What a culture (or the majority of a culture) thinks is right is right— for them. However, a moral reformer challenges the conventional beliefs of his or her own culture. For example, Martin Luther King, Jr., said that segregation was wrong. According to relativism, this can only mean that segregation is considered wrong by his culture, which was obviously false in the American South in the 1950s. Of course King was not claiming that his culture *regarded* segregation as wrong. He was making the very different claim that segregation *was* wrong. (Indeed, if his culture already believed that segregation was wrong, he would not have had to demonstrate and go to jail for his beliefs!) Relativism simply cannot make sense of the claims of moral reformers. Since we do understand the claims of moral reformers, and at least sometimes are influenced by them, it seems that relativism cannot be true.

Despite these considerations, ethical relativism holds sway with many people, perhaps because the alternative seems terribly arrogant. One often hears the following sort of argument: "How can anyone say that another person's values are wrong? Who are you to tell me that you're right and I'm wrong? What makes you an authority? Everyone has a right to an opinion." However, we must be careful here. To say that everyone has a right to an opinion is not to say that every opinion is right. One can certainly agree that people have a right to their moral views without being a relativist. Indeed, if we think that everyone has the right to an opinion, we are *not* relativists. For "everyone has the right to an opinion" is itself a moral value. According to relativism, this moral value (like any other) is only true for societies that believe it. But not all cultures accept freedom of thought as a basic value. What if a culture believes in complete conformity of thought, and in brutal suppression of nonconformity? What if they practice conversion by the sword? Can we say that they are wrong to do this, that they ought to be tolerant? Not if we are relativists. Tolerance, then, is not a value that relativists can consistently promote, for tolerance, like all other moral values, is only right in cultures that think it right.

Finally, relativism not only prevents us from criticizing the brutal and intolerant practices of others, it also does not permit us to criticize our own past. We cannot say that slavery or child labor or the oppression of women were mistakes, since this implies an objective moral standard according to which we can evaluate our past practices. There is no moral progress, only moral change. This is another reason for rejecting ethical relativism, at least in its most extreme form.

At the same time, relativism has two things to recommend it, which we believe can be incorporated into a nonrelativist approach. First, the relativist is right to point out that morality occurs in a cultural context. Before presuming to judge another culture's practices and beliefs, we would do well to try to understand them "from the inside." We may still decide ultimately that a practice is wrong, but we are not entitled to make this judgment without understanding the practice in context. Second, relativism encourages multiple perspectives on and solutions to moral problems. Both of these insights are present in "multiculturalism." As we understand it, multiculturalism is *not* an uncritical acceptance of the values and practices of all other cultures. Rather, it is the awareness that there are a range of different ways to live, which offer different solutions to the problems faced by human beings, combined with a recognition that our own solutions—practices, institutions, values, and moral rules—may not be the best ones. Multiculturalism is a welcome corrective to an unfortunate tendency of Western civilization to assume superiority and to dismiss other ways of life as inferior and backward.

One can, however, be a multiculturalist without being a relativist. Indeed, it is only if one *rejects* relativism that one can meaningfully say such things as, "Our culture's attitude toward nature is domineering, exploitative, and wasteful. We could learn something from Native Americans." Multiculturalism requires an open mind toward the customs and beliefs of other cultures, but such open-mindedness need not, and should not, be uncritical. It is entirely consistent with a conception of morality as amenable to rational considerations, and the conviction that there can be better or worse moral justifications.[5]

MORAL THEORIES AND PERSPECTIVES

How are we to assess moral reasons and arguments? Intuitively, most of us can probably recognize good—or especially bad—moral reasoning, but in complicated situations we are often left wondering whether a consideration is pertinent. Is assisted suicide wrong because it helps someone to kill himself or herself, and killing is wrong? Or is it right because it helps someone do what he or she reasonably wants to do, and thus promotes autonomy? To answer questions of this sort, we need "a framework within which agents can reflect on the acceptability of actions and can evaluate moral judgments and moral character."[6] Such a framework is known as an "ethical theory."

---

5. Robert K. Fullinwider, "Ethnocentrism and Education in Judgment," *Report from the Institute for Philosophy & Public Policy* 14 (1994): 6–11. See also Charles Taylor et al., *Multiculturalism and "The Politics of Recognition"* (Princeton, NJ: Princeton University Press, 1992); and Amy Gutmann, "The Challenge of Multiculturalism in Political Ethics," *Philosophy and Public Affairs* 22, no. 3 (Summer 1993): 171–206.

6. Tom Beauchamp and James F. Childress, *The Principles of Biomedical Ethics,* 4th ed. (New York: Oxford University Press, 1994), 44.

Traditionally, ethical theories tend to be reductionist; that is, they offer one idea as the key to morality, and attempt to reduce everything to that one idea. For example, classical utilitarians maintain that right actions are those that promote the greatest happiness of the greatest number, while Kantians tell us that right actions are those that can be consistently willed universally. Each theory claims to have discovered the single, overarching standard of morality or right action. In a typical introduction to ethical theory class, each theory is presented and subjected to devastating criticism. The unfortunate result is that students frequently conclude that all of the theories are wrong—or worse, are pretentious nonsense.

In recent years, a number of philosophers have come to doubt that any normative theory can plausibly claim to be *the* correct theory. It may be that moral reality is sufficiently complex that any one theory gives only partial insight. Utilitarians are certainly right that achieving human happiness is an important goal of morality, but nonconsequentialists are also right in insisting, first, that other values such as justice and autonomy are also important, and second, that these values cannot be reduced to happiness. We conclude that it is a mistake to view the various theoretical alternatives as mutually exclusive claims to moral truth. Instead, we should view them as important but partial contributions to a comprehensive, although necessarily fragmented, moral vision.

Utilitarianism

Jeremy Bentham (1748–1832) and John Stuart Mill (1806–1873) are generally credited with developing the first detailed and systematic formulation of the ethical theory known as "utilitarianism." The heart of utilitarianism is "the greatest happiness principle," which, as Mill puts it, "holds that actions are right in proportion as they tend to promote happiness; wrong as they tend to produce the reverse of happiness."[7] The greatest happiness principle is also known as the principle of utility. The utility of an action is determined by its tendency to produce

or promote happiness. Actions that result in happiness have positive utility; those that create misery have negative utility. Clearly, many actions can create both conditions. An act that is pleasurable now (not going to the dentist) can cause considerable suffering later on; and often the happiness of some persons (car thieves) is purchased at the expense of unhappiness for others. The right action is the one that, on balance, promotes the most happiness, or the greatest amount of pleasure over pain.

The first thing to note about utilitarianism is that it is a "consequentialist" theory. That is, it judges the rightness and wrongness of an action by its consequences, or what will happen if the action is or is not performed. Second, utilitarianism's theory of value says that good consequences are those that produce or promote happiness or pleasure, bad consequences those that produce or promote the reverse. As we will see, both consequentialism and utilitarianism's theory of value have lately come under attack.

There are several advantages to utilitarianism. It provides us with a decision procedure for deciding what to do: namely, whichever action produces, on balance, the greatest net amount of happiness. Moreover, happiness is alleged to be something empirical, something both measurable and comparable. In principle, therefore, utilitarianism provides definite answers to the question of how we ought to act.

Features of Utilitarianism As we indicated earlier, utilitarianism is a form of consequentialism, and thus it holds that the results of actions are the *only* relevant feature in assessing actions. Considerations of an agent's intentions, feelings, or convictions are seen as irrelevant to the question, "What is the right thing to do?" Similarly, utilitarianism regards the question of whether a given course of action conforms to established social norms or ethical codes as relevant only to the extent that such conformity has a bearing on the production of happiness or unhappiness. Departing from established social codes typically has adverse consequences for the rule-breaker, and these consequences must be considered in deciding whether departing from the norm is the right thing to do.

Another important feature of utilitarianism is its impartiality. The utilitarian does not say, "The goodness of an action is determined by the amount

---

7. John Stuart Mill, *Utilitarianism* (New York: Liberal Arts Press, 1957), 10.

of happiness it produces *for me*." Rather, the good is determined by the overall net happiness achieved. The utilitarian considers his or her own happiness, but no more and no less than the happiness of others. In weighing the effects of an action, utilitarianism maintains that we must take into consideration all of the parties concerned and that all parties shall be given equal consideration. Thus, utilitarianism is committed to the value of equality.

How far does this equality extend? In the nineteenth century, women were not considered the equals of men. Women were largely under the control of their fathers before marriage, and their husbands after. They could not vote, and their ability to own property was greatly restricted. Mill rejected such inequality. He supported equal rights for women and opposed slavery. Indeed, Mill thought that any creature capable of being happy or miserable—"all sentient creation so far as possible"—was deserving of moral concern. Contemporary utilitarians, like Peter Singer, have argued that nonhuman animals should count equally with humans, and that therefore painful experimentation on animals is wrong.

Utilitarianism has been influential not only in expanding our notion of "who counts" morally, but also in focusing attention on long-term, as well as short-term, results. Many decisions and actions performed today have an impact on the future. Remoteness in time is not, in principle, a reason to ignore a consequence, any more than is remoteness in space (although, of course, our knowledge about the future is less certain than our knowledge of the present). This is particularly important when we think of issues such as genetic engineering and gene therapy, which may have a profound impact on the genetic makeup of people in future generations. Utilitarianism espouses a prudent moral doctrine that requires us to think carefully about what we should do, and to consider not only the immediate effects of our actions, but also their long-term consequences.

To summarize the advantages of utilitarianism, first, it reduces vagueness by providing a single criterion of right action: namely, the promotion of human happiness. Moreover, happiness, whether understood as pleasure or as preference satisfaction, is something that can be empirically measured. Utilitarianism thus provides an objective standard for judging whether an action is right or wrong, and a method for resolving moral disputes. Finally, and more importantly, the principle of utility is derived from the very point of morality, which is to improve the lot of human beings living together. Morality does not relate to the satisfaction of some abstract or arbitrary code; rather, it relates to the improvement of the human condition, which means alleviating suffering and increasing happiness.

That the point of morality is to promote human welfare may seem boringly obvious, but it was regarded as quite radical in the nineteenth century, and not only because of its egalitarian implications. In addition, the focus on human happiness seemed to conflict with Christian teachings; for example, those teachings espousing the value of suffering. As we noted earlier, anesthesia during childbirth was condemned in the nineteenth century as unnatural and contrary to biblical teachings ("In sorrow shalt thou bring forth children"). Even today the suffering of terminally ill patients is valued by some Catholic theologians, who regard the opportunity to identify with and participate in Christ's suffering on the cross as a positive good. Utilitarians are likely to have little patience with such views. Utilitarianism regards suffering and sacrifice as having moral value only if they promote overall happiness. Suffering and sacrifice have no intrinsic moral worth.

Objections to Utilitarianism   Utilitarianism has been subjected to numerous objections, four of which we will consider here. One objection is to utilitarianism's theory of value: namely, the claim that happiness is the greatest good, the ultimate end. Critics have maintained that this theory leaves out many other "goods," such as health, friendship, creativity, intellectual attainment, and so forth. Mill agreed that these things are all valuable, but argued that they are valuable because they contribute to a happy life, one as rich as possible in enjoyment and as free as possible from pain. However, it remains questionable whether all values are commensurable; that is, whether all values can be reduced to happiness, however happiness is interpreted. And even if it were possible to reduce the plurality of values to a single value, happiness, is it possible to compare and weigh the happiness of one person against that of another?

What if an action will make one person intensely happy but leave several people somewhat depressed? Exactly how are we to arrive at the right utilitarian solution? Moreover, some people feel things more intensely than others. Should we pay attention to the strength of desires? On the one hand, it seems that we should, since the intensity of an individual's happiness or unhappiness affects the total amount, and utilitarianism tells us to maximize happiness. On the other hand, this gives an advantage to the passionate over the phlegmatic that seems to violate Bentham's dictum that everyone counts for one, nobody for more than one.

A second objection to utilitarianism is that it requires us to calculate the probable consequences of every action, and this task is impossible. The sheer calculations alone would prevent anyone from doing anything. In response, it should be noted that both Bentham and Mill thought of utilitarianism primarily as a guide to legislative policy, rather than as a guide to individual behavior. No one thinks it unreasonable to ask for impact studies on the likely consequences of legislation. These are sometimes called "cost–benefit" analyses, and they are the direct descendants of classical utilitarianism.

Being utilitarians in our private lives does not mean that we must calculate all the consequences of every act, which would be impossible. Instead, we can rely on what Mill calls secondary principles, like "Don't lie," and "Don't harm others." We know from centuries of experience that adherence to these secondary principles promotes the greatest happiness for all, while departure from them causes insecurity and misery.

A more recent criticism of utilitarianism (or consequentialism generally) concerns the theory of responsibility it implies. For nonconsequentialists, it can be very significant whether an outcome occurs because of something *I did*, whereas for consequentialists all that matters ultimately is *what happens*. This has led some consequentialists to reject a time-honored distinction in medicine, the distinction between killing and "letting die." Many doctors believe that it is permissible for them to stop treatment when death is desirable; for example, in the case of a terminally ill patient in a great deal of pain who wants to die. However, they think

it would be wrong (as well as illegal) actively to kill a patient in that same situation. Utilitarians, by contrast, are likely to regard killing and letting die as morally equivalent, since the outcome—a desirable death—is achieved in both cases (see Part 3, Section 6).

A final major criticism of utilitarianism is that it is inadequate as a moral theory because it conflicts with some of our most basic moral intuitions.

> Suppose we could greatly increase human happiness and diminish misery by occasionally, and perhaps secretly, abducting derelicts from city streets for use in fatal but urgent medical experiments. If utilitarian considerations were decisive, this practice might well be justifiable, even desirable. Yet it is surely wrong. Such a case suggests that we cannot always explain good and bad simply in terms of increasing or decreasing overall happiness.[8]

A utilitarian might respond by denying the premise that we could in fact promote the greatest happiness by abducting derelicts for medical experiments. He or she might argue that this fails to take into consideration all the negative side effects of such a policy: the impossibility of keeping it secret, the terror of the derelicts not yet abducted, the risk of mistake and abuse, the psychological effect on the doctors performing the experiments, etc. It is precisely because of such long-range negative consequences that policies like informed consent are rational from a utilitarian viewpoint. Still, it seems possible that, in special circumstances, the good effects could outweigh the bad. Some utilitarians will acknowledge that in such circumstances it would be right to use derelicts in fatal medical experiments (while reminding us that such circumstances are extremely unlikely to obtain, and it is even less likely that we can be sure that they do). However, they maintain that the fact that this practice would conflict with many people's deeply held moral convictions is not a worthwhile criticism of utilitarianism. Many utilitarians are quite skeptical of "deeply held moral convictions," which they regard as often no more than irrational superstitions.

---

8. Christina and Fred Sommers, eds., *Vice and Virtue in Everyday Life: Introductory Readings in Ethics*, 2nd ed. (San Diego, CA: Harcourt Brace Jovanovich, 1989), 80.

Others, attracted by the virtues of utilitarianism, are nevertheless disturbed by the possibility of conflicts with justice and other basic moral practices, such as telling the truth and keeping promises. Rule-utilitarianism may be seen as one attempt to counter this objection.

Rule-Utilitarianism versus Act-Utilitarianism

Mill left unresolved the question whether the greatest happiness principle is to be applied to specific acts or to general kinds of acts. It has been suggested that if we apply the principle to kinds of acts, we can avoid some of the criticisms of utilitarianism. The version of utilitarianism that is primarily concerned with the consequences of specific acts has become known as "act-utilitarianism," while the version primarily concerned with the consequences of general policies is called "rule-utilitarianism."

Act-utilitarianism tells us to apply the principle of utility directly to the particular act in question. Suppose a doctor is faced with the question whether it would be morally right to help a terminally ill patient to die. An act-utilitarian would seek to determine which alternative in this particular case would maximize happiness and/or minimize suffering. Relevant considerations would include the possibility of recovery, whether the patient really wanted to die or was in a depression that might be alleviated, the impact on the patient's family, the impact on the doctor, and so forth.

By contrast, rule-utilitarianism uses the principle of utility not to decide which acts to perform or avoid, but rather to formulate and justify moral rules. The correct moral rules are those that promote the greatest happiness of the greatest number. Faced with a decision about how to act, rule-utilitarianism tells us that we are not to appeal directly to the principle of utility. Rather, we are to consider whether this action falls under a rule that is justified by the principle of utility. Rule-utilitarianism would direct Dr. Brody to ask whether a general rule permitting assisted suicide would maximize happiness. Here, an important consideration would be whether such a practice would start us down a "slippery slope" and threaten the lives of terminally ill patients who do not really want to die, but who, for various reasons, are either afraid of being a burden to their families, or have families that want to get rid of them. Thus, a rule-utilitarian might argue that while helping *this* patient die might maximize happiness (or minimize misery), it would nevertheless be wrong, because the consequences of a general policy of assisting suicide would be disastrous.

The difference between act- and rule-utilitarianism is *not* that only the latter appeals to moral rules. Both act- and rule-utilitarians use rules to guide their behavior. Rather, the difference lies in the way each group regards moral rules. For the act-utilitarian, rules are *summaries of past experience*. They're what we might call "rules of thumb": handy guides to the future based on past experience. Since it's often difficult to know what will maximize happiness in a particular situation, and since people are likely to be prejudiced by their own self-interest in their calculations, rules help us decide what to do.

Rules are regarded differently by rule-utilitarians. Rules are not just devices to help us figure out what will maximize happiness in a particular case. The rules themselves are justified on the grounds that having these particular rules maximizes happiness. But once we decide what the best rules are (that is, which ones are most likely to maximize happiness over the long run), then those are the rules we should follow, even if following them in a particular situation doesn't maximize happiness.

Thus, the rule-utilitarian can apparently avoid the sorts of situations that make act-utilitarianism unsatisfactory to many. In brief, the rule-utilitarian agrees with the act-utilitarian that the value of just practices resides in their tendency to promote happiness; but he will not agree that it is permissible to perform an unjust act in order to maximize happiness.

Is Rule-Utilitarianism an Improvement over Act-Utilitarianism?   Act-utilitarians make this criticism of rule-utilitarianism: It makes no sense for a utilitarian to insist that a rule that will have less than optimal consequences should be followed simply because the rule maximizes happiness *in general.* J. J. C. Smart gives the following example. A good rule of thumb in a chess game is that you shouldn't sacrifice your queen for a pawn. But if, in a particular game of chess, you could checkmate your opponent by sacrificing your queen for a pawn, it would be absurd to stick dogmatically to the "Never sacrifice your queen for a pawn" rule. Smart thinks rule-utilitarianism is guilty of the same absurdity. Just as checkmating your opponent is the whole point of chess, so maximizing happiness is the whole point of utilitarian morality. It would not be rational from the standpoint of utility to refuse to break a moral rule when by doing so you could maximize welfare. For this reason, Smart calls rule-utilitarianism "superstitious rule worship."[9]

A related objection to rule-utilitarianism is that it collapses into act-utilitarianism. For whenever an act-utilitarian would say it was right to *break* a moral rule, it seems that the rule-utilitarian would generally agree, but instead say that the rule should be *modified*. Suppose, for example, that the only way to save someone's life is by telling a lie. An act-utilitarian would say that it was right to lie in such circumstances. But what would a rule-utilitarian say? That it is wrong to lie, knowing that the result will be an avoidable death? Surely not. A rule-utilitarian would say that the original rule, "Don't lie," is too crude. A better rule would be, "Don't lie, except to save a life." Moreover, it is likely that there is more than one exception to the "Don't lie" rule. That is, the rule most likely to maximize happiness probably allows for several situations in which lying is morally right. But now it seems that whatever would lead the act-utilitarian to break the rule would lead the rule-utilitarian to modify the rule. Thus, the two versions give exactly the same advice; they are "extensionally equivalent," so rule-utilitarianism cannot be an improvement over act-utilitarianism. On the other hand, if the rule-utilitarian holds fast to the original rule, even when modifying it would have better results, he or she deviates from utilitarianism and is guilty of Smart's charge of "rule-worship."

In response, a rule-utilitarian might say that the criticism of extensional equivalence reflects a naive view of the operation of social rules and policies. While the considerations that lead an act-utilitarian to break a rule in a particular case can perhaps be articulated, it is much less easy to formulate a general policy that covers all the relevant exceptions. Consider the case study with which we began. A rule-utilitarian would not only consider whether it would be right for Dr. Brody to help Mr. Lasken kill himself, but also whether doctors generally ought to be able to make decisions of this kind. For it is clear that this is not a one-of-a-kind situation; there are lots of Jim Laskens and Deborah Brodys. Should doctors make such decisions on a case-by-case basis? That approach has the advantage of allowing the individual doctor to decide whether the patient's pain outweighs the general rule against killing. The disadvantage of that approach, however, is that most people, including doctors, are not perfect happiness optimizers. There are bound to be mistakes. Some patients who are not terminally ill will be killed, as will some who could have been helped with psychiatric treatment or better pain medicine. Some doctors may be unduly influenced by relatives who want the patient's life to be over when the patient does not. More disturbing, in times of cost-cutting, might there not be a tendency to regard the terminally ill as "expendable" and not worth spending money on, even if a sick individual does not want to die? The problem is not so much that we cannot say when assisted suicide would and would not be justified (though this too is difficult to specify in advance); rather, it is that the practice of this policy on a large scale may result in many unnecessary and undesirable deaths. The question, then, is whether the need for such a policy is outweighed by the risk of mistake and abuse. These rule-utilitarian considerations do not seem to be captured by an act-utilitarian approach, which looks only at the consequences of a specific act. Therefore, rule-utilitarianism does not collapse into act-utilitarianism.

Nevertheless, rule-utilitarianism acknowledges that it is, in principle, possible that a practice we ordinarily think of as completely immoral (such as slavery) might, in unusual circumstances, promote the greatest happiness and would therefore be right. Moreover, the factor that determines whether a practice maximizes happiness (for example, whether the number of people made miserable was sufficiently small) seems morally irrelevant. How can it be right to ride roughshod over the rights of a few people simply to make the majority happy? It is considerations of this kind that lead some people to

---

9. J. J. C. Smart, "Extreme and Restricted Utilitarianism," in *Theories of Ethics*, edited by Philippa Foot (Oxford: Oxford University Press, 1967), 177.

reject utilitarianism altogether and opt for something completely different.

Kantian Ethics

Utilitarian ethics has a strong appeal. The utilitarian says, "*Surely* consequences are terribly important. Whenever we act, we are trying to bring about certain states of affairs and avoid others. It is right to bring about happiness, and wrong to create misery. How can there be any other criterion of right and wrong? What *makes* lying and cheating wrong, if not that they cause misery?"

At the same time, it seems that there are some things we must not do, even if doing them would accomplish great good. What if we could maximize happiness by deliberately hurting innocent people or by violating their rights? Surely this would be wrong. It seems to matter not just *what* happens, but *how* it comes about.

Kantian ethics, so titled from its most illustrious exponent Immanuel Kant (1724–1804), captures this intuitive conviction. Whereas Mill said that the right act is the one with the best consequences, Kant argued that consequences can never make an action right or wrong. An action that brings about the greatest amount of happiness might still be wrong. Good consequences can never make a wrong action right, and one must never act wrongly in order to bring about good consequences. In other words, the ends do not justify the means.

In addition to rejecting consequentialism, Kant also rejects the view that pain is intrinsically bad and pleasure intrinsically good. According to Kant, the badness of pain depends on whether it is deserved. It is morally right that the wicked should suffer and morally wrong that they should prosper. Kant rejects the utilitarian view that the pleasure experienced by a sadist is an intrinsic good, albeit one which can be outweighed by the suffering of his victim. The sadist's pleasure has absolutely no moral worth. Indeed, pain and pleasure, which play so prominent a role in utilitarian ethics, have a relatively minor role in Kantian ethics. As we saw earlier, Mill and Bentham extended moral concern to all sentient beings. By contrast, Kant considers our capacity to experience pleasure and pain as fairly insignificant morally. Of far greater importance is

our rationality: our ability to think, to plan our lives, to be motivated by abstract considerations. This is allegedly what separates us from the rest of creation, giving human beings a central and special moral status. As animals, we are subject to the laws of nature, physical and psychological. However, unlike other animals, human beings are rational beings, or persons.

For Kant, rational beings have a special moral standing because of their ability to act on the basis of reason and to conform their behavior to the moral law. Kant argues that many of the common ends that people pursue, such as health, wealth, education, and the like, are valuable only because of their place in the projects of rational beings. In contrast, the value of persons does not depend on the way they fit into the projects of other rational beings. Persons have intrinsic worth and must be treated as ends in themselves and not merely as a means to some other end. Because the source of this dignity lies in rational nature, Kant also argues that morality requires that all persons must be treated equally.

To contrast the value of persons as ends in themselves with the value of the ends that depend on the projects of persons, Kant says that rational beings possess dignity, as opposed to a use-value. Consider the way that Kant differs from the consequentialist over the question of whether it would be morally right to prevent the deaths of five innocent people, each of whom needs an organ transplant, by killing another innocent person and distributing his or her vital organs. According to utilitarianism, this would be right, since it results in a net gain of four lives. Of course, this reasoning fails to take into consideration the side effects we mentioned earlier in the theoretical use of derelicts in urgent medical experiments. For a utilitarian, the moral question turns on whether the negative side effects outweigh the benefit of saving four lives. On a Kantian approach, however, to kill an innocent person for his or her organs is a paradigm case of treating a person as a mere means, and could never be justified. The fact that the killing is done from altruistic motives, or that it would result in a net saving of lives, does not change the fact that it would be murder, which is intrinsically wrong. Kant did not claim that we should *ignore* the consequences of actions; that would be absurd. Other things being equal, we should of course try to bring about good consequences, if we can do so without doing anything morally wrong. We should consider the consequences of a proposed action only after determining that the action is morally permissible.

How then are we to identify morally permissible and impermissible actions? Most people already have a pretty good idea of the kinds of actions that are wrong. We learn to distinguish right from wrong from our parents, teachers, and playmates. We know that lying, breaking promises, cheating, stealing, and hurting others are wrong—and if someone does not know these things by the time he or she is seven or eight, a course in moral philosophy is unlikely to be of help. What a moral theory can do is provide an explanation of *why* these things are wrong. What makes them wrong? As we've seen, the utilitarian explanation is that the actions we normally regard as wrong—lying, cheating, stealing, killing—promote unhappiness. The trouble with this explanation is that it seems possible, in a particular case, that no one gets hurt by an act of lying or cheating, or that the negative consequences of such an act are outweighed by the positive. Suppose I can get away with cheating without anyone finding out; would that make it morally acceptable? Kant would say of course not, it's still cheating. The important thing is not the consequences of the act, but the kind of act it is. An action could bring about the best nonmoral consequences—for instance, save the most number of lives, make the most people happy—and still be morally wrong because it is unjust or dishonest.

Another reason Kant rejects consequentialism is that what happens is often not within our control and so is not something for which we can be praised, blamed, or held at all responsible. A physician may administer a drug that kills a patient due to unknown and unforeseeable side effects. Though the outcome is disastrous, surely the physician does not act immorally. Kant holds that if you act rightly, you are not responsible for any bad effects that occur. (Utilitarians distinguish between rightness and moral blameworthiness. They say that what the physician did was wrong, though it was not his fault and he should not be *blamed*.)

According to Kant, the fact that an action is likely to promote happiness or human welfare has nothing to do with whether anyone has a moral duty to do it. Duty must be entirely independent of consequences, for if it were otherwise, moral imperatives could only be "hypothetical." That is, they would tell us only, "*If* you want to achieve *x*, then do *y*." If someone does not want to achieve *x*, or does not care if *x* occurs, then he or she has no reason to do *y*. Morality, Kant held, is clearly *not* like this. Morality tells us, "Do *y*, whatever you may happen to want or feel." In other words, morality yields "categorical," rather than mere hypothetical, imperatives.

Imperatives (commands) can be either hypothetical or categorical, depending on the implicit principle contained within them. For example, "Treat people with respect" is a hypothetical imperative if the rationale for respecting others is to gain their friendship. Interpreted as a hypothetical imperative, this maxim tells us to treat others with respect *if* we want their friendship. However, some people do not care about gaining others' friendship. If "Treat others with respect" were only a hypothetical imperative, it would not apply to those who are indifferent to others. Since morality is clearly not conditional in this way, however, Kant argued that morality cannot consist of hypothetical imperatives. Instead, morality consists of categorical imperatives: commands that are valid for rational agents as such, independent of the feelings and desires they happen to have. Moreover, because morality consists of these categorical imperatives devoid of empirical content, it can have necessity; it can tell us what we *must* do, what we are obligated to do, what it is our duty to do.

To find out whether a proposed action is consistent with duty, and morally permissible, the right question to ask, Kant says, is not "What are the likely consequences of doing (or not doing) this action?" but rather, "*Can I, as a rational agent, consistently will that everyone in a similar situation should act this way?*" If we convert this question into an imperative, we get "Act always on that maxim (or principle) that you can consistently will as a principle of action for everyone similarly situated." Kant calls this rule the "categorical imperative," and it is the foundation of his ethical system. If the proposed action is one that would be wrong if done generally, then the particular action is wrong, too—even if it would not, in the case at hand, have harmful consequences. What matters is that the maxims of these actions cannot be consistently universalized. While it may seem entirely abstract and formal, universalization is, in part, a mechanism for ensuring equal respect for persons. It achieves this by not allowing us to make exceptions of ourselves, but requires us always to act only on principles that we could consistently will that everyone follow.

Kant thought that consistency and universality are clearly part of our concept of morality and duty. In trying to explain why we ought to do certain things (like voting) or refrain from doing others (like cheating), we are liable to ask, "What would happen if everyone acted that way?" But note that we do not regard it as a rebuttal if it is pointed out that not everyone *will* act that way. Universalization requires us to abstract from the actual circumstances and to refrain from making exceptions of ourselves. This test of right action is considered so important that many moral philosophers hold that a person "has a morality" only if that person is willing to universalize his or her moral judgments.[10]

Universalization is only one aspect of Kantian ethics. Equally important is Kant's insistence that persons must always be treated as "ends in themselves" and never merely as means. This means that in our dealings with others, we are to realize that they have their own goals, aims, and projects. We are never to treat other people as if they do not matter or count, or as if they exist simply to fulfill our purposes. This Kantian idea is reflected in the insistence that patients and research subjects must give informed consent before they can be treated or used in experiments. We also show respect for persons by telling them the truth, even when such knowledge might be painful, and by allowing them to make their own moral choices, even when we think they will choose unwisely. Thus, Kantian ethics has been a strong force against the medical paternalism that held sway until fairly recently.

If a proposed action fails either the universalization test or the respect for persons test, then it is contrary to duty and must not be done. Kantian ethics can help us determine what we must not do; but how are we to decide what we should do? For

often in deciding what to do, we are faced with a range of alternatives, none of which conflict with duty and all of which are morally permissible. Kantian ethics does not provide a decision procedure for deciding which out of all morally permissible acts is the right act. It thus gives the individual a great deal more latitude than does utilitarianism, which commands us to choose the act that has the best consequences. At the same time, Kantian ethics gives proportionately less guidance. This can be viewed as a deficiency, but it can also be viewed as an advantage, in that it allows for more individual autonomy.

How would a Kantian resolve Dr. Brody's dilemma? May Dr. Brody end the life of a suffering and seriously ill patient who requests such help? To answer this question, we need to ask whether it is morally permissible for Mr. Lasken to engineer his own death. For no one can have a duty to help another person do something that is morally wrong. Thus, we first have to consider the question of the morality of suicide. Kant himself thought that suicide violated the categorical imperative. His argument is as follows: Suicides kill themselves to spare themselves the pain of living. However, the desire to avoid pain is intrinsic to self-preservation. Committing suicide is thus acting from both self-preservation and self-destruction at the same time, and so is self-contradictory. Kant's argument here seems extremely murky. It is far from clear why it is self-contradictory to prefer death to life under horrible conditions.

Does suicide violate the requirement of respect for persons? Persons are worthy of respect, according to Kant, because they are ends in themselves. This rather obscure formulation alludes to the fact that persons are not mere things which are simply subject to natural laws, but rather rational agents with their own goals and ends. Moreover, rational natures are capable of assessing their own goals and desires, of deciding whether they want to pursue a certain goal or have a particular desire. (Philosophers call these wants about wants "second-order desires.") This ability to assess our desires and goals, and to act on those assessments, makes us *autonomous*. Autonomy, for Kant, is not simply a matter of the ability to make choices (as it is often portrayed in the medical context). Autonomy is the ability to formulate and follow laws that we would

---

10. See, for example, William Frankena, *Ethics,* 2nd ed. (Englewood Cliffs, NJ: Prentice Hall, 1972), 113–114.

be willing to have everyone follow, that is, universal laws. It is because human beings are autonomous that they have dignity and are worthy of respect.

Would acceding to Mr. Lasken's request to be killed violate the principle of respect for humanity, and thus be contrary to duty? Certainly, pressuring Mr. Lasken to die, or taking advantage of his vulnerable situation, would be ruled out by Kantian ethics. As Onora O'Neill puts it, "We use others as *mere means* if what we do reflects some maxim *to which they could not in principle consent.*"[11] Deception, coercion, and exploitation are all wrong because they treat others as mere means. We are assuming, however, that Mr. Lasken genuinely wants to die and is not being deceived, coerced, or exploited. Does helping him die fail to respect his humanity? A possible Kantian objection might be that in choosing to die in order to avoid pain, the prospective suicide treats himself as merely a sentient being, no more than an animal. In creating a maxim that derives solely from his animal nature, he fails to respect his own humanity or rational nature. However, Mr. Lasken might respond that he wants to end his life, and to get Dr. Brody's help in doing so, not simply to avoid pain, but also to avoid the certain deterioration of his mental powers, the subsequent loss of rationality, and the gradual erosion of his own sense of dignity and meaning. This reasoning should have considerable weight from a Kantian perspective. Kant's absolute opposition to rational suicide seems more a product of the conventional morality of his time than a requirement of the categorical imperative in either of its formulations.

It appears that a Kantian, even if not the historical Kant, could in principle support assisted suicide and voluntary euthanasia as promoting autonomy and self-determination. On the other hand, it is possible that a policy of voluntary euthanasia would lead to the devaluing of human life, and ultimately the nonvoluntary killing of the weak, the vulnerable, and the poor. If so, this would violate the values of autonomy and respect for persons, which would

lead Kantians to oppose euthanasia. (Remember that Kantians do not ignore consequences; they simply do not regard consequences themselves as determinative of right and wrong.)

Thus, we may expect to find Kantians—as well as utilitarians—on both sides of the euthanasia issue, depending on their factual predictions and their conceptions of basic moral concepts, such as autonomy and personhood. This conclusion will be discouraging for anyone who expects ethical theories to provide handy-dandy formulas for resolving moral issues. But ethical theories are not meant to provide formulas; instead, they provide frameworks for trying to reach workable solutions to complex and difficult questions.

Social Contract Theory

Any ethical theory must answer two fundamental questions. The first is about the content of our moral obligations: What are we required to do? The second is about our motivation for acting: Why are we required to do it? The social contract approach to ethics gives related answers to these questions. Our obligations are determined by the agreements we have made, and we ought to fulfill our obligations because we have agreed to them.[12]

There are two basic forms of contemporary social contract theory. Philosopher Will Kymlicka explains their difference this way:

> One approach stresses a natural equality of physical power, which makes it mutually advantageous for people to accept conventions that recognize and protect each other's interests and possessions. The other approach stresses a natural equality of moral status, which makes each person's interests a matter of common or impartial concern. This impartial concern is expressed in agreements that recognize each person's interests and moral status.[13]

Kymlicka calls proponents of the mutual advantage theory "Hobbesian contractarians," and proponents of the impartial theory "Kantian contractarians,"

---

11. Onora O'Neill, "The Moral Perplexities of Famine and World Hunger," in *Matters of Life and Death: New Introductory Essays in Moral Philosophy,* 2nd ed., edited by Tom Regan (New York: Random House, 1986), 322.

12. Will Kymlicka, "The Social Contract Tradition," in *A Companion to Ethics,* edited by Peter Singer (Oxford: Basil Blackwell, 1993), 186.

13. Ibid., 188.

because Hobbes and Kant inspired and foreshadowed these two forms of contract theory.

Hobbesian Contractarianism   Hobbesian contractarianism is a form of moral nihilism in its rejection of objective (or real) moral values. There is nothing inherently right or wrong about the goals one chooses to pursue, or the means one uses to pursue these goals. However, unless there are restrictions on the goals people pursue and the means by which they pursue them, the world is a threatening, dangerous place. Everyone is better off restricting his or her own liberty to injure others, so long as the others do likewise. Harming others is not inherently wrong in this view, but it is to our mutual advantage to accept conventions that define such harm as wrong.[14]

Hobbesian contractarianism replicates a good deal of ordinary morality, but not all of it. For one thing, it is clear that there is no mutual advantage in bargaining with those who are too weak to pose a threat of retaliation. Thus, Hobbesian contractarianism leaves out defenseless human beings, such as babies and those who are disabled.[15] This departure from everyday morality is no argument against Hobbesian contractarianism since, as Kymlicka points out, the theory denies that we have any natural duties to others; it is, as we said, a form of moral nihilism. Hobbesian contractarianism may be the best we can do in a world without natural duties or objective values.[16]

How would a Hobbesian contractarian approach the problem of doctor-assisted suicide? The question is whether it is to everyone's mutual advantage to allow doctors to kill (or help die) their terminally ill patients who request such help. On the one hand, it would appear irrational to rule out an option that a great many people apparently wish to have at the end of life. On the other hand, when we become terminally ill, we do not want doctors killing us for cost-control, to convenience our relatives, and so on. Thus, the Hobbesian contractarian analysis looks a great deal like a rule-utilitarian analysis.

Kantian Contractarianism   The best-known exponent of Kantian contractarianism is John Rawls. According to Rawls, people matter not because they can harm or benefit others (as in the Hobbesian view), but because they are ends in themselves (as Kant held). Everyone is entitled to equal consideration, and this basic notion of equality gives rise to a natural duty to promote a just society. A just society is one based on fair principles. However, the social contract approach creates a problem in attempting to derive fair principles. The problem is that, in a bargaining situation, the strong have a clear advantage over the weak, which is intuitively unfair. Rawls's solution to the problem of natural inequality is a hypothetical social contract whereby a society chooses its basic social principles from the standpoint of "the original position."

In the original position, all parties are under a "veil of ignorance." That is, while they know that they are human and have basic human needs, they are deprived of all knowledge of their special characteristics. No one knows if he or she is rich or poor, black or white, male or female, or politically liberal or conservative. This ignorance prevents people from tailoring social principles to their own advantage.

In the original position, each contractor is motivated by self-interest; that is, each is trying to do the best for himself or herself. But since no one knows what his or her position in society eventually will be, this self-interest amounts to acting impartially. To promote my own good, I must put myself in the shoes of every member of society and see what promotes his or her good, since I may end up being any one of these members.[17] It would be contrary to my own self-interest to choose a society that permitted slavery, since I might be a slave. Of course, it might turn out that I get to be a master, in which case I would be better off living in a slave-owning society. However, one cannot know one's place in advance. Rawls thinks that it would be irrational to opt for a slave-owning society, since being a slave in a slave-owning society is much worse than living as a free person in a society that prohibits slavery. Similarly, individuals in the original position could not choose a caste system, since they might turn out to

---

14. Ibid., 189.

15. David Gauthier, *Morals by Agreement* (Oxford: Oxford University Press, 1986), 286.

16. Kymlicka, "The Social Contract Tradition," 191 (see note 12).

17. Ibid., 192.

be untouchables; they could not choose a male-dominated society, since they might turn out to be women. The very arrangements we intuitively reject as unfair turn out to be irrational from the perspective of the original position.

Rawls goes on to argue that rational people in the original position would choose two basic principles to guide and determine the institutions of their society. The first principle is a principle of liberty. It maintains that everyone is to have as much liberty as possible, consonant with everyone else's having the same amount of liberty. This principle would be chosen from the standpoint of the original position because it would be irrational to choose a principle that gives some people more liberty than others. After all, you might end up being one of the people with less liberty.

The second principle is a principle of equality. It has two parts. The first part is a principle of distribution, often referred to as the "difference principle." It says that all goods should be equally distributed, except where an unequal distribution makes everyone, especially the worst off, better off. Why would choosers in the original position opt for equal distribution? Because if you don't know your position in society, it would be irrational to choose a distribution in which some have enormous wealth and others are impoverished. True, you might be Donald Trump, but it's better to forgo the chance for great wealth than to risk being impoverished. At the same time, it would be irrational to insist on absolute equal distribution if an unequal distribution would make everyone better off. (For example, it is in the best interests of the worst off to have an adequate supply of well-trained brain surgeons who are paid much more than the average person, if this inequality is the necessary incentive for them to set aside so many years for training.)

The second part of the principle of equality is a principle of equality of opportunity. Everyone is to have equal opportunity in achieving the various offices and roles in society; they are all to be open to everyone. Rawls's principle of fair equality of opportunity has been used by Norman Daniels as the basis for a universal right to health care.[18] The basic idea is that sickness and disability prevent us from functioning normally and deprive us of the opportunity to compete on an equal basis with others for the goods in society. While we can strive to keep ourselves healthy through various means (e.g., abstaining from smoking, following a low-fat diet, exercising regularly), for the most part, we have no control over becoming sick or disabled. Those who are sick or disabled are therefore at a considerable and unfair disadvantage. Those who do not get the medical attention that can restore "normal species-functioning" are thus doubly disadvantaged, first by "nature's lottery," and second by social arrangements that give some, but not others, access to health care. If equal opportunity is to be a reality, we must guarantee universal access to health care. Moreover, the concept of "normal species-functioning" is a guide for what kinds of treatment should be provided. Vaccination and eyeglasses are obvious candidates, while cosmetic surgery is not.

Rawls requires that his principle of liberty take precedence over his principle of equality. He states that the claims of liberty must be satisfied before social and economic inequalities can be contemplated, and that departures from the principle of equal liberty cannot be justified or made good by greater social and economic advantages.[19] The elements of the principle of equality are similarly ordered: Rawls sees that genuinely fair equality of opportunity (as opposed to merely formal access) must be guaranteed before we can address ourselves to social or economic inequalities.

If we compare Rawls's vision of "justice as fairness" with utilitarianism, we see some striking differences. The most dramatic difference concerns the respective theories of the "good" and the "right," and the way these important moral concepts are related. Utilitarian theories define the good independently of the right: First the good is defined as happiness, then the right is defined as that which maximizes happiness. Because justice is defined as a function of utility, it cannot limit the claims of utility. By contrast, Rawls sees the concepts of right and justice as preceding the concept of the good.[20] He

---

18. See Norman Daniels, *Just Health Care* (Cambridge: Cambridge University Press, 1985).

19. John Rawls, *A Theory of Justice* (Cambridge, MA: Harvard University Press, 1971), 61.
20. Ibid., 31.

states that for desires to have any value or to play any role in ethical calculations, they must accord with the principles of justice.

Rawls's theory of justice has been criticized as embodying problematic notions of rationality—in particular, a fundamental aversion to risk. Why assume that a rational person behind the veil of ignorance would opt for the equality of the difference principle? A gambler might be willing to take a relatively small risk of being impoverished for the chance of becoming very wealthy. Is this obviously irrational? A related criticism is that the contract does no real work. As we have seen, and as Rawls acknowledges, there can be different interpretations of the original position. A risk-aversive interpretation, which yields the difference principle, is not the only possible one. According to Rawls, we decide which interpretation of the original position is most suitable by determining which interpretation yields principles that match our convictions of justice. But, as Kymlicka points out, "if each theory of justice has its own account of the contracting situation, then we have to decide *beforehand* which theory of justice we accept, in order to know which description of the original position is suitable."[21] If this is so, then the contract cannot be used to establish the correct theory of justice. Nevertheless, contracting from an original position has some useful purposes. The veil of ignorance is a vivid expression of the moral requirement of our commitment to others, and of putting ourselves in their shoes. It dramatizes the claim that we would accept a certain principle, however it affected us. As Kymlicka says, "In these and other ways, the contract device illuminates the basic ideas of morality as impartiality, even if it cannot help defend those ideas."[22]

So how would a Kantian contractarian, or Rawlsian, approach Dr. Brody's dilemma? The principle of liberty requires that each individual have the maximum liberty possible, consistent with equal liberty for others. That requirement seems to argue in favor of allowing people to choose the time and manner of their death at the end of their life, in order to avoid great suffering, as well as financial loss for their families. At the same time, Rawls is concerned to protect the weak and vulnerable who cannot bargain on their own behalf. That would militate against a policy that could have a discriminatory impact on elderly, disabled, and poor people. Thus, a Rawlsian would be likely to approve of a policy of doctor-assisted suicide if it promoted the value of individual autonomy, but not if it violated equal respect for persons. (Rawls's own view on physician-assisted suicide is given in "The Philosophers' Brief" in Part 3, Section 6.)

RELIGIOUS ETHICS

We noted previously that religious ethics is one of the parent disciplines of bioethics. We are not suggesting that "religious ethics" is an ethical theory in the same sense as utilitarianism and Kantian ethics; religious beliefs do not, in general, imply any one particular ethical orientation. Some Christians take a utilitarian approach, while others have views closer to Kantianism. Although there are certainly ethical directives inherent in religious belief (e.g., "Do unto others as you would be done by"), each of these directives can be compatible with very different ethical theories.

Some religious traditions have been more influential than others in bioethics; for example, Roman Catholic moral thought. One reason for this influence is that the Roman Catholic Church is characterized by considerable unanimity. There is, on a number of issues, an official Church doctrine—this is not generally true of Protestantism, which has a great many denominations, or Judaism, which is divided into Orthodox, Conservative, Reform, and Reconstructionist. Another reason for the more powerful influence of Roman Catholicism is that it includes a well-developed, written body of thought on medical-moral issues, which has had considerable influence on prevailing attitudes (even among many non-Catholics), as well as on legal doctrine regarding a wide range of biomedical ethical issues. Lastly, the Catholic tradition includes an alternative ethical theory—known as natural law ethics—that provides principles for interpreting the general ethical directives of the Christian faith.

Natural Law Theories

Natural law theorists offer an account of the human good and ethical duty that contrasts sharply with

---

21. Kymlicka, "The Social Contract Tradition," 193 (see note 12).

22. Ibid.

the views of both utilitarianism and Kantianism on these issues. Utilitarianism defines the good in terms of happiness or the satisfaction of desire, while Kant repudiated all ethical theories based in any way upon desire or inclination. In contrast to utilitarianism, natural law ethicists insist that the human good cannot be reduced to a mere function of what people happen to desire. In this view, things are not good because we desire them; rather, we desire them, or should desire them, because they are good.

But natural law ethics is also opposed to Kantian ethics in that it is based on a conception of human nature. Kant insists that the categorical imperative must be empty of all empirical content; otherwise it could not have the necessity characteristic of the moral law. But what else, if not a concern for human welfare, can ethics possibly be founded upon, and how can it have any motivational force? Why, asks the natural law theorist, should we desire to be moral in the first place and follow the dictates of morality, unless such behavior holds out some prospect of promoting human well-being and happiness?

Natural law theorists thus agree with utilitarians that ethics must be grounded in a concern for the human good. But they agree with Kantians that the good cannot be defined simply in terms of what people "happen" to want. Instead, there is a good for human beings that, based on their nature, is objectively desirable.

Catholic theologians conceive of natural law as the law inscribed by God into the nature of things—as a species of divine law. According to this conception, the Creator endows all things with certain potentialities or tendencies that serve to define their natural end; the fulfillment of a thing's natural tendencies constitutes the specific "good" of that thing. The natural potential of an acorn is to become an oak. But what is the natural potential of human beings? Like Kant, the natural law theorist focuses on what makes human beings distinctive, what separates us from the rest of the natural world—namely, the ability to reason. Through our ability to reason, we can participate actively in God's plan. However, natural law ethics is distinct from Kantian ethics in that natural law ethicists do not attempt to empty their theories of all empirical content. On the contrary, our moral obligations are derived from a conception of

the good life for human beings. For example, the Catholic Church opposes both abortion and birth control because these are inconsistent with a conception of sexuality as expressed within monogamous marriage only, and primarily oriented toward its natural end or purpose, procreation.

The most general moral precept of the natural law is "do good and avoid evil." Evil must always be avoided, even if avoiding evil will bring about great harm. As St. Paul put it, "Do not evil that good may come." The commission of an evil deed, such as the murder of an innocent person, can never be condoned, even if it is intended to advance the noblest of ends.

The Doctrine of the Double Effect

The doctrine of the double effect (DDE) was formulated in response to the recognition that an act may have both a good and a bad effect. Are we to shun such an action because of its bad effect? For example, administering morphine to a dying cancer patient may be necessary to ease his or her pain, but it may also depress respiration and hasten death. Must a doctor refrain from using the most effective pain medication because it might also kill the patient? Would this count as "doing evil (causing death) that good (relieving pain) may come"?

According to Catholic doctrine, the permissibility of the action depends largely on whether the bad effect is intended, or merely foreseen and permitted to happen. In addition, it must also be the case that

1. The act itself is not intrinsically wrong.
2. The good effect is produced directly by the action and not by the bad effect.
3. The good effect is sufficiently desirable to compensate for allowing the bad effect.[23]

Applying these conditions, the use of pain-relieving drugs that may also shorten life can be justified. The physician's purpose is not to kill, but rather to ease pain, although he or she foresees that death is a possible, or even likely, result. Giving drugs for pain relief is not intrinsically wrong; indeed, it is a central function of the physician. The

---

23. "Double Effect," *New Catholic Encyclopedia.*

good effect—the relief of pain—is produced directly by the administering of the drug, and not by the bad effect: namely, the patient's death. And lastly, when a patient is both terminally ill and suffering, the desirability of relieving suffering compensates for the shortening of his or her life. Thus, the DDE can be a useful tool for justifying an action that has a bad effect.

Double-effect reasoning has sometimes been incorrectly and speciously used. Someone who shoots a person at point-blank range cannot use the DDE to mitigate his or her responsibility, saying, "I didn't mean to kill him, only to get him out of the way." One is guilty of killing a person even if death is not desired in itself, but only as a means to achieve an end. A Michigan jury used such specious reasoning in their acquittal of Dr. Jack Kevorkian, who was accused of violating the state's assisted-suicide law when he helped a terminally ill man die by carbon monoxide poisoning. The law made an exception for physicians who administer pain-relieving drugs that may cause death. The jury accepted Kevorkian's argument that he did not intend to cause the man's death, but only to relieve his suffering. This reasoning, however, is a perversion of the DDE. Carbon monoxide, unlike morphine, is never offered as a means of pain relief. It has no medical use at all. It causes death, and death causes cessation of pain, but this is bringing about the good effect by means of the bad effect, which violates the second condition of the DDE. Thus, the DDE cannot be used to justify Dr. Kevorkian's act or to sustain his claim that he did not intend to cause the man's death. After the acquittal, law professor Yale Kamisar characterized the jury's decision as "confused." However, it seems likely that the decision was less the result of confusion about the appropriate application of double-effect reasoning, and more the result of their belief that Dr. Kevorkian was *right* in doing what he did and should not be punished.

Critics of the DDE argue that the principle is confusing and difficult to apply. It is not always easy to know whether a result is intended or merely foreseen, or whether it is brought about (impermissibly) by means of the bad effect or (permissibly) by the morally neutral action. The concepts of "means" and "intention" need to be made clearer before the DDE can give clear guidance.

Some theorists doubt that the DDE has moral significance even if it can be clearly and correctly applied. They note that the whole point of the doctrine is to avoid the counterintuitive implications of an absolutist ethic that insists that some acts (like directly causing the death of an innocent person) are absolutely wrong, regardless of reason or context. However, why should we assimilate garden-variety murder with causing the death of a terminally ill patient who wants to die? The solution, these critics say, is to recognize that causing death is not always wrong. If death is desirable, why should it make any difference *how* death is brought about—whether indirectly, by pain relief, or directly, by carbon monoxide?

Ordinary versus Extraordinary Treatment

Another influential distinction devised by Catholic medical ethicists is the distinction between "ordinary" and "extraordinary" treatment. Ordinary treatment is considered obligatory, while there is no obligation to provide extraordinary treatment. How are these two types of treatment to be best defined?

This question is complicated because there are various different grounds that have been used to distinguish ordinary and extraordinary treatments. For example, "ordinary" treatment may be viewed as routine or standard care, while "extraordinary" treatment is considered unusual. This distinction has the advantage of providing an empirical definition, based on current medical practice. However, it is not clear that this basis has moral significance. If a treatment is helpful to a patient, what difference does it make that it is unusual, or even unique? For this reason, some people prefer to think of the distinction between ordinary and extraordinary treatment as being a distinction between "beneficial" and "nonbeneficial" treatment.

Understood this way, the ordinary–extraordinary distinction is context dependent. Treatment such as a respirator may be ordinary in one context (e.g., to sustain a patient through a severe bout with a respiratory disease), but extraordinary in another (e.g., to sustain the life of a severely brain-damaged patient in a persistent vegetative state [PVS]). This makes the normative assumption that a PVS individual is not benefited by continued existence with no hope of recovery to consciousness. Someone who regards biological life itself as valuable will not agree that the use of a respirator to sustain the life of a PVS patient is "nonbeneficial," and so will not classify the treatment as extraordinary. However, this reasoning raises serious doubts about the usefulness of the distinction. If our moral views determine whether a treatment is to be classified as ordinary or extraordinary, the distinction itself cannot provide moral guidance.

Despite this difficulty, doctors and laypeople alike often use terms like "extraordinary" and "heroic" to characterize treatment they regard as inappropriate. Rather than regarding these classifications as morally significant in themselves, it is important to understand the moral presuppositions lying behind them. It is these presuppositions—not the shorthand labels that stand for them—that need discussion and debate (see *"In the Matter of Claire C. Conroy,"* Part 3, Section 4).

"RIGHTS-BASED" APPROACHES

The idea that, simply by virtue of being human, people can have rights regardless of the legal system under which they live, has ancient roots. The Stoic philosophers recognized the possibility that actual human laws might be unjust. They contrasted conventional laws with an unvarying natural law to which everyone had access through individual conscience and by which actual laws could be judged.[24] Later, the spread of the Roman Empire provided a system of law that applied to all people, whatever their tribe, race, or nationality. Christianity also incorporated the idea of natural law as the paramount standard by which all social institutions and laws should be judged.

However, neither the ancient Greeks, nor the Romans, nor the medieval Christians made the transition to natural rights. The notion of natural rights had its heyday in the seventeenth century, with writers like Grotius, Pufendorf, and Locke. Rights also played a crucial role in the American and French revolutions in the late eighteenth century.

However, states Brenda Almond, "In the nineteenth and early twentieth centuries, . . . appeal to rights was eclipsed by movements such as utilitarianism and Marxism, which could not, or would not, accommodate them."[25]

Appeal to natural rights revived in the aftermath of World War II, during the Nuremberg trials. Some theorists argued that since the actions of the accused were not contrary to German law (indeed, were required by it), the trials had no legal basis, but were merely a cynical attempt by the victors to punish the losers. Others maintained that the trials were a return to principles of legality and justice in the aftermath of Nazi barbarism, and that these principles have their foundation in both international and natural law.

Natural or human rights unquestionably occupy an important role in contemporary international moral and political debate. Apartheid, the death penalty, and female genital mutilation, to take just a few examples, have all been condemned as violations of human rights. Discussions of abortion, euthanasia, access to health care, the treatment of animals and the environment, and our obligations to future generations are typically framed in terms of conflicting moral rights.

Some see "rights talk" as unnecessary and vague. Bentham regarded the notion of moral—as opposed to legal—rights as "nonsense," and the notion of natural rights as "nonsense on stilts."[26] According to Bentham and other legal positivists, legal rights can be explained as claims that will be upheld by the power of the state. Legal rights can be identified because they stem from legislative acts or judicial decisions. So-called moral rights have no such legitimation, and it is partly for this reason that positivists regard them as empty rhetoric. According to utilitarianism, to say that someone has a moral right to something is only a shorthand way of saying that he or she *ought* to have it, and ought to be protected in his or her possession of it. There is, then, a role for

---

24. Brenda Almond, "Rights," in *A Companion to Ethics,* edited by Peter Singer (Oxford: Basil Blackwell, 1993), 259.

25. Ibid.

26. From *Anarchical Fallacies: Being an Examination of the Declaration of Rights Issued During the French Revolution.* Cited in Ronald Dworkin, *Taking Rights Seriously* (Cambridge, MA: Harvard University Press, 1977), 184.

moral rights in utilitarianism, but it is completely derivative from the principle of utility. To some extent, rights can serve as barriers against the application of overall utility. For example, utilitarians might, on grounds of utility, take property rights very seriously. They will agree that individuals should not be deprived of their property, unless this is essential to the general welfare, and even then there should be compensation. In other words, while utilitarians reject the Lockean idea of a "natural right to property," they are likely to agree that there are good utilitarian reasons to create something very like our existing system of property rights.

Rights-based critics of utilitarianism maintain that its conception of rights gives insufficient protection to individuals, whose happiness may be sacrificed for the benefit of the many. In *Taking Rights Seriously*, Ronald Dworkin offers a penetrating critique of the positivist analysis of law, as well as the utilitarian morality intimately linked to it. Rather than seeing rights as a device to achieve net utility, Dworkin sees rights as "trumps," as claims that supersede other kinds of claims. Similarly, Robert Nozick conceives of rights as "side constraints," which place limits on the things we may do to achieve goals.

In *Anarchy, State, and Utopia*, Nozick presents a libertarian view that is fundamentally opposed to utilitarianism.[27] He thus joins Kant, Rawls, and Dworkin in this opposition, holding that an action that is unfair or that violates someone's rights cannot be right, even if it does achieve the greatest net happiness. Happiness might be maximized by forcing people to volunteer their time to work in hospitals, or by making them donate blood or spare kidneys, but they have no obligation to do so according to Nozick; indeed, they have a right not to do so.

Nozick is equally opposed to Rawls's contractarianism. The central question of distributive justice is, "How should the goods of society be distributed?" According to Nozick, this question misconceives the issue because it implies that the goods of society—money, property, services—are there

simply to be distributed, like manna fallen from the heavens. Instead, these goods already belong to people who have invested their labor in them, been given them, or traded something for them. Taking goods away from those who are entitled to them violates their rights, and so is fundamentally unfair.

Another important feature of libertarianism is the distinction between negative and positive rights. Libertarians maintain that the only rights are negative rights: rights to be left alone, rights not to be interfered with. They reject positive rights—rights to be helped—because recognition of such rights would infringe on the freedom of individuals to spend their time and money as they choose. An example of a positive right is a right to an education. Libertarians oppose taxation generally on the grounds that it deprives individuals of their legitimate property; thus, they oppose taxation for the creation and support of public schools. However, they recognize the need for an army to defend a country from foreign enemies, for a police force to protect citizens against aggression and attack, and for a legal system to uphold contractual agreements. Taxation to support these purposes is regarded as legitimate.

Libertarians reject the idea of a right to health care, since health care is regarded as a positive right—a right to be given certain treatment. However, it is not clear why they assume this distinction to have such moral significance. If it is legitimate to tax people for a police force that will protect their lives, why isn't it equally legitimate to tax people to provide them with health care, which is also often necessary for survival?

Perhaps the biggest objection to libertarianism is that it works to the disadvantage of those who, through no fault of their own, are born into poverty. Poverty limits people's life chances. The poor typically get substandard health care, inferior schools, and inadequate housing. These disadvantages make it unlikely that they will have an equal opportunity to obtain the goods of society: jobs, money, and material goods. Rawls attempts to compensate for life's initial unfairness, but libertarianism reinforces it.

In a rights-based approach, the fundamental question in our opening case study would be whether Mr. Lasken has a right to end his life, and to ask his doctor for help in doing so. Those who

---

27. Robert Nozick, *Anarchy, State, and Utopia* (New York: Basic Books, 1974).

oppose voluntary euthanasia and physician-assisted suicide maintain that Lasken has no such right. They see a distinction between the established right to refuse medical treatment and an affirmative right to seek help in dying. However, this interpretation was disputed for the first time by a federal judge on May 3, 1994, when Judge Barbara F. Rothstein found Washington State's assisted-suicide law unconstitutional. Rothstein held that the law places an undue burden on the Fourteenth Amendment interests of terminally ill, mentally competent patients. Moreover, she found that the law "unconstitutionally distinguishes between two similarly situated groups," namely, those on life support and those not on life support. Washington permits terminally ill patients to hasten their deaths by allowing removal of life-support systems, yet bars physicians from giving medication that would bring about the same results. Rothstein wrote that from "a constitutional perspective, the court does not believe that a distinction can be drawn between refusing life-sustaining medical treatment, and physician-assisted suicide by an uncoerced, mentally competent, terminally ill adult."[28]

Rights play an important role in moral discourse. Without the notion of individual rights, it would be difficult—if not impossible—to express our convictions about informed consent, protections for research subjects, and other such issues. However, this should not lead us to conclude that the application of individual rights is always appropriate, or that such rights are the only relevant factors.

The area of treatment refusal presents an obviously inappropriate instance of invoking the right to self-determination. Suppose that a patient enters an emergency room screaming from the pain of severe burns. The attending physicians conclude that, although her burns are serious, she will recover if given immediate and sustained treatment. Suddenly the patient, on the verge of shock, rebuffs the efforts of the medical staff on the grounds that she has a right to "die with dignity." Clearly, in this sort of case it would be wrong for the medical staff to honor the claimed right to refuse treatment. Not only is the woman mistaken in her belief that she is about to die, regardless of treatment, but her capacity for self-determination has itself been substantially impaired or temporarily eclipsed by her recent trauma. To honor her refusal would be tantamount to treating this incompetent person as though she were competent, with morally disastrous results.

The previous example demonstrates limits to the scope of the right of self-determination, namely, that it should be restricted to competent individuals. Conflicts between individual rights and the welfare of other persons—including, on occasion, the welfare of the entire community—constitute another set of problematic issues of libertarianism. For example, some libertarians argue that people should have the right to do whatever they please, so long as they do not violate anyone's rights. On a small-scale, interpersonal level, this principle is extremely problematic. Imagine a jilted lover who decides on impulse to marry another woman, not because he loves her, but merely to spite the woman who rejected him. We might all agree that this man has a right to marry whomever he chooses, but is "having a right" the same as "doing the right thing"? Obviously not, since the decision to marry out of spite will predictably inflict great suffering upon his unsuspecting bride.

On a broader social scale, libertarians often assert that individual freedom should include the right to shoot heroin, smoke crack cocaine, and take any other accurately labeled drug, so long as an individual freely chooses to do so. If our liberty is to mean anything, so the argument goes, it must encompass the right to take risks. To allow the government to decide what we may or may not put into our own bodies is to give up control over them. It is analogous to slavery.[29]

The trouble with a libertarian approach to the drug problem is that it ignores social consequences and focuses only on individual rights. Drugs have destroyed many inner-city neighborhoods. Some of the related problems—such as crime due to illegal trafficking—might be solved by legalization, but

---

28. *National Law Journal* (May 16, 1994): A6.

29. Walter Block, "Drug Prohibition: A Legal and Economic Analysis," in *Drugs, Morality, and the Law*, edited by Steven Luper-Foy and Curtis Brown (New York: Garland), 199–216.

not all of them would. Drug addiction has contributed to a skyrocketing rate of child abuse and neglect, because addicts—especially crack addicts—make notoriously poor parents. In addition, drug abuse by pregnant women is connected with dramatic increases in infant mortality, congenital syphilis, and HIV-positive infants. Serious students of the drug problem realize that hard questions remain even after the right of the individual to go to the devil has been invoked. What, for example, is the causal connection, if any, between unemployment, poverty, and ghetto conditions on the one hand, and hard drug addiction on the other? Would not an important consideration be if widespread use of drugs could be shown to reinforce racism and poverty? When unthinkingly waved as a trump, the right to self-determination can mask injustice and justify inequity.

We also need to ask what the effect of legalization on access and consumption would be. Some say that it would have little effect, since it is already so easy to obtain drugs in certain areas. At the same time, it should be remembered that three times as many Americans abuse alcohol as use illegal drugs, largely because of availability. From a public health perspective, if the end result of legalization is higher addiction rates, this is a serious argument against it. Astonishingly, this consideration has no bearing at all on a libertarian view. For the libertarian, the level of addiction in society is irrelevant; the only thing that matters is whether the individual has made a free and voluntary decision to use drugs. Once again, the individual's freedom is everything, and the impact on society is ignored.[30]

Rights are important, for they protect individuals from—as Mill called it—"the tyranny of the majority." Nevertheless, an overemphasis on rights can sometimes exacerbate conflict. For example, to justify criminal punishment of women who use drugs during pregnancy, conservatives appeal to fetal rights. At the other extreme, some feminists and civil libertarians insist that a woman has a right to control her own body during pregnancy, regardless of the harm she causes to her future child. A recognition that mother and fetus are a unit, whose interests are

generally promoted together, might be preferable to a rigid rights-based approach.

COMMUNITARIAN ETHICS

For all their differences, Hobbes, Mill, Kant, Rawls, Gauthier, and Nozick share the belief, bequeathed to us by the Enlightenment philosophers of the eighteenth century, that people should find moral rules in the application of reason to practical conduct. For this tradition, which we shall call "liberal individualism," ethical truth must be sought not in the vagaries of history, tradition, and religious faith, but rather in the universal tenets of rationality. Whether ethical norms are conceived in terms of enlightened self-interest, maximized utility, or the recognition of autonomy and human rights, they are viewed by this tradition as objective and universal, applicable to all times and places.

Another important theoretical strand connecting these theorists is their commitment to the individual as the unique focal point of moral concern. In utilitarianism, the collective preferences of each individual determine right and wrong. Everyone is to count as one, and nobody for more than one. However, the interest of the community as a whole may conflict with any particular individual's interest. Thus, a perennial problem for utilitarianism is the conflict between individual rights and the welfare of society as a whole. By contrast, "rights-based" Kantian and contractarian moral theory, as well as Nozick's brand of libertarianism, are committed to the notion that the rights and dignity of the individual should never (or rarely) be sacrificed to the interests of the larger society. Indeed, the whole point of social organization, of the "social contract," according to this tradition is the advancement of the *individual's* interests, rights, and happiness.

An important corollary of this view is the claim that, since different individuals will naturally have different values and conflicting visions of the good life, a truly liberal society will not—indeed cannot justifiably—adopt any particular conception of the good life to the exclusion or diminution of others.[31]

---

30. Bonnie Steinbock, "Drug Prohibition: A Public-Health Perspective," in *Drugs, Morality, and the Law*, 233–234.

31. Ronald Dworkin, "Liberalism," in *A Matter of Principle* (Cambridge, MA: Harvard University Press, 1985), 181–204.

Thus, a liberal society must remain "neutral" with regard to these competing conceptions of value and the good. To do otherwise—for example, by imposing a religion-based test on what kind of literature people should be allowed to read—amounts to a serious form of tyranny.

This ethical consensus on rationalism and individualism has had a profound impact on the development of contemporary biomedical ethics. Recently, however, the consensus has been challenged by a number of critics who can usefully, if somewhat uneasily, be lumped under the common banner of "communitarianism."[32] According to communitarian ethical theorists, all of our guiding ethical norms, rules, principles, theories, and virtues can be traced to distinct ethical traditions and ways of life. They argue that it is impossible for us to "bootstrap" ourselves outside of time and space in order to discover some eternal realm of ethical insight. Rather, they claim, history, tradition, and concrete moral communities are the real wellsprings of our moral thought, judgment, and action. As Aristotle put it, we are social beings; our values, our conceptual schemes, our very identities are engendered, shaped, and nurtured within the confines of community.

Within this countertradition, ethical truth is thus particular, not universal. In contrast to the liberal claim that society must remain neutral vis-à-vis competing conceptions of the good life, communitarians argue that if any progress is to be made on a host of public controversies, ranging from pornography to the treatment of dying patients, we will have to begin not with abstract statements of rights, nor with an attempt to promote the good of all by promoting the good of each, but rather with some conception of common meanings, with a vision of what we take to be a "good society." Necessarily, our conception of this good society will crucially depend upon our own history, traditions, institutions, and customs.

Communitarians reject both the rationalism of liberalism's approach to method and their claim to value neutrality. In opposition to individualistic utilitarianism, they offer the idea of a "common good." That is, where utilitarianism looks to the welfare of all individuals taken together, communitarianism looks to the *shared* values, ideals, and goals of a community. Where utilitarianism asks, "Which policies will produce the greatest happiness, on balance, of all of the individuals in society?" communitarianism asks, "Which policies will promote the kind of community in which we want to live?" The difference is subtle, but real. Against rights-based approaches, communitarians reject the penchant for elevating the individual above the social group or community. According to communitarians, the tendency of liberalism to focus so insistently on individual rights—to the exclusion of other social interests—can give rise to circumstances that a good society would not, and should not, tolerate.[33] Take, for example, the practice of some very large corporations with deep community roots—firms employing thousands of workers in relatively small cities—of simply pulling up stakes to search for cheaper labor markets in Mexico. In a society that gives pride of place to rights of ownership, such companies are given total freedom of movement; but the social costs of such rights and freedom can be enormous and often devastating to the affected communities, adding to unemployment, poverty, and the disintegration of neighborhoods and families. A good society, it is argued, would focus not only on individual rights, but also on the good of the larger community.

The dominance of liberal individualism within bioethics has recently been challenged on a number of fronts. Daniel Callahan has brought a communitarian perspective to debates over health care

32. See, for example, Alasdair MacIntyre, *After Virtue* (Notre Dame, IN: University of Notre Dame Press, 1981). Reprinted in *Contemporary Moral Problems*, 4th ed., edited by James E. White (St. Paul, MN: West, 1994). See also Michael Sandel, *Liberalism and the Limits of Justice* (Cambridge: Cambridge University Press, 1982); Charles Taylor, "Atomism," in *Philosophical Papers*, vol. 2 (Cambridge: Cambridge University Press, 1982); Michael Walzer, *Spheres of Justice* (New York: Basic Books, 1983); Shlomo Avineri and Avner de-Shalit, eds., *Communitarianism and Individualism* (Oxford: Oxford University Press, 1992); and, for a good general overview, Stephen Mulhall and Adam Swift, *Liberals and Communitarians* (Oxford: Basil Blackwell, 1992).

33. See, for example, Mary Ann Glendon, *Rights Talk: The Impoverishment of Political Discourse* (New York: Free Press, 1991).

issues, such as rationing and reform (see Part 2, Section 2). According to Callahan, the combination of our desire to provide universal access to care, the burgeoning cost of high-tech medicine, and the sharp rise in the elderly population force some very hard choices that may decide who will live. Instead of starting, in standard liberal fashion, with individual wants, needs, interests, and rights, Callahan urges us to begin by asking what kind of society we wish to have—or as one of his book titles puts it, "What kind of life?"[34] To get at this big question, Callahan must confront some other very difficult and controversial questions, such as, What ought to be the goals and virtues of elderly persons? Should they seek individual happiness, or devote themselves to the education and welfare of future generations? And what ought to be the goals of medicine at various stages of the life cycle? Should medicine seek, at great expense, to forestall death for the very old with the latest high-tech devices, or should it merely try to provide dignified terminal *care?* Clearly, all this talk about goals and virtues necessarily implicates us in a quest for common meanings and values. Rather than ruling such questions off-limits due to the strictures of liberal neutrality, Callahan claims simply that we *must* address them as a community if we are to act responsibly. Failure to do so, thus allowing each person to chart his or her own course, could well vindicate individual freedom of elderly persons at the expense of the young.

How might a communitarian interpret our case of physician-assisted suicide? This is a difficult question to answer in light of the remarkable diversity among communitarian thinkers. For communitarians such as Alasdair MacIntyre, the emphasis upon history, traditional practices, and virtues leads to the wholesale abandonment of liberal individualism and the embrace of a rather "conservative" political agenda. More moderate communitarians,

on the other hand, some of whom are politically quite "progressive," stress the importance of social meanings and communal values while attempting to preserve a more modest role for the language of individual rights.

Some communitarians, then, might approach the case of Dr. Brody and Mr. Lasken by stressing the customary and time-honored prohibition of assisted suicide and euthanasia in all Western societies. They might argue that, in spite of individuals' strong claims to liberty in this area, the claims of society are stronger. The needs of many suicidal patients might well be met in ways other than by killing them, and society will be a better place if it acknowledges the sanctity and inviolability of human life. A similar argument might be mounted by physicians who could point to their own traditional professional commitments and values: "We heal; we don't kill. That's who we are as doctors; that's how we have always been."

An alternative communitarian reading of the case might reach the same conclusion, but for very different reasons. One could argue, for example, that even though individuals have a powerful claim of self-determination in this matter, the social costs of allowing a right of assisted suicide in a society distinguished by widespread poverty, lack of access to health care, and discrimination against vulnerable minority groups would be prohibitive. While the first communitarian response to our case has a distinctly conservative political flavor, the second might issue from a highly progressive, even Marxist, critique of existing social relationships.

An overall evaluation of communitarianism is an exceedingly complicated matter, due to the disparate character of the theorists and theories lumped under its banner. For the purposes of this brief introduction, however, we venture the following conclusions and recommendations. (1) We agree with the claim that all ethical principles, rules, and virtues grow out of concrete historical traditions and derive their meaning and weight from those traditions. Thus, although our moral principles might extend very far indeed in both space and time, they are not the products of disembodied "reason." (2) The emphasis upon the communal dimension of our moral lives should be viewed as a welcome corrective to the largely asocial invocation of individual rights. We should worry a lot more

---

34. Daniel Callahan, *What Kind of Life?* (New York: Simon and Schuster, 1990). See also his *Setting Limits* (New York: Simon and Schuster, 1987). For a recent attempt to develop a comprehensive communitarian theory of bioethics, focusing specifically on end-of-life and access to health care issues, see Ezekiel Emanuel, *The Ends of Human Life: Medical Ethics in a Liberal Polity* (Cambridge, MA: Harvard University Press, 1991).

about the "ecology of rights,"[35] the kind of society, neighborhood, and family life within which rights are developed and claimed.

On the negative side, (3) the more hardcore communitarians' wholesale rejection of liberal rights in favor of traditional practices and virtues is especially problematic. Curbing the socially destructive invocation of property rights is one thing, but limiting the freedom of individuals, in the name of communal values, to read pornography, obtain contraceptives, have abortions, or engage in homosexual relationships is, to us, a more disturbing prospect.[36] Finally, (4) it must be noted that an emphasis upon community, neighborhood, family, and traditional values will always express a preference for some *particular conception* of family, neighborhood, and community. For minority groups and women struggling to assert their own, quite varied, conceptions of individual and cultural identity, the communitarian impulse must learn to appreciate and respect such differences within our increasingly cosmopolitan societies.[37]

FEMINIST ETHICS

Just as communitarianism started as a critique of certain assumptions in liberal theory, so too the idea of a feminist ethic stems, in part, from a critique of traditional ethical theories as representing the experiences of men, not women. Feminist approaches to morality seek to correct this underlying bias.

Feminism is not a monolithic theory; thus, there is no one definition of "feminist ethics." Rather, feminism incorporates a variety of social and political beliefs, and there are even differing conceptions of feminism itself. All varieties of feminism are characterized by a concern for the welfare of all women, and a belief that women have historically been—and continue to be—oppressed by patriarchal societies. As Alison Jaggar writes, "Feminist

approaches to ethics are distinguished by their explicit commitment to rethinking ethics with a view to correcting whatever forms of male bias it may contain."[38] They all seek to unmask and challenge the oppression, discrimination, and exclusion that women have faced. Feminist approaches to ethics are political, in the sense that they are keenly aware of imbalances of power between women and men, rich and poor, healthy and disabled, white people and people of color, and first world and third world peoples.

Feminist approaches to ethics are also marked by attention to the so-called private sphere, including reflection on intimate relations, such as affection and sexuality, which were ignored by modern moral theory until quite recently. Finally, feminist ethics, rather than seeing women as less fully developed versions of men, insists on taking the moral experience of all women seriously. Modern feminists also warn against the tendency to make generalizations about "women" based on the experience of the relatively small group of middle-class white women. Many feminists today emphasize that sexual oppression is only one form of oppression, and that all forms—whether based on gender, class, race, or disability—must be acknowledged and fought.

Some issues, such as abortion and reproductive technology, are traditionally conceived as "women's issues," and many feminists have written on these topics. However, feminist approaches to bioethics are not limited to this sphere; feminist thought has influenced thinking about the health professional–patient relationship, informed consent, experimental trials, disability, access to health care, and other issues.[39]

One issue that divides feminists is whether virtue is "gendered"; that is, whether there are

---

35. Mary Ann Glendon, *Rights Talk*, 136–144 (see note 33).

36. See Amy Gutmann, "Communitarian Critics of Liberalism," *Philosophy and Public Affairs* 14 (1985): 308–322.

37. See Iris Marion Young, *Justice and the Politics of Difference* (Princeton, NJ: Princeton University Press, 1990); and Marilyn Friedman, "Feminism and Modern Friendship: Dislocating the Community," *Ethics* 99 (1989): 275–290.

38. Alison M. Jaggar, "Feminist Ethics: Some Issues for the Nineties," in *Contemporary Moral Problems*, 4th ed., edited by James E. White (St. Paul, MN: West, 1994), 61.

39. See Susan Wolf, ed., *Feminism and Bioethics: Beyond Reproduction* (New York: Oxford University Press, 1995); Helen B. Holmes and Laura Purdy, eds., *Feminist Perspectives in Medical Ethics* (Bloomington: Indiana University Press, 1992); and Susan Sherwin, *No Longer Patient* (Philadelphia: Temple University Press, 1992).

virtues that are specifically female and male. Many feminists reject this approach, as the idea of "feminine virtues"—including selflessness, devotion to family needs, and submissiveness to men—has long been linked with the oppression of women. Nevertheless, many nineteenth-century women, including many who were concerned with women's emancipation, believed not only that there were specifically female virtues, but also that women were morally superior to men and that society could be transformed through the influence of women. Today, some feminists regard many of the evils of society—war, violence, racism, the destruction of the environment—as the result of specifically male faults, such as aggression.[40] They believe that the "feminine" virtues of kindness, generosity, helpfulness, and sympathy can serve as a corrective to these evils.

A related issue on which feminists divide is the meaning of sexual equality. Are men and women treated equally when they are treated the same? Jaggar states that "By the end of the 1960s, most feminists in the United States had come to believe that the legal system should be sex-blind, that it should not differentiate in any way between women and men."[41] However, this version of equality does not always promote women's interests. A notorious example is "no-fault" divorce settlements that divide family property equally between husband and wife. Here, equal distribution leaves many women much worse off financially, because women—who often shoulder most of the family responsibilities, such as housework and caring for children—typically have much lower job qualifications and less work experience than men. Divorce settlements that do not take social realities into account are egregiously unfair, and moreover reinforce sexual inequality. At the same time, the alternative way of seeking equality, by providing women with special legal protection, appears to promote sexual stereotypes.

Feminists continue to debate the correct interpretation of equality, even while some feminists reject the entire concept of equality as part of an "ethic of justice" that is characteristically masculine, relying

on rules and abstracting from particular, concrete situations, instead of responding to immediately perceived needs.[42] Such feminists suggest an alternative "ethic of care,"[43] stressing connectedness, the importance of human relationships, empathy, and an acknowledgment of dependency. It shares with virtue ethics the conviction that undue emphasis on moral rules obscures the crucial role of moral insight, virtue, and character in determining how to deal with ethical issues.

Some feminists have claimed that the ethic of caring fails to give enough attention to moral principles. Virginia Held reminds us that "an absence of principles can be an invitation to capriciousness."[44] Moreover, issues such as economic justice "cry out for relevant principles. Although caring may be needed to motivate us to act on such principles, the principles are not dispensable."[45] Without such principles, the claims of those unrelated to us, or different from us, may go unheeded. Furthermore, it is not clear that an ethic of care would ensure the rights of women to equality and fair treatment.[46]

The emphasis on the importance of emotions is seen by many (and not just feminists) as a welcome balance to the sort of moral theory that completely ignores feeling. At the same time, taking emotion as a guide can often degenerate into a "do what feels good" kind of subjective relativism.[47] The problem of relativism remains a difficult one for feminism. On the one hand, many feminists join with postmodernists and communitarians in rejecting the Enlightenment notion of a universal morality, valid for all people at all times and places. This notion ignores the particularity most feminists regard as essential

---

40. Mary Daly, *Gyn/Ecology: The Metaethics of Radical Feminism* (Boston: Beacon Press, 1978).

41. Jaggar, "Feminist Ethics," 63 (see note 38).

42. Ibid., 64.

43. Carol Gilligan, *In a Different Voice: Psychological Theory and Women's Development* (Cambridge, MA: Harvard University Press, 1982); Nell Noddings, *Caring: A Feminine Approach to Ethics and Moral Education* (Berkeley: University of California Press, 1984).

44. Virginia Held, "Feminism and Moral Theory," in *Contemporary Moral Problems*, 4th ed., edited by James E. White (St. Paul, MN: West, 1994), 75.

45. Ibid.

46. Ibid., 76. See also Joan Tronto, *Moral Boundaries: A Political Argument for an Ethic of Care* (New York: Routledge, 1993).

47. Jaggar, "Feminist Ethics," 68 (see note 38).

and too long ignored by Western ethics. On the other hand, feminists are understandably concerned that their critique of the oppression of women not be dismissed as a single point of view.[48]

The problem of relativism for feminists is poignantly posed by the practice of clitoridectomy, or female "circumcision." This practice, common among certain groups in Africa, involves the excision of the clitoris. Sometimes the vulva is sewn up as well. The clitoris is removed to reduce sexual pleasure and remove temptation to sexual activity; the lips of the vulva are sewn up to ensure that the young woman will remain a virgin until her marriage. The circumcision is usually done when a girl reaches puberty, although it is also often performed on very young children. It is performed without anesthesia, using unsterilized razor blades, while the girl is held down by older women. It frequently causes life-threatening blood loss and infection. It can lead to painful intercourse, infertility, and difficult childbirth.

> Ironically, the frigidity or infertility caused by the mutilation leads many husbands to shun their brides . . . . Doctors throughout Africa recognize the harmful effects of female circumcision but feel powerless to stop a practice so entrenched in custom and tradition. Many organizations are campaigning against it, and the new African Charter on the Rights of Children includes items condemning circumcision. Governments in Sudan and elsewhere have passed laws against it, but they are seldom enforced.[49]

Despite this opposition, many Africans continue to regard female circumcision as an important cultural and religious ritual.

The practice of female circumcision poses a dilemma for feminists. On the one hand, feminism is committed to multiculturalism, that is, to the view that no culture has a monopoly on the right way to live, and that the voices of all people must be heard. On the other hand, feminists must reject a practice they regard as patently contrary to the interests of women. Not only is clitoridectomy painful and dangerous, but its justification stems from suppositions antithetical to feminist thought: that women are male

property, that female virginity must be preserved, that women ought not to have sexual feelings, that adultery is a male prerogative, and so forth. Is there a way out of the dilemma, a way to remain faithful to feminist ideals without rejecting multiculturalism?

We think that there is a way out. As suggested earlier, we need to develop an interpretation of multiculturalism that does not imply relativism. Keeping an open mind about the practices of other cultures, and attempting to understand them "from within," does not commit us to unqualified acceptance of these practices, particularly when they conflict with our deepest values and principles. For feminists, a core value is the conviction that women are full human persons, entitled to equality and justice. Clitoridectomy is not compatible with the recognition of women as free and equal members of society; indeed, it contributes to women's oppression, and is thus opposed by many African women and men. Western feminists can support these Africans in this struggle, and not be guilty of arrogance, smugness, or cultural imperialism.

VIRTUE ETHICS

In light of the problems facing consequentialist and deontological moral theories, the last fifty years or so have witnessed a growing interest in what is called "virtue ethics." Virtue ethics does not represent a single distinctive moral theory. Rather, it is a label for a family of moral theories that are specially concerned with or that give special priority to the role of the virtues in the moral life. In fact, one of the main challenges facing theories of this kind is to differentiate themselves from the moral theories we have already discussed. After all, a utilitarian like Mill will value the moral virtues on the grounds that they motivate those who possess them to reliably perform actions that maximize the overall good. Contractarians like Hobbes will value them because of the way they contribute to our ability to cooperate with one another and to form a stable community.[50] In fact, virtue plays a central role in

---

48. Ibid., 67.

49. *Time* (Fall 1990), 39. Cited in Joel Feinberg, *Freedom and Fulfillment: Philosophical Essays* (Princeton, NJ: Princeton University Press, 1992), 199.

50. For an analysis of the role of moral virtues in Hobbes's moral philosophy and a contrast of this view with those of Plato and Aristotle, see Alex John London, "Virtue and Consequences: Hobbes on the Value of the Moral Virtues," *Social Theory and Practice* (Spring 1998).

Kant's moral philosophy. For Kant, the good will is the only thing unconditionally good, and virtue is what makes the good will good. Virtue is the strength of the will's commitment to performing actions from the motive of duty, and it is, therefore, the condition for the goodness of anything the will does. To begin with, then, it will be useful to mark a very general contrast between the role the virtues play in these moral theories and the more central place they occupy in virtue ethics.

According to an act-consequentialist moral theory, the right action is the one that produces the best consequences. In order to be practically useful, such theories must provide us with a meaningful account of the relevant consequences and how they are to be calculated or measured. Similarly, according to a deontological moral theory, the right action is the one specified by a particular rule of some sort. In order to be of any practical benefit, such theories must supply us with the appropriate set of rules or with some procedure or criteria by which we can generate the relevant rules. In contrast, the right action in a virtue–theoretic account is the one that the virtuous person would perform. In order to be practically useful, this sort of theory must tell us who the virtuous people are and it must give us an account of the nature and number of whatever virtues it recognizes.[51] Unlike consequentialist or rule-based theories, then, virtue ethics begins with an account of the moral virtues and then links the possession of these traits to the ability to reliably perform certain kinds of actions and, importantly, to an inability to perform certain others. As a result, moral theories in this family may differ in the kinds of things they count as virtues and vices, the number of virtues and vices they recognize, their reasons why the virtues are valuable, and the relationship of the virtues to right actions.

Contemporary virtue ethicists tend to see themselves as carrying on or working within a tradition of moral philosophy that begins with Aristotle. According to Aristotle, the priorities reflected in the choices we make in our lives reveal our conception of the good life, or human flourishing—what Aristotle calls *"eudaimonia."* We may disagree about the nature of the good life, but we can all agree that it is around some conception of happiness or doing well that we structure our various activities and give a distinctive shape to our lives. As a result, a central question for Aristotle is, What is the best life for a person to lead?

For Aristotle, a candidate for this highest good must not be something that others bestow upon us. Rather, it must be proper to its possessor and not easily taken away (1095b26-27).[52] Because honor or fame fail both of these tests, the life dedicated to their pursuit is ruled out as a candidate for the good life. Similarly, any candidate for the highest good must be a final good in the sense that we choose other things for the sake of it, but we don't choose it for the sake of anything else (1097a30). As a result, the life of money making is ruled out. In addition, the candidate must be self-sufficient in the sense that the presence of it alone makes life desirable and worth living (1097b ff). In Aristotle's view, the virtues of temperance, courage, justice, wisdom, and practical reason represent the excellent states of our emotional and intellectual faculties. Because each of these traits represents the proper development of some human faculty, they are valuable for themselves (1097b2-5, 1144a1-7). But Aristotle believes that the virtues are also valuable for the activities that they produce and that happiness, or the highest human good, is a life of activity that consists in the exercise of such well-developed emotional and intellectual faculties under the guidance of our distinctly human capacity for rationality.

To cultivate the virtues, however, one must first perform actions that are noble and good. Noble and just actions have a kind of symmetry or balance about them—they are a mean between unacceptable extremes—and the only way to cultivate character states that share this symmetry is to repeatedly perform virtuous actions. To understand

---

51. This way of contrasting virtue ethics with consequentialist and deontological moral theories is explained at length by Rosalind Hursthouse in "Normative Virtue Ethics," in *How Should One Live One's Life?* edited by Roger Crisp (New York: Oxford University Press, 1996), 19–36.

52. These numbers refer to the page and line numbers of Bekker's edition of Aristotle's works. They are the standard method of citing particular passages in the works of Aristotle and can be found in the margins of the text of most translations.

what is right, noble, and just, however, one must have received a proper upbringing. One must have cultivated good habits, such as consideration for others, truthfulness, and self-control, because one becomes just and temperate by first doing just and temperate things. But virtue isn't simply a matter of practice or mere habit. Rather, it is only by acting in certain ways that we can come to understand what is noble and just and why this is so. Those who lack appropriate role models or guardians to instruct them will be unable to appreciate these things. Furthermore, Aristotle thinks that right, noble, and just actions are of such a diverse nature that they cannot be adequately captured by a set of rules or decision procedures. As a result, one cannot rely solely on some external theory or decision principle to determine which actions one ought to perform. To reliably perform the right action, one must cultivate the virtues for oneself and rely on one's experience and ability to appreciate and judge such things for oneself.

This does not mean that one will not be able to explain why something was the right thing to do given a particular situation. To the contrary, the virtuous person will be able to bring out the salient features of a situation and to say why some action is morally acceptable. This ability to appreciate the facts of a situation and to justify acting in one way rather than another, however, is quite different from the ability to give a general and practically useful account of the features that are morally important to situations in general and of what makes an action right and noble such that nonvirtuous people could use this account as a guide to action. For Aristotle, the only reliable way to understand what must be done, and to ensure that one is sufficiently willing to act on this understanding, is to become a just person oneself.

In this reading of Aristotle, the virtues play a central role in his ethical theory for several reasons. First, because they represent the excellent states of important human emotional and intellectual capacities, they are valuable in their own right. Second, the virtues play an important role in human flourishing, since the exercise of these well-developed states of our faculties is what Aristotle regards as happiness, or *eudaimonia*. Third, the virtues play an important epistemological role in the good life—namely, without the virtues, one will not fully understand what makes an action noble and just, or be able to appreciate the morally relevant factors of complicated situations. Fourth, the moral virtues provide the motivation for consistently performing the right actions since the person who possesses them will not only understand what makes them noble and just, but will also take pleasure in acting well and will do so for its own sake and not for the sake of some external consideration. Those who lack the proper upbringing will regard such actions as painful, to be done only to avoid punishment or to gain some advantage, such as obtaining money, power, or friends.

Some contemporary versions of virtue ethics differ from Aristotle on one or more of these points. For example, Aristotle says that the right action is the one that the virtuous person would perform because the virtuous person "judges each thing rightly" and "things appear to him as they truly are," so that what sets the virtuous person apart from others is that "he sees the truth in each thing, being himself the norm and measure of the noble and the pleasant" (1113a26-35 cf. 1176a12-19). We can use the virtuous person as a standard or measure of what is right because she understands why some action is right and just and can be counted on to reliably perform such actions. The virtuous person is thus an epistemological guide to determining which actions are right. But the rightness of those actions is not a product of the fact that they are the actions virtuous people would perform, although some contemporary virtue theorists embrace this view.

According to these theorists, the virtues are of primary importance to the moral life because they are the primary locus of moral value. As such, the virtuous are the norm and measure of what is right and good precisely because actions derive whatever moral value they possess from their relationship to the virtues. If an action is one that the virtuous person would perform, then this makes the action right and just.[53] The value of the action is therefore determined by the judgment of the virtuous person. One major problem for a view of this sort lies in

---

53. A version of this view can be found in Rosalind Hursthouse, "Virtue Theory and Abortion," *Philosophy & Public Affairs* 20 (1991): 223–246.

explaining the grounds on which virtuous agents make their initial judgment. On what grounds do they decide whether an action is the right one? Certainly it cannot be simply because it is the action they did in fact choose. This would make their judgment seem arbitrary and capricious. But if it is because it is the action they *should* choose, then we want to know what it is about the action that makes it worthy of choice. In either case it looks like such a theory will either turn out to be arbitrary and unhelpful or it will have to advert to some explanation of the value of an action that reaches beyond its relation to the judgment of the virtuous themselves.

Similarly, many contemporary virtue ethicists differ from Aristotle in rejecting the view that the virtues are excellent states of our cognitive and affective faculties. For example, Alasdair MacIntyre argues that the virtues should not be thought of as timeless, human excellences. Rather, they are acquired human qualities that allow us to achieve goods internal to those cultural roles and practices that can be shaped into a coherent vision of the good life within a particular community.[54] As such, cultural traditions, community membership, and role obligations play a crucial part in determining which kinds of human qualities are virtues and what kinds of activities count as virtuous activities.

In MacIntyre's view, Dr. Brody has to ask herself whether assisting in suicide is consistent with the goods that are internal to the practice of medicine in late twentieth-century America and the obligations that she has taken on in her role as physician. On the one hand, Dr. Brody is committed to ameliorating pain and suffering, but she is also aware that doctors have traditionally conceived of themselves as the agents of health, not death. She also knows that there may be considerable consequences to a choice to assist Mr. Lasken's suicide, and she has to weigh these consequences against her own well-being and self-interest. Is it fair that Mr. Lasken cannot receive help in ending his suffering until his condition degenerates to the point that his life is being sustained by machines, the support of which it might then be permissible to

withdraw? Is it acceptable for her to lie or dissemble in order to help Mr. Lasken and avoid going to jail, or to comfort or assuage him if she decides not to come to his aid?

These are difficult questions, and the fact that virtue ethics does not provide us with easy answers to them is not peculiar to this ethical theory. Even so, critics are generally nonplussed by the advice to do whatever the virtuous person would do, especially in situations where compassion, fidelity, courage, prudence, and self-interest seem to be at odds with one another. What critics demand is some way of ranking the virtues and their hold on us so that people like Dr. Brody will know how to negotiate such conflicts. In the eyes of critics, without such a ranking, virtue ethics will never entirely substitute for a more principled approach.

Yet the fact that the virtue ethicist relies on the good judgment of the virtuous person to negotiate such apparent conflicts should not detract from the fact that the consequentialist and the deontologist face very similar problems. The consequentialist must provide Dr. Brody with an account of the relevant consequences and with a procedure by which to weigh or measure them without running afoul of our deepest intuitions about this case. Similarly, the deontologist must produce a set of rules or decision procedures flexible enough to accommodate the nuances of the situation. So it appears that with each of these theories as well, Dr. Brody is going to have to exercise her deliberative skills to do what is right for Mr. Lasken and for herself.

Nevertheless, the virtue-based approach to cases like this does have certain advantages. For example, it brings out a variety of prima facie concerns, each of which makes a serious claim on us and demands that we apply ourselves to finding a judicious way to address each of them as best we can. It also brings out the way in which a physician must be committed to her patients and to her craft. The goal and goods of medicine require physicians to take chances for their patients—to have the courage to attend to them even when this may conflict with their own self-interest. Willingness to expose oneself to risk, including disease and sickness, is part of what it means to be a physician. As Arnold Relman puts it, "the risk of contracting the patient's disease is one of the risks that is inherent in the profession of medicine. Physicians who are not willing to

---

54. Alasdair MacIntyre, *After Virtue*, 2nd ed. (Notre Dame, IN: University of Notre Dame Press, 1984), 191.

accept that risk . . . ought not to be in the practice of medicine."[55] Although there are limits to the duty to put oneself at risk, a virtue-based approach establishes a strong presumption in favor of the duty to treat over doctors' rights to decide whom to treat and what risks to take.[56] Indeed, one of the shortcomings of a narrowly contractualist approach to the doctor-patient relationship, an approach that specifies numerous duties *within* that relationship, is its silence on the question of whether doctors have moral and professional obligations to *establish* relationships with needy, dangerous, or HIV-infected patients.

NONMORAL CONSIDERATIONS

The dizzying array of moral theories and perspectives presented above make it hard enough to decide how to act in a given situation. We suggested that it is not a question of determining which moral theory is correct; all of them contribute to an extraordinarily complex moral reality. Still, in deciding what to do, one must decide when utilitarian considerations should prevail, or when one ought to adhere to absolutist principles; when to appeal to principles and when to seek guidance in virtues; when to abide by universal, impartial considerations and when to concentrate on personal relationships and feelings.

As if the moral dimension of decision making were not complicated enough, there is another dimension we have not so far discussed: the "non-moral" dimension. How should we think about the political, personal, prudential, economic, or legal implications of our actions? According to one school of thought, moral reasons are the "best" reasons; they always "trump" other considerations. Thus, if it would be morally right to do something, then one ought to do it, even if it would have adverse non-moral consequences. More recently, philosophers

like Bernard Williams[57] and Susan Wolf[58] have argued that one is sometimes entirely justified in overriding impartial moral reasons to pursue a significant personal goal or defining relationship. Conceivably, many of the considerations left out of traditional ethics can be recovered if we take seriously the idea, advocated by feminists and others, that personal relations and feelings are as important to ethics as universal and impartial principles. Nevertheless, however broadly ethics is conceived, there will always be the possibility of conflict between moral and nonmoral considerations. In such cases, how are we to decide what to do?

Consider, once again, Dr. Brody. Suppose she decides that the morally right thing to do is to help Mr. Lasken. Helping him is breaking the law. She could be prosecuted and go to jail; even if she is not convicted, she could lose her license to practice medicine. It seems clear that these are important considerations and that it would be absurd (as opposed to noble) for Dr. Brody to completely ignore them. Whether her personal risk should override her view of the morally right action depends, in part, on the degree of the risk. If the risks of discovery, prosecution, and punishment are sufficiently low, and if she believes that it is morally right to help Mr. Lasken, Dr. Brody should perhaps be willing to risk legal and professional repercussions. In other situations, doing the morally right thing might ask too much of a person. The hard thing in life is having the wisdom to figure out when nonmoral actions are justified.

MODES OF MORAL REASONING

The previous survey of moral theories suggests the richness and diversity of our repertoire of ethical language and concepts. The task for this section is to show how these disparate and sometimes conflicting elements of morality figure into the moral judgments that we make. What should we *do* with all this ethical "raw material"?

---

55. *Cardiovascular News* (August 1987): 7.

56. Norman Daniels argues that a virtue-based approach to the question of the duty to treat implies a contractualist theory. See "Duty to Treat or Right to Refuse?" *Hasting Center Report* 21, no. 2 (1991): 36–46.

57. Bernard Williams, *Ethics and the Limits of Philosophy* (Cambridge, MA: Harvard University Press, 1985).

58. Susan Wolf, "Moral Saints," *Journal of Philosophy* (August 1982): 419–439.

Many of the enumerated theoretical perspectives—such as utilitarianism, Kantianism, and rights-based theories—articulate basic moral values, principles, and rules at a fairly high level of abstraction. We are told, for example, to maximize happiness, respect persons, honor patients' rights to confidentiality, and so on. But we are also told—for example, by the partisans of an ethic of care—to de-emphasize such abstractions in favor of a heightened caring responsiveness to individual people and situations. An important question arises, then, about precisely how these generalities are, or should be, brought to bear in specific cases. In the language of the philosophical tradition, it is a question about the relationship between the universal and the particular.

This is also a question about the nature of moral justification. In pointing out the importance of happiness, personhood, rights, virtues, caring, and so on, each of these theories contributes to our search for ethical *warrants* or reasons that tend to *justify* our actions. When called upon to justify or defend individual actions or social policies, how do—or how should—we respond? Insofar as it makes sense to pursue ethical certitude about our actions, where does such certitude lie: in our philosophical or religious theories, in our pretheoretical convictions of right and wrong generated by our history and culture, or perhaps in some combination of these two areas?

The Principles Approach

One tempting response to these questions is to hold that justification in ethics is a matter of deducing the best and most comprehensive ethical theory from the foregoing list, and deriving this theory's correct conclusions. Thus, one should throw in his or her lot with, say, utilitarianism or Kantianism and then "apply" this theoretical framework to the facts at hand. Understood in this way, bioethics has been described as a kind of "applied ethics," as though philosophers and theologians do all the ethical heavy lifting, while others simply apply their findings to this or that set of factual circumstances. Tempting as it is in its simplicity, this conception of bioethics must nevertheless be rejected.

First, although this approach identifies philosophical theory as the ultimate locus of moral

certitude, it is far from clear what the "best and most comprehensive" ethical theory is. Indeed, after centuries of moral debates, we still disagree, sometimes vehemently, about justice and the nature of the good life. Second, as we have seen in the application of various theories to our case of physician-assisted suicide, theories are often stated at such a high level of generality (e.g., "Maximize happiness," "Respect persons") that they are capable of generating contradictory answers to the same moral questions. Third, this way of understanding "theory" (i.e., as an abstract construction built upon one or two overarching values) tends to obscure the extraordinary richness and diversity of the moral life. So, even if one of the enumerated "standard" theories were miraculously to attract a consensus, the result would be more impoverishing than liberating. To repeat, ethical theories as we understand them are best viewed as partial perspectives on a complex moral reality.

A powerful alternative to theory-driven approaches to bioethics emphasizes the role in moral reasoning of a small cluster of middle-level ethical principles. Instead of pursuing difficult and highly divisive foundational issues, the partisans of the "principles approach" (or "principlism") begin with our common moral experience and the manifest importance of keeping a short list of moral duties. Originally developed by Tom Beauchamp and James Childress in their justly influential book *The Principles of Biomedical Ethics*,[59] and later endorsed by prestigious governmental ethics commissions,[60] the method of principlism rapidly became the dominant mode of "doing bioethics" in the United States.

Stated in their popular tongue-twisting, Latinate formulations, these norms include the principles of autonomy, beneficence, nonmaleficence, and justice. In simpler terms, the core principles of bioethics bid us to (1) respect the capacity of individuals to choose their own vision of the good life and act accordingly;

---

59. Beauchamp and Childress, *The Principles of Biomedical Ethics* (see note 6).

60. National Commission for the Protection of Human Subjects of Biomedical and Behavioral Research, *The Belmont Report: Ethical Principles and Guidelines for the Protection of Human Subjects of Research* (Washington, DC: U.S. Government Printing Office, 1978).

(2) foster the interests and happiness of other persons and of society at large; (3) refrain from harming other persons; and (4) act fairly, distribute benefits and burdens in an equitable fashion, and resolve disputes by means of fair procedures.

In contrast to the partisans of applied moral theory, who tend to reduce the sources of normative guidance and criticism to a single overarching value (for example, Kantian respect for persons or the maximization of utility), the principlists settle for a small cluster of "middle level" norms, each one consistent with a number of ethical theories, no one of which enjoys automatic supremacy over the others. They reject the notion that serious moral conflict can always be resolved by appeal to a higher moral standard provided by some ultimate theory. Instead, they frankly admit the necessity of "weighing and balancing" the various principles against one another in each concrete moral situation.

While each principle articulates a serious moral duty, these duties are not absolute. They are, in the words of the late philosopher W. D. Ross, prima facie obligations.[61] This means that the ethical principles are indeed binding, but on any given occasion one principle may eclipse another with which it conflicts. So we say that a given principle is binding prima facie, or "at first blush," but that in the final analysis, all things having been considered, the pull of another principle might turn out to be even stronger. Importantly, however, even when a principle is outweighed, it usually continues to exert a strong moral pull on our behavior; it does not simply become irrelevant.

The conflict between the demands of confidentiality and the protection of public health in the context of AIDS provides a useful example of how principlism could be applied. On the one hand, physicians swear an oath to uphold the confidentiality of their patients. Since Hippocrates, this duty has been utterly central to the vocation of physicians. Without assurances that their often embarrassing secrets are safe with the doctor, patients will be reluctant to speak frankly about their symptoms or medical history, and in some cases may avoid

seeking medical attention to the detriment of their condition. A doctor's violations of confidentiality thus might be seen as violating the principles of beneficence and nonmaleficence.

The principle of autonomy provides further warrant for a doctor's confidentiality. Patients have a right to determine who knows what about their medical history. When physicians or nurses share this information with others who do not have a legitimate medical need to know, they rob their patients of control over information that is rightfully theirs. Combined, then, the principles of autonomy, beneficence, and nonmaleficence make an exceedingly strong case for respecting patient confidentiality.

But now suppose that you are a physician caring for a bisexual male infected with the HIV/AIDS virus. Your patient admits to having regular unprotected sex with his fiancée, who does not suspect his HIV status, yet he insists upon absolute confidentiality out of a (well-founded) fear of losing her. On one hand, you feel the pull of your duty to respect confidentiality; but, on the other hand, your patient's behavior is placing another human being in mortal peril and you are in a unique position to protect this unsuspecting, vulnerable person.

This ethical dilemma, discussed at greater length in Part 1, Section 3, effectively illustrates the prima facie character of the principles approach. As a physician, you are clearly bound by your duty of confidentiality, but you are also bound to prevent grave harm to highly vulnerable people, especially when you are in a unique position to do so. According to principlism, you cannot simply invoke a supreme value that always wins; you must instead undertake the difficult task of weighing and balancing conflicting values. In this case, you might decide that the principle of autonomy is outweighed by the prevention of harm to others. The risk is great, the projected harm exceedingly grave, and your patient's insistence upon his autonomy might be discounted as self-contradictory and hypocritical in light of his irresponsible disregard of his fiancée's autonomy, as well as her life.

On balance, then, your prima facie duty to respect your patient's confidentiality might fall short as a duty *all things considered* in this particular situation. But this does not mean either that these rival concerns will always prevail in similar circumstances or

---

61. W. D. Ross, *The Right and the Good* (Oxford: Clarendon Press, 1930).

that confidentiality simply becomes irrelevant once it is outweighed. If your patient is an HIV-infected woman who (credibly) claims that her abusive, drug-taking, and possibly HIV-infected boyfriend will kill her should he discover her secret, you will most likely find another way to solve the problem than by violating your patient's confidentiality. And even when you decide that, all things considered, confidentiality must yield to another principle, such as the prevention of harm, confidentiality continues to exert moral influence by setting the terms of legitimate disclosure. Even though the bisexual's fiancée has a right to know the truth, the same cannot be said of his employer, the other patients in your waiting room, or the members of your weekly poker game.

Objections to the Principles Approach

In spite of its enormous success, the method of principlism has recently been criticized on a number of fronts. Although some of these objections lack merit, others pose important challenges to principlism. As we shall see, principlism has nevertheless proved itself remarkably adaptive in responding to many of these complaints.[62]

1. Principlism Is Mechanistic and Vacuous. Although astute commentators like Beauchamp and Childress have wielded principlism in a thoughtful, carefully nuanced, and fruitful manner, in less-skilled hands this method has tended to degenerate into a ritualistic incantation of empty abstractions. Bioethical literature abounds with superficial claims that "the principle of autonomy (or of beneficence, or of the 'best interests' of the patient) *requires* that we do such and such." The problem with this common locution is that it ignores the difficulty (or the vacuousness) of passing immediately from very abstract statements of principle to very concrete conclusions about what to do here and now. Quite apart from the vexing problem of rank

ordering *competing* principles in morally complex situations, we first have to determine what these abstract formulations of principle actually mean.

What does it mean, for example, to invoke the moral principle that caregivers should always seek the best interests of all patients, including severely impaired newborns? How are the interests of such a child to be assessed, and according to which conception of the good? Some argue that life is sacred and that continued life is always in the child's interest; others contend that a life of constant suffering is not a life worth living; while still others advance a conception of the good based on more complex notions of human flourishing and dignity, which might sanction nontreatment decisions even given the absence of pain and suffering.[63]

Whatever the merit of these individual suggestions, the point is that unless we *interpret* "the principles of bioethics," they will merely play the role of empty "chapter headings,"[64] doing little, if any, actual work in moral analysis. Unless we furnish principles with a definite shape and content—*Which* principle of justice? *Which* conception of autonomy?—they will merely lend a patina of objectivity to bioethical debates while masking the need to pin down arguments and choices defining the substance of those principles.

2. Principlism Founders on the Problem of Moral Conflict. Other critics call attention to principlism's inability or unwillingness to provide a rationally defensible framework for settling conflicts between competing principles. Clearly, such critics have a point here. Unlike utilitarians or Rawlsians who could settle, at least to their own satisfaction, the inevitable conflicts of the moral life using some overarching principle of "lexical ordering," the principlists forthrightly admit that their moral principles do not come with preestablished theoretical weights; consequently, conflicts have to be settled through a subtle process of weighing and balancing of principles in the midst of real cases, an approach to

---

62. The following account of the role of principles and cases in moral argument is based upon John Arras's more extensive discussion in "Principles and Particularity: The Roles of Cases in Bioethics," *Indiana Law Journal* 69, no. 4 (Symposium on Emerging Paradigms in Bioethics, Fall 1994): 983–1014.

63. See Ezekiel Emanuel, *The Ends of Human Life,* 70–87 (see note 34).

64. K. Danner Clouser and Bernard Gert, "A Critique of Principlism," *Journal of Medicine and Philosophy* 15 (1990): 227.

conflict resolution that some philosophers regard as excessively subjective. We believe, however, that there is wisdom in the principlists' modesty. Their critics have neither established the clear superiority of any monistic theory, such as utilitarianism, nor have they produced a convincing account of why, within more pluralistic systems, certain favored values such as utility or liberty should *always* prevail over all other competing values in a myriad of convoluted real-world situations.

3. Principlism Is Deductivistic. Another group of critics, the partisans of a more "case-driven" mode of analysis, object to the apparently unidirectional movement from principles to cases within principlism. While later editions of Beauchamp and Childress's *The Principles of Bioethics* address this criticism, earlier editions gave the distinct impression that theory justifies principles, that principles justify moral rules, and that rules justify moral judgments in particular cases.[65]

This top-down conception of moral reasoning has been faulted for ignoring the pivotal role of intuitive, case-based judgments of right and wrong. To be sure, the judgments in question are not to be confused with just any responses to cases, no matter how prejudiced, ill-considered, or subject to coercion they might be. Rather, the critics have in mind something more akin to John Rawls's notion of "considered" moral judgments[66] (i.e., those judgments about whose genesis and moral rectitude we feel most confident, such as that slavery is wrong). It is precisely these judgments, they claim, that give concrete meaning, definition, and scope to our moral principles, thus providing us with critical leverage in refining their articulation.

The ultimate point of this criticism is that the relationship between principles and cases is dialectical or reciprocal: The principles provide normative guidance and the cases provide considered judgments that, in turn, help shape the principles, which then provide more precise guidance. Another way of putting this, following Rawls's terminology, is

that principles and cases exist together in creative tension or reflective equilibrium.[67] One can thus insist on a robust role for principles in moral reasoning without being committed to a top-down or deductivistic approach.[68]

Casuistry or "Case-Based" Reasoning

The renaissance of casuistry, or "case-based" reasoning, in practical ethics has stressed the pivotal role of the particularity of cases while deemphasizing the role of theory and routinized appeals to the principles of bioethics.[69] According to its leading proponents, a casuistical method must begin with a typology or grouping of cases around paradigmatic instances of a moral rule or principle. In the area of research ethics, for example, the atrocities of Nazi medicine still serve to exemplify unethical dealing with human subjects. From this signal case, one then branches out to analogous cases of greater complexity and difficulty, such as research on children or the demented elderly, proceeding by a method akin to "moral triangulation." As one goes from case to case, responding to the particularities of different settings, treatments, and categories of research subjects, principles emerge and become increasingly refined and complex.

Crucially, the casuists contend that whatever "weight" a principle might have vis-à-vis competing principles must be determined not in the abstract, but rather in response to the particularities of

---

65. Beauchamp and Childress, *The Principles of Biomedical Ethics* (New York: Oxford University Press, 1979), 5.

66. Rawls, *A Theory of Justice*, 47 (see note 19).

67. Ibid., 20ff, 48–50.

68. The principlists' response to this line of criticism has been to embrace it, over time, with increasing forthrightness and enthusiasm. Although they may have been slower than others to discern the formative and critical roles of case analysis with regard to principles and theories, Beauchamp and Childress (4th ed.) now embrace reflective equilibrium as *the* methodology of principlism, and emphatically denounce deductivism for precisely the same reasons given by their critics. See Chapters 1–2 (see note 6).

69. See, for example, Albert Jonsen and Stephen Toulmin, *The Abuse of Casuistry* (Berkeley: University of California Press, 1988); John D. Arras, "Getting Down to Cases: The Revival of Casuistry in Bioethics," *Journal of Medicine and Philosophy* 16 (1991): 29–51; and Baruch Brody, *Life and Death Decision Making* (New York: Oxford University Press, 1988).

individual cases.[70] Suppose, for example, that physicians and nurses at a nursing home wish to study the refusal to eat of many elderly patients with Alzheimer's disease. Further suppose that informed consent to participate in the study cannot be expected from this impaired patient population. According to the dictates of our paradigm case—for example, the infamous and lethal experiments of the Nazi doctors—the principle of respect for persons always requires the free and informed consent of the research subject. But according to the casuists, whether the principle of autonomy should prevail over the principle of beneficence in nursing home research—a result that many consider the primary lesson of Nazi research atrocities—will be determined in the context of a nuanced investigation into the "who" (enslaved ethnic populations vs. patients with Alzheimer's disease); the "what" (experiments designed to kill vs. studying and filming patients' eating behaviors); the "where" (death camps vs. a regulated nursing home with a competent research review board); and the "when" (after capture and before execution vs. after the consent of family, the loss of decision-making capacity, and the approval and ongoing oversight of an ethics committee). Rather than assigning a timeless relative weight to a certain principle, casuistry holds that the weight lies in the details. In this hypothetical situation, a proposed protocol might be so far removed from our paradigm of unethical research, and the potential benefits to future patients might be so great, that our moral approval may be justified even without the patient's consent.

Presented in this way, the casuistical method obviously has much in common with the method of the common law. Indeed, given the pivotal and ubiquitous role of legal cases in the recent history of bioethics—a history punctuated by such names as Karen Quinlan, Claire Conroy, and Nancy Cruzan (Part 3, Section 4)—it was entirely natural for bioethicists to begin drawing parallels between case-based reasoning in ethics and in law. In both

casuistry and law, we seem to reason from the bottom up (from specific cases to fleshed-out principles) rather than from the top down (as in most versions of applied ethics); the principles themselves are consequently "open textured," always subject to further revision and specification; and our final judgments usually turn on a fine-grained analysis of the particularities of the case.

To many ethicists, this account of reasoning in both ethics and law accurately describes how we actually think, both in clinical situations and in the classroom; that is, we tend to see cases, which serve as a kind of shorthand, as exemplars for moral analysis and assessment. "This is a Quinlan-type case, except instead of a ventilator the issue is a feeding tube (or antibiotics, or the sustainment of minimal conscious awareness, or a family insisting that everything be done, etc.). How does each different variable alter the case? Is it so different that it should dictate an alternative result?" Instead of ritualistically invoking the mantra of principles, casuistic ethicists thus urge us all to conform our rhetoric to our actual practice.

Just as the casuists insist that the weight of principles resides in the details, they also insist that moral certainty resides in our responses to paradigmatic cases, rather than in abstractions of theory or principle. We are much more confident in our knowledge that torturing and killing Jews to learn about hypothermia is wrong than we are in our assessment of which moral theory or constellation of moral principles best explains why. We would, in fact, be much more likely to switch our allegiance to a different moral theory or set of principles than to change our judgment on what the Nazi doctors did. Indeed, were a moral theory to approve of the Nazis' experiments, we would most likely take that specific judgment as sufficient reason to reject the theory.

Although some extreme casuists reject principles entirely, more moderate versions of casuistry make room for principles, theories, and cultural norms, while still insisting on the priority of the particular. Instead of imposing a false choice between principles and responses to cases, these ethicists envision, in the words of Martha Nussbaum, a "process of loving conversation between rules and concrete responses, general conceptions and unique cases, in which the general articulates the particular and

---

70. Albert Jonsen, "Of Balloons and Bicycles, or the Relationship between Ethical Theory and Practical Judgment," *Hastings Center Report* 21 (1991): 14–16.

is in turn further articulated by it."[71] Principles play a role, then, but rarely—if ever—as mere axioms from which to deduce moral conclusions. Indeed, whatever validity or usefulness general principles might have depends upon the insight, moral sensitivity, and casuistical skill that mediate their "application" to the particulars of a case.

At this point it should be clear that principlism and the emerging paradigm of casuistry are not necessarily as antithetical as their respective partisans often suggest. On the contrary, chastened principlists who have abandoned deductivism, and moderate casuists who admit a role for principles and general norms, could endorse Nussbaum's dictum with equal enthusiasm; it is, after all, just another way of calling for reflective equilibrium between principles and cases.

According to this emerging consensus, then, moral justification lies not in the correspondence between our moral theories and some sort of moral bedrock, such as nature or God's will; rather, justification resides in the coherence or "fit" among the whole network of our considered judgments and the principles and rules that emanate from them. Insofar as our most confident moral judgments cohere with the system of norms built upon them, they can be considered justified. Contrary to deductivism, moral certainty does not lie in either principles or theory; and contrary to extreme casuistry, certainty does not lie only in our responses to paradigmatic cases. Instead, we believe that any moral certitude lies at the intersection between our abstract norms and our responses to cases.

Judgments that conflict with well-established moral norms, even judgments that might have once seemed unassailable, should be subjected to further scrutiny. Even though it might have once been "plain as day" that African Americans deserve second-class status or that doctors should never assist patients to commit suicide, the principles of respect for persons or individual autonomy might well prompt us to rethink—and in some cases reject—what was once thought to be our moral bedrock. By the same token, as we have seen, principles develop out of reflection on our considered judgments and acquire their precise meaning and weight within the crucible of contextualized judgments.

It should be noted, however, that even though we speak of reflective "equilibrium" and the "system" of coherent judgments and general norms, the moral life will always be more dynamic and less tidy than these terms imply. The uneasy balance between particular judgments and general norms will most likely never reach equilibrium. Our considered judgments are in a state of constant, if glacially slow, flux, and our concepts, principles, and rules are always merely provisional—always subject to further expansion in scope, specification of meaning, and fluctuation in importance vis-à-vis other general norms. The best we can hope for, then, is a constant striving for greater and greater coherence. Complete coherence—a total seamless system of morality—is most likely beyond our grasp, kept out of reach by both the limitations of our mental capacities and the inherent fragmentation among the values that constitute our complicated moral lives.

---

71. Martha Nussbaum, "The Discernment of Perception: An Aristotelian Conception of Private and Public Rationality," in *Love's Knowledge: Essays on Philosophy and Literature* (New York: Oxford University Press, 1990), 95.

PART ONE

FOUNDATIONS OF THE HEALTH PROFESSIONAL– PATIENT RELATIONSHIP

The success of scientific medicine, the growing impersonality of the medical setting, and the rise of consumerism—together with the recent emergence of managed care—have combined to shake the foundations of the traditional doctor–nurse–patient relationship. The burgeoning number of medical malpractice suits alone provides eloquent testimony of profound changes taking place both in our expectations of medical science and in our awareness of patients' rights. What responsibilities and rights *should* attach to the roles of nurse, doctor, and patient? And how should health professionals think about the inevitable conflicts of duty that arise from the intersection of their specific roles? Part 1 is devoted to the exploration of these questions. Although clarifying the moral foundations of the health professional–patient relationship is an interesting and important task in its own right, the resolution of these basic issues will also shed welcome light on the biomedical problems raised in subsequent parts of the text.

AUTONOMY, PATERNALISM, AND MEDICAL MODELS

The relationship between health professionals and patients is mediated in complex ways by an array of values and social norms. Sometimes these norms are explicit and overt, as when physicians take an oath to look after the welfare of their patients. In many cases, however, these values remain largely implicit and unarticulated, embedded in the culture and the institutions in which we work, learn, or live, and in the roles that persons inhabit within those institutions. Sometimes sociologists, social psychologists, anthropologists, and other social scientists seek to understand these norms, to explain their origins and the myriad ways in which they actually shape the expectations, responses, emotions, and other dispositions of the persons who are affected by them. Understanding this factual information is also of fundamental importance for bioethics, because medicine and the biosciences are not isolated fields that operate on an ideal frictionless plane. They are concrete social activities that take place within specific institutions, with their own histories and traditions.

For the ethicist, however, this information is not the end of the inquiry. Rather, it provides the background against which a more fundamental set of questions is posed: How *ought* we to think about the bond uniting health care providers and patients? How *ought* we to organize the larger concrete social institutions in which this bond is forged? What are the values that *ought* to shape the way people perceive and respond to others in these settings? Consider the different values implicit in the metaphors that have been used to describe the relationship between health care providers and patients: parent–child, teacher–student, seller–buyer, priest–penitent, oppressor–victim, friends, contractors. Understanding, for example, that a particular way of conceiving of the "patient" shapes the way we are disposed to perceive and respond to persons so labeled is but one extremely important step in a process of critical reflection in which latent norms are made explicit so that they can be discussed and evaluated publicly. The choice between these and other possible "models" of the provider–patient relationship will profoundly shape both our outlook on medical ethics generally and our views on particular controversies.

Not long ago, the patient–provider relationship was conceived almost exclusively in terms of a patient-centered consequentialism that traced its roots back to the Hippocratic tradition. Section 1 begins with the formative text of this tradition. If we turn to the Hippocratic oath, we see that the doctor pledges to "apply dietetic measures for the benefit of the sick according to [his] ability and judgment," and he promises to keep his patients from "harm and injustice." This "moral core" of the oath admirably commits the physician above all else to the health and well-being of his patients—as opposed, for example, to the advancement of medical science, profits, or cost containment. Unlike utilitarianism, a form of consequentialism that instructs agents to evaluate the consequences of their actions for some large social group, patient-centered consequentialism enjoins providers to evaluate their conduct based on its consequences for the welfare of the individual patient. Perhaps the most controversial element of traditional Hippocratic ethics, however, is the way it identifies the patient's welfare with physical health. This strikingly narrow way of thinking about a person's welfare allows the patient to be conceived of as a largely passive recipient of the physician's expert ministrations which are determined by the principles of his art and his own "ability and judgment."

On this model, physicians are thought to be better suited to make health-related decisions for their patients than are the patients themselves because the patient's welfare is defined in terms of physical health, a subject about which physicians and other health professionals have special technical knowledge. As a result, the medical tradition based on this oath has hardly considered lying or shielding the patient from the truth a form of "injustice," as the following passage from the "Decorum," another Hippocratic text, strikingly shows: "Perform [these duties] calmly and adroitly, concealing most things

from the patient while you are attending to him. Give necessary orders with cheerfulness and serenity, turning his attention away from what is being done to him; sometimes reprove sharply and emphatically, and sometimes comfort with solicitude and attention, revealing nothing of the patient's future or present condition."

This model, however, is highly paternalistic because it entails that health care providers can legitimately restrict or dictate the conduct of even competent adults for the sake of that person's own good. On the traditional model, the physician's duty to tell the truth to patients is subordinated to, and derived from, the more fundamental duty to "do no harm." If, in the physician's judgment, telling the truth would result in depression or otherwise adversely impact the care of a patient, then the physician would be duty bound to withhold such information.

In the 1960s and 1970s, however, the prevailing paternalism of American medicine was subjected to increased public scrutiny as a broad range of reform movements encouraged the public to question the authority of many dominant social institutions and the values imbedded in the roles those institutions assigned to persons. Also during these decades, a number of prominent research scandals came to light in which physicians had performed medical experiments on vulnerable populations such as the indigent, elderly patients of the Jewish Chronic Disease Hospital who were injected with live cancer cells without their consent, the mentally disabled children of the Willowbrook State School who were purposefully infected with hepatitis, or the 600 poor, African American males whose syphilis was deliberately left untreated for forty years so that a generation of physician researchers could study the natural history of the disease (see Part 5, Section 1). High-profile revelations like these fueled distrust of the authority wielded by the medical profession, and out of the resulting scrutiny there emerged a trenchant and multifaceted critique of medical paternalism.

The question of truth-telling became a lightning rod for criticism as an increasingly skeptical public began to question the assumptions of traditional medical practice. Some critics attempted to refute the paternalistic approach to truth-telling on its own terms, by demonstrating through opinion polls and empirical research that many patients want to be told the truth. Contrary to the assumption that physicians are well qualified to assess the risks and benefits of withholding the truth, it was argued that they rarely possess good evidence for their customary refusal to disclose the truth and that they have no special training to make such difficult value-laden decisions regarding what is really best for patients and their families. As Alan Goldman points out in "The Refutation of Medical Paternalism," this view equates welfare with physical health, ignoring the fact that how people value health is itself shaped by their broader values and life projects. Doctors and patients do not always share the same values or aim at the same treatment goals. Whereas many physicians tend to regard the extension of life as the predominant value, their patients might well value the quality of their future life more than its quantity.

On a more fundamental level, though, Goldman argues that paternalism fails to recognize the independent value of self-determination and the respect that people are entitled to as "choosing beings." Because the traditional view leaves no room for self-determination as an important aspect of a patient's welfare, it fails to treat patients as the *moral* equals of their physicians by denying them the information they need to make informed decisions about their own person. Without sufficient information upon which to base a judgment, a patient's consent to treatment will not be informed, and in the absence of informed consent a patient's self-determination is effectively thwarted. From this perspective, the physician always has a strong duty to be truthful with patients—a duty that is grounded ultimately on the patient's dignity as a choosing being. All the various tried and true forms of deceit—from outright lying, to withholding information, to using medical jargon ("no need to worry; it's just a little carcinoma")—undermine the status of the patient as an autonomous agent.

In the vast majority of cases, respecting patient autonomy by engaging the patient's own powers of deliberation, choice, and agency is not just consistent with the desire to benefit the patient, but is itself a means of doing so. As a result, the importance of respect for autonomy is widely recognized in contemporary medicine and can fairly be described as the cornerstone of contemporary bioethics. Nevertheless, this does not mean that many of the central

views and values of the Hippocratic tradition have disappeared. Rather, they persist even today, only they tend now to be expressed, not in direct opposition to the value of respect for autonomy, but within the debate over what it means to respect autonomy in practice and where to draw the boundaries where the pursuit of this goal should give way to other values such as beneficence or nonmaleficence.

This is illustrated nicely in the case study "Beneficence Today, or Autonomy (Maybe) Tomorrow?" in which a health care team disagrees over whether to wake a heavily sedated patient on a ventilator in order to inform her that she has terminal cancer and perhaps less than three months to live. For Bernice S. Elger, the fact that waking Monica may cause her physical distress and informing her of her terminal condition may cause psychological pain is of secondary importance in comparison to the need to give her a chance to make informed decisions about how she wants to face her illness and order her life in her remaining days. In contrast, Jean-Claude Chevrolet likens waking Monica and asking her to choose between several bleak options to subjecting her to a pointless medical intervention. For Chevrolet, Monica's situation is so bleak that her best interests would not be served by subjecting her to physical and mental anguish under the name of respect for her autonomy.

In this instance, Elger and Chevrolet agree that in ordinary situations, health care providers cannot legitimately restrict or dictate the conduct of competent adults for the sake of that person's own good. Their disagreement thus presupposes a common rejection of traditional medical paternalism. For Chevrolet, however, this is an extraordinary case. His suggestion that waking Monica to get her consent would be analogous to administering a pointless treatment harkens back to the well-worn idea in Hippocratic ethics that information ought to be treated like any other tool in the physician's black bag; it should be used sparingly and only to advance therapeutic goals. If Chevrolet thinks that this is a case in which it does not make sense to pursue the goal of facilitating patient autonomy, it may be because he conceives of the value of this goal in terms of its ultimate contribution to patient welfare. In most cases, respect for autonomy is an important element in achieving the more fundamental aim of ministering to the welfare of the patient, but not in this case. Similarly, if Elger thinks that it does make sense to try to facilitate Monica's ability to make important decisions about the end of her life, it may be because she thinks that the contribution of autonomy to patient welfare outweighs the physical and emotional distress that will come with it. Alternatively, however, it may be that Elger gives independent weight to the value of autonomy, quite apart from its contribution to patient welfare, and that her commitment to wake Monica is rooted not in a concern for her state of being (i.e., for her welfare), but for Monica as a person.

Placing respect for autonomy at the core of the provider–patient relationship represents the ideal of treating both providers and patients as responsible moral agents capable of making important decisions that will have a bearing on their lives. This has given rise to a model of the provider–patient relationship based on the metaphor of a contract or covenant. Contrary to the paternalistic or Hippocratic model, the patient is the party within the "contractual" relationship charged with making important value-laden decisions that will affect the overall direction of treatment. The physician is responsible for presenting the available treatment options to the patient and carrying out the details of the agreed-upon plan of care with professional expertise. Importantly, the physician retains his or her moral integrity within the contractual model and is not reduced to a mere "body mechanic" or "engineer" doing the bidding of patients. Since a contractual relationship is a two-way street, the physician may decide to terminate the relationship if, for example, the patient makes unreasonable demands or is flagrantly noncompliant with treatment (Veatch 1972). This contractual understanding of the physician–patient relationship has proven to be a powerful counterpoint to traditional physician ethics.

One of the most attractive features of the contractual model is its commitment to the fundamental moral equality of doctors and patients. Yet precisely this commitment is at the heart of one of the central challenges to this model. In "Why Doctors Should Intervene" Terrence F. Ackerman argues that defining features of the contractual model are insensitive to the "transforming effects of illness." In order to fully respect patients as moral equals, Ackerman argues, physicians will have to be far more active in influencing not only the decision-making process of individual patients, but potentially the dynamics of the family or the institutional context in which patients make those decisions.

Ackerman singles out two features of the contractual model for special scrutiny. The first is the idea that the primary responsibility of physicians is to provide patients with the information that they need in order to make the relevant decision. The second is the idea that apart from serving as a knowledge resource, physicians respect the autonomy of patients by not interfering in the process of deliberation through which the patient arrives at a final decision.

These features are problematic, Ackerman argues, because they ignore profound respects in which sickness and disease can dampen and impede the ability of ill people to marshal the cognitive, affective, and social capabilities that they need in order to make decisions that accurately reflect the application of their own values and priorities to their particular situation. For instance, denial, depression, guilt, fear, and even the desire not to give up hope can impede the ability of patients to process information effectively. This can be exacerbated by having to absorb large amounts of information that may be complex or technical and, therefore, completely foreign to the patient.

Similarly, illness can also impair the ability of patients to arrive at decisions that accurately reflect their own values and priorities. Illness can be overwhelming. On top of pain and fatigue that may be associated with the underlying condition, medical intervention itself can involve unpleasant, painful, and even humiliating experiences. In order to cope with so many physical and emotional challenges, patients sometimes may seek to abdicate important decisions to others, such as family members or physicians themselves. Or, alternatively, when patients become dependent on familiar for care and for emotional or financial support, it can be difficult to prevent the values and priorities of those family members from crowding out, or supplanting, the values of the patient.

For Ackerman, respect for autonomy therefore requires physicians to be more than information delivery devices. They have to recognize the potential for abuse that is created by the practical inequalities that characterize their relationships with their patients. Physicians have more knowledge than patients. They often face lower affective and intellectual barriers to decision making and fewer institutional hurdles to self-governance. In order to treat their patients as their moral equals in the face of these practical inequalities, physicians may have to actively support patient decision making in a way that fosters or brings about greater patient autonomy.

Ackerman is not recommending a return to the old paternalism of Hippocratic medicine. But proponents of the contractual model may nevertheless be uncomfortable with the more attenuated form of paternalism latent in the idea that "the goal of the therapeutic relationship is the 'development' of the patient" and that in this respect, at least, the "doctor patient interaction is not unlike the parent-child or teacher-student relationship."

The idea that the value of respecting patient autonomy is richer and more complex than is captured by simple juxtapositions of "autonomy versus paternalism" is explored further by Ezekiel J. and Linda L. Emanuel in "Four Models of the Physician–Patient Relationship." The Emanuels present a typology of various models of the physician–patient relationship, including (1) the paternalistic model, (2) the informative model, (3) the interpretive model, and (4) the deliberative model. They also point out that all of the previous models, excluding, of course, all frankly coercive approaches, accept some notion of autonomy, ranging from the mere acceptance of the doctor's recommendations to the more robust notion of moral learning and development in the deliberative model. Although there are few proponents of bald-faced paternalism today, there remains widespread debate about the nature and limits of autonomy, how it should be related to other aspects of a person's welfare, and how to respect it in the complex world of contemporary medicine.

Important threads of this debate are illustrated by the Emanuels. While their first model is the familiar Hippocratic approach, the second and third together constitute what others would call the "contractual approach." Their version of the informative model, however, makes a sharp distinction between facts and values, assigning the patient the role of decision maker concerning values and relegating the physician to the role of providing expert factual information to the patient. In this respect, it deviates

from standard conceptions of the contractual model because it tends to reduce the physician to a mere tool of the patient's wishes.

The interpretive model, like the standard contractual approach, lodges final decision-making authority in the patient, but it emphasizes the problematic nature of discovering what the patient's values and preferences really are. Advocates of the contractual model often seem to assume, quite erroneously, that patients always know exactly how they feel and what they want in enormously complex and emotionally trying circumstances. In this interpretive model, by contrast, the doctor's role is analogous to that of a counselor who engages the patient in a mutual effort to understand what the patient's values really are and to discern which medical interventions will best advance those values.

The Emanuels' deliberative model encompasses the information-sharing and interpretive efforts of the previous models, but goes one controversial step further in recommending that the patient choose the "best" or "most admirable" course involving health-related values. Here the doctor's role is that of a teacher or moral guide who, though shunning coercive methods, recommends to the patient the medically best choice. For example, instead of simply laying out all the pros and cons of gluttony and smoking, a "deliberative" physician will directly recommend that the patient eat in moderation and stop smoking altogether. The directive aspect of their favored deliberative model, however, remains a point of controversy. Many readers might well wonder how physicians are to distinguish in-practice recommendations based upon "health-related values," which are permitted in this model, from those recommendations based on the physician's personal moral code, which are not permitted.

At the other extreme, one must avoid holding an overintellectualized and one-dimensional view of what it means to be autonomous. The Emanuels' deliberative model treats patients and physicians as moral equals, capable of reflecting together on the values that are relevant to a decision and justifying; their decision to ultimately allow certain values to drive a particular decision. This model embodies important insights about the power of reasoning and shared reflection to shape an individual's decision-making process. But in practice, individual patients may not either possess the argumentative skills and intellectual bent required by this model or welcome the challenge of defending their values to their clinician.

There remains significant room for debate, therefore, about which of these models best facilitates autonomy and avoids backdoor paternalism. One might consider, therefore, how likely it is that patients already endorse a fairly robust array of health-related values such that clarifying these values, as the interpretive model requires, might help the patient determine their importance in relation to the patient's other values. One might then consider how the deliberations required by the deliberative model would be carried out in practice and then consider which is likely to go the farthest toward enhancing the effective autonomy of patients in actual practice.

INFORMED CONSENT AND TRUTH-TELLING

The ethical cornerstone of the contractual and interpretive models is their insistence that the patient should make value-laden decisions bearing on his or her body and future life. The philosophical basis for this position is based on two distinct values: advancement of the patient's well-being and respect for the patient's autonomy. Partisans of the contractual and interpretive models contend that the patient, if adequately informed, is usually the best judge of his or her own best interests and should therefore possess the ultimate decision-making authority. Moreover, as Goldman points out, most of us value the ability to make decisions on our own behalf, quite apart from the consequences.

This ethical ideal of self-determination has received legal sanction in the doctrine of informed consent. As articulated by Justice Cardozo in a justly celebrated formulation in the case of *Schloendorff* v. *Society of New York Hospital* (1914), "Every adult human being of adult years and sound mind has a right to determine what shall be done with his own body." In order to consent freely, the patient must not be subject to any coercion or undue influence; and in order that the patient's consent be *informed*, the patient must, as we shall see in the readings, receive adequate information on which to base his or her choice. A final threshold condition for informed

consent, in the words of Cardozo, is that the patient have a "sound mind" (a requirement that is addressed in Part 3, Section 2).

How much information is required in order to render the patient's consent truly informed? The law's attempt to answer this difficult question can be found in the 1972 California Supreme Court case of *Cobbs* v. *Grant*.

Mr. Cobbs, the plaintiff, had the misfortune of experiencing a number of remote "maloccurrences" incidental to his original surgery for a peptic ulcer. Since none of his physicians had warned him of any of these risks, Mr. Cobbs sued on the ground that his right to informed consent had been violated.

At the time he brought suit, however, the hapless Mr. Cobbs had little reason to think that his claim would hold up in court. In determining the scope of a physician's duty to inform patients, most American jurisdictions had adopted a "professional standard" approach that placed lay claimants at a severe disadvantage. Under this rule, a physician's conduct in disclosing information was to be judged by the standards actually observed by members of the local medical community. If it was not common practice to disclose a given risk, then the patient could not recover damages for breach of informed consent. Under this legal doctrine, good medical practice (as defined by the local medical community) made good law.

Mr. Cobbs sued nonetheless, arguing that the "professional standard" approach placed too much discretion in the hands of physicians. Happily for Mr. Cobbs, he again found himself on the cutting edge, but this time of a revolution in the law of informed consent. His case, *Cobbs* v. *Grant*, along with several others decided in the early 1970s, made the patient's right of self-determination the measure of the doctor's duty to reveal. Doctors were found to have a duty to disclose "all information relevant to a meaningful decisional process." Instead of asking "What do physicians ordinarily disclose around here?" the *Cobbs* court asked, "What information would a competent patient need to make a reasonable decision?"

In response to those critics who debunk the informed consent requirement as a sheer impossibility, presiding Judge Mosk noted that a "minicourse" in medicine is not required, nor is a useless list of remote minor risks. Simply put, the patient must be told what a reasonable person would need to know about the procedure and its attendant risks in order to make a rational decision on the basis of his or her own values. In a passage strongly influenced by the contractual model, Mosk noted that the physician's expert *medical function* is limited to describing the nature of the procedure and its risks; the actual decision must incorporate those risks, must weigh them against a patient's values, hopes, and fears, and must therefore be left to the patient.

Against this historical background, Section 2 begins with a case study. In "Antihypertensives and the Risk of Temporary Impotence: A Case Study in Informed Consent," John D. Arras illustrates how difficult problems of information sharing are not limited to complex surgical cases such as *Cobbs.* Even in the more mundane setting of primary care medicine physicians may face difficult decisions about how much information to disclose to patients and about how best to convey such information to specific individuals. This case asks whether a physician should inform a patient with high blood pressure that a cheap and effective medication also poses a very small risk of inducing temporary impotence, a risk that might be magnified by the very act of informing the patient.

In his article "Informed Consent—Must It Remain a Fairy Tale?" Jay Katz contends that the ethical ideal of self-determination at the core of informed consent has been resisted by medicine and distorted by the law. Contrary to those who view the advent of informed consent as the triumph of patient autonomy over medical paternalism, Katz shows how the framework of malpractice law has systematically betrayed the ethical ideal of self-determination out of deference to medical professionalism. Notwithstanding a brief flirtation with autonomy in cases like *Cobbs,* Katz argues that the law has fallen far short of its promise in reshaping the doctor–patient relationship. At most, he says, the law has created an expanded *duty to warn* rather than a more supportive context for patient decision making.

Although Katz would agree with critics who charge that the law's capacity for fundamental reform of the doctor–patient relationship is quite limited, and that real progress will most likely come (if at all) from a different kind of medical education, he nevertheless claims that the doctrine

of informed consent ha[...] and disturbing questi[...] sion. In particular, I[...] whether their oppo[...] stems not merely fro[...] tence to handle harsh tru[...], [...] their own deep-seated reluctance to admit [...] widespread existence of medical uncertainty both to their patients and to themselves. For Katz, the ethical ideal of informed consent, as opposed to its legalistic trappings, is an appeal to the medical profession to discover new ways of relating to patients, new modes of communication that might foster hope on the basis of mutual respect rather than deceit.

Two features of Katz's article are particularly noteworthy. First, in stark contrast to courts and physicians, who tend to view informed consent either as a mere recitation of potential risks or, worse yet, as the signing of a form, Katz envisions true informed consent as a kind of searching conversation between patient and physician. Second, Katz is aware of the extent to which illness itself can pose an obstacle to this kind of decision-making process. But he is also profoundly sensitive to the myriad psychological, social, and institutional forces that make such searching conversations psychologically burdensome and institutionally inefficient for physicians. In this respect, he is careful to point out that having the correct doctrine of informed consent does not mean that one therefore has an adequate strategy for effecttuting the relevant conversational exchanges between actual individuals in concrete cases.

As several of the readings in this section highlight, caregivers must find a delicate balance between being a source of strength and support to patients and a champion of the patient's health interests while at the same time actively facilitating and respecting the autonomous decision making of patients. As Katz insightfully notes, crucial to this balance is the capacity of health care providers to recognize and to come to terms with their own human limitations and fallibility, both on a personal, psychological level, as well as on an institutional and professional level.

The importance of coming to terms with one's human limitations is powerfully illustrated by Francoise Baylis in "Errors in Medicine: Nurturing Truthfulness." In this analysis, Baylis explores in detail of the psychological, social, and institutional dynamics that prevent many health care providers from openly disclosing the occurrence of medical errors to their patients. These dynamics are emblematic of the way that individual caregivers struggle, often in isolation, with their own fallibility and with a medical culture that tends to treat errors as moral as well as technical failures.

A recent report on medical errors issued by the Institute of Medicine estimated that between 44,000 and 98,000 people die in U.S. hospitals annually as a result of medical errors. If these figures are accurate, medical mistakes surpass motor vehicle accidents, breast cancer, and AIDS as a cause of death in the United States. As a result, the Institute of Medicine report has generated a maelstrom of controversy and brought a public spotlight to the question of whether and to what extent medical professionals are obligated to disclose the occurrence of mistakes to patients or their families. It has also raised the issue of how mistakes ought to be dealt with inside the medical profession.

Disclosing medical mistakes can isolate a caregiver, making him or her subject to recrimination and scapegoating from colleagues while opening up the possibility of litigation from patients. In fact, many health professionals avoid disclosing mistakes to patients out of a fear of being sued, even though many patients report that a key factor in their decision to litigate was the perception that caregivers were being less than candid with them. Undoubtedly, the pursuit of individual excellence is a laudable and exemplary goal, but the activities of physicians, nurses, and other caregivers are often structured by larger systems, protocols, or routines that it may be possible to redesign in order to minimize the likelihood of error. The process of examining and testing these systems can only begin, however, with the recognition of deficiencies, and this will require a change in the way the medical profession and the public it serves think about fallibility. Sweeping mistakes under the institutional rug can foster a perception of concealment and incubate resentment that may erode public trust and rob health care teams of their best chance to learn and improve.

Profound social, psychological, and institutional hurdles to truth-telling can arise in almost any clinical setting. These difficulties can be ampli-fied and exacerbated, however, when patients and physicians occupy different cultural traditions and therefore bring divergent expectations to the clinical setting.

At a very general level, cultural diversity can be seen as posing what we will call "strategic" and "substantive" challenges. Strategic challenges are what Katz has in mind when he argues that having the correct doctrine of informed consent does not automatically translate into an adequate strategy for implementing that doctrine in concrete situations between real people. That is, cultural differences can create novel practical obstacles to achieving the goals that Katz and others see as fundamental elements of the physician–patient relationship, such as respect for individual autonomy as embodied in the ideal of free and informed consent.

In "Bioethics in a Different Tongue: The Case of Truth-Telling," Leslie J. Blackhall, Gelya Frank, Sheila Murphy and Vicki Michel illustrate how cultural differences often go deeper than differences in custom, manner, language, and dress. They can include differences in fundamental values and ends such that patients and physicians may not automatically pursue the same goals in the clinical encounter. Cultural diversity poses a substantive challenge to effective communication when patients and their caregivers differ over fundamental values such as the relative importance of individual autonomy and familial harmony.

For example, Blackhall and colleagues found that Korean American and Mexican American patients were more likely to view the explicit disclosure of a patient's diagnosis or prognosis as a form of cruelty and as something that might even hasten the patient's demise. According to Blackhall and colleagues, European Americans and African Americans tend to see the dignity and worth of persons as emanating from their capacity for free and autonomous choice, whereas Korean Americans or Mexican Americans are more likely to view the self as one element within a larger family unit whose value and identify is intimately connected to its place in that larger network of relationships. When dealing with patients from these cultural backgrounds, therefore, the physician may be faced with more than the strategic challenge of educating the patient and the larger family unit. The physician may be confronted with a substantive challenge to the value of patient autonomy by a culture in which individual autonomy is circumscribed by or subordinated to the autonomy of the larger family unit. In this case, the physician must find a way to live up to his or her own moral commitments while also respecting the patient by respecting the cultural practices and values with which the patient identifies.

At the same time, Blackhall and colleagues are quick to point out that cultural groups themselves are not monolithic. Often cultures are a composite of diverse traditions, each of which may differ in its values and priorities. In addition, however, when communities become increasingly diverse it is also more likely that individuals in those communities may identify with or straddle several cultural communities. So physicians must walk a fine line between the Scylla of outright cultural relativism and the Charybdis of disrespect for legitimate cultural difference. On the one hand, they must try to educate themselves about the various norms and values that are common to ethnic and cultural groups in their area. On the other hand, they must simultaneously resist the urge to reduce individuals to cultural stereotypes.

In "Offering Truth," Benjamin Freedman takes up the question of how to balance these competing goals without sacrificing the physician's commitment to respecting *individual* autonomy. Freedman notes that even when it is possible to locate a particular individual within a determinate cultural tradition, individuals may differ in the extent to which they identify with and endorse the dominant norms within that tradition. Although it is important to recognize that cultures provide the context in which individuals forge common bonds of meaning and commitment, it is equally important to recognize that individuals can endorse distinctive interpretations of common cultural traditions or embrace unique configurations of those values. Similarly, that individuals sometimes seek to reform the norms of their culture illustrates that group membership and explicit cultural identification do not exclude critical moral reflection.

Freedman therefore emphasizes the epistemological dilemma facing the clinician: In order to show respect for the patient's wishes, one must have a sense of what those wishes are. Freedman's solution to this problem is, in effect, to approach cultural differences as though they are fundamentally strategic

challenges. This approach enables caregivers to focus on finding a way to interact with the individual patient that allows the caregiver to live up to moral obligations to the patient in a way that also respects the values and preferences of that patient. To meet these competing goals, Freedman argues that autonomous persons may decide that they want to be shielded from the truth or that they want to delegate responsibility for their care to loved ones. Rather than a zero-sum game, Freedman argues that responsible providers can offer patients the opportunity to decide how much of the truth they want to be told and that this represents a reasonable middle ground between unjustified paternalism and a conception of respect for autonomy that bludgeons unprepared or vulnerable patients with blunt discussions of difficult news.

As Blackhall and colleagues note, some cultures are "high-context" cultures, meaning that individuals are expected to infer some information from social context and other forms of indirect communication, rather than having that information stated explicitly. Freedman's proposal relies heavily on the provider's ability to engage in this kind of indirect communication, especially when it comes to inferring the patient's preferences.

Although Freedman's proposal is surely well advised and sensible, it has its limitations. In particular, proponents of the interpretive model of the provider–patient relationship discussed in the previous section will likely point out that it leaves little room to determine whether the patient's desire not to learn the truth reflects that person's authentic value commitments or one of the many psychological or social dynamics illustrated by Ackerman and Katz. Similarly, proponents of the deliberative model will press further, and want to know whether the patient would continue to endorse this preference after due reflection. Ultimately, these issues boil down to an inescapable question: To what degree is the value of autonomy something that is culturally relative and to what degree does it reflect a human right, universal in its scope and applicability?

One of the common themes uniting the articles in this section is that the moral ideal of informed consent is at best a kind of moral skeleton; it dictates that the relationship between patients and their caregivers should have a certain structure and functionality. In order to work in actual practice, however, this skeleton must be attached to tendons of personal commitment, muscles of mutual trust, and the flesh and blood of genuine compassion and concern.

CONFLICTING PROFESSIONAL ROLES AND RESPONSIBILITIES

The relationship between health professionals and patients provides the background against which the foregoing controversies are set. This might lead some readers to conclude that this context provides the sole source of the health professional's moral obligations. Such a conclusion, however, would be seriously mistaken. Although the Hippocratic tradition in medicine would have us believe that the physician's only obligation is to his or her patient, such a view ignores the complex relationships that obtain between health workers, as members of distinctive professions, and the social and cultural settings in which those professions exist. Even a cursory look at the Hippocratic oath belies this convenient image. Before the "moral core" of the oath in which the physician pledges to keep the sick from "harm and injustice," the physician binds himself to honor "him who has taught me this art as equal to my parents and to live my life in partnership with him, and if he is in need of money to give him a share of mine." Already in this ancient document there is an awareness of responsibilities that physicians incur, not in their role as healers, but insofar as they are members of a particular profession.

It is a fact of contemporary professional life that the health professional's obligations to his or her patients often conflict with duties to other parties—such as other members of the health care team, the patient's family, other patients, or persons who might be harmed in some way by the patient. In addition, physicians and other health professionals are increasingly employed by large institutions such as the armed forces, prisons, insurance companies, and corporations—whose goals have more to do with killing, retribution, and profits than with healing. When health workers act as "double agents" on behalf of both patients and agencies of social control, how should they resolve the inevitable conflicts of loyalty stemming from their conflicting roles? While we might think it appropriate for company physicians to report workers who pose a health hazard to other employees or to the public at large, what are we to think when psychiatrists are required to warn third parties about the violent tendencies of their patients, or when physicians are asked to administer capital punishment by means of lethal injections?

Section 3 explores some of the diverse social commitments, contexts, and entanglements that give rise to these conflicts. It begins with an examination of some of the complex ways in which the bonds of trust between patients and health care providers, and in particular, the provider's obligation to maintain patient confidentiality, come into conflict with the imperative to protect the basic interests of third parties.

The obligation on the part of health professionals to maintain the confidentiality of patient information is grounded in part in the patient's right to control sensitive information about himself or herself—for example, the right to privacy. Just as patients have a right to decide what happens to their bodies, they have a right to keep certain facts about themselves private. It is also grounded in the vital protection it provides, both to the interests of patients and to the very existence of the health professional-patient relationship. Due to the sensitive nature of the information shared in the medical context, patients are highly vulnerable to serious harm should that information fall into the hands of others. This is especially true of persons suffering from conditions that may be stigmatized by negative social stereotypes or associations. Given the still pervasive discrimination against persons who are HIV positive, for instance, medical confidentiality helps shield patients from the loss of employment, insurance, and important human relationships.

Perhaps the most important function of confidentiality is to maintain the very possibility of a productive relationship between physicians and patients. If prospective patients distrust the willingness of physicians to keep secrets, they may not seek help in the first place. Even if they do enter into a treatment relationship, a lack of trust will often prevent patients from revealing important but potentially embarrassing information about clinical signs and symptoms. The caregiver's ability to heal and guide the patient thus depends on the maintenance of trust, but in the absence of confidentiality there can be no trust. Hence, confidentiality is a basic requirement of medical practice.

Although some might claim that this duty imposes an *absolute* requirement of fidelity to patients, it can conflict with equally compelling values and obligations, such as the duty to protect innocent third parties from harm. In the famous *Tarasoff* case, for example, psychotherapists were found to have a positive *legal duty* to violate confidentiality in order to protect a young woman, Tatiana Tarasoff, from the murderous intentions of their patient, Prosenjit Poddar. The California Supreme Court ruled that the public interest in safety and the peril to the woman's life outweighed the medical values of confidentiality and free communication between therapist and patient. Given the presence of a "determinate threat," the court ruled that therapists had a duty to exercise "reasonable care" to protect the intended victim.

In the *Tarasoff* case, the severity of the threatened harm was very grave (i.e., death), but its predictability became the point of heated debate within both the court and the psychiatric profession. Recognizing the difficulty of predicting dangerous behavior, the court merely required therapists to exercise "that reasonable degree of skill, knowledge, and care ordinarily possessed and exercised [by therapists] under similar circumstances." But critics of the court contended that psychiatrists and psychologists possessed no special "professional skill" of predicting violence and claimed that the court's ruling would prompt therapists to vastly overestimate the likelihood of violence.

The problems associated with accurately predicting possible harms to third parties arise again in "Please Don't Tell!" For commentator Leonard Fleck, the likelihood that Consuela would contract HIV from caring for her brother Carlos is too remote to license breaching Carlos's confidentiality in order to inform her of his HIV-positive status. Instead, health professionals can discharge their duty to exercise reasonable care by instructing Consuela in the use of universal precautions; providing her with the necessary gloves, masks, goggles, and gowns; and insisting that she practice these measures when caring for Carlos.

Fleck is quick to note that, while members of the health care team treating Carlos have an obligation to

safeguard information about his HIV-positive status and his sexual orientation, his sister would be under no such obligation, even though she would be acting as his nurse. For commentator Marcia Angell, however, the fact that Consuela is providing a service that normally would be provided by the health system entitles her to be informed of information that is material to her choice to care for her brother. In fact, Angell worries that not informing Consuela of her brother's HIV status would constitute a form of deception and would rob her of the chance to decide for herself what risks she is willing to assume in caring for her brother. Beneath Angell's assessment of this case lurks a tension between fulfilling the special duties that health professionals owe to their patients and fulfilling one's more general moral obligations to persons as such. Protecting Carlos's confidentiality respects his right to privacy. But is it achieved at the cost of deceiving or acting paternalistically toward Consuela, who is not a patient in this case, but who will be assuming the responsibilities of caring for Carlos at home?

Even if we conclude that medical professionals may set aside their oath of confidentiality in such cases, they will still have to confront a number of problems as they exercise their discretion or duty to warn. For example, when should efforts to persuade be abandoned and confidentiality finally violated? To whom does the provider owe this duty—only to named family members or named sexual partners or more broadly to friends and associates or all sexual partners the patient may have (with the added obligation to discover the identities of these persons)? As we consider the concrete implications of questions like these, the worries expressed by Justice Clark in the striking dissent to the majority in *Tarasoff* become more salient. In particular, will the imposition of a duty to warn deter those who are most in need of help from seeking it? Justice Clark's essentially rule-consequentialist argument is that a duty to violate the confidentiality of dangerous persons will most likely lead to more violence, not less, and that continued contact with health care professionals and voluntary persuasion are the best strategies for dealing with most conflicts between confidentiality and possible harms to third parties.

These cases pit the confidentiality of one patient against possible harms to nonpatient third parties. Advances in genetics and information sciences, however, may challenge the way we think about the provider–patient relationship as they expand the scope of the personal information that can be gathered in the health care setting, and the number of people regarded as "patients." In "Disclosing Misattributed Paternity" Lainie Friedman Ross discusses the ethical issues that arise when genetic tests for heritable medical conditions reveal that the male partner in a relationship is not the biological father of a child. As Ross notes, several recent studies show that genetic counselors are extremely reluctant to inform the male partner of misattributed paternity, even though his genetic material was used in the testing process and the resulting information may have important implications for his future procreative choices. Although, in such cases, each party contributes genetic material for testing, do genetic counselors have separate obligations to protect the confidentiality of each party individually? Even if they do, does the obligation to respect the woman's confidentiality justify withholding information from the male party that was gained in part through testing of his genetic material? To what extent, if any, should the decisions of counselors in these cases be based on estimates of the likely consequences that disclosing such information will have on the relationship between, or the individual well-being of, the persons involved? Similarly, how, if at all, should our deliberations about these issues take account of gender inequalities that persist in contemporary American culture?

When multiple persons with possibly diverging interests have the status of patient in a single case, as previously discussed, medical professionals may struggle to honor, for each patient, some of the very moral commitments that help define their professional role. When a patient poses a credible threat to the welfare of other persons, the health professional's obligation to the individual patient conflicts with the general duty to prevent significant harm where possible—a duty that may apply to the health professional as a person, but that many believe is a duty that applies directly to the professional as such.

A different kind of moral conflict arises when the individual medical professional embraces moral values, on a personal level, that conflict with one or more of the moral obligations associated with his or her social role. This gives rise to what is commonly called a conflict of conscience. Conflicts of conscience are often treated as purely personal moral dilemmas, since they primarily involve a conflict between an individual's personal moral views and that same individual's commitment to the goals, ends, and values of their particular professional role. Although this is certainly a fundamental component of conflicts of conscience, this view does not capture the important social aspect to such conflicts.

In particular, conflicts of conscience have an important social aspect to them because they often involve a conflict between several broader, social commitments that are embraced by liberal democratic communities. On the one hand, for example, most liberal democratic communities are committed to meeting fundamental health needs of community members by fostering a social division of labor in which certain rights and duties are assigned to particular individuals. In the medical arena, physicians, nurses, pharmacists, and others are granted special rights—such as the right to diagnose and treat injury and illness, to dispense controlled substances, and to bill for such services at a fair price—in return for assuming certain social obligations. Which obligations attach to different professional roles can be seen as at least partly a function of the role that that the profession in question is supposed to serve in the larger social division of labor.

Physicians, for example, are traditionally regarded as having what the philosopher Charles Fried called a "duty of personal care" to safeguard and advance the interests of each individual patient to the best of one's ability (Fried 1974). On this view, the patient's medical need, which is often accompanied by a certain degree of personal vulnerability, combines with the physician's expertise concerning health matters to produce a *fiduciary* relationship; that is, a relationship in which the physician is morally bound to elevate the interests of the patient above other competing concerns. Not only does the fiduciary nature of this relationship generate a legitimate expectation on the part of patients that their physician will put their interests before the physician's personal interest, it also generates a societal expectation that physicians, as health professionals, can be relied on to advance the interests of sick and injured persons.

On the other hand, liberal democratic communities are also committed to respecting the personal liberty of each community member, including the liberty to pursue a reasonable life plan that is distinctive, in the sense that its values may not be widely embraced by others. In the rejection of medical paternalism we see this social commitment manifest from the standpoint of the patient. Patients should be free to use their own judgment to decide how their health interests, narrowly conceived, relate to their broader personal goals and commitments. In conflicts of conscience, this same social commitment applies to medical professionals themselves. That is, liberal democratic communities are also committed to ensuring that the liberties of the individuals who "inhabit" important professional roles are not *unduly* or *unfairly* limited.

To some degree, what constitutes an undue or an unfair limitation on the liberties of the persons who fill important professional roles can be inferred from the obligations of those social roles. For example, the very claim that the physician has a fiduciary relationship with the patient entails that it is not unfair to limit the liberties of medical professionals from engaging in kinds of relationships—such as having sexual relationships with their patients—that have a significant potential to compromise the integrity of that relationship. In difficult cases, the problem lies in ascertaining how to define the boundary of an undue or an unjust limitation when there is a stronger case for the importance of the value that competes with the physician's fiduciary duties.

In "The Limits of Conscientious Objection—May Pharmacists Refuse to Fill Prescriptions for Emergency Contraception?" Julie Cantor and Ken Baum explore both the social and personal aspects of this issue for another class of medical professionals, pharmacists. Recently, some pharmacists have refused to honor valid prescriptions for emergency contraception on the ground that doing so violates their personal moral beliefs about the wrongness of using such medications. As Cantor and Baum emphasize, however, pharmacists have also advanced a claim to having the status, like physicians and nurses, of health professionals. With the rights that distinguish pharmacists from mere merchants or dispensers of prescription drugs, come corollary duties to advance the interests of their clients. The difficult question,

therefore, lies in delineating the acceptable balance between the requirements of the pharmacist's professional obligations, respecting the liberty of conscience of individual pharmacists, and also ensuring that the public can still rely on pharmacists to safeguard their personal interests without impinging unduly or unjustly on the moral and legal reproductive rights of patients.

After assessing the arguments on each side of the issue, Cantor and Baum conclude that an absolute right to conscientious objection and an absolute prohibition of such a right are equally untenable. They are therefore driven to a kind of middle ground in which public policy strives to accommodate the reasonable interests of each party. On the side of clients, this includes ensuring that there is open disclosure by pharmacies and by pharmacists of their objections to filling certain prescriptions and a legitimate claim to be referred in a timely manner to another pharmacy or pharmacist who will fill their valid prescription. On the part of pharmacists this means honoring their right not to fill certain prescriptions, so long as the exercise of this right on the part of individual pharmacists does not result in an undue hardship on the part of their clients.

Whether such a middle road is sustainable in practice will depend on several factors. For instance, it will depend on the number of pharmacists who make conscientious refusals and the willingness of such individuals and their employers to refer clients in a timely fashion to other pharmacists who will honor their valid prescription.

One position that Cantor and Baum's compromise does not support, and which seems to be at odds not only with the fiduciary nature of the pharmacist's professional role but also with fundamental values of liberal political communities, is the position that individual pharmacists should have the right not to assist their clients in finding another provider who will honor their prescription or to refrain from assisting them in other ways, such as by transferring the prescription to that provider. Here, the line between liberal democratic respect for the right of individual conscience seems to give way to the fiduciary nature of the medical professional's role, combined with the liberal democratic goal of ensuring that the social division of labor safeguards the basic interests of every community member.

What is at issue, therefore, is a right of individual refusal, and not a right of medical professionals to impede or obstruct their clients from exercising their moral and legal rights.

At bottom, one of the fundamental issues raised in this case concerns the degree to which the personal values of medical professionals must take a backseat to their professional obligations. Perhaps nowhere is this conflict exemplified in as raw or as pure a form than in cases where serving the interests of one's patients, or fulfilling one's social obligations as a guardian of health in general, requires medical professionals to put their own life at risk.

The significance of this question has been driven home for U.S. residents by at least two high-profile events. First, in the aftermath of the terrorist attack on the United States on September 11, 2001, the American public and its national leaders have been alarmed by the possibility that a major U.S. population center might be the subject of chemical or biological attack. This has generated intense interest in the question of whether health care professionals have an obligation to respond to situations in which the nature, scope, and etiology of an attack or an outbreak is either clouded in uncertainty or known to be particularly hazardous.

Second, heightened awareness of vulnerabilities of population centers to chemical and biological attack has also helped sensitize the public to the dangers of communicable disease more generally. The outbreak of severe acute respiratory syndrome (SARS) in 2002 and the subsequent emergence of avian influenza have made salient the possibility that wealthy nations of the developed world may be vulnerable to a global pandemic of communicable disease. This realization has crystallized the public's uncertainty about, and resolve to bolster, the willingness of medical professionals to attend to the afflicted and to ensure that the medical and public health infrastructure of affected communities operate in service of the public trust.

Three readings in this section dramatize the stakes at issue in this context for a wide range of parties. In "SARS Plague: Duty of Care or Medical Heroism?" Dessmon YH Tai presents a powerful narrative of his experience as director of the National SARS Intensive Care Unit during the March 2003 SARS outbreak in Singapore. Although the SARS outbreak was ultimately contained and the scope of its toll limited, it remains a signal event for several reasons. As Tai notes, the outbreak and subsequent spread of SARS created widespread fear that was rooted in both the high morality rates associated with infection and the almost complete lack of information surrounding the condition. This created a situation in which the dedication of trained medical professionals was essential to protecting the public's health, but in which medical professionals became socially stigmatized, to some degree, as potential carriers of an unknown contagion, and were forced to make difficult personal choices about their own health and safety, fidelity to their individual families, and their obligations as medical professionals. Ultimately, 21 percent of SARS victims worldwide were health care workers. In some countries, health care workers constituted over half of the national deaths from the disease.

Woven through Tai's narrative are values ranging from the role-related obligations of medical professionals, the personal imperatives of virtues such as courage and fidelity, the tensions within the virtue of fidelity itself between fidelity to community and fidelity to family, and the tremendous sense of individual pride or guilt that different agents experienced in the aftermath of the decisions they made. Salient also is, on the one hand, a recognition of the profound value of the efforts and sacrifices of medical professionals to the eventual containment of the SARS plague and, on the other hand, a reluctance to affirm explicitly that medical professionals have an obligation—an affirmative duty—to perform in the manner that some have described as "heroic."

The tension involved in this dual attitude is emphasized by Ezekiel J. Emanuel in "The Lessons of SARS." In particular, Emanuel notes the medical profession's mixed history of embracing a duty to care when it conflicts with the personal safety of the individual caregiver. During the 1980s, for example, a number of very vocal U.S. physicians asserted that their liberty right, codified as a professional right in Principle VI of the American Medical Association's Code of Medical Ethics, to choose whom to accept as a client made it permissible to decline to treat HIV/AIDS patients. In particular, Principle VI of the AMA's code holds that "a physician shall, in the provision of appropriate patient care, except in emergencies, be free to choose whom to serve, with whom to associate, and the environment in which to provide medical care" (Ameican medical association 2002, xii). Moreover, the substance of this principle has been present in the AMA's code of ethics since 1912 (Clark 2005).

As Emanuel notes, the reaction of both the general public and the medical profession itself to this response to the plight of HIV-positive patients was vociferous and unfavorable. In its wake the medical profession appeared to reaffirm the physician's duty to care for HIV/AIDS patients, and for those in medical need more generally. Emanuel emphasizes the importance of maintaining this commitment in the face of a potential pandemic. Yet there remains some uncertainty about how individual care providers will respond in the face of the next "SARS." Prompted by concerns about preparedness for biological and chemical attack, a recent study by Alexander and Wynia (2003) found that 80 percent of respondents reported a willingness to treat patients in situations of an uncertain level of risk. Alternatively, 20 percent or one-fifth of respondents were unwilling to treat patients under such conditions and just under half (44 percent) disagreed with the claim that "physicians have an obligation to care for patients in epidemics even if doing so endangers the physician's health."

The case study "What Should the Dean Do?" poses the question of the limits of professional obligation in a slightly different context. During the SARS epidemic in Taiwan, SARS patients were treated at teaching hospitals where medical students routinely round and carry out a variety of clinical duties. The deans of many of the medical schools affiliated with such hospitals received calls from parents and politicians requesting that medical students either be excused from school or be kept from contact with SARS patients. In asking what the dean should do, this case complicates the previously discussed conflict between professional obligations and personal safety since medical students are in a very real sense not fully members of the medical profession.

Noting the high risks associated with SARS and the fact that medical students are still students, Gregory L. Eastwood argues that students should be excused from activities that would bring them into contact with SARS patients. Central to this argument is the claim that professionals' moral duties

emanate from their professional expertise and from the fact it is precisely this expertise that students lack. Daniel Fu-Chang Tsai and Ding-Shinn Chen take a different position. Noting that senior medical students—what they refer to as "acting interns'— already shoulder significant clinical responsibilities, they defend a tiered policy that excuses only junior medical students from interactions with SARS patients. Rather than requiring senior students to participate in the direct care of SARS patients, however, these authors defend a policy of allowing senior students the opportunity to decide for themselves whether or not to participate in such activities. James Dwyer defends the latter idea in an even more general form. Noting the importance of helping students understand the commitments of the profession they are joining and to cultivate such commitments on a personal level, Dwyer would leave the choice to the students as a group.

As these articles illustrate, both the moral foundation for the duty to care and for the public's expectation that medical professionals will honor this obligation lies in the social role of the medical professions as committed to protecting and advancing individual and public health. Moreover, it is the medical professional's special knowledge or expertise that forges the connection between the profession's social role and the individual medical professional's duty to care.

A different kind of professional conflict arises when the community asks medical professionals to participate in activities that some feel are at odds, not simply with the individual values of the person who inhabits the professional role, but with the moral mission of the profession itself.

As Atul Gawande points out in "When Law and Ethics Collide—Why Physicians Participate in Executions" of the thirty-eight states in the United States with the death penalty, seventeen require the participation of physicians in execution in execution and all but three permit it. Yet such participation on the part of physicians is expressly forbidden by the code of ethics of the AMA; the American Nurses Association (ANA) code of ethics takes a similar position on the participation of nurses. According to the AMA, what is at stake is not an issue of the personal views of individual physicians about the morality of capital punishment. The 1992 Code of Medical Ethics states that "an individual's opinion on capital punishment is the personal moral decision of the individual." What is at stake, rather, is the social role of the physician "as a member of a profession dedicated to preserving life when there is hope of doing so" that is undermined by the participation of physicians in even legally authorized execution.

Gawande provides a portrait of several physicians and a nurse who have, with varying degrees of reluctance, participated in executions. One striking feature of their stories is how little bearing an individual's view about the morality of capital punishment appears to have on their willingness to participate in the process. Some appear ambivalent about the question. Dr. D is opposed to the death penalty, viewing it as "inhumane, immoral, and pointless," although he has participated in at least six executions. Gawande himself admits to being, if not a supporter of the death penalty, at least sympathetic to it. Yet he vigorously opposes the participation of physicians and nurses as morally wrong.

For Gawande, as for the AMA and other professional associations, participation of physicians and nurses in executions undermines the moral core of the medical profession. Their position is that society vests medical professionals with a certain authority and trust because of the profession's commitment to advancing health, minimizing suffering, and providing knowledgeable, humane care. Using the physician's expert knowledge as an instrument of punishment subverts these goals and is antithetical to the aspirations of medicine.

For Dr. D, however, one of the most salient reasons for his involvement in capital punishment stems precisely from his commitment to care for the dying. From a pragmatic standpoint, what difference does it make if the patient is dying from cancer, or because of a sentence made by a court, in accordance, with the law, to be carried out by prison officials? In both cases a person is going to die and Dr. D has the knowledge and ability to ease their suffering. From his standpoint, it is precisely his commitment to core values of the medicine that leads him to participate in executions, over his own objections to the death penalty.

Gawande is skeptical of this analogy. What kind of relationship can physicians have with their patients when in many cases the inmate and his or her family are prohibited from knowing the identity of the participating physician? Moreover, in most

clinical relationships, the physician's activities are directed at serving the health interests of patients, as they are understood in light of that person's larger goals and commitments. In the case of capital punishment, the physician's actions are directed by the ends of the state, and are geared ultimately at securing the inmate's death. Moreover, Gawande emphasizes that 'the hand that more gently places the IV, more carefully times the bolus of potassium, is also the hand of death.' This image is meant to underscore the fact that the state is seeking to use the trappings, as well as the tools, of medicine to make the intentional and deliberate killing of another human more sanitary, more "clinical,' and therefore more palatable. But, for Gawande, beneath these trappings is the unvarnished reality that, though they may kill more efficiently and with less suffering, physicians who participate in executions are killing other persons.

For some, however, Gawande's response to Dr. D may be a bit too quick. A position similar to the one expressed by Dr. D is fleshed out and defended at greater length by Kenneth Baum in "To Comfort Always': Physician Participation in Executions." Baum takes the title of his article from an aphorism according to which "the task of medicine is to cure sometimes; to relieve often, and to comfort always.' His central claim is that the core values of the medical profession, or at least the core commitment to comfort and to relieve suffering where possible, provide powerful support for the claim that physicians should play an active role in executions.

One of Baum's central arguments is that the position of Gawande and of the AMA is out of step with the best philosophical conception of the relationship between doctors and patients. He claims, for example, that "what is important is not that physicians stave off death, but that they tailor their actions, as much as possible, to the interests of their patients and the realities and necessities of their circumstances." As we saw in the readings from Section 1, part of the argument rejecting medical paternalism involves a rejection of view that physicians are, or should be, singularly committed to the health of patients in complete isolation from the way that the patient views health in relation to his or her other interests. Baum is leveraging this fact in order to argue that participation in executions can be consistent with the physician's commitment to his or her patient, given the fact that the patient is going to die and given that the patient likely has an interest in avoiding unnecessary pain and suffering.

In fact, one of Baum's more extreme arguments holds that it is those who refuse to participate that betray their professional obligation by letting larger social concerns take precedence over their commitment to provide comforting care to patients. As Gawande's portraits themselves illustrate, the involvement of a skilled physician in an execution by lethal injection can be the difference between botched procedures that cause unnecessary and potentially excruciating pain or relatively fast, relatively painless death that respects the dignity of the criminal as the state carries out its sentence.

Against the idea that by participating in executions physicians are abandoning or even subverting their commitment to health well-being by becoming killers, Baum argues that the physician participation in executions is *analytically* no different from what happens routinely on oncology wards. That is, on the oncology ward physicians sometimes hasten the death of patients in the course of providing diligent comfort care. In such cases it is widely recognized that the physician is not responsible for killing the patient, the cancer is. So too, Baum argues, in the execution chamber it is not the physician who kills the patient, but the state. The physician is involved solely to minimize suffering during a death that would have occurred anyway, but which would have involved a greater risk of unnecessary suffering without the physician's involvement. So Baum's response to Gawande might be that the hand of death in this case is the hand of the state, and that it is against this reality that the physician intervenes to provide a more comfortable death.

It is important to see that Baum does not want to cast many of his most important arguments as about the conflict between state power and the boundaries of physician duties as medical professionals. Rather, he presents them as growing out of the fundamentally patient-centered nature of the professional's moral obligations. But it is also important to recognize that these arguments require that we take certain social facts—such as the fact that an otherwise healthy person is going to die because of an act of state—as practical realities, or givens. Only from this perspective can physicians and other medical professionals be required to

adapt their perspective to one of compassionately shepherding the patient through the dying process.

It is worth contrasting this case with another in which the interests of the state and the interests of the patient conflict. "Dialysis for a Prisoner of War" is a case study in which U.S. military forces capture an enemy combatant who is diagnosed with renal failure. In this case, the prisoner refuses dialysis on the ground that he would rather die than live as a prisoner of the United States. When the military nephrologists asks her commanding officer for guidance, the issue is passed up the chain of command until, ultimately, the secretary of defense orders that dialysis be initiated because the prisoner is believed to possess information that could be valuable to the war effort. In this case, the fidelity of the nephrologists to the interests of her patient is pitted against her position as an officer in the military and its interests in keeping her patient alive.

In their analysis, Daniel Zupan, Gary Solis, and Richard Schoonhoven highlight the extent to which this case falls within a gray area of international law. Most of the treatise to which the United States is a signatory deal with the obligation to provide medical care to prisoners of war (POWs) and do not address the question of honor refusals of care. In this respect, given the military rationale for keeping the POW alive and the silence of international law on this issue, they argue that forced dialysis could be permitted. However, they recognize that such a position could not be justified under domestic U.S. law or medical ethics, where the informed wishes of patients to refuse even life-sustaining care must be honored out of respect for the patient's dignity and autonomy. In the face of this larger conflict between the domestic attitude toward respect for autonomy and the dignity of humanity, and the silence of international and military law, they ultimately side with the former.

As George Annas correctly points out, this puts the military nephrologists in the position of having to disobey a direct order from a superior. While Annas agrees that the POW's wishes must be honored, he thinks that it was wrong of the nephrologists to abdicate her authority as a physician by submitting this decision to her superiors. For Annas, the initial moral breach in this case occurs when the nephrologist turns over to military personnel what Annas views as fundamentally a medical decision.

To his lights, this represents a case of inappropriately subordinating the physician's commitment to human rights to the ends of military expediency.

It is somewhat ironic, perhaps, that both commentators agree in this case that the weight of the ethical arguments support the permissibility of honoring the wishes of the prisoner, knowing full well that doing so will hasten his preventable death. How should we reconcile this with the case of the domestic prisoner sentenced to death? If the cases must be treated differently, then what are the salient differences between them? If they are not significantly different in their key features, then what is a coherent policy that would cover them both?

REFERENCES

Alexander, G. C., and M. K. Wynia. 2003. Ready and willing?: Physician preparedness and willingness to treat potential victims of bioterrorism. *Health Affairs* 22 (5): 189–197.

American Medical Association. 2002. *Code of medical ethics: Current opinions.* Chicago: AMA Press.

Clark, Chalmers C. 2005. In harm's way: AMA physicians and the duty to treat. *Journal of Medicine and Philosophy* 30:65–87.

Fried, C. 1974. *Medical experimentation: Personal integrity and social policy.* New York: Elsevier.

Veatch, Robert M. June 1972. Models for medicine in a revolutionary age. *Hastings Center Report* 2:5–7.

AUTONOMY, PATERNALISM, AND MEDICAL MODELS

THE HIPPOCRATIC OATH

I swear by Apollo Physician and Asclepius and Hygieia and Panaceia and all the gods and goddesses, making them my witness, that I will fulfil according to my ability and judgment this oath and this covenant:

To hold him who has taught me this art as equal to my parents and to live my life in partnership with him, and if he is in need of money to give him a share of mine, and to regard his offspring as equal to my brothers in male lineage and to teach them this art—if they desire to learn it—without fee and covenant; to give a share of precepts and oral instruction and all the other learning to my sons and to the sons of him who has instructed me and to pupils who have signed the covenant and have taken an oath according to the medical law, but to no one else.

I will apply dietetic measures for the benefit of the sick according to my ability and judgment; I will keep them from harm and injustice.

I will neither give a deadly drug to anybody if asked for it, nor will I make a suggestion to this effect. Similarly I will not give to a woman an abortive remedy. In purity and holiness I will guard my life and my art.

I will not use the knife, not even on sufferers from stone, but will withdraw in favor of such men as are engaged in this work.

Whatever houses I may visit, I will come for the benefit of the sick, remaining free of all intentional injustice, of all mischief and in particular of sexual relations with both female and male persons, be they free or slaves.

What I may see or hear in the course of the treatment or even outside of the treatment in regard to the life of men, which on no account one must spread abroad, I will keep to myself holding such things shameful to be spoken about.

If I fulfil this oath and do not violate it, may it be granted to me to enjoy life and art, being honored with fame among all men for all time to come; if I transgress it and swear falsely, may the opposite of all this be my lot.

From Edelstein, Ludwig. *Ancient Medicine.* p. 6 © 1967 The Johns Hopkins University Press.

THE REFUTATION OF MEDICAL PATERNALISM

Alan Goldman

In the case of doctors the question is whether they have the authority to make decisions for others that they would lack as nonprofessionals. The goal of providing optimal health treatment may be seen to conflict in some circumstances with the otherwise overriding duties to tell the patient the truth about his condition or to allow him to make decisions vitally affecting his own interests. Again the assumption of the profession itself appears to be that the doctor's role is strongly differentiated in this sense. The Principles of Medical Ethics of the American Medical Association leaves the question of informing the patient of his own condition up to the professional judgment of the physician, presumably in relation to the objective of maintaining or improving the health or well-being of the patient.[1] I shall concentrate upon these issues of truth telling and informed consent to treatment in the remainder of this chapter. They exemplify our fundamental issue because the initially obvious answer to the question of who should make decisions or have access to information vital to the interests of primarily one person is that person himself.[2]

Rights are recognized, we have said, partially to permit individuals control over their own futures. Regarding decisions vital to the interests of only particular individuals, there are three main reasons why such decisions should normally be left to the individuals themselves, two want-regarding and one ideal-regarding. First is the presumption of their being the best judges of their own interests, which may depend upon personal value orderings known only to them. There is often a temptation for others to impose their own values and preferences, but this would be less likely to produce satisfaction for the individuals concerned. The second reason is

the independent value of self-determination, at least in regard to important decisions (in medical contexts decisions may involve life and death alternatives, affect the completion of major life projects, or affect bodily integrity). Persons desire the right or freedom to make their own choices, and satisfaction of this desire is important in itself. In addition, maximal freedom for individuals to develop their own projects, to make the pivotal choices that define them and to act to realize them, allows for the development of unique creative personalities, who become sources of new value in the goods they create and that they and others enjoy.

Resentment as well as overall harm is therefore generally greater when caused by a wrong, even if well-meaning, decision of another than when caused to oneself. There is greater chance that the other person will fail to realize one's own values in making the decision, and, when this happens, additional resentment that one was not permitted the freedom to decide. Thus, since individuals normally have rights to make decisions affecting the course of their lives and their lives alone, doctors who claim authority to make medical decisions for them that fall into this self-regarding category are claiming special authority. The normally existing right to self-determination implies several more specific rights in the medical context. These include the right to be told the truth about one's condition, and the right to accept or refuse or withdraw from treatment on the basis of adequate information regarding alternatives, risks and uncertainties. If doctors are permitted or required by the principle of providing optimal treatment, cure or health maintenance for patients sometimes to withhold truth or decide on their own what therapeutic measures to employ, then the Hippocratic principle overrides important rights to self-determination that would otherwise obtain, and the practice of medicine is strongly role differentiated.

This is clear enough in the case of informed consent to therapy; it should be equally clear in the case of withholding truth, from terminally ill patients for

From *The Moral Foundations of Professional Ethics* by Alan Goldman, Rowman and Littlefield, 1980. Reprinted by permission of the publisher.

Editors' note: Some text and author's notes have been cut. Students who want to read the article in its entirety should consult the original.

example. The right violated or overridden when truth is withheld in medical contexts is not some claim to the truth per se, but this same right to self-determination, to control over decisions vital to the course of one's life. In fact, it seems on the face of it that there is a continuum of medical issues in which this right figures prominently. These range from the question of consent to being used as a subject in an experiment designed primarily to benefit others, to consent to treatment intended as benefit to the patient himself, to disclosure of information about the patient's condition. In the first case, that of medical experimentation, if the consent of subjects is required (as everyone these days admits it is), this is partly because the duty not to harm is stronger than the duty to provide benefits. Hence if there is any risk of harm at all to subjects, they cannot be used without consent, even if potential benefits to others is great. But consent is required also because the right to self-determination figures independently of calculations of harms and benefits. Thus a person normally ought not to be used without his consent to benefit others even if he is not materially harmed. This same right clearly opposes administration of treatment to patients without their consent for their own benefit. It opposes as well lying to patients about their illnesses in order to save them distress.

What is at least prima facie wrong with lying in such cases is that it shifts power to decide future courses of action away from the person to whom the lie is told.[3] A person who is misinformed about his own physical condition may not complete certain projects or perform certain actions that he would choose to perform in full knowledge. If a person is terminally ill and does not know it, for example, he may fail to arrange his affairs, prepare himself for death, or may miss opportunities to complete projects or seek certain experiences always put off before. Being lied to can reduce or prevent from coming into view options that would otherwise be live. Hence it is analogous to the use of force, perhaps more coercive than the use of force in that there is not the same chance to resist when the barrier is ignorance. The right to know the truth in this context then derives from the right to make for oneself important decisions relating primarily to one's own welfare and to the course of one's life. If the doctor's authority is to be augmented beyond that of any nonprofessional, allowing him to override these

important rights in contexts in which this is necessary to prevent serious harm to the patient's health, then his position appears to meet in a dramatic way our criteria for strong role differentiation.

THE CASE FOR MEDICAL PATERNALISM

Since the primary rights in potential conflict with the presumed fundamental norm of medical ethics are rights of patients themselves, and since the norm seeks to serve the health needs of patients themselves, arguments in favor of strong role differentiation in this context are clearly paternalistic. We may define paternalism as the overriding or restricting of rights or freedoms of individuals for their own good. It can be justified even for competent adults in contexts in which they can be assumed to act otherwise against their own interests, values, or true preferences. Individuals might act in such self-defeating ways from ignorance of the consequences of their actions, from failure to weigh the probabilities of various consequences correctly, or from irrational barriers to the operation of normal short-term motivations. Paternalistic measures may be invoked when either the individual in question, or any rational person with adequate knowledge of the situation, would choose a certain course of conduct, and yet this course is not taken by the individual solely because of ignorance, carelessness, fear, depression, or other uncontroversially irrational motives.[4]

Paradigm Cases

It will be useful in evaluating arguments for strong role differentiation for doctors to look first at criteria for justified paternalism in nonmedical cases, in order to see then if they are met in the medical context. In approaching the controversial case of withholding truth from patients, we may begin with simpler paradigm cases in which paternalistic behavior is uncontroversially permissible or required. We can derive a rule from these cases for the justification of such conduct and then apply the rule to decide this fundamental question of medical ethics.

The easiest cases to justify are those in which a person is acting against even his immediate desires out of ignorance: Dick desires to take a train to New York, is about to board the train for Boston on the other side of the platform, and, without time to warn him, he can only be grabbed and shoved in the other direction. Coercing him in this way is paternalistic, since it overrides his right of free movement for his own good. "His own good" is uncontroversial in interpretation in this easiest case. It is defined by his own clearly stated immediate and long-range preferences (the two are not in conflict here). Somewhat more difficult are cases in which persons voluntarily act in ways inconsistent with their long-range preferences: Jane does not desire to be seriously injured or to increase greatly her chances of serious injury for trivial reasons; yet, out of carelessness, or just because she considers it a nuisance and fails to apply statistical probabilities to her own case, she does not wear a helmet when riding a motorcycle. Here it might be claimed that, while her action is voluntary in relation to trivial short-term desires, it is nevertheless not fully voluntary in a deeper sense. But to make this claim we must be certain of the person's long-range preferences, of the fact that her action is inconsistent with these preferences (or else uncontroversially inconsistent with the preferences of any rational person). We must predict that the person herself is likely to be grateful in the long run for the additional coercive motivation. In this example we may assume these criteria to be met. For rational people, not wearing a helmet is not an essential feature in the enjoyment of riding a motorcycle, even if people ride them primarily for the thrill rather than for the transportation. The chances are far greater that a rider will at some time fall or be knocked off the cycle and be thankful for having a helmet than that one will prefer serious head injury to the inconvenience of wearing protection that can prevent such injury. Therefore we may justifiably assume that a person not wearing a helmet is not acting in light of her own true long-range values and preferences.

As the claim that the individual's action is not truly voluntary or consistent with his preferences or values becomes more controversial, additional criteria for justified paternalism must come into play. They become necessary to outweigh the two considerations mentioned earlier: the presumption that individuals know their own preferences best (that interference will be more often mistaken than

not), and that there is an important independent value to self-determination or individual freedom and control (the latter being true both because persons value freedom and because such freedom is necessary to the development of genuinely individual persons). The additional criteria necessary for justifying paternalism in more controversial cases relate to the potential harm to the person from the action in question: it must be relatively certain, severe, and irreversible (relative to the degree of coercion contemplated). These further criteria are satisfied as well in the case of motorcycle helmets, because the action coerced is only a minor nuisance in comparison to the severity of potential harm and the degree of risk.

It is important for the course of the later argument to point out that these additional criteria relating to the harm that may result from self-regarding actions need not be viewed in terms of a simple opposition between allowing freedom of action and preventing harm. It is not simply that we can override a person's autonomy when in our opinion the potential harm to him from allowing autonomous decision outweighs the value of his freedom. His right to self-determination, fundamental to individuality itself, bars such offsetting calculations. The magnitude of harm is rather to be conceived as *evidence* that the person is not acting in accord with *his own* values and preferences, that he is not acting autonomously in the deepest sense. A rights-based moral theory of the type I am assuming as the framework for this study will view the autonomy of the individual as more fundamental than the particular goods he enjoys or harms he may suffer. The autonomous individual is the source of value for those other goods he enjoys and so not to be sacrificed for the sake of them. The point here is that cases of justified paternalism, even where the agent's immediate or short-term preferences are overridden, need not be viewed as reversing that order of priority.

Criteria for justified paternalism are also clearly satisfied in certain medical contexts, to return to the immediate issue at hand. State control over physician licensing and the requirement that prescriptions be obtained for many kinds of drugs are medical cases in point. Licensing physicians prevents some quacks from harming other persons, but also limits these persons' freedom of choice for their own good. Hence it is paternalistic. We may assume that no rational person would want to be treated by a quack or to take drugs that are merely harmful, but that many people would do so in the absence of controls out of ignorance or irrational hopes or fears. While controls impose costs and bother upon people that may be considerable in the case of having to see a doctor to obtain medication, these are relatively minimal in comparison to the certainty, severity and irreversibility of the harm that would result from drugs chosen by laymen without medical assistance. Such controls are therefore justified, despite the fact that in some cases persons might benefit from seeing those who could not obtain licenses or from choosing drugs themselves. We can assume that without controls mistakes would be made more often than not, that serious harm would almost certainly result, and that people really desire to avoid such harm even given additional costs.

There is another sense too in which paternalistic measures here should not be viewed as prevention of exclusively self-regarding harm by restriction of truly autonomous actions. The harm against which laymen are to be protected in these cases, while deriving partly from their own actions in choosing physicians or drugs, can be seen also as imposed by others in the absence of controls. It results from the deception practiced by unqualified physicians and unscrupulous drug manufacturers. Hence controls, rather than interfering with autonomous choice by laymen, help to prevent deceptive acts of others that block truly free choice.[5] This is not to say that some drugs now requiring prescriptions could not be safely sold over the counter at reduced cost, or that doctors have not abused their effective control over entrance to the profession by restraining supply in relation to demand, maintaining support for exorbitant prices. Perhaps controls could be imposed in some other way than by licensing under professional supervision. This issue is beyond our scope here. The point for us is that some such restraints appear to be necessary. Whichever form they take, they will be paternalistic, justifiably so, in their relation to free patient choice.

We have now defined criteria for justified paternalism from considering certain relatively easy examples or paradigm cases. The principal criterion is that an individual be acting against *his own* predominant long-range value preferences, or that a

strong likelihood exist that he will so act if not prevented. Where either clause is controversial, we judge their truth by the likelihood and seriousness of the harm to the person risked by his probable action. It must be the case that this harm would be judged clearly worse from the point of view of the person himself than not being able to do what we prevent him from doing by interfering. Only if the interference is in accord with the person's real desires in this way is it justified. Our question now is whether these criteria are met in the more controversial medical cases we are considering, those of doctors' withholding truth or deciding upon courses of treatment on their own to prevent serious harm to the health of their patients.

Application of the Criteria to Medical Practice

The argument that the criteria for justified paternalism are satisfied in these more controversial medical cases begins from the premise that the doctor is more likely to know the course of treatment optimal for improving overall health or prolonging life than is his patient. The patient will be comparatively ignorant of his present condition, alternative treatments, and risks, even when the doctor makes a reasonable attempt to educate him on these matters. More important, he is apt to be emotional and fearful, inclined to hold out false hope for less painful treatments with little real chance of cure, or to despair of the chance for cure when that might still be real. In such situations it again could be claimed, as in the examples from the previous subsection, that patient choice in any event would not be truly voluntary. A person is likely to act according to his true long-range values only when his decision is calm, unpressured, and informed or knowledgeable. A seriously ill person is unlikely to satisfy these conditions for free choice. Choice unhindered by others is nevertheless not truly free when determined by internal factors, among them fear, ignorance, or other irrational motivation, which result in choice at variance with the individual's deeper preferences. In such circumstances interference is not to be criticized as restrictive of freedom.

The second premise states that those who consult doctors really desire to be cured above all else.

Health and the prolonging of life may be assumed (according to this argument) to have priority among values for any rational person, since they are necessary conditions for the realization of almost every other personal value. While such universally necessary means ought to have priority in personal value orderings, persons may again fail to act on such orderings out of despair or false hope, or simply lack of knowledge, all irrational barriers to genuinely voluntary choice. When they fail to act rationally in medical contexts, the harm may well be serious, probable and irreversible. Hence another criterion for justified paternalism appears to be met; we have another sign that the probable outcome in these circumstances of unhindered choice is not truly desired, hence the choice not truly voluntary.

While it is possible that a doctor's prognosis might be mistaken, this can be argued to support further rather than weaken the argument for paternalism. For if the doctor is mistaken, this will infect the patient's decision-making process as well, since his appreciation of the situation can only fall short of that of his source of information. Furthermore, bad prognoses may tend to be self-fulfilling when revealed, even if their initial probability of realization is slight. A positive psychological attitude on the part of the patient often enhances chances for cure even when they are slight; and a negative attitude, which might be incurred from a mistaken prognosis or from fear of an outcome with otherwise low probability, might increase that probability. In any case it can be argued that a bad prognosis is more likely to depress the patient needlessly than to serve a positive medical purpose if revealed. The doctor will most likely be able to convince the patient to accept the treatment deemed best by the doctor even after all risks are revealed. The ability to so convince might well be conceived as part of medical competence to provide optimal treatment. If the doctor knows that he can do so in any case, why needlessly worry or depress the patient with discussion of risks that are remote, or at least more remote or less serious than those connected with alternative treatments? Their revelation is unlikely to affect the final decision, but far more likely to harm the patient. It therefore would appear cruel for the doctor not to assume responsibility for the decision or for remaining silent on certain of its determining factors.

Thus all the criteria for justified paternalism might appear to be met in the more controversial cases as well. The analogies with our earlier examples appear to support overriding the patient's right to decide on the basis of the truth by the fundamental medical principle of providing optimal care and treatment. Let us apply this argument more specifically to . . . the case of withholding truth when no other medical decisions remain to be made, when the question is what to tell the terminally ill patient for example. Here recognition of an absolute right of the patient is likely to result in needless mental suffering and even in some cases hasten death. The dying patient is likely to realize at a certain point that he is dying without having to be informed. If he does realize it, blunt and open discussion of the fact may nevertheless be depressing. What appear to be pointless deceptive games played out between patients and relatives in avoiding such discussion may actually express delicate defense mechanisms whose solace may be destroyed by the doctor's intrusion. When the doctor has no reason to predict such detrimental effects, then perhaps he ought to inform. But why do so when this is certain to cause needless additional suffering or harm? To do so appears not only wrong, but cruel.

We certainly are justified in lying to a person in order to prevent serious harm to another. If I must lie to someone in order to save the life of another whom the first person might kill if told the truth (even if the killing would be nonintentional), there is no doubt at all that I should tell the lie or withhold the information. Rights to be told the truth are not absolute, but, like all rights, must be ordered in relation to others. If I may lie to one person to save another from harm, why not then when the life of the person himself might be threatened or seriously worsened by the truth, as it might be in the medical contexts we are considering? Why should the fact that only one person is involved, that only the person himself is likely to be harmed by the truth, alter the duty to deceive or withhold information in order to prevent the more serious harm? If it is replied that when only one person is involved, that person is likely to know the best course of action for himself, the answer is that in medical contexts this claim appears to be false. The doctor is likely to be better informed than the patient about his condition and the optimal treatments for it.

Thus there are two situations in which the doctor's duty not to harm his patient's health or shorten his life might appear to override otherwise obtaining rights of the patients to the full truth. One is where the truth will cause direct harm—depression or loss of continued will to live. The other is where informing may be instrumentally harmful in leading to the choice of the wrong treatment or none at all. Given that information divulged to the patient may be harmful or damaging to his health, may interfere with other aspects of optimal or successful treatment, it is natural to construe what the doctor tells the patient as an aspect of the treatment itself. As such it would be subject to the same risk-benefit analysis as other aspects. Doctors must constantly balance uncertain benefits and risks in trying to provide treatment that will maximize the probability of cure with least damaging side effects. Questions regarding optimal treatment are questions for medical expertise. Since psychological harm must figure in the doctor's calculations if he is properly sensitive, since it may contribute as well to physical deterioration, and since what he says to a patient may cause such harm, it seems that the doctor must construe what he *says* to a patient as on a par with what he *does* to him, assuming full responsibility for any harm that may result. Certainly many doctors do so conceive of questions of disclosure. A clear example of this assimilation to questions regarding treatment is the following:

> From the foregoing it should be self-evident that what is imparted to a patient about his illness should be planned with the same care and executed with the same skill that are demanded by any potentially therapeutic measure. Like the transfusion of blood, the dispensing of certain information must be distinctly indicated, the amount given consonant with the needs of the recipient, and the type chosen with the view of avoiding untoward reactions.[6]

When the patient places himself in the care of a physician, he expects the best and least harmful treatment, and the physician's fundamental duty, seemingly overriding all others in the medical context, must be to provide such treatment. Indeed the terminology itself, "under a physician's care," suggests acceptance of the paternalistic model of strong role differentiation. To care for someone is to provide first and foremost for that person's welfare.[7]

The doctor ministers to his patient's needs, not to his immediate preferences. If this were not the case, doctors would be justified in prescribing whatever drugs their patients requested. That a person needs care suggests that, at least for the time being, he is not capable of being physically autonomous; and given the close connection of physical with mental state, the emotional stress that accompanies serious illness, it is natural to view the patient as relinquishing autonomy over medical decisions to the expert for his own good. Being under a physician's care entails a different relationship from that involved in merely seeking another person's advice.

THE REFUTATION OF MEDICAL PATERNALISM

In order to refute an argument, we of course need to refute only one of its premises. The argument for medical paternalism, stripped to its barest outline, was:

1. Disclosure of information to the patient will sometimes increase the likelihood of depression and physical deterioration, or result in choice of medically inoptimal treatment.
2. Disclosure of information is therefore sometimes likely to be detrimental to the patient's health, perhaps even to hasten his death.
3. Health and prolonged life can be assumed to have priority among preferences for patients who place themselves under physicians' care.
4. Worsening health or hastening death can therefore be assumed to be contrary to patients' own true value orderings.
5. Paternalism is therefore justified: doctors may sometimes override patients' prima facie rights to information about risks and treatments or about their own conditions in order to prevent harm to their health.

The Relativity of Values: Health and Life

The fundamentally faulty premise in the argument for paternalistic role differentiation for doctors is that which assumes that health or prolonged life must take absolute priority in the patient's value orderings. In order for paternalistic interference to be justified, a person must be acting irrationally or inconsistently with his own long-range preferences. The value ordering violated by the action to be prevented must either be known to be that of the person himself, as in the train example, or else be uncontroversially that of any rational person, as in the motorcycle helmet case. But can we assume that health and prolonged life have top priority in any rational ordering? *If* these values could be safely assumed to be always overriding for those who seek medical assistance, then medical expertise would become paramount in decisions regarding treatment, and decisions on disclosure would become assimilated to those within the treatment context. But in fact very few of us act according to such an assumed value ordering. In designing social policy we do not devote all funds or efforts toward minimizing loss of life, on the highways or in hospitals for example.

If our primary goal were always to minimize risk to health and life, we should spend our entire federal budget in health-related areas. Certainly such a suggestion would be ludicrous. We do not in fact grant to individuals rights to minimal risk in their activities or to absolutely optimal health care. From another perspective, if life itself, rather than life of a certain quality with autonomy and dignity, were of ultimate value, then even defensive wars could never be justified. But when the quality of life and the autonomy of an entire nation is threatened from without, defensive war in which many lives are risked and lost is a rational posture. To paraphrase Camus, anything worth living for is worth dying for. To realize or preserve those values that give meaning to life is worth the risk of life itself. Such fundamental values (and autonomy for individuals is certainly among them), necessary within a framework in which life of a certain quality becomes possible, appear to take precedence over the value of mere biological existence.

In personal life too we often engage in risky activities for far less exalted reasons, in fact just for the pleasure or convenience. We work too hard, smoke, exercise too little or too much, eat what we know is bad for us, and continue to do all these things even when informed of their possibly fatal effects. To doctors in their roles as doctors all this may appear irrational, although they no more act always to preserve their own health than do the rest of us. If certain risks to life and health are irrational,

others are not. Once more the quality and significance of one's life may take precedence over maximal longevity. Many people when they are sick think of nothing above getting better; but this is not true of all. A person with a heart condition may decide that important unfinished work or projects must take priority over increased risk to his health; and his priority is not uncontroversially irrational. Since people's lives derive meaning and fulfillment from their projects and accomplishments, a person's risking a shortened life for one more fulfilled might well justify actions detrimental to his health. . . .

To doctors in their roles as professionals whose ultimate concern is the health or continued lives of patients, it is natural to elevate these values to ultimate prominence. The death of a patient, inevitable as it is in many cases, may appear as an ultimate defeat to the medical art, as something to be fought by any means, even after life has lost all value and meaning for the patient himself. The argument in the previous section for assuming this value ordering was that health, and certainly life, seem to be necessary conditions for the realization of all other goods or values. But this point, even if true, leaves open the question of whether health and life are of ultimate, or indeed any, intrinsic value, or whether they are valuable *merely* as means. It is plausible to maintain that life itself is not of intrinsic value, since surviving in an irreversible coma seems no better than death. It therefore again appears that it is the quality of life that counts, not simply being alive. Although almost any quality might be preferable to none, it is not irrational to trade off quantity for quality, as in any other good.

Even life with physical health and consciousness may not be of intrinsic value. Consciousness and health may not be sufficient in themselves to make the life worth living, since some states of consciousness are intrinsically good and others bad. Furthermore, if a person has nothing before him but pain and depression, then the instrumental worth of being alive may be reversed. And if prolonging one's life can be accomplished only at the expense of incapacitation or ignorance, perhaps preventing lifelong projects from being completed, then the instrumental value of longer life again seems overbalanced. It is certainly true that normally life itself is of utmost value as necessary for all else of value, and that living longer usually enables one to complete more projects and plans, to satisfy more desires and derive more enjoyments. But this cannot be assumed in the extreme circumstances of severe or terminal illness. Ignorance of how long one has left may block realization of such values, as may treatment with the best chance for cure, if it also risks incapacitation or immediate death.

Nor is avoidance of depression the most important consideration in such circumstances, as a shallow hedonism might assume. Hedonistic theories of value, which seek only to produce pleasure or avoid pain and depression, are easily disproven by our abhorrence at the prospect of a "brave new world," or our unwillingness, were it possible, to be plugged indefinitely into a "pleasure machine." The latter prospect is abhorrent not only from an ideal-regarding viewpoint, but, less obviously, for want-regarding reasons (for most persons) as well. Most people would in fact be unwilling to trade important freedoms and accomplishments for sensuous pleasures, or even for the illusion of greater freedoms and accomplishments. As many philosophers have pointed out, while satisfaction of wants may bring pleasurable sensations, wants are not primarily *for* pleasurable sensations, or even for happiness more broadly construed, per se. Conversely, the avoidance of negative feelings or depression is not uppermost among primary motives. Many people are willing to endure frustration, suffering, and even depression in pursuit of accomplishment, or in order to complete projects once begun. Thus information relevant to such matters, such as medical information about one's own condition or possible adverse effects of various treatments, may well be worth having at the cost of psychological pain or depression.

The Value of Self-Determination

We have so far focused on the inability of the doctor to assume a particular value ordering for his patient in which health, the prolonging of life, or the avoidance of depression is uppermost. The likelihood of error in this regard makes it probable that the doctor will not know the true interests of his patient as well as the patient himself. He is therefore less likely than the patient himself to make choices in accord with that overall interest, and paternalistic assumption of authority to do so is therefore unjustified.

There is in addition another decisive consideration mentioned earlier, namely the independent value of self-determination or freedom of choice. Personal autonomy over important decisions in one's life, the ability to attempt to realize one's own value ordering, is indeed so important that normally no amount of other goods, pleasures or avoidance of personal evils can take precedence. This is why it is wrong to contract oneself into slavery, and another reason why pleasure machines do not seem attractive. Regarding the latter, even if people were willing to forgo other goods for a life of constant pleasure, the loss in variety of other values, and in the creativity that can generate new sources of value, would be morally regrettable. The value of self-determination explains also why there is such a strong burden of proof upon those who advocate paternalistic measures, why they must show that the person would otherwise act in a way inconsistent with his own value ordering, that is, irrationally. A person's desires are not simply evidence of what is in his interest—they have extra weight.

Especially when decisions are important to the course of our lives, we are unwilling to relinquish them to others, even in exchange for a higher probability of happiness or less risk of suffering. Even if it could be proven, for example, that some scientific method of matching spouses greatly increased chances of compatibility and happiness, we would insist upon retaining our rights over marriage decisions. Given the present rate of success in marriages, it is probable that we could in fact find some better method of matching partners in terms of increasing that success rate. Yet we are willing to forgo increased chances of success in order to make our own choices, choices that tend to make us miserable in the long run. The same might be true of career choices, choices of schools, and others central to the course of our lives. Our unwillingness to delegate these crucial decisions to experts or computers, who might stand a better chance of making them correctly (in terms of later satisfactions), is not to be explained simply in terms of our (sometimes mistaken) assumptions that we know best how to satisfy our own interests, or that we personally will choose correctly, even though most other people do not. If our retaining such authority for ourselves is not simply irrational, and I do not believe it is, this can only be because of the great independent value of self-determination. We value the exercise of free choice itself in personally important decisions, no matter what the effects of those decisions upon other satisfactions. The independent value of self-determination in decisions of great personal importance adds also to our reluctance to relinquish medical decisions with crucial effects on our lives to doctors, despite their medical expertise.

Autonomy or self-determination is independently valuable, as argued before, first of all because we value it in itself. But we may again add to this want-regarding or utilitarian reason a second ideal-regarding or perfectionist reason. What has value does so because it is valued by a rational and autonomous person. But autonomy itself is necessary to the development of such valuing individual persons or agents. It is therefore not to be sacrificed to other derivative values. To do so as a rule is to destroy the ground for the latter. Rights in general not only express and protect the central interests of individuals (the raison d'être usually emphasized in their exposition); they also express the dignity and inviolability of individuality itself. For this reason the most fundamental right is the right to control the course of one's life, to make decisions crucial to it, including decisions in life-or-death medical contexts. The other side of the independent value of self-determination from the point of view of the individual is

the recognition of him by others, including doctors, as an individual with his own possibly unique set of values and priorities. His dignity demands a right to make personal decisions that express those values. . . .

NOTES

1. American Medical Association, *Principles of Medical Ethics.*
2. I restrict discussion for the time being to competent adults. I assume for now that if they have rights to information or to make their own decisions in medical contexts, then parents or guardians, not doctors, have these same rights in relation to children or the mentally incapacitated.
3. Compare Sissela Bok, *Lying* (New York: Pantheon, 1978), pp. 18–19.
4. See Gerald Dworkin, "Paternalism," in R. Wasserstrom, ed., *Morality and the Law* (Belmont, Cal.: Wadsworth, 1971).
5. Compare Norman Cantor, "A Patient's Decision to Decline Life-Saving Medical Treatment: Bodily Integrity Versus the Preservation of Life," in T. Beauchamp and S. Perlin, eds., *Ethical Issues in Death and Dying* (Englewood Cliffs, N.J.: Prentice-Hall, 1978), pp. 208–209.
6. Bernard Meyer, "Truth and the Physician," in Beauchamp and Perlin, eds., op. cit., p. 160.
7. Compare A. R. Jonsen, "Do No Harm: Axiom of Medical Ethics," *Philosophy and Medicine* 3 (1977): 27–41, p. 30.

BENEFICENCE TODAY, OR AUTONOMY (MAYBE) TOMORROW?

Monica, a forty-nine-year-old divorced mother of two children in their early twenties, was admitted to the hospital for acute respiratory insufficiency on a Friday evening. She is a heavy smoker and had experienced dyspnea for several weeks previously, but had not sought medical advice. Chest x-ray revealed several abnormalities and a bronchoscopy was scheduled for Monday morning.

From *Hastings Center Report* 30, no. 1 (January–February 2000): 18–19. Reprinted by permission of The Hastings Center.

On Saturday evening Monica's difficulty breathing worsened and during a heavy cough of sudden onset she became cyanotic and nearly lost consciousness. The physician on call performed an emergency intubation and transferred her to the intensive care unit, where she was heavily sedated. On Sunday, a bronchoscopy was performed, revealing a large, tumor-like mass in her trachea. Biopsies were taken from the mass, and from a palpable lymph node. On Monday the pathologist confirmed the presence of tumor cells and a diagnosis was made of a poorly differentiated squamous cell carcinoma of the lungs metastatic to the lymph node.

The multidisciplinary treatment team agreed that the tumor is inoperable (by either surgery or laser) and chemotherapy and radiation therapy are of unproven benefit. Monica cannot be extubated because the tumor will immediately obstruct her airway, and tracheostomy would be very risky—and probably not feasible—given the size of the tumor. Implanting a stent would also be difficult with so advanced a tumor. The team believes Monica's life expectancy is no more than three months.

The team discussed the following alternatives for Monica's care: they could withdraw life-sustaining measures; continue mechanical ventilation and heavy sedation but not treat any complications, such as infection, that arise; persuade (or coerce) the surgeon to implant a stent without consulting Monica; or wake Monica so that the team could discuss the diagnosis and prognosis with her and ascertain her preferences among the treatment alternatives.

The team is concerned that Monica will not really be able to make an informed, autonomous decision if they wake her. They worry that being intubated without sedation will impose further suffering for Monica, only to allow them to impart a grim prognosis. Should they wake her, or should they make treatment decisions on her behalf?

COMMENTARY

Bernice S. Elger

When Monica lost consciousness she knew only that she was in the hospital to be treated for an acute lung problem. We do not know why she did not seek treatment earlier—did she perhaps fear lung cancer? Even if she did, she cannot be supposed to be aware of the severity of her illness and of the small amount of time left to her to live.

The principle of autonomy, so central to modern biomedical ethics, clearly dictates that Monica should have the opportunity to decide about her future. While there are limits to imposing suffering on patients in order to grant them autonomy in decisionmaking, only patients themselves can know exactly what those limits are. Would Monica prefer to be awakened from sedation at all? If so, would she want to participate in the medically, ethically, and psychologically difficult decision about her treatment options?

Reducing sedation in an intubated patient like Monica in order to allow her to be informed about her situation and to communicate her preferences will induce significant physical and psychological suffering. The coughing and vomiting reflex caused by the tube cannot be completely inhibited and makes the patient very uncomfortable. Learning in such a difficult moment that she is going to die soon of lung cancer is likely to be very painful psychologically. Monica's willingness to accept this suffering will depend on her individual threshold of pain and her ability to cope with both pain and learning that she is near death. Perhaps even more importantly, it will depend on whether there are important things in her life that she would like to accomplish before she dies. Many patients would like at least to say goodbye to their loved ones or clarify a relationship after a recent dispute. Monica might want to make a will or indicate how and by whom her affairs should be handled after her death.

Monica, it seems, has not previously expressed preferences about end of life care either in a living will or orally to a relative, friend, or physician, and there is no way to know her desire except by waking her. Discussion with her children or someone else who knows her well might be helpful, but individuals in close emotional contact with patients in situations like Monica's can too easily be influenced by an overwhelming desire to protect the patient from suffering. In the absence of written or oral directives, not waking Monica would be an unjustified form of hard paternalism.

The harm done to her by waking her should be kept to a minimum. She should know her diagnosis and prognosis, and that she can at any time delegate decisionmaking power to another person and receive sedating medication. Without the attempt, she would not be in a good position to know how it feels to be on a ventilator while conscious and whether she is able to tolerate this for the sake of a last contact with her family and friends.

At this stage it is not necessary to tell her the details about heroic or experimental treatment options. Only if Monica chooses to participate in decisions about her care must she then choose between refusing or accepting aggressive therapy at all, and if she wants treatment, how aggressive her care should be. One could imagine her, for example, wanting the surgeon to attempt to place a stent, even if chances of success are slim, to enable her to spend her last days more comfortably and gain time to think about her future.

When deciding about Monica's participation in the treatment decision, caregivers are right to be concerned about whether she will truly be competent to make decisions in this complex situation. If we accept a sliding scale of competency, however, we can make the case that she can be the ultimate decisionmaker: since there is no clearly "best" alternative among the treatment possibilities, Monica will not be in a position of asking doctors to do something "irrational" or "dangerous" and thus will not have to "prove" her competency on the highest standards. Physicians concerned about the distress of asking Monica to make a decision on her own could also recommend the treatment that a majority of the team has decided is most adequate in her situation and ask Monica whether she consents.

Monica has a right to be informed to a degree that she herself determines according to her ability and willingness to cope with suffering. The team should wake her. Unless she declares that she does not want to know, she should be told that the decision she faces is difficult and that at any time she may designate another person or group to make decisions in her place.

COMMENTARY

Jean-Claude Chevrolet

Strong arguments can be made justifying the preeminence of autonomy in any situation and they seem easily accepted by anyone, at least on theoretical grounds. Nonetheless, Monica's caregivers, even after a thorough discussion of the ethical dimensions of the situation, and after having obtained expert medical opinions, could not see concretely how to proceed. They could not immediately accept causing what they believed would be a great amount of suffering to their patient for what they estimated to be a very poor result—that is, to offer benefits primarily to others, including Monica's family and other associates—without any certainty that this suffering could lead to an autonomous decision by Monica herself.

The question for Monica's caregivers, then, is whether autonomy becomes overvalued when it conflicts with other values, and what the conditions are or should be for applying the "therapeutic privilege" of not informing Monica of her diagnosis and prognosis in her own best interest. When the possibility was discussed of waking Monica so that she could decide what to do next, her physicians and nurses were really afraid that when faced with physical suffering and a horrible prognosis, she would not in fact be in any position to make an autonomous decision on any possible issue. They worried that the conditions for autonomous choice— that is, being able to act intentionally, with understanding, and without controlling influences—simply could not be met in this situation.

Of course, not respecting Monica's autonomy must be well justified because it clearly represents a decision that could be characterized as strong paternalism. The caregivers have to be sure, of course, that their own psychological distress in the case of waking Monica for respecting her autonomy and asking her to choose between several horrible options would not influence their own medical and ethical judgment. If this could not be assumed or were not the case, the real ethical dilemma would indeed be the clash between autonomy and beneficence. But Monica faces so short a life expectancy, and the quality of that life can be presumed to be so miserable, that caregivers may ask whether waking her just for the purpose of letting her choose among her horrible options isn't similar to the use of extraordinary means—that is, therapeutic tools and resources that have no reasonable chance of succeeding and could even be considered malpractice. They might ask whether the best analogy isn't to withholding a pointless treatment, in which case Monica's best interest could not be served by clinging to the ethical principle of autonomy.

It takes courage to decide that waking Monica only to impose on her a question that is impossible to answer, in conditions that could not permit sound judgment, is not the ethically best course of action. But Monica's best interests will not be served by a charade of autonomy.

WHY DOCTORS SHOULD INTERVENE

Terrence F. Ackerman

Patient autonomy has become a watchword of the medical profession. According to the revised 1980 AMA Principles of Medical Ethics, no longer is it permissible for a doctor to withhold information from a patient, even on grounds that it may be harmful. Instead the physician is expected to "deal honestly with patients" at all times. Physicians also have a duty to respect the confidentiality of the doctor-patient relationship. Even when disclosure to a third party may be in the patient's interests, the doctor is instructed to release information only when required by law. Respect for the autonomy of patients has given rise to many specific patient rights—among them the right to refuse treatment, the right to give informed consent, the right to privacy, and the right to competent medical care provided with "respect for human dignity."

While requirements of honesty, confidentiality, and patients rights are all important, the underlying moral vision that places exclusive emphasis upon these factors is more troublesome. The profession's notion of respect for autonomy makes noninterference its essential feature. As the Belmont Report has described it, there is an obligation to "give weight to autonomous persons' considered opinions and choices while refraining from obstructing their actions unless they are clearly detrimental to others" [see Part 6 Section 1]. Or, as Tom Beauchamp and James Childress have suggested, "To respect autonomous agents is to recognize with due appreciation their own considered value judgments and outlooks even when it is believed that their judgments are mistaken." They argue that people "are entitled to autonomous determination without limitation on their liberty being imposed by others."

When respect for personal autonomy is understood as noninterference, the physician's role is dramatically simplified. The doctor need be only an honest and good technician, providing relevant information and dispensing professionally competent care. Does noninterference really respect patient autonomy? I maintain that it does not,

From *Hastings Center Report* 12, no. 4 (August 1982): 14–17. Reprinted by permission of The Hastings Center.

Editors' note: An author's notes have been cut. Students who want to follow up on sources should consult the original article.

because it fails to take account of the transforming effects of illness.

"Autonomy," typically defined as self-governance, has two key features. First, autonomous behavior is governed by plans of action that have been formulated through deliberation or reflection. This deliberative activity involves processes of both information gathering and priority setting. Second, autonomous behavior issues, intentionally and voluntarily, from choices people make based upon their own life plans.

But various kinds of constraints can impede autonomous behavior. There are physical constraints—confinement in prison is an example—where internal or external circumstances bodily prevent a person from deliberating adequately or acting on life plans. Cognitive constraints derive from either a lack of information or an inability to understand that information. A consumer's ignorance regarding the merits or defects of a particular product fits the description. Psychological constraints, such as anxiety or depression, also inhibit adequate deliberation. Finally, there are social constraints—such as institutionalized roles and expectations ("a woman's place is in the home," "the doctor knows best") that block considered choices.

Edmund Pellegrino suggests several ways in which autonomy is specifically compromised by illness:

> In illness, the body is interposed between us and reality—it impedes our choices and actions and is no longer fully responsive. . . . Illness forces a reappraisal and that poses a threat to the old image; it opens up all the old anxieties and imposes new ones—often including the real threat of death or drastic alterations in lifestyle. This ontological assault is aggravated by the loss of . . . freedoms we identify as peculiarly human. The patient . . . lacks the knowledge and skills necessary to cure himself or gain relief of pain and suffering. . . . The state of being ill is therefore a state of "wounded humanity," of a person compromised in his fundamental capacity to deal with his vulnerability.

The most obvious impediment is that illness "interposes" the body or mind between the patient and reality, obstructing attempts to act upon cherished plans. An illness may not only temporarily obstruct long-range goals; it may necessitate permanent and drastic revision in the patient's major activities, such as working habits. Patients may also need to set limited goals regarding control of pain, alteration in diet and physical activity, and rehabilitation of functional impairments. They may face considerable difficulties in identifying realistic and productive aims.

The crisis is aggravated by a cognitive constraint—the lack of "knowledge and skills" to overcome their physical or mental impediment. Without adequate medical understanding, the patient cannot assess his or her condition accurately. Thus the choice of goals is seriously hampered and subsequent decisions by the patient are not well founded.

Pellegrino mentions the anxieties created by illness, but psychological constraints may also include denial, depression, guilt, and fear. I recently visited an eighteen-year-old boy who was dying of a cancer that had metastasized extensively throughout his abdomen. The doctor wanted to administer further chemotherapy that might extend the patient's life a few months. But the patient's nutritional status was poor, and he would need intravenous feedings prior to chemotherapy. Since the nutritional therapy might also encourage tumor growth, leading to a blockage of the gastrointestinal tract, the physician carefully explained the options and the risks and benefits several times, each time at greater length. But after each explanation, the young man would say only that he wished to do whatever was necessary to get better. Denial prevented him from exploring the alternatives.

Similarly, depression can lead patients to make choices that are not in harmony with their life plans. Recently, a middle-aged woman with a history of ovarian cancer in remission returned to the hospital for the biopsy of a possible pulmonary metastasis. Complications ensued and she required the use of an artificial respirator for several days. She became severely depressed and soon refused further treatment. The behavior was entirely out of character with her previous full commitment to treatment. Fully supporting her overt wishes might have robbed her of many months of relatively comfortable life in the midst of a very supportive family around which her activities centered. The medical staff stalled for time. Fortunately, her condition improved.

Fear may also cripple the ability of patients to choose. Another patient, diagnosed as having a cerebral tumor that was probably malignant, refused life-saving surgery because he feared the cosmetic effects of neurosurgery and the possibility of neurological damage. After he became comatose and new evidence suggested that the tumor might be benign, his family agreed to surgery and a benign tumor was removed. But he later died of complications related to the unfortunate delay in surgery. Although while competent he had agreed to chemotherapy, his fears (not uncommon among candidates for neurosurgery) prevented him from accepting the medical intervention that might have secured him the health he desired.

Social constraints may also prevent patients from acting upon their considered choices. A recent case involved a twelve-year-old boy whose rhabdomyosarcoma had metastasized extensively. Since all therapeutic interventions had failed, the only remaining option was to involve him in a phase 1 clinical trial. (A phase 1 clinical trial is the initial testing of a drug in human subjects. Its primary purpose is to identify toxicities rather than to evaluate therapeutic effectiveness.) The patient's course had been very stormy and he privately expressed to the staff his desire to quit further therapy and return home. However, his parents denied the hopelessness of his condition, remaining steadfast in their belief that God would save their child. With deep regard for his parents' wishes, he refused to openly object to their desires and the therapy was administered. No antitumor effect occurred and the patient soon died.

Various social and cultural expectations also take their toll. According to Talcott Parsons, one feature of the sick role is that the ill person is obligated ". . . . to seek *technically competent* help, namely, in the most usual case, that of a physician and to *cooperate* with him in the process of trying to get well." Parsons does not describe in detail the elements of this cooperation. But clinical observation suggests that many patients relinquish their opportunity to deliberate and make choices regarding treatment in deference to the physician's superior educational achievement and social status ("Whatever you think, doctor!"). The physical and emotional demands of illness reinforce this behavior.

Moreover, this perception of the sick role has been socially taught from childhood—and it is not easily altered even by the physician who ardently tries to engage the patient in decision making. In ?? when patients are initially asked to participate in the decision-making process, some exhibit considerable

confusion and anxiety. Thus, for many persons, the institutional role of patient requires the physician to assume the responsibilities of making decisions.

Ethicists typically condemn paternalistic practices in the therapeutic relationship, but fail to investigate the features that incline physicians to be paternalistic. Such behavior may be one way to assist persons whose autonomous behavior has been impaired by illness. Of course, it is an open moral question whether the constraints imposed by illness ought to be addressed in such a way. But only by coming to grips with the psychological and social dimensions of illness can we discuss how physicians can best respect persons who are patients.

RETURNING CONTROL TO PATIENTS

In the usual interpretation of respect for personal autonomy, noninterference is fundamental. In the medical setting, this means providing adequate information and competent care that accords with the patient's wishes. But if serious constraints upon autonomous behavior are intrinsic to the state of being ill, then noninterference is not the best course, since the patient's choices will be seriously limited. Under these conditions, real respect for autonomy entails a more inclusive understanding of the relationship between patients and physicians. Rather than restraining themselves so that patients can exercise whatever autonomy they retain in illness, physicians should actively seek to neutralize the impediments that interfere with patients' choices.

In *The Healer's Art*, Eric Cassell underscored the essential feature of illness that demands a revision in our understanding of respect for autonomy:

> If I had to pick the aspect of illness that is most destructive to the sick, I would choose the loss of control. Maintaining control over oneself is so vital to all of us that one might see all the other phenomena of illness as doing harm not only in their own right but doubly so as they reinforce the sick person's perception that he is no longer in control.

Cassell maintains, "The doctor's job is to return control to his patient." But what is involved in "returning control" to patients? Pellegrino identifies two elements that are preeminent duties of the physician: to provide technically competent care

: MS
 clear.

and to fully inform the patient. The noninterference approach emphasizes these factors, and their importance is clear. Loss of control in illness is precipitated by a physical or mental defect. If technically competent therapy can fully restore previous health, then the patient will again be in control. Consider a patient who is treated with antibiotics for a routine throat infection of streptococcal origin. Similarly, loss of control is fueled by lack of knowledge—not knowing what is the matter, what it portends for life and limb, and how it might be dealt with. Providing information that will enable the patient to make decisions and adjust goals enhances personal control.

If physical and cognitive constraints were the only impediments to autonomous behavior, then Pellegrino's suggestions might be adequate. But providing information and technically competent care will not do much to alter psychological or social impediments. Pellegrino does not adequately portray the physician's role in ameliorating these.

How can the doctor offset the acute denial that prevented the adolescent patient from assessing the benefits and risks of intravenous feedings prior to his additional chemotherapy? How can he deal with the candidate for neurosurgery who clearly desired that attempts be made to restore his health, but feared cosmetic and functional impairments? Here strategies must go beyond the mere provision of information. Crucial information may have to be repeatedly shared with patients. Features of the situation that the patient has brushed over (as in denial) or falsely emphasized (as with acute anxiety) must be discussed in more detail or set in their proper perspective. And the physician may have to alter the tone of discussions with the patient, emphasizing a positive attitude with the overly depressed or anxious patient, or a more realistic, cautious attitude with the denying patient, in order to neutralize psychological constraints.

The physician may also need to influence the beliefs or attitudes of other people, such as family members, that limit their awareness of the patient's perspective. Such a strategy might have helped the parents of the dying child to conform with the patient's wishes. On the other hand, physicians may need to modify the patient's own understanding of the sick role. For example, they may need to convey that the choice of treatment depends not merely upon the physician's technical assessment, but on the quality of life and personal goals that the patient desires.

Once we admit that psychological and social constraints impair patient autonomy, it follows that physicians must carefully assess the psychological and social profiles and needs of patients. Thus, Pedro Lain-Entralgo insists that adequate therapeutic interaction consists in a combination of "objectivity" and "cooperation." Cooperation "is shown bypsychologically reproducing in the mind of the doctor, insofar as that is possible, the meaning the patient's illness has for him.' Without such knowledge, the physician cannot assist patients in restoring control over their lives. Ironically, some critics have insisted that physicians are not justified in acting for the well-being of patients because they possess no "expertise" in securing the requisite knowledge about the patient. But knowledge of the patient's psychological and social situation is also necessary to help the patient to act as a fully autonomous person.

BEYOND LEGALISM

Current notions of respect for autonomy are undergirded by a legal model of doctor-patient interaction. The relationship is viewed as a typical commodity exchange—the provision of technically competent medical care in return for financial compensation. Moreover, physicians and patients are presumed to have an equal ability to work out the details of therapy, *provided that* certain moral rights of patients are recognized. But the compromising effects of illness, the superior knowledge of physicians, and various institutional arrangements are also viewed as giving the physician an unfair power advantage. Since the values and interests of patients may conflict with those of the physician, the emphasis is placed upon noninterference.

This legal framework is insufficient for medical ethics because it fails to recognize the impact of illness upon autonomous behavior. Even if the rights to receive adequate information and to provide consent are secured, affective and social constraints impair the ability of patients to engage in contractual therapeutic relationships. When people are sick, the focus upon equality is temporally misplaced. The goal of the therapeutic relationship is the "development" of the patient—helping to resolve the underlying physical (or mental) defect, and to deal with cognitive, psychological, and social constraints in order to restore autonomous functioning. In this sense, the doctor-patient interaction is not unlike the parent-child or teacher-student relationship.

The legal model also falls short because the therapeutic relationship is not a typical commodity exchange in which the parties use each other to accomplish mutually compatible goals, without taking a direct interest in each other. Rather, the status of patients as persons whose autonomy is compromised constitutes the very stuff of therapeutic art. The physician is attempting to alter the fundamental ability of patients to carry through their life plans. To accomplish this delicate task requires a personal knowledge about and interest in the patient. If we accept these points, then we must reject the narrow focus of medical ethics upon noninterference and emphasize patterns of interaction that free patients from constraints upon autonomy.

I hasten to add that I am criticizing the legal model only as a *complete* moral framework for therapeutic interaction. As case studies in medical ethics suggest, physicians and patients *are* potential adversaries. Moreover, the disability of the patient and various institutional controls provide physicians with a distinct "power advantage" that can be abused. Thus, a legitimate function of medical ethics is to formulate conditions that assure noninterference in patient decision making. But various positive interventions must also be emphasized, since the central task in the therapeutic process is assisting patients to reestablish control over their own lives.

In the last analysis, the crucial matter is how we view the patient who enters into the therapeutic relationship. Cassell points out that in the typical view ". . . the sick person is seen simply as a well person with a disease, rather than as qualitatively different, not only physically but also socially, emotionally, and even cognitively." In this view, ". . . the physician's role in the care of the sick is primarily the application of technology . . . and health can be seen as a commodity." But if, as I believe, illness renders sick persons "qualitatively different," then respect for personal autonomy requires a therapeutic interaction considerably more complex than the noninterference strategy.

Thus the current "Principles of Medical Ethics" simply exhort physicians to be honest. But the crucial requirement is that physicians tell the truth in a way, at a time, and in whatever increments are necessary to allow patients to effectively use the information in adjusting their life plans. Similarly, respecting a patient's refusal of treatment maximizes autonomy only if a balanced and thorough deliberation precedes the decision. Again, the "Principles" suggest that physicians observe strict confidentiality. But the more complex moral challenge is to use confidential information in a way that will help to give the patient more freedom. Thus, the doctor can keep a patient's report on family dynamics private, and still use it to modify attitudes or actions of family members that inhibit the patient's control.

At its root, illness is an evil primarily because it compromises our efforts to control our lives. Thus, we must preserve an understanding of the physician's art that transcends noninterference and addresses this fundamental reality.

FOUR MODELS OF THE PHYSICIAN-PATIENT RELATIONSHIP

Ezekiel J. Emanuel and Linda L. Emanuel

During the last two decades or so, there has been a struggle over the patient's role in medical decision making that is often characterized as a conflict between autonomy and health, between the values of the patient and the values of the physician. Seeking to curtail physician dominance, many have advocated an ideal of greater patient control. Others question this ideal because it fails to acknowledge the potentially imbalanced nature of this interaction when one party is sick and searching for security, and when judgments entail the interpretation of technical information. Still others are trying to delineate a more mutual relationship. This struggle shapes the expectations of physicians and patients as well as the ethical and legal standards for the physician's duties, informed consent, and medical malpractice. This struggle forces us to ask, What should be the ideal physician-patient relationship?

We shall outline four models of the physician-patient interaction, emphasizing the different understandings of (1) the goals of the physician-patient interaction, (2) the physician's obligations, (3) the role of patient values, and (4) the conception of patient autonomy. To elaborate the abstract description of these four models, we shall indicate the types of response the models might suggest in a clinical situation. Third, we shall also indicate how these models inform the current debate about the ideal physician-patient relationship. Finally, we shall evaluate these models and recommend one as the preferred model.

As outlined, the models are Weberian ideal types. They may not describe any particular physician-patient interactions but they highlight, free from complicating details, different visions of the essential characteristics of the physician-patient interaction. Consequently, they do not embody minimum ethical or legal standards, but rather constitute regulative ideals that are "higher than the law" but not "above the law."

THE PATERNALISTIC MODEL

First is the *paternalistic* model, sometimes called the parental or priestly model. In this model, the physician-patient interaction ensures that patients receive the interventions that best promote their health and well-being. To this end, physicians use their skills to determine the patient's medical condition and his or her stage in the disease process and to identify the medical tests and treatments most likely to restore the patient's health or ameliorate pain. Then the physician presents the patient with selected information that will encourage the patient to consent to the intervention the physician considers best. At the extreme, the physician authoritatively informs the patient when the intervention will be initiated.

The paternalistic model assumes that there are shared objective criteria for determining what is best. Hence the physician can discern what is in the patient's best interest with limited patient participation. Ultimately, it is assumed that the patient will be thankful for decisions made by the physician even if he or she would not agree to them at the time. In the tension between the patient's autonomy and well-being, between choice and health, the paternalistic physician's main emphasis is toward the latter.

In the paternalistic model, the physician acts as the patient's guardian, articulating and implementing what is best for the patient. As such, the physician has obligations, including that of placing the patient's interest above his or her own and soliciting the views of others when lacking adequate knowledge. The conception of patient autonomy is patient assent, either at the time or later, to the physician's determinations of what is best.

From *Journal of the American Medical Association* 267, no. 16 (April 22/29, 1992): 2221–2226. Copyright © 1992 American Medical Association.

Editors' note: Some authors' notes have been cut. Students who want to follow up on sources should consult the original article.

THE INFORMATIVE MODEL

Second is the *informative* model, sometimes called the scientific, engineering, or consumer model. In this model, the objective of the physician-patient interaction is for the physician to provide the patient with all relevant information, for the patient to select the medical interventions he or she wants, and for the physician to execute the selected interventions. To this end, the physician informs the patient of his or her disease state, the nature of possible diagnostic and therapeutic interventions, the nature and probability of risks and benefits associated with the interventions, and any uncertainties of knowledge. At the extreme, patients could come to know all medical information relevant to their disease and available interventions and select the interventions that best realize their values.

The informative model assumes a fairly clear distinction between facts and values. The patient's values are well defined and known; what the patient lacks is facts. It is the physician's obligation to provide all the available facts, and the patient's values then determine what treatments are to be given. There is no role for the physician's values, the physician's understanding of the patient's values, or his or her judgment of the worth of the patient's values. In the informative model, the physician is a purveyor of technical expertise, providing the patient with the means to exercise control. As technical experts, physicians have important obligations to provide truthful information, to maintain competence in their area of expertise, and to consult others when their knowledge or skills are lacking. The conception of patient autonomy is patient control over medical decision making.

THE INTERPRETIVE MODEL

The third model is the *interpretive* model. The aim of the physician-patient interaction is to elucidate the patient's values and what he or she actually wants, and to help the patient select the available medical interventions that realize these values. Like the informative physician, the interpretive physician provides the patient with information on the nature of the condition and the risks and benefits of possible interventions. Beyond this, however, the interpretive physician assists the patient in elucidating and articulating his or her values and in determining what medical interventions best realize the specified values, thus helping to interpret the patient's values for the patient.

According to the interpretive model, the patient's values are not necessarily fixed and known to the patient. They are often inchoate, and the patient may only partially understand them; they may conflict when applied to specific situations. Consequently, the physician working with the patient must elucidate and make coherent these values. To do this, the physician works with the patient to reconstruct the patient's goals and aspirations, commitments and character. At the extreme, the physician must conceive of the patient's life as a narrative whole, and from this specify the patient's values and their priorities. Then the physician determines which tests and treatments best realize these values. Importantly, the physician does not dictate to the patient; it is the patient who ultimately decides which values and course of action best fit who he or she is. Neither is the physician judging the patient's values; he or she helps the patient to understand and use them in the medical situation.

In the interpretive model, the physician is a counselor, analogous to a cabinet minister's advisory role to a head of state, supplying relevant information, helping to elucidate values, and suggesting what medical interventions realize these values. Thus the physician's obligations include those enumerated in the informative model but also require engaging the patient in a joint process of understanding. Accordingly, the conception of patient autonomy is self-understanding; the patient comes to know more clearly who he or she is and how the various medical options bear on his or her identity.

THE DELIBERATIVE MODEL

Fourth is the *deliberative* model. The aim of the physician-patient interaction is to help the patient determine and choose the best health-related values that can be realized in the clinical situation. To this end, the physician must delineate information on the patient's clinical situation and then help elucidate the types of values embodied in the available options. The physician's objectives include suggesting why certain health-related values are more worthy and should be aspired to. At the extreme, the physician and patient engage in deliberation about what kind of health-related values the patient could and ultimately should pursue. The physician discusses only health-related values, that is, values that affect or are affected by the patient's disease and treatments; he or she recognizes that many elements of morality are unrelated to the patient's disease or treatment and beyond the scope of their professional relationship. Further, the physician aims at no more than moral persuasion; ultimately, coercion is avoided, and the patient must define his or her life and select the ordering of values to be espoused. By engaging in moral deliberation, the physician and patient judge the worthiness and importance of the health-related values.

In the deliberative model, the physician acts as a teacher or friend, engaging the patient in dialogue on what course of action would be best. Not only does the physician indicate what the patient could do, but, knowing the patient and wishing what is best, the physician indicates what the patient should do—what decision regarding medical therapy would be admirable. The conception of patient autonomy is moral self-development; the patient is empowered not simply to follow unexamined preferences or examined values, but to consider, through dialogue, alternative health-related values, their worthiness, and their implications for treatment.

COMPARING THE FOUR MODELS

Importantly, all models have a role for patient autonomy; a main factor that differentiates the models is their particular conceptions of patient autonomy. Therefore, no single model can be endorsed because it alone promotes patient autonomy. Instead the models must be compared and evaluated, at least in part, by evaluating the adequacy of their particular conceptions of patient autonomy.

The four models are not exhaustive. At a minimum, there might be added a fifth: the *instrumental* model. In this model, the patient's values are irrelevant; the physician aims for some goal independent of the patient, such as the good of society or the furtherance of scientific knowledge. The Tuskegee

syphilis experiment and the Willowbrook hepatitis study [see Part 6, Section 1] are examples of this model. As the moral condemnation of these cases reveals, this model is not an ideal, but an aberration. Thus we have not elaborated it herein.

A CLINICAL CASE

To make tangible these abstract descriptions and to crystallize essential differences among the models, we will illustrate the responses they suggest in a clinical situation, that of a 43-year-old premenopausal woman who has recently discovered a breast mass. Surgery reveals a 3.5-cm ductal carcinoma with no lymph node involvement that is estrogen receptor positive. Chest roentgenogram, bone scan, and liver function tests reveal no evidence of metastatic disease. The patient was recently divorced and has gone back to work as a legal aide to support herself. What should the physician say to this patient?

In the paternalistic model a physician might say, "There are two alternative therapies to protect against recurrence of cancer in your breast: mastectomy or radiation. We now know that the survival with lumpectomy combined with radiation therapy is equal to that with mastectomy. Because lumpectomy and radiation offers the best survival and the best cosmetic result, it is to be preferred. I have asked the radiation therapist to come and discuss radiation treatment with you. We also need to protect you against the spread of the cancer to other parts of your body. Even though the chance of recurrence is low, you are young, and we should not leave any therapeutic possibilities untried. Recent studies involving chemotherapy suggest improvements in survival without recurrence of breast cancer. Indeed, the National Cancer Institute (NCI) recommends chemotherapy for women with your type of breast cancer. Chemotherapy has side effects. Nevertheless, a few months of hardship now are worth the potential added years of life without cancer."

In the informative model, a physician might say, "With node-negative breast cancer there are two issues before you: local control and systemic control. For local control, the options are mastectomy or lumpectomy with or without radiation. From many studies we know that mastectomy and lumpectomy with radiation result in identical overall survival, about 80 percent 10-year survival. Lumpectomy without radiation results in a 30 percent to 40 percent chance of tumor recurrence in the breast. The second issue relates to systemic control. We know that chemotherapy prolongs survival for premenopausal women who have axillary nodes involved with tumor. The role for women with node-negative breast cancer is less clear. Individual studies suggest that chemotherapy is of no benefit in terms of improving overall survival, but a comprehensive review of all studies suggests that there is a survival benefit. Several years ago, the NCI suggested that for women like yourself, chemotherapy can have a positive therapeutic impact. Finally, let me inform you that there are clinical trials, for which you are eligible, to evaluate the benefits of chemotherapy for patients with node-negative breast cancer. I can enroll you in a study if you want. I will be happy to give you any further information you feel you need."

The interpretive physician might outline much of the same information as the informative physician, then engage in discussion to elucidate the patient's wishes, and conclude, "It sounds to me as if you have conflicting wishes. Understandably, you seem uncertain how to balance the demands required for receiving additional treatment, rejuvenating your personal affairs, and maintaining your psychological equilibrium. Let me try to express a perspective that fits your position. Fighting your cancer is important, but it must leave you with a healthy self-image and quality time outside the hospital. This view seems compatible with undergoing radiation therapy but not chemotherapy. A lumpectomy with radiation maximizes your chance of surviving while preserving your breast. Radiotherapy fights your breast cancer without disfigurement. Conversely, chemotherapy would prolong the duration of therapy by many months. Further, the benefits of chemotherapy in terms of survival are smaller and more controversial. Given the recent changes in your life, you have too many new preoccupations to undergo months of chemotherapy for a questionable benefit. Do I understand you? We can talk again in a few days."

The deliberative physician might begin by outlining the same factual information, then engage in a conversation to elucidate the patient's values, but

continue, "It seems clear that you should undergo radiation therapy. It offers maximal survival with minimal risk, disfigurement, and disruption of your life. The issue of chemotherapy is different, fraught with conflicting data. Balancing all the options, I think the best one for you is to enter a trial that is investigating the potential benefit of chemotherapy for women with node-negative breast cancer. First, it ensures that you receive excellent medical care. At this point, we do not know which therapy maximizes survival. In a clinical study the schedule of follow-up visits, tests, and decisions is specified by leading breast cancer experts to ensure that all the women receive care that is the best available anywhere. A second reason to participate in a trial is altruistic; it allows you to contribute something to women with breast cancer in the future who will face difficult choices. Over decades, thousands of women have participated in studies that inform our current treatment practices. Without those women, and the knowledge they made possible, we would probably still be giving you and all other women with breast cancer mastectomies. By enrolling in a trial you participate in a tradition in which women of one generation receive the highest standard of care available but also enhance the care of women in future generations because medicine has learned something about which interventions are better. I must tell you that I am not involved in the study; if you elect to enroll in this trial, you will initially see another breast cancer expert to plan your therapy. I have sought to explain our current knowledge and offer my recommendation so you can make the best possible decision."

Lacking the normal interchange with patients, these statements may seem contrived, even caricatures. Nevertheless, they highlight the essence of each model and suggest how the objectives and assumptions of each inform a physician's approach to his or her patients. Similar statements can be imagined for other clinical situations such as an obstetrician discussing prenatal testing or a cardiologist discussing cholesterol-reducing interventions.

THE CURRENT DEBATE AND THE FOUR MODELS

In recent decades there has been a call for greater patient autonomy or, as some have called it, "patient sovereignty," conceived as patient *choice* and *control* over medical decisions. This shift toward the informative model is embodied in the adoption of business terms for medicine, as when physicians are described as health care providers and patients as consumers. It can also be found in the propagation of patient rights statements, in the promotion of living-will laws, and in rules regarding human experimentation. For instance, the opening sentences of one law state: "The Rights of the Terminally Ill Act authorizes an adult person to *control* decisions regarding administration of life-sustaining treatment. . . . The Act merely provides one way by which a terminally-ill patient's *desires* regarding the use of life-sustaining procedures can be legally implemented" (emphasis added). Indeed, living-will laws do not require or encourage patients to discuss the issue of terminating care with their physicians before signing such documents. Similarly, decisions in "right-to-die" cases emphasize patient control over medical decisions. As one court put it:

> The right to refuse medical treatment is basic and fundamental. . . . Its exercise requires no one's approval. . . . [T]*he controlling decision belongs to a competent informed patient.* . . . It is not a medical decision for her physicians to make. . . . It *is a moral and philosophical decision that, being a competent adult, is [the patient's] alone.*[1] (emphasis added)

Probably the most forceful endorsement of the informative model as the ideal inheres in informed consent standards. Prior to the 1970s, the standard for informed consent was "physician based." Since 1972 and the *Canterbury* case, however, the emphasis has been on a "patient-oriented" standard of informed consent in which the physician has a "duty" to provide appropriate medical facts to empower the patient to use his or her values to determine what interventions should be implemented.

> True consent to what happens to one's self is the informed exercise of a choice, and that entails an opportunity to evaluate knowledgeably the options available and the risks attendant upon each. . . . [I]*t is the prerogative of the patient, not the physician, to determine for himself the direction in which his interests seem to lie.* To enable the patient to chart his course understandably, some familiarity with the therapeutic alternatives and their hazards becomes essential.[2] (emphasis added)

SHARED DECISION MAKING

Despite its dominance, many have found the informative model somewhat "arid." The President's Commission and others contend that the ideal relationship does not vest moral authority and medical decision-making power exclusively in the patient but must be a process of shared decision making constructed around "mutual participation and respect." The President's Commission argues that the physician's role is "to help the patient understand the medical situation and available courses of action, and the patient conveys his or her concerns and wishes." Brock and Wartman[3] stress this fact-value "division of labor"—having the physician provide information while the patient makes value decisions—by describing "shared decision making" as a collaborative process

> in which both physicians and patients make active and essential contributions. Physicians bring their medical training, knowledge, and expertise—including an understanding of the available treatment alternatives—to the diagnosis and management of patients' conditions. Patients bring knowledge of their own subjective aims and values, through which risks and benefits of various treatment options can be evaluated. With this approach, selecting the best treatment for a particular patient requires the contribution of both parties.

Similarly, in discussing ideal medical decision making, Eddy[4] argues for this fact-value division of labor between the physician and patient as the ideal:

> It is important to separate the decision process into these two steps. . . . The first step is a question of facts. The anchor is empirical evidence. . . . [T]he second step is a question not of facts but of personal values or preferences. The thought process is not analytic but personal and subjective. . . . [I]t is the patient's preferences that should determine the decision. . . . Ideally, you and I [the physicians] are not in the picture. What matters is what Mrs. Smith thinks.

This view of shared decision making seems to vest the medical decision-making authority with the patient while relegating physicians to technicians "transmitting medical information and using their technical skills as the patient directs." Thus, while the advocates of "shared decision making" may aspire toward a mutual dialogue between physician and patient, the substantive view informing their ideal reembodies the informative model under a different label.

Other commentators have articulated more mutual models of the physician-patient interaction. Prominent among these efforts is Katz's *The Silent World of the Doctor and Patient*. Relying on a Freudian view in which self-knowledge and self-determination are inherently limited because of unconscious influences, Katz views dialogue as a mechanism for greater self-understanding of one's values and objectives. According to Katz, this view places a duty on physicians and patients to reflect and communicate so that patients can gain a greater self-understanding and self-determination. Katz's insight is also available on grounds other than Freudian psychological theory and is consistent with the interpretive model.

OBJECTIONS TO THE PATERNALISTIC MODEL

It is widely recognized that the paternalistic model is justified during emergencies when the time taken to obtain informed consent might irreversibly harm the patient. Beyond such limited circumstances, however, it is no longer tenable to assume that the physician and patient espouse similar values and views of what constitutes a benefit. Consequently, even physicians rarely advocate the paternalistic model as an ideal for routine physician-patient interactions.

OBJECTIONS TO THE INFORMATIVE MODEL

The informative model seems both descriptively and prescriptively inaccurate. First, this model seems to have no place for essential qualities of the ideal physician-patient relationship. The informative physician cares for the patient in the sense of competently implementing the patient's selected interventions. However, the informative physician lacks a caring approach that requires understanding what the patient values or should value and how his or her illness impinges on these values. Patients seem to expect their physician to have a caring approach; they deem a technically proficient but detached physician as deficient, and properly condemned. Further, the informative physician is proscribed from giving a recommendation for fear of imposing his or her will on the patient and thereby competing for the decision-making control that has been given to the patient. Yet, if one of the essential qualities of the ideal physician is the ability to assimilate medical facts, prior experience of similar situations, and intimate knowledge of the patient's view into a recommendation designed for the patient's specific medical and personal condition, then the informative physician cannot be ideal.

Second, in the informative model, the ideal physician is a highly trained subspecialist who provides detailed factual information and competently implements the patient's preferred medical intervention. Hence, the informative model perpetuates and accentuates the trend toward specialization and impersonalization within the medical profession.

Most importantly, the informative model's conception of patient autonomy seems philosophically untenable. The informative model presupposes that persons possess known and fixed values, but this is inaccurate. People are often uncertain about what they actually want. Further, unlike animals, people have what philosophers call "second-order desires," that is, the capacity to reflect on their wishes and to revise their own desires and preferences. In fact, freedom of the will and autonomy inhere in having "second-order desires" and being able to change our preferences and modify our identities. Self-reflection and the capacity to change what we want often require a "process" of moral deliberation in which we assess the value of what we want. And this is a process that occurs with other people who know us well and can articulate a vision of who we ought to be that we can assent to. Even though changes in health or implementation of alternative interventions can have profound effects on what we desire and how we realize our desires, self-reflection and deliberation play no essential role in the informative physician-patient interaction. The informative model's conception of autonomy is incompatible with a vision of autonomy that incorporates second-order desires.

OBJECTIONS TO THE INTERPRETIVE MODEL

The interpretive model rectifies this deficiency by recognizing that persons have second-order desires and dynamic value structures and placing the elucidation of values in the context of the patient's medical condition at the center of the physician-patient interaction. Nevertheless, there are objections to the interpretive model.

Technical specialization militates against physicians cultivating the skills necessary to the interpretive model. With limited interpretive talents and limited time, physicians may unwittingly impose their own values under the guise of articulating the patient's values. And patients, overwhelmed by their medical condition and uncertain of their own views, may too easily accept this imposition. Such circumstances may push the interpretive model toward the paternalistic model in actual practice.

Further, autonomy viewed as self-understanding excludes evaluative judgment of the patient's values or attempts to persuade the patient to adopt other values. This constrains the guidance and recommendations the physician can offer. Yet in practice, especially in preventive medicine and risk-reduction interventions, physicians often attempt to persuade patients to adopt particular health-related values. Physicians frequently urge patients with high cholesterol levels who smoke to change their dietary habits, quit smoking, and begin exercise programs before initiating drug therapy. The justification given for these changes is that patients should value their health more than they do. Similarly, physicians are encouraged to persuade their human immunodeficiency virus (HIV)–infected patients who might be engaging in unsafe sexual practices either to abstain or, realistically, to adopt "safer sex" practices. Such appeals are not made to promote the HIV–infected patient's own health, but are grounded on an appeal for the patient to assume responsibility for the good of others. Consequently, by excluding evaluative judgments, the interpretive model seems to characterize inaccurately ideal physician-patient interactions.

OBJECTIONS TO THE DELIBERATIVE MODEL

The fundamental objections to the deliberative model focus on whether it is proper for physicians to judge patients' values and promote particular health-related values. First, physicians do not possess privileged knowledge of the priority of health-related values relative to other values.

Indeed, since ours is a pluralistic society in which people espouse incommensurable values, it is likely that a physician's values and view of which values are higher will conflict with those of other physicians and those of his or her patients.

Second, the nature of the moral deliberation between physician and patient, the physician's recommended interventions, and the actual treatments used will depend on the values of the particular physician treating the patient. However, recommendations and care provided to patients should not depend on the physician's judgment of the worthiness of the patient's values or on the physician's particular values. As one bioethicist put it:

> The hand is broken; the physician can repair the hand; therefore the physician must repair the hand—as well as possible—without regard to personal values that might lead the physician to think ill of the patient or of the patient's values. . . . [A]t the level of clinical practice, medicine should be value-free in the sense that the personal values of the physician should not distort the making of medical decisions.[5]

Third, it may be argued that the deliberative model misconstrues the purpose of the physician-patient interaction. Patients see their physicians to receive health care, not to engage in moral deliberation or to revise their values. Finally, like the interpretive model, the deliberative model may easily metamorphose into unintended paternalism, the very practice that generated the public debate over proper physician-patient interaction.

THE PREFERRED MODEL AND THE PRACTICAL IMPLICATIONS

Clearly, under different clinical circumstances, different models may be appropriate. Indeed, at different times, all four models may justifiably guide physicians and patients. Nevertheless, it is important to specify one model as the shared, paradigmatic reference; exceptions to use other models would not be automatically condemned, but would require justification based on the circumstances of a particular situation. Thus, it is widely agreed that in an emergency where delays in treatment to obtain informed consent might irreversibly harm the patient, the paternalistic model correctly guides physician-patient interactions. Conversely, for patients who have clear but conflicting values, the interpretive model is probably justified. For instance, a 65-year-old woman who has been treated for acute leukemia may have clearly decided against reinduction chemotherapy if she relapses. Several months before the anticipated birth of her first grandchild, the patient relapses. The patient becomes torn about whether to endure the risks of reinduction chemotherapy in order to live to see her first grandchild or whether to refuse therapy, resigning herself to not seeing her grandchild. In such cases, the physician may justifiably adopt the interpretive approach. In other circumstances, where there is only a one-time physician-patient interaction without an ongoing relationship in which the patient's values can be elucidated and compared with ideals, such as in a walk-in center, the informative model may be justified.

Descriptively and prescriptively, we claim that the ideal physician-patient relationship is the deliberative model. We will adduce six points to justify this claim. First, the deliberative model more nearly embodies our ideal of autonomy. It is an oversimplification and distortion of the Western tradition to view respecting autonomy as simply permitting a person to select, unrestricted by coercion, ignorance, physical interference, and the like, his or her preferred course of action from a comprehensive list of available options. Freedom and control over medical decisions alone do not constitute patient autonomy. Autonomy requires that individuals critically assess their own values and preferences; determine whether they are desirable; affirm, upon reflection, these values as ones that should justify their actions; and then be free to initiate action to realize the values. The process of deliberation integral to the deliberative model is essential for realizing patient autonomy understood in this way.

Second, our society's image of an ideal physician is not limited to one who knows and communicates to the patient relevant factual information and competently implements medical interventions. The ideal physician—often embodied in literature, art, and popular culture—is a caring physician who integrates the information and relevant values to make a recommendation and, through discussion, attempts to persuade the patient to accept this recommendation as the intervention that best promotes his or her overall well-being. Thus, we expect the best physicians to engage their patients in

evaluative discussions of health issues and related values. The physician's discussion does not invoke values that are unrelated or tangentially related to the patient's illness and potential therapies. Importantly, these efforts are not restricted to situations in which patients might make "irrational and harmful" choices but extend to all health care decisions.

Third, the deliberative model is not a disguised form of paternalism. Previously there may have been category mistakes in which instances of the deliberative model have been erroneously identified as physician paternalism. And no doubt, in practice, the deliberative physician may occasionally lapse into paternalism. However, like the ideal teacher, the deliberative physician attempts to *persuade* the patient of the worthiness of certain values, not to *impose* those values paternalistically; the physician's aim is not to subject the patient to his or her will, but to persuade the patient of a course of action as desirable. In the *Laws*, Plato[6] characterizes this fundamental distinction between persuasion and imposition for medical practice that distinguishes the deliberative from the paternalistic model:

> A physician to slaves never gives his patient any account of his illness. . . . [T]he physician offers some orders gleaned from experience with an air of infallible knowledge, in the brusque fashion of a dictator. . . . The free physician, who usually cares for free men, treats their disease first by thoroughly discussing with the patient and his friends his ailment. This way he learns something from the sufferer and simultaneously instructs him. Then the physician does not give his medications until he has persuaded the patient; the physician aims at complete restoration of health by persuading the patient to comply with his therapy.

Fourth, physician values are relevant to patients and do inform their choice of a physician. When a pregnant woman chooses an obstetrician who does not routinely perform a battery of prenatal tests or, alternatively, one who strongly favors them; and when patients seek an aggressive cardiologist who favors procedural interventions or one who concentrates therapy on dietary changes, stress reduction, and life-style modifications, they are, consciously or not, selecting a physician based on the values that guide their medical decisions. And, when disagreements between physicians and patients arise, there are discussions over which values are more important and should be realized in medical care. Occasionally, when such disagreements undermine the physician-patient relationship and a caring attitude, a patient's care is transferred to another physician. Indeed, in the informative model the grounds for transferring care to a new physician is either the physician's ignorance or incompetence. But patients seem to switch physicians because they do not "like" a particular physician or that physician's attitude or approach.

Fifth, we seem to believe that physicians should not only help fit therapies to the patients' elucidated values, but should also promote health-related values. As noted, we expect physicians to promote certain values, such as "safer sex" for patients with HIV or abstaining from or limiting alcohol use. Similarly, patients are willing to adjust their values and actions to be more compatible with health-promoting values. This is in the nature of seeking a caring medical recommendation.

Finally, it may well be that many physicians currently lack the training and capacity to articulate the values underlying their recommendations and persuade patients that these values are worthy. But, in part, this deficiency is a consequence of the tendencies toward specialization and the avoidance of discussions of values by physicians that are perpetuated and justified by the dominant informative model. Therefore, if the deliberative model seems most appropriate, then we need to implement changes in medical care and education to encourage a more caring approach. We must stress understanding rather than mere provisions of factual information in keeping with the legal standards of informed consent and medical malpractice; we must educate physicians not just to spend more time in physician-patient communication but to elucidate and articulate the values underlying their medical care decisions, including routine ones; we must shift the publicly assumed conception of patient autonomy that shapes both the physician's and the patient's expectations from patient control to moral development. Most important, we must recognize that developing a deliberative physician-patient relationship requires a considerable amount of time. We must develop a health care financing system that properly reimburses—rather than penalizes—physicians for taking the time to discuss values with their patients.

CONCLUSION

Over the last few decades, the discourse regarding the physician-patient relationship has focused on two extremes: autonomy and paternalism. Many have attacked physicians as paternalistic, urging the empowerment of patients to control their own care. This view, the informative model, has become dominant in bioethics and legal standards. This model embodies a defective conception of patient autonomy, and it reduces the physician's role to that of a technologist. The essence of doctoring is a fabric of knowledge, understanding, teaching, and action, in which the caring physician integrates the patient's medical condition and health-related values, makes a recommendation on the appropriate course of action, and tries to persuade the patient of the worthiness of this approach and the values it realizes. The physician with a caring attitude is the ideal embodied in the deliberative model, the ideal that should inform laws and policies that regulate the physician-patient interaction.

Finally, it may be worth noting that the four models outlined herein are not limited to the medical realm; they may inform the public conception of other professional interactions as well. We suggest that the ideal relationships between lawyer and client, religious mentor and laity, and educator and student are well described by the deliberative model, at least in some of their essential aspects.

NOTES

1. *Bouvia v. Superior Court*, 225 Cal Rptr 297 (1986).
2. *Canterbury v. Spence*, 464 F2d 772 (D.C. Cir 1972).
3. Brock DW, Wartman SA. When competent patients make irrational choices. *N Engl J Med.* 1990; 322: 1595–1599.
4. Eddy DM. Anatomy of a decision. *JAMA.* 1990; 263:441–443.
5. Gorovitz S. *Doctors' Dilemmas: Moral Conflict and Medical Care.* New York, NY: Oxford University Press Inc; 1982:chap 6.
6. Plato; Hamilton E, Cairns H, eds; Emanuel EJ, trans. *Plato: The Collected Dialogues.* Princeton, NJ: Princeton University Press; 1961:720 c–e.

INFORMED CONSENT AND TRUTH-TELLING

ANTIHYPERTENSIVES AND THE RISK OF TEMPORARY IMPOTENCE: A CASE STUDY IN INFORMED CONSENT

John D. Arras

Dr. Sylvia Kramer pondered what she would tell Robert Williams on his next visit to her primary care clinic. Mr. Williams was an affable 40-year-old African-American, and one of Dr. Kramer's favorite patients. He had recently remarried, and enjoyed telling his doctor about his two young stepdaughters. The problem that brought him to this inner-city clinic was high blood pressure, which was first diagnosed by Dr. Kramer a year ago, during her first year as a resident in family medicine. Mr. Williams's blood pressure had then measured 180/103: not frightening numbers, to be sure, but still very much on the high side of "mild hypertension." If his blood pressure were not lowered, Mr. Williams could anticipate some serious related health problems, such as an increased risk of stroke.

Dr. Kramer's initial recommendation to Mr. Williams was that he attempt to control his weight and blood pressure through a regimen of regular exercise and a sensible diet low in salt and fat. She had recalled one of her mentor's lectures on hypertension: "No need to burden your patients with expensive drugs with side effects when they can solve the problem on their own through good behavior." Although Mr. Williams had achieved some lowering of his blood pressure during the ensuing months, down to 160/95, this improvement still left him in the marginal zone and was, in any case, short-lived. His blood-pressure readings were now consistently elevated. On his last visit, he had expressed some frustration to Dr. Kramer that, try as he might, no amount of exercise or diet seemed to be working.

Given Mr. Williams's lack of progress, Dr. Kramer was considering prescribing a common diuretic, hydrochlorothiazide, as the second line of defense against his hypertension. This particular drug, she knew, has a long history as a cheap and highly effective remedy. The price tag, 5 cents per pill, was particularly attractive to Dr. Kramer, who realized that her clinic patients often

This case study has benefited from helpful discussions with my brother, Ernest Arras, M.D., and from the careful scrutiny of several physician-colleagues at Montefiore Medical Center, including Michael Alderman, Ellen Cohen, Tom McGinn, and Doug Shenson.

had a hard time paying for some of the more "high-tech" and high-priced hypertension medications that had been flooding the market in recent years.

Notwithstanding its relative safety, efficacy, and affordability, this particular drug still posed problems. First, it had a tendency to leech potassium from the body. She could address that problem by prescribing bananas. The second problem, a more serious matter, was a risk of causing impotence in males. The risk was small, however: only about 3 to 5 percent of men who took the pill were likely to be affected, and the impotence was easily reversible. One simply had to stop taking the drug for this side effect to disappear.

Dr. Kramer pondered the question of what "informed consent" should mean in this situation. In particular, she wondered whether she had an obligation to inform Mr. Williams of the risk of temporary impotence when recommending that he start with this diuretic. While this risk was certainly a lot less worrisome than the remote possibility of death attendant upon many medical and surgical procedures, it was still significant. If Mr. Williams, a newlywed, were to experience an unexpected and unexplained episode of sexual dysfunction, he would no doubt be extremely upset and anxious about it. Dr. Kramer, the product of a family-medicine training program committed to the value of patient self-determination, initially felt that she should share all the risks that Mr. Williams would likely consider relevant to his decision. Cost was certainly a factor, but so was his sex life. He should have the right, she reasoned, to make his own trade-offs among competing values. If sexual dysfunction is high on his list of things to avoid, especially at this time in his marriage, he might be willing to pay extra for another drug.

Still somewhat uncomfortable with her conclusion, Dr. Kramer asked the advice of Dr. Robert Black, a senior physician in her program. Dr. Black registered total disbelief upon hearing the resident's plan of action. "Look," he said, "I'm a staunch supporter of patients' rights, autonomy, and all that, but this is just ridiculous. The risk is quite low, entirely reversible, and consider this: if you share this possible side effect with your patient, this little bit of truth is likely to make him extremely anxious about what could happen. You've heard of the Hawthorne effect, haven't you? Telling him about the risk of impotence could actually make Mr. Williams so worried that he would become impotent at your suggestion. I've been practicing medicine for fifteen years, and I've never told a patient about this sort of thing beforehand. If Mr. Williams comes back to you in a couple of weeks complaining about his sex life, you can deal with it then. But in the meantime, don't make a counterproductive fetish of informed consent. Lighten up!"

At this point, Dr. Kramer was truly puzzled. If she were to be entirely honest with her patient, she might end up doing him harm, and all for a very remote and reversible risk. On the other hand, it still bothered her to hide a fact from her patient that she suspected he would consider significant. He was, moreover, a rather shy man, especially about sexual matters. Dr. Kramer was not entirely confident that, should a problem develop, Mr. Williams would feel comfortable talking with a young female physician about his sexual "failure." He might just conclude that it was his or his new wife's fault, not the result of the drug, and live with impaired sexual function for some time.

How should Dr. Kramer resolve her ethical conflict? Should she (a) have a serious discussion with Mr. Williams about the small risk of temporary impotence, (b) casually mention the risk, perhaps using medical jargon, but only in passing along with many other minor risks, (c) withhold information about this particular risk until the patient complained of sexual dysfunction, or (d) withhold the information at first, but inquire specifically at a later date about the patient's sex life?

INFORMED CONSENT—MUST IT REMAIN A FAIRY TALE?

Jay Katz

I. THE PREHISTORY OF INFORMED CONSENT IN MEDICINE

The idea that, prior to any medical intervention, physicians must seek their patients' informed consent was introduced into American law in a brief paragraph in a 1957 state court decision,[1] and then elaborated on in a lengthier opinion in 1960.[2] The emerging legal idea that physicians were from now on obligated to share decisionmaking authority with their patients shocked the medical community, for it constituted a radical break with the silence that had been the hallmark of physician-patient interactions throughout the ages. Thirty-five years are perhaps not long enough for either law or medicine to resolve the tension between legal theory and medical practice, particularly since judges were reluctant to face up to implications of their novel doctrine, preferring instead to remain quite deferential to the practices of the medical profession.

Viewed from the perspective of medical history, the doctrine of informed consent, if taken seriously, constitutes a revolutionary break with customary practice. Thus, I must review, albeit all too briefly, the history of doctor-patient communication. Only then can one appreciate how unprepared the medical profession was to heed these new legal commands. But there is more: Physicians could not easily reject what law had begun to impose on them, because they recognized intuitively that the radical transformation of medicine since the age of medical science made it possible, indeed imperative, for a doctrine of informed consent to emerge. Yet, bowing to the doctrine did not mean accepting it. Indeed, physicians could not accept it because,

for reasons I shall soon explore, the nature of informed consent has remained in the words of Churchill, "an enigma wrapped in a mystery."

Throughout the ages physicians believed that they should make treatment decisions for their patients. This conviction inheres in the Hippocratic Oath: "I swear by Apollo and Aesculepius [that] I will follow that system of regimen which according to *my* ability and judgment *I* consider for the benefit of *my* patients. . . ."[3] The patient is not mentioned as a person whose ability and judgment deserve consideration. Indeed, in one of the few references to disclosure in the Hippocratic Corpus, physicians are admonished "to [conceal] most things from the patient while attending to him; [to] give necessary orders with cheerfulness and serenity, . . . revealing nothing of the patient's future or present condition."[4] When twenty-five centuries later, in 1847, the American Medical Association promulgated its first Code of Ethics, it equally admonished patients that their "obedience . . . to the prescriptions of [their] physician should be prompt and implicit. [They] should never permit (their) own crude opinions . . . to influence [their] attention to [their physicians]."[5]

The gulf separating doctors from patients seemed unbridgeable both medically and socially. Thus, whenever the Code did not refer to physicians and patients as such, the former were addressed as "gentlemen" and the latter as "fellow creatures." To be sure, caring for patients' medical needs and "abstain[ing] from whatever is deleterious and mischievous"[6] was deeply imbedded in the ethos of Hippocratic medicine. The idea that patients were also "autonomous" human beings, entitled to being partners in decisionmaking, was, until recently, rarely given recognition in the lexicon of medical ethics. The notion that human beings possess individual human rights, deserving of respect, of course, is of recent origin. Yet, it antedates the twentieth century and therefore could have had an impact on the nature and quality of the physician-patient relationship.

From *Journal of Contemporary Health Law and Policy,* 10:67. Used with permission. Deletions approved by the author.

Editors' note: Some text and, author's notes have been cut. Students who want to read the article in its entirety should consult the original.

It did not. Instead, the conviction that physicians should decide what is best for their patients, and, therefore, that the authority and power to do so should remain vested in them, continued to have a deep hold on the practices of the medical profession. For example, in the early 1950s the influential Harvard sociologist Talcott Parsons, who echoed physicians' views, stated that the physician is a technically competent person whose competence and specific judgments and measures cannot be competently judged by the layman and that the latter must take doctors' judgments and measures on "authority."[7] The necessity for such authority was supported by three claims:

First, *physicians' esoteric knowledge, acquired in the course of arduous training and practical experience, cannot be comprehended by patients.* While it is true that this knowledge, in its totality, is difficult to learn, understand and master, it does not necessarily follow that physicians cannot translate their esoteric knowledge into language that comports with patients' experiences and life goals (i.e., into language that speaks to quality of future life, expressed in words of risks, benefits, alternatives and uncertainties). Perhaps patients can understand this, but physicians have had too little training and experience with, or even more importantly, a commitment to, communicating their "esoteric knowledge" to patients in plain language to permit a conclusive answer as to what patients may comprehend.

Second, *patients, because of their anxieties over being ill and consequent regression to childlike thinking, are incapable of making decisions on their own behalf.* We do not know whether the childlike behavior often displayed by patients is triggered by pain, fear, and illness, or by physicians' authoritarian insistence that good patients comply with doctors' orders, or by doctors' unwillingness to share information with patients. Without providing such information, patients are groping in the dark and their stumbling attempts to ask questions, if made at all, makes them appear more incapable of understanding than they truly are.

We know all too little about the relative contributions which being ill, being kept ignorant, or being considered incompetent make to these regressive manifestations. Thus, physicians' unexamined convictions easily become self-fulfilling prophesies. For example, Eric Cassell has consistently argued that

illness robs patients of autonomy and that only subsequent to the act of healing is autonomy restored.[8] While there is some truth to these contentions, they overlook the extent to which doctors can restore autonomy prior to the act of healing by not treating patients as children but as adults whose capacity for remaining authors of their own fate can be sustained and nourished. Cassell's views are reminiscent of Dostoyevsky's Grand Inquisitor who proclaimed that "at the most fearful moments of life," mankind is in need of "miracle, mystery and authority."[9] While, in this modern age, a person's capacity and right to take responsibility for his or her conduct has been given greater recognition than the Grand Inquisitor was inclined to grant, it still does not extend to patients. In the context of illness, physicians are apt to join the Grand Inquisitor at least to the extent of asserting that, while patients, they can only be comforted through subjugation to miracle, mystery and authority.

Third, *physicians' commitment to altruism is a sufficient safeguard for preventing abuses of their professional authority.* While altruism, as a general professional commitment, has served patients well in their encounters with physicians, the kind of protection it does and does not provide has not been examined in any depth. I shall have more to say about this later on. For now, let me only mention one problem: Altruism can only promise that doctors will try to place their patients' medical needs over their own personal needs. Altruism cannot promise that physicians will know, without inquiry, patients' needs. Put another way, patients and doctors do not necessarily have an identity of interest about matters of health and illness. Of course, both seek restoration of health and cure, and whenever such ends are readily attainable by only one route, their interests indeed may coincide.

In many physician-patient encounters, however, cure has many faces and the means selected affect the nature of cure in decisive ways. Thus, since quality of life is shaped decisively by available treatment options (including no treatment), the objectives of health and cure can be pursued in a variety of ways. Consider, for example, differences in value preferences between doctors and patients about longevity versus quality of remaining life. Without inquiry, one cannot presume identity of interest. As the surgeon Nuland cogently observed:

"A doctor's altruism notwithstanding, his agenda and value system are not the same as those of the patient. That is the fallacy in the concept of beneficence so cherished by many physicians."[10]

II. THE AGE OF MEDICAL SCIENCE AND INFORMED CONSENT

During the millennia of medical history, and until the beginning of the twentieth century, physicians could not explain to their patients, or—from the perspective of hindsight—to themselves, which of their treatment recommendations were curative and which were not. To be sure, doctors, by careful bedside observation, tried their level best "to abstain from what is deleterious and mischievous," to help if they could, and to be available for comfort during the hours, days or months of suffering. Doing more curatively, however, only became possible with the advent of the age of medical science. The introduction of scientific reasoning into medicine, aided by the results of carefully conducted research, permitted doctors for the first time to discriminate more aptly between knowledge, ignorance and conjecture in their recommendations for or against treatment. Moreover, the spectacular technological advances in the diagnosis and treatment of disease, spawned by medical science, provided patients and doctors with ever-increasing therapeutic options, each having its own particular benefits and risks.

Thus, for the first time in medical history it is possible, even medically and morally imperative, to give patients a voice in medical decisionmaking. It is possible because knowledge and ignorance can be better specified; it is medically imperative because a variety of treatments are available, each of which can bestow great benefits or inflict grievous harm; it is morally imperative because patients, depending on the lifestyle they wish to lead during and after treatment, must be given a choice.

All this seems self-evident. Yet, the physician-patient relationship—the conversations between the two parties—was not altered with the transformation of medical practice during the twentieth century. Indeed, the silence only deepened once laboratory data were inscribed in charts and not in patients' minds, once machines allowed physicians' eyes to gaze not at patients' faces but at the numbers they displayed, once x-rays and electrocardiograms began to speak for patients' suffering rather than their suffering voices.

What captured the medical imagination and found expression in the education of future physicians, was the promise that before too long the diagnosis of patients' diseases would yield objective, scientific data to the point of becoming algorithms. *Treatment*, however, required subjective data from patients and would be influenced by doctors' subjective judgments. This fact was overlooked in the quest for objectivity. Also overlooked was the possibility that greater scientific understanding of the nature of disease and its treatment facilitated better communication with patients. In that respect contemporary Hippocratic practices remained rooted in the past.

III. THE IMPACT OF LAW

The impetus for change in traditional patterns of communication between doctors and patients came not from medicine but from law. In a 1957 California case,[11] and a 1960 Kansas case,[12] judges were astounded and troubled by these undisputed facts: That without any disclosure of risks, new technologies had been employed which promised great benefits but also exposed patients to formidable and uncontrollable harm. In the California case, a patient suffered a permanent paralysis of his lower extremities subsequent to the injection of a dye, sodium urokan, to locate a block in the abdominal aorta. In the Kansas case, a patient suffered severe injuries from cobalt radiation, administered, instead of conventional x-ray treatment, subsequent to a mastectomy for breast cancer. In the latter case, Justice Schroeder attempted to give greater specifications to the informed consent doctrine, first promulgated in the California decision: "To disclose and explain to the patient, in language as simple as necessary, the nature of the ailment, the nature of the proposed treatment, the probability of success or of alternatives, and perhaps the risks of unfortunate results and unforeseen conditions within the body."[13]

From the perspective of improved doctor-patient communication, or better, shared decisionmaking, the fault lines inherent in this American legal doctrine are many:

One: The common law judges who promulgated the doctrine restricted their task to articulating new and more stringent standards of liability whenever physicians withheld material information that patients should know, particularly in light of the harm that the spectacular advances in medical technology could inflict. Thus, the doctrine was limited in scope, designed to specify those minimal disclosure obligations that physicians must fulfill to escape *legal* liability for alleged nondisclosures. Moreover, it was shaped and confined by legal assumptions about the objectives of the laws of evidence and negligence, and by economic philosophies as to who should assume the financial burdens for medical injuries sustained by patients.

Even though the judges based the doctrine on "Anglo-American law['s] . . . premise of thorough-going self-determination,"[14] as the Kansas court put it, or on "the root premise . . . fundamental in American jurisprudence that 'every human being of adult years and sound mind has a right to determine what shall be done with his own body,'"[15] as the Circuit Court for the District of Columbia put it in a subsequent opinion, the doctrine was grounded not in battery law (trespass), but in negligence law. The reasons are many. I shall only mention a compelling one: Battery law, based on unauthorized trespass, gives doctors only one defense—that they have made adequate disclosure. Negligence law, on the other hand, permits doctors to invoke many defenses, including "the therapeutic privilege" not to disclose when in their judgment, disclosure may prove harmful to patients' welfare.

[A] recent opinion illustrate[s] the problems identified here.* . . . [T]he Court of Appeal of California, in a groundbreaking opinion, significantly reduced the scope of the therapeutic privilege by requiring that in instances of hopeless prognosis (the most common situation in which the privilege has generally been invoked) the patient be provided with such information by asking, "If not the physician's duty to disclose a terminal illness, then whose?"[16] The duty to disclose prognosis had never before been identified specifically as one of

the disclosure obligations in an informed consent opinion.

Thus, the appellate court's ruling constituted an important advance. It established that patients have a right to make decisions not only about the fate of their bodies but about the fate of their lives as well. The California Supreme Court, however, reversed. In doing so, the court made too much of an issue raised by the plaintiffs that led the appellate court to hold that doctors must disclose "statistical life expectancy information."[17] To be sure, disclosure of statistical information is a complex problem, but in focusing on that issue, the supreme court's attention was diverted from a more important new disclosure obligation promulgated by the appellate court: the duty to inform patients of their dire prognosis. The supreme court did not comment on that obligation. Indeed, it seemed to reverse the appellate court on this crucial issue by reinforcing the considerable leeway granted physicians to invoke the therapeutic privilege exception to full disclosure: "We decline to intrude further, either on the subtleties of the physician-patient relationship or in the resolution of claims that the physician's duty of disclosure was breached, by requiring the disclosure of information that may or may not be indicated in a given treatment context."[18]

Two: The doctrine of informed consent was not designed to serve as a *medical* blueprint for interactions between physicians and patients. The medical profession still faces the task of fashioning a "doctrine" that comports with its own vision of doctor-patient communication and that is responsive both to the realities of medical practices in an age of science and to the commands of law. . . . Thus, disclosure practices only changed to the extent of physicians disclosing more about the risks of a proposed intervention in order to escape legal liability.

Three: Underlying the legal doctrine there lurks a broader assumption which has neither been given full recognition by judges nor embraced by physicians. The underlying idea is this: That from now on patients and physicians must make decisions jointly, with patients ultimately deciding whether to accede to doctors' recommendations. In *The Cancer Ward*, Solzhenitsyn captured, as only a novelist can, the fears that such an idea engenders. When doctor Ludmilla Afanasyevna was challenged by her patient, Oleg Kostoglotov, about physicians'

---

*Editor's note: The case is *Arato* v. *Avedon*.

ERRORS IN MEDICINE: NURTURING TRUTHFULNESS

Françoise Baylis

In "When a Physician Harms a Patient by a Medical Error," Finkelstein and colleagues maintain that patients have a right to the truth and that physicians have a corresponding obligation to be truthful. In their view, when an erroneous act or omission results in an adverse outcome for the patient, the physician should truthfully disclose the medical error, offer the patient a sincere apology, and explore the option of financial compensation. In the abstract, this seems reasonable—and some might even argue uncontestable. Why then is it not common practice for physicians to routinely discuss their errors with their patients? In this article, I will critically examine some of the reasons given by physicians for nondisclosure or partial disclosure, and then consider what the medical profession should do to foster more respectful, open, and honest communication about errors with patients.

WHY DON'T PHYSICIANS DISCUSS MEDICAL ERRORS WITH PATIENTS?

One reason for silence on the part of physicians, as regards not only their own "errors" but those of their colleagues, is genuine uncertainty about whether a particular adverse outcome is the result of an error.

Case 1

A 47-year-old woman is admitted to the gynecology service with suspected ovarian disease. She has a complicated past medical history, including four previous surgical interventions in the lower abdomen and adhesions. She is extremely distressed and very upset over the prospect of another operation. The surgeon considers the options and decides to try laparoscopic surgery as the least traumatic intervention possible. The procedure becomes

extremely difficult because of the adhesions and the woman's obesity. The surgeon accidentally nicks the posterior aspect of the bladder. Postoperatively the woman suffers an episode of abdominal sepsis.

In this case there is an unanticipated, unintentional outcome that harms the patient, but is there an error?

Not all harms that result from medical interventions (for example, sepsis, prolonged pain, prolonged hospitalization, additional therapy, permanent disability, death) are due to medical error. For example, some harms are a manifestation of naturally occurring statistical risk. Patients may perceive these harms as errors (especially if the informed-consent process is flawed and the patient does not understand and accept the possibility of an adverse outcome), but these harms are anticipated and predictable for a patient population, and ultimately they are unavoidable.

Medical errors, on the other hand, are avoidable. In general, errors occur when a planned act or omission fails to achieve its intended outcome and this failure has nothing to do with chance or inherent risk. In medicine, errors can happen because a physician doesn't know something she should know, doesn't properly execute a requisite clinical skill, or doesn't bring together the facts of a case in a manner that promotes good judgment. Such errors may be due to circumstances beyond the physician's control, such as unrealistic workloads, stress, and sleep loss. Alternatively, they may be the result of inadvertence, or they may be due to inexperience, ignorance, inability, or impairment.

Determining that a particular unfortunate outcome is the result of an avoidable medical error is not always an easy task. Medical mishaps (including errors) are often multifactorial—in a certain set of circumstances, a sequence or cluster of actions and decisions by different people combine in unfortunate ways that result in unintentional harm. Further, the view that a particular act or omission constitutes a medical error very much depends upon the social, professional, and cultural contexts in which the determination is made. Which is to say that there is an element of subjectivity in naming certain misadventures as errors and in determining levels of culpability. In the case described above it is debatable whether there was error and, if so, whether the error was due to substandard clinical skills or poor judgment in proceeding with laparoscopic instead of conventional surgery.

A second reason why capable, well-meaning physicians are loathe to disclose medical errors to patients is a belief that in many (perhaps most) cases, full disclosure serves no useful purpose—it only increases patients' anxiety and suffering, and contributes to a loss of confidence in the physician in particular and in the profession in general. At least two responses are possible here. First, in some instances, the belief is false—disclosure will not increase anxiety and suffering, nor undermine confidence. Errors can be more or less serious, more or less complex, more or less blameworthy. With minor errors (that is, errors with trivial or limited harmful consequences for patients)—which are the majority of medical errors[1]—increased anxiety and loss of confidence is an unlikely consequence of disclosure. To believe otherwise is to engage in elaborate self-deception, characterizing nondisclosure as "in the best interest" of patients.

Case 2

A four-year-old girl is admitted for investigation of a persisting anemia. There is careful discussion by the healthcare team of the need to plan these investigations well and to take no more blood than necessary. The clinical clerk is left to write the orders after rounds; inadvertently she orders some blood work for this child that was intended for the patient in the next room. When discovered, it is estimated that 10 ccs of blood were taken unnecessarily.

In other instances, as when there are serious errors or a series of minor errors, the concerns about increased anxiety and loss of confidence are accurate. This is not only a likely response, but arguably an appropriate one. Physicians or systems that are prone to serious errors are deserving of skepticism and distrust.

Case 3

A 58-year-old male is admitted for investigation and treatment of persistent hypertension. The junior resident admitting the patient finds a blood pressure of 240/190. He diagnoses this as malignant hypertension and initiates immediate treatment on the ward. A precipitous drop in the patient's blood pressure goes unnoticed in the absence of appropriate monitoring equipment. The man suffers a moderately severe stroke.

While physicians may express concerns about patients' anxiety, suffering, and loss of confidence, in cases with serious adverse consequences for patients, nondisclosure is typically motivated by self-interest or the interests of colleagues (for example, concerns about professional relationships with other physicians, diminished professional reputation owing to a perception of incompetence, fear of disciplinary proceedings or litigation). Efforts to cloak these interests in the "patient's best interest" are, at best, disingenuous.

A third reason why patients are not always truthfully told that there has been a medical error is fear of litigation. Of the many possible reasons given by physicians for nondisclosure, this is likely the most common. Many physicians believe that disclosure of a mistake and an apology will expose them to the risk of legal liability, and they fear not only the possibility of a successful suit but also the process involved (for example, stress and time). This belief, however, is false. Studies have reported that "the absence of explanations, a lack of honesty, [and] the reluctance to apologize," are factors that significantly influence a patient's decision to pursue legal action.[2] As well, physicians' fears are misplaced. Patients usually don't sue decent, capable physicians for their medical errors when the errors are openly discussed with them. Further, while it is reasonably easy for patients to threaten a suit (and for this reason there are many unmeritorious claims), the fact is that few negligently injured patients sue. For example, the recent Harvard Medical Practice Study of New York hospitals found that seven to eight times as many patients suffered negligent injuries as filed malpractice claims.[3] Also, one of the investigators with the Harvard Study who compared hospital files with litigated actions found that fewer than 2 percent of negligent adverse outcomes resulted in claims.[4]

Now in general terms, each of these reasons for less-than-full-disclosure of a medical error—uncertainty regarding the characterization of "error," concern for patients' well-being, and fear of litigation—may account for specific instances of nondisclosure or partial disclosure. They do not in themselves, however, account for the general lack of honesty with patients about medical errors. I want to suggest here that the more encompassing reason for nondisclosure or partial disclosure of medical error is widespread acceptance (if not endorsement) of the practice.

Early in their careers, physicians learn to "manage" medical errors; the coping mechanisms used include denial, discounting, and distancing.[5] Minor errors are typically denied, and this denial may involve negating the concept of error, repressing actual errors, and redefining errors as nonerrors. When the errors are of such magnitude that they cannot be denied, there may be an effort to discount personal responsibility, and externalize blame. And finally, when the physician can no longer deny or discount an error, distancing mechanisms are utilized in which human fallibility and the inevitability of error are embraced in an effort to temper feelings of guilt. At the same time that physicians are socialized into ways of coping with their medical errors, they observe entrenched practice that does not include routine disclosure of medical errors to patients.

In fact, the medical profession, the healthcare institutions in which physicians practice, medical liability insurers, and medical colleagues tolerate, expect, and sometimes actively encourage nondisclosure of medical errors. And so, the physician who discloses an error (and thereby displaces the myth of the infallible physician) must not only risk whatever negative responses may come from the patient (for example, anger, a lawsuit), but she must also risk a loss of personal confidence and self-esteem, diminished professional authority and reputation, as well as a loss of referrals and income. Typically, she risks these consequences alone, and possibly in the face of powerful opposition from colleagues and the profession. In this climate, many physicians who are inclined to be truthful are "led astray by fear or a drive for self-preservation."[6] Truth-telling appears to them to require an act of heroism, the duty to disclose having moved from

the realm of the obligatory to the superogatory. This brings me to a discussion of the profession's moral obligations in the face of physicians' silence about medical errors.

In my view, it is not sufficient to shine the moral light on decent, capable physicians and instruct them on their moral duty to disclose their medical errors without, at the same time, attending to the broader social context in which physicians are being directed to be truthful. Such attention suggests that changes to the structure and culture of medicine are needed to empower the capable (yet fallible) physician who is inclined to be truthful. In my view, such changes can be initiated by attending to the reasons for nondisclosure briefly outlined above.

WHAT SHOULD THE PROFESSION DO TO ENCOURAGE HONEST DISCLOSURE OF MEDICAL ERRORS?

First, it is important to provide a collegial and supportive environment in which (possible) medical errors can be discussed openly and honestly with colleagues. Such open discussion could provide a useful forum in which to determine whether an unfortunate outcome is or is not the result of a medical error. In those cases where it is determined that there has been a medical error, helpful suggestions could be made as to ways in which the error could be honestly explained without causing undue anxiety or a loss of confidence. Anecdotally, many physicians report that peer review committees and morbidity and mortality rounds are not always constructive arenas in which to explore errors and plan for their avoidance. Too often the focus is on the attribution of blame, which explains some of the defensiveness frequently exhibited by physicians. Conscientious and competent physicians who are responsible for, or have contributed to, an adverse outcome already experience anguish, guilt, and self-doubt. It is not contempt, but rather support and understanding, that will help them to acknowledge their errors and give them the confidence to discuss these with their patients.

Second, the profession might remind physicians that patients will experience emotions other than (or in addition to) anxiety, if (when) they discover that they have been lied to or misled by their physicians. Truthfulness is a cornerstone of the physician-patient relationship; lying is disrespectful and breeds mistrust and contempt.

Third, the profession might explore ways in which the determination of negligence could be dealt with separately from the issue of compensation. The arguments around comprehensive no-fault medical insurance schemes, where compensation is based on the fact that the patient has suffered an unintended or unexpected injury attributable to medical care (without regard to cause), are too numerous and complex to discuss here. There are important potential advantages, but also significant limitations.[7] The medical profession needs to participate actively in the ongoing process of tort reform with particular attention to what is best for patients, not just physicians.

Finally, attention must be directed toward the profession's obligation to create an environment in which truthfulness with patients regarding medical errors is an expected, common, everyday occurrence. Medicine is not error-free, yet in subtle ways the profession still promotes and reinforces the false belief that physicians are infallible. If the ideal physician is socially constructed as one who doesn't make mistakes, then the real physician who errs may be seen as uniquely fallible. Errors, however, are an "inevitable accompaniment of the human condition, even among conscientious professionals with high standards."[8] More specifically, "mistakes are inevitable in the practice of medicine because of the complexity of medical knowledge, the uncertainty of medical predictions, time pressures, and the need to make decisions despite limited or uncertain knowledge."[9]

The medical profession knows but has yet to accept this reality, as evidenced by the fact that there are all kinds of mechanisms in place to punish and reprimand those who err, but there are few mechanisms to praise and reward those who are truthful with their patients in disclosing their errors. Similarly there is little praise for those who are truthful about the errors of their colleagues. In fact, physicians who dare to report the error(s) of others are usually not revered for "doing the right thing" in the face of serious obstacles, but more typically are cast in the role of traitor.

In closing, the medical profession has a moral obligation to ensure that truth-telling not "fall outside the notion of duty and seem to go beyond it."[10] Truth-telling should not be the mark of the heroic physician, but rather a distinguishing feature of all decent physicians. If the profession is to meet this obligation it cannot continue to tacitly reinforce the status quo, but must strive to make changes that will clearly show physicians that honesty is valued. This will require important changes to both the structure and culture of medicine.

NOTES

1. L.L. Leape, "Error in Medicine," *Journal of the American Medical Association* 272, no. 23 (1994): 1851–57.
2. C. Vincent, M. Young, and A. Philips, "Why Do People Sue Doctors? A Study of Patients and Relatives Taking Legal Action," *Lancet* 343 (1994): 1609–13.
3. Harvard Medical Practice Study Group, *Patients, Doctors, and Lawyers: Medical Injury, Malpractice Litigation, and Patient Compensation in New York* (Cambridge, Mass.: Harvard Medical Practice Study Group, 1990), 6. See also, P.C. Weiler et al., *A Measure of Malpractice* (Cambridge, Mass.: Harvard University Press, 1993), 69–71.
4. T.A. Brennan, "An Empirical Analysis of Accidents and Accident Law: The Case of Medical Malpractice Law," *St. Louis University Law Journal* 36 (1992): 823, at 847.
5. T. Mizrahi, "Managing Medical Mistakes: Ideology, Insularity and Accountibility Among Internists-in-Training," *Social Science and Medicine* 19, no. 2 (1984): 135–46.
6. J.O. Urmson, "Saints and Heroes," in *Moral Concepts*, F. Feinberg, ed. (Oxford, England: Oxford University Press, 1996), 60–73.
7. L.N. Klar, "Tort and No-Fault," *Health Law Review* 5, no. 3 (1997): 2–8; R.E. Astroff, "Show Me the Money! Making the Case for No-Fault Medical Malpractice Insurance," *Health Law Review* 5, no. 3 (1997): 9–17; and "Medical Accidents," in D. Dewees, D. Duff, and M. Trebilcock, *Exploring the Domain of Accident Law. Taking the Facts Seriously* (New York: Oxford University Press, 1996), 95–187.
8. See note 1 above.
9. A.W. Wu et al., "Do House Officers Learn from Their Mistakes?" *Journal of the American Medical Association* 265, no. 16 (1991): 2089–94.
10. See note 6 above.

BIOETHICS IN A DIFFERENT TONGUE: THE CASE OF TRUTH-TELLING

Leslie J. Blackhall, Gelya Frank, Sheila, Murphy, and Vicki Michel

INTRODUCTION

The study discussed in this paper began with the concern that much of bioethics was a top-down affair. The ethical problems surrounding end-of-life care and the solutions to these problems have been defined by professionals (like the authors) who are mainly white, middle-class people with advanced educational degrees and good (or at least decent) health insurance. When we looked at care at the end of life, we were concerned about excessive, burdensome, and futile medical technology and with the right to chose and, especially, to refuse treatments. Advance care directives were invented to address these problems, to ensure that patients' rights to refuse excessive care were preserved when they were so demented or comatose that they were unable to communicate, or even know, what those wishes were. Having decided what the problem was (too much futile care at the end of life) and the solution (advance care directives), much space then was devoted in the literature on bioethics to promoting these documents. However, most studies that look at the use of advance directives, even those studies with interventions designed to increase accessibility, show that relatively few people actually have completed a directive.

The reasons why people do not complete advance directives are many and complex, but one reason may be that the concerns of bioethics professionals about care at the end of life are not necessarily those most important to all segments of the population. For example, it is questionable whether patients,

many of whom have no health insurance, who receive care at major urban hospitals are worried about getting too much medical care at the end of life. At these hospitals, their experience is more likely to be a fight for every bit of medical attention they receive, not fending off excessive care. Also, in the clinical experience of one of us (L.J.B.), it is not uncommon for patients and their families, particularly recent immigrants, to seem puzzled by, if not downright hostile to, attempts to involve them in end-of-life decisions.

Observations and reflections such as these led us to undertake a study to look at attitudes concerning end-of-life care among elderly people of different ethnicities. The purpose of this study was to examine and compare the attitudes and life experiences of people from African-American, European-American, Korean-American, and Mexican-American ethnic groups with respect to topics such as truth-telling, patient autonomy, advance care directives, and forgoing life support. This paper presents qualitative data from the portion of the study that dealt with the issue of truth-telling.

METHODS

This study used a combination of quantitative and qualitative research methodologies. After preliminary interviews, a review of the existing literature, and consultation with medical anthropologists who were expert in the groups we were studying, we developed a survey instrument designed to measure attitudes toward three main areas in end-of-life care: truth-telling and patient autonomy, advance decision making (such as advance care directives), and forgoing life support. This instrument then was translated into Spanish and Korean and pilot tested in all three languages. We recruited 200 subjects aged 65 and older from each of our four groups at 31 different senior citizen centers in the Los Angeles, California, area. (Elderly subjects were chosen because they

Leslie J. Blackhall, Geyla Frank, Sheila Murphy and Vicki Michel. Bioethics in a Different Tongue: The Case of Truth-Telling. Journal of Urban Health, 78/1 (March 2001): p. 59–71. Publisher: Springer.

Editors' note: Most authors' notes have been cut. Students who want to follow up on sources should consult the original article.

were more likely to have personal experience caring for a seriously ill or dying loved one.)

Interviews were conducted by an interviewer of the same ethnicity and the language of choice of the subject was used. Methodology for this part of the study has been reported elsewhere. With respect to truth-telling, our survey presented respondents with the case of a sick person who had been diagnosed with metastatic cancer by a doctor; we asked, "Should the doctor tell the patient that they have cancer?" In the next question, we stated that the doctor believed the patient would die of the cancer, and we asked, "Should the doctor tell the patient that he or she is going to die of the cancer?"

The second phase of this study began when the survey data were collected, and a preliminary analysis was completed. Medical anthropologists with expertise in the areas regarding our four groups then conducted in-depth ethnographic interviews with 10% of the original group. The purpose of these interviews was to illuminate and enrich our understanding of the findings from the survey data, to help explain seeming contradictions in that data, and to allow our subjects to speak their minds on issues of concern to them that we might have missed in our survey.

Subjects were selected using standard case sampling; however, in each group, we interviewed at least two subjects whose responses on the survey were atypical. This step was done to obtain insight into the diversity within groups. Within each group of typical or atypical cases, respondents were selected further for personal experiences with serious illness of self or family (as recorded in the survey), articulateness (as reported by survey interviewer), demographic characteristic (socioeconomic status, gender, and religion), and willingness to participate in a second interview. Participants were paid $25 for their time.

The qualitative interview guide was structured according to a standard set of domains and sections. Direct questions, conversational probes, and scenarios based on hypothetical cases were used to elicit open-ended responses about experiences and attitudes related to end-of-life care. All interviews (which averaged 1.5 hours long) were tape recorded and transcribed verbatim. Korean and Spanish language transcripts were translated into English, and the transcriptions and translations were checked

and edited by the anthropologist who conducted the interview. In discussions among the principal investigators and the anthropologist interviewers, the interviews were read and analyzed for emerging themes.

RESULTS

The data from this survey have been published elsewhere;[1] they are reviewed only briefly here. Almost all of the African-American and European-American subjects in our study believed that patients should be told the truth about a diagnosis of cancer (87% and 89%, respectively). Only 47% of Korean-Americans and 65% of Mexican-Americans believed in telling the truth about the diagnosis. With respect to telling the truth about a terminal prognosis, again the European-American and African-American respondents were much more likely to believe in open disclosure, with 63% of African-American and 69% of European-American subjects agreeing that a patient should be told. Only 33% of the Korean-American and 48% of the Mexican-American subjects agreed with telling a terminally ill patient about the patient's prognosis. Among the Mexican-American and Korean-American respondents, more years of education, higher income, younger age, and the ability to speak and read English predicted a positive attitude toward truth-telling.* Statistical analysis of the data, controlling for variables such as income, education, and access to care, revealed that ethnicity was the most important factor contributing to attitudes toward truth-telling.

---

*This was particularly important in the Mexican-American group, which was divided into two groups, one that spoke and read English and got their news from English-language media. The group generally had a higher socioeconomic status. The attitudes of those in this group on the survey tended to look more like those of the European-American group. The second group of Mexican-Americans spoke, read, and thought in Spanish; had a generally lower socioeconomic status; and had attitudes that were more negative toward truth-telling. The Korean-American group was much less diverse. In general, this group had immigrated to Los Angeles from Korea more recently, and few of them spoke English.

Although large differences among the attitudes of our groups with respect to truth-telling are apparent from the survey data, the reasons for these differences cannot be determined from the survey responses alone. For this reason, in the ethnographic interviews, we repeated the case and asked not only whether should the patient be told, but also why. Why is it okay or not okay to tell? If it generally is not okay to tell, does that include you? Would you want to be kept in the dark? Have you ever had the experience of telling or not telling the truth to a relative or friend? The remainder of this article presents the results of our analysis of these ethnographic interviews; these results have not been published previously. The themes that emerged from the interviews are presented below; quotations from subjects are included to illustrate each point. In the sections that follow, subjects are identified by RP (research participant) number and ethnicity (EA, European-American; AA, African-American; MA, Mexican-American; KA, Korean-American).

Themes

Patient Autonomy: "Because It's Me" Among the European-American and African-American subjects, the theme that emerged most frequently was that patients in general and the subjects themselves should know the truth because, as RP 001 (EA) put it, "I'd want to know the worst because it's me; I would have to face it." For the participants holding this belief, information about their bodies is theirs to know, good or bad, simply because it is *their* body.

Although the knowledge of a terminal prognosis may be distressing, if you are not told, someone else is making decisions that are properly yours, and this lack of control is even more distressing than the bad news. As RP 008 (EA) said, "If there's anything wrong with me, tell me; it's my decision what to do. . . . I happen to be a person that wants to control my destiny as much as I can." Even if there is nothing that can be done to cure the disease, the knowledge itself is a form of power. To be the owner of your own body and life, you need to know about yourself. RP 259 (AA) stated this succinctly: "I want to know everything about me." It is a patient's right to know this information and the doctor's duty to tell it since "the person was intelligent enough to go to the

doctor because he knew something was wrong, and he wanted to know what was wrong with him" (RP 263, AA). This complex of ideas, which is consistent with the patient autonomy model of bioethics, was mentioned by almost every African-American and European-American respondent interviewed. Many qualified their support for truth-telling with the idea that some people were not able to handle such information: "Some people, it would frighten them very much" (RP 022, EA). However, even those who worried that some were too fragile to hear the truth seemed to feel that most people could and should be told their diagnosis and prognosis, and that doctors should err on the side of truth-telling. The Korean-American and Mexican-American subjects, as we show below, were more likely to see truth-telling as cruel and potentially harmful rather than empowering, and they rarely mentioned the idea of a "right" to the truth.

You Know Anyway Related to the idea of truth as a right of the patient is the idea that patients will know, intuitively, that they are very sick or even dying, so there is no harm in telling them. RP 133 (EA) put it this way: "I think we have a sense of our bodies, and you know something's wrong, and it's better . . . to know exactly what," RP 108 (EA) said. "The person has a right to know, and I think internally a person has a feeling as to what the prognosis might be." The right to know is connected to the ability to know for these subjects. "It's my life, and I ought to know. 'Cause you got a feeling anyway. You know" (RP 301, AA). Ownership of your body gives you a right to truthful information; it also gives you the ability to sense this information before it is told. In comparison, some of the Korean-American and Mexican-American subjects agreed that the patient will know, but for these participants, this was a reason not to tell the patient the truth. "You don't have to tell the person about such a thing because, unless the person is a dummy, he or she will figure it out" (RP 451, KA).

Getting Your Things in Order One of the most common reasons given by our European-American respondents for wanting to know the truth about a terminal prognosis was so they could get their "things" in order. This rationale was much less common in our other groups. As RP 008 (EA) put it, doctors should tell the truth because "so many people don't have wills or anything else." "We feel that you need to take care of your business . . . make provisions for those who need to have provisions made for them. To me that's simply manly" (RP 22, EA). By getting your things in order, you can ensure that your family is cared for or, at the very least, prevent them from being burdened with complex financial matters after your death:

> You settle your affairs. You've got to have a trust or a will . . . and let your wife know where everything is, and go over the things with your kids and your family so you know that by the time I'm gone this is what's here and you do this and you do that. (RP 171, EA)

A subtext here is the desire to exert control in the face of an uncontrollable process, death. In this way, one could almost link the desire to complete a will prior to death with the desire to complete a living will prior to becoming incompetent. Both are attempts to extend the reach of one's control into situations in which, by definition, one otherwise is unable to exert any control. This interpretation is supported by the fact that, when our respondents were asked about living wills or durable power of attorney for health care, they frequently discussed the concepts of living trust and durable power of attorney for financial matters. At first, it seemed that our respondents were confusing the two concepts, but when pushed by our interviewers, it became clear that these two concepts simply were linked very tightly in their minds. Both types of document usually were completed in the same place (an attorney's office), often at the same time, and were saturated with complex meanings that revolved around the themes of mortality, burdensomeness, and control.

Get It Right with God   When asked about truth-telling, some of our subjects discussed the issue as one having religious or spiritual significance. According to this idea, you should know the truth so that you can get it right with God. This theme was mentioned most frequently by our African-American respondents. If you know the truth, you have time to "get right with the good Lord . . . so when you die, your soul is saved" (RP 347, AA). "There are too many things a person has to do with his life at that point, to be in ignorance of his

death . . . he has to go to his minister and . . . make whatever peace you have to make with your minister" (RP 252, AA). Even in the face of this knowledge, "When the Lord is with you, the devil can't do you no harm" (RP 289, AA).

Getting it right with God does not necessarily mean simply preparing your soul for death. If your doctor tells you that you have cancer, you have an opportunity to bring the problem to God, whose healing powers are greater than a doctor's. "I got another doctor, that's Doctor Jesus" (RP 201, AA). "[I would want him to tell me] because . . . I got another doctor I would go to that's the master of the universe, and let him tell me what to think about it" (RP 208, AA). If you know the truth, "you can prepare for it . . . ask your God [if you can live a longer life]" (RP 280, AA). "I want to know, can he help me; if he can't, tell me. If he can't help me, I go to the next person; that's the man above" (RP 364, AA). These answers reflect the belief that doctors are fallible and frequently can not know whether a patient will live or die. Only God is capable of having that kind of knowledge. As RP 289 (AA) said, "I wouldn't care if he told me because it wouldn't make it true. . . . I believe in the Lord just because he [the doctor] said you're going to die next week, I never will believe nothing like that." "Some [doctors] they say that, and they come out of it" (RP 280, AA). Doctors have one kind of knowledge and power; God another. "The doctors say what . . . the afflictions of the righteous is, but God delivers them out of it all" (RP 201, AA).

Interestingly, this theme of needing to know the truth so that one could become closer to God either for healing or for absolution simply was not mentioned by any of the subjects in the European-American group. This was a religiously diverse group that included (in roughly equal numbers) Protestants, Catholics, and Jews. Only one of our Korean-American subjects, a deeply religious convert to Christianity, mentioned this rationale: "Yes, I would [want to know the truth]. Then, I could repent for my sins before God" (RP 409, KA). Several of the Mexican-American subjects made similar comments: "I would not want to be deceived. . . . I would put myself in God's hands; I would repent for all my sins and for the bad things I have done" (RP 607, MA).

It Is Cruel to Tell In contrast to the European-American and African-American subjects, most of our Korean-American and Mexican-American subjects did not perceive the truth (especially the truth about a fatal prognosis) as empowering. Rather than envisioning the patient as an autonomous agent who needs information to make decisions and maintain control and dignity, the Mexican-American and Korean-American respondents viewed the patient as sick, weak, and in need of protection by the doctor and the family. Telling the truth in this context was seen as cruel. "Tell him [the patient] that he is getting better . . . because we should not be so cruel as to tell him, 'You are going to die, and it will be on such and such a day'" (RP 607, MA). Instead, it is kinder to "give him hope, console him . . . [so he can] always have hope that he will get better" (RP 607, MA).

> Anyway, the patient will die, so what is the use of saying you are going to die of cancer, right? The doctor should say, "You are okay; you will be fine. . . . Just take the medicine which will get you better." He shouldn't say that you have cancer so that you will die in a few months. Isn't that common sense? (RP 414, KA)

When one of our anthropologists commented to a Korean-American subject that, in America, most people were informed of their diagnosis and prognosis, the subject replied, "Yes, they are, because this allows patients to be prepared for death, but it must be very painful for those patients" (RP 447, KA). The benefit of "being prepared" here is seen as insufficient to outweigh the pain caused by knowledge of the truth. Of a son dying with liver cancer, one Korean-American respondent stated, "We just couldn't tell him because it was cruel" (RP 451, KA). She went on to illustrate this by telling how her son had guessed that he had cancer and had been very distressed:

> Holding on to me, he cried very, very sadly, saying, "Mother, I do not remember that I have done anything bad to others in my whole life. I do not know how I got stricken with this bad disease." . . . So, both he and I cried to the last drop of our tears.

This mother felt guilty that she had not been able to protect her son from the truth and did her best to make up for it: "After that, I comforted him so that he would not give up hope on himself."

Most of these subjects agreed not only that the truth should be withheld in general, but also that they would not want to know it themselves: "If they tell me . . . I have the terminal cancer, I will become more depressed because my life is coming to an end" (RP 605, MA). "I wouldn't [want to know]. . . . I would be afraid of dying" (RP 640, MA). One of our Korean-American subjects told us that, for many years, her children had hidden from her the knowledge that a surgical procedure was for cancer, and she stated, "My children did a good thing for me, not a bad thing. If I had researched what it was, then it would be bad for everyone" (RP 480, KA, after a cone biopsy).

Many of the respondents, especially the Korean-American respondents, were aware that patients often come to know the truth even if they are not told directly. As one subject put it, "The patient in critical condition could get an idea of what she or he has by the doctor's attitude. However, there is a difference in knowing about one's disease from guessing and from confirmation by others. I feel I don't want to know about my impending death . . . without hope, one cannot live. . . . So anyone who says that she or he wants to know about having a disease is out of their minds because the knowing itself is painful. If the patients have more stress, their lives are shortened" (RP 414, KA). This is discussed in more detail below; here, we just note that knowing, or rather guessing, is better than being told directly because it allows for some ambiguity and for the possibility of hope.

If You Know You Die Faster The truth not only is distressing according to these respondents, but also it potentially is harmful, even fatal. "It's not good to tell people what's wrong with them because they die sooner. . . . I told the doctor not to tell him" (RP 605, MA). "If the spreading cancer didn't kill her, the fear would" (RP 640, MA). One respondent told us the story of his brother, who died of cancer in rural Mexico. The truth had been kept carefully from him until almost the end of his life, when he happened to come by a mirror and see himself. Seeing how wasted he looked, he realized his condition. After that, according to his brother, "He never recuperated. . . . That is when he gave up. I think that [noticing how grave the illness is] is very bad for a deathly ill patient. If he has something to pick him up, his life is prolonged" (RP 666, MA). One of our Korean-American subjects brought his wife from Seoul, Korea, to Sacramento, California, for treatment without informing her of her condition: "We kept it a tight secret. . . . If she knew, she would not be able to live longer because of the fear" (RP 447, KA).

Some People Can't Take It   These themes, that the truth is cruel and harmful to patients, could be found in the transcripts of European-American and African-American subjects as well. Here, it almost always took the form of a statement that the truth is harmful for *some* people: "Some people just are not able, for whatever reason, to deal with unpleasant facts" (RP 007, EA). This almost always was qualified: "But, in general, I think you've got to level with people." (This statement was made by a man who felt that he could take it, but was not sure about his wife.) In this view, some people will not be able to cope after they receive such bad news; for these few, the truth is not empowering, but disabling. "Some people fall apart over nothing. And if the doctor knows the patient at all, he should be able to determine whether this person could handle it or not" (RP 259, AA). Some even admitted that they were one of the ones who couldn't take it: "I think it depends on the person. Some people can take the news better than others. . . . I'm a worrywart, and they tell me that; all positive things I would throw out of my mind" (RP 258, AA).

Not the Truth, but Hope   Although superficially the attitudes of our Korean-American and Mexican-American subjects toward the truth seemed identical, there were differences between them. As we reviewed the data from our Mexican-American subjects, we were confused initially by what seemed to be a contradictory and ambiguous attitude toward the truth in many of the transcripts. For example, one of our Mexican-American subjects told us that, "It is my opinion that the truth must always be told [to everyone]. . . . I would want the doctor to tell me directly" (RP 658, MA). However, speaking of a cousin with cancer, she told this story:

> She suffered a lot . . . and always asked me, "Isn't it true that I have cancer?" I told her, "C'mon, what cancer? It's not cancer." . . . It would have been more suffering if she had known what she had. (RP 658, MA)

A respondent (RP 666, MA) (mentioned above), said, "I think that [noticing how grave the illness is] is very bad for a deathly ill patient," about his brother, who died after looking in a mirror. Further in that same transcript, this respondent said that, "Knowing the truth helps to make you feel better because you can look for a way to cheer up and not get to the end of the road like the doctors thought" (RP 666, MA). When asked by our anthropologist how a doctor should tell a patient the truth, he replied:

> He would tell you gently [saying], "Now, we are going to do everything in our hands so you feel better; however, we will not stop you from dying, but the 2 or 3 days you have left should be happy, and don't think about leaving because maybe it won't happen." (RP 666, MA)

That is, the doctor should tell the patient that the patient will die in 2 or 3 days, but at the same time tell the patient that maybe they aren't going to die at all.

Another subject (RP 730) answered an emphatic "Yes" to the truth-telling question and at first denied that people die faster when they are told ("Those are just rumors"), but later told us that the patient should not be told about the prognosis: "It's better not to tell them that part to encourage her so that she thinks she's going to live more than she will actually live" (RP 730, MA).

Some of these seeming contradictions simply may be an expression of the complexity of the subject. However, the perceived contradictory nature of these answers actually may be another variant of the top-down problem mentioned above. At the start of this study, the authors identified an ethical problem: truth-telling. The issue for us was whether the doctor should tell the truth. But, for these subjects, it appears that the more appropriate ethical category is "hope," and the issue is whether the doctor and family take away hope. Taking away hope is prohibited because it is cruel and because it makes the patient die faster. The truth is not the main issue; the truth can be told as long as it is told in such a way as not to remove hope. You can tell the patient that he or she is going to die as long as you tell the patient that he or she might not die. This is why telling the prognosis is so much worse than telling the diagnosis.

As long as you tell the patient that the cancer can be cured, it is not so bad to tell the patient that they have cancer.

This interpretation is supported by two respondents in the Mexican-American group who actually had cancer. One of them had lung cancer. One of them had lung cancer. He agreed that people should be told the truth about their diagnosis, as he was. However, he admitted that he wouldn't want to know about a terminal prognosis: "No [don't tell me]. . . . It would torment me" (RP 615, MA). As far as could be determined from his description, he had only palliative (not curative) treatment (draining pleural effusions), but was convinced he was cured, or as he put it, "The tumor is dry" (RP 615, MA). (This case will be discussed in detail in a future paper.) The patient was told the truth about his diagnosis, but given hope.

Another respondent, with head and neck cancer, had a similar story. When asked if it was appropriate to tell the truth, he stated, "Oh, yes, because then [they could] connect me to a machine instead of having surgery and giving me therapy and X-rays. . . . He [the doctor] told me that it was going to get better with the machines" (RP 754, MA). Later, when asked about being told the prognosis, he said it was okay "for the doctor to tell me, but so that I won't become discouraged, to tell me that I am [going to live longer] even though I am not." Tell me the truth about my dying, but tell it in such a way that I do not have to face it without hope that I will live.

Hyodo and Nunchi   For the Korean-American subjects, the issue of truth-telling was tied to the concepts of *hyodo* and *nunchi*. Hyodo is usually translated as filial piety. It refers to the duties that family members owe each other, particularly the duties that grown children owe to their parents. One of these duties, as noted above, is the duty of the family to take care of sick relatives, to take care of the relatives' physical needs, and to take care of the relatives' physical needs, and to take care of the relatives' emotional needs by protecting them from the cruel and harmful truth. One example of good hyodo was mentioned above regarding the women who was kept in the dark about the reason for her cone biopsy (RP 480, KA). Another, more extreme, example was given by a subject whose wife was taken to open-heart surgery without her or her husband's

knowledge: "She had it done without [us] knowing about it" (RP 419, KA). (Amazingly, this was done in a Los Angeles hospital.) The husband who told this story offered it as an example of good hyodo. Another of our Korean-American subjects stated that, "It is okay for me to know my disease, but what can I do for her [my wife] when she knows she has cancer? . . . It can't be possible; I can't do it. She would like to know . . . but she shouldn't [be informed]" (RP 576, KA). Since almost all of our respondents felt that doctors should check with the family prior to telling a patient the truth and because of hyodo the family cannot tell even those who wanted to know that they had cancer, it makes it very unlikely that the patient will be told the truth. This brings us to the concept of nunchi.

Nunchi is translated frequently as a guess or a hunch, but it might also be translated as nonverbal communication. Your daughter tells you that you are getting better, that nothing is seriously wrong with you. On the other hand, you feel very ill, and you are going to the doctor all the time to get medications intravenously. By nunchi, you figure out that you have cancer. This concept, therefore, relates to the idea that people often know their diagnosis and prognosis without being told. Several of our respondents stated that they would want to know the truth, but that they would not expect to be told. Instead, if they did come to know it, it would be by nunchi. When asked if he would want to know the truth, one subject replied, "I would like to know it; I should." Later, however, in response to the question, "Do you think a doctor should inform his patients who have incurable diseases regardless of their age?" he answered, "The doctor wouldn't tell it to his patient directly, but the patient would be aware of it indirectly. Patients have to know. . . . The patients somehow end up knowing it [by nunchi]" (RP 517, KA).

Another subject (RP 489) stated:

As a patient, of course, I would want to know what I've got, but I doubt whether the doctor and the family would tell me the truth. They would not. If I were to hear the truth, the shock would be severe. . . . In terms of shock, not to inform seems better. . . . Telling you you have cancer, and it will be difficult to save your life gives a big shock, doesn't it? That's why the doctor should keep it a secret to the patient while informing the family of the fact; this may be the rule.

The patient wants to know, but does not expect that the doctor or family will tell him or her. If they care for the patient at all, they will try to keep it from him or her.

Learning by nunchi is more acceptable, as discussed above, because it leaves room for hope and perhaps because it comforts you to know that your doctor and children love you enough to try to give you hope. "if he told it to the patient, the patient would die more quickly. . . . I would try to know it, but he [the doctor] had better not tell me" (RP 563, KA). When speaking of their family members, even those who wanted to know the truth flatly stated that they would never tell a loved one:

> It is okay for me to know my disease, but what can I do for her [my wife] when she knows she has cancer? [How would I comfort her?] . . . It can't be possible, I can't do it. She would like to know . . . . but she shouldn't [be informed]. (RP 576, KA)

What Does It Mean to Tell?   This discussion of nunchi brings up the question, What does it mean to tell? As we can see from above, some of the Korean-American subjects who said they would like to be told actually meant they would like to learn the truth by nunchi, by nonverbal communication. The truth may also be told indirectly. One of our interviewers, who was from South America, told us how she learned that her mother had cancer. The doctor put her arm around her and said, "Your mother is very sick, and you must take very good care of her." The interviewer felt that this was a completely adequate disclosure. Later, when the mother was close to death, the doctor let slip the word "cancer," not to the mother, but to the interviewer's sister. Both felt that this had been a rude and insensitive thing to do.

A hospice patient from El Salvador of one of us (L.J.B.) provides another example of indirect communication. This man knew he had cancer; however, his family insisted he be shielded from the truth about his prognosis. The patient agreed with this. He asked that his son be in charge of learning all information and making all decisions about his care. However, the patient let the hospice team know that, before he died, he wanted to go back to El Salvador. A time came when he was told that he should go back to El Salvador. He was never told he was dying, but the information was conveyed. Even the patient mentioned above (RP 615, MA)

with lung cancer, who insisted that his cancer was cured since the "tumor is dry," by his action (making funeral plans, etc.) indicated that he had knowledge, on some level, about his actual situation.

This communication style is characteristic of what are sometimes referred to as "high-context" cultures. In a high-context culture, such as that of Korea, Japan, or Mexico, one is expected to infer from the social context many things without being told explicitly. Information is conveyed by nonverbal or indirect means. In low-context cultures, such as those of Germany and much of America, information is conveyed directly with detail and precision. Patients from low-context cultures who want to know the truth will expect to be told with this type of explicitness. The same is not necessarily true for patients from high-context cultures.

This may explain a situation that several oncologists have described to one of the authors (L.J.B.). If a doctor is asked directly by a patient from a culture such as that of Korea, usually considered high context, about his prognosis, the oncologist answers frankly. At the next visit, the patient complains, "How could you have said that to me? Don't you care about my feelings?" The patient is appalled that the doctor would be so direct. Instead of hearing, "You probably have 2 or 3 months to live," he was expecting to hear something like, "We are doing everything we can, but you are very, very sick."

Thus, people vary not only in whether they want to know the truth, but also in their understanding of what constitutes "telling."

CONCLUSION

This study of 800 elderly subjects showed that major differences exist in the way people of different ethnicities view the issue of truth-telling. One of the core differences, around which many of the themes circled, is the question of how the truth affects the terminally ill patient. On one hand, the truth can be seen as an essential tool that allows the patient to maintain a sense of personal agency and control. Seen in this light, telling the truth, however painful, is empowering. On the other hand, the truth can be seen as traumatic and demoralizing, sapping the patient of hope and the will to live. For those who hold this view, truth-telling is an act of cruelty.

In fact, many, if not most, of our subjects held both views. They differed in the relative weight given to each view. In weighing the positive benefits of the truth versus its potential to harm, the deciding factor seems to be the way the self is understood. Are we mainly autonomous agents whose dignity and worth come from the individual choices we make with our lives, or is our most important characteristic the web of social relations in which we exist? If we hold the former view (as most of our African-American and European-American respondents did), then lack of access to the truth is almost dehumanizing since it strips us of our ability to make choices, without which we are something less than fully human. If, however, we tend to see ourselves not as individuals, but as a part of a larger social network (as was more common in the Mexican-American and Korean-American groups), then the notion of personal choice loses something of its force, and we may expect that those close to us will act on our behalf to protect and nurture us in our time of need.

The second meta-theme that emerged from these data has to do with the many meanings of telling. When we began this study, we assumed that there were two possibilities: The truth could be told to or withheld from the patient. This is how the survey instrument was designed; respondents had to answer yes or no to questions about telling the diagnosis and prognosis to a patient with terminal cancer. However, many of our subjects, particularly in the Mexican-American and Korean-American groups, had a view with more nuances of how the patient could be told, or could come to know, the truth. According to these respondents, the truth could be told vaguely, partially; could be understood without telling, by context and hints; or could be known by nunchi. These types of telling allow for ambiguity and therefore for hope. This adds another layer of complexity to the issue of truth-telling and

calls into question not only whether, but also how, we should tell the truth and even what telling and the truth mean.

Limitations to these data should be noted. As with all qualitative studies, a relatively small number of subjects were interviewed (80, or 10% of the 800 survey respondents). Although we attempted to pick subjects for the ethnographic interviews whose survey responses were consonant with the norm of their ethnic group, as well as some who disagreed for comparison, it is inevitable that some points of view were not represented. Furthermore, this project focused on elderly people from only four ethnic groups in urban Southern California. We cannot know how other age or ethnic groups or those in more rural locations would respond.

Finally, it is important to note the danger of stereotyping. Data like these that compare the differences in attitudes among groups cannot be used to predict the attitudes of any individual within one of those groups. People can, and frequently do, disagree with the norms of their culture. However, if we do not try to understand how people of different backgrounds think, we will fail to examine our most deeply held beliefs. Instead, we may end up thinking that these unexamined attitudes are self-evident, in need of no justification: common sense. To some degree, this may have happened with bioethics. Beliefs commonly held in the European-American culture about individuality, self-determination, and the importance of maintaining control too often have been treated as if they were universal ethical principles. Only by allowing diverse voices to speak, and hearing the sometimes surprising things they have to say, can we ensure that we are addressing the real concerns of the communities we serve.

REFERENCE

1. Hare J, Nelson C. Will outpatients complete living wills? A comparison of two interventions. *J Gen Intern Med.* 1991;6:41–46.

OFFERING TRUTH
One Ethical Approach to the Uninformed Cancer Patient

Benjamin Freedman

Medical and social attitudes toward cancer have evolved rapidly during the last 20 years, particularly in North America.[1,2] Most physicians, most of the time, in most hospitals, accept the ethical proposition that patients are entitled to know their diagnosis. However, there remains in my experience a significant minority of cases in which patients are never informed that they have cancer or, although informed of the diagnosis, are not informed when disease progresses toward a terminal phase. Although concealment of diagnosis can certainly occur in cases of other terminal or even nonterminal serious illnesses, it seems to occur more frequently and in more exacerbated form with cancer because of the traditional and cultural resonances of dread associated with cancer.

These cases challenge our understanding of and commitment to an ethical physician-patient relationship. In addition, they are observably a significant source of tension between health-care providers. When the responsible physician persists in efforts to conceal the truth from patients, consultant physicians, nurses, social workers, or others may believe that they cannot discharge their functions responsibly until the patient has been told. Alternatively, when a treating physician decides to inform the patient of his or her diagnosis, strong resistance from family members who have instigated a conspiracy of silence may be anticipated.

This article outlines one approach, employed in my own ethical consultations and at some palliative care services or specialized oncology units. This approach, offering truth to patients with cancer, affords a means of satisfying legal and ethical norms of patient autonomy, ameliorating conflicts between families and physicians, and acknowledging the cultural norms that underlie family desires.

From *Archives of Internal Medicine* 153, no. 5 (1993): 572–576. Reprinted with permission of the American Medical Association.

COMMON FEATURES OF CASES

Mrs A is a woman in her 60s with colon cancer, with metastatic liver involvement and a mass in the abdomen. She is not expected to survive longer than weeks. Other than a course of antibiotics, which she was just about to complete, no active treatment is indicated or intended. She is alert. She knows that she has an infection; her family refuses to inform her that she has cancer. The precipitating cause of the ethical consultation, requested by the newly assigned treating physician (Dr H), is his ethical discomfort with treating Mrs A in this manner.

When one is confronted with a case of concealment, it is worth wondering how it came about that everyone but the patient has been told of the diagnosis, so that similar situations may be avoided in the future. Often, a diagnosis is defined in the course of surgery and disclosed to waiting relatives; this may most appropriately be handled by a prior understanding with the patient, communicated to the family, as to whether and how much they will be told before the patient awakens. But there are at least two other major ways in which a situation of concealment might develop.

A patient might be admitted in medical crisis, at a time when he or she is obtunded and incapable of being informed of his or her condition and treatment options. Law and ethics alike require that the medical team inform and otherwise deal with the person who is most qualified to speak on the patient's behalf (usually, the next of kin), until the patient has recovered enough to speak for himself or herself. Unfortunately for this plan, though, a patient will often fail to cross, at one moment, the bright line from incompetent to competent. Consequently, patterns of communicating with the relative instead of with the patient may persist beyond the intended period. Such situations have their own momentum. Later disclosure to the patient will need to deal both with the burden of providing bad news and with the fact that this information has been concealed from the patient up to that point.

A second typical way in which concealment develops is the following. A patient with close family ties is always attended by a relative (commonly, spouse or child) at medical appointments. Before a firm diagnosis is established, that relative manages to elicit a promise from the physician not to tell the patient should the tests show that the patient has cancer. Faced with a distraught and deeply caring relative, the physician goes along, at least as a temporizing tactic, only to discover, as described above, how the situation develops its own inertia. The cycle may be broken in a number of ways. Sometimes the physician simply decides to call a halt to concealment; often the patient's care is transferred to another physician who has not been a party to the conspiracy, as had happened with Mrs A.

> As clinical ethicist, I met with Dr H and the relevant family members (husband, daughter, and son). Most of the discussion was held with the son; the husband, a first-generation Greek-Canadian immigrant, knows little English and was at any rate somewhat withdrawn. As expected, they are a close family, deeply solicitous of the patient, and convinced that she will suffer horribly were she to be told she has cancer. They confirmed my sense that the Greek cultural significance of cancer equals death—something that in this case is in all likelihood true.
>
> At this time the family was willing to sign any document we wanted them to, assuming all responsibility for the decision to conceal the truth from Mrs A. "Do us this one favor" was a plea that punctuated the discussion.

Although other factors, such as the context of treatment and the patient's own idiosyncratic personality, may cause the same kind of problem in communication, my experience suggests the situation is often, as here, mediated by cultural factors. As one text on ethnic factors in family counseling puts it, "Greek Americans do not believe that the truth shall make you free, and the therapist should not attempt to impose the love of truth upon them."[3] (And compare Dalla-Vorgia et al.[4]) I often find other immigrant families of Mediterranean or Near Eastern origin reacting similarly, for example, Italian families and those of Sephardic Jews who have immigrated from Morocco. In all cases, in my experience, there is a special plea on the part of families to respect their cultural pattern and tradition. Health-care providers often feel the force of

this claim and its corollary: informing the patient would be an act of ethical and cultural imperialism. Moreover, the family not uncommonly feels strongly enough that legal action is threatened unless their wishes are respected. Mrs A's family, in fact, threatened to sue at one point when they were told that Mrs A's diagnosis would be revealed.

TELLING FAMILIES WHY THE PATIENT SHOULD BE INFORMED

By the time a clinical ethical consultation is requested, the situation has often become highly charged emotionally. In addition to the unpleasantness of threats of legal action, there may have been some physical confrontation.

> Mrs S was a Sephardic woman in her 70s with widespread metastatic seedings in the pleura and pericardium from an unknown primary tumor. Her family insisted that she not be informed of her diagnosis and prognosis. Suffering from a subjective experience of apnea, she was to have a morphine drip begun to alleviate her symptoms. The family physically expelled the nurse from the room. If their mother were to learn she was getting morphine, they said, she would deduce that her situation was grave.

Such aberrant behavior cannot fairly be understood without realizing that these families may be acting out of uncommonly deep concern for the well-being of the patient, as they (perhaps misguidedly) understand it. The health-care team shares the same ultimate goal, to care for the patient in a humane, decent, caring manner. This commonality can serve as the basis for continuing discussion, as in the above case of Mrs A, the Greek patient.

> Discussion with the family was long and meandering. The usual position of the health-care team was explained in some detail: patients in our institution are generally told their diagnosis; we are accustomed to telling patients that they have cancer, and we know how to handle the varied normal patient reactions to this bad news; patients do not (generally) kill themselves immediately on being told, or die a voodoo death, in spite of the family's fears and cultural beliefs about patient reaction to this diagnosis. Patients have a right to this information and may have the need to attend to any number of tasks pending death: to say goodbye, to make arrangements, to complete unfinished business. As her

illness progresses, decisions will likely need to be made about further treatment, for example, of infections or blockages that develop. Already, one of Mrs A's kidneys is blocked and her urine is backing up. If the mass should obstruct her other kidney, for example, should a catheter be placed directly into the kidney or not? These decisions of treatment management for dying patients are dreadful and should if possible be made by the patient, with awareness of her choices and prospects. In addition, Mrs A is very likely already suspicious that she is gravely ill, and we have no means of dealing with her fears without the ability to speak to her openly. Finally, the fears that the family expresses about the manner of informing her—"How can we tell our mother, 'You have cancer, it will kill you in weeks'"—are groundless: she must be told that she is very ill, but we would never advise telling her she has a period of x weeks to live—a statement that is never wise or medically sound-nor will we try to remove her hope.

The physician or other health-care provider may be primarily motivated by the ethical principle of respect for patient autonomy, grounding a patient's right to know of his or her situation, choices, and likely fate. Connected with this may be the correct belief that any consent to treatment that the patient provides without having an opportunity to learn the reason for that treatment is legally invalid. To be properly informed, consent must be predicated on information about the nature and consequences of treatment, which must in turn be understood in the context of the patient's illness. A patient cannot validly consent to the passing of a tube into the kidney without being informed that her urinary tract is blocked, or of the reason for that blockage.

These reasons, so determinative for the physician, often carry no weight with the family. In Mrs A's case, for example, the family pledged to sign anything we would like to free us of liability. Our response, that their willingness cannot affect either our moral or legal obligation, which vests in the patient directly, was similarly unpersuasive; nonetheless, it was a fact and had to be said.

The direct negative impact on the patient's care and comfort that results from her being left in the dark represents more in the way of common ground between family and health-care provider. It is often quite clear that failure to reveal the truth causes a variety of unfortunate psychosocial results.

As in all such cases, we highlighted for Mrs A's family the strong possibility that she already suspects she is ill and dying of cancer but is unable to speak about this with them because all of us, in our concealment and evasions, had not given her "permission" to broach the topic. Mrs A is dying, but there are things worse than dying, for example, dying in silence when one needs to speak.

It is also important to emphasize to families that the patient may have "unfinished business" that he or she would like to complete. For example, after one of my earliest consultations of this nature, the patient in question chose to leave the hospital for several weeks to revisit his birthplace in Greece.

Finally, it is sometimes the case that the failure to discuss with the patient his or her diagnosis can directly result in inadequate or inappropriate medical care. Mrs S, above, was denied adequate comfort measures because the institution of morphine might tip her off to her condition. In another case, the son and daughter-in-law of a patient insisted that she not receive chemotherapy for an advanced but treatable blood cancer so that she would be spared the knowledge of her disease and the side effects of treatment. In such cases, great injury is added to the insult of withholding the truth from a patient. Often, it is this prospect that serves as the trigger to mobilize the health-care team to seek an ethical consultation.

OFFERING TRUTH TO THE UNINFORMED PATIENT WITH CANCER

A patient's knowledge of diagnosis and prognosis is not all-or-nothing. It exists along a continuum, anchored at one end by the purely theoretical "absolute ignorance" and at the other by the unattainable "total enlightenment." Actual patients are to be found along this continuum at locations that vary in response to external factors (verbal information, nonverbal clues, etc) as well as internal dynamics, such as denial.

The approach called here "offering truth" represents a brief dance between patient and health-care provider, a pas de deux, that takes place within that continuum. When offering truth to the patient with cancer, rather than simply ascertaining that the patient is for the moment lucid, and then proceeding to explain all aspects of his or her condition and treatment, both the physician(s) and I attempt repeatedly to ascertain from the patient how much he or she wants to know. In dealing with families who insist that the patient remain uninformed, I explain this approach, a kind of compromise between the polar stances. I also explain that sometimes the results are surprising, as indeed happened with Mrs A.

> In spite of all the explanations we provided to Mrs A's family of the many reasons why it might be best to speak with her of her illness, they continued to resist. Mrs A, the son insisted, would want all the decisions that arise to be made by the physicians, whom they all trusted, and the family itself.
>
> If their assessment of Mrs A is correct, I pointed out, we have no problem. Dr H agrees with me that while Mrs A has a *right* to know, she does not have a *duty* to know. We would not force this information on her—indeed, we cannot. Patients who do not want to know will sometimes deny ever having been told, however forthrightly they have been spoken to. So Mrs A will be offered this information, not have it thrust on her—and if they are right about what she wants, and her personality, she will not wish to know.
>
> Mrs A was awake and reasonably alert, although not altogether free of discomfort (nausea). She was told that she had had an infection that was now under control, but that she remains very ill, as she herself can tell from her weakness. Does she have any questions she wants to ask; does she want to talk? She did not. We repeated that she remains very ill and asked if she understands that— she did. Some patients, it was explained to her, want to know all about their disease—its name, prognosis, treatment choices, famous people who have had the disease, etc—while others do not want to know so much, and some want to leave all of the decisions in the hands of their family and physicians. What would she like? What kind of patient is she? She whispered to her daughter that she wants to leave it alone for now.
>
> That seemed to be her final word. We repeated to her that treatment choices would need to be made shortly. She was told that we would respect her desire, but that if she changed her mind we could talk at any time; and that, in any event, she must understand that we would stay by her and see to her comfort in all possible ways. She signified that she understood and said that we should deal with her children. Both Dr H and I understood this as explicitly authorizing her children to speak for her with respect to treatment decisions.

The above approach relies on one simple tactic: a patient will be offered the opportunity to learn the truth, at whatever level of detail that patient desires. The most important step in these attempts is to ask questions of the patient and then listen closely to the patient's responses. Since the discussion at hand concerns how much information the patient would like to receive, here, unlike most physician-patient interchanges, the important decisions will need to be made by the patient.

Initiating discussion is relatively easy if the patient is only recently conscious and responsive; it is more difficult if a conspiracy of silence has already taken effect. The conversation with the patient might be initiated by telling him or her that at this time the medical team has arrived at a fairly clear understanding of the situation and treatment options. New test results may be alluded to; this is a fairly safe statement, since new tests are always being done on all patients. These conversational gambits signal that a fresh start in communication can now be attempted. (At the same time it avoids the awkwardness of a patient's asking, "Why haven't you spoken to me before?")

The patient might then be told that, before we talk about our current understanding of the medical situation, it is important to hear from the patient himself or herself, so that we can confirm what he or she knows or clear up any misunderstanding that may have arisen. The patient sometimes, with more than a little logic, responds, "Why are you asking me what is wrong? You're the doctor, you tell me what's wrong." A variety of answers are possible. A patient might be told that we have found that things work better if we start with the patient's understanding of the illness; or that time might be saved if we know what the patient understands, and go from there; or that whenever you try to teach someone, you have to start with what they know. Different approaches may suggest themselves as more fitting to the particular patient in question. The important thing is to begin to generate a dynamic within which the patient is speaking and the physician responding, rather than vice versa. Only then can the pace of conversation and level of information be controlled by the patient. The structure of the discussion, as well as the content of what the physician says, must reinforce the message: We are now establishing a new opportunity to talk and question, but you as the patient will have to tell us how much you want to know about your illness.

The chief ethical principle underlying the idea that patients should be offered the truth is, of course, respect for the patient's personal autonomy. By holding the conversation, the patient is given the opportunity to express autonomy in its most robust, direct fashion: the clear expression of preference. Legal systems that value autonomy will similarly protect a physician who chooses to offer truth and to respect the patient's response to that offer; "a medical doctor need not make disclosure of risks when the patient requests that he not be so informed."[5] A patient's right to information vests in that patient, to exercise as he or she desires; so that a patient's right to information is respected no less when the patient chooses to be relatively uninformed as when full information is demanded.[6] This stance is entirely consistent with the recent adoption of the widely noted (and even more widely misconstrued) Patient Self-Determination Act.[7] The major innovation this entails has been to involve institutions in the process of informing patients of their rights. However, the Patient Self-Determination Act has not changed state laws about informed consent to treatment in any way,[8] and as such the basic question here addressed—a physician's responsibility to inform patients of their diagnoses—remains entirely unaffected.

When offering truth, we are forced to recognize that patients' choices should be respected not because we or others agree with those choices (still less, respected *only* when we agree with those choices), but simply because those are the patient's choices. Indeed, the test of autonomy comes precisely when we personally disagree with the path the patient had chosen. If, for example, patient choice is respected only when the patient chooses the most effective treatment, when respecting those choices we would be respecting only effective therapeutics, not the person who has chosen them.

Many physicians hold to the ideal of an informed, alert, cooperative, and intelligent patient. But the point of offering truth—rather than inflicting it—is to allow the patient to choose his or her own path. As a practical matter, of course, it could scarcely be otherwise. A physician with fanatic devotion to informing

patients can lecture, explain, even harangue, but cannot force the patient to attend to what the physician is saying, or think about it, or remember it.

Families need to confront the same point. Ambivalence and conflict are often observed among family members concerning whether the patient who has not been informed "really" knows (or suspects, etc), and by offering the patient the opportunity to speak, this issue may be settled. More fundamentally, though, the concealing family—which is after all characterized by deep concern for the patient's well-being—will rarely (has never, in my experience to date) maintain that even if the patient demands to know the truth, the secret should still be kept. The family rather relies on the patient's failure to make this explicit demand as his or her tacit agreement to remain ignorant. Families can be helped to see that there may be many reasons for the patient's failure to demand the truth (including the fact that the patient may believe the lies that have been offered). If the patient wishes to remain in a state of relative ignorance, he or she will tell us that when asked; and if the patient states an explicit desire to be informed, families will find it hard to deny his or her right to have that desire respected.

Some families, naturally enough, suspect chicanery, that this approach is rigged to get the patient to ask for the truth. To them I respond that my experience proves otherwise: to my surprise and that of the physicians, some patients ask to leave this in the family's hands; to the surprise of families, some patients who seemed quietistic in fact strongly wish to be told the truth (which many of them had already suspected). We cannot know what the patient wants until we ask, I tell them, and we all want to do what the patient wants.

Having held the discussion, it is important to move on to its resolution as soon as possible.

I met with Mrs S's children, together with a nurse, medical resident, and medical student, for about an hour and a half; the treating oncologist also made a brief appearance. The discussion featured a lengthy and eloquent exposition by the resident of why Mrs S needs to be spoken to, and a passionate and equally eloquent appeal by one son to respect the different culture from which they come. Finally, I introduced the idea that we offer her the truth, and then follow her lead. This was agreed to by the family, and I left.

The medical student thanked me some days later and told me the rest of the story. The tension that had existed between health-care team and family had largely dissipated; as the student put it, "People were able to look each other in the eye again." Mrs S was lucid but fatigued that evening; for that reason, and probably because they had already spent so much time talking at our meeting, the family delayed the agreed-on discussion. Unexpectedly, Mrs S did not survive the night.

CONCLUSION

The problem of the uninformed patient with cancer can be described in many different ways, for example, as faulty physician-patient communication; as an obstacle to good medical care; as a cause of stress among hospital staff; and as a failure to respect patient autonomy. A dimension at least as important as these, but rarely acknowledged, is the clash it may represent between diverse cultures and their basic moral commitments.

The approach presented above reflects an effort to maintain accepted standards of the physician-patient relationship while respecting the cultural background and requirements of families. This form of respect involves reasonable accommodation to these cultural expectations but should not be confused with uncritical acquiescence. The critical question is, perhaps, this: How should we react to a family that refuses to allow the patient an offering of truth, that maintains that discussion itself to be contrary to cultural norms? Under those circumstances, I believe the offering must be made notwithstanding family demands. My reasons have as much to do with my beliefs about the nature of ethnic and religious moral norms themselves as with the view that in cases of conflict, our public morality (as concretized in law) should prevail.

First, I believe that members of a cultural community are as prone to mistaking what their own norms require of them as we within the broader culture are to mistaking our own moral obligations. The norm of protecting the patient clearly requires rather than prohibits disclosure in some cases, including some described above, to prevent physical

or psychological damage or to enable some final task to be consummated. All of the factors that we recognize sometimes to derange our own moral judgment—inertia, ill-grounded prejudices and generalizations, lack of the courage to confront unpleasant situations, and many more—may operate as powerfully in deranging the views of those from another culture. Their initial sense of what ethics require may, that is, be mistaken, from the point of view of their own norms as well as those of modern, Western, secular culture.

Second, even if a family's judgment of what their culture requires is accurate, we must not presume that a patient like Mrs A will choose, in extremis, to abide by her own cultural norms. Like any immigrant, she may have adopted the norms of broad society, or, acculturated to some lesser degree, she may act according to some hybrid set of values. Concretely, the offering of truth is about her diagnosis; symbolically, it is a process that allows her to declare her own preference regarding which norms shall be respected and how.

A last word is in order about the view implicit in this approach regarding the nature of a bioethical consultation. As these cases illustrate, patients, families, and health-care professionals come to a meeting from different moral worlds, as well as different backgrounds and biographies; and these worlds involve not simply rights and privileges, but duties as well. A successful consultation attempts to clarify on behalf of the different parties their own moral principles and associated moral commitments. It needs to proceed from the premise that all present ultimately share a common goal: the well-being of the patient.

REFERENCES

1. Oken D. What to tell cancer patients: a study of medical attitudes. *JAMA.* 1961;175:1120–1128.
2. Novack DH, Plumer R, Smith RL, Ochitil H, Morrow GR, Bennett JM. Changes in physicians' attitudes toward telling the cancer patient. *JAMA.* 1979;241:897–900.
3. Welts EP. The Greek family. In: McGoldrick MM, Pearce JK, Giordano J. *Ethnicity and Family Therapy.* New York, NY: Guilford Press; 1982:269–288.
4. Dalla-Vorgia P, Katsouyanni K, Garanis TN, et al. Attitudes of a Mediterranean population to the truth-telling issue. *J Med Ethics.* 1992;18:67–74.

5. *Cobbs v Grant*, 502 P2d 1 (Cal 1972) (a similar provision for a patient's right to waive being informed was established by the Supreme Court of Canada in *Reibl v Hughes* 2SCR 880 [1980]).

6. Freedman B. The validity of ignorant consent to medical research. *IRB Rev Hum Subjects Res.* 1982;4(2):1–5.

7. The Patient Self Determination Act, sections 4206 and 4751 of the Omnibus Reconciliation Act of 1990, Pub L 101-508.

8. McCloskey E. Between isolation and intrusion: the Patient Self Determination Act. *Law Med Health Care.* 1991;19:80–82.

CONFLICTING PROFESSIONAL ROLES AND RESPONSIBILITIES

VITALY TARASOFF ET AL. V. THE REGENTS OF THE UNIVERSITY OF CALIFORNIA ET AL., DEFENDANTS AND RESPONDENTS

551 P.2d 334, 17 Cal.3d 425, Supreme Court of California, In Bank. July 1, 1976.

TOBRINER, Justice.

On October 27, 1969, Prosenjit Poddar killed Tatiana Tarasoff. Plaintiffs, Tatiana's parents, allege that two months earlier Poddar confided his intention to kill Tatiana to Dr. Lawrence Moore, a psychologist employed by the Cowell Memorial Hospital at the University of California at Berkeley. They allege that on Moore's request, the campus police briefly detained Poddar, but released him when he appeared rational. They further claim that Dr. Harvey Powelson, Moore's superior, then directed that no further action be taken to detain Poddar. No one warned plaintiffs of Tatiana's peril.

> Plaintiffs can state a cause of action against defendant therapists for negligent failure to protect Tatiana.

The second cause of action can be amended to allege that Tatiana's death proximately resulted from defendants' negligent failure to warn Tatiana or others likely to apprise her of her danger. Plaintiffs contend that as amended, such allegations of negligence and proximate causation, with resulting damages, establish a cause of action. Defendants, however, contend that in the circumstances of the present case they owed no duty of care to Tatiana or her parents and that, in the absence of such duty, they were free to act in careless disregard of Tatiana's life and safety.

In analyzing this issue, we bear in mind that legal duties are not discoverable facts of nature, but merely conclusory expressions that, in cases of a particular type, liability should be imposed for damage done. As stated in *Dillon* v. *Legg:*

> The assertion that liability must . . . be denied because defendant bears no "duty" to plaintiff "begs the essential question—whether the plaintiff's interests are entitled to

legal protection against the defendant's conduct. . . . [Duty] is not sacrosanct in itself, but only an expression of the sum total of those considerations of policy which lead the law to say that the particular plaintiff is entitled to protection."

In the landmark case of *Rowland* v. *Christian*, Justice Peters recognized that liability should be imposed "for an injury occasioned to another by his want of ordinary care or skill" as expressed in section 1714 of the Civil Code. Thus, Justice Peters, quoting from *Heaven* v. *Pender* stated:

> whenever one person is by circumstances placed in such a position with regard to another . . . that if he did not use ordinary care and skill in his own conduct . . . he would cause danger of injury to the person or property of the other, a duty arises to use ordinary care and skill to avoid such danger.

We depart from "this fundamental principle" only upon the "balancing of a number of considerations"; major ones

> are the foreseeability of harm to the plaintiff, the degree of certainty that the plaintiff suffered injury, the closeness of the connection between the defendant's conduct and the injury suffered, the moral blame attached to the defendant's conduct, the policy of preventing future harm, the extent of the burden to the defendant and consequences to the community of imposing a duty to exercise care with resulting liability for breach, and the availability, cost and prevalence of insurance for the risk involved.

The most important of these considerations in establishing duty is foreseeability. As a general principle, a "defendant owes a duty of care to all persons who are foreseeably endangered by his conduct, with respect to all risks which make the conduct unreasonably dangerous." As we shall explain, however, when the avoidance of foreseeable harm requires a defendant to control the conduct of another person, or to warn of such conduct, the common law has traditionally imposed liability only if the defendant bears some special relationship to the dangerous person or to the potential victim. Since the relationship between a therapist and his patient satisfies this requirement, we need not here decide whether foreseeability alone is sufficient to create a duty to exercise reasonable care to protect a potential victim of another's conduct.

Although, as we have stated above, under the common law, as a general rule, one person owed no duty to control the conduct of another, nor to warn those endangered by such conduct, the courts have carved out an exception to this rule in cases in which the defendant stands in some special relationship to either the person whose conduct needs to be controlled or in a relationship to the foreseeable victim of that conduct. Applying this exception to the present case, we note that a relationship of defendant therapists to either Tatiana or Poddar will suffice to establish a duty of care; as explained in section 315 of the Restatement Second of Torts, a duty of care may arise from either

> (a) a special relation . . . between the actor and the third person which imposes a duty upon the actor to control the third person's conduct, or (b) a special relation . . . between the actor and the other which gives to the other a right of protection.

Although plaintiffs' pleadings assert no special relation between Tatiana and defendant therapists, they establish as between Poddar and defendant therapists the special relation that arises between a patient and his doctor or psychotherapist. Such a relationship may support affirmative duties for the benefit of third persons. Thus, for example, a hospital must exercise reasonable care to control the behavior of a patient which may endanger other persons. A doctor must also warn a patient if the patient's condition or prescribed medication renders certain conduct, such as driving a car, dangerous to others.

Although the California decisions that recognize this duty have involved cases in which the defendant stood in a special relationship both to the victim and to the person whose conduct created the danger, we do not think that the duty should logically be constricted to such situations. Decisions of other jurisdictions hold that the single relationship of a doctor to his patient is sufficient to support the duty to exercise reasonable care to protect others against dangers emanating from the patient's illness. The courts hold that a doctor is liable to persons infected by his patient if he negligently fails to diagnose a contagious disease or, having diagnosed the illness, fails to warn members of the patient's family.

Since it involved a dangerous mental patient, the decision in *Merchants Nat. Bank & Trust Co. of Fargo*

v. *United States* comes closer to the issue. The Veterans Administration arranged for the patient to work on a local farm, but did not inform the farmer of the man's background. The farmer consequently permitted the patient to come and go freely during nonworking hours; the patient borrowed a car, drove to his wife's residence and killed her. Notwithstanding the lack of any "special relationship" between the Veterans Administration and the wife, the court found the Veterans Administration liable for the wrongful death of the wife.

In their summary of the relevant rulings Fleming and Maximov conclude that

> case law should dispel any notion that to impose on the therapists a duty to take precautions for the safety of persons threatened by a patient, where due care so requires, is in any way opposed to contemporary ground rules on the duty relationship. On the contrary, there now seems to be sufficient authority to support the conclusion that by entering into a doctor-patient relationship the therapist becomes sufficiently involved to assume some responsibility for the safety, not only of the patient himself, but also of any third person whom the doctor knows to be threatened by the patient.[1]

Defendants contend, however, that imposition of a duty to exercise reasonable care to protect third persons is unworkable because therapists cannot accurately predict whether or not a patient will resort to violence. In support of this argument amicus representing the American Psychiatric Association and other professional societies cites numerous articles which indicate that therapists, in the present state of the art, are unable reliably to predict violent acts; their forecasts, amicus claims, tend consistently to overpredict violence, and indeed are more often wrong than right. Since predictions of violence are often erroneous, amicus concludes, the courts should not render rulings that predicate the liability of therapists upon the validity of such predictions.

The role of the psychiatrist, who is indeed a practitioner of medicine, and that of the psychologist who performs an allied function, are like that of the physician who must conform to the standards of the profession and who must often make diagnoses and predictions based upon such evaluations. Thus the judgment of the therapist in diagnosing emotional disorders and in predicting whether a patient presents a serious danger of violence is comparable to the judgment which doctors and professionals must regularly render under accepted rules of responsibility.

We recognize the difficulty that a therapist encounters in attempting to forecast whether a patient presents a serious danger of violence. Obviously we do not require that the therapist, in making that determination, render a perfect performance; the therapist need only exercise "that reasonable degree of skill, knowledge, and care ordinarily possessed and exercised by members of [that professional specialty] under similar circumstances." Within the broad range of reasonable practice and treatment in which professional opinion and judgment may differ, the therapist is free to exercise his or her own best judgment without liability; proof, aided by hindsight, that he or she judged wrongly is insufficient to establish negligence.

In the instant case, however, the pleadings do not raise any question as to failure of defendant therapists to predict that Poddar presented a serious danger of violence. On the contrary, the present complaints allege that defendant therapists did in fact predict that Poddar would kill, but were negligent in failing to warn.

Amicus contends, however, that even when a therapist does in fact predict that a patient poses a serious danger of violence to others, the therapist should be absolved of any responsibility for failing to act to protect the potential victim. In our view, however, once a therapist does in fact determine, or under applicable professional standards reasonably should have determined, that a patient poses a serious danger of violence to others, he bears a duty to exercise reasonable care to protect the foreseeable victim of that danger. While the discharge of this duty of due care will necessarily vary with the facts of each case, in each instance the adequacy of the therapist's conduct must be measured against the traditional negligence standard of the rendition of reasonable care under the circumstances. As explained in Fleming and Maximov,

> the ultimate question of resolving the tension between the conflicting interests of patient and potential victim is one of social policy, not professional expertise. . . . In sum, the therapist owes a legal duty not only to his patient, but also to his patient's would-be victim and is subject in both respects to scrutiny by judge and jury. . . .

The risk that unnecessary warnings may be given is a reasonable price to pay for the lives of possible victims that may be saved. We would hesitate to hold that the therapist who is aware that his patient expects to attempt to assassinate the President of the United States would not be obligated to warn the authorities because the therapist cannot predict with accuracy that his patient will commit the crime.

Defendants further argue that free and open communication is essential to psychotherapy; that "Unless a patient . . . is assured that . . . information [revealed by him] can and will be held in utmost confidence, he will be reluctant to make the full disclosure upon which diagnosis and treatment . . . depends." The giving of a warning, defendants contend, constitutes a breach of trust which entails the revelation of confidential communications.

We recognize the public interest in supporting effective treatment of mental illness and in protecting the rights of patients to privacy, and the consequent public importance of safeguarding the confidential character of psychotherapeutic communication. Against this interest, however, we must weigh the public interest in safety from violent assault. The Legislature has undertaken the difficult task of balancing the countervailing concerns. In Evidence Code section 1014, it established a broad rule of privilege to protect confidential communications between patient and psychotherapist. In Evidence Code section 1024, the Legislature created a specific and limited exception to the psychotherapist-patient privilege:

> There is no privilege . . . if the psychotherapist has reasonable cause to believe that the patient is in such mental or emotional condition as to be dangerous to himself or to the person or property of another and that disclosure of the communication is necessary to prevent the threatened danger.

We realize that the open and confidential character of psychotherapeutic dialogue encourages patients to express threats of violence, few of which are ever executed. Certainly a therapist should not be encouraged routinely to reveal such threats; such disclosures could seriously disrupt the patient's relationship with his therapist and with the persons threatened. To the contrary, the therapist's obligations to his patient require that he not disclose a confidence unless such disclosure is necessary to avert danger to others, and even then that he do so discreetly, and in a fashion that would preserve the privacy of his patient to the fullest extent compatible with the prevention of the threatened danger.

The revelation of a communication under the above circumstances is not a breach of trust or a violation of professional ethics; as stated in the Principles of Medical Ethics of the American Medical Association (1957), section 9: "A physician may not reveal the confidence entrusted to him in the course of medical attendance . . . *unless he is required to do so by law or unless it becomes necessary to protect the welfare of the individual or of the community.*" (Emphasis added.) We conclude that the public policy favoring protection of the confidential character of patient-psychotherapist communications must yield to the extent to which disclosure is essential to avert danger to others. The protective privilege ends where the public peril begins.

Our current crowded and computerized society compels the interdependence of its members. In this risk-infested society we can hardly tolerate the further exposure to danger that would result from a concealed knowledge of the therapist that his patient was lethal. If the exercise of reasonable care to protect the threatened victim requires the therapist to warn the endangered party or those who can reasonably be expected to notify him, we see no sufficient societal interest that would protect and justify concealment. The containment of such risks lies in the public interest. For the foregoing reasons, we find that plaintiffs' complaints can be amended to state a cause of action against defendants Moore, Powelson, Gold, and Yandell and against the Regents as their employer, for breach of a duty to exercise reasonable care to protect Tatiana.

CLARK, Justice, dissenting.
Overwhelming policy considerations weigh against imposing a duty on psychotherapists to warn a potential victim against harm. While offering virtually no benefit to society, such a duty will frustrate psychiatric treatment, invade fundamental patient rights and increase violence.

The importance of psychiatric treatment and its need for confidentiality have been recognized by this court. . . .

Assurance of confidentiality is important for three reasons.

DETERRENCE FROM TREATMENT

First, without substantial assurance of confidentiality, those requiring treatment will be deterred from seeking assistance. It remains an unfortunate fact in our society that people seeking psychiatric guidance often tend to become stigmatized. Apprehension of such stigma—apparently increased by the propensity of people considering treatment to see themselves in the worst possible light—creates a well-recognized reluctance to seek aid. This reluctance is alleviated by the psychiatrist's assurance of confidentiality.

FULL DISCLOSURE

Second, the guarantee of confidentiality is essential in eliciting the full disclosure necessary for effective treatment. The psychiatric patient approaches treatment with conscious and unconscious inhibitions against revealing his innermost thoughts. "Every person, however well-motivated, has to overcome resistances to therapeutic exploration. These resistances seek support from every possible source and the possibility of disclosure would easily be employed in the service of resistance." Until a patient can trust his psychiatrist not to violate their confidential relationship," the unconscious psychological control mechanism of repression will prevent the recall of past experiences."[2]

SUCCESSFUL TREATMENT

Third, even if the patient fully discloses his thoughts, assurance that the confidential relationship will not be breached is necessary to maintain his trust in his psychiatrist—the very means by which treatment is effected. "[T]he essence of much psychotherapy is the contribution of trust in the external world and ultimately in the self, modelled upon the trusting relationship established during therapy."[3] Patients will be helped only if they can form a trusting relationship with the psychiatrist. All authorities appear to agree that if the trust relationship cannot be developed because of collusive communication between the psychiatrist and others, treatment will be frustrated.

Given the importance of confidentiality to the practice of psychiatry, it becomes clear the duty to warn imposed by the majority will cripple the use

and effectiveness of psychiatry. Many people, potentially violent—yet susceptible to treatment—will be deterred from seeking it; those seeking it will be inhibited from making revelations necessary to effective treatment; and, forcing the psychiatrist to violate the patient's trust will destroy the interpersonal relationship by which treatment is effected.

VIOLENCE AND CIVIL COMMITMENT

By imposing a duty to warn, the majority contributes to the danger to society of violence by the mentally ill and greatly increases the risk of civil commitment—the total deprivation of liberty—of those who should not be confined. The impairment of treatment and risk of improper commitment resulting from the new duty to warn will not be limited to a few patients but will extend to a large number of the mentally ill. Although under existing psychiatric procedures only a relatively few receiving treatment will ever present a risk of violence, the number making threats is huge, and it is the latter group—not just the former—whose treatment will be impaired and whose risk of commitment will be increased.

Both the legal and psychiatric communities recognize that the process of determining potential violence in a patient is far from exact, being fraught with complexity and uncertainty.[4] In fact, precision has not even been attained in predicting who of those having already committed violent acts will again become violent, a task recognized to be of much simpler proportions.

This predictive uncertainty means that the number of disclosures will necessarily be large. As noted above, psychiatric patients are encouraged to discuss all thoughts of violence, and they often express such thoughts. However, unlike this court, the psychiatrist does not enjoy the benefit of overwhelming hindsight in seeing which few, if any, of his patients will ultimately become violent. Now, confronted by the majority's new duty, the psychiatrist must instantaneously calculate potential violence from each patient on each visit. The difficulties researchers have encountered in accurately predicting violence will be heightened for the practicing psychiatrist dealing for brief periods in his office with heretofore nonviolent patients. And, given that the decision not to warn or commit must always be made at the psychiatrist's civil peril, one can expect most doubts will be resolved in favor of the psychiatrist protecting himself.

Neither alternative open to the psychiatrist seeking to protect himself is in the public interest. The warning itself is an impairment of the psychiatrist's ability to treat, depriving many patients of adequate treatment. It is to be expected that after disclosing their threats, a significant number of patients, who would not become violent if treated according to existing practices, will engage in violent conduct as a result of unsuccessful treatment. In short, the majority's duty to warn will not only impair treatment of many who would never become violent, but worse, will result in a net increase in violence.[5]

NOTES

1. Fleming and Maximov, *The Patient or His Victim: The Therapist's Dilemma* (1974) 62 Cal.L.Rev. 1025, 1030.
2. Butler, *Psychotherapy and Griswold: Is Confidentiality a Privilege or a Right?* (1971) 3 Conn.L.Rev. 599, 604.
3. Dawidoff, *The Malpractice of Psychiatrists* (1966) Duke L.J. 696, 704.
4. A shocking illustration of psychotherapists' inability to predict dangerousness, cited by this court in *People v. Burnick, supra,* 14 Cal.3d 306, 326–327, fn. 17, 121 Cal.Rptr. 488, 535 P.2d 352, is cited and discussed in Ennis, *Prisoners of Psychiatry: Mental Patients, Psychiatrists, and the Law* (1972): "In a well-known study, psychiatrists predicted that 989 persons were so dangerous that they could not be kept even in civil mental hospitals, but would have to be kept in maximum security hospitals run by the Department of Corrections. Then, because of a United States Supreme Court decision, those persons were transferred to civil hospitals. After a year, the Department of Mental Hygiene reported that one-fifth of them had been discharged to the community, and over half had agreed to remain as voluntary patients. During the year, only 7 of the 989 committed or threatened any act that was sufficiently dangerous to require retransfer to the maximum security hospital. Seven correct predictions out of almost a thousand is not a very impressive record. Other studies, and there are many, have reached the same conclusion: psychiatrists simply cannot predict dangerous behavior." (*Id.* at p. 227.) Equally illustrative studies are collected in Rosenhan, *On Being Sane in Insane Places* (1973) 13 Santa Clara Law. 379, 384; Ennis & Litwack, *Psychiatry and the Presumption of Expertise: Flipping Coins in the Courtroom, supra,* 62 Cal.L.Rev. 693, 750–751.

5. The majority concedes that psychotherapeutic dialogue often results in the patient expressing threats of violence that are rarely executed. (*Ante,* p. 441, p. 27 of 131 Cal.Rptr., p. 347 of 551 P.2d.) The practical problem, of course, lies in ascertaining which threats from which patients will be carried out. As to this problem, the majority is silent. They do, however, caution that a therapist certainly "should not be encouraged routinely to reveal such threats; such disclosures could seriously disrupt the patient's relationships with his therapist and with the persons threatened." (*Id.*)

Thus, in effect, the majority informs the therapists that they must accurately predict dangerousness—a task recognized as extremely difficult—or face crushing civil liability. The majority's reliance on the traditional standard of care for professionals that "therapist need only exercise 'that reasonable degree of skill, knowledge, and care ordinarily possessed and exercised by members of [that professional specialty] under similar circumstances'" (*ante,* p. 438, p. 25 of 131 Cal.Rptr., p. 345 of 551 P.2d) is seriously misplaced. This standard of care assumes that, to a large extent, the subject matter of the specialty is ascertainable. One clearly ascertainable element in the psychiatric field is that the therapist cannot accurately predict dangerousness, which, in turn, means that the standard is inappropriate for lack of a relevant criterion by which to judge the therapist's decision. The inappropriateness of the standard the majority would have us use is made patent when consideration is given to studies, by several eminent authorities, indicating that "[t]he chances of a second psychiatrist agreeing with the diagnosis of a first psychiatrist 'are barely better than 50–50; or stated differently, there is about as much chance that a different expert would come to some different conclusion as there is that the other would agree.'" (Ennis & Litwack, *Psychiatry and the Presumption of Expertise: Flipping Coins in the Courtroom, supra,* 62 Cal.L.Rev. 693, 701, quoting Ziskin, Coping With Psychiatric and Psychological Testimony, 126.) The majority's attempt to apply a normative scheme to a profession which must be concerned with problems that balk at standardization is clearly erroneous.

In any event, an ascertainable standard would not serve to limit psychiatrist disclosure of threats with the resulting impairment of treatment. However compassionate, the psychiatrist hearing the threat remains faced with potential crushing civil liability for a mistaken evaluation of his patient and will be forced to resolve even the slightest doubt in favor of disclosure or commitment.

PLEASE DON'T TELL!

The patient, Carlos R., was a twenty-one-year-old Hispanic male who had suffered gunshot wounds to the abdomen in gang violence. He was uninsured. His stay in the hospital was somewhat shorter than might have been expected, but otherwise unremarkable. It was felt that he could safely complete his recovery at home. Carlos admitted to his attending physician that he was HIV-positive, which was confirmed.

At discharge the attending physician recommended a daily home nursing visit for wound care. However, Medicaid would not fund this nursing visit because a care-

From *Hastings Center Report* (November–December 1991): 39–40. Reprinted by permission of The Hastings Center.

giver lived in the home who could adequately provide this care, namely, the patient's twenty-two-year-old sister Consuela, who in fact was willing to accept this burden. Their mother had died almost ten years ago, and Consuela had been a mother to Carlos and their younger sister since then. Carlos had no objection to Consuela's providing this care, but he insisted absolutely that she was not to know his HIV status. He had always been on good terms with Consuela, but she did not know he was actively homosexual. His greatest fear, though, was that his father would learn of his homosexual orientation, which is generally looked upon with great disdain by Hispanics.

Would Carlos's physician be morally justified in breaching patient confidentiality on the grounds that he had a "duty to warn"?

COMMENTARY

Leonard Fleck

If there were a home health nurse to care for this patient, presumably there would be no reason to breach confidentiality since the expectation would be that she would follow universal precautions. Of course, universal precautions could be explained to the patient's sister. In an ideal world this would seem to be a satisfactory response that protects both Carlos's rights and Consuela's welfare. But the world is not ideal.

We know that health professionals, who surely ought to have the knowledge that would motivate them to take universal precautions seriously, often fail to take just such precautions. It is easy to imagine that Consuela could be equally casual or careless, especially when she had not been specifically warned that her brother was HIV-infected. Given this possibility, does the physician have a duty to

warn that would justify breaching confidentiality? I shall argue that he may not breach confidentiality but he must be reasonably attentive to Consuela's safety. Ordinarily the conditions that must be met to invoke a duty to warn are: (1) an imminent threat of serious and irreversible harm, (2) no alternative to averting that threat other than this breach of confidentiality, and (3) proportionality between the harm averted by this breach of confidentiality and the harm associated with such a breach. In my judgment, none of these conditions are satisfactorily met.

No one doubts that becoming HIV-infected represents a serious and irreversible harm. But, in reality, is that threat imminent enough to justify breaching confidentiality? If we were talking about two individuals who were going to have intercourse on repeated occasions, then the imminence condition would likely be met. But the patient's sister will be caring for his wound for only a week or two, and wound care does not by itself involve any exchange of body fluids. If we had two-hundred and forty surgeons operating on two-hundred and forty HIV-infected patients, and if each of those surgeons nicked himself while doing surgery, then the likelihood is that only one of them would become HIV-infected. Using this as a reference point, the likelihood of this young woman seroconverting if her intact skin comes into contact with the blood of this patient is very remote at best.

Moreover in this instance there are alternatives. A frank and serious discussion with Consuela about the need for universal precautions, plus monitored, thorough training in correct wound care, fulfills what I would regard as a reasonable duty to warn in these circumstances. Similar instructions ought to be given to Carlos so that he can monitor her performance. He can be reminded that this is a small price for protecting his confidentiality as well as his sister's health. It might also be necessary to provide gloves and other such equipment required to observe universal precautions.

We can imagine easily enough that there might be a lapse in conscientiousness on Consuela's part, that she might come into contact with his blood. But even if this were to happen, the likelihood of her seroconverting is remote at best. This is where proportionality between the harm averted by the breach and the harm associated with it comes in. For if confidentiality were breached and she were informed of his HIV status, this would likely have very serious consequences for Carlos. As a layperson with no

professional duty to preserve confidentiality herself, Consuela might inform other family members, which could lead to his being ostracized from the family. And even if she kept the information confidential, she might be too afraid to provide the care for Carlos, who might then end up with no one to care for him.

The right to confidentiality is a right that can be freely waived. The physician could engage Carlos in a frank moral discussion aimed at persuading him that the reasonable and decent thing to do is to inform his sister of his HIV status. Perhaps the physician offers assurances she would be able to keep that information in strict confidence. The patient agrees. Then what happens? It is easy to imagine that Consuela balks at caring for her brother, for fear of infection.

Medicaid would still refuse to pay for home nursing care because a caregiver would still be in the home, albeit a terrified caregiver. Consuela's response may not be rational, but it is possible. If she were to react in this way it would be an easy "out" to say that it was Carlos who freely agreed to the release of the confidential information so now he'll just have to live with those consequences. But the matter is really more complex than that. At the very least the physician would have to apprise Carlos of the fact that his sister might divulge his HIV status to some number of other individuals. But if the physician impresses this possibility on Carlos vividly enough, Carlos might be even more reluctant to self-disclose his HIV status to Consuela. In that case the physician is morally obligated to respect that confidentiality.

COMMENTARY

Marcia Angell

It would be wrong, I believe, to ask this young woman to undertake the nursing care of her brother and not inform her that he is HIV-infected.

The claim of a patient that a doctor hold his secrets in confidence is strong but not absolute. It

can be overridden by stronger, competing claims. For example, a doctor would not agree to hold in confidence a diagnosis of rubella, if the patient were planning to be in the presence of a pregnant woman without warning her. Similarly, a doctor would be justified in acting on knowledge that a patient planned to commit a crime. Confidentiality should, of course, be honored when the secret is entirely personal, that is, when it could have no impact on anyone else. On the other hand, when it would pose a major threat to others, the claim of confidentiality must be overridden. Difficulties arise when the competing claims are nearly equal in moral weight.

In this scenario, does Consuela have any claims on the doctor? I believe she does, and that her claims are very compelling. They stem, first, from her right to have information she might consider relevant to her decision to act as her brother's nurse, and, second, from the health care system's obligation to warn of a possible risk to her health. I would like to focus first on whether Consuela has a right to information apart from the question of whether there is in fact an appreciable risk. I believe that she has such a right, for three reasons.

First, there is an element of deception in *not* informing Consuela that her brother is HIV-infected. Most people in her situation would want to know if their "patient" were HIV-infected and would presume that they would be told if that were the case. (I suspect that a private nurse hired in a similar situation would expect to be told—and that she would be.) At some level, perhaps unconsciously, Consuela would assume that Carlos did not have HIV infection because no one said that he did. Thus, in keeping Carlos's secret, the doctor implicitly deceives Consuela—not a net moral gain, I think.

Second, Consuela has been pressed to provide nursing care in part because the health system is using her to avoid providing a service it would otherwise be responsible for. This fact, I believe, gives the health care system an additional obligation to her, which includes giving her all the information that might bear on her decision to accept this responsibility. It might be argued that the information about her brother's HIV infection is not relevant, but it is patronizing to make this assumption. She may for any number of reasons, quite apart from the risk of transmission, find it important to know that he is HIV-infected.

Finally, I can't help feeling that this young woman has already been exploited by her family and that the health care system should not collude in doing so again. We are told that since she was twelve, she has acted as "mother" to a brother only one year younger, presumably simply because she is female, since she is no more a mother than he is. Now she is being asked to be a nurse, as well as a mother, again presumably because she is female. In this context, concerns about the sensibilities of the father or about Carlos's fear of them are not very compelling, particularly when they are buttressed by stereotypes about Hispanic families. Furthermore, both his father and his sister will almost certainly learn the truth eventually.

What about the risk of transmission from Carlos to Consuela? Many would—wrongly, I believe—base their arguments solely on this question. Insofar as they did, they would have very little to go on. The truth is that no one knows what the risk would be to Consuela. To my knowledge, there have been no studies that would yield data on the point. Most likely the risk would be extremely small, particularly if there were no blood or pus in the wound, but it would be speculative to say how small. We do know that Consuela has no experience with universal precautions and could not be expected to use them diligently with her brother unless she had some sense of why she might be doing so. In any case, the doctor has no right to decide for this young woman that she should assume a risk, even if he believes it would be remote. That is for her to decide. The only judgment he has a right to make is whether *she* might consider the information that her brother is HIV-infected to be relevant to her decision to nurse him, and I think it is reasonable to assume she might.

There is, I believe, only one ethical way out of this dilemma. The doctor should strongly encourage Carlos to tell his sister that he is HIV-infected or offer to do it for him. She could be asked not to tell their father, and I would see no problem with this. I would have no hesitation in appealing to the fact that Carlos already owes Consuela a great deal. If Carlos insisted that his sister not be told, the doctor should see to it that his nursing needs are met in some other way. In sum, then, I believe the doctor should pass the dilemma to the patient: Carlos can decide to accept Consuela's generosity—in return for which he must tell her he is HIV-infected (or ask the doctor to tell her)—or he can decide not to tell her and do without her nursing care.

DISCLOSING MISATTRIBUTED PATERNITY

Lainie Friedman Ross

INTRODUCTION

Genetic counseling is the process by which individuals are informed about the risks to themselves and/or their offspring of genetic diseases and susceptibilities. The counseling provides information about genetic conditions, their inheritance, short- and long-term implications, and, when relevant, procreative options. To promote "client autonomy," geneticists and genetic counselors emphasize information giving and truth telling. Yet there are situations in which genetic counselors do not disclose pertinent information to all involved parties. The focus of this paper is on one such situation: the case of "non-paternity" or misattributed paternity. In 1990, Dorothy Wertz, John C. Fletcher, and John Mulvihill reported on an international study conducted in 1985–6 in which 1,053 M.D. and Ph.D. geneticists in 18 nations analyzed frequent ethical dilemmas in medical genetics. One case depicted a child with an autosomal recessive disorder for which carrier testing was possible and accurate. Genetic workup revealed that her husband was not the biological father. Of the 677 respondents, 96% believed that "protection of the mother's confidentiality overrode disclosure of true paternity."[1] Of these, 81% said they would tell the woman alone; 13% would tell the couple that they were both genetically responsible, and 2% would ascribe the child's disorder to a new mutation which was unrepeatable. The same question was asked by Deborah Pencarinha, Nora K. Bell, Janice G. Edwards, and Robert

G. Best in a 1989 survey of non-doctoral genetic counselors, and their results were even more uniform. Pencarinha *et al.* surveyed 545 counselors. Of the 199 respondents, 98.5% said that they would not disclose misattributed paternity to the male partner in order "to preserve patient confidentiality."[2] Because of their similarity of views, I will refer to both groups when I use the term "counselor."

This practice of the counselors contradicts the recommendations of the President's Commission for the Study of Ethical Problems in Biomedical and Behavioral Research (1983) which studied the question of misattributed paternity. The President's Commission recommended that misattributed paternity be disclosed to both partners.[3] In 1994, however, the Committee on Assessing Genetic Risks of the Institute of Medicine (IOM) recommended that only the woman be informed and that misattributed paternity should not be disclosed to her partner.[4] The IOM's major justification was similar to the rationale given by the genetic counselors: "Genetic testing should not be used in ways that disrupt families."

From Lainie Friedman Ross, "Disclosing Misattributed Paternity," *Bioethics*, Blackwell Publishers.

Editors' note: Some author's notes have been cut. Students who want to follow up on sources should consult the original article.

1. Dorothy Wertz, John C. Fletcher, and John J. Mulvihill, "Medical Geneticists Confront Ethical Dilemmas: Cross-cultural Comparisons among 19 Nations," *American Journal of Human Genetics* 1990; 46; 1202.

2. Deborah F. Pencarinha, Nora K. Bell, Janice G. Edwards, and Robert G. Best, "Ethical Issues in Genetic Counseling: A Comparison of M.S. Counselor and Medical Geneticist Perspectives," in *Journal of Genetic Counseling* 1992; 1(1); 23.

3. President's Commission for the Study of Ethical Problems in Medicine and Biomedical and Behavioral Research, *Screening and counseling for genetic conditions: the ethical, social, and legal implications of genetic screening, counseling, and education programs.* Washington D.C.: U.S. Government Printing Office, 1983, pp. 60–1.

4. Committee on Assessing Genetic Risks, Institute of Medicine, *Assessing Genetic Risks: Implications for Health and Social Policy*, ed. Lori B. Andrews, Jane E. Fullarton, Neil A. Holtzman, and Arno G. Motulsky. Washington D.C.: National Academy Press, 1994. The Committee reiterated this position several times (see pages 6, 23, 38, 70, 100, 127, 163, and 175). Of note is that the Committee did add that there may be "*rare* circumstances that warrant such disclosure" (p. 100), but they did not elaborate about what such circumstances might entail.

In this paper I evaluate and criticize the policy recommended by the IOM and practiced by most counselors in which only the woman is informed about the genetic results of misattributed paternity. I consider whether non-disclosure to either or both partners is consistent with the standards and goals of genetic counselors, and whether the genetic counselor can choose not to disclose this information to the partner based on such concerns as preservation of the family and protection of the woman. I also consider what obligations counselors have to children, a topic ignored to date in the literature.

I   THE PRINCIPLES OF GENETIC COUNSELING

Genetic textbooks often cite the rate of misattributed paternity as 10–15%. This number is not based on published evidence. The data that do exist are based on nonrepresentative populations and any extrapolation is problematic. Rather, as the various published studies show, the rate of misattributed paternity is likely to vary between countries, age groups, cultural or ethnic groups, and socioeconomic classes.

Despite the lack of data on how often misattributed paternity occurs, the empirical studies cited above reveal that there is a consensus on how to deal with this occurrence. Both the studies by Wertz *et al.* and Pencarinha *et al.* found that over 95% of counselors would not inform the woman's partner that he is not the biological father.

Given the goals and standards of genetic counseling, the almost unanimous agreement not to disclose misattributed paternity to the male partner is initially surprising. As enumerated by Fraser in 1974, the prime goal of genetic counseling is to promote "client autonomy": to help clients "to understand their options and to choose the course of action which seems most appropriate to them in view of their risk and their family goals and act in accordance with that decision."[5] To achieve client autonomy requires "full disclosure" of information

in a "non-directive" manner. Counselors place great emphasis on full disclosure because they realize that different information will have different meaning and different impact on different patients. They also emphasize a non-directive approach in which counselors attempt to give their clients information objectively and allow the clients to come to a decision that is most consonant with their own values and beliefs. The assumption is that all decisions are equally valid. The counselors' goal is to help their clients define what is best for themselves. Genetic counselors pride themselves on helping their clients reach their own decisions and not to impose their own values on their clients.

Who are the clients of the genetic counselor? Consider, first, the scenario in which a couple presents for genetic counseling because their first child has a congenital condition which their pediatrician believes to be genetic. The couple may seek genetic counseling to clarify their child's diagnosis, to understand their future procreative risks, or to undergo prenatal testing and diagnosis. The genetic counselor begins by taking a family history from both the woman and her partner, and when necessary, draws blood from each family member to ascertain the child's diagnosis, its mode of inheritance, and/or its risk of reoccurrence in future children. Genetic tests done on the blood samples provide information about the child, and about each partner as the parent of the child, as individuals, and as a couple. As such, it would seem that both parents and the child are the counselor's clients. Similarly, when a couple presents for in-utero testing of their potential child, both parents and the potential child would seem to be clients even though the procedure is done exclusively on the woman and the fetus. The two cases have morally relevant differences. In the first scenario, each partner has the right to refuse or consent to testing and they make this same decision on behalf of their child. In the second scenario, the woman alone has final authority on whether or not the procedure is performed because prenatal testing requires that she undergo an invasive diagnostic procedure. But in both scenarios, the information that is obtained is relevant to all the parties. As such, information ought to be disclosed to the family. The decision to inform only the woman of unanticipated misattributed paternity implies that

---

5. F.C. Fraser, "Genetic Counseling," *American Journal of Human Genetics* 1974; 26: 636–59.

the counselor considers the woman alone to be her client, or at least the primary client. This conflicts with the already established counselor-client relationships and the counselor's obligations to *each* of her clients.[6]

If both adult partners seek genetic counseling, then both partners are clients of the genetic counselor. As such, the counselor has a duty to both of them. True disclosure of the findings are relevant to both of them. The purpose of genetic counseling is to disclose as much information as possible to the clients so that they can reach their own decisions. If both the woman and man are clients, then the counselor ought to respect each partner's right to know his or her genetic endowment and the genetic endowment of their child. The decision to conceal misattributed paternity is not consistent with such respect. Rather, the virtually unanimous consensus to disclose misattributed paternity only to the woman implies that counselors consider the woman alone to be their client. While it is and should be the case that pregnant women have ultimate decision making authority over their own body with regard to prenatal testing and whether to continue or terminate a pregnancy, information obtained about the fetus or about a child is not the exclusive property of the woman and the counselor. To argue that only women should be informed is to imply that men are second-class citizens in genetic testing. Non-disclosure shows a lack of respect for the male partner as a person, as a client interested in his own genetic make-up, and as a parent interested in his child's genetic endowment.

Failure to disclose misattributed paternity to the male partner assumes that the woman has a greater interest than her partner in the true genetic explanation of the child's genetic disease. In cases of autosomal recessive diseases, if the partner is the child's biological father, then he is a carrier for the disease and has 50% responsibility for his child's illness. If he is not the biological father, then he is not responsible, but another man is. This is not meant to assign blame, but only to explain the genetic basis

of the child's illness and to help the parents make future informed procreative decisions. To deny the partner the knowledge of his true carrier status, or to mislead the partner into believing that his child's illness involved a mutation, is to deny the partner the knowledge of his and/or his child's genetic endowment. If the couple is deciding whether to have another child, the genetic knowledge that a second child is not at risk may be all that is necessary. But what if the parents separate and the partner becomes involved with another woman? He may be reluctant to have more children based on false and incomplete genetic information: genetic information that was supplied by a health care professional. And he may have informed his siblings of his carrier status provoking unnecessary testing or worry on their part.

The decision to conceal misattributed paternity from the partner and to inform the woman confidentially of this finding is contrary to the standards of full-disclosure and non-directiveness. While disclosure of misattributed paternity to the woman empowers her with relevant information regarding her child's parentage based on accurate genetic data and protects and promotes her privacy, it reflects a value judgement as to what each partner ought to know. The unknowing partner is left in the dark as the health care team helps his wife conceal the child's true genetic identity. The male partner's autonomy as an active decision maker is violated because he is denied relevant information.

II   DISCLOSURE OF MISATTRIBUTED PATERNITY TO THE MOTHER ALONE

Current practice in genetic counseling supported by the IOM's recent recommendation is to disclose misattributed paternity to the mother alone. The main reason cited in the studies and reiterated by the IOM is the preservation of the family. In this section, I argue that this reason is inappropriate for genetic counselors. The goal of family preservation is a proper goal of marriage and family counselors, not of genetic counselors, particularly when this can only be achieved by deceiving one of her clients. Instead I argue that non-disclosure of misattributed paternity is deceptive and immoral.

---

6. Judith L. Benkendorf, Nancy P. Callanan, Rose Grobstein, Susan Schmerler, and Kevin T. FitzGerald. "An Explication of the National Society of Genetic Counselors (NSGC) Code of Ethics," *Journal of Genetic Counseling* 1992; 1(1): 31–9.

The surveys' responses and the IOM's recommendation presume that the preservation of the family is a legitimate goal of geneticists and genetic counselors. Genetic counselors are neither trained to be nor hired to be marriage counselors. The decision to withhold sensitive information regarding biology presumes that disclosing misattributed paternity would be detrimental to the family, a claim that has not been empirically proven. It is possible (even probable) that disclosure may be disruptive to the family, but it is also possible that disclosure may give the family an opportunity to confront their problems head-on. Even if it were true that disclosure would disrupt the family, the question still remains whether the counselor should decide not to disclose information in an effort to preserve the family. That may be the counselor's goals; but it may not be the goal of the partners. This may be their opportunity to confront the meaning of their relationship and to decide whether or not to separate. What is best for the couple must be determined by the couple. As such, the counselor's decision not to disclose false paternity is contrary to her emphasis on being non-directive.

If preserving the family is a valid goal of geneticists and genetic counselors, then it is questionable whether the policy of disclosing misattributed paternity to the mother promotes this goal. Consider, for example, one possible scenario of false paternity. Mr. and Mrs. A are married for seven years. Their son, age 5, has cystic fibrosis (CF). They state that the illness has caused great strain on their marriage. They are now reconciled and Mrs. A is pregnant. They want to know if this child has CF. Given the need for genetic linkage testing in CF,[7] the counselor gets blood samples from Mr. and Mrs. A and their older

son. The results are inconclusive because Mr. A is not the biological father of their older son. The counselor's disclosure of false paternity to Mrs. A may set back their reconciliation. Even if Mrs. A knew that the child could be her lover's child, she may have convinced herself that her husband is the true father. However if she is informed of the false paternity, she will harbor a secret that could have wide implications on her marriage and on the well-being of the family. This secret knowledge could renew marital tension and discord. She may neglect or abuse the child who is a constant reminder of her past infidelity. As such, it may be better for the marriage if Mrs. A were not informed about the child's true parentage. Disclosure to the mother alone may or may not promote the preservation of the family: its impact will depend on the specific details of the particular family.

Consider, further, what it means to fail to disclose misattributed paternity to the woman's partner. Presently, if genetic testing is inconclusive because the putative father is not the biological father, virtually all geneticists and genetic counselors tell the couple that testing was inconclusive. A counselor may fudge the truth and assert that the tests have not been informative with regard to future risk. Alternatively, a counselor may falsely claim that the first child's genetic disease was caused by a rare mutation and that the risk of another affected offspring is negligible. In general, the putative father is never told that he is not the biological father of the affected infant. The woman, however, will be informed about the false paternity in a confidential meeting at a future date and time.

Failure to disclose misattributed paternity to the partner, then, is not merely a lack of full disclosure but requires active deception. The problem with the counselor's decision to actively deceive the partner is that the partner is her client as well. The counselor's action assumes that health care professionals should decide what information is relevant or important to their clients. Traditionally physicians did unilaterally decide whether or not to divulge sensitive information to patients. In the 1960s such practices were questioned and publicly condemned as immoral. The reaction of physicians was a rapid change in disclosure policies. Whereas in the 1950s and 1960s, most physicians did not disclose the diagnosis of cancer to their patients, today such disclosure is commonplace.

---

7. Cystic Fibrosis is an autosomal recessive illness which means that a child can only be affected if both parents are carriers and pass that gene onto the child. Because there are many mutations for the genes for Cystic Fibrosis, genetic testing can require determining the particular mutation that each parent has. This requires examining the chromosomes of each parent against the child's chromosomes to determine the particular CF genes (linkage testing). In contrast, sickle cell anemia is an autosomal recessive illness which is caused by only one mutation for which direct testing exists. As such, it is unnecessary to link the chromosomes in sickle cell testing.

Failure to inform the partner of misattributed paternity can also be rejected on deontological grounds: the physician-patient or counselor-client relationship is or should be based on trust and shared decision making. Failure to disclose this information to the male partner prevents him from real participation in decision making. Some men who learn that their children are not biologically their own may want to divorce or separate. Counselors may have legitimate concerns that partners may not want to support a child that they did not sire, but counselors do not have moral responsibility for ensuring the monetary support of children. Rather it is presumptuous for them to think that they are.

The decision to preserve the woman's privacy means that these children will not be informed of their true parentage. How could a child be told that his biological father is not his social father if his social father is not told this as well? Problems may arise, then, if the child's actual biological father has a transmittable genetic illness. Imagine, for example, that the biological father has Huntington's Chorea. If the mother chooses not to inform her child of his true parentage, her son will not know that he is at risk, because as far as he knows, his family history is negative in that regard. He may not learn the truth until after he has sired a family. Likewise, a mother may not choose to tell her daughter that all of her true paternal biological aunts died from breast cancer in their early 30s and that she should undergo mammography beginning at age 20. As genetic diseases become more amenable to treatment, accurate genetic information becomes more relevant to the child's health care.

III   NON-DISCLOSURE TO EITHER PARENT

An alternative to the present-day policy of disclosure to the woman alone is a policy in which counselors would not disclose unanticipated misattributed paternity to either parent. Unlike the policy of unilateral disclosure to the woman and unilateral deception of her partner, this can be achieved without using a deception through a policy of "if they don't ask, I won't tell." According to such a policy, the counselors would only divulge that information which the couple specifically requested. Such a

policy must be rejected because it is contrary to the educative and resourceful roles to which counselors aspire. Counselors cannot limit their disclosure to information about which their clients directly ask, because part of counseling is to educate clients to know what to ask, and to tell clients what they would have wanted to ask, had they known more genetics.

One rationale for a policy in which neither parent is informed about the finding of misattributed paternity is that the family has not asked about paternity, and the finding is incidental. The family came in to understand their future risk of conceiving an affected child and the finding of false paternity was an incidental finding. Much information is determined in genetic studies, and not all information obtained from genetic testing is revealed as it is the counselor's job to inform the family of genetic risks, not to give them a full degree in genetics. But the information about whether one is or is not a child's biological parent is *never* incidental. Genetic counselors fear the impact of false paternity on marriage precisely because such knowledge is *not* incidental.

If counselors have an obligation to preserve the integrity of their clients' families, then they may decide that family integrity is best achieved if they fail to reveal false paternity to either partner. First, as I argued above, I do not believe that preservation of families is an appropriate goal of genetic counselors. Second, I do not believe that non-disclosure to both parties will necessarily promote family integrity. Recall Mr. and Mrs. A. They may suspect that their first child is not biologically related to Mr. A. They may be embarrassed and decide not to divulge this information freely, but wait and see what the genetic tests reveal. If the counselor were to confirm their suspicion, they may be relieved to learn that Mr. A is not a carrier of the CF gene and that their future progeny are not at risk. If the counselor fails to disclose the false paternity, the couple may undergo an amniocentesis to avoid another child with CF. As such, the non-disclosure results in an unnecessary amniocentesis which risks the woman's and the fetus' health and well-being. This is unacceptable: a counselor *cannot* permit an unnecessary test with known serious risks to prevent a possible but unproven threat to a marriage. In addition, an iatrogenic complication to either the woman or the fetus may cause unanticipated (as well as avoidable) marital discord. Thus, the counselor's attempt to preserve family integrity may backfire. Since counselors do not know the consequences of revealing misattributed paternity, they should not ground their actions on speculative consequences. Rather, counselors must judge the morality of their actions only on the basis of whether their actions comply with their moral duties. Deception is contrary to their obligations to tell the truth and to give their clients accurate information: it cannot be morally justified.

A policy of bilateral non-disclosure is also dangerous because no one in the family knows the true genetic history of their child. This may place the child at risk for knowable, potentially treatable, diseases. Again, imagine that the true biological father has a strong family history of early-onset breast cancer. If the mother knows that her lover and not her husband is the true father, she may encourage her daughter to get breast cancer mammography screening at a much younger age than is generally done in the general population.

A policy of bilateral non-disclosure also leaves the couple at risk for future decisions based on false information. The parents may choose not to have further children based on this inaccurate knowledge. And the parents' siblings may suffer needlessly thinking that they themselves or their children are at risk. Moreover, the decision not to disclose may cause a backlash if the parents learn of the false paternity in another setting (e.g. the child needs a kidney transplant and histocompatibility testing[8] reveals misattributed paternity). What response can the counselor give when both parents converge on her and demand to know what right she had to decide what information they needed?

The failure of a counselor to tell either party of the child's true parentage implies that the counselor believes that the genetic makeup of the clients and their child is not the clients' exclusive property. It implies that the counselor who has analyzed their DNA is the rightful proprietor who can do with it what she wants. Such a claim contradicts the moral

and legal standards of disclosure for health care professionals.[9]

If a major goal of genetic counselors is to disclose relevant information to their clients, then the finding of misattributed paternity must be disclosed to both partners because it is relevant to their clients' identity and procreative decisions. Failure to disclose misattributed paternity to either partner leaves the family and the individual members at unnecessary and unjustifiable risk.

IV   DISCLOSURE OF MISATTRIBUTED PATERNITY TO BOTH PARENTS

What are the arguments in favor of full disclosure to both parents, particularly the partner who has been routinely overlooked? First, the partner has come to a health professional for information about himself and his child. His genetic background is his, and like all genetic counseling clients, he should be given as much accurate information as possible. It also seems obvious that it is relevant from the partner's perspective to know that the child is not genetically his. Genetic counselors should not speculate as to what the partner will choose to do with this information. To determine that it is better for him not to know detracts from the counselor's main goal of promoting client autonomy.

Another argument in favor of disclosure is the acknowledgement that the relationship is already characterized by deception and this may give the family an opportunity to confront their problems or to redefine the terms of their relationship. While full disclosure may be disruptive to the family, whether this happens and the extent of the disruption will depend on many factors unique to the family which the counselors cannot predict. The family has sought genetic information: it is the geneticist's responsibility to inform them of this as accurately as possible. The information, however, should not be divulged acrimoniously. Rather the information must be given in a sensitive non-judgmental manner that will help to minimize undue harm. The counselor can assess how, when, and in what context to

---

8. Histocompatibility refers to the compatibility (similarity) of one's immunological status to another. It is genetically determined. A child has 50% histocompatibility with each genetic parent.

9. See, for example, *Canterbury v Spence* 464 F.2d 772 (D.C. Cir. 1972).

divulge this information. She may choose to have a therapist present to enable the family to address their feelings. But ultimately she must inform them of the genetic evidence of misattributed paternity because this is integral to their relationship and identities. This is not to deny that the truth will be painful. But this is true of many medical diagnoses. Outside of the genetic context, it is no longer acceptable for physicians to fail to disclose the true nature of their patients' conditions:[10] the same should be true with genetic information.

Full disclosure to both partners is consonant with the belief that genetic counselors have responsibility to all their competent adult clients. Genetic information is not the counselor's property which she can divulge as she sees fit. It is the property of her clients. Full disclosure empowers the partners so that they can choose how best to use this information. It also makes possible the disclosure of the child's true parentage at some future date.

V   OBJECTIONS TO BILATERAL DISCLOSURE

My recommendation of full disclosure to both partners is in conflict with the practices of virtually all geneticists and genetic counselors. Many reviewers were also troubled by my recommendation. The three most common objections to my proposal are that bilateral disclosure: 1. places the woman and child at physical risk; 2. places the woman at psychological risk; and 3. fails to respect the woman's right to privacy. Let me respond to each objection in turn.

First, I do not mean to downplay the *potential* threat to some women and children if misattributed paternity is determined and revealed. But there are no data to support this concern. And in fact, the dominant theme in the family counseling literature is that the woman's behavior has no causal influence on the man's decision to batter, but rather, that the problem lies exclusively in the man.[11]

This is not meant to minimize the serious medical and social issue of domestic violence. Data show that 30% of married American women will experience at least one violent episode in their lifetime and similar data exist in other Western countries. Furthermore 50% of female homicides are perpetrated by male intimates. There are also data to show that abusive men are sexually possessive and jealous. But the relationship of abuse and infidelity has not been extensively examined. In a search of the medical, philosophical and sociological literature between 1975–1995, I was able to locate only two studies which examined this issue. One study found a correlation between wife infidelity and spousal abuse, but it could not prove whether men are abusive because women are unfaithful, or whether women are unfaithful because their partners are abusive. The second reference focused on the more narrow issue of domestic homicide. It stated that men kill their partners more frequently than women kill their partners, and the reasons given for spousal homicides are different. Women invariably kill male partners after years of abuse whereas men kill their female partners for a variety of reasons including revelations of infidelity.

Would my conclusions be different if the data revealed that men became even more aggressive/homicidal upon learning of misattributed paternity? Probably not. Such a finding would underscore the need for policies and programs that educate the public regarding the wide range of information that genetic testing can reveal so that at-risk women would avoid such testing to protect themselves and their children. However, I do not believe it would justify a policy of non-disclosure given that most men do not and would not abuse their partners.

A second concern is the psychological risk that a policy of bilateral disclosure may produce. Imagine that a couple comes in for genetic testing and the counselor explains the wide spectrum of information that genetic testing can and will determine: from extra chromosomes to chromosomal deletions, from false paternity to mistaken identity, from lethal conditions which present in infancy (e.g. Tay Sachs) to those which present in adulthood (e.g. Alzheimer's). Genetic counselors need to help clients decide what information they want to obtain and what information they would rather not have.

10. See, for example, *Arato v. Avedon* 5 Cal. 4th 1172, 23 Cal. Rptr.2d 131, 858 P.2d 598 (1993).

11. See, for example, Douglas Sprenkle, "Wife Abuse Through the Lens of 'Systems Theory,'" *The Counseling Psychologist* 1994: 22(4): 598–602; and Morton Stenchever and Diane Stenchever, "Abuse of Women: An Overview," *Women's Health Issues* 1991; 1(4): 187–192.

If the counselor raises the possibility of unanticipated findings to the couple prior to testing, then the woman is in a bind because it is only her infidelity which can be discovered and revealed: How can the woman, at that point, ask to know the risk of their future children, but not be told about misattributed paternity? Such a request would be an admission of previous infidelity.

One solution would be to better educate the public-at-large regarding what genetic testing can and cannot determine. More specifically, education regarding genetic testing could be emphasized during prenatal care. I would even accept a policy whereby when an appointment for genetic counseling was sought, a counselor would contact the female partner confidentially and inform her in a precounseling session about the potential for misattributed paternity so that she can choose not to undergo testing. This would permit women to decide in an uncoerced non-threatening environment whether or not this is a risk and whether or not this is a risk that they want to confront.

Of course, a decision to back out of testing may still raise suspicions and several readers have argued that my solution does not protect the woman from the psychological risk that revelations about her other sexual relationships may create. How would I resolve the difficulty for her? My response is that it is not my responsibility to do this. The woman, through her voluntary actions, has placed herself in this quandary. If a woman voluntarily has sexual relationships with another man, then her decision should incorporate the risk of discovery both during the affair and afterwards, particularly if a child may be conceived in the process. To argue that women need to be protected by a blanket policy of deception towards their partners suggests that women are not capable of taking responsibility for their actions and their consequences. This suggests that women are not competent to make autonomous decisions regarding sexual relationships (that they are incompetent) and that third-party protection (paternalism) is appropriate and necessary. I reject these conclusions.

Nevertheless, it is true that the risk of disclosure is asymmetrical. The testing can only reveal the woman's infidelities. But conception is also asymmetrical. Only women can be 100% confident of a genetic relationship to the child. As such, gestation

is both a privilege and a responsibility. Women need to know that genetic testing can reveal misattributed paternity so that decisions which relate to sexual relationships, reproduction, and genetic counseling are informed. Some women who have had more than one partner may be in denial that these concerns pertain to them, but that does not change the fact that they are responsible for their decisions.

The third objection asks why I perceive disclosure purely as an issue of truth-telling and not as an issue regarding respect for the privacy of the woman. My answer is in the framing of the question. This paper addresses the issue of who has the right to genetic information in the scenario when *both* partners come to the counselor for testing and counseling. My argument is that when both partners are clients of the counselor, they both have the right to the genetic information. In reality, the vast majority of clients are pregnant women, many of whom come alone. In those cases, testing of the woman and the fetus are her decision and her partner does not have any claims to the counselor's disclosures unless she consents to it. But when a couple elects for genetic testing and does not limit the requested information, then the counselor has a moral obligation to disclose the test results to both adult clients.

VI   COUNSELOR'S OBLIGATIONS TO THE CHILD

The question of whether the genetic counselor has obligations to reveal misattributed paternity directly to the child is complex. Three reasons to favor disclosure are 1. its role in health care screening, diagnosis, and treatment; 2. its role in procreative decisions, and 3. the importance of genetic identity to one's self-identity. Two reasons to favor non-disclosure are 1. that such knowledge may threaten the parent-child relationship; and 2. that it might threaten the integrity of the family. Which reasons are stronger depend on how one weighs the advantages and disadvantages. Presently, in medical care involving children, parents are empowered to make many decisions on their child's behalf, and to determine what is in their child's best interest, all things considered. In their calulations, parents are allowed to balance the competing and conflicting needs of other family members provided that their decision is not abusive or harmful to the child. While I believe that the genetic counselors have an obligation to the child, I would argue that the counselors should defer to the parents as to when and how the child is to be informed about his true biological identity. Counselors fulfill their obligation by encouraging the parents to disclose the truth about the child's genetic identity to the child when they deem it appropriate. The counselor should also offer to counsel the child directly, but should respect the parents' decision not to reveal false paternity at this time. Likewise, if the child is an infant or otherwise unable to understand the genetic facts, then counseling of the child must be deferred. The counselor should offer to be available at a future time, but he should respect those families who choose to deal with this privately. While the counselor has an obligation to encourage the parents to reveal this information to the child, he or she is not empowered to confront the child, now or in the future, without parental permission. Parents are the guardians of their children. While deceiving one's child regarding his or her genetic identity is morally problematic, to compel parents to tell the truth about genetic parentage is to intrusively interfere into the private family. The counselor's right to interfere in the family is and ought to be limited. It does not and should not extend this far.

VII   CONCLUSION

In conclusion, I support the 1983 recommendation of the President's Commission. I believe that the arguments favor disclosure of false paternity to both partners. Men as well as women have a valid interest in knowing the true biological parentage of their legal children. The impact that disclosure of false paternity will have on men, women and families is unknown. Geneticists and genetic counselors must present the data in a responsible yet sensitive way, but the couple ought to be the ultimate arbiter of what to do with their genetic information (including the issue of whether or not to inform the child of his true parentage).

My proposal should not be interpreted to support routine paternity testing or to encourage genetic testing in cases where false paternity is a potential issue. My point is that deception of either adult partner by the counselor is not morally justified and will only further erode the trust which our patients and clients have in the health care profession. The recent recommendation of the Institute of Medicine regarding misattributed paternity is misconceived.

SARS PLAGUE: DUTY OF CARE OR MEDICAL HEROISM?

Dessmon YH Tai

INTRODUCTION

SARS has been described as a Chinese plague because it emerged from the colourful markets of wild animals and the exotic kitchens of Guangdong, southern China in mid-November 2002. In late February 2003, the Metropole Hotel in Hong Kong became the epicentre where SARS crossed intercontinental boundaries through rapid air travel, affecting mainly Asian countries. Hence it has also been labeled an Asian plague. Singapore was the fifth most severely SARS-afflicted country, with 238 cases after China (5327), Hong Kong (1755), Taiwan (346) and Canada (251).[1]

HEALTHCARE WORKERS AND SARS

Worldwide, about 21% (1706/8096) of SARS victims were healthcare workers (HCWs).[2] The percentage of HCWs was highest in Vietnam (57%), Canada (43%) and Singapore (41%), followed by Hong Kong (22%), Taiwan (20%) and mainland China (19%).[3]

From *Annals Academy of Medicine Singapore* 35 (2006): 374–378. Published by permission of The Annals Academy of Medicine, Singapore.

Editors' note: Two sections of the article have been revised by the author and some notes have been cut. Students who want to follow up on sources should consult the original.

In Singapore, three-quarters of infection occurred in hospitals or nursing homes. Tan Tock Seng Hospital (TTSH) was designated the national SARS hospital on 22 March 2003. As Director of medical intensive care unit (MICU) in TTSH, I became the Director of the National SARS ICU by default. I'll never forget that shocking one-week belated birthday present, mixed with conflicting feelings of responsibility, pride and that all-too human fear of the unknown. Being in the frontline, I hid my fear behind my N95 mask. I had to set an example of courage and confidence for others to follow. Medicine being my vocation, I told myself that I could not turn my back on my responsibilities, however dangerous, especially in the thick of an unprecedented national crisis.

FEAR OF THE UNKNOWN AND DEATH

Initially, SARS was an unknown microbiological enemy. We were grappling in the dark with this highly contagious, deadly disease. We raced against time to try to outwit the virus before it overwhelmed us. We knew we were gambling with our lives. As one French lung specialist in Hanoi eloquently expressed, *"We were not playing with fire—the fire was playing with us. We faced death. We played bridge with it, but it was not a virtual partner."*

Every day, when we arrived in hospital for work, we had to gear up, physically, psychologically and emotionally, for another day of battle. We could not escape from hard facts such as these: 1 in 5 patients required ICU care and about half of ICU patients died.

Within the jaws of death, many of us stopped having physical contact with our family and loved ones, as we just could not risk passing the infection to them in case we had been infected. One nurse shared that she had stopped kissing her child so that others could continue to do so. I stayed in a separate room from my wife during the epidemic.

The fear of death was intensified by the close proximity to and personal identification with our previously healthy colleagues, who had been struck down by SARS and were dying in our own ICU. We had a very touching and special experience of the fragility of life and the sudden imminence of our mortality. I could fully empathise with Dr Vu Hoang Thu from Hanoi, who said, *"We were scared. But we did not have a choice; we had to work, to care for*

our colleagues. Those in good health saw others fall sick and their health deteriorate. We cried a lot. But we had to encourage them; and for some, lie to them, about the progress of the illness. What we lived through, it was like a war. Without force, without solidarity, we would not have been able to get through it."

A TTSH medical social worker made up her mind to help colleagues combat SARS without consulting her husband and 3 children. She wrote in a letter to her family, *"Forgive me for my decision to help my colleagues fight SARS, which may hurt you or bring the possible risk of disease back home . . . I hope you remember that I love all of you very much."*

We knew that dying from SARS was a very lonely affair because of the need for strict isolation to prevent transmission. Nobody wanted to die in this lonely manner, isolated from their loved ones. Dr Carlo Urbani, aged 46, was not spared a similar fate. The world is indebted to this SARS warrior, who first alerted the medical community about this new infectious disease.[4] Dr Scott Dowell, a WHO doctor who attended to Dr Urbani in Bangkok, aptly said, *"To be by yourself in a strange country, in a room full of people in spacesuits who cannot touch you . . . That is not a good way to die."*

Our worst nightmare became a reality when our colleague, a 27-year-old medical officer, died on 7 April 2003. We lost a total of 5 HCWs to SARS in Singapore: 2 doctors, 1 nursing officer, 1 nursing aide and 1 hospital attendant.

During the SARS Commemoration Ceremony on 22 July 2003, among the 4000 who gathered to remember the 33 victims were widows and widowers. One mother, who had lost her husband, had brought her young daughter, said, *"I want her to remember that (her dad died while looking after patients). I also want her to know that she can live on because there are children who have lost a mother."*[5]

The then Prime Minister Goh Chok Tong, during the SARS Commemoration Ceremony that moved many to tears, commended these HCWs. *"There is nothing more noble. There is nothing more humbling."*[6]

MEDICAL PLAGUE

Fighting this scourge was a very traumatic experience for HCWs. They risked their lives fighting a previously unknown enemy, yet they faced discrimination from the public. For example, nurses in uniform were given suspicious stares, or kept at a distance by the public in buses or Mass Rapid Transit (MRT) trains.[7] Some foreign HCWs living in Housing and Development Board (HDB) flats found leaflets in their letterboxes stating: *"TTSH staff are not allowed to use lifts."*

The SARS crisis had become a medical plague. One citizen wrote to The Straits Times, the largest circulating English local newspaper, *"I read with tears in my eyes to see that you have to make arrangements to stay elsewhere, get ostracized by family, friends and society, are unable to show love and care to your family members . . . Some of you even have to sign on insurance policies, write a will, in case anything happens. Only you will know how it feels to be outcast by the very society that you're serving."*

Is the accepted norm of professional responsibility for HCWs to be ready to sacrifice their lives for patients they do not even know during epidemics? In reality, the medical profession will always carry an inherent occupational risk of being infected by their patients even during normal times.

Many HCWs struggled to choose between their instinct of self-preservation (fear of contracting SARS and dying) and their professional duty as HCWs. In our personal capacity, each one of us is still a parent, spouse and child. Faced with the risk of contracting the bug and facing death, despite taking all the necessary precautions, our personal duties to loved ones usually take an overwhelming priority over our professional duties. Our ex-PM Goh praised the HCWs who soldiered on to treat SARS patients as valiant people. *"To get the nurses and doctors to work with SARS patients is a feat. I really admire the dedication and professionalism of our hospital workers."*[8]

The Hippocratic Oath embodies the doctors' moral identity by providing a broad ethical framework for the conduct and practice of doctors.[9] Although the Pledge has been modified since the 1948 Geneva declaration adopted by the World Medical Association, 3 important obligations remain, namely *"duty to the public, duty to the patient and duty to the profession."*

At the Singapore Medical Council Physician's Pledge Affirmation Ceremony on 7 May 2005, Dr Balaji Sadasivan, Senior Minister of State, Ministry of Information, Communications and the Arts and Health, aptly said: *"The practice of medicine is a calling. It is a calling in which your heart will be exercised as much as your mind. Your call is to be with those who*

suffer . . . Nothing will sustain you more potently than the power to recognise in your humdrum routine, the true poetry of life—the poetry of the commonplace, of the ordinary man, of the plain, toil-worn woman, with their loves and their joys, their sorrows and their griefs."[10]

Dr Carlo Urbani helped accept the Nobel Peace Prize for Doctors Without Borders in 1999. He eloquently exemplified this calling in his speech: *"Health and dignity are indissociable in human beings. It is a duty to stay close to victims and guarantee their rights."*[11]

COURAGE

Courage, HCWs realised, was not the absence of fear. Instead, it was a devotion to duty which became so powerful it overcame all fear of adversity. TTSH's Chief Executive Officer, Dr Lim Suet Wun, recalled: *"The doctors and nurses were just as fearful as anybody else . . . They were aware of the risks yet they went right in to take care of SARS patients."*[12]

Even foreign HCWs stood shoulder to shoulder with their Singaporean colleagues throughout the crisis.[13] They could have simply returned home. One foreign HCW said, *"At the end of the day, this is my job; and it is like a war, you don't leave your colleagues to fight it alone."*

There was a very high level of camaraderie and determination to give our utmost despite the high risks involved. We trusted our lives with our comrades-in-arms. There was never a question of giving up the battle.

Professor Low Cheng Hock, Associate Dean of TTSH, broke down in tears and said: *"We are a nation in tears, but tears of love . . . tears that will galvanise the medical profession as we rise to the challenges ahead."*[14]

HEROES AND COWARDS

Theoretically, heroes are admired. But their loved ones would rather grow old with an ordinary person than live with the memory of a dead hero. Honestly, who is not afraid to die? But the sad fact was that we had to be prepared to die in the course of our professional duties.

In a study on the psychological impact of SARS on HCWs in Singapore, fear was the most commonly reported emotion. This was not surprising as prior to 12 March 2003, the disease did not even have a name. The utter lack of knowledge of this new disease meant that we did not know about the aetiological agent, its mode of transmission, its natural history or effective therapy. It was terrifying to turn up for work daily and face an unseen lethal enemy while none of us could yet be certain about the efficacy of protective measures. In addition, there was the haunting fear of acquiring and spreading the disease to families, friends and colleagues. Helplessness prevailed as anyone could fall victim to the disease in the line of duty.

Love of life also includes love of self, not just love for others. The HCW's autonomy in making their own decision to take either a break from intensive physical and emotional burdens or to soldier on in their job should be respected. It is within their human right. In some countries (including Singapore), frontline warriors of SARS were honoured as heroes.[15] Concurrently, punishment was suggested, such as the threat of withdrawing the professional licenses of those who refused to turn up for work in Taiwan. Between the hero and coward labels, there must be sufficient space in a developed and cultured society to practice humanism to every human being in any kind of crisis. For those HCWs who resigned because of SARS, they had *"made a personal decision when they realised that this is not the profession for them."*[16]

Two weeks after the recognition of the syndrome and the implementation of full protective measures, not a single SARS ICU staff was infected from 17 March 2003.[17] This testimony to the effectiveness of our protective gear was a crucial and potent psychological antidote to our anxiety about the safety of our work environment. To be a well-equipped and well-prepared, combat-ready professional is more useful than being a dead hero.

What factors made HCWs continue *"to give their heart and soul to the battle, even when their colleagues fall victim to the deadly virus"* and to even *"step foot outside the security of their home every day"*?[18] Firstly, it was their professional commitment to duty. Secondly, a sense of altruism and self-sacrifice was very strong when facing the uncertainty of this new disease. A study from Hong Kong reported that at least 90% of the respondents who survived the SARS catastrophe believed themselves to be more altruistic because the diversion of attention and energy to helping others helped them to conquer their own feelings of powerlessness and regain a sense of control over other aspects of life.[19] Thirdly, an adequate supply of protective gear[20] and medical insurance coverage for all HCWS and their families were crucial for their physical and psychological well-being. Fourthly, messages of gratitude and encouragement from relatives, friends and strangers were morale boosters.[21] Emotional support and positive affirmations from fellow HCWs were also useful. Lastly, many found calm and peace entrusting themselves to their gods.

CONCLUSION

This SARS scourge will go down in history as one of our darkest moments but it was also one of our finest triumphs. Being in the medical profession, caring for patients is one of our expected responsibilities. On the other hand, as public citizens, HCWs have the right to resign when they feel that their responsibilities to their families should take priority over that to their patients. This microbiological battle has been a great humbling experience, in which our healthcare community has epitomised their Hippocratic Oath through their acts of selfless behaviour, sacrifice, and love. Many HCWs now have a renewed appreciation for the meaning, nobility and importance of their profession.[22]

Dr Lim Suet Wun said: *"Somebody has to do it. We have been designated and entrusted to do it. We will do it to the best of our ability . . ."*[23] For the frontline SARS HCWs who had soldiered on despite the risk, it was the "badge of honour" that they chose to wear.

This scourge forced each HCW to make a personal decision: whether caring for patients against great odds, would be their chosen profession and vocation. Many chose to live up to their Hippocratic Oath.

REFERENCES

1. World Health Organization. Summary of probable SARS cases with onset of illness from 1 November 2002 to 31 July 2003 (based on data as of 31 December 2003). Available at: http://www.who.int/csr/sars/country/table2004_04_21/en/index.html. Accessed 16 November 2005.

2. Ibid.

3. Ibid.

4. Cox News Service. WHO doctor Carlo Urbani warned the public of SARS but succumbed to the virus in a Bangkok hospital. The Straits Times 6 April 2003; p 32, col 2–6.

5. Cheong SW, Soh N, Ng J. Not one dry eye . . . Video moved 4,000 who gathered to remember the 33 victims. The Straits Times 23 July 2003; p H2, col 1–6.

6. Long S. Tributes, tears for SARS heroes. The Straits Times 23 July 2003; p 1, col 1–7.

7. Ng C. A nurse's sadness: when a hospital uniform keeps people away . . . Today 3 April 2003; p 8, col 1–3.

8. Khalik S. PM Goh praises "valiant" doctors and nurses. The Straits Times 7 April 2003; p 4, col 5–7.

9. Nambiar RM. Physician's Pledge taking Ceremony—7th May 2005—Prof Raj M Nambiar. SMC In-Touch December 2005:4–7.

10. The Singapore Medical Council. Speech by Dr Balaji Sadasivan. SMC In-Touch December 2005:1–3.

11. Cox News Service, WHO doctor Carlo Urbani.

12. Anonymous. Pat on the back from TTSH's CEO, Dr Lim Suet Wun. A Special Supplement of together@NHG May/Jun 2003; p 3, col 1.

13. Cheong SW, Soh N, Ng J. PM lauds foreign medical 'warriors' who didn't walk away. The Straits Times 23 July 2003; p H3, col 1–7.

14. Frances J. Remembering an atypical man. Today 2 June 2003; p 1, col, 1–4, and p 2, col 2–3.

15. Chee YC. Heroes and heroines of the war on SARS. Singapore Med J 2003; 44:221–8.

16. Lee CW. SARS hospital's badge of honour. Today 2 April 2003; p 3, col 1–3.

17. Loo S, Tai DY, Tai HY, Ang B, Soon M, Leong HN, et al. Effective protective measures for healthcare workers in an intensive care unit dedicated for patients with severe acute respiratory syndrome. Ann Acad Med Singapore 2003;32(Suppl):S79.

18. Koh A. Medical heroism . . . The Straits Times 7 April 2003; p 17, col 1–2.

19. Tam CW, Pang EP, Lam LC, Chiu HF. Severe acute respiratory syndrome (SARS) in Hong Kong in 2003: stress and psychological impact among frontline healthcare workers. Psychol Med 2004; 34:1197–204.

20. Ibid.

21. Chee, Heroes and heroines.

22. Tam et al., Severe acute respiratory syndrome.

23. Lee, SARS hospital's badge of honour.

THE LESSONS OF SARS

Ezekiel J. Emanuel

Many people wonder whether all of the international attention heaped on the severe acute respiratory syndrome (SARS) has been misdirected. As of 11 July 2003, there were just 8437 cases of SARS worldwide, leading to 813 deaths. While each of these deaths is a tragedy, the numbers pale in comparison to the numbers of deaths caused by HIV infection, malaria, and tuberculosis, not to mention more mundane but more deadly infectious diseases such as pneumococcal pneumonia and diarrhea. In 2002, 40 million people worldwide were infected with HIV. Five million had newly contracted the disease during that year, and approximately 3.1 million died of AIDS. Similarly, malaria afflicts over 400 million people world wide each year and causes approximately 2 million deaths. The corresponding figures for tuberculosis are 8 million cases and 2 million deaths. Indeed, even in local contexts, the impact of SARS on mortality rates is much less significant than that of these other diseases. In the United States, over 750 people die of tuberculosis each year and over 14000 die of AIDS; in contrast, none of the 73 U.S. patients who have contracted SARS have died of the disease. In Canada, 81 persons died of tuberculosis in 2000 and about 400 died of AIDS, substantially more than the 39 deaths among the 438 patients with SARS (250 probable cases and 188 suspected cases).

From *Annals of Internal Medicine* 139 (2003): 589–591. Reprinted by permission of the Annals of Internal Medicine. *Editors' note:* Most author's notes have been cut. Students who want to follow up on sources should consult the original article.

Among the many reasons for the disproportionate response to SARS are its high mortality rate compared with other respiratory infections, its rapid spread across the globe, and the remarkable sleuthing that identified the etiologic virus and decoded its genome in just a handful of days. But novelty may be the most powerful force behind all the public attention. Despite its continued threat, West Nile virus, which dominated the media just a few years ago, now receives minimal coverage, and the outbreak of monkeypox in the midwestern United States already seems to have eclipsed SARS in the headlines. Nevertheless, for all the disproportionate attention, the focus on SARS has taught some invaluable lessons that will have long-term positive effects on health care.

One is that the SARS epidemic has better prepared the world's public health authorities for a major influenza or other pandemic. For many years, public health officials have been worrying about a repeat of the great influenza pandemic of 1918 and 1919. In less than a year, between 20 and 40 million people, 1% to 2% of the world's entire population, died. In most European countries, the mortality rate was 2.5%; in other places, it reached 5%. Over one quarter of the U.S. population was infected, and some 675000 people died, 10 times the number of Americans who died fighting in World War I. As 1 commentator noted, the influenza pandemic decreased the average life span in the United States by 10 years. Two characteristics of the flu were even scarier than just the sheer numbers of dead. First, it did not kill only the old and infirm; nearly 43000 young and fit U.S. servicemen suffocated from the fluid in their lungs. The second was the speed with which death overtook the victim. People who looked fine one day were dead the next. In recent decades, public health workers have been trying to prevent a pandemic of comparable magnitude by sequencing the genome of the 1918 influenza virus strain and by linking early monitoring systems to strategies for rapid vaccine development and dissemination.

As the SARS epidemic spread, many feared that it was the long-dreaded second coming. Luckily it was not. Nevertheless, SARS severely tested the capacity of the worldwide public health system to respond rapidly and decisively. Moreover, it tested each country's integrity in reporting data as well as the emergency response plans of each country, city, and hospital. The SARS epidemic focused a harsh light on the Chinese public health system and the deadly consequences of suppressing health care information. Simultaneously, it illuminated the efficient Vietnamese response and the value of strict quarantines. Local public health departments and hospitals throughout the world had to reevaluate and strengthen their measures for handling infectious emergencies, quarantining patients, and ensuring the safety of other hospitalized patients. The lessons learned have—and will continue to have—an impact beyond refining the response to SARS. The epidemic has highlighted the developing public health gaps in tuberculosis, HIV infection, and other communicable diseases as China has privatized medical services. These disparities may now receive much-needed attention. Thus, a benefit of SARS has been to mobilize resources for the worldwide public health infrastructure, which is necessary for addressing rapidly spreading, deadly respiratory infections. It is hoped that this awakening will lessen the impact of the next pandemic and perhaps even avert it.

A closely related lesson is the necessity of global cooperation in containing infectious diseases. For those who are unconvinced by the ongoing saga of HIV infection and AIDS, SARS is a forceful reminder that everyone has a personal health interest in what happens in other countries. Living in a rich, developed country does not protect people from emerging infections. Borders, oceans, and other natural barriers are not what they once were. Housing, farming techniques, food handling and transportation arrangements, sexual practices, public health measures, and even political practices in developing countries around the globe can adversely affect health everywhere. Isolationist attitudes will not protect a country that participates in the global economy and transportation system. Working with other countries, supporting international development institutions, and providing development aid are likely to be critical to protecting the health of people in developed countries. If a passion for distributed justice cannot induce us to care for people living in poor countries, then self-interest in our own health should engage us in improving their living standards lest we become infected by diseases that emerge there.

Another lesson from the SARS epidemic relates to the internal morality of medicine. Carlo Urbani, a physician from the World Health Organization, responded to a new respiratory infection at the Vietnam French Hospital in Hanoi. Dr. Urbani determined that the new respiratory infection was SARS, warned the world about it, and worked tirelessly to help the hospital staff care for the patients by developing an isolation ward, quarantining the hospital, and helping the country cope with the contagion. Less than 4 weeks after responding to the first case of SARS, Dr. Urbani died of the disease. His dedication was not unique. More than half of the first 60 reported cases of SARS involved health care workers who had come into contact with SARS patients. Indeed, apart from the very first case, all of the people who died in Vietnam were doctors and nurses. Nearly a quarter of all patients with SARS in Hong Kong were health care workers. In Canada, of the 141 probable cases of SARS diagnosed between 23 February and 14 May 2003, 92 (65%) involved health care workers. Despite deadly peril, physicians and nurses tirelessly cared for patients with SARS.

This reaffirmation of health care workers' duty to care for the sick at the risk of death is amazing. It did not have to be this way. The history of physicians' responses to other contagions is mixed. Galen is reported to have fled from Rome during a plague in 166. Although in the 14th century some physicians stayed and cared for the sick, most responded to the Black Death by fleeing. Defoe indicates in *A Journal of the Plague Years*—a novelistic chronicle about London's great plague of 1665—that most physicians were called "deserters." In the mid-19th century, nascent professional organizations began to articulate the physician's ethical obligation to care for the sick during epidemics. The SARS epidemic tested the dedication of a medical profession that might have been weakened by increasing commercialization, poor morale, an emerging preference for easier professional lifestyles, and the pervasive self-centered individualism of the larger society. In light of these worldwide trends, it would have been disappointing but perhaps not surprising if physicians refused to care for highly infectious patients spreading a deadly virus. That they continued to care despite personal risk is one of the ennobling—and, it is hoped, enduring—legacies of the SARS epidemic.

Nearly 20 years ago, when the HIV and AIDS epidemic was erupting, physicians expressed what some commentators called "profound reluctance and concern" about caring for any of the "4-H" patients: homosexuals, hemophiliacs, Haitians, and heroin addicts. Indeed, while many thousands of health care workers cared for these patients despite uncertain risks, many others vocally refused to do so. Saying that the patients somehow deserved the disease because of their lifestyles or that "accidental injuries [were] inevitable,"[1] many claimed that "no one can condemn a doctor for not taking on a patient with AIDS." Prompted by such views, medical and dental societies convened panels to debate the issue. These discussions concluded by reaffirming that devotion to caring for the sick is what distinguishes health professionals from lawyers, teachers, and businesspeople.[2,3] This moral ideal defines the core element of being a medical professional. The obligation is not chosen; it is inseparable from the choice to become a doctor. To reject this ethical ideal is to reject the profession.

The logic of this view became so irrefutable that, against its own tenet that doctors should be free to choose their patients, the American Medical Association's Council on Ethical and Judicial Affairs declared that " a physician may not ethically refuse to treat a patient whose condition is within the physician's current realm of competence solely because the patient is seropositive [for HIV]. Ultimately, this thinking came to dominate the medical profession in the late 1980s and was inculcated through hospital practices and training programs. It simply became ethically and professionally unacceptable for health care workers to refuse to treat a patient with HIV infection or AIDS.

Health care workers educated with this ethos responded with dedication to the SARS epidemic. This response does not mean that physicians and nurses caring for patients with SARS were not concerned. They asked questions, wondering how much risk they needed to take, how to deal with uncertainty in deciding about interventions, and what they—and, more important, their hospital administrators—could do to reduce the risks. But proceeding with caution is different from refusing to care for patients, different from declaring that health care workers are not obliged to risk their lives for patients with SARS, and different from threatening to quit practicing rather than care for such patients. Thus, in dealing with SARS, the health professions have reaffirmed Dr. Urbani's model of physicians' dedication to caring for the sick. They have rejected a "me first" philosophy.

Affirming health care workers' ethical duty to care for the sick imposes a correlative duty on health care administrators and senior physicians to quickly develop and deploy procedures to maximize the safety of frontline physicians and nurses. The gloves, eye shields, and other paraphernalia that are now routine did not exist 20 years ago. While it took many years to develop and implement these measures in response to HIV and AIDS, the response to SARS took just a handful of weeks. Canadian health and hospital administrators in particular seem to have done an extraordinary job deploying maximal protective measures, including N95 respirators, negative air pressure examining rooms, long-sleeved gowns, redesigned traffic flow patterns to ensure minimal contact with suspected case-patients, and adequate quarantines of health care workers with suspected SARS. These measures doubtless stressed hospital facilities and health care workers and may not be perfect. However, their proven efficacy in reducing the risk for transmission made it easier to hold physicians to their obligation to care for patients despite personal risk.

Malaria, HIV infection, tuberculosis, and a host of other deadly infections are more devastating than SARS. However, while its novelty focused disproportionate attention on SARS, the attention has been of incalculable value. These lessons—the importance of the public health infrastructure throughout the world, the importance of improving health and living conditions in developing countries, the reaffirmation of the moral center of the medical profession, and the urgent need to implement measures that minimize risks to health care workers—are valuable far beyond SARS. Indeed, they may help to focus worldwide attention on the global threat of both long-standing and emerging infections.

REFERENCES

1. Viets J. Surgeon urges AIDS tests for her colleagues. San Francisco Chronicle. 16 February 1989:1.
2. Emanuel EJ. Do physicians have an obligation to treat patients with AIDS? N Engl J Med. 1988; 318:1686–90. [PMID: 3374540]
3. Freedman B. Health professions, codes, and the right to refuse HIV-infectious patients. Hastings Cent Rep. 1988; 18:S20–5. [PMID: 11650067]

WHAT SHOULD THE DEAN DO?

Acoronavirus that normally occurs in some nonhuman animals infected humans and caused what came to be called severe acute respiratory syndrome (SARS). In 2003, not long after the initial infections occurred in Guandong, China, SARS spread to almost thirty countries. By the time the disease was contained, about eight thousand people had contracted the virus, and approximately eight hundred had died.

The course of the disease in Taiwan was typical. The first cases were people who returned to Taiwan from China. Health care professionals tried to identify and isolate these people to prevent transmission, and for two months this seemed to work. Then a series of outbreaks originating in seven different hospitals led to many more infections. By the end of the epidemic, Taiwan had about four hundred confirmed cases of SARS.

At the beginning of the outbreak, no one knew how infectious SARS was and what course the disease would take. The evidence at the time suggested a respiratory infection with a mortality rate of about 10 percent. Transmission of SARS appeared to be airborne, both through large droplets and tiny droplet nuclei, implying that incidental as well as close proximity to infected patients might result in transmission. The rate of infection in hospitals was high, and around 30 to 40 percent of reported cases were health care workers.

At this time, when knowledge was limited and fear was strong, the dean of each medical school in Taiwan had to consider the role of students during the epidemic. Many parents and even some politicians called to ask that medical students be excused from school or kept from contact with patients until the outbreak ended. Each dean listened to these requests, consulted with various people, and reviewed the facts before making a decision.

What should the dean decide? What is the ethically appropriate role for medical students during an epidemic?

COMMENTARY

Gregory L. Eastwood

The dean must make a decision that will affect many lives and perhaps save some of them. If she allows her students to help in the care of SARS patients, some of them may contract SARS and die. Without question, the dean must be troubled by the prospect of placing her students in a situation that exposes them to a significant risk of severe illness or death. She has undoubtedly heard from students, parents, faculty, community leaders, the press, and others, all expressing opinions and trying to influence her decision. She should consider their input and share with them her view of the situation; but in the end, she should make it clear that she will decide herself, and that her decision will apply to all her students.

More than twenty-five hundred years ago, Hippocrates declared, "The health and life of my patients will be my first consideration." More than nine hundred years ago, the rabbi-physician Moses Maimonides said, "I have been appointed to watch over the life and death of my fellow human beings." These principles, enduring today, mean that the physician's obligation to the patient outweighs obligations to self, and the physician's responsibility to the patient encompasses the full continuum of life, including death's approach.

The ethical obligation of physicians to place the patient's welfare before their own may be modified by particular circumstances. During past epidemics,

some physicians have tried to suspend their obligations to care for patients presenting risks to their own health by invoking duty to self, family, or future patients. Also, physicians vary in their abilities to care for certain diseases—for example, the skills of emergency medicine physicians and specialists in infectious diseases would be more relevant in the care of patients with SARS than those of radiologists or pathologists.

However, the question here is not what the ethical and professional obligations of fully trained physicians competent to treat SARS patients are, but rather what the dean should require of students in this situation. To paraphrase Maimonides, the dean has been appointed to watch over the lives of her students, and arguably their welfare should be her primary consideration.

What applies to fully trained, competent physicians may help inform the dean's decision but must be modified by several pragmatic considerations. She should ask, How are medical students similar to fully trained physicians, and how do they differ? Certainly we expect students to be committed to the medical profession and to behave in accordance with its ethical principles. In fact, as students enter many medical schools in the United States, they take an oath that declares their patients' welfare will be their primary concern.

Yet I believe there is an important difference between medical students and physicians: students do not yet have the requisite knowledge, skills, and experience to be of meaningful use in the care of

From *Hastings Center Report* 36 (July–August 2006). Reprinted by permission of The Hastings Center.

patients with SARS. Further, participation in the care of patients by medical students is primarily for the students' educational benefit, not the patients'. The dean should ask, Will the educational experience that my students have in helping to care for SARS patients outweigh the risk to their health and lives? I doubt it.

What are the dean's options? She could have the students carry out all clinical duties, but the risk to students, despite instruction in dealing with SARS patients, is still unacceptably high. She could suspend all clinical rotations and remove the students from all patient contact, but there is no compelling reason to take such a drastic measure and interrupt

all forms of clinical education. She could allow the students to make individual choices or a collective decision about whether to care for SARS patients, but by doing so, she would surrender her ethical, professional, and supervisory responsibilities.

The best option is to have the students carry on with their clinical duties, but not to allow them in the vicinity of patients with possible or probable SARS. It is highly likely that some students will acquire SARS if they are exposed to SARS patients, and the risk to the students of severe illness or death outweighs any educational benefit to the students or clinical benefit to the patients.

COMMENTARY

Daniel Fu-Chang Tsai and Ding-Shinn Chen

The SARS epidemic in Taiwan took the lives of four senior nurses, one laboratory technician, and two first-year residents. These deaths—especially those of the two inexperienced doctors—shocked Taiwan. Parents of many medical students, concerned about their children's safety, asked that they be excused from all clinical duties. Since the Ministry of Education cautioned teaching hospitals against letting medical students participate in the direct care of SARS patients, some schools called back their students from teaching hospitals or allowed them to make individual choices about whether to remain in clinical settings.

Our medical school, National Taiwan University College of Medicine, took a nuanced but principled course. After graduating high school, medical students in Taiwan spend seven years finishing their degree. The fifth and sixth years are devoted to clerkships, and the seventh year is devoted to internships. (To avoid confusion with the U.S. system, we will refer to seventh year students as acting interns or senior students, not as interns.) Although clerks and acting interns are both medical students, their clinical responsibilities vary greatly. We decided to give clerks assignments that took them off the wards, but to require acting interns to carry

out their clinical duties with some modifications. Of course, all acting interns received special training in infection control, sterile technique, and use of protective equipment.

After making this decision, the dean of our school (one of the authors of this commentary) received many phone calls from frightened parents who tried to persuade him to change the policy for senior students. He reassured them that precautions would be taken to keep students safe. About 60 percent of the parents accepted this; 20 percent recognized it very reluctantly; and 20 percent rejected it and pressured him to change his mind.

The dean resisted this pressure by explaining his view of medical professionalism. Acting interns have historically been part of the health care team at our school and have a duty to participate in clinical settings. Although they are still students needing skills and experience, they have taken an oath and committed themselves to the profession. To develop mature and reliable doctors, professional attitudes should be fostered as well as clinical skills. Acting interns abandoning all clinical duties in the face of the risk posed by SARS would be similar to soldiers fleeing the battlefield in the face of combat. Senior students might not be fully competent to fight the enemy, but they must contribute to the team and prepare themselves to treat patients with the SARS virus. In addition, to excuse residents and acting interns from duty would have a negative impact on nurses, lab technicians, and all other health care workers and trainees.

We decided to modify the obligations of acting interns by not requiring them to participate in the direct care of SARS patients. Medical schools have an interest in protecting their junior staff from the harm caused by a new and poorly understood disease. Therefore, sending in more experienced hands first and modifying the duties of acting interns is a sensible and justifiable way to prepare acting interns. When they are more competent to

care for SARS patients, they can undertake standard responsibilities.

In reaching our decision, we tried not only to emphasize doctors' responsibilities, but also to allow for some individual autonomy. By allowing acting interns to decide whether to engage in the direct care of SARS patients, we encouraged them to cultivate a genuine concern for patient welfare and a sense of responsibility and human compassion. According to Confucian ethics, this is the way to develop "humaneness" (jen) in doctors. As members of a profession that has promised "to cure, to care, to comfort," acting interns should be encouraged, but not forced, to participate in the care of SARS patients.

COMMENTARY

James Dwyer

We usually think of the dean's office as a well-furnished room in the administration building. But as the etymology of the word suggests, an office is also a constellation of duties. In this case, three important duties stand out. First, the dean must see that students develop the knowledge, skills, habits, and attitudes they need to be excellent doctors. Second, she must protect their physical and psychological wellbeing. And third, she must ensure that students, residents, and faculty contribute to patient care. All the dean's duties should be animated by a desire to make medicine more effective, accessible, and caring.

The problem in this case arises because various duties come into conflict. A recently emerged infectious illness like SARS provides a rich opportunity for students to study a new disease, develop clinical skills, cultivate appropriate habits, adopt compassionate attitudes, and contribute to patient care. But this opportunity also poses a danger—students may become sick and die.

My own view is that health care professionals have a special and important role to play in caring for the sick and dying. When people commit themselves to this social role, they have a duty to accept

a reasonable level of occupational risk, even if what counts as reasonable is open to further discussion. Medical students have made a commitment and therefore share this duty. Although we need to take into account their skill level and to train and supervise them so that they are not exposed to unnecessary and unreasonable risks, we do not need to dilute the ethical duty.

If I were the dean, I would set aside three days for reflection and deliberation on the question, Should medical students carry out their usual clinical assignments during this outbreak? To decide, students would need to learn more about infectious diseases, study ethics, consult with various people, and discuss the matter in groups. I would speak to the class and express my views, but so would many others, such as experts in infectious diseases, philosophers, concerned parents, and doctors who have accepted the risks. Arguments and analysis are important, but so are narratives of those who have nobly served. Of course, the students could also listen to and respond to narratives of people who fled to avoid the risk of infectious disease. After a robust deliberation, I would let the students decide as a group; because this decision is more akin to a political decision than a consumer choice, it should be a collective one. If the students decide to retreat to the classroom, so be it. If they decide to stay and serve, good for them.

Most ethical decisions worth deliberating have both an analytical element and a creative one. We try to analyze the relevant features and norms to find the best decision, but we also fashion a creative response that expresses values and hopes for the future. My approach aims to help students realize and shape the meaning of their profession. Here the term "realize" has two important senses: to understand and to actualize. It is vitally important to understand the moral meaning of our social roles

and undertakings. But it is equally important to shape those meanings and put them into practice. Realizing moral meaning is the deepest form of ethics education.

My approach also fosters an appropriate kind of participatory democracy. Many people will dismiss the idea that a dean would or should be concerned with participatory democracy, but I'm not so cynical. Part of the dean's office is to listen to many voices, to enable people to contribute more fully to joint enterprises, and to encourage better responses to problems. Encouraging participation is one way for the dean to shape the future of medical practice—a future that will call upon us to respond in better ways to outbreaks of infectious diseases.

THE LIMITS OF CONSCIENTIOUS OBJECTION—MAY PHARMACISTS REFUSE TO FILL PRESCRIPTIONS FOR EMERGENCY CONTRACEPTION?

Julie Cantor and Ken Baum

Health policy decisions are often controversial, and the recent determination by the Food and Drug Administration (FDA) not to grant over-the-counter status to the emergency contraceptive Plan B was no exception. Some physicians decried the decision as a troubling clash of science, politics, and morality. Other practitioners, citing safety, heralded the agency's prudence. Public sentiment mirrored both views. Regardless, the decision preserved a major barrier to the acquisition of emergency contraception—the need to obtain and fill a prescription within a narrow window of efficacy. Six states have lowered that hurdle by allowing pharmacists to dispense emergency contraception without a prescription.[1–6]

From *New England Journal of Medicine* 351, no. 19 (November 4, 2004): 2008–2012. Copyright © 2004 Massachusetts Medical Society. All rights reserved.

Editors' note: Most authors' notes have been cut. Students who want to follow up on sources should consult the original article.

In those states, patients can simply bypass physicians. But the FDA's decision means that patients cannot avoid pharmacists. Because emergency contraception remains behind the counter, pharmacists can block access to it. And some have done just that.

Across the country, some pharmacists have refused to honor valid prescriptions for emergency contraception. In Texas, a pharmacist, citing personal moral grounds, rejected a rape survivor's prescription for emergency contraception.[7] A pharmacist in rural Missouri also refused to sell such a drug,[8] and in Ohio, Kmart fired a pharmacist for obstructing access to emergency and other birth control.[9] This fall, a New Hampshire pharmacist refused to fill a prescription for emergency contraception or to direct the patron elsewhere for help. Instead, he berated the 21-year-old single mother, who then, in her words, "pulled the car over in the parking lot and just cried,"[10] Although the total number of incidents is unknown, reportsof pharmacists who refused to dispense emergency contraception date back to 1991 and show no sign of abating.

Though nearly all states offer some level of legal protection for health care professionals who refuse to provide certain reproductive services, only Arkansas, Mississippi, and South Dakota explicitly protect pharmacists who refuse to dispense emergency and other contraception. But that list may grow. In past years, legislators from nearly two dozen states have taken "conscientious objection"—an idea that grew out of wartime tension between religious freedom and national obligation and was co-opted into the reproductive-rights debate of the 1970s—and applied it to pharmacists. One proposed law offers pharmacists immunity from civil lawsuits, criminal liability, professional sanctions, and employment repercussions. Another bill, which was not passed, would have protected pharmacists who refused to transfer prescriptions.

This issue raises important questions about individual rights and public health. Who prevails when the needs of patients and the morals of providers collide? Should pharmacists have a right to reject prescriptions for emergency contraception? The contours of conscientious objection remain unclear. This article elucidates those boundaries and offers a balanced solution to a complex problem. Because the future of over-the-counter emergency contraception is in flux, this issue remains salient for physicians and their patients.

ARGUMENTS IN FAVOR OF A PHARMACIST'S RIGHT TO OBJECT

Pharmacists Can and Should Exercise Independent Judgment

Pharmacists, like physicians, are professionals. They complete a graduate program to gain expertise, obtain a state license to practice, and join a professional organization with its own code of ethics. Society relies on pharmacists to instruct patients on the appropriate use of medications and to ensure the safety of drugs prescribed in combination. Courts have held that pharmacists, like other professionals, owe their customers a duty of care. In short, pharmacists are not automatons completing tasks; they are integral members of the health care team. Thus, it seems inappropriate and condescending to question a pharmacist's right to exercise personal judgment in refusing to fill certain prescriptions.

Professionals Should Not Forsake Their Morals As A Condition of Employment

Society does not require professionals to abandon their morals. Lawyers, for example, choose clients and issues to represent. Choice is also the norm in the health care setting. Except in emergency departments, physicians may select their patients and procedures. Ethics and law allow physicians, nurses, and physicians assistants to refuse to participate in abortions and other reproductive services. Although some observers argue that active participation in an abortion is distinct from passively dispensing emergency contraception, others believe that making such a distinction between active and passive participation is meaningless, because both forms link the provider to the final outcome in the chain of causation.

Conscientious Objection Is Integral to Democracy

More generally, the right to refuse to participate in acts that conflict with personal ethical, moral, or religious convictions is accepted as an essential element of a democratic society. Indeed, Oregon acknowledged this freedom in its Death with Dignity Act, which allows health care providers, including pharmacists, who are disquieted by physician-assisted suicide to refuse involvement without fear of retribution. Also, like the draftee who conscientiously objects to perpetrating acts of death and violence, a pharmacist should have the right not to be complicit in what they believe to be a morally ambiguous endeavor, whether others agree with that position or not. The reproductive-rights movement was built on the ideal of personal choice; denying choice for pharmacists in matters of reproductive rights and abortion seems ironic.

ARGUMENTS AGAINST A PHARMACIST'S RIGHT TO OBJECT

Pharmacists Choose to Enter a Profession Bound by Fiduciary Duties

Although pharmacists are professionals, professional autonomy has its limits. As experts on the profession of pharmacy explain, "Professionals are expected to exercise special skill and care to place the interests of their clients above their own immediate interests." When a pharmacist's objection directly and detrimentally affects a patient's health, it follows that the patient should come first. Similarly, principles in the pharmacists' code of ethics weigh against conscientious objection. Given the effect on the patient if a pharmacist refuses to fill a prescription, the code undermines the right to object with such broadly stated objectives as "a pharmacist promotes the good of every patient in a caring, compassionate, and confidential manner," "a pharmacist respects the autonomy and dignity of each patient," and "a pharmacist serves individual, community, and societal needs."[11] Finally, pharmacists understand these fiduciary obligations when they choose their profession. Unlike conscientious objectors to a military draft, for whom choice is limited by definition, pharmacists willingly enter their field and adopt its corresponding obligations.

Emergency Contraception Is Not an Abortifacient

Although the subject of emergency contraception is controversial, medical associations, government agencies, and many religious groups agree that it is not akin to abortion. Plan B and similar hormones have no effect on an established pregnancy, and they may operate by more than one physiological mechanism, such as by inhibiting ovulation or creating an unfavorable environment for implantation of a blastocyst. This duality allowed the Catholic Health Association to reconcile its religious beliefs with a mandate adopted by Washington State that emergency contraception must be provided to rape survivors. According to the association, a patient and a provider who aim only to prevent conception follow Catholic teachings and state law. Also, whether one believes that pregnancy begins with fertilization or implantation, emergency contraception cannot fit squarely within the concept of abortion because one cannot be sure that conception has occurred.

Pharmacists' Objections Significantly Affect Patients' Health

Although religious and moral freedom is considered sacrosanct, that right should yield when it hinders a

patient's ability to obtain timely medical treatment. Courts have held that religious freedom does not give health care providers an unfettered right to object to anything involving birth control, an embryo, or a fetus. Even though the Constitution protects people's beliefs, their actions may be regulated. An objection must be balanced with the burden it imposes on others. In some cases, a pharmacist's objection imposes his or her religious beliefs on a patient. Pharmacists may decline to fill prescriptions for emergency contraception because they believe that the drug ends a life. Although the patient may disapprove of abortion, she may not share the pharmacist's beliefs about contraception. If she becomes pregnant, she may then face the question of abortion—a dilemma she might have might have avoided with the morning-after pill.

Furthermore, the refusal of a pharmacists to fill a prescription may place a disproportionately heavy burden on those with few options, such as a poor teenager living in a rural area that has a lone pharmacy. Whereas the savvy urbanite can drive to another pharmacy, a refusal to fill a prescription for a less advantaged patient may completely bar her access to medication. Finally, although Oregon does have an opt-out provision in its statute regulating assisted suicide, timing is much more important in emergency contraception than in assisted suicide. Plan B is most effective when used within 12 to 24 hours after unprotected intercourse. An unconditional right to refuse is less compelling when the patient requests an intervention that is urgent.

Refusal Has Great Potential for Abuse and Discrimination

The limits to conscientious objection remain unclear. Pharmacists are privy to personal information through prescriptions. For instance, a customer who fills prescriptions for zidovudine, didanosine, and indinavir is logically assumed to be infected with the human immunodeficiency virus (HIV). If pharmacists can reject prescriptions that conflict with their morals, someone who believes that HIV-positive people must have engaged in immoral behavior could refuse to fill those prescriptions. Similarly, a pharmacist who does not condone extramarital sex might refuse to fill a sildenafil prescription for an unmarried man. Such objections go beyond "conscientious" to become invasive. Furthermore, because a pharmacist does not know a patient's history on the basis of a given prescription, judgments regarding the acceptability of a prescription may be medically inappropriate. To a woman with Eisenmenger's syndrome, for example, pregnancy may mean death. The potential for abuse by pharmacists underscores the need for policies ensuring that patients receive unbiased care.

TOWARD BALANCE

Compelling arguments can be made both for and against a pharmacist's right to refuse to fill prescriptions for emergency contraception. But even cogent ideas falter when confronted by a dissident moral code. Such is the nature of belief. Even so, most people can agree that we must find a workable and respectful balance between the needs of patients and the morals of pharmacists.

Three possible solutions exist: an absolute right to object, no right to object, or a limited right to object. On balance, the first two options are untenable. An absolute right to conscientious objection respects the autonomy of pharmacists but diminishes their professional obligation to serve patients. It may also greatly affect the health of patients, especially vulnerable ones, and inappropriately brings politics into the pharmacy. Even pharmacists who believe that emergency contraception represents murder and fell compelled to obstruct patients' access to it must recognize that contraception and abortion before fetal viability remain legal nationwide. In our view, state efforts to provide blanket immunity to objecting pharmacists are misguided. Pharmacies should follow the prevailing employment-law standard to make reasonable attempts to accommodate their employees' personal beliefs. Although neutral policies to dispense medications to all customers may conflict with pharmacists' morals, such policies are not necessarily discriminatory, and pharmacies need not shoulder a heightened obligation of absolute accommodation.

Complete restriction of a right to conscientious objection is also problematic. Though pharmacists voluntarily enter their profession and have an obligation to serve patients without judgment, forcing them to abandon their morals imposes a heavy toll. Ethics and law demand that a professional's morality not interfere with the provision of care in life-or-death situations, such as a ruptured ectopic

pregnancy. Whereas the hours that elapse between intercourse and the intervention of emergency contraception are crucial, they do not meet that strict test. Also, patients who face an objecting pharmacist do have options, even if they are less preferable than having the prescription immediately filled. Because of these caveats, it is difficult to demand by law that pharmacists relinquish individual morality to stock and fill prescriptions for emergency contraception.

We are left, then, with the vast middle ground. Although we believe that the most ethical course is to treat patients compassionately—that is, to stock emergency contraception and fill prescriptions for it—the totality of the arguments makes us stop short of advocating a legal duty to do so as a first resort. We stop short for three reasons: because emergency contraception is not an absolute emergency, because other options exist, and because, when possible, the moral beliefs of those delivering care should be considered. However, in a profession that is bound by fiduciary obligations and strives to respect and care for patients, it is unacceptable to leave patients to fend for themselves. As a general rule, pharmacists who cannot or will not dispense a drug have an obligation to meet the needs of their customers by referring them elsewhere. This idea is uncontroversial when it is applied to common medications such as antibiotics and statins; it becomes contentious, but is equally valid, when it is applied to emergency contraception. Therefore, pharmacist who object should, as a matter of ethics and law, provide alternatives for patients.

Pharmacists who object to filling prescriptions for emergency contraception should arrange for another pharmacist to provide this service to customers promptly. Pharmacies that stock emergency contraception should ensure, to the extent possible, that at least one nonobjecting pharmacist is on duty at all times. Pharmacies that do not stock emergency contraception should give clear notice and refer patients elsewhere. At the very least, there should be a prominently displayed sign that says, "We do not provide emergency contraception. Please call Planned Parenthood at 800-230-PLAN (7526) or visit the Emergency Contraception Web site at www.not-2-late.com for assistance." However, a direct referral to a local pharmacy or pharmacist who is willing to fill the prescription is preferable. Objecting pharmacists should also redirect prescriptions for emergency contraception that are received by telephone to another pharmacy known to fill such prescriptions. In rural areas, objecting pharmacists should provide referrals within a reasonable radius.

Notably, the American Pharmacists Association has endorsed referrals, explaining that "providing alternative mechanisms for patients . . . ensures patient access to drug products, without requiring the pharmacist or the patient to abide by personal decisions other than their own." A referral may also represent a break in causation between the pharmacist and distributing emergency contraception, a separation that the objecting pharmacist presumably seeks. And, in deference to the law's normative value, the rule of referral also conveys the importance of professional responsibility to patients. In areas of the country where referrals are logistically impractical, professional obligation may dictate providing emergency contraception, and a legal mandate may be appropriate if ethical obligations are unpersuasive.

Inevitably, some pharmacists will disregard our guidelines, and physicians—all physicians—should be prepared to fill gaps in care. They should identify pharmacies that will fill patient's prescriptions and encourage patients to keep emergency contraception at home. They should be prepared to dispense emergency contraception or instruct patients to mimic it with other birth-control pills. In Wisconsin, family-planning clinics recently began dispensing emergency contraception, and the state set up a tool-free hotline to help patients find physicians who will prescribe it. Emergency departments should stock emergency contraception and make it available to rape survivors, if not all patients.

In the final analysis, education remains critical. Pharmacists may have misconceptions about emergency contraception. In one survey, a majority of pharmacists mistakenly agreed with the statement that repeated use of emergency contraception is medically riskly. Medical misunderstandings that lead pharmacists to refuse to fill prescriptions for emergency contraception are unacceptable. Patients, too, may misunderstand or be unaware of emergency contraception. Physicians should teach patients about this option before the need arises, since patients may understand their choices better

when they are not under stress. Physicians should discuss emergency contraception during office visits, offer prescriptions in advance of need, and provide education through pamphlets or the Internet. Web sites such as www.not-2-late.com allow users to search for physicians who prescribe emergency contraception by ZIP Code, area code, or address, and Planned Parenthood offers extensive educational information at www.plannedparenthood.org/library/birhtcontrol/ec.html, including details about off-label use of many birth-control pills for emergency contraception.

Our principle of a compassionate duty of care should apply to all health care professionals. In a secular society, they must be prepared to limit the reach of their personal objection. Objecting pharmacists may choose to find employment opportunities that comport with their morals—in a religious community, for example—but when they pledge to serve the public, it is unreasonable to expect those in need of health care to acquiesce to their personal convictions. Similarly, physicians who refuse to write prescriptions for emergency contraception should follow the rules of notice and referral for the reason previously articulated: the beliefs of health care providers should not trump patient care. It is difficult enough to be faced with the consequences of rape or of an unplanned pregnancy; health care providers should not make the situation measurably worse.

Former Supreme Court Chief Justice Charles Evans Hughes called the quintessentially American custom of respect for conscience a "happy tradition"— happier, perhaps, when left in the setting of a draft objection than when pitting one person's beliefs against another's reproductive health. Ideally, conflicts about emergency contraception will be rare, but they will occur. In July, 11 nurses in Alabama resigned rather than provide emergency contraception in state clinics.[12] As patients understand their birth-control options, conflicts at the pharmacy counter and in the clinic may become more common. When professionals' definitions of liberty infringe on those they choose to serve, a respectful balance must be struck. We offer one solution. Even those who challenge this division of burdens and benefits should agree with our touchstone—although health professionals may have a right to object, they should not have a right to obstruct.

NOTES

1. Alaska Admin. Code tit. 12, §52.240 (2004).
2. Cal. Bus. & Prof. Code §4052 (8) (2004).
3. Hawaii Rev. Stat §461-1 (2003).
4. N. M. Admin. Code §16.19.26.9 (2003).
5. Wash. Rev. Code §246-863-100 (2004).
6. Me. Rev. Stat. Ann. tit. 32, §§13821-13825 (2004).
7. Pharmacist refuses pill for victim. Chicago Tribune. February 11, 2004:C7.
8. Simon S. Pharmacists new players in abortion debate. Los Angeles Times. March 20, 2004:A18.
9. Sweeney JF. May a pharmacist refuse to fill a prescription? Plain Dealer. May 5, 2004:E1.
10. Associated Press. Pharmacist refuses to fill morning after prescription. (Accessed October 14, 2004, at http://www.thechamplainchannel.com/wnne/3761928/detail.html.)
11. American Pharmacists Association. Code of ethics for pharmacists: preamble. (Accessed October 14, 2004, at http://www.aphanet.org/pharmcare/ethics.html.)
12. Elliott D. Alabama nurses quite over morning-after pill. Presented on All Things Considered. Washington, D. C.: National Public Radio, July 28, 2004 (transcript).

WHEN LAW AND ETHICS COLLIDE—WHY PHYSICIANS PARTICIPATE IN EXECUTIONS

Atul Gawande

On February 14, 2006, a U. S. District Court issued an unprecedented ruling concerning the California execution by lethal injection of murderer Michael Morales. The ruling ordered that the state have a physician, specifically an anesthesiologist, personally supervise the execution, or else drastically change the standard protocol for lethal injections.[1] Under the protocol, the anesthetic sodium thiopental is given at massive doses that are expected to stop breathing and extinguish consciousness within one minute after administration; then the paralytic agent pancuronium is given, followed by a fatal dose of potassium chloride.

The judge found, however, that evidence from execution logs showed that six of the last eight prisoners executed in California had not stopped breathing before technicians gave the paralytic agent, raising a serious possibility that prisoners experienced suffocation from the paralytic, a feeling much like being buried alive, and felt intense pain from the potassium bolus. This experience would be unacceptable under the Constitution's Eighth Amendment protections against cruel and usual punishment. So the judge ordered the state to have an anesthesiologist present in the death chamber to determine when the prisoner was unconscious enough for the second and third injections to be given—or to perform the execution with sodium thiopental alone.

The California Medical Association, the American Medical Association (AMA), and the American Society of Anesthesiologists (ASA) immediately and loudly opposed such physician participation as a clear violation of medical ethics codes. "Physicians are healers, not executioners," the ASA's president told reporters. Nonetheless, in just two days, prison officials announced that they had found two willing anesthesiologists. The court agreed to maintain their anonymity and to allow them to shield their identities from witnesses. Both withdrew the day before the execution, however, after the Court of Appeals for the Ninth Circuit added a further stipulation requiring them personally to administer additional medication if the prisoner remained conscious or was in pain.[2] This they would not accept. The execution was then postponed until at least May, but the

From *New England Journal of Medicine* 354, no. 12 (March 23, 2006): 1221–1229. Copyright © 2004 Massachusetts Medical Society. All rights reserved.

Editors' note: Some text has been cut. Students who want to read the article in its entirety should consult the original.

court has continued to require that medical professionals assist with the administration of any lethal injection given to Morales.

This turn of events is the culmination of a steady evolution in methods of execution in the United States. On July 2, 1976, in deciding the case of *Gregg v. Georgia,* the Supreme Court legalized capital punishment after a decade-long moratorium on executions. Executions resumed six months later, on January 17, 1977, in Utah, with the death by firing squad of Gary Gilmore for the killing of Ben Bushnell, a Provo motel manager.

Death by firing squad, however, came to be regarded as too bloody and uncontrolled. (Gilmore's heart, for example, did not stop until two minutes afterward, and shooters have sometimes weakened at the trigger, as famously happened in 1951 in Utah when the five riflemen fired away from the target over Elisio Mares's heart, only to hit his right chest and cause him to bleed slowly to death.[3]

Hanging came to be regarded as still more inhumane. Under the best of circumstances, the cervical spine is broken at C2, the diaphragm is paralyzed, and the prisoner suffocates to death, a minutes-long process.

Gas chambers proved no better: asphyxiation from cyanide gas, which prevents cells from using oxygen by inactivating cytochrome oxidase, took even longer than death by hanging, and the public revolted at the vision of suffocating prisoners fighting for air and then seizing as the hypoxia worsened. In Arizona, in 1992, for example, the asphyxiation of triple murderer Donald Harding took 11 minutes, and the sight was so horrifying that reporters began crying, the attorney general vomited, and the prison warden announced he would resign if forced to conduct another such execution.[4] Since 1976, only 2 prisoners have been executed by firing squad, 3 by hanging, and 12 by gas chamber.[5]

Electrocution, thought to cause a swifter, more acceptable death, was used in 74 of the first 100 executions after *Gregg.* But officials found that the electrical flow frequently arced, cooking flesh and sometimes igniting prisoners—postmortem examinations frequently had to be delayed for the bodies to cool—and yet some prisoners still required repeated jolts before they died. In Alabama, in 1979, for example, John Louis Evans III was still alive

after two cycles of 2600 V; the warden called Governor George Wallace, who told him to keep going, and only after a third cycle, with witnesses screaming in the gallery, and almost 20 minutes of suffering did Evans finally die.[6] Only Florida, Virginia, and Alabama persisted with electrocutions with any frequency, and under threat of Supreme Court review, they too abandoned the method.

Lethal injection now appears to be the sole method of execution accepted by courts as humane enough to satisfy Eighth Amendment requirements—largely because it medicalizes the process. The prisoner is laid supine on a hospital gurney. A white bedsheet is drawn to his chest. An intravenous line flows into his or her arm. Under the protocol devised in 1977 by Dr. Stanley Deutsch, the chairman of anesthesiology at the University of Oklahoma, prisoners are first given 2500 to 5000 mg of sodium thiopental (5 to 10 times the recommended maximum), which can produce death all by itself by causing complete cessation of the brain's electrical activity followed by respiratory arrest and circulatory collapse. Death, however, can take up to 15 minutes or longer with thiopental alone, and the prisoner may appear to gasp, struggle, or convulse. So 60 to 100 mg of the paralytic agent pancuronium (10 times the usual dose) is injected one minute or so after the thiopental. Finally, 120 to 240 meq of potassium is given to produce rapid cardiac arrest.

Officials liked this method. Because it borrowed from established anesthesia techniques, it made execution like familiar medical procedures rather than the grisly, backlash-inducing spectacle it had become. (In Missouri, executions were even moved to a prison-hospital procedure room.) It was less disturbing to witness. The drugs were cheap and routinely available. And officials could turn to doctors and nurses to help with technical difficulties, attest to the painlessness and trustworthiness of the technique, and lend a more professional air to the proceedings.

But medicine balked. In 1980, when the first execution was planned using Dr. Deutsch's technique, the AMA passed a resolution against physician participation as a violation of core medical ethics. It affirmed that ban in detail in its 1992 Code of Medical Ethics. Article 2.06 states, "A physician, as a member of a profession dedicated to preserving life when there is hope of doing so, should not be a participant in a legally authorized execution," although an individual physician's opinion about capital punishment remains "the personal moral decision of the individual." It states that unacceptable participation includes prescribing or administering medications as part of the execution procedure, monitoring vital signs, rendering technical advice, selecting injection sites, starting or supervising placement of intravenous lines, or simply being present as a physician. Pronouncing death is also considered unacceptable, because the physician is not permitted to revive the prisoner if he or she is found to be alive. Only two actions were acceptable: provision at the prisoner's request of a sedative to calm anxiety beforehand and certification of death after another person had pronounced it.

The code of ethics of the Society of Correctional Physicians establishes an even stricter ban: "The correctional health professional shall . . . not be involved in any aspect of execution of the death penalty." The American Nurses Association (ANA) has adopted a similar prohibition. Only the national pharmacists' society, the American Pharmaceutical Association, permits involvement, accepting the voluntary provision of execution medications by pharmacists as ethical conduct.

States, however, wanted a medical presence. In 1982, in Texas, Dr. Ralph Gray, the state prison medical director, and Dr. Bascom Bentley agreed to attend the country's first execution by lethal injection, though only to pronounce death. But once on the scene, Gray was persuaded to examine the prisoner to show the team the best injection site.[7] Still, the doctors refused to give advice about the injection itself and simply watched as the warden prepared the chemicals. When he tried to push the syringe, however, it did not work. He had mixed all the drugs together, and they had precipitated into a clot of white sludge. "I could have told you that," one of the doctors reportedly said, shaking his head.[8] Afterward, Gray went to pronounce the prisoner dead but found him still alive. Though the doctors were part of the team now, they did nothing but suggest allowing time for more drugs to run in.

Today, all 38 death-penalty states rely on lethal injection. Of 1012 murderers executed since 1976, 844 were executed by injection.[9] Against vigorous opposition from the AMA and state medical societies, 35

of the 38 states explicitly allow physician participation in executions. Indeed, 17 require it: Colorado, Florida, Georgia, Idaho, Louisiana, Mississippi, Nevada, North Carolina, New Hampshire, New Jersey, New Mexico, Oklahoma, Oregon, South Dakota, Virginia, Washington, and Wyoming. To protect participating physicians from license challenges for violating ethics codes, states commonly provide legal immunity and promise anonymity. Nonetheless, several physicians have faced such challenges, though none have lost their licenses as yet.[10] And despite the promised anonymity, several states have produced the physicians in court to vouch publicly for the legitimacy and painlessness of the procedure.

States have affirmed that physicians and nurses— including those who are prison employees—have a right to refuse to participate in any way in executions. Yet they have found physicians and nurses who are willing to participate. Who are these people? And why do they do it?

It is not easy to find answers to these questions. The medical personnel are difficult to identify and reluctant to discuss their roles, even when offered anonymity. Among the 15 medical professionals I located who have helped with executions, however, I found 4 physicians and 1 nurse who agreed to speak with me; collectively, they have helped with at least 45 executions. None were zealots for the death penalty, and none had a simple explanation for why they did this work. The role, most said, had crept up on them.

Dr. A has helped with about eight executions in his state. He was extremely uncomfortable talking about the subject. Nonetheless, he sat down with me in a hotel lobby in a city not far from where he lives and told me his story.

Almost 60 years old, he is board certified in internal medicine and critical care, and he and his family have lived in their small town for 30 years. He is well respected. Almost everyone of local standing comes to see him as their primary care physician— the bankers, his fellow doctors, the mayor. Among his patients is the warden of the maximum-security prison that happens to be in his town. One day several years ago, they got talking during an appointment. The warden complained of difficulties staffing the prison clinic and asked Dr. A if he would be willing to see prisoners there occasionally. Dr. A said he would. He'd have made more money in his own clinic—the prison paid $65 an hour—but the prison was important to the community, he liked the warden, and it was just a few hours of work a month. He was happy to help.

Then, a year or two later, the warden asked him for help with a different problem. The state had a death penalty, and the legislature had voted to use lethal injection exclusively. The executions were to be carried out in the wardens' prison. He needed doctors, he said. Would Dr. A help? He would not have to deliver the lethal injection. He would just help with cardiac monitoring. The warden gave the doctor time to consider it.

"My wife didn't like it," Dr. A told me. "She said, 'Why do you want to go there?' But he felt torn. "I knew something about the past of these killers." One of them had killed a mother of three during a convenience-store robbery and then, while getting away, shot a man who was standing at his car pumping gas. Another convict had kidnapped, raped, and strangled to death an 11-year-old girl. "I do not have a very strong conviction about the death penalty, but I don't feel anything negative about it for such people either. The execution order was given legally by the court. And morally, if you think about the animal behavior of some of these people. . . . " Ultimately, he decided to participate, he said, because he was only helping with monitoring, because he was needed by the warden and his community, because the sentence was society's order, and because the punishment did not seem wrong.

At the first execution, he was instructed to stand behind a curtain watching the inmate's heart rhythm on a cardiac monitor. Neither the witnesses on the other side of the glass nor the prisoner could see him. A technician placed two IV lines. Someone he could not see pushed the three drugs, one right after another. Watching the monitor, he saw the sinus rhythm slow, then widen. He recognized the peaked T waves of hyperkalemia followed by the fine spikes of ventricular fibrillation and finally the flat, unwavering line of an asystolic arrest. He waited half a minute, then signaled to another physician who went out before the witnesses to place his stethoscope on the prisoner's unmoving chest. The doctor listened for 30 seconds and then told the warden the inmate was dead. Half an hour later, Dr. A was

released. He made his way through a side door, past the crowd gathered outside, and headed home.

In three subsequent executions there were difficulties, though, all with finding a vein for an IV. The prisoners were either obese or past intravenous drug users, or both. The technicians would stick and stick and, after half an hour, give up. This was a possibility the warden had not prepared for. Dr. A had placed numerous lines. Could he give a try?

OK, Dr. A decided. Let me take a look.

This was a turning point, though he didn't recognize it at the time. He was there to help, they had a problem, and so he would help. It did not occur to him to do otherwise.

In two of the prisoners, he told me, he found a good vein and placed the IV. In one, however, he could not find a vein. All eyes were on him. He felt responsible for the situation. The prisoner was calm. Dr. A remembered the prisoner saying to him, almost to comfort him, "No, they can never get the vein." The doctor decided to place a central line. People scrambled to find a kit.

I asked him how he placed the line. It was like placing one "for any other patient," he said. He decided to place it in the subclavian vein, because that is what he most commonly did. He opened the kit for the triple-lumen catheter and explained to the prisoner everything he was going to do. I asked him if he was afraid of the prisoner. "No," he said. The man was perfectly cooperative. Dr. A put on sterile gloves, gown, and mask. He swabbed the man's skin with antiseptic.

"Why?" I asked.

"Habit," he said. He injected local anesthetic. He punctured the vein with one stick. He checked to make sure he had good, nonpulsatile flow. He threaded the guidewire, the dilator, and finally the catheter. All went smoothly. He flushed the lines, secured the catheter to the skin with a stitch, and put a clean dressing on, just as he always does. Then he went back behind the curtain to monitor the lethal injection.

Only one case seemed to really bother him. The convict, who had killed a policeman, weighed about 350 pounds. The team placed his intravenous lines without trouble. But after they had given him all three injections, the prisoner's heart rhythm continued. "It was an agonal rhythm," Dr. A said. "He was dead," he insisted. Nonetheless, the rhythm continued. The team looked to Dr. A. His explanation of what happened next diverges from what I learned from another source. I was told that he instructed that another bolus of potassium be given. When I asked him if he did, he said, "No, I didn't. As far as I remember, I didn't say anything. I think it may have been another physician." Certainly, however, all boundary lines had been crossed. He had agreed to take part in the executions simply to pronounce death, but just by being present, by having expertise, he had opened himself to being called on to do steadily more, to take responsibility for the execution itself. Perhaps he was not the executioner. But he was darn close to it.

I asked him whether he had known that his actions—everything from his monitoring the executions to helping officials with the process of delivering the drugs—violated the AMA's ethics code. "I never had any inkling," he said. And indeed, the only survey done on this issue, in 1999, found that just 3 percent of doctors knew of any guidelines governing their participation in executions.[11] The humaneness of the lethal injections was challenged in court, however. The state summoned Dr. A for a public deposition on the process, including the particulars of the execution in which the prisoner required a central line. His local newspaper printed the story. Word spread through his town. Not long after, he arrived at work to find a sign pasted to his clinic door reading, "THE KILLER DOCTOR." A challenge to his medical license was filed with the state. If he wasn't aware of the AMA's stance on the issue earlier, he was now.

Ninety percent of his patients supported him, he said, and the state medical board upheld his license under a law that defined participation in executions as acceptable activity for a physician. But he decided that he wanted no part of the controversy anymore and quit. He still defends what he did. Had he known of the AMA's position, though, "I never would have gotten involved," he said. . . .

The medical people most wary of speaking to me were those who worked as full-time employees in state prison systems. Nonetheless, two did agree to speak, one a physician in a Southern state prison and the other a nurse who had worked in a prison out West. Both were less uncertain about being involved in executions than Dr. A or Dr. B.

The physician, Dr. C, was younger than the others and relatively junior among his prison's doctors. He did not trust me to keep his identity confidential, and I think he worried for his job if anyone found out about our conversation. As a result, although I had independent information that he had participated in at least two executions, he would speak only in general terms about the involvement of doctors. But he was clear about what he believed.

"I think that if you're going to work in the correctional setting, [participating in executions] is potentially a component of what you need to do," he said. "It is only a tiny part of anything that you're doing as part of your public health service. A lot of society thinks these people should not get any care at all." But in his job he must follow the law, and it obligates him to provide proper care, he said. It also has set the prisoners' punishment. "Thirteen jurors, citizens of the state, have made a decision. And if I live in that state and that's the law, then I would see it as being an obligation to be available."

He explained further. "I think that if I had to face someone I loved being put to death, I would want that done by lethal injection, and I would want to know that it is done competently."

The nurse saw his participation in fairly similar terms. He had fought as a Marine in Vietnam and later became a nurse. As an Army reservist, he served with a surgical unit in Bosnia and in Iraq. He worked for many years on critical care units and, for almost a decade, as nurse manager for a busy emergency department. He then took a job as the nurse-in-charge for his state penitentiary, where he helped with one execution by lethal injection.

It was the state's first execution by this method, and "at the time, there was great naïveté about lethal injection," he said. "No one in that state had any idea what was involved." The warden had the Texas protocol and thought it looked pretty simple. What did he need medical personnel for? The warden told the nurse that he would start the IVs himself, though he had never started one before.

"Are you, as a doctor, going to let this person stab the inmate for half an hour because of his inexperience?" the nurse asked me. "I won't." He said, "I had no qualms. If this is to be done correctly, if it is to be done at all, then I am the person to do it."

This is not to say that he felt easy about it, however. "As a Marine and as a nurse . . ., I hope I will never become someone who has no problem taking another person's life." But society had decided the punishment and had done so carefully with multiple judicial reviews, he said. The convict had killed four people even while in prison. He had arranged for an accomplice to blow up the home of a county attorney he was angry with while the attorney, his wife, and their child were inside. When the accomplice turned state's evidence, the inmate arranged for him to be tortured and killed at a roadside rest stop. The nurse did not disagree with the final judgment that this man should be put to death.

The nurse took his involvement seriously. "As the leader of the health care team," he said, "it was my responsibility to make sure that everything be done in a way that was professional and respectful to the inmate as a human being." He spoke to an official with the state nursing board about the process, and although involvement is against the ANA's ethics code, the board said he could do everything except push the drugs.

So he issued the purchase request to the pharmacist supplying the drugs. He did a dry run with the public citizen chosen to push the injections and with the guards to make sure they knew how to bring the prisoner out and strap him down. On the day of the execution, the nurse dressed as if for an operation, in scrubs, mask, hat, and sterile gown and gloves. He explained to the prisoner exactly what was going to happen. He placed two IVs and taped them down. The warden read the final order to the prisoner and allowed him his last words. "He didn't say anything about his guilt or his innocence," the nurse said. "He just said that the execution made all of us involved killers just like him."

The warden gave the signal to start the injection. The nurse hooked the syringe to the IV port and told the citizen to push the sodium thiopental. "The inmate started to say, 'Yeah, I can feel . . .' and then he passed out." They completed the injections and, three minutes later, he flatlined on the cardiac monitor. The two physicians on the scene had been left nothing to do except pronounce the inmate dead.

I have personally been in favor of the death penalty. I was a senior official in the 1992 Clinton presidential campaign and in the administration, and in that role I defended the President's stance in support of capital punishment. I have no illusions that the death penalty deters anyone from murder. I also have great concern about the ability of our justice system to avoid putting someone innocent to death. However, I believe there are some human beings who do such evil as to deserve to die. I am not troubled that Timothy McVeigh was executed for the 168 people he had killed in the Oklahoma City bombing, or that John Wayne Gacy was for committing 33 murders. The European Union refuses to participate in any way in the trial of Saddam Hussein because of the court's insistence on allowing the death penalty as a possible punishment, but given Hussein's role in the massacre of more than 100,000 people, the European position only puzzles me.

Still, I have always regarded involvement in executions by physicians and nurses as wrong. The public has granted us extraordinary and exclusive dispensation to administer drugs to people, even to the point of unconsciousness, to put needles and tubes into their bodies, to do what would otherwise be considered assault, because we do so on their behalf—to save their lives and provide them comfort. To have the state take control of these skills for its purposes against a human being—for punishment—seems a dangerous perversion. Society has trusted us with powerful abilities, and the more willing we are to use these abilities against individual people, the more we risk that trust. The public may like executions, but no one likes executioners.

My conversations with the physicians and the nurse I had tracked down, however, rattled both of these views—and no conversation more so than one I had with the final doctor I spoke to. Dr. D is a 45-year-old emergency physician. He is also a volunteer medical director for a shelter for abused children. He works to reduce homelessness. He opposes the death penalty because he regards it as inhumane, immoral, and pointless. And he has participated in six executions so far.

About eight years ago, a new jail was built down the street from the hospital where he worked, and it had an infirmary "the size of our whole emergency room." The jail needed a doctor. So, out of curiosity as much as anything, Dr. D began working there. "I found that I loved it," he said. "Jails are an underserved niche of health care." Jails, he pointed out, are different from prisons in that they house people who are arrested and awaiting trial. Most are housed only a few hours to days and then released.

"The substance abuse and noncompliance is high. The people have a wide variety of medical needs. It is a fascinating population. The setting is very similar to the ER. You can make a tremendous impact on people and on public health." Over time, he shifted more and more of his work to the jail system. He built a medical group for the jails in his area and soon became an advocate for correctional medicine.

Three years ago, the doctors who had been involved in executions in his state pulled out. Officials asked Dr. D if his group would take the contract. Before answering, he went to witness an execution. "It was a very emotional experience for me," he said. "I was shocked to witness something like this." He had opposed the death penalty since college, and nothing he saw made him feel any differently. But, at the same time, he felt there were needs that he as a correctional physician could serve.

He read about the ethics of participating. He knew about the AMA's stance against it. Yet he also felt an obligation not to abandon inmates in their dying moments. "We, as doctors, are not the ones deciding the fate of this individual," he said. "The way I saw it, this is an end-of-life issue, just as with any other terminal disease. It just happens that it involves a legal process instead of a medical process. When we have a patient who can no longer survive his illness, we as physicians must ensure he has comfort. [A death-penalty] patient is no different from a patient dying of cancer—except his cancer is a court order." Dr. D said he has "the cure for this cancer"—abolition of the death penalty—but "if the people and the government won't let you provide it, and a patient then dies, are you not going to comfort him?"

His group took the contract, and he has been part of the medical team for each execution since. The doctors are available to help if there are difficulties with IV access, and Dr. D considers it their task to ensure that the prisoner is without pain or suffering through the process. He himself provides the cardiac monitoring and the final determination of death. Watching the changes on the two-line electrocardiogram tracing, "I keep having that reflex as an ER doctor, wanting to treat that rhythm," he said. Aside from that, his main reaction is to be sad for everyone involved—the prisoner whose life has led to this, the victims, the prison officials, the doctors. The team's payment is substantial—$18,000—but he donates his portion to the children's shelter where he volunteers.

Three weeks after speaking to me, he told me to go ahead and use his name. It is Dr. Carlo Musso. He helps with executions in Georgia. He didn't want to seem as if he was hiding anything, he said. He didn't want to invite trouble, either. But activists have already challenged his license and his membership in the AMA, and he is resigned to the fight. "It just seems wrong for us to walk away, to abdicate our responsibility to the patients," he said.

There is little doubt that lethal injection can be painless and peaceful, but as courts have recognized, this requires significant medical assistance and judgment—for placement of intravenous lines, monitoring of consciousness, and adjustments in medication timing and dosage. In recent years, medical societies have persuaded two states, Kentucky and Illinois, to pass laws forbidding physician participation in executions. Nonetheless, officials in each of these states intend to continue to rely on medical supervision, employing nurses and nurse-anesthetists instead. How, then, to reconcile the conflict between government efforts to ensure a medical presence and our ethical principles forbidding it? Are our ethics what should change?

The doctor's and nurse's arguments for competence and comfort in the execution process do have some force. But however much they may wish to be there for an inmate, it seems clear that the inmate is not really their patient. Unlike genuine patients, an inmate has no ability to refuse the physicians' "care"—indeed, the inmate and his family are not even permitted to know the physician's identity. And the medical assistance provided primarily serves the government's purpose—not the inmate's needs as a patient. Medicine is being made an instrument of punishment. The hand of comfort that more gently places the IV, more carefully times the bolus of potassium, is also the hand of death. We cannot escape this truth. The ethics codes seem right.

It is this truth that persuades me that we should seek a legal ban on the participation of physicians and nurses in executions. And if it turns out that executions cannot then be performed without, as the courts put it, "unconstitutional pain and cruelty," the death penalty should be abolished.

It is far from clear that a society that punishes its most evil murderers with life imprisonment is worse off than one that punishes them with death. But a society in which the government actively subverts core ethical principles of medical practice is patently worse off for it. The government has shown willingness to use medical skills against individuals for its own purposes—having medical personnel assist in the interrogation of prisoners, for example, place feeding tubes for force-feeding them, and help with executing them. As medical abilities advance, government interest in our skills will only increase. Preserving the integrity of our ethics could not be more important.

The four physicians and the nurse I spoke to all acted against long-standing principles of their professions. Their actions have made our ethics codes effectively irrelevant in society. Yet, it must be said, most took their moral duties seriously. It is worth reflecting on this truth as well.

The easy thing for any doctor or nurse is simply to follow the written rules. But each of us has a duty not to follow rules and laws blindly. In medicine, we face conflicts about what the right and best actions are in all kinds of areas: relief of suffering for the terminally ill, provision of narcotics for patients with chronic pain, withdrawal of care for the critically ill, abortion, and executions, to name just a few. All have been the subject of professional rules and government regulation, and at times those rules and regulations will be wrong. We will then be called on to make a choice. We must do our best to choose intelligently and wisely.

Sometimes? however, we will be wrong—as I think the doctors and nurses are who have used their privileged skills to make possible 844 deaths by lethal injection thus far. We each should then be prepared to accept the consequences. Unlike Dr. Musso, however, nearly all these doctors and nurses have sought to keep their actions hidden in order not to face the consequences. In the final analysis, I think this is what makes their actions seem particularly troubling. We cannot blame them for their impulse to hide. But we cannot admire them either.

NOTES

1. Michael Angelo Morales v. Roderick Q. Hickman, No. C 06 219 J F. (Dist. Ct. Northern Dist. of Cal. February 14, 2006).
2. Michael Angelo Morales v. Roderick Q. Hickman, No. CV 06 00926 JF (9th Cir. February 20, 2006).
3. Trombley S. The execution protocol: inside America's capital punishment industry. New York: Crown, 1992.
4. Solotaroff I. The last face you'll ever see: the private life of the American death penalty. New York: Harper Collins, 2001:7.
5. Death Penalty Information Center execution database. Accessed March 1, 2006, at http://www.deathpenaltyinfo.org/executions. php.
6. Trombley, The execution protocol.
7. Breach of trust: physician participation in executions in the United States. Philadelphia: American College of Physicians, 1994.
8. Trombley, The execution protocol.
9. Death Penalty Information Center execution database.
10. Norbut M. Complaint cites Georgia doctors who took part in executions. American Medical News. July 4, 2005:1.
11. Farber NJ, Aboff BM, Weiner J, Davis EB, Boyer EG, Ubel PA. Physicians' willingness to participate in the process of lethal injections for capital punishment. Ann Intern Med 2001;135:884–8.

"TO COMFORT ALWAYS":[†] PHYSICIAN PARTICIPATION IN EXECUTIONS

Ken Baum

INTRODUCTION

Physician participation in the implementation of the death penalty is a highly contentious issue, spawning voluminous professional and academic debate. Society has long provided a role for physicians in the execution process, but as the death penalty has become more and more medicalized, the appropriate contours of such participation have come under increasing scrutiny. Should physicians be present at executions? Should they oversee the execution process? Should they deliver lethal injections or pronounce death? Social consensus on these pressing issues is imperative in order to guide legislation and remove current roadblocks to appropriate physician involvement.

Resolution is particularly crucial at a time when debate concerning the institution of capital punishment is experiencing renewed intensity. Recently, politicians, physicians, and the media have pulled the death penalty back into the national spotlight. Governor Ryan's moratorium on executions in Illinois (the result of numerous DNA-confirmed wrongful convictions), the start of George W. Bush's presidential administration, and the recent federal executions of Timothy McVeigh and Juan Raul Garza after a thirty-eight-year hiatus on federal executions have focused the public's attention on many aspects of our capital punishment system.

At both its 2000 and 2001 annual meetings, the American Medical Association (AMA) considered, but ultimately rejected, a resolution calling upon the entire medical profession to support a moratorium on all executions until questions regarding the availability of

DNA evidence and the quality of legal representation are resolved. Arguably more important are the results of a recent survey of American physicians finding that, despite the norms adopted by the AMA and other professional societies, the majority of physicians approve of physician participation in executions.[1]

Further, the media, seizing this opportunity, has flooded the public with articles and television shows questioning the accuracy, fairness, and morality of capital punishment in America. The nation appears to be reassessing the institution of capital punishment, and central to that evaluation is the appropriate role for the scientific community, and particularly the medical profession, in the accurate and ethical implementation of that punishment.

Unique circumstances and compelling arguments exist both for and against continued physician participation in executions, making any choice about participation a difficult one. This article critically examines the relevant ethical, legal, and policy arguments that bear on this decision. By doing so, it comes to the conclusion that, taken as a whole, all perspectives speak in favor of an active role for physicians in the lethal injection process, conditioned, in every case, on the wishes of the condemned. However, current legal tensions between state death penalty statutes and medical practice acts stand in the way, creating an unnecessary and unwarranted ethical bind for physicians. Although most death penalty statutes provide for or even require physician participation in executions, many current medical practice acts allow physicians to be subjected to professional discipline for such actions. Although the negative effect of this threat of sanction and delicensure is difficult to quantify, it increases as our system of capital punishment becomes more and more medicalized.

.   .   .

[†]From the quote, widely attributed to sixteenth-century French surgeon Ambroise Pare, "The task of medicine is to cure sometimes, to relieve often, and to comfort always."

Reprinted by permission of *New York University Journal of Legislation & Public Policy*.

Editors' note: Some text and author's notes have been cut. Students who want to read the article in its entirety should consult the original.

---

1. Neil Farber et al., *Physicians' Attitudes about Involvement in Lethal Injection for Capital Punishment*, 160 Archives Internal Med. 2912 (2000).

I   BACKGROUND

A. What Is "Participation"?

Before discussing whether or not physicians should participate in lethal injections and other forms of capital punishment, we must first define what "participation" means in this context. For the purposes of this article, physician participation refers only to actions taken as part of the actual execution process, as opposed to physician involvement in earlier stages of the criminal justice system, such as trials and sentencing hearings. The following actions are illustrative of the sort of physician participation in capital punishment envisioned by this article, but are not inflexible or exhaustive—details will necessarily depend on context. First are preparatory actions taken prior to the scheduled date of the execution, such as examining the condemned to determine whether any medical condition might interfere with the execution process, examining the condemned's medical records to determine and prescribe an appropriate lethal pharmacological regimen, or supervising the arrangement of medical supplies needed for the execution. Second are preparatory actions taken immediately prior to the execution, like preparing syringes with lethal solution, supervising attachment of a heart monitor to the condemned, locating appropriate veins for insertion of catheters that will deliver the lethal solution, or inserting the catheters. Next are supervisory or direct actions during the execution itself, including beginning the flow of the lethal solution, monitoring the flow of lethal solution, and monitoring the vital signs of the condemned. Finally, there are conclusory actions taken after the execution, most notably pronouncing death.[2]

B. History of Physician Participation in Executions

Physician participation in the death penalty is not novel. To the contrary, the medical establishment has had a long and storied history of involvement in both the evolution and implementation of capital punishment. While that participation may initially seem macabre, the impetus for physicians who have chosen to participate in the execution process has always been to ease the suffering of the condemned.

At the end of the eighteenth century, during the French Revolution, Dr. Joseph Ignace Guillotine developed the machine of the same name in an attempt to civilize the practice of capital punishment. Dr. Guillotine, a respected and dedicated physician, and a notable opponent of the death penalty, felt that his invention was a more humane alternative to contemporary approaches such as hanging because it was quick, relatively painless, and highly effective. The French surgeon Dr. Antoine Louis, who was likewise concerned with making capital punishment more humane and egalitarian, improved upon the guillotine's design by changing the blade's shape from crescent to diagonal, resulting in a cleaner incision.

Similarly, in 1887, a commission of American physicians lobbied for electrocution as a more humane alternative to hanging, claiming that hanging was imprecise, undignified, and unnecessarily unpleasant for criminals. In fact, two American physicians, Dr. Carlos MacDonald and Dr. E.C. Spitzka, supervised the first use of the electric chair as a method of execution. More recently, physicians played integral roles in the adoption and acceptance of lethal injections as the new standard of practice in capital punishment. Again, physicians were on hand to play prominent roles in the first executions by lethal injection.

It is perhaps because of the medical profession's extensive and intimate relationship with capital punishment policies that the death penalty has generally taken increasingly controlled, precise, and medicalized forms. This influence is most striking today, now that lethal injection is the mandatory or optional method of execution in the majority of states with capital punishment. This new method not only furthers the march towards more precise and painless forms of execution, but it incorporates what is otherwise a standard medical procedure as its foundation.

---

2. Alternatively, the AMA's Council on Ethical and Judicial Affairs has defined physician participation in executions to include three categories of actions: (1) actions that "directly cause the death of the condemned," such as administering the lethal injection itself; (2) actions that "assist, supervise, or contribute to the ability of another individual to directly cause the death of the condemned," such as prescribing the necessary drugs; and (3) actions that "could automatically cause an execution to be carried out on a condemned prisoner," including determinations of death during an execution. *Council Report, supra* note 1, at 368.

Whether this employment of the medical profession's tools in the realm of capital punishment is beneficial—and to whom—is debatable and is further addressed in Part II. For now, it is enough to acknowledge that the medicalization of capital punishment has taken place, and has done so in large part because of the active role that physicians have historically played in the implementation of the death penalty. It is from this perspective that we must approach the question of the appropriate role for physicians in future executions.

II ARGUMENTS FOR AND AGAINST PHYSICIAN PARTICIPATION IN EXECUTIONS

A. Ethical Arguments Against Physician Participation

Opponents of physician participation in the death penalty argue that doctors are healers, and as such, active participation by physicians in executions would be irreconcilable with their basic ethical code. The medical profession has an implicit understanding with the public that it will employ its tools and skills only for the betterment of individual and public health. Therefore, using their healing skills to serve as the harbingers of death appears to be contrary to medicine's most cherished ideals, and seems to violate the physician's fiduciary role to act in the best interests of the patient.

Such a position finds substantial support in both ancient and modern medical ethics. The Hippocratic Oath, while over 2000 years old, remains one of the most well-known and frequently cited sources of professional ideals for practicing physicians. Popularly attributed to physicians of the Hippocratic tradition who dominated Greek medicine near 400 B.C., the Oath's language broadly condemns any physician action taken with the intent of causing harm or death: "I will prescribe regimen for the good of my patients according to my ability and my judgment and never do harm to anyone. To please no one will I prescribe a deadly drug, nor give advice which may cause his death."

Modern ethical treatments of medical practice stress similar disdain for actions that knowingly present harm to patients or contribute to death. That sentiment, embodied by the ideal of nonmaleficence, remains a cornerstone of current bioethical ideology. The American Medical Association, the most powerful political faction within the profession, continues to oppose an active role for physicians in the execution process. In its statement on the ethics of physician participation in executions, the AMA's Council on Ethical and Judicial Affairs (CEJA) pronounced: "A physician, as a member of a profession dedicated to preserving life when there is hope of doing so, should not be a participant in a legally authorized execution."

In 1994, physician and human rights organizations published an in-depth review and ethical analysis of physician participation in executions which concluded that, beyond the Hippocratic Oath's and the AMA's general prohibitions, proscription of physician participation is justified on more specific grounds that outweigh its potential beneficial effects:

> Although physician participation in some instances may arguably reduce pain, there are many countervailing arguments. First, the purpose of medical involvement may not be to reduce harm or suffering, but to give the surface appearance of humanity. Second, the physician presence also serves to give an aura of medical legitimacy to the procedure. Third, in the larger picture, the physician is taking over some of the responsibility for carrying out the punishment and in this context, becomes the handmaiden of the state as executioner. In return for possible reduction of pain, the physician, in effect, acts under the control of the state, doing harm.[3]

Acknowledging that someone must oversee the technical aspects of executions, those opposed to physician participation assert that other non-physician personnel could serve as able substitutes. Lethal injections are not technically difficult. They merely consist of inserting intravenous lines, administering a drug through those lines, monitoring vital signs, and pronouncing death. It requires little more than training in basic blood-drawing and monitoring. Therefore, other allied health professionals, such as nurses or physician assistants (PAs), or a new class of medical technicians trained specifically for such situations, could fill this role, leaving physicians to fulfill their ethical obligations.

---

3. Breach Of Trust, *supra* note 1, at 38.

B. Ethical Arguments for Physician Participation

"The task of medicine is to cure sometimes, to relieve often, to comfort always." That is the ethical ideal to which physicians should aspire. Physicians' deepest obligation is to their patients' interests and wishes. While it is true that the preservation of life is an important maxim for medical practitioners, it is neither always the paramount ethical value nor always in the best interests of the patient. The preservation of life must, therefore, yield at times to other objectives, such as the treatment of extreme suffering. Such is the logic of the ethical acceptance of withholding and withdrawing life-sustaining treatment to relieve pain and suffering. Doing so hastens, and arguably even causes, death. But for some patients, death is a welcome alternative to a slowly deteriorating life of agony. More generally, contemporary legal theory and medical ethics both sanction the Double Effect Doctrine, which holds that actions undertaken for beneficent purposes, such as the amelioration of suffering, may be morally permissible even if they foreseeably contribute to death. Ethical ideologies such as the Hippocratic tradition that categorically preclude physician actions that contribute to death fail to appreciate this distinction, and thus miss the mark.

For many other reasons, it seems unreasonable to rely on the Hippocratic Oath as a rigid and ultimate source of ethical guidance. For one, the foremost historian on the Oath has concluded that it has never been representative of prevailing thought in medical ethics, and was never intended to be an absolute standard for medical conduct. In fact, the Oath was likely the product of a small, nontraditional Greek sect of Pythagorean physicians. Further, regardless of its role in ancient medical practice, the Oath's broad mandates make it anachronistic and antithetical to modern medical practice and ethics. For instance, it explicitly forbids abortion, restricts the practice of medicine to men, and prohibits physicians from ever breaching patient confidentiality, despite the well-established obligation of modern day physicians to do so in various situations. Blindly clinging to its "Do no harm" ideology in the face of so many other clearly inapplicable edicts without critically examining its justification disserves both the profession and the public.

More fundamentally, it is inaccurate to conceive of medical ethics as being driven by a single imperative, such as "Preserve life" or "Do no harm." Instead, it requires balancing a number of independent interests and objectives. Sometimes the totality of the circumstances will call for the preservation of life, sometimes it will not. In many situations, hastening death is harmful and contrary to the patient's best interests, but in other instances it is the only compassionate thing that can be done. What is important is not that physicians stave off death, but that they tailor their actions, as much as possible, to the interests of their patients and the realities and necessities of the circumstances. The practice of medicine is a therapeutic *and* compassionate enterprise, dedicated to furthering human dignity and well-being beyond the myopic goal of simply preserving life. The relevant question then changes: What should the caring physician do to best comfort an individual being executed?

Operating within this reality, it is not clear that physician participation in executions is contrary to either the patient's interests or the doctor's ethical obligations. As the AMA states, "A physician, as a member of a profession dedicated to preserving life *when there is hope of doing so*, should not be a participant in a legally authorized execution." But here, there is no such hope. This is a patient who is going to die. By the time physicians become involved in the actual execution process, prisoners have exhausted all appeals and the state has assigned an execution date. Barring intervention by the governor or the Supreme Court, the death of the condemned is a forgone conclusion. Condemned death row inmates are, for all practical purposes, terminally ill patients, albeit under a nontraditional definition of the term, and deserve to be treated as such. Therefore, physicians should do what any compassionate physician would do for a dying patient—preside over the condemned's final moments to minimize complications and suffering, and maximize the patient's comfort until the end of his life. Physicians are expected to provide these services to all others facing imminent death. Why should they deny comforting care to the condemned? It is the physician who abandons his or her patient by failing to provide such comforting care who truly violates the ethical code of the profession.

By contrast, physicians who care for condemned prisoners at their executions are models for other doctors and medical students. They poignantly illustrate the physician's obligation not to abandon the dying. To desert these individuals in their most vulnerable hour would be antithetical to the beneficent ideals of medical practice. Physicians are ethically obligated to help their patients, and considering the circumstances, all that can be done here is to ensure the condemned's comfort and minimize their suffering. The caring physician can prescribe and prepare a lethal pharmacological regimen compatible with the condemned's unique medical condition, and assure that the drugs are given in the correct order, thereby minimizing the chance that the condemned will regain consciousness during the lethal injection and suffer the unimaginable horror of conscious asphyxiation. The physician can locate appropriate veins and insert the catheters so that the condemned will not suffer the pain and humiliation of multiple needle punctures by inept technicians. The physician can monitor vital signs during the injection to guarantee that death, and not some irreversible condition of brain damage, is achieved. That is the ethical role for the compassionate physician—to help a patient in need and provide the only source of comforting care still available.

Even the narrower proposition that physicians should not participate in the *involuntary* death of a patient (i.e., a death against the patient's wishes) lacks reason and rationality. Quite commonly, and necessarily, physicians are actively involved in involuntary deaths. How often does the terminal cancer patient or gun shot victim really "want" to die? Granted, for some, acceptance of impending death is achieved, but this is quite different from what we think of as "voluntary." Yet we acknowledge the ethical propriety of physician involvement, even palliative actions that hasten death, in such cases. It is not the mere participation in involuntary deaths by physicians that bothers us, but participation motivated by any desire other than to maximize comfort and minimize suffering for the individual, such as a desire to force an involuntary death upon an individual.

There is no rational distinction between the dying patient and the condemned criminal, *if* one accepts the patient-centered conception of medical ethics espoused above. In neither the hospital nor the execution chamber does the physician kill the patient—in one, it is the disease or trauma, in the other, it is the state. Put differently, in neither case is the physician a "but for" cause of death—death would take place regardless of whether the physician was involved or not. And if the physician is ultimately ethically obligated to the patient, why should it matter what the underlying cause of death is? In all end-of-life situations, where there is no hope of survival, the physician's role is to minimize suffering and maximize comfort for the patient. Therefore, it is the condemned patient who suffers when the medical establishment arbitrarily chooses to turn its back on, and withhold its experience and wisdom from, this subset of the patient population. The only relevant achievement of such categorical abandonment is increased suffering for the condemned patient, and, ethically, this cannot be tolerated.

The only rule that one can derive from the classic ethical prohibition of physician participation in executions that is consistent with a patient-centered theory of medical ethics is the following: A physician should not participate in the death of a patient, whether voluntary or involuntary, if such participation is against the wishes of that patient. Any other rule necessarily fosters irrationality, discrimination, and a departure from the core tenets of medical ethics. The condemned should be free to request or refuse physician oversight, and the individual physician should be free to choose to participate in executions or not to do so. But the medical profession should not, based on political beliefs and flawed conceptions of ethical practice, deprive condemned patients of this last choice and physicians of the leeway to carry out that wish. Paternalism practiced for the benefit of patients is problematic, but paternalism practiced to the detriment of patients is unacceptable.

True, physician participation may have the consequence of providing a surface appearance of humanity or adding an aura of medical legitimacy to the execution process. This is undoubtedly a troubling proposition, and one worthy of significant consideration. But this is a concern with the death penalty itself, not physician participation. The unease that underlies this potential whitewashing of the core identity of the death penalty concerns the morality of any state-sanctioned taking of life, not the involvement of physicians in carrying out that penalty. The physician's obligation is to the patient, not to the political agenda of special interest groups—not even to the American Medical Association. And although it is sometimes difficult to distinguish intent (when is participation intended to ameliorate suffering and when does it aim to aid in execution?), the AMA has stated in the execution context that, "[T]here is no alternative at this time than to rely upon the treating physician to exercise judgment in deciding when and to what extent treatment is necessary to reduce suffering."

Further, although less trained personnel could oversee the execution process, experience proves that without the benefit of compassionate physician oversight, condemned patients sometimes endure unnecessary pain and suffering. Media accounts have detailed numerous instances in which poorly trained execution technicians botched seemingly basic medical procedures, leading to excruciating pain and prolonged suffering for the condemned. Maybe these procedures are more difficult than they appear. Or maybe the stress of the situation leads to errors in the procedures. Regardless, physicians have more extensive training and experience acting under the pressure of imminent death than any other class of health practitioners. Participation by skilled physicians could likely protect many of the condemned from unnecessary mishaps. Further, there is a lack of logic underlying the assertion that, although it is inappropriate for physicians to play this role, nurses or PAs could alternatively do so. Why are other health professionals any less dedicated to the ethical ideals of medical practice, whatever those might be, than physicians? Why shouldn't the same ethical arguments and constraints apply to them?

Logic and consistency also argue for physician participation. Doctors routinely use their medical skills to contribute to the capital punishment process. Physicians facilitate the gathering of evidence when they pump victims' stomachs or draw blood from detained suspects for DNA or other testing. They regularly testify in criminal trials and capital sentencing hearings. They restore the mentally ill to competence in the process leveling the last barrier to execution.

Some may argue that participation at these earlier stages is somehow ethically distinct from participation in the final process, but such arbitrary and emotionally-based distinctions have little merit. Participation in any stage of a capital case is ethically equivalent, as it may always be a "but for" cause of

execution. To argue otherwise blurs the line between emotion and logic. Were it not for a DNA test based on a physician's blood-draw or the psychiatrist's testimony that the accused is competent to stand trial, there would be no conviction, and thus no execution. Likewise, were it not for the pharmacological restoration of competency, there would be no execution. Such conduct differs temporally from direct participation in executions, but not ethically. In all cases, there is at least the possibility that the physician's conduct will facilitate an execution. Prohibiting physicians from fulfilling their ethical obligations of care and compassion at the end of the criminal process—when their patients need them the most—while ignoring that physicians play integral roles throughout that process is arbitrary and irrational. There is no reasoned way to draw this bright line across time.

C. Policy Arguments Against Physician Participation

Opponents of physician participation in executions argue that such involvement will erode the public's trust in the medical profession. According to this argument, the credibility of the profession is undermined when its members take actions that directly conflict with its central mission. As former AMA Executive Vice President James Todd, M.D., put it, "When the healing hand becomes the hand inflicting the wound, the world is turned inside out."[4] Blurring the line between healer and executioner, then, will allegedly compromise future interactions between the medical profession and the public, as patients will question their physicians' motives and loyalties.

Opponents of physician participation also note that in the recent physician-assisted suicide case of *Washington v. Glucksberg*, the United States Supreme Court asserted that states "ha[ve] an interest in protecting the integrity and ethics of the medical profession." This interest presumably arises from states' obligation to promote the safety and well-being of their citizens. Some might argue that in furtherance

---

4. James Todd, Address at Opening of *The Worth of the Human Being: Medicine in Germany 1918–1945* (Nov. 5, 1992), *quoted in* BREACH OF TRUST, *supra* note 1, at 38.

of this interest, legislatures should explicitly prohibit physicians from taking actions, such as participating in executions, which have the potential to jeopardize the public-physician relationship.

In addition, some have argued that physicians should not be "prostituting medical knowledge and skills" to legitimize "the nonbeneficent goals of the state." They argue that by turning to medicalized forms of execution like lethal injection, and by having the medical profession lend its credibility to the execution process, pro-capital punishment groups are distorting public perception of the death penalty. The process becomes more palatable, but no less inhumane. Some go so far as to argue that this subversion of medicine's caring ethic for the furtherance of the state's criminal justice system is highly reminiscent of, and equally inappropriate as, the role that Nazi physicians played in covering up and rationalizing the atrocities of the Holocaust.

D. Policy Arguments for Physician Participation

Despite the initial appeal of the preceding policy arguments, further reflection casts serious doubts on their merits. While there is a trust between the public and the medical profession, physician participation in executions will not undermine that trust. First, such actions are not incompatible with the physician's role when properly conceived of as that of a compassionate healer, as opposed to a zealous advocate of the preservation of life under all circumstances. Second, there is no empirical evidence to support the conclusion that physician participation in executions is detrimental to the best interests of the public.

Although the *Glucksberg* Court did indeed assert that states have an interest in protecting the integrity and ethics of the medical profession, it stopped there. The Court merely acknowledged the existence of the opinion *by others* that certain behaviors, like physician-assisted suicide, *could* adversely affect the medical community's image and *perhaps* harm the public. But it did not take that view as its own, and with good reason.

The argument that physician involvement in execution harms the public by eroding its trust in the medical establishment is unsupported and over-stated. Does the presence of a priest at a parishioner's execution erode the public's trust in the church? Certainly not. The mere involvement of a priest in an execution says nothing about either the priest's or the church's feelings about the death penalty. The clergy's involvement is intended to minimize the suffering of the condemned, not contribute to the punishment. The public recognizes that distinction, and its trust in religious institutions has not wavered as a result of clergy participation in executions. The same should hold true for physicians, even if they play a more direct role in the execution process than the clergy.

Like the clergy, physicians who participate in executions do not make political statements about the death penalty, and they do not blur the line between healing and harming. Rather, such participation reinforces the medical profession's compassion for all human beings—even those sentenced to death. By overseeing the execution process, physicians fulfill their ethical obligation to ensure that society carries out its medicalized executions as humanely and painlessly as possible.

In fact, one could credibly argue that physicians are more likely to erode public trust by *refusing* to participate in executions than by participating. The public could view a blanket refusal by physicians to assist a dying prisoner as medical abandonment in the patients' greatest hour of need. This is particularly so for penitentiary staff physicians who have already established doctor-patient relationships with the condemned. The refusal to care for certain patients—those who are sentenced to death—undergoing medically related procedures (i.e., lethal injections) could taint the public's view of the medical profession. Prisoners, too, are deserving of compassionate and competent medical care.

The public's trust in physicians is built on the profession's unswerving commitment to the medical interests of its patients, regardless of the circumstances. It is worth repeating: "The task of medicine is to cure sometimes, to relieve often, to comfort always." This is the ultimate expression of the medical establishment's altruistic ideal, and it underscores the point that the doctor-patient relationship does not end on death row. Without question, states have an interest in maintaining the ethics of the medical profession. But allowing medical ethics boards to professionally sanction physicians for providing comfort care to condemned prisoners contradicts this interest.

The lack of evidence of any such detrimental effect on public trust is also highly instructive. As noted previously, the medical establishment has consulted for and participated in state ordered executions for centuries. But in the face of all this intermingling of medicine and capital punishment, we have yet to see erosion in the doctor-patient or doctor-public relationship as a consequence. There is no reason to believe that continued active participation in lethal injections, in the name of compassion and comfort, will be any different. In fact, the one court that has directly addressed this issue, a California court of appeals, concluded that there is no evidence that such conduct "has in any way affected the trusting quality of the doctor-patient relationship for the population at large."

Further, analogies between physician participation in American executions and the role of Nazi doctors in the Holocaust fail to appreciate crucial differences between the two contexts. First and foremost, the democratic nature of our system of government and our treatment of capital punishment undercuts analogies to the dictatorial political environment of Nazi Germany. The citizens of the United States democratically chose the death penalty, and the majority of citizens continue to support its use. Here, the state's objective is to carry out the will of the people, not usurp it. Second, our legal system and the rights guaranteed to citizens by our Constitution, such as the Fourteenth Amendment's due process guarantees and the Sixth Amendment's right to a trial by an impartial jury, provide protections that were not available to Holocaust victims. We do not arbitrarily choose whom to execute. Third, as this article suggests, physicians should willingly participate in executions only if their participation is consistent with the wishes of the condemned. They should not force their way into the execution chamber. Because the decision on physician participation lies with the condemned patient, any analogies to Nazi physicians are fundamentally flawed. This emotional appeal to a terrible tragedy in world history may be powerful, but it is unfounded and exaggerated.

Our democratic governance structure has further implications for arguments against physician participation, particularly those that are based on philosophical or moral disapproval of capital punishment itself. If an individual opposes the death penalty, he or she can and should support legislation and candidates that are similarly opposed. The same is true for physicians. But what physicians should not do is refuse, on professional grounds, to participate in executions in order to subvert the democratic will of the people. Doctors are healers, not politicians, and the medical establishment should not exert its political power to the detriment of its patients. To be sure, physicians may lobby against the death penalty. But if the death penalty is to be undermined, it should be done democratically or constitutionally, not through the strong-arm politics of physicians or other professional groups. And as long as state ordered executions persist, physicians' primary ethical obligation is to make them as painless and humane as possible for the condemned.

. . .

CONCLUSION

Few social conventions evoke more visceral and polemical reactions than capital punishment. The involuntary termination of an individual life is permanent and final. Reflexive opposition to healers' participation, of any kind, is to be expected because of the grave, contentious, and irreversible nature of an execution. But a patient-centered theory of medical ethics demands a more probing analysis.

The current trend towards lethal injection as the preferred method of execution presents an opportunity for physicians to participate in the evolution and implementation of capital punishment in this country while still maintaining their role as comforting caregivers. Despite reasonable and legitimate concerns, ethical, legal, and public policy considerations all suggest that physicians should embrace this opportunity to extend their comforting capabilities to the condemned. Physicians should not, as urged by the dominant professional societies, abandon these patients for the sake of political posturing. External influences have already fractured the modern doctor-patient relationship; professional politics should not compromise patient care in the execution chamber.

Further, legislatures should remove the ambiguity that currently plagues statutes concerning physician participation in capital punishment in a way that explicitly permits physician involvement in the execution process. This resolution will benefit the condemned, the profession, and society at large. It is clear that preventable mishaps occur during executions, particularly lethal injections. Competent medical oversight by physicians can ensure that these mishaps are minimized as much as they possibly can be. Prisoners killed by the state are entitled to such competent oversight—no one should be sentenced to a botched execution.

DIALYSIS FOR A PRISONER OF WAR

United States Special Forces capture a combatant in the mountains of Eastern Afghanistan whom they believe has vital information that would help lead to the arrest of a major suspected terrorist. He is transferred to a U.S. military hospital at an undisclosed location. The physicians at the hospital soon discover that he is suffering from renal failure, and they prepare to provide dialysis. The combatant refuses, however, stating that he would rather die than live as a prisoner of the United States.

Uncertain how to proceed, the military nephrologist asks her commanding officer for guidance. The question of whether to override the prisoner's refusal of treatment is quickly relayed up the military hierarchy. Two days later, the Secretary of Defense delivers the order to initiate dialysis, despite the prisoner's refusal. The order cites as justification the pressing national security interest in keeping the prisoner alive for a thorough interrogation that would lead to the arrest of an important terrorist suspect. Is the decision the right course of action?

COMMENTARY

Daniel Zupan, Gary Solis, and Richard Schoonhoven

This case is difficult to decide. Most of the international legal resources seem to suggest that the individual, who we presume is an enemy prisoner of war—an EPW—could be treated. The United States in this case has complied with its 1949 Geneva POW Convention responsibilities to admit and treat prisoners of war. However, his demand not to undergo medical treatment takes us outside the Geneva conventions. If the patient were an American combatant, we would rely on the Supreme Court's holding in *In re Quinlan* that a competent adult has a right to refuse life-saving medical treatment, but Supreme Court rulings do not apply to foreign-situated

non-citizens. Nor does a U.S.-ratified human rights treaty exist that bears on this point.

The traditional law of armed conflict also does not render treatment unacceptable. First, dialysis is unlikely to cause unnecessary suffering—one of the law of armed conflicts's four core concepts—because the suffering caused would *not* be clearly disproportionate to the military advantage gained, namely, significant military intelligence. Further, the core concept of military necessity tells us that measures not *forbidden* by international law are *lawful* if they are indispensable for securing the enemy's prompt submission, and this may describe the military intelligence here. So, providing life-saving care over an EPW's objection contradicts neither ratified international law nor the conventional law of armed conflict.

From *Hastings Center Report* 34, no. 6 (November–December 2004). Reprinted by permission of The Hastings Center.

Nor is providing dialysis in this case contrary to the two 1977 Additional Protocols (APs) to the 1949 Geneva Conventions, which have been signed but not ratified by the United States (and ratified by most of the rest of the world—161 of 191 nations, including most of our major allies). Article 11.5 of AP I, applicable to international armed conflicts, states that detainees "have the right to refuse any surgical operation," but dialysis does not fall within either the letter or spirit of that article. Article 10.2 of AP II, applicable to internal conflicts, specifies that "Persons engaged in medical activities shall [not] be compelled to perform acts. . . . contrary to . . . the rules of medical ethics. . . . " Disregarding the EPW's wishes may conflict with the nephrologist's view of medical ethics that a patient's wishes should always be honored.

In any event, this is not an AP II situation, and the United States has ratified neither of the APs. In short, we believe that disregarding the EPW's wishes to forego dialysis presents no violation of domestic, international, or battlefield law. However, we feel that the case's complexity warrants reliance on a moral perspective over a legal one. Also, our legal analysis might be different if the EPW had refused dialysis on religious or moral grounds. Moreover, it might be that we should afford the EPW the same basic rights that we afford our domestic criminals, whether he refuses dialysis on religious grounds or because he wishes not to be a prisoner.

If the moral analysis should be decisive, then the Supreme Court's ruling in the Quinlan case applies here, and, military necessity notwithstanding, we should abide by the prisoner's wishes because the Court's legal ruling can be seen as representing a moral principle related to the dignity of humanity, something we respect even in criminals,

and therefore in an EPW. With both criminals and EPWs, for example, we rule out torture. This consideration reveals the limits of what we can do, even for purposes of military necessity.

Much controversy revolves around what we may or may not do to an EPW in the current war on terror; controversy exists concerning what does or does not constitute torture. In order to keep our moral bearings in the face of ambiguity and the mounting pressure of military necessity, we should abide by the standards of domestic law, at least with respect to basic human rights, if not for all civil rights. If a certain procedure is permitted under domestic law, it should be permissible in the case of an EPW. If the procedure is prohibited under domestic law, it should be prohibited in the case of an EPW. Such a methodology would be consistent with the United States' legal and moral commitments.

We offer a final observation about how the moral analysis could be extended. We assume that there would be no qualms about preventing a prisoner from committing suicide simply because he did not want to be in our custody. If this is right, then comparing the similarities and differences between refusal of treatment and suicide might clarify further the moral requirements of this case. Dialysis is similar to preventing suicide in that it requires intervention on our part. On the other hand, dialysis arguably differs from preventing suicide in that it interferes with the "natural" course of events while preventing suicide protects it, although such appeals are notoriously hard to make. As it stands, our conviction is that the case is morally ambiguous, and that in such situations, we should take our lead from domestic law, on the grounds that domestic law is built around our most compelling moral principles and that these principles should prevail.

COMMENTARY

George Annas

Battlefield bioethics is much more intense and potentially conflicted than "civilian" bioethics; nonetheless, the core duties of physicians are substantially identical. At the outset, the question in this case admits a simple answer, which follows the Geneva Conventions. A captured combatant is a prisoner of war. Prisoners of war are entitled to medical treatment as detailed in the Geneva Conventions (III) and the two protocols. Prisoners are no longer combatants, and military physicians must treat sick prisoners just as they would treat sick or wounded members of their own military units or wounded civilians. Moreover, the protocols, which are part of international customary law, include a noncontroversial section that prohibits any physician from being punished "for carrying out medical activities compatible with medical ethics." POWs cannot be coerced into answering any questions beyond their name, rank, and serial number. Applying the Geneva Conventions principles, the POW should have the same right to refuse treatment that an American civilian would have. Since medical ethics would prohibit forced treatment under these circumstances, so would the Geneva Conventions, Geneva III, Article 17 also prohibits "any form of coercion" from being "inflicted on prisoners of war to secure from them any information of any kind whatever." In short, the POW's right to refuse treatment should be honored, though the nephrologist would be justified to review the refusal periodically with the prisoner-patient.

The simple and correct treatment decision was not made, however, because the nephrologist undermined her role as a physician by deciding not on medical ethics, but on military considerations by referring it up the chain of command. This illustrates the physician-soldier's ever-present dual loyalty problem in wartime: is the physician first and foremost a physician, whose primary loyalty must be to patients; or is the physician first and foremost a military officer, whose primary loyalty and duty is to the military mission? These dual loyalties do not always conflict, but in this case they do, and the two competing ethics cannot be reconciled. Following medical ethics, acting in the POW's best interests would have required further exploration of motivation and of the alternative treatments available, and these discussions, and the ultimate treatment decision, would have been made in the context of the doctor-patient relationship. Once the nephrologist determined that her obligations were primarily to the military, she referred the decision to her superior officers, who had no firsthand knowledge of the patient's medical condition and whose primary interest was in fulfilling the military mission. The nephrologist should not have been surprised that, having asked her superior officers to answer her question for her, ultimately a non-medical superior, the Secretary of Defense, made a military decision and ordered her to carry it out. Under these circumstances she must under military rules initiate dialysis or face court martial.

If she decides to carry out the order, and the prisoner either refuses to agree or actively resists, then to the extent that physical force, drugs, or the threat of them are necessary to restrain the prisoner to make the treatment possible, the "treatment" would amount to torture and abuse under the Geneva Conventions, and the nephrologist would be obligated (under both the Conventions and the basic rules governing medical officers in the United States military) to cease attempting to perform dialysis at this point. I believe torture is never permissible: it is wrong as a matter of morality and international human rights law and laws of war, and (taking a utilitarian point of view) because it virtually never produces accurate information. Some commentators mistakenly make an exception for circumstances that do not exist in this case or any other in the real world, sometimes called "supreme necessity," when torture will almost certainly result in saving the entire country, winning the war, or saving the lives of many innocent people.

This case illustrates the dual loyalty problem that the military could and should solve by adopting a clear doctrine stating that the ethical obligation of a military physician is always to act in the best interests of the patient (with the patient's consent)—military, civilian, and captured enemy alike.

RECOMMENDED SUPPLEMENTARY READING

GENERAL WORKS

Ahronheim, Judith C., Jonathan D., Moreno, and Connie Zuckerman. *Ethics in Clinical Practice.* 2nd ed. Gaithersburg, MD: Aspen, 2000.

Annas, George J. *Standard of Care: The Law of American Bioethics.* Oxford: Oxford University Press, 1993.

Beauchamp, Tom L., and James F. Childress. *Principles of Biomedical Ethics.* 5th ed. New York: Oxford University Press, 2001.

Benjamin, Martin, and Joy Curtis. *Ethics im Nursing.* New York: Oxford University Press, 1992.

Burt, Robert. *Taking Care of Strangers.* New York: Free Press, 1979.

Campbell, Alastair, Max Charlesworth, Grant Gillett and Gareth Jones. *Medical Ethics.* New York: Oxford University Press, 1997.

Caplan, Arthur. *If I Were a Rich Man Could I Buy a Pancreas?* Bloomington: Indiana University Press, 1992.

Cassell, Eric. *The Nature of Suffering and the Goals of Medicine.* New York: Oxford University Press, 1991.

Childress, James F. *Practical Reasoning in Bioethics.* Bloomington: Indiana University Press, 1997.

Crigger, Bette-Jane, ed. *Cases in Bioethics.* 3rd ed. New York: St. Martin's Press, 1998.

Downie, R. S., and Kenneth C. Calman. *Healthy Respect: Ethics in Health Care.* New York: Oxford University Press, 1994.

Dubler, Nancy, and David Nimmons. *Ethics on Call.* New York: Crown, 1992.

Dworkin, Roger B. *Limits: The Role of the Law in Bioethical Decision Making.* Bloomington: Indiana University Press, 1996.

Englehardt, H. Tristam, Jr. *The Foundations of Bioethics.* 2nd ed. New York: Oxford University Press, 1996.

Fried, C. *Medical Experimentation: Personal Integrity and Social Policy.* New York: Elsevier, 1974.

Gert, Bernard. Charles M. Culver and K. Danner Clouser. *Bioethics: A Return to Fundamentals.* New York: Oxford University Press, 1997.

Groopman, Jerome. *How Doctors Think.* Boston: Houghton Mifflin, 2007.

Herbert, Philip. *Doing Right: A Practical Guide for Physicians and Medical Trainees.* New York: Oxford University Press, 1996.

Holms, Helen, and Laura Purdy, eds. *Feminist Perspectives in Medical Ethics.* Bloomington: Indiana University Press, 1992.

Jonsen, Albert. *The New Medicine and the Old Ethics.* Cambridge, MA: Harvard University Press, 1990.

Kass, Leon. *Toward a More Natural Science.* New York: Free Press, 1985.

Kuhse, Helga, and Peter Singer. *A Companion to Bioethics.* Oxford: Basil Blackwell, 1998.

Macklin, Ruth. *Mortal Choices: Bioethics in Today's World.* New York: Pantheon Books, 1987.

May, Thomas. *Bioethics in a Liberal Society: The Political Framework of Bioethics Decision Making.* Baltimore: Johns Hopkins University Press, 2002.

May, William F. *The Patient's Ordeal.* Bloomington: Indiana University Press, 1991.

McGee, Glenn, ed. *Pragmatic Bioethics.* Nashville, TN: Vanderbilt University Press, 1999.

Moreno, Jonathan D. *Deciding Together.* New York: Oxford University Press, 1995.

Pence, Gregory. *Classic Cases in Medical Ethics: Accounts of Cases That Have Shaped Medical Ethics, with Philosophical, Legal, and Historical Backgrounds.* Berkshire: McGraw-Hill Humanities, 2003.

Polansky, Ronald, and Mark Kuczewski, eds. *Bioethics: Ancient Themes in Contemporary Issues.* Cambridge, MA: MIT Press, 2000.

Reynolds, Richard, and John, Stone, eds. *On Doctoring.* Washington DC: Free Press, 2001.

Rothman, David J. *Strangers at the Bedside: A History of How Law and Bioethics Transformed Medical Decision Making.* New York: Basic Books, 1991.

Steinbock, Bonnie. *The Oxford Handbook of Bioethics.* New York: Oxford University Press, 2007.

Tong, Rosemarie. *Feminist Approaches to Bioethics.* Boulder, CO: Westview Press, 1997.

Veatch, Robert M. *A Theory of Medical Ethics.* New York: Basic Books, 1981.

AUTONOMY, PATERNALISM, AND MEDICAL MODELS

Agich, George J. *Autonomy and Long-Term Care.* Oxford: Oxford University Press, 1993.

Blustein, Jeffrey. "Doing What the Patient Orders: Maintaining Integrity in the Doctor-Patient Relationship." *Bioethics* 7, no. 4 (1993): 289–314.

Bok, Sissela. *Lying.* New York: Pantheon Books, 1978.

———. *Secrets: On the Ethics of Concealment and Revelation.* New York: Pantheon Books, 1982.

———. *Common Values.* Columbia: University of Missouri Press, 1995.

Brennan, Troy A. *Just Doctoring: Medical Ethics in the Liberal State.* Berkeley: University of California Press, 1991.

Brody, Howard. *The Healer's Power.* New Haven, CT: Yale University Press, 1992.

Churchill, Larry R. "Reviving a Distinctive Medical Ethic." *Hastings Center Report* (May–June 1989): 28–34.

Collopy, Bart J., Nancy Dubler, and Connie Zuckerman. "The Ethics of Home Care: Autonomy and Accommodation." *Hastings Center Report* (March–April 1990): S1–S16.

Dworkin, Gerald. *The Theory and Practice of Autonomy.* Cambridge: Cambridge University Press, 1988.

Fan, Ruiping. "Self-Determination vs. Family-Determination: Two Incommensurable Principles of Autonomy." *Bioethics* 11 (1997): 309–322.

Halper, Thomas. "Privacy and Autonomy: From Warren and Brandeis to Roe and Cruzan." *Journal of Medicine and Philosophy* 21, no. 2 (April 1996): 121–135.

"Healthcare Relationships: Ties That Bind." *Cambridge Quarterly of Healthcare Ethics* 3, no. 1 (Winter 1994): 1–82.

Kant, Immanuel. "On the Supposed Right to Lie from Altruistic Motives." In *Critique of Practical Reason,* trans. L. W. Beck. Chicago: University of Chicago Press, 1949.

Kleinig, John. *Paternalism.* Totowa, NJ: Rowman and Allanheld, 1984.

Kultgen, John. *Autonomy and Intervention: Paternalism in the Caring Life.* New York: Oxford University Press, 1995.

Levi, Benjamin H. *Respecting Patient Autonomy.* Urbana: University of Illinois Press, 1999.

Lidz, Charles, Lynn Fischer, and Robert M. Arnold. *The Erosion of Autonomy in Long-Term Care.* Oxford: Oxford University Press, 1992.

May, William F. "Code, Covenant, Contract, or Philanthropy." *Hastings Center Report* 5 (December 1975): 29–38.

O'Neill, Onora. *Autonomy and Trust in Bioethics.* Cambridge: Cambridge University Press, 2002.

Pellegrino, Edmund D., and David C. Thomasma. *For the Patient's Good: The Restoration of Beneficence in Health Care.* New York: Oxford University Press, 1988.

Quill, Timothy E., and Howard Brody. "Physician Recommendations and Patient Autonomy: Finding a Balance between Physician Power and Patient Choice." *Annals of Internal Medicine* 125, no. 9 (1996): 763–769.

Schermer, M. *The Different Faces of Autonomy: Patient Autonomy in Ethical Theory and Hospital Practice.* New York: Springer, 2003.

Schneider, Carl E. *The Practice of Autonomy: Patients, Doctors, and Medical Decisions.* New York: Oxford University Press, 1998.

Shelp, Earl E., ed. *Virtue and Medicine.* Dordrecht, Holland: D. Reidel, 1985.

Strasser, Mark. "The New Paternalism." *Bioethics* 7, no. 2 (1988): 103–117.

Tauber, Alfred I. *Patient Autonomy and the Ethics of Responsibility.* Boston: MIT Press, 2005.

VanDeVeer, Donald. *Paternalistic Intervention: The Moral Bounds of Benevolence.* Princeton, NJ: Princeton University Press, 1986.

Veatch, Robert M. "Models for Medicine in a Revolutionary Age." *Hastings Center Report* 2 (June 1972): 5–7.

INFORMED CONSENT AND TRUTH-TELLING

Appelbaum, Paul S., Charles W., Lidz, and Alan Meisel. *Informed Consent: Legal Theory and Clinical Practice.* New York: Oxford University Press, 1987.

Berg, Jessica, Paul Appelbaum Charles Lidz, and Lisa Parker. *Informed Consent: Legal Theory and Clinical Practice.* 2nd ed. New York: Oxford University Press, 2001.

Brock, Dan. *Life and Death: Philosophical Essays in Biomedical Ethics.* New York: Cambridge University Press, 1993.

Cassell, Eric J. *Talking with Patients: Vol. 1. The Theory of Doctor-Patient Communication* and *Vol. 2. Clinical Technique:* Cambridge, MA: MIT Press, 1985.

Faden, Ruth, and Tom Beauchamp. *A History and Theory of Informed Consent.* New York: Oxford University Press, 1986.

Geller, Gail et al. "'Decoding' Informed Consent." *Hastings Center Report* (March–April 1997): 28–33.

"In Case of Emergency: No Need for Consent." *Hastings Center Report* (symposium, January– February 1997): 7–12.

Katz, Jay. *The Silent World of Doctor and Patient.* New York: Free Press, 1984.

Kuczewski, Mark G. "Reconceiving the Family: The Process of Consent in Medical Decisionmaking." *Hastings Center Report* (March–April 1996): 30–37.

Marta, Jan. "A Linguistic Model of Informed Consent." *Journal of Medicine and Philosophy* 21, no. 1 (February 1996): 41–60.

President's Commission for the Study of Ethical Problems in Medicine and Biomedical and Behavioral Research. Making Health Care Decisions: The Ethical and Legal Implications of Informed Consent in the Patient-Practitioner Relationship. Washington, DC: U.S. Government Printing Office, 1982.

Schuck, Peter H. "Rethinking Informed Consent." *Yale Law Journal* 103 (1994): 899 ff.

Veatch, Robert M. "Abandoning Informed Consent." *Hastings Center Report* (March–April 1995): 5–12.

CONFLICTING PROFESSIONAL ROLES AND RESPONSIBILITIES

Agich, George J., ed. *Responsibility in Health Care.* Dordrecht, Holland: D. Reidel, 1982.

Angell, Marcia. "The Doctor as Double Agent." *Kennedy Institute of Ethics Journal* 3, no. 3 (September 1993): 279.

Balint, John, Robert Baker, Martin Strosberg, and Sean Philpott, eds. *Ethics and Epidemics: Vol. 9. Advances in Bioethics.* Stamford, CT: JAI Press, 2006.

Chandrasekhar, C. A. "Rx for Drugstore Discrimination: Challenging Pharmacy Refusals to Dispense Prescription Contraceptives under State Public Accommodations Laws." *Albany Law Review* 70, no. 1 (2006): 55–115.

"Conflicts of Interest in Health Care." *American Journal of Law and Medicine* 21, nos. 2 and 3 (1995).

Danis, Marion, and Larry Churchill, "Automomy and the Common Weal." *Hastings Center Report* (January–February 1991): 25–31.

"The Ethics of Medical Mistakes: Historical, Legal, and Institutional Perspectives." *Kennedy Institute of Ethics Journal* 11, no. 2 (June 2001).

Fleischman, A. R., and A. Sikora. "Physician Participation in Capital Punishment: A Question of Professional Integrity." *Journal of Urban Health* 76, no. 4 (December 1999): 400–408.

Fost, Norman. "Ethical Issues in Whistleblowing." *Journal of the American Medical Association* 286, no. 5 (September 5, 2001): 1079.

Gawande, Atul. *Complications: A Surgeon's Notes on an Imperfect Science.* New York: Picador, 2003.

Gray, Bradford H. The Profit Motive and Patient Care: The Changing Accountability of Doctors and Hospitals. Cambridge, MA: Harvard University Press, 1991.

———, ed. *For-Profit Enterprise in Health Care.* Washington, DC: National Academy Press, 1986.

"Health Care Capitated Payment Systems." *American Journal of Law and Medicine* 22, nos. 2 and 3 (1996).

Hoy, E. W. "Change and Growth in Managed Care." *Health Affairs* 10 (Winter 1991): 19.

Kohn, L. T., J. M., Corrigan, and M. S., Donaldson, eds. *To Err Is Human: Building a Safer Health System.* Washington, DC: National Academy Press, 2000.

Latham, Stephen R. "Regulation of Managed Care Incentive Payments to Physicians." *American Journal of Law and Medicine* 22, no. 4 (1996): 399–432.

Macklin, Ruth. *The Enemies of Patients.* New York: Oxford University Press, 1993, chapter 7.

Martin, Julia A., and Lisa K. Bjerknes, "The Legal and Ethical Implications of Gag Clauses in Physician Contracts." *American Journal of Law and Medicine* 22, no. 4 (1996): 433–476.

Menzel, Paul T. "Double Agency and the Ethics of Rationing Health Care: A Response to Marcia Angell." *Kennedy Institute of Ethics Journal* 3, no. 3 (1993): 293–302.

Orentlicher, David. "Health Care Reform and the Patient-Physician Relationship." *Health Matrix: Journal of Law-Medicine* 5, no. 1 (1995): 141–180.

Rajendram, Pam R. "Ethical Issues Involved in Disclosing Medical Errors." *Journal of the American Medical Association* 286, no. 5 (September 5, 2001): 1078.

Ries, Nola M. "Public Health Law and Ethics: Lessons from SARS and Quarantine." *Health Law Review* 13, no. 1 (December 22, 2004): 3–7.

Ragon, S. A. "A Doctor's Dilemma: Resolving the Conflict between Physician Participation in Executions and the AMA's Code of Medical Ethics." *University of Dayton Law Review* 20, no. 3 (Spring 1995): 975–1007.

Rodwin, Marc A. *Medicine, Money and Morals: Physicians' Conflicts of Interest.* New York: Oxford University Press, 1993.

Rubin, Susan B., and Laurie, Zoloth, eds. *Margin of Error: The Necessity, Inevitability and Ethics of Mistakes in Medicine and Bioethics.* Hagerstown, MD: University Publishing Group, 2000.

Spece, Roy G., Jr., David S., Shimm, and Allen E., Buchanan, eds. *Conflicts of Interest in Clinical Practice and Research.* New York: Oxford University Press, 1996.

Wicclair, M. R. "Pharmacies, Pharmacists, and Conscientious Objection." *Kennedy Institute of Ethics Journal* 16, no. 3 (September 2006): 225–250.

Wolf, Susan M. "Health Care Reform and the Future of Physician Ethics." *Hastings Center Report* 24, no. 2 (March–April 1994): 28–41.

Wusthoff, Courtney J. "Medical Mistakes and Disclosure: The Role of the Medical Student," *Journal of the American Medical Association* 286, no. 5 (September 5, 2001): 1080–1081.

ALLOCATION, SOCIAL JUSTICE, AND HEALTH POLICY

Even if we believe that all men and women are "created equal," it's hard to deny that we are not equal with regard to health. Some of us, the winners in the "natural lottery," are blessed with good health and live to a ripe old age without the meddling of physicians and nurses. Others are born with catastrophic diseases requiring massive amounts of high-technology medicine merely to survive painfully from day to day.

It is also hard to deny that we are not equal with regard to availability of health care. Some are fortunate enough to work for employers who can offer a generous health benefits package or are wealthy enough to either purchase outright all the health care they want or to buy enough insurance to cover their needs. Others, the unemployed as well as those who work part time or for small businesses that cannot afford to offer health benefits, go without health insurance and many of the poorest members of our population cannot afford adequate nutrition, housing, and clothing, let alone insurance for health care. These losers in the "social lottery"—the working poor, the child in the welfare hotel, the impoverished person living with AIDS, the unemployed farmer—often have desperate needs for care that go unmet.

Although attempts have been made to provide a social safety net for the poor, for those poor enough to meet the definition of poverty stipulated by their state-run Medicaid programs, access to health care is often an entitlement in name only. Since most states reimburse only a small fraction of physicians' usual rates, very few of them are willing to treat Medicaid patients. With the notable exception of some extraordinarily devoted physicians, those who do accept such patients are often poorly qualified and offer substandard care in large, impersonal practices featuring "turnstile" medical attention. Hospitals that deal with a predominantly Medicaid population are notoriously understaffed and undersupplied. Patients are regularly subjected to long waiting periods for necessary treatments during which their conditions may badly deteriorate. And these treatments are often delivered through dangerously antiquated technology. At one Brooklyn hospital, a cancer unit's decrepit radiation unit was nicknamed "the killer" due to its tendency to destroy roughly equal portions of both cancerous and healthy tissue. Yet across the street at the university-affiliated hospital, the insured "paying customers" benefited from state-of-the-art technology and care.

Those who are not poor enough to qualify for Medicaid, yet are too poor to afford private health insurance, pose perhaps the greatest challenge both to our nation's emerging health policy and to our collective moral conscience. Numbering roughly (at this writing) 46–47 million people, these uninsured individuals must either go without treatment entirely or obtain care from chaotic emergency rooms. Journalist Laurie Kaye Abraham provides a compelling and poignant account of the uninsured:

> [They are] often in advanced stages of treatable disease, with undiagnosed diabetes attacking their kidneys, or even breast tumors large enough to break through their skin. Their conditions certainly are

emergencies now but emergencies that . . . did not necessarily have to be. They got so sick waiting, waiting,
waiting, because they had no health insurance and did
not think they could afford a doctor until they *really*
needed one. And even when things went bad enough
that they *really* needed one, they still feared they could
not afford it—who knows how expensive a doctor's
visit will be?—so they stumbled into the emergency
room instead. There, the clerks ask if you have insurance but will not draw in their breath when you say
you do not, will not ask you to wait while they confer
with someone else, will not, cannot, turn you away.
(Abraham 1993, 96)

The first section of Part 2 asks how we should think
about these inequalities in both the natural and
social lotteries. Are they merely instances of misfortune that should elicit pity and perhaps charity, or
are they injustices that society has an obligation to
rectify? Additionally, Part 2 focuses on a related but
nevertheless distinct question of public policy: If
these inequalities are sufficiently problematic from
the moral point of view that they require rectification, what should the target or goal of this rectification be? Should it focus on providing community
members with a certain amount or level of health
care? Or, given the extent to which conditions of
sickness and disease are rooted in larger social
inequalities, such as poverty, lack of access to
healthy food, and unsafe living environments,
should society focus instead on reducing social
inequalities relating to these so-called social determinants of health?

Whereas Section 1 situates our thinking about
issues of health and health care in a larger philosophical context, Section 2 examines some of the
hard choices forced upon society by the confluence
of an ever-expanding demand for health care, high-
cost technology, and the rise of managed care and
other cost-constraining strategies. When goods and
resources are scarce, and not everyone can receive
as much of a good as they need, society must face
thorny questions about how to ration goods or services fairly. Despite a widespread perception to the
contrary, issues of priority setting and allocating
scarce resources are a fundamental component of
every health care system. Section 2 also shows how
such questions are brought into stark relief in the
context of preparing for the next outbreak of pandemic influenza.

Section 3 focuses on questions relating to one
specific scarce resource, namely, transplantable
human organs. It considers the extent to which such
allocation decisions should be made by, or should
be isolated from, market mechanisms.

Finally, Section 4 returns to a broader question
relating to justice and health. In particular, the readings in this section address the staggering health
disparities between the global poor and members of
affluent, developed nations and asks whether these
are tragic misfortunes, or whether they constitute
an injustice that must be rectified. Together the readings in this section bring the reader back to some of
the questions laid out in Section 1 concerning the
implications for different conceptions of moral
equality on the way we think about the distribution of health and health care, not just within
a particular society, but across national boundaries
as well.

JUSTICE, HEALTH, AND HEALTH CARE

How healthy a person is, whether he or she is born
with a debilitating disorder or is susceptible to various cancers or conditions, is determined in large
part by a host of factors that are beyond one's control. Some of these factors constitute what we might
call a "natural" lottery in the sense that they are the
product of inherited genetic traits and of the operation, or failure, of various biological mechanisms.
Other factors are the result of a social lottery: maternal health habits (which are highly correlated with
the level of maternal education, which in turn is
correlated with socioeconomic status), environmental factors such as the presence of toxins, and
whether one's neighborhood provides an ecological
niche for diseases such as malaria.

All of these factors can influence the health status of an individual before he or she is in a position
to make important life choices. Moreover, the presence or absence of many of these factors plays a crucial role in determining which life choices will
remain open to an individual. For instance, whether
one lives to make a decision in adolescence about
whether or not to smoke depends significantly on
whether one is born in a country like Finland where
the rate of infant mortality is 3.6 for every 1,000
births (just over a third of a percent), or Sierra Leone

where infant mortality is a staggering 283 deaths per 1,000 births (just under 30 percent).

The primary question addressed in Section 1 is whether social inequalities in health are unjust or merely unfortunate—a failure of charity or a violation of rights—and how these inequalities should be addressed. The President's Commission for the Study of Ethical Problems in Medicine and Biomedical and Behavioral Research confronts this question in the domestic U.S. context in its report *An Ethical Framework for Access to Health Care.*

According to the commission, health problems can significantly affect the range of social opportunities that are open to an individual. Moreover, many health problems are caused by factors that are beyond the control of the individuals they affect. As a result, the commission argues that health problems, and the restrictions on opportunity that they produce, are often undeserved. They argue further that the factors that cause health problems are often difficult to predict and to prevent, that they are widely, but unevenly distributed in society, and that their effects on individuals are often costly to ameliorate.

As a result, the commission concludes that the free market alone cannot be counted on to meet these crucial needs and that society therefore has an obligation to help meet them. Providing access to health care represents the natural mechanism through which society should discharge this obligation. The commission views health care as being different from other consumer goods in that it is crucially related to one's level of well-being, helping ward off pain, suffering, and premature death. Like education, health care is necessary to achieve equal opportunity in society. And health care is freighted with "interpersonal significance." As the philosopher Michael Walzer puts it, failure to obtain needed health care in our society is not merely dangerous; it is also degrading, signaling a lack of full citizenship (Walzer 1983).

The commission insists, however, that this social obligation is not unlimited; it must be discharged with an eye to the costs and burdens to society in meeting it. Moreover, the fact that society is morally obligated to provide some care does not mean that everyone is entitled to an equal amount of health care or to health care of equal quality. In other words, not all *inequalities* in access to health care constitute *inequities*. So long as everyone is guaranteed access to

an "acceptable level" or, as others have put it, to a "decent level" of health care, society will have lived up to its moral obligation.

Although the approach of the President's Commission lacks the rigor of a sustained philosophical analysis, it is particularly significant in at least two respects. First, it illustrates quite naturally the intimate connection in the minds of many between health problems and health care as the social mechanism through which those problems should be addressed.

Second, it assembles a broad array of cogent arguments in favor of a right to health care. Interestingly, however, the commission self-consciously retreated from the vocabulary of rights in attempting to frame its notion of a social duty, a move that has prompted a good deal of criticism from philosophers (Arras 1984; Bayer 1984). If society has a strong duty to ensure that every citizen has access to at least a decent level of health care, why not conclude that each citizen has a moral right, as opposed to a legal right, against the government to that level of care?

A more focused and philosophical approach can be found in Norman Daniels's work titled "Equal Opportunity and Health Care." Like the President's Commission, Daniels first attempts to explain what is special about health needs. As opposed to mere preferences we may have for fine wines or top-of-the-line stereo speakers, our health needs are special in that they relate to our ability to function as normal members of our biological species. If our ability to function normally is impaired—for example, because of a broken arm or cancer cells colonizing our bodies—Daniels observes that we will then be unable to enjoy our fair share of what he calls the "normal opportunity range" for our society. In other words, illness prevents us from enjoying the range of opportunities—to be, for instance, an athlete, a businessperson, or a lawyer—that we would have been able to access or take advantage of, given our natural endowment of talents and skills. Daniels contends that this lack of equal opportunity will not be viewed as "merely unfortunate" in any society that is committed to providing equal opportunity to its members.

Daniels also makes the natural move from the importance of health needs to the importance of health care. Just as we say that children deprived of a decent education are robbed of their right to equal opportunity, so Daniels concludes that people deprived of adequate health care in our society are treated unjustly.

Although Daniels is firmly committed to viewing access to health care as a matter of justice, he too denies that a right to health care would entitle everyone to all the health care that they might want or need. First, our right to health care covers only deviations from normal species functioning, not idiosyncratic desires for nose jobs or tummy tucks. Second, although health needs are special compared to goods normally distributed on the free market, they are not so important that society must give them absolute priority over all other needs or go broke trying. Other important interests besides health care—such as needs for good schooling, housing, nutrition, and jobs—must also figure in any robust conception of equal opportunity; so the task for public policy is to weigh and balance all these higher-level interests in fashioning a just *system* that protects equal opportunity. On this view, access to health care is seen as vitally important, but not so uniquely important that making it available to all can threaten to break the societal bank.

A very different view of the importance of health and health care is articulated by the philosopher H. Tristram Englehardt, Jr. in "Freedom and Moral Diversity: The Moral Failures of Health Care in the Welfare State." Engelhardt is a self-described postmodernist and a libertarian who rejects the fundamental assumptions behind most liberal egalitarian theories of health care justice. His postmodernism derives from his conviction that in the modern world there is no one correct or canonical answer to the question of what constitutes justice and equality. People from different cultures and religious or philosophical traditions define these key notions in radically different ways. This is a crucial problem for allocating health care in a pluralistic society, because any scheme for allocating such care must of necessity implicate one or another such vision of justice and the good life.

Engelhardt's libertarianism stems from his conviction that free and equal individuals should not be coerced into accepting, much less paying for, the views of others bearing on such basic but ultimately unresolvable questions as the morality of abortion, physician-assisted suicide, the desirability of organ transplants, and the true nature of equality and social justice. In the face of such important and unresolvable questions, libertarians like Engelhardt insist that individuals must remain free from societal or governmental interference to make their own choices about such matters. Thus, although it might be perfectly appropriate, even praiseworthy, for many individuals to band together and pool their extra resources to make health care more available to poor and unfortunate persons, libertarians insist that no one should be forced to give away his or her resources for the benefit of others. Access to health care thus remains either a matter of buying and selling on the free market or a matter of charity; failure to access adequate amounts of health care will thus be viewed by libertarians as perhaps unfortunate, but not as unjust.

It follows that for Engelhardt the notion of a right to health care is both unfounded and positively dangerous. Unfounded because it must rely on some debatable and not universally endorsed understanding of justice; and dangerous because it would necessarily impinge on the rights and lifestyles of those who embrace other visions of the good life. Although Engelhardt concedes that society might possess a moral warrant to tax its citizens for various purposes, including the provision of some level of health care for its citizens in need, he steadfastly resists the notion that this societal choice is demanded by anyone's corresponding entitlement.

In addition to engaging liberal egalitarian claims, such as those of Daniels and the President's Commission, on the level of political philosophy, Engelhardt offers some practical suggestions for making health care more widely available without foundering on the prohibitions of his postmodern libertarianism. One way to provide greater access to the poor without implicating controversial views of justice and the good life, he contends, would be to establish a voucher system. Given a fund of public monies earmarked for humanitarian purposes, society could distribute health care vouchers to individuals in need who could redeem them at the health system of their choice. Thus, instead of imposing, say, a single view of abortion and euthanasia on all of society, we could leave it up to individuals to cash in their vouchers at avowedly pro-choice or pro-life health plans as they saw fit. This way, Engelhardt suggests, poor individuals could obtain expanded access without any accompanying "welfare rights," and without the state imposing a single, "official" morality on everyone.

Engelhardt's approval of taxation for purposes other than maintaining a so-called nightwatchman state consisting solely of police, army, courts, and so forth, appears to deviate from orthodox libertarian doctrine, which views all such taxation as forms of theft and forced labor. Likewise, his claim that individual autonomy must be universally respected in a world of moral diversity would seem to contradict the thoroughgoing relativism of more robust versions of postmodernism. Still, his critique of welfare rights raises important questions bearing on the legitimacy of state health policies and the wisdom of many practical interventions that the partisans of more egalitarian theories cannot ignore.

Whatever the outcome of the argument between liberal egalitarians like Daniels and libertarians like Engelhardt, it remains true that the notion of a right to health, or to some level of health care, has only a limited usefulness. Supposing we were to endorse such a right; what would it mean? And how would it help us answer the tough questions facing health policy experts, legislators, and society at large today (Brody 1991)?

At most, as Daniels acknowledges, a right to health care would mean that every citizen had an entitlement to an unspecified amount of health care (a decent minimum) within an overall entitlement to equal opportunity. Since health care needs must ultimately be balanced against other compelling opportunity-related needs, such as nutrition, schooling, and housing, it is impossible to say in the abstract exactly to what kind and amount of health care each person is entitled. Do individuals have a right, for example, to expensive experimental treatments, psychotherapy, organ transplants, AIDS therapies, and so on? The mere stipulation of a right to health care does not appear to be very helpful in coming to grips with these and other crucial questions of health care policy. In each case, we have to ask, How great is the need, how many people will be affected, how likely the harm, how expensive the treatment or diagnostic test, and what are the alternative uses to which our scarce public funds could be put? (See Section 2.)

There is, however, a more fundamental reason to rethink the emphasis that has been placed on establishing and then honoring a right to health care. This challenge targets the assumption, common among political liberals, that the proper response to ameliorating health needs and their adverse effects on individual opportunity is via the mechanism of health care. Recently, there has been a convergence of evidence from a variety of sources linking a range of social factors to the health status of individuals. More important, there is significant evidence that these factors help explain health inequalities that persist even in the face of universal access to medical care. In other words, even in wealthy countries in which there is a system of universal access to health care there is evidence that those who have higher incomes and who enjoy greater social status are healthier than those in less affluent groups of a lower social status.

Some of this evidence is cataloged in the World Health Organization's "Social Determinants of Health: The Solid Facts." One of the first claims in this report is that there is a health gradient that tracks the social gradient. That is, within socially stratified countries—even those such as England, where there is a system of universal access to health care—people who occupy the highest social classes have better health outcomes than those in the middle class, who, in turn, have better health outcomes than those in the lower social classes.

The report claims that there are multiple causes of this health gradient. It surveys the effects that stress has on the immune system and identifies various ways in which social environments and policies can cause some groups to experience greater stress burdens than others. It examines the extent to which the social and material circumstances in which children are conceived, incubated, and born can materially affect their health for years to come. It also details how social exclusion, poor job security, lack of effective social support mechanisms, addiction and substance abuse, and access to proper nutrition all constitute important social determinants of individual health.

In each case the report makes important policy recommendations. Taken together, these recommendations are stunning in their focus and implications. With few exceptions, they focus predominantly on enhancing social support mechanisms for all community members, including access to education, proper nutrition, child care, psychological services, and a plethora of other programs for reducing social inequalities.

In "Why the United States Is Not Number One in Health," Ichiro Kawachi argues that it is precisely a lack of access to these so-called social determinants of health that explains why the United States compares so poorly to other developed countries on key health measures. Although the United States accounts for only about 4.5 percent of the world's population, its roughly $12 trillion gross domestic product (GDP) (in 2005 estimates of purchasing power parity) accounts for 20 percent of the $60 trillion global GDP. As Kawachi notes, U.S. expenditures account for about half of all the money spent on medical care across the globe. One might expect that in return for the 14.5 percent of its GDP (in 2002 dollars) that it spends on health care, the world's wealthiest nation would have the best health outcomes. Yet this is not the case.

Kawachi argues that three factors that are commonly cited as causing these shortcomings do not withstand careful scrutiny. The idea that the bad genes of certain members of the U.S. population— predictably, the bad genes of minority populations— are the culprit is undermined by the fact when you look at populations in other countries that share the genetic ancestry of U.S. populations, those foreign populations often have better health outcomes than their U.S. counterparts. Similarly, he argues that it is difficult to lay blame at the feet of individuals for their poor health behaviors, since many such behaviors are initiated in childhood, and because these behaviors themselves can be seen as responses to environmental factors that are overrepresented in poor and minority neighborhoods. Advertisements for cigarettes, for example, are often highly concentrated in poor and minority neighborhoods and are designed with cartoon characters that disproportionately attract children and adolescents.

Finally, Kawachi also argues that lack of access to universal health care cannot explain the poor performance of the United States on important health measures. Part of the argument for this claim hinges on the fact that the health gradient tracks the social gradient even in countries with universal access to health care. Kawachi is quick to argue that universal access to health care can be part of the cure for U.S. health problems, but that lack of access to health care is not the cause of their persistence.

The root cause, according to Kawachi, is the high degree of social inequality that characterizes the United States. Although CEO salaries continue to skyrocket and the top 1 percent of the country continues to accumulate ever greater stores of wealth, the poor and the working class have seen their economic prospects stagnate or even decline. From this vantage point, universal access to health care represents the proverbial finger in the dyke of social inequality. While health care can alleviate the most immediate effects of sickness, injury, and disease, it cannot remediate the social inequalities that provide the ecological niche in which higher rates of morbidity and mortality thrive.

Together, these two articles provide a profound challenge to contemporary liberal egalitarian theories. This is because political liberals like John Rawls and Norman Daniels hold that social inequalities in wealth are permissible so long as they work to the advantage of the worst off. The idea behind this position is that allowing those who are willing to take risks, to innovate, and who are energetic and competitive to keep a significant share of the wealth they generate provides an incentive to innovate. This in turn creates goods, services, and information that can be used to make life better for everyone—think of innovations such as the personal computer, the cell phone, and medical advances such as antibiotics. These thinkers do, however, support progressive tax schemes that serve to redistribute a portion of the wealth from the best off to the worst off, thereby ensuring that social inequalities work to the advantage of the latter.

If, as Daniels claims, health has special ethical significance because of its impact on individual opportunities, and if, as the public health literature appears to show, those in lower classes lead shorter and more painful lives than those in higher classes, then liberal egalitarians may have to rethink the level of relative socioeconomic inequality that can be permitted to exist within a just political system. That is, if the health gradient increases with the social gradient, so that the worst off live shorter lives and suffer greater health burdens than the more affluent, then justice may require a much greater reduction in the degree of inequality that can be tolerated in a just society.

In "Justice, Health, and Healthcare," Norman Daniels addresses these implications. He argues, first, that when properly understood Rawls's theory of justice would prohibit many of the social inequalities that he sees as responsible for the differential health status of the rich and the poor. This is because Rawls's theory holds that each citizen has an equal right to "the most extensive scheme of equal basic liberties compatible with a similar scheme of liberties for all." The "basic liberties" that he refers to here include civil and political liberties such as freedom of thought and expression, freedom of association, and the political freedoms that are associated with the rule of law. They also include the liberty to choose one's occupation, where this choice can be made against a background of diverse opportunities. With respect to these basic liberties, therefore, Rawls is what we might call a strict egalitarian: Each individual has a right to the largest share of these liberties that is consistent with the recognition of the same right for every other citizen.

Rawls then adopts what he refers to as the "difference principle" to govern other basic goods, including income and wealth, and the "social bases of self respect." The difference principle holds, in part, that inequalities in this last set of goods—social and economic inequalities—must be to the greatest benefit of the least advantaged members of society.

According to Daniels, Rawls's theory is more demanding than many may realize, since making social inequalities work to the greatest benefit of the least advantaged would require taxing a substantial portion of the wealth of the best off in order to fund a much more robust system of education, job training, environmental health and safety, and so on.

Whether social and economic inequalities that remain after the application of the difference principle would be justified within this framework remains controversial. On the one hand, Rawls explicitly permits social inequalities in income and wealth. On the other hand, his theory is highly idealized and explicitly assumes equal health status. Because social and economic inequalities appear to bring with them inequalities in health in real communities, it may be that even Rawlsian political liberals would have to give up the difference principle in favor of a more strict egalitarianism about income and wealth.

Both Daniels and Kawachi make a special point of emphasizing that although establishing universal access to health care will not eliminate the existence of a social gradient in health, it remains an important social goal nonetheless. Yet, this view is not without some controversy.

In "Opportunity Is Not the Key," Gopal Sreenivasan argues that if we agree with Daniels and the President's Commission that the importance of health care lies in its ability to secure for individuals their fair share of the normal opportunity range, and if we take seriously the importance of the social determinants of health on individual opportunity, then the link between opportunity and access to health care is severed. The reason is simply that the social determinants of health are so important that they overwhelm the impact of medical care on opportunity.

For Sreenivasan, if what we care about is individual opportunity, then fair-minded social planners could not justify the large social expenditures that would be necessary to provide universal access to health care. The reason is simply that these resources would have a greater impact on individual health, and therefore on equality of opportunity, if they were diverted to reducing social inequalities in education, income, and control over one's work environment. Moreover, the justification for this latter claim emanates precisely from the literature on the social determinants of health, which indicates that health inequalities tied to social inequalities persist even in the presence of universal access to health care. Given that resources are limited, and given that health inequalities persist in the face of universal access to health care, why would a fair-minded social planner ever dedicate scarce social resources to funding a social entitlement to health care when that money could be applied directly to ameliorating the social inequalities that create the underlying ecological niche in which social inequalities in health persist?

ALLOCATING SCARCE RESOURCES

Section 2 takes up some of the vexing allocation problems confronting health policy experts, legislators, and consumers today. The common focus of these policy case studies is the need to make difficult choices in a context of fiscal scarcity (Morreim 1995). If we had unlimited amounts of money, there would be no need to ration health care; but as we all know, money and resources are scarce and health care is expensive, so we cannot afford to satisfy everyone's preferences and needs for health care. Even if we can reach consensus that there is a right to health care, we must still learn to assign priorities—a tricky business. Who should be saved when all cannot be saved? Which groups of people and which treatments and diagnostic techniques should be given highest priority? The articles in this section are intended to give the reader a lively sense of the issues in this area. They are, however, only a small sample of the many complex and difficult questions facing our nation as we struggle to contain health care costs while expanding access to the millions of people whose health needs currently go unmet.

Americans do not like to hear about rationing health care. The term conjures up images of tightwad insurance companies or government bureaucrats deciding that some lives are worth less than others. One of the charges that in 1994 helped scuttle the ill-fated Clinton plan for health care reform was the claim that it would necessitate rationing. Well aware of the unpopularity of this notion, the Clinton administration actually forbade its 500 consultants to use the word "rationing" in any correspondence or official documents.

The fact remains, however, that we have always rationed health care in one way or another. By far, the most widespread method has also been the most morally suspect: rationing care by ability to pay. But we have also rationed organ transplants, intensive care unit beds, and other life-sustaining medical treatments. There are, however, important differences between these traditional forms of rationing and what is happening today under managed care organizations (MCOs). When the poor and uninsured failed to receive needed care, it seemed not to be the result of an official social policy; their inability to access care was the result of structural features of the existing health care system and, consequently, was often treated as though it was a fact of nature. And when patients died of liver or heart failure on a waiting list for an organ transplant, it was usually due to a natural shortage of organs, not to a decision on anyone's part that these lives were simply too expensive to save. So we developed a complicated attitude with regard to rationing: On the one hand, we grew accustomed to the tacit and limited rationing we permitted while fiercely resisting the explicit, publicly imposed rationing, respectively, by doctors on paying customers and by bureaucrats on the poor.

Managed care has changed all this. Operating essentially within closed systems of shared financial resources, MCOs must ration health care on a daily

basis. Money spent on expensive but marginally effective treatments cannot be used for other purposes within an MCO, so difficult choices must be made. Under this new dispensation, rationing is explicit; it is implemented by physicians at the bedside; it targets insured populations by restricting potentially beneficial services; and it is justified by fiscal scarcity, rather than by natural shortages (Eddy 1996; Morreim 1995). The notion that rationing would be entirely unnecessary if we could only cut the fat by reorganizing our wasteful health care system has been disproven by history and the fact of scarcity. The question now is not, Shall we ration care? It is, rather, *How* shall we ration, by what principles and processes, and how may we do so without seriously compromising justice and patients' rights?

Setting health care priorities, however, has proven to be a difficult matter. Consider the case of women with advanced breast cancer for whom standard chemotherapies have failed to effect a remission of the disease. Having exhausted proven medical alternatives, these women frequently seek out investigational or experimental alternatives in the hope of staving off imminent death. Throughout the decade of the nineties, an extremely expensive experimental procedure known as high-dose chemotherapy followed by autologous bone marrow transplantation (or HDC-ABMT) was thought to hold out tremendous promise as a possible means of helping these desperate women. As Alex John London explains in "Bone Marrow Transplants for Advanced Breast Cancer: The Story of Christine deMeurers," decisions about providing promising but expensive treatments frequently have to be made when there are no definitive answers about the treatment's efficacy. Costing well over $100,000 per patient, HDC-ABMT was offered at many hospitals and cancer centers to women who saw this highly invasive and onerous treatment as their last best hope of staving off death. Most of these women were relatively young, in their twenties and thirties, and many had families who depended on them. Waiting for the results of rigorous clinical trials to accumulate would have meant foregoing an expensive, but promising option. To the managed care companies who were being asked to pay for these costly last-ditch efforts, however, it would not have been a responsible use of scarce resources to spend such large amounts of money without sufficient evidence that HDC-ABMT might succeed where standard therapies had failed.

In light of more recent clinical research, it now seems clear that HDC-ABMT is not superior to standard chemotherapy (Mello and Brennan 2001). This information was not available a decade ago, however, and while the results of this more recent research may dissolve the dilemma about providing access to this particular intervention, there is no shortage of new investigational treatments appearing on the horizon. As a result, we are left with the same general ethical questions, even if they now apply to different treatments. Should insurance providers be forced to pay for promising interventions whose therapeutic merits have yet to be fully measured or vindicated? Is it unconscionably hard-hearted to deny persons a last chance at remission or cure—no matter how remote— merely to save money?

Following the narrative of Christine deMeurers, a woman who fought valiant battles against both her MCO and her encroaching terminal breast cancer, London attempts to put this health policy debate into proper perspective. Rejecting an all-or-nothing perspective on such so-called last-chance therapies, London attempts to focus our attention on the crucial questions we must ask and the procedures we must establish to come to a just and stable resolution of this difficult issue.

The difficult question of how to ration health care in cases like this is taken up by Ronald Dworkin in "Justice and the High Cost of Health." Dworkin argues that the high cost of health care in the United States stems at least in part from the fact that those who make the spending decisions—patients in consultation with their physicians—are often shielded from the direct financial consequences of those decisions. Rather, the costs of these decisions are born by third-party payers, then passed on to employers, and ultimately on to plan members.

Another reason for the high cost of health care stems from the widespread acceptance of what Dworkin calls the rescue principle. This principle has two components. First, health and long life are viewed as fundamental goods in the sense that one's ability to enjoy any other good is conditional on being healthy and alive. Second, because health is a fundamental good for every individual, fairness demands that health care be distributed on the basis of medical need so that the life prospects for some

are not unfairly restricted because of their inability to pay.

Undoubtedly, the rescue principle has strong appeal for people like Christine deMeurers who believe that their last best option for extending their lives lies in an expensive and unproven technology. Moreover, as Dworkin notes, this is the principle on which communities often act when stories about such desperate people make it into the spotlight and communities band together to try to save the imperiled individual.

Although the values embodied in the rescue principle are noble, Dworkin argues that the principle itself is "almost wholly useless" for making decisions about how to allocate health care resources when not all health needs can be met. In essence, he argues that no matter how much we identify with individuals in need, and no matter how much we recognize that we may one day find ourselves in their situation, the resources of the community are sufficiently limited that we simply cannot meet the health needs of every community member.

The problem, therefore, is how to respect the equality of persons and allocate health resources fairly without breaking the bank. Dworkin's solution is what he refers to as the "prudent insurance ideal." This is an ideal because it begins with an idealized situation of fairness. Imagine a situation in which resources are fairly distributed to community members, in which every community member has perfect information about medical matters, and in which no individual faces higher insurance costs because of differences in his or her health baseline. Within this context Dworkin asks the deliberator to consider what portion of their resources prudent individuals would spend on health insurance and what kind of coverage those individuals would purchase.

Although Dworkin admits that there are many cases in which it is not clear what prudent deliberators would do, he argues persuasively that there are nevertheless genuine risks or situations for which no prudent agent would insure. For instance, he argues that a prudent deliberator would not purchase a policy that would pay to keep the individual alive in a persistent vegetative state (PVS). No prudent deliberator would do this because the resources that would have to be spent on such a policy would be better spent on other goals or ends that the patient might pursue while active and able.

It is likely that similar consequences would result from applying this model to the case of Christine deMeurers. Prudent deliberators would pay for a generous package of preventative services because they reduce the likelihood of winding up with advanced breast cancer in the first place. But they would not dedicate larger sums of money to pay for access to unproven interventions, should they wind up with advanced breast cancer. The rationale for this conclusion is quite simple. An ideally situated prudent deliberator would seek to minimize the chance of ending up with end-stage breast cancer and then use her remaining resources on other goals or ends that she values.

In this model, when the prudent deliberator finds herself in the situation of having advanced breast cancer she can endorse, at least in principle, the decision not to cover such last-chance treatments because she can recognize that it would not have been prudent to insure against such a threat under the ideal conditions that Dworkin lays out. The claim, therefore, is that even those who ultimately are denied care because of decisions dictated by this model can recognize those decisions as fair.

In effect, Dworkin's approach to rationing is to define a just allocation of health care resources as whatever prudent individuals would choose from within an idealized choice situation. This approach has two fundamental strengths. First, it can legitimately claim to treat all individuals equally, not in outcome, but in being free to allocate a fair share of resources across their various goals and priorities, both health related and not. Second, this approach attempts to avoid one of the features that many find most objectionable about health care rationing, namely, the imposition by government bureaucrats of rationing decisions on some individuals for the benefit of others. Dworkin is trying to show that, at least under ideal conditions, each of us would *choose* to have our care rationed. His approach thus appeals to a Kantian ideal of rational self-determination in place of the utilitarian, aggregationist methods usually linked with rationing. This is why he can claim that rationing is not only compatible with justice, it is demanded by it.

At the heart of Dworkin's approach is an ideal of ensuring that individuals are treated equally, not in terms of the outcomes they enjoy, but in terms of their ability to make decisions about how to allocate

their resources among their various goals and priorities. This suggests another approach to rationing health care that does not rely on the various idealizations required by Dworkin's approach.

In particular, actual individuals routinely make concrete choices that have a material impact on their health. Some individuals explicitly choose healthy lifestyles. They eat healthy foods, exercise regularly, and avoid excessive alcohol or tobacco use. When they have a problem, they seek prompt medical attention, are scrupulous about taking their medications, and play an active role in shaping their care plan. Others make different choices. They gravitate toward unhealthy food, lead sedentary lifestyles, and have problems with alcohol or smoking.

As a result of these different choices, individuals increase or reduce their risks of encountering significant health problems. If health care resources are scarce, however, and if we are committed to making rationing decisions in a way that is consistent with showing equal regard for all individuals, is it fair for society to provide equal levels of care for individuals who have not taken equal care to avoid sickness, injury, or disease?

For many, showing equal respect for individuals essentially involves holding those individuals responsible for their choices and decisions. This emphasis on personal responsibility is playing an increasing role in both private and public decisions about health care. For instance, in May 2006 West Virginia received permission from the federal government to proceed with one of the largest experiments in personal accountability in health care.

As Robert Steinbrook explains in "Imposing Personal Responsibility for Health," under the redesign of West Virginia's Medicaid program, healthy children and adults who meet the state's eligibility requirements will be enrolled in a basic program that provides a reduced package of benefits in comparison with the previous plan. However, if they are willing to sign a Medicaid Members Agreement in which they pledge to do their "best to stay healthy," and to take a variety of particular steps toward this goal, then they will be entitled to a slightly expanded package of benefits. To retain this expanded package of benefits, participants must show up for doctors' visits, take their medications, read medical information that is given to them, and take various other steps to stay healthy.

The moral rationale for making personal responsibility for health a centerpiece of health rationing is outlined by Alexander W. Cappelen and Ole Frithjof Norheim in "Responsibility in Health Care: A Liberal Egalitarian Approach." They also lay out five important objections to this kind of approach. For example, they point out that different individuals can often make the same poor choices without experiencing equally deleterious health outcomes. Whether poor choices result in health problems is itself a function of factors that are beyond the control of the agent, such as differences in genetic predisposition, differences in environmental factors, differences in social or interpersonal circumstances, and brute luck. Given the fundamental role of such mediating factors—factors that are often beyond the agent's ability to control— is it fair to hold these parties responsible for their differential health outcomes?

Additionally, Cappelen and Norheim note that policies that seek to treat agents equally by making medical coverage conditional on estimations of the degree to which the patient is responsible for his or her own medical problems can inadvertently generate important inequalities in other domains. In particular, many egalitarians hold that all democratic citizens are entitled to equal social and political liberties. But policies that focus on personal responsibility for health are likely to result in broader forms of social exclusion and discrimination that would have a negative impact on the basic rights and liberties of the affected individuals.

As a result, Cappelen and Norheim reject social policies that would hold individuals responsible for the health consequences of their various choices. Instead, they argue that individuals ought to be held responsible for their choices, regardless of whether they result in adverse or beneficial health effects. They argue that the way to hold individuals responsible for their choices is to levy a special tax on social activities that are known to be associated with poor health outcomes. Large taxes on cigarettes and alcoholic beverages, for example, raise the cost of these products, thereby creating a disincentive to habitual use. They also generate a revenue stream that could be used to fund the provision of health care. The goal is to ensure that those who take socially salient risks are also contributing additional resources to the health care system, since it is precisely the members of these groups who are at increased risk of encountering significant health problems.

As several of the articles in this and previous sections illustrate, there are many competing approaches to the rationing of health care, each of which appeals to slightly different moral and political values. Additionally, even if we could agree to an approach such as Dworkin's, we would still face difficult questions about who should be entitled to participate in either public or private insurance schemes. This decision, however, has significant implications for how many people have to share the same economic pie.

Our apparent inability to reach consensus on such basic but seemingly intractable questions of distributive principles leads Norman Daniels and James Sabin to concentrate on the fairness of our procedures for resolving such knotty questions. In "Last-Chance Therapies and Managed Care: Pluralism, Fair Procedures, and Legitimacy," they suggest that if we cannot always agree at the level of principles, then perhaps our best bet is to design various procedural mechanisms that will yield results that are "just enough."

Keying on the example of HDC-ABMT for advanced breast cancer, Daniels and Sabin report on a variety of "exemplary practices" adopted by managed care plans in the wake of the bad publicity, adverse court decisions, and legislative mandates noted by London. Instead of relying on unilateral denials of care, as in the case of Christine deMeurers, to resolve the tension between the efficient use of resources and the desperate appeals of patients for last-chance therapies, many MCOs are now resorting to such procedural solutions as outside review panels and internal appeals mechanisms that emphasize constructive deliberation and dialogue. By openly experimenting with a variety of such strategies while remaining tolerant of the differing value orientations they represent, Daniels and Sabin hope to "move [us] along a learning curve towards a more patient-centered, cost-effective and ethical health care system." By bringing such tensions and disagreements out into the open where they can be rationally and respectfully discussed among subscribers, patients, physicians, and managers, MCOs will have to acknowledge that such questions are not merely technical and economic, but also deeply political.

In the previous section we examined the broad outlines of the debate concerning whether health is a sufficiently important social good that communities should pool their collective resources in an effort to try to safeguard and to advance the health interests of their constituent members. A similar issue reemerges at a lower level in the context of rationing health resources. In particular, there remains a heated debate in some quarters about who should be recognized as a "community member" and therefore entitled to receive community subsidized health services.

In "Illegal Immigrants, Health Care, and Social Responsibility," James Dwyer examines what he refers to as "nationalist" arguments for restricting illegal immigrants from receiving health benefits and "humanist" arguments for extending those benefits to all who need them. In each case, Dwyer argues that the most common, and often the most intuitive, stances on this issue are inadequate. Frequently, they are based on misconceptions about the extent to which illegal immigrants make a social contribution to the communities in which they live, the reasons that they immigrate, their plight and condition, and so on. Similarly, he argues that these positions often move too quickly from premises about professional obligations or the fact that illegal aliens have broken the law to normative conclusions about whether they should receive access to subsidized health services.

The upshot of this analysis is to undermine simple, sound-bite solutions to a complex problem and to situate the issue within a richer context of facts and within a broader context of social and political philosophy. Although Dwyer does not defend his positive position in depth, he lays the groundwork for an argument that grants illegal immigrants access to health care based on the value of reciprocity. That is, because illegal immigrants often fill an important economic niche, taking some of the dirtiest, most difficult, and sometimes demeaning jobs, often for low pay and long hours, fairness may require granting them access to the social services necessary to sustain their health and welfare. Ultimately, however, it is up to the reader, relying on the material from Section 1, to construct a more detailed and more nuanced position on this important issue.

Section 2 concludes with a pair of articles that drive home the significance and the urgency of health care rationing in a particularly pointed way. Each year, as millions of Americans line up for an annual influenza vaccination there is some uncertainty about how much vaccine will be available and about how bad that year's flu season will be. According to the Centers for Disease Control and Prevention (CDC), each year anywhere from 5 to 20 percent of the U.S. population contracts the flu. This results in more than 200,000 people being hospitalized and about 36,000 deaths, mostly among the very old and the very young.

Periodically, however, the influenza virus mutates into a significantly more virulent and lethal strain. In 1918–1919 the so-called Spanish flu killed approximately 500,000 Americans and is estimated to have killed as many as 50 million people worldwide. The Spanish flu was also remarkable in another respect: Unlike the common flu that takes the heaviest toll on the very young and the very old, the Spanish flu preyed heavily on healthy, young individuals. Subsequent flu pandemics occurred in 1957 with the so-called Asian flu and in 1968 with the Hong Kong flu.

Currently the global health community is vigilantly monitoring the status of the H5N1 strain, commonly known as avian flu. Given the laws of probability and the propensity of the influenza virus to mutate, the question is not so much whether there will be another global flu pandemic but, rather, when it will occur.

As John D. Arras points out in "Rationing Vaccine During An Avian Influenza Pandemic: Why It Won't Be Easy," preparation for the next outbreak of pandemic flu must involve a frank and broad-based discussion of who should receive the vaccine, once one is finally made available, when not all can.

During normal or "interpandemic" flu seasons CDC guidelines indicate that the very young and the very old should be given priority access to the annual flu vaccine. This strategy is supported by a principle that gives priority to those who are most vulnerable. But this may not be an appropriate strategy in the face of a pandemic. In particular, as Arras argues, an outbreak on the scale of the 1918 Spanish flu could effectively send the country's social and economic infrastructure into disarray. In this case, it may actually be self-defeating to allocate scarce doses of a vaccine to the very old and the very young, since these are populations that depend heavily on care from persons in other age categories. But if those caregivers are felled in large numbers, the social supports on which the old and the young depend may collapse.

For this reason it may make sense to give priority to those in their prime for whom the vaccine is most likely to have a beneficial effect. Such a strategy is supported by a principle of maximizing the medical benefit of the scarce medical resource. But if quantities of the vaccine are severely limited—as they surely will be for most of the first year of the outbreak—then such a strategy may be too diffuse. That is, it may make sense to give priority to personnel who play essential roles within society's basic health and social infrastructure. This would give priority to first responders—such as police, paramedics, physicians, and public health workers—as well as to other government employees. Such an allocation scheme would be supported by a kind of social triage principle according to which, when not all can be saved, those who play the most important role in keeping the social infrastructure of the community functioning should be saved first.

Arras canvases a range of additional allocation strategies and their underlying moral justifications. He also illustrates the palpable ways in which these principles conflict, so that the requirements of one can only be satisfied at the expense of the others. For Arras, the problem is not that none of these strategies and principles is sufficiently compelling. The problem, rather, is that each is especially compelling and that there is no single definitive standpoint from which one of these options should be prioritized over the others.

In the end, Arras argues that what is needed is a broad-based, process-oriented approach to this question modeled on the approach of Daniels and Sabin (see Section 2). The idea is that community members must decide together which set of values and priorities best captures their collective set of priorities so that the resulting strategy will be one that is recognized as politically legitimate.

Arras's article provides a detailed context in which deliberative methods, like those outlined by Daniels and Sabin, can be applied and their merits assessed. One particular question to consider is this: If Arras is correct and each of the strategies and principles for rationing that he considers has a compelling rationale and makes a legitimate claim on us, how will the process-oriented approach of Daniels and Sabin produce consensus at the community level? If the idea is that these claims are so compelling that individuals will not be able to provide a definitive justification for giving priority to one over the others, why will it be easier for a group of individuals to do this? If the idea is, instead, that some strategies and principles will have greater appeal to different people, then how will the group not simply recapitulate the divided commitments of its constituent members? If the question cannot be decided on the basis of the best argument, then will it ultimately come down to a vote? Is this a question that should ultimately be decided by majority vote?

In "Who Should Get Influenza Vaccine When Not All Can?" Ezekiel J. Emanuel and Alan Wertheimer attempt to justify adopting one rationing strategy over its competitors. They argue that in emergency situations the commitment to recognize the moral equality of each community member should translate into a commitment to ensure, as far as possible, that each has the opportunity to live through all of life's stages. However, they modify this view in an interesting and controversial way. They argue that priority should be given to those individuals who have already made a substantial investment in their lives. The idea is that two-year-olds, for example, have not yet developed robust goals and commitments, and begun to pursue a set of projects and plans that will span the course of the rest of their lives. In contrast, the seventeen-year-old is fully enmeshed in precisely this project.

In the view of Emanuel and Wertheimer, therefore, after those who play key roles in manufacturing and distributing the flu vaccine, and frontline health care workers, priority should be given to those between thirteen and forty years old because they have already invested heavily in their current lives and they have the longest time left to live.

Whether the arguments in support of this view are sufficiently compelling that they will be able to support a broad-based social consensus remains to be seen. But together these articles illustrate in a microcosm both the dire necessity of rationing health care resources and of doing so in a way that can be justified both to those who will receive priority and, perhaps most important, to those who will not.

ORGAN TRANSPLANTATION: ACQUISITION AND ALLOCATION

In different ways the readings of the previous sections illustrate some of the challenges involved in devising a health care system that treats individuals as moral equals and addresses appropriate health needs without becoming either fiscally profligate or unfairly parsimonious. Section 3 returns to these questions in the context of acquiring and allocating organs for transplantation.

At the start of 2007 there were just over 94,000 individuals in the United States in line for an organ transplant (United Network for Organ Sharing n.d.). About three-quarters of these, some 69,590 people, were waiting for a kidney transplant. In 1998 about 80 percent of the organs used for kidney transplant came from deceased donors, so-called cadaveric organs. The remaining 20 percent were obtained from living donors. Although the number of transplants involving cadaveric organs has gradually increased, the most dramatic increase has occurred in the number of transplants involving living donors. Since 2000, between 34 and 42 percent of all kidney transplants were from living donors. The total number of kidney transplants in the United States performed in any given year reached a high in 2005 of 16,481. Yet this figure represents only about 20 percent of the number of people who are currently on the waiting list. As a result, roughly eighteen Americans die each day waiting for an organ transplant of some kind.

In the United States, the procurement and allocation of organs is coordinated by a single, centralized institution known as the United Network for Organ Sharing (UNOS). Patients in need of a transplant are evaluated at a transplant hospital and, if appropriate, are signed onto a wait list. Organs are allocated to the first recipient on the list who represents the best match for the organ. Who represents the best match is determined by a range of factors including blood and tissue type, size of the organ, the urgency of the recipient's condition, time spent on the wait list, and distance between the donor and the recipient. Because organs are usually allocated locally, many patients visit several transplant hospitals in order to join the wait list in several places. However, not all patients can afford the time or the considerable expense required to do this.

Currently in the United States, organ donation is conceived according to the paradigm of the gift. That is, individuals must decide to make a gift of life to others in need, either by agreeing to donate their organs after their death, or by agreeing to donate while they are alive. In the United States, as in many other developed countries, the system of organ acquisition is configured on an opt-in basis. This means that individuals must opt-in in order to donate their organs.

In the face of the dramatic imbalance between supply and those who need organs to survive, Janet Radcliffe-Richards and colleagues argue that the gift model of organ acquisition is unjustly restrictive. They argue, instead, that there are compelling reasons to permit a market in human organs in which donors would be allowed to sell, for example, one of their kidneys.

The central line of argument advanced by these authors is that prohibiting the sale of organs is what we might call "Pareto inferior": It leaves both the potential donor and the potential recipient worse off. Recipients are prevented from receiving organs they need to survive, and donors are denied the opportunity to engage in a profitable transaction. Against the argument that a market in human organs is effectively an engine for exploiting the poorest and most vulnerable members of society, Radcliffe-Richards and colleagues respond that the poor and the vulnerable would be willing to sell their organs only if it represented the best option available to them. How, they ask, does preventing the poor and the vulnerable from taking the best option open to them advance their interests? This question is especially important when we take into account the fact that the poor are likely to use the proceeds from such a sale to sustain their own life, and the lives of those who depend on them. In some cases, the ability or inability to sell one's organ could amount to a difference between life and death for each of the parties to the transaction.

The arguments advanced by these authors would also seem to permit a cross-national market in organs. Consider that approximately 1.1 billion people worldwide live on less than $1 a day in a condition the World Bank refers to as extreme poverty. About another billion people live on less than $2 a day. Allowing for a cross-national market in organs could provide a significant income stream for the global poor, while at the same time providing wealthy citizens of developed countries with a scarce, life-saving resource. In "An Ethical Market in Human Organs," Charles A. Erin and John Harris echo the sentiments of Radcliffe-Richards and colleagues. However, Erin and Harris add some important practical details about constraints that would need to be in place in order to make a market in human organs ethically acceptable. In particular, they would confine markets to self-governing political units, such as the European Union or the United States, and forbid cross-network transactions. They would also permit only a single agency—funded through tax dollars or some other cost-sharing mechanism—to purchase organs so that all organs could be purchased and allocated in a centrally coordinated way. In this way, although individuals will be paid for selling their organs, recipients will not be able to purchase them. Presumably, this restriction is intended to preserve an allocation scheme that gives highest priority to medical need.

For those who are convinced by the arguments of Radcliffe-Richards and colleagues, the proposal of Erin and Harris may seem too restrictive. In particular, such an objection might be leveled at the prohibition against mutually beneficial sales of organs between the global rich and the global poor. For others, however, even this more modest proposal is ethically suspect.

In "Body Values: The Case Against Compensating for Transplant Organs," Donald Joralemon and Phil Cox argue that even limited markets in organs violate some of our most deeply held convictions about the relationship between the body and the self. The cornerstone of their view is the fundamentally Kantian claim that persons ought not to be treated as commodities that can be bought and sold and whose value can be quantified in terms of their usefulness to others. As they see it, the way that we procure organs from living donors is both determined by and expressive of our attitude toward the value of the "donor." Allowing the sale of organs commodifies not just the organs in question, but the persons from whom those organs must be removed.

By extension, they argue that there is widespread evidence that most people do not view even corpses as biological material that has market-based use value. Rather, corpses continue to be seen for

some time as the physical remnant of the person; and it is this intimate connection between the body and personhood that explains the persistence of everything from elaborate burial rituals to the reluctance of many physicians to become organ donors.

Joralemon and Cox also attempt to rebut the arguments of critics such as Radcliffe-Richards and colleagues. For example, they argue that there is a fundamental difference between what it may be rational for an individual to do in a desperate situation, and how basic social institutions governing a particular activity ought to be configured. For example, it would almost certainly be rational for individuals facing death, or for the parents of a child facing death, to sell themselves into slavery if doing so would save either their lives or the life of their child. Yet, they argue, this fact does not entail that social institutions should be configured to permit, let alone to facilitate, such transactions.

Additionally, Joralemon and Cox attack the consistency of the utilitarian arguments that provide the moral urgency for taking practically any step necessary to increase the supply of viable organs. They argue that taking seriously the imperative to maximize the number of lives saved—as these utilitarian arguments do—undercuts the moral foundation for organ transplantation itself. That is, they claim that the roughly $6 billion spent each year to save a few thousand lives in the United States could save significantly larger numbers of people if it were directed at exceedingly low cost vaccinations for diseases that takes the lives of hundreds of thousands annually. From a utilitarian perspective, therefore, consistency would require allocating scarce resources away from highly cost-ineffective organ transplant procedures altogether.

Several important disagreements emerge from this exchange. For Erin and Harris, the fact that organ donors are practically the only individuals who do not make money from the practice of organ transplantation represents an inefficiency in an economic system and carries a moral lesson. The inefficiency lies in the disequilibrium between supply and demand. The moral lesson is that if transplant surgeons get paid—and they are usually quite highly paid—and nobody questions their moral motivations, then perhaps paying donors would be an acceptable way of bring supply into equilibrium with demand.

From the Kantian perspective of Joralemon and Cox, in contrast, the act of gifting one's organs, or the organs of one's deceased loved one, to someone in need is a highly ethical act. But it is also a kind of act that cannot be purchased, because assigning a price to it fundamentally changes the nature of the transaction. It is analogous to the difference between sexual encounters that manifest love and devotion, and those that are the end product of a financial negotiation. While society has important, nonconsequentialist reasons to support moral acts of the former kind, they argue that it has equally weighty reasons to prohibit degrading transactions of the latter stripe. From a utilitarian perspective, such a prohibition may seem inefficient. But Joralemon and Cox argue that this utilitarian perspective has much more dramatic and far-reaching consequences than their proponents realize. In particular, this utilitarian perspective would ultimately reject the inefficiency of dedicating significant social resources to such a highly cost-ineffective medical intervention as organ transplantation.

POVERTY, HEALTH, AND JUSTICE BEYOND NATIONAL BORDERS

The final section of Part 2 returns to an issue that has surfaced in several articles in previous sections and that will surface again in Part 6, Section 3. The issue concerns the severity of social and economic inequalities that divide the comparatively healthy citizens of affluent, developed countries and the burgeoning populations of the global poor.

To get a sense of just how steep these inequalities are, consider that in 1998 the combined assets of the world's three wealthiest *individuals* were greater than the combined gross national products of all 50 least developed countries (LDCs). Similarly, the combined assets of the world's 200 richest individuals in 1998 was equivalent to the combined assets of 41 percent of the world's population (United Nations Development Program 1999). The bottom half of the world's population owns barely 1 percent of global wealth.

The majority of LDCs are in sub-Saharan Africa, one of the only regions of the world that in 2003 was poorer than it was twenty-five years earlier. In 2005 there were 18,000 deaths from HIV/AIDS in all of

North America. That same year there were about 2.4 million deaths from HIV/AIDS in sub-Saharan Africa (World Health Organization 2005). Africa alone is home to some 70 percent of the world's HIV-positive individuals, even though the continent contains only about 10 percent of the world's population (Fauci 1999). Similarly, of the 3.5 million deaths from pneumonia each year, 99 percent take place in developing countries where pneumonia claims the lives of more children than any other infectious disease. Deaths from pneumonia are increasingly rare events in developed counties where populations are properly nourished, have access to clean water and sanitation, and low-cost antibiotics that are widely available. Although a five-day regimen of antibiotics costs 0.27 U.S. dollars—literally pocket-change for an American—it is more than a day's income for the roughly 1 billion people who live below the World Bank's threshold of severe poverty. Similarly, because of poor sanitation and contaminated drinking water, diarrhea-related diseases such as cholera, dysentery, typhoid fever, and rotavirus claim the lives of nearly 2 million children under the age of five every year. In contrast, such infections are much less likely to occur in developed countries and are more easily treated when they do.

As Joralemon and Cox mention in the previous section, utilitarian moral theorists have argued persuasively that the residents of the affluent nations of the developed world have a moral duty to aid those among the global poor who suffer and die under the terrible yoke of sickness and disease. The ground for this duty lies in the utilitarian's single moral principle—maximize the aggregate social utility.

For utilitarians, the moral significance of national boundaries depends, like all other things, on the extent to which their recognition advances or detracts from the overall amount of welfare in the world. In contrast, political liberals from the social contract tradition tend to see national boundaries as imbued with greater moral significance, to the extent that they demarcate peoples who have formed a shared social and political life together under a common institutional order.

Most contemporary social contract theorists, however, are hypothetical contractarians. That is, they view the social contract, not as an explicit agreement that citizens of a particular community actually make, but as a philosophical construct that such citizens would agree too under specified conditions. It is therefore worth considering what the implications of the material from Section 1 are when the context of inquiry is expanded to the global realm. Because the world is increasingly connected at an institutional, social, and economic level, should the social contract be conceived of in a more cosmopolitan way so that it includes representatives from the global community?

Adopting such a cosmopolitan perspective would surely have radical implications. For example, the fact that a child born in Sierra Leone is 100 times more likely to die in infancy than a child born in Finland is the result of the combined natural and social lotteries. If this inequality has a significant impact on individual opportunity—which it surely does—and if social institutions should be designed to benefit the worst off, then surely the wealthy nations of the developed world would have a duty to transfer significant resources toward the project of safeguarding the health and basic social opportunities of the global poor.

As we saw in Section 1, libertarians would balk at such a proposal. For such theorists, the plight of the global poor may be tragic, but severity alone is not sufficient to generate a duty to aid. Even libertarians recognize, however, that individuals have an affirmative duty, known as a duty of reparation or rectification, to aid those whom they have harmed. In "Responsibilities for Poverty-Related Illness," Thomas W. Pogge argues that members of wealthy, developed nations not only owe a duty of rectification to the global poor, but that this duty takes precedence over some of the medical needs of their compatriots.

Pogge's position rests on two pillars. The first is the claim that those who are involved in configuring social institutions that materially affect the health of those whose lives they regulate have an obligation to ensure that those institutions are configured to minimize their harmful effects. The second is that the moral reasons for helping a foreigner whose health has been adversely affected by an institutional order that one has helped shape or construct are stronger than the moral reasons for helping one's own community members whose poor health status does not stem from the effects of such an institutional order.

For Pogge, severe poverty represents the key pathway through which a variety of domestic and international institutions create and perpetuate the poor health of the world's poor. Similarly, democratic governance represents the link between the activities of these institutions and the majority of persons living in the developing world. For Pogge, that is, if the citizens to whom elected officials are accountable made creating a more just international order a policy priority, their elected leaders would march in line. Since they have not pushed for such policies, Pogge argues that they bear some responsibility for the adverse toll that the resulting institutional order exacts from the health of the global poor.

Pogge's position is both demanding and startling, and its implications are far-reaching. Consider, for example, the discussion from the previous section in which it was suggested that a transnational market in human organs might provide a mutually beneficial opportunity for "trade" between the global rich and the global poor. Such a proposal appears most plausible only under the assumption that the global rich do not already owe the global poor some form of aid or assistance, the provision of which would make selling one's organ a less attractive economic "opportunity." On Pogge's account, however, the global rich have exactly such obligations to the global poor and these obligations stem, not from the unvarnished severity of the plight of those at the bottom of the global heap or from a general duty to maximize aggregate welfare, but from the way in which the former are complicit in the institutional arrangements that helped cause the desperate situation of the latter.

In "Do We Owe the Global Poor Assistance or Rectification?" Mathias Risse disputes one of the central premises of Pogge's argument. He argues that the global order has not harmed the global poor and that, in fact, it has brought about one of the most stunning advances in prosperity in the history of humankind. Risse's case rests primarily on two points.

First, in the period before the industrial revolution a much more equal global economic situation existed—everyone was relatively poor. Over the course of the next two hundred years the division of labor, along with advances in materials and machinery, created an engine for economic growth unprecedented in human history. The industrial revolution created a rising tide of economic prosperity that lifted all boats. True, the nautical metaphor is inapt, since some boats rose higher than others. But even sub-Saharan Africa experienced a period of more or less sustained economic growth.

Second, Risse claims that the kind of counterfactual comparisons that Pogge's arguments require simply cannot be made. How is it possible to know what would have transpired in African nations had they never come under colonial rule? While Risse admits that colonial rule was surely problematic, he thinks that we simply cannot know whether contemporary Africans would be better off had that rule never taken place. In the face of these two facts, Risse concludes that affluent members of developed countries do not, in fact, owe the global poor duties of rectification—at least not for the reasons that Pogge advances.

In evaluating this exchange, readers would do well to consider whether Pogge's central objection is incompatible with Risse's observation that all regions of the world are better off now than they were two hundred years ago. It is not clear that Pogge is committed to denying this claim. Similarly, readers should consider carefully what kind of counterfactual claims Pogge's arguments require. Do they require wholesale assessments of what the world would have looked like without colonial rule, or merely the evaluation of particular policies and institutional structures? After all, Risse might be correct in his assertion that the World Trade Organization (WTO) represents a significant advance over the previous GATT treatise, but this may not undermine Pogge's central claim that concrete aspects of the WTO harm the global poor because there are viable alternative ways of structuring that international institution that would be more effective at reducing global poverty.

REFERENCES

Abraham, Laurie K. 1993. *Mama might be better off dead: The failure of health care in urban America.* Chicago: University of Chicago Press.

Arras, John. 1984. Retreat from the right to health care: The President's Commission and access for health care. *Cardozo Law Review* 6:321–345.

Bayer, Ronald. 1984. Ethics, politics, and access to health care: A critical analysis of the President's Commission. *Cardozo Law Review* 6:303–320.

Brody, Baruch. 1991. Why the right to health care is not a useful concept for policy debates. In *Rights to health care*, ed. T. J. Bole III and W. B. Bondeson. Netherlands: Kluwer Academic.

Eddy, David M. 1996. *Clinical decision making: From theory to practice.* Sudbury, MA: Jones and Bartlett.

Fauci, A. S. 1999. The AIDS epidemic: Considerations for the 21st century. *New England Journal of Medicine* 314 (14): 1046–1050.

Mello, Michelle M., and Troyen A. Brennan. 2001. The controversy over high-dose chemotherapy with autologous bone marrow transplant for breast cancer. *Health Affairs* 20 (5): 101–117.

Morreim, E. Haavi. 1995. *Balancing act: The new medical ethics of medicine's new economics.* Washington, DC: Georgetown University Press.

United Nations Development Program. 1999. *Human development report 1999.* New York: Oxford University Press: 38.

United Network for Organ Sharing. n.d. Retrieved from UNOS Web site, http://www.unos.org/data/about/viewDataReports.asp.

Walzer, Michael. 1993. *Spheres of justice: A defense of pluralism and equality.* New York: Basic Books.

World Health Organization. December 2005. *AIDS epidemic update.* Geneva, Switzerland: United Nations Program on HIV/AIDS and World Health Organization: 3.

JUSTICE, HEALTH, AND HEALTH CARE

AN ETHICAL FRAMEWORK FOR ACCESS TO HEALTH CARE

President's Commission for the Study of Ethical Problems in Medicine and Biomedical and Behavioral Research

The prevention of death and disability, the relief of pain and suffering, the restoration of functioning: these are the aims of health care. Beyond its tangible benefits, health care touches on countless important and in some ways mysterious aspects of personal life that invest it with significant value as a thing in itself. In recognition of these special features, the President's Commission was mandated to study the ethical and legal implications of differences in the availability of health services. In this Report to the President and Congress, the Commission sets forth an ethical standard: access for all to an adequate level of care without the imposition of excessive burdens. It believes that this is the standard against which proposals for legislation and regulation in this field ought to be measured. . . .

In both their means and their particular objectives, public programs in health care have varied over the years. Some have been aimed at assuring the productivity of the work force, others at protecting particularly vulnerable or deserving groups, still others at manifesting the country's commitment to equality of opportunity. Nonetheless, most programs have rested on a common rationale: to ensure that care be made accessible to a group whose health needs would otherwise not be adequately met.

The consequence of leaving health care solely to market forces—the mechanism by which most things are allocated in American society—is not viewed as acceptable when a significant portion of the population lacks access to health services. Of course, government financing programs, such as Medicare and Medicaid as well as public programs that provide care directly to veterans and the military and through local public hospitals, have greatly improved access to health care. These efforts, coupled with the expanded availability of private health insurance, have resulted in almost 90% of Americans having

Editors' note: Some text and notes have been cut. Students who want to read the article in its entirety should consult the original.

some form of health insurance coverage. Yet the patchwork of government programs and the uneven availability of private health insurance through the workplace have excluded millions of people. The Surgeon General has stated that "with rising unemployment, the numbers are shifting rapidly. We estimate that from 18 to 25 million Americans—8 to 11 percent of the population—have no health insurance coverage at all." Many of these people lack effective access to health care, and many more who have some form of insurance are unprotected from the severe financial burdens of sickness. . . .

Most Americans believe that because health care is special, access to it raises special ethical concerns. In part, this is because good health is by definition important to well-being. Health care can relieve pain and suffering, restore functioning, and prevent death; it can enhance good health and improve an individual's opportunity to pursue a life plan; and it can provide valuable information about a person's overall health. Beyond its practical importance, the involvement of health care with the most significant and awesome events of life—birth, illness, and death—adds a symbolic aspect to health care: it is special because it signifies not only mutual empathy and caring but the mysterious aspects of curing and healing.

Furthermore, while people have some ability— through choice of life-style and through preventive measures—to influence their health status, many health problems are beyond their control and are therefore undeserved. Besides the burdens of genetics, environment, and chance, individuals become ill because of things they do or fail to do—but it is often difficult for an individual to choose to do otherwise or even to know with enough specificity and confidence what he or she ought to do to remain healthy. Finally, the incidence and severity of ill health is distributed very unevenly among people. Basic needs for housing and food are predictable, but even the most hardworking and prudent person may suddenly be faced with overwhelming needs for health care. Together, these considerations lend weight to the belief that health care is different from most other goods and services. In a society concerned not only with fairness and equality of opportunity but also with the redemptive powers of science, there is a felt obligation to ensure that some level of health services is available to all.

There are many ambiguities, however, about the nature of this societal obligation. What share of health costs should individuals be expected to bear, and what responsibility do they have to use health resources prudently? Is it society's responsibility to ensure that every person receives care or services of as high quality and as great extent as any other individual? Does it require that everyone share opportunities to receive all available care or care of any possible benefit? If not, what level of care is "enough"? And does society's obligation include a responsibility to ensure both that care is available and that its costs will not unduly burden the patient?

The resolution of such issues is made more difficult by the spectre of rising health care costs and expenditures. Americans annually spend over 270 million days in hospitals, make over 550 million visits to physicians' offices, and receive tens of millions of X-rays. Expenditures for health care in 1981 totaled $287 billion—an average of over $1225 for every American. Although the finitude of national resources demands that trade-offs be made between health care and other social goods, there is little agreement about which choices are most acceptable from an ethical standpoint. In this chapter, the Commission attempts to lay an ethical foundation for evaluating both current patterns of access to health care and the policies designed to address remaining problems in the distribution of health care resources. . . .

THE SPECIAL IMPORTANCE OF HEALTH CARE

Although the importance of health care may, at first blush, appear obvious, this assumption is often based on instinct rather than reasoning. Yet it is possible to step back and examine those properties of health care that lead to the ethical conclusion that it ought to be distributed equitably.

Well-Being

Ethical concern about the distribution of health care derives from the special importance of health care in promoting personal well-being by preventing or relieving pain, suffering, and disability and by avoiding loss of life. The fundamental importance of the latter is obvious; pain and suffering are also experiences that people have strong desires to avoid, both because of the intrinsic quality of the experience and because of their effects on the capacity to pursue and achieve other goals and purposes. Similarly, untreated disability can prevent people from leading rewarding and fully active lives.

Health, insofar as it is the absence of pain, suffering, or serious disability, is what has been called a primary good, that is, there is no need to know what a particular person's other ends, preferences, and values are in order to know that health is good for that individual. It generally helps people carry out their life plans, whatever they may happen to be. This is not to say that everyone defines good health in the same way or assigns the same weight or importance to different aspects of being healthy, or to health in comparison with the other goods of life. Yet though people may differ over each of these matters, their disagreement takes place within a framework of basic agreement on the importance of health. Likewise, people differ in their beliefs about the value of health and medical care and their use of it as a means of achieving good health, as well as in their attitudes toward the various benefits and risks of different treatments.

Opportunity

Health care can also broaden a person's range of opportunities, that is, the array of life plans that is reasonable to pursue within the conditions obtaining in society.[1] In the United States equality of opportunity is a widely accepted value that is reflected throughout public policy. The effects that meeting (or failing to meet) people's health needs have on the distribution of opportunity in a society become apparent if diseases are thought of as adverse departures from a normal level of functioning. In this view, health care is that which people need to maintain or restore normal functioning or to compensate for inability to function normally. Health is thus comparable in importance to education in determining the opportunities available to people to pursue different life plans.

Information

The special importance of health care stems in part from its ability to relieve worry and to enable patients to adjust to their situation by supplying reliable information about their health. Most people do not understand the true nature of a health problem when it first develops. Health professionals can then perform the worthwhile function of informing people about their conditions and about the expected prognoses with or without various treatments. Though information sometimes creates concern, often it reassures patients either by ruling out a feared disease or by revealing the self-limiting nature of a condition and, thus, the lack of need for further treatment. Although health care in many situations may thus not be necessary for good physical health, a great deal of relief from unnecessary concern—and even avoidance of pointless or potentially harmful steps—is achieved by health care in the form of expert information provided to worried patients. Even when a prognosis is unfavorable and health professionals have little treatment to offer, accurate information can help patients plan how to cope with their situation.

The Interpersonal Significance of Illness, Birth, and Death

It is no accident that religious organizations have played a major role in the care of the sick and dying and in the process of birth. Since all human beings are vulnerable to disease and all die, health care has a special interpersonal significance: it expresses and nurtures bonds of empathy and compassion. The depth of a society's concern about health care can be seen as a measure of its sense of solidarity in the face of suffering and death. Moreover, health care takes on special meaning because of its role in the beginning of a human being's life as well as the end. In spite of all the advances in the scientific understanding of birth, disease, and death, these profound and universal experiences remain shared mysteries that touch the spiritual side of human nature. For these reasons a society's commitment to health care reflects some of its most basic attitudes about what it is to be a member of the human community.

THE CONCEPT OF EQUITABLE ACCESS TO HEALTH CARE

The special nature of health care helps to explain why it ought to be accessible, in a fair fashion, to all. But if this ethical conclusion is to provide a basis for evaluating current patterns of access to health care and proposed health policies, the meaning of fairness or equity in this context must be clarified. The concept of equitable access needs definition in its two main aspects: the level of care that ought to be available to all and the extent to which burdens can be imposed on those who obtain these services.

Access to What?

"Equitable access" could be interpreted in a number of ways: equality of access, access to whatever an individual needs or would benefit from, or access to an adequate level of care.

Equity as Equality It has been suggested that equity is achieved either when everyone is assured of receiving an equal quantity of health care dollars or when people enjoy equal health. The most common characterization of equity as equality, however, is as providing everyone with the same level of health care. In this view, it follows that if a given level of care is available to one individual it must be available to all. If the initial standard is set high, by reference to the highest level of care presently received, an enormous drain would result on the resources needed to provide other goods. Alternatively, if the standard is set low in order to avoid an excessive use of resources, some beneficial services would have to be withheld from people who wished to purchase them. In other words, no one would be allowed access to more services or services of higher quality than those available to everyone else, even if he or she were willing to pay for those services from his or her personal resources.

As long as significant inequalities in income and wealth persist, inequalities in the use of health care can be expected beyond those created by differences in need. Given people with the same pattern of preferences and equal health care needs, those with greater financial resources will purchase more health care. Conversely, given equal financial resources, the different patterns of health care preferences that typically exist in any population will result in a different use of health services by people with equal health care needs. Trying to prevent such inequalities would require interfering with people's liberty to use their income to purchase an important good like health care while leaving them free to use it for frivolous or inessential ends. Prohibiting people with higher incomes or stronger preferences for health care from purchasing more care than everyone else gets would not be feasible, and would probably result in a black market for health care.

Equity as Access Solely According to Benefit or Need Interpreting equitable access to mean that everyone must receive all health care that is of any benefit to them also has unacceptable implications. Unless health is the only good or resources are unlimited, it would be irrational for a society—as for an individual—to make a commitment to provide whatever health care might be beneficial regardless of cost. Although health care is of special importance, it is surely not all that is important to people. Pushed to an extreme, this criterion might swallow up all of society's resources, since there is virtually no end to the funds that could be devoted to possibly beneficial care for diseases and disabilities and to their prevention.

Equitable access to health care must take into account not only the benefits of care but also the cost in comparison with other goods and services to which those resources might be allocated. Society will reasonably devote some resources to health care but reserve most resources for other goals. This, in turn, will mean that some health services (even of a lifesaving sort) will not be developed or employed because they would produce too few benefits in relation to their costs and to the other ways the resources for them might be used.

It might be argued that the notion of "need" provides a way to limit access to only that care that confers especially important benefits. In this view, equity as access according to need would place less severe demands on social resources than equity according to benefit would. There are, however, difficulties with the notion of need in this context. On the one hand, medical need is often not narrowly defined but refers to any condition for which medical treatment might be effective. Thus, "equity as access according to need" collapses into "access according to whatever is of benefit."

On the other hand, "need" could be even more expansive in scope than "benefit." Philosophical and economic writings do not provide any clear distinction between "needs" and "wants" or "preferences." Since the term means different things to different people, "access according to need" could become "access to any health service a person wants." Conversely, need could be interpreted very narrowly to encompass only a very minimal level of services—for example, those "necessary to prevent death."

Equity as an Adequate Level of Health Care
Although neither "everything needed" nor "everything beneficial" nor "everything that anyone else is getting" are defensible ways of understanding equitable access, the special nature of health care dictates that everyone have access to *some* level of care: enough care to achieve sufficient welfare, opportunity, information, and evidence of interpersonal concern to facilitate a reasonably full and satisfying life. That level can be termed "an adequate level of health care." The difficulty of sharpening this amorphous notion into a workable foundation for health policy is a major problem in the United States today. This concept is not new; it is implicit in the public debate over health policy and has manifested itself in the history of public policy in this country. In this chapter, the Commission attempts to demonstrate the value of the concept, to clarify its content, and to apply it to the problems facing health policymakers.

Understanding equitable access to health care to mean that everyone should be able to secure an adequate level of care has several strengths. Because an adequate level of care may be less than "all beneficial care" and because it does not require that all needs be satisfied, it acknowledges the need for setting priorities within health care and signals a clear recognition that society's resources are limited and that there are other goods besides health. Thus, interpreting equity as access to adequate care does not generate an open-ended obligation. One of the chief dangers of interpretations of equity that require virtually unlimited resources for health care is that they encourage the view that equitable access is an impossible ideal. Defining equity as an adequate level of care for all avoids an impossible commitment of resources without falling into the opposite error of abandoning the enterprise of seeking to ensure that health care is in fact available for everyone.

In addition, since providing an adequate level of care is a limited moral requirement, this definition also avoids the unacceptable restriction on individual liberty entailed by the view that equity requires equality. Provided that an adequate level is available to all, those who prefer to use their resources to obtain

care that exceeds that level do not offend any ethical principle in doing so. Finally, the concept of adequacy, as the Commission understands it, is society-relative. The content of adequate care will depend upon the overall resources available in a given society, and can take into account a consensus of expectations about what is adequate in a particular society at a particular time in its historical development. This permits the definition of adequacy to be altered as societal resources and expectations change.

With What Burdens?

It is not enough to focus on the care that individuals receive; attention must be paid to the burdens they must bear in order to obtain it—waiting and travel time, the cost and availability of transport, the financial cost of the care itself. Equity requires not only that adequate care be available to all, but also that these burdens not be excessive.

If individuals must travel unreasonably long distances, wait for unreasonably long hours, or spend most of their financial resources to obtain care, some will be deterred from obtaining adequate care, with adverse effects on their health and well-being. Others may bear the burdens, but only at the expense of their ability to meet other important needs. If one of the main reasons for providing adequate care is that health care increases welfare and opportunity, then a system that required large numbers of individuals to forego food, shelter, or educational advancement in order to obtain care would be self-defeating and irrational.

The concept of acceptable burdens in obtaining care, as opposed to excessive ones, parallels in some respects the concept of adequacy. Just as equity does not require equal access, neither must the burdens of obtaining adequate care be equal for all persons. What is crucial is that the variations in burdens fall within an acceptable range. As in determining an adequate level of care, there is no simple formula for ascertaining when the burdens of obtaining care fall within such a range. . . .

A SOCIETAL OBLIGATION

Society has a moral obligation to ensure that everyone has access to adequate care without being subject to excessive burdens. In speaking of a societal obligation the Commission makes reference to society in the broadest sense—the collective American community. The community is made up of individuals, who are in turn members of many other, overlapping groups, both public and private: local, state, regional, and national units; professional and workplace organizations; religious, educational, and charitable organizations; and family, kinship, and ethnic groups. All these entities play a role in discharging societal obligations.

The Commission believes it is important to distinguish between society, in this inclusive sense, and government as one institution among others in society. Thus the recognition of a collective or societal obligation does not imply that government should be the only or even the primary institution involved in the complex enterprise of making health care available. It is the Commission's view that the societal obligation to ensure equitable access for everyone may best be fulfilled in this country by a pluralistic approach that relies upon the coordinated contributions of actions by both the private and public sectors.

Securing equitable access is a societal rather than a merely private or individual responsibility for several reasons. First, while health is of special importance for human beings, health care—especially scientific health care—is a social product requiring the skills and efforts of many individuals; it is not something that individuals can provide for themselves solely through their own efforts. Second, because the need for health care is both unevenly distributed among persons and highly unpredictable and because the cost of securing care may be great, few individuals could secure adequate care without relying on some social mechanism for sharing the costs. Third, if persons generally deserved their health conditions or if the need for health care were fully within the individual's control, the fact that some lack adequate care would not be viewed as an inequity. But differences in health status, and hence differences in health care needs, are largely undeserved because they are, for the most part, not within the individual's control.

Uneven and Unpredictable Health Needs

While requirements for other basic necessities, such as adequate food and shelter, vary among people within a relatively limited range, the need for health care is distributed very unevenly and its occurrence at any particular time is highly unpredictable. One study shows 50% of all hospital billings are for only 13% of the patients, the seriously chronically ill.

Moreover, health care needs may be minor or overwhelming, in their personal as well as financial impact. Some people go through their entire lives seldom requiring health care, while others face medical expenses that would exceed the resources of all but the wealthiest. Moreover, because the need for care cannot be predicted, it is difficult to provide for it by personal savings from income. . . .

WHO SHOULD ENSURE THAT SOCIETY'S OBLIGATION IS MET?

In this country, the chief mechanism by which the cost of health care is spread among individuals is through the purchase of insurance. Another method of distributing health care costs is to rely on acts of charity in which individuals, such as relatives and care givers, and institutions assume responsibility for absorbing some or all of a person's health care expenses. These private forces cannot be expected to achieve equitable access for all, however. States and localities have also played important roles in attempting to secure health care for those in need. To the extent that actions of the market, private charity, and lower levels of government are insufficient in achieving equity, the responsibility rests with Federal government. The actual provision of care may be through arrangements in the private sector as well as through public institutions, such as local hospitals.

Market Mechanisms in Health Care

One means societies employ for meeting needs for goods and services that individuals cannot produce by themselves is the complex legal and economic mechanism known as a market. When health care is distributed through markets, however, an acceptable distribution is not achieved; indeed, given limitations in the way markets work, this result is practically inevitable.

The Inability to Ensure Adequate Care   First, many people lack the financial resources to obtain access to adequate care. Since American society encompasses a very wide range in income and wealth, distributing goods and services through markets leads to large differences in their consumption. The variations in need for health care do not, however, match variations in ability to purchase care. The market response to variable risk is insurance. Insurance has long existed for certain calamities—such as fire damage to property—and in the past 30 years, a huge market in health insurance has developed that enables people to share some of the financial risk of ill health. The relevant question for determining equity of access thus becomes: Is everyone able to afford access to adequate care through some combination of insurance and direct payment?

Admittedly, "ability to afford" is an ambiguous concept, given different attitudes toward risk and the importance of health care, and, even more important, possibly insufficient information about the likelihood of ill health and about the possible effects of care. For example, people may want an adequate level of care and may be able to afford to pay for it, but they may lack information about the amount of coverage needed to secure adequate care. As a result, the insurance market may not do a good job of providing plans that actually do protect people adequately. And, of course, some people who can afford to pay for their health care (and who would if they knew they would have to go without it otherwise) fail to make sufficient provisions because they rely on others not being willing to let them suffer. Furthermore, the cost of basic health insurance (which does not even guarantee financial access to adequate care in all cases) is high enough to place it beyond the reach of many families by *any* reasonable standard of affordability. Ironically, those who need the most care will find it most difficult to obtain it, both because their disease or disability impairs their opportunities for accumulating financial resources and because insurers will charge them higher rates. . . .

A Right to Health Care?

Often the issue of equitable access to health care is framed in the language of rights. Some who view health care from the perspective of distributive justice argue that the considerations discussed in this chapter show not only that society has a moral obligation to provide equitable access, but also that

every individual has a moral right to such access. The Commission has chosen not to develop the case for achieving equitable access through the assertion of a right to health care. Instead it has sought to frame the issues in terms of the special nature of health care and of society's moral obligation to achieve equity, without taking a position on whether the term "obligation" should be read as entailing a moral right. The Commission reaches this conclusion for several reasons: first, such a right is not legally or constitutionally recognized at the present time; second, it is not a logical corollary of an ethical obligation of the type the Commission has enunciated; and third, it is not necessary as a foundation for appropriate governmental actions to secure adequate health care for all.

Legal Rights   Neither the Supreme Court nor any appellate court has found a constitutional right to health or to health care. However, most Federal statutes and many state statutes that fund or regulate health care have been interpreted to provide statutory rights in the form of entitlements for the intended beneficiaries of the program or for members of the group protected by the regulatory authority. . . .

Moral Obligations and Rights   The relationship between the concept of a moral right and that of a moral obligation is complex. To say that a person has a moral right to something is always to say that it is that person's due, that is, he or she is morally entitled to it. In contrast, the term "obligation" is used in two different senses. All moral rights imply corresponding obligations, but, depending on the sense of the term that is being used, moral obligations may or may not imply corresponding rights. In the broad sense, to say that society has a moral obligation to do something is to say that it ought morally to do that thing and that failure to do it makes society liable to serious moral criticism. This does not, however, mean that there is a corresponding right. For example, a person may have a moral obligation to help those in need, even though the needy cannot, strictly speaking, demand that person's aid as something they are due.

The government's responsibility for seeing that the obligation to achieve equity is met is independent of the existence of a corresponding moral right to health care. There are many forms of government involvement, such as enforcement of traffic rules or taxation to support national defense, to protect the environment, or to promote biomedical research, that do not presuppose corresponding moral rights but that are nonetheless legitimate and almost universally recognized as such. In a democracy, at least, the people may assign to government the responsibility for seeing that important collective obligations are met, provided that doing so does not violate important moral rights.

As long as the debate over the ethical assessment of patterns of access to health care is carried on simply by the assertion and refutation of a "right to health care," the debate will be incapable of guiding policy. At the very least, the nature of the right must be made clear and competing accounts of it compared and evaluated. Moreover, if claims of rights are to guide policy they must be supported by sound ethical reasoning and the connections between various rights must be systematically developed, especially where rights are potentially in conflict with one another. At present, however, there is a great deal of dispute among competing theories of rights, with most theories being so abstract and inadequately developed that their implications for health care are not obvious. Rather than attempt to adjudicate among competing theories of rights, the Commission has chosen to concentrate on what it believes to be the more important part of the question: What is the nature of the societal obligation, which exists whether or not people can claim a corresponding right to health care, and how should this societal obligation be fulfilled?[2]

MEETING THE SOCIETAL OBLIGATION

How Much Care Is Enough?

Before the concept of an adequate level of care can be used as a tool to evaluate patterns of access and efforts to improve equity, it must be fleshed out. Since there is no objective formula for doing this, reasonable people can disagree about whether particular patterns and policies meet the demands of adequacy. The Commission does not attempt to spell out in detail what adequate care should include. Rather it frames the terms in which those who discuss or critique health care issues can consider ethics as well as economics, medical science, and other dimensions.

Characteristics of Adequacy   First, the Commission considers it clear that health care can only be judged adequate in relation to an individual's health condition. To begin with a list of techniques or procedures, for example, is not sensible: A CT scan for an accident victim with a serious head injury might be the best way to make a diagnosis essential for the appropriate treatment of that patient; a CT scan for a person with headaches might not be considered essential for adequate care. To focus only on the technique, therefore, rather than on the individual's health and the impact the procedure will have on that individual's welfare and opportunity, would lead to inappropriate policy.

Disagreement will arise about whether the care of some health conditions falls within the demands of adequacy. Most people will agree, however, that some conditions should not be included in the societal obligation to ensure access to adequate care. A relatively uncontroversial example would be changing the shape of a functioning, normal nose or retarding the normal effects of aging (through cosmetic surgery). By the same token, there are some conditions, such as pregnancy, for which care would be regarded as an important component of adequacy. In determining adequacy, it is important to consider how people's welfare, opportunities, and requirements for information and interpersonal caring are affected by their health condition.

Any assessment of adequacy must consider also the types, amounts, and quality of care necessary to respond to each health condition. It is important to emphasize that these questions are implicitly comparative: The standard of adequacy for a condition must reflect the fact that resources used for it will not be available to respond to other conditions. Consequently, the level of care deemed adequate should reflect a reasoned judgment not only about the impact of the condition on the welfare and opportunity of the individual but also about the efficacy and the cost of the care itself in relation to other conditions and the efficacy and cost of the care that is available for them. Since individual cases differ so much, the health care professional and patient must be flexible. Thus adequacy, even in relation to a particular health condition, generally refers to a range of options.

The Relationship of Costs and Benefits   The level of care that is available will be determined by the level of resources devoted to producing it. Such allocation should reflect the benefits and costs of the care provided. It should be emphasized that these "benefits," as well as their "costs," should be interpreted broadly, and not restricted only to effects easily quantifiable in monetary terms. Personal benefits include improvements in individuals' functioning and in their quality of life, and the reassurance from worry and the provision of information that are a product of health care. Broader social benefits should be included as well, such as strengthening the sense of community and the belief that no one in serious need of health care will be left without it. Similarly, costs are not merely the funds spent for a treatment but include other less tangible and quantifiable adverse consequences, such as diverting funds away from other socially desirable endeavors including education, welfare, and other social services.

There is no objectively correct value that these various costs and benefits have or that can be discovered by the tools of cost/benefit analysis. Still, such an analysis, as a recent report of the Office of Technology Assessment noted, "can be very helpful to decisionmakers because the process of analysis gives structure to the problem, allows an open consideration of all relevant effects of a decision, and forces the explicit treatment of key assumptions." But the valuation of the various effects of alternative treatments for different conditions rests on people's values and goals, about which individuals will reasonably disagree. In a democracy, the appropriate values to be assigned to the consequences of policies must ultimately be determined by people expressing their values through social and political processes as well as in the marketplace.

Approximating Adequacy   The intention of the Commission is to provide a frame of reference for policymakers, not to resolve these complex questions. Nevertheless, it is possible to raise some of the specific issues that should be considered in determining what constitutes adequate care. It is important, for example, to gather accurate information about and compare the costs and effects, both favorable and unfavorable, of various treatment or management options. The options that better serve the goals that make health care of special importance should be assigned a higher value. As already noted, the assessment of costs must take two factors

into account: the cost of a proposed option in relation to alternative forms of care that would achieve the same goal of enhancing the welfare and opportunities of the patient, and the cost of each proposed option in terms of foregone opportunities to apply the same resources to social goals other than that of ensuring equitable access.

Furthermore, a reasonable specification of adequate care must reflect an assessment of the relative importance of many different characteristics of a given form of care for a particular condition. Sometimes the problem is posed as: What *amounts* of care and what *quality* of care? Such a formulation reduces a complex problem to only two dimensions, implying that all care can readily be ranked as better or worse. Because two alternative forms of care may vary along a number of dimensions, there may be no consensus among reasonable and informed individuals about which form is of higher overall quality. It is worth bearing in mind that adequacy does not mean the highest possible level of quality or strictly equal quality any more than it requires equal amounts of care; of course, adequacy does require that everyone receive care that meets standards of sound medical practice.

Any combination of arrangements for achieving adequacy will presumably include some health care delivery settings that mainly serve certain groups, such as the poor or those covered by public programs. The fact that patients receive care in different settings or from different providers does not itself show that some are receiving inadequate care. The Commission believes that there is no moral objection to such a system so long as all receive care that is adequate in amount and quality and all patients are treated with concern and respect. . . .

NOTES

1. Norman Daniels, *Health Care Needs and Distributive Justice*, 10 Phil. & Pub. Aff. 146 (1981).
2. Whether the issue of equity is framed in terms of individual rights or societal obligation, it is important to recall that society's moral imperative to achieve equitable access is not an unlimited commitment to provide whatever care, regardless of cost, individuals need or that would be of some benefit to them. Instead, society's obligation is to provide adequate care for everyone. Consequently, if there is a moral right that corresponds to this obligation, it is limited, not open-ended.

EQUAL OPPORTUNITY AND HEALTH CARE

Norman Daniels

A natural place to seek principles of justice for regulating health-care institutions is by examining different general theories of justice. Libertarian, utilitarian, and contractarian theories, for example, each support more general principles governing the distribution of rights, opportunities, and wealth, and these general principles may bear on the specific issue of health care. But there is a difficulty with this strategy. In order to apply such general theories to health care, we need to know what kind of a social good health care is. An analysis of this problem is not provided by general theories of justice. One way to see the problem is to ask whether health-care services, say personal medical services, should be viewed as we view other commodities in our society. Should we allow inequalities in the access to health-care services to vary with whatever economic inequalities are permissible according to more general principles of distributive justice? Or is health care "special" and not to be assimilated with other commodities, like cars or personal computers, whose distribution we allow to be governed by market exchanges among economic unequals?

Is health care special? To answer this question, we must see that not all preferences individuals have—and express, for example, in the marketplace—are of equal moral importance. When we judge the importance to society of meeting someone's preferences we use a restricted measure of well-being. We do not simply ask, how much does the person want something? Or, how happy an individual will be if he gets it? Rather, we are concerned whether the preference is for something that affects well-being in certain fundamental or important ways (cf. Scanlon 1975). Among the kinds of preferences to which we give special weight are those that meet certain important

categories of need. Among these important needs are those necessary for maintaining normal functioning for individuals, viewed as members of a natural species. Health-care needs fit this characterization of important needs because they are things we need to prevent or cure diseases and disabilities, which are deviations from species-typical functional organization ("normal functioning" for short).

This preference suggests health care may be special in this restricted sense: Health care needs are important to meet because they affect normal functioning. But there is still a gap in our answer: Why give such moral importance to health-care needs merely because they are necessary to preserve normal functioning? Why is preserving normal functioning of special moral importance? The answer lies in the relationship between normal functioning and opportunity, but to make the relationship clear, I must introduce the notion of a normal opportunity range.

The *normal opportunity range* for a given society is the array of life plans reasonable persons in it are likely to construct for themselves. The normal range is thus dependent on key features of the society—its stage of historical development, its level of material wealth and technological development, and even important cultural facts about it. This dependency is one way in which the notion of normal opportunity range is socially relative. Facts about social organization, including the conception of justice regulating its basic institutions, will also determine how that total normal range is distributed in the population. Nevertheless, that issue of distribution aside, normal functioning provides us with one clear parameter affecting the share of the normal range open to a given individual. It is this parameter that the distribution of health care affects.

The share of the normal range open to individuals is also determined in a fundamental way by their talents and skills. Fair equality of opportunity does not require opportunity to be equal for all persons. It requires only that it be equal for persons with similar skills and talents. Thus individual shares of the normal range will not in general be *equal*, even when they are *fair* to the individual. The general principle of fair equality of opportunity does not imply leveling individual differences. Within the general theory of justice, unequal chances of success which derive from unequal talents may be compensated for in other ways. I can now state a fact at the heart of my approach: Impairment of normal functioning through disease and disability restricts individuals' opportunities relative to that portion of the normal range their skills and talents would have made available to them were they healthy. If individuals' fair shares of the normal range are the arrays of life plans they may reasonably choose, given their talents and skills, then disease and disability shrinks their shares from what is fair.

Of course, we also know that skills and talents can be undeveloped or misdeveloped because of social conditions, for example, family background or racist educational practices. So, if we are interested in having individuals enjoy a fair share of the normal opportunity range, we will want to correct for special disadvantages here too, say through compensatory educational or job-training programs. Still, restoring normal functioning through health care has a particular and *limited* effect on an individual's shares of the normal range. It lets them enjoy that portion of the range to which a full array of skills and talents would give them access, assuming that these too are not impaired by special social disadvantages. Again, there is no presumption that we should eliminate or level individual differences: These act as a baseline constraint on the degree to which individuals enjoy the normal range. Only where differences in talents and skills are the results of disease and disability, not merely normal variation, is some effort required to correct for the effects of the "natural lottery."

One conclusion we may draw is that impairment of the normal opportunity range is a (fairly crude) measure of the relative importance of health-care needs, at least at the social or macro level. That is, it will be more important to prevent, cure, or compensate for those disease conditions which involve a greater curtailment of an individual's share of the normal opportunity range. More generally, this relationship between health-care needs and opportunity suggests that the principle that should govern the design of health-care institutions is a principle guaranteeing fair equality of opportunity.

The concept of equality of opportunity is given prominence in Rawls's (1971) theory of justice, and it has also been the subject of extensive critical discussion. I cannot here review the main issues (see Daniels 1985, Chapter 3), nor provide a full justification for the principle of fair equality of opportunity. Instead, I shall settle for a weaker, conditional claim, which suffices for my purposes. Health-care institutions should be among those governed by a principle of fair equality of opportunity, provided two conditions obtain: (1) an acceptable general theory of justice includes a principle that requires basic institutions to guarantee fair equality of opportunity, and (2) the fair equality of opportunity principle acts as a constraint on permissible economic inequalities. In what follows, for the sake of simplicity, I shall ignore these provisos. I urge the fair equality of opportunity principle as an appropriate principle to govern macro decisions about the design of our health-care system. The principle defines, from the perspective of justice, what the moral *function* of the health-care system must be—to help guarantee fair equality of opportunity. This relationship between health care and opportunity is the fundamental insight underlying my approach.

My conditional claim does not depend on the acceptability of any particular general theory of justice, such as Rawls's contractarian theory. A utilitarian theory might suffice, for example, if it were part of an ideal moral code, general compliance with which produced at least as much utility as any alternative code (cf. Brandt 1979). That utilitarian theory could then be extended to health care through the analysis provided by my account. Because Rawls's is the main general theory that has incorporated a fair equality of opportunity principle, I have elsewhere suggested in some detail (Daniels 1985, Chapter 3) how it can be extended, with minor modifications, to incorporate my approach. These details need not distract us here.

The fair equality of opportunity account has several important implications for the issue of access to health care. First, the account is compatible with, though it does not imply, a multitiered health-care system. The basic tier would include health-care services that meet health-care needs, or at least important needs, as judged by their impact on opportunity range. Other tiers might involve the use of health-care services to meet less important needs or other preferences, for example, cosmetic surgery. Second, the basic tier, which we might think of as a "decent basic minimum," is characterized in a principled way, by reference to its impact on opportunity. Third, there should be no obstacles—financial, racial, geographical—to access to the basic tier. (The account is silent about what inequalities are permissible for higher tiers within the system.) Social obligations are focused on the basic tier.

The fair equality of opportunity account also has implications for issues of resource allocation. First, I have already noted that we have a crude criterion—impact on normal opportunity range—for distinguishing the importance of different health-care needs and services. Second, preventive measures that make the distribution of risks of disease more equitable must be given prominence in a just health-care system. Third, the importance of personal medical services, despite what we spend on them, must be weighed against other forms of health care, including preventive and public health measures, personal care and other long-term-care services. A just distribution of health-care services involves weighing the impact of all of these on normal opportunity range. This point has specific implications for the importance of long-term care, but also for the introduction of new high-cost technologies, such as artificial hearts, which deliver a benefit to relatively few individuals at very great cost. We must weigh new technologies against alternatives and judge the overall impact of introducing them on fair equality of opportunity—which gives a slightly new sense to the term "opportunity cost."

This account does not give individuals a basic right to have all of their health-care needs met. Rather, there are social obligations to provide individuals only with those services that are part of the design of a system which, on the whole, protects equal opportunity. If social obligations to provide appropriate health care are not met, then individuals are definitely wronged. Injustice is done to them. Thus, even though decisions have to be made about how best to protect opportunity, these obligations nevertheless are not similar to imperfect duties of

beneficence. If I could benefit from your charity, but you instead give charity to someone else, I am not wronged and you have fulfilled your duty of beneficence. But if the just design of a health-care system requires providing a service from which I could benefit, then I am wronged if I do not get it.

The case is similar to individuals who have injustice done to them because they are discriminated against in hiring or promotion practices on a job. In both cases, we can translate the specific sort of injustice done, which involves acts or policies that impair or fail to protect opportunity, into a claim about individual rights. The principle of justice guaranteeing fair equality of opportunity shows that individuals have legitimate claims or rights when their opportunity is impaired in particular ways—against a background of institutions and practices which protect equal opportunity. Health-care rights in this view are thus a species of rights to equal opportunity.

The scope and limits of these rights—the entitlements they actually carry with them—will be relative to certain facts about a given system. For example, a health-care system can protect opportunity only within the limits imposed by resource scarcity and technological development for a given society. We cannot make a direct inference from the fact that an individual has a right to health care to the conclusion that this person is entitled to some specific health-care service, even if the service would meet a health-care need. Rather, the individual is entitled to a specific service only if it is or ought to be part of a system that appropriately protects fair equality of opportunity. . . .

REFERENCES

Brandt, R. 1979. *A Theory of the Good and the Right*. Oxford: Oxford University Press.

Daniels, N. 1985. "Family Responsibility Initiatives and Justice Between Age Groups." *Law, Medicine, and Health Care* 13(4):153–159.

Rawls, J. 1971. *A Theory of Justice*. Cambridge, MA: Harvard University Press.

Scanlon, T. M. 1975. "Preference and Urgency." *Journal of Philosophy* 77(19):655–669.

FREEDOM AND MORAL DIVERSITY: THE MORAL FAILURES OF HEALTH CARE IN THE WELFARE STATE

H. Tristram Engelhardt, Jr.

I.   AN INTRODUCTION: BEYOND EQUALITY

In his 1993 health-care reform proposal, Bill Clinton offered health care as a civil right. If his proposal had been accepted, all Americans would have been guaranteed a basic package of health care. At the same time, they would have been forbidden to provide or purchase better basic health care, as a cost of participating in a national system to which they were compelled to contribute. A welfare entitlement would have been created and an egalitarian ethos enforced.[1] This essay will address why such egalitarian proposals are morally unjustifiable, both in terms of the establishment of a uniform health-care welfare right, and in terms of the egalitarian constraints these proposals impose against the use of private resources in the purchase of better-quality basic health care, not to mention luxury care.

In framing health-care welfare policy, one must address people's fears of being impoverished while at risk of death and suffering when medicine can offer a benefit. Simultaneously, one must confront significantly different understandings of the appropriate use of medicine, the claims of justice, and the meaning of equality. Any approach to providing health care for those who cannot afford it must come to terms with the substantial disagreements that separate individuals and communities regarding provision of health care by the state. In addition, the attempt to frame a uniform policy must confront the nonegalitarian consequences of human freedom. To be free is to make choices that have nonegalitarian results.

From *Social Philosophy and Policy* 14, no. 2 (Summer 1997): 180–196. Reprinted with permission from Cambridge University Press.

Editors' note: Some author's notes have been cut. Students who want to follow up on sources should consult the original article.

I shall argue that our disagreements about equality, fairness, and justice have a depth similar to that of our disagreements about contraception, abortion, third-party-assisted reproduction, and physician-assisted suicide, in that they are not resolvable in general secular moral terms. The lesson of the postmodern era is that there are as many secular accounts of equality, justice, and fairness as there are religious groups, sects, and cults.[2] There is no principled basis for choosing a particular content-full account as canonical. As a consequence, establishing a particular content-full notion of equality, fairness, and justice in health care is the secular equivalent of establishing, for a secular national health-care system, the Roman Catholic proscriptions regarding contraception: it would be morally arbitrary and without secular moral justification. Consequently, there are robust secular moral limitations on the establishment of particular views of equality, limitations resulting from the centrality of human persons as the source of secular moral authority. There are good grounds for holding that current health-care policies, such as those embodied in Medicare, which forbid recipients from paying more for better basic care from participating physicians while coercing them to contribute to this program, are immoral. I argue in this essay that welfare rights in health care, if they are to be established, should be recognized as the creations of limited governmental insurance policies and not as expressions of foundational rights to health care or claims of equality or fairness.[3]

II.   MEDICAL WELFARE: TEMPTATIONS AND DISAGREEMENTS IN THE FACE OF FINITUDE

Health care claims attention because of the dramatic ways in which medicine and the biomedical sciences address our finitude, vulnerability, and mortality.

Political support for the governmental provision of health care often involves the view that to deny someone health care is to deny him or her protection against suffering, disease, disability, and death. The suppressed premise is that such a denial would be unfair. This view has difficulties. First, one must show how and why needs generate rights. Second, unlike food, clothing, and shelter, which can be provided at relatively minimal costs while still being sufficient for health and life, health care frequently confronts disabilities, diseases, disorders, and threats of death that cannot be overcome even with maximum medical efforts and the costs they involve. Often, illness can be cured only in part, suffering ameliorated only to some extent, disabilities remedied only to some degree, and death postponed only for a short time. In many cases, no matter how much one does, more resources could have been invested with some benefit for some recipients or possible recipients of health care. Just as ever more resources could be invested in avoiding accidental injuries and deaths by improving workplace safety, or invested in diminishing highway deaths by licensing only those cars that have front and side air bags as well as the front-end collision protection available in luxury cars, so, too, in medicine more resources could always be invested in preventive and curative endeavors without ever being fully successful against our finite, vulnerable, and mortal condition. Death and suffering are inescapable, so that we must decide what finite effort we should make to postpone death and avoid some suffering. We must ask whether there is secular moral authority coercively to impose one particular approach and whether it may be an egalitarian one.

The human condition itself conspires against discovering a generally convincing understanding of what should count as a basic adequate package of health-care services. First, there is the problem that medical knowledge is limited and probabilistic. Practicing medicine requires accepting that all life is a gamble, that medicine is a part of life, and that therefore health-care professionals must gamble with the suffering, disability, and death of all whom they treat. Moreover, resources that one might use to improve knowledge and technology are themselves limited. On the one hand, there is not enough money to avoid all suffering, disability, and death. On the other hand, there is not enough knowledge to know with certainty when particular interventions will succeed or fail. As a result, given the finitude of resources and the indefinite range of threats to well-being and life, investments in protection against suffering, disability, and death must take into account probabilities of success and failure. Investments must be limited and one must gamble.

To gamble, one must be willing to lose. Suppose that, as a matter of public policy, one has decided that in order to make good use of resources, one will not provide resources to the poor for a particular intervention—even when it might offer some protection against suffering, disability, and death—because the costs, probability of failure, and/or likely poor quality of results outweigh the possible benefits. In such a case, one must be willing to allow people to experience suffering, disability, and death when the resources are not available. One must also confront the circumstance that those with sufficient resources will purchase protection against death and suffering which is not available to all. In short, since ever more resources could always be invested in health care with some positive benefit, one faces two especially troubling policy questions: (1) May a basic, less-than-optimal package of health care be established for the poor? (2) May individuals, communities, and organizations use their own funds and energies to secure for themselves even better basic protection, as well as supplementary protection, against death and suffering? If secular morality (a) cannot reveal a content-full canonical morality that requires an egalitarian health-care policy, but (b) rather reveals that individuals are the source of secular moral authority, then one will need to endorse a national health-care policy that accepts both moral diversity and inequality.

III.   BAD LUCK, UNFAIRNESS, AND INEQUALITY

If the authority of persons over themselves is morally legitimate, then individuals will, through their free choices, set limits to the realization of government-endorsed visions of the good and of human flourishing. Among the goods with which freedom will collide are those of equality and long life. To be free in any way that allows one to pursue particular goods or goals despite risks of death or disability is to be free to place oneself at risk of needing additional health care. To be free in any way that allows the acquisition of wealth as well as the giving and receiving of funds, valuables, and labor is to be free in ways that produce inequalities in opportunity and outcome. If the authority of governments is derived from the free consent of citizens, then citizens can freely limit governmental authority by withholding consent. Freedom brings into question the plausibility of a uniform and equal basic health-care entitlement. Insofar as people are free and have their own resources, some will take greater risks than others and some will purchase better protection than many can afford. Beyond that, one faces other persistent inequalities and a significant diversity of views about how one should respond to inequalities.

All will die, though some will die in their youth and others will live long lives. Inequality in health is, for many, especially vexing, since it involves significant differences in suffering and length of life. Still, differences in health status are not, on average, dramatically related to the level of access to high-cost health care. Cross-national comparative data concerning health-care investments and life expectancies suggest that differences in access to high-technology medicine pale in importance when compared to differences attributable to gender, income, and genetic luck. Women outlive men, the rich outlive the poor, and high-status individuals tend to outlive low-status individuals. For example, in the United Kingdom men and women in 1991 had life expectancies at birth of 73.2 and 78.8 years, respectively, while those in the United States had life expectancies of 72.0 and 78.9 years, respectively, though the United Kingdom invested $1,151 per person for health care, 7.1 percent of its gross domestic product, in comparison with the United States, which invested $3,094 per person, 13.6 percent of its gross domestic product. At age 80, the life expectancy was 6.3 years for men and 8.3 years for women in the United Kingdom, versus 7.2 years for men and 9.1 years for women in the United States. Though the differences in resource investment for health care likely express themselves in these differences in life expectancies at age 80, in absolute terms the differences due to gender still outweighed the differences between the two systems.

Given these data, a national health-care policy which focused on equality in mortality outcomes would most plausibly direct energies toward developing new ways to address the health needs of men and toward preventing pediatric deaths.

Indeed, for egalitarians concerned with equality in life expectancies, a cross-national examination of life-expectancy outcomes by gender would seem to mandate a major commitment to the increased study of diseases of men, an increase in the representation of men in research protocols, and the development of better treatments for life-threatening conditions facing men. Such egalitarians would also favor the prevention of pediatric deaths over improvements in geriatric medicine, because of the robust inequalities in life presented, say, in the comparison between having a life span of twelve years versus one of seventy-two years. If one invokes an expository device such as John Rawls's original position,* one can easily imagine a characterization of the contractors such that they would regard those dying young as the least well-off, and would therefore direct energies against pediatric life-threatening conditions before directing resources to geriatric care, other than perhaps comfort care. A somewhat similar case can be made for directing medical research toward diseases afflicting the poor and persons of low status. In short, a dedicated pursuit of equality in mortality expectations should give priority to medical research and treatment development for men, children, the poor, and persons of low status.

Not all will agree with this approach, either in detail or in its foundations. Since we do not share one concrete morality, the very energies which direct our concerns toward medical issues separate us into disagreeing communities of moral commitment. Disputes regarding bioethics and health-care policy cut to the moral quick regarding equality, not only because individuals and communities differ with respect to the weight assigned to equality interests, but also because of the moral ambiguity of the term itself. If one is to develop an egalitarian policy, one must establish the importance and compelling moral authority of a particular form or understanding of equality. The difficulty is that our understandings of the importance of equality differ substantially.

To appreciate the force of these differences, one might imagine three worlds. The first world has ten

---

Editors' note: See the Introduction.

people in it, each with six units of goodness or utility. In a second world there are nine people with six units of goodness or utility and one person with ten units. If one is on principle an egalitarian of outcomes, one will regard the second world as worse than the first, even though no one is worse off and the total amount of utility or goodness is greater. If one is morally concerned to rectify the inequalities of the second world, one will incline to what can be characterized as an egalitarianism of envy. That is, one will want all persons to be made equal, even when some have more without dispossessing those who have less. This attitude toward equality can be understood as a form of envy in the sense of an endorsed discontent with the good fortune of others, holding unequalizing good fortune to be unfair, even if it is not at the expense of others. Inequality in and of itself is regarded as a circumstance to be rectified in preference to and in priority over other goods or right-making conditions. Finally, one can consider a third world with nine people with six units of goodness or utility and one person with only one unit. If one wishes to improve the lot of the tenth person as cheaply and efficiently as possible, not because the person's share is unequal, but because that person lacks important goods and satisfactions, one can be characterized as endorsing an egalitarianism of altruism. One is not, in principle, concerned that some have more. Instead, one has sympathy for those who, in having less, lack a good.[4]

How one regards the inequalities presented in the descriptions of these three worlds is important for assessing how one regards inequalities in health care and elsewhere. This is especially significant for health-care policy, given that major differences in per-capita investments in health care across nations do not lead to dramatic differences in mortality expectations, once one has achieved a rather modest level of investment (e.g., Greece does very well with $452 of health care per person).[5] One must look to other considerations for the special place of equality in debates regarding health-care policy. Perhaps the special place given to equality in health care depends on (1) the ways in which medicine is felt to bear on our finitude, in particular, on the postponement of death and the blunting of suffering, as well as (2) the difficulties of steadfastly refusing to commit communal funds to rescue persons with expensive health

needs, even when (a) some individuals with disposable resources may decide to have themselves treated when they have such needs, and (b) individuals without the funds demand such treatment. If one is to set limits on public health-care expenditures when it has been decided that the costs of such interventions on average outweigh the benefits, while recognizing the authority of persons to make choices about themselves and to use their resources as they wish, one must commit oneself to opposing high-cost last-minute state attempts at medical rescue for the poor and one must accept inequalities in access to health care.

Even if one were resolved to set egalitarian limits on health-care expenditures, one would still be confronted with a diversity of equalities. One would need a basis in principle for choosing among: an equality of opportunity in using one's own resources to pursue one's own health-care goals; an equality of opportunity supported by governmental funds in the acquisition of health care; an equality of opportunity supported by governmental funds and by proscriptions against unbalancing this equality by private purchases.[6] If one pursued an equality of outcome rather than an equality of opportunity, one would need to choose among: an equality of outcome supported by research and treatment directed toward avoiding the premature death of men, children, etc.; an equality of outcome directed toward equalizing the likelihood of suffering, including the use of nonvoluntary euthanasia; an equality of outcome directed toward equalizing wealth, etc. One would also need a basis for choosing among conflicting views of governmental authority that could be invoked in the coercive realization of a particular ethos of health-care delivery. Does the government have the moral authority only to ensure that the provision of health care will be honest and nonfraudulent? Does the government also have the moral authority to ensure that everyone receives the health care that the government deems to be appropriate? Does the government have the secular moral authority to forbid the rich from leaving the country in order to purchase better health care abroad?

At stake also are conflicting views of what it is for the state to own the resources which politicians might wish to redistribute for egalitarian purposes, and what it is for individuals and groups to have holdings independently of the state. For example, does one own resources because one has produced them or has been given those resources by those who have produced them? Or does one only own resources if such entitlements conform to a governmentally endorsed understanding of a desirable or right distribution of resources? For that matter, why are communal claims to possess resources advantaged over those made by individuals? In addition, one must decide what counts as just, fair, right, and good. For example, do needs generate rights, so that if resources are not available to meet health-care needs, such a state of affairs is unfair? Or are some outcomes simply unfortunate without being unfair? For instance, if certain screening programs can decrease the risk of developing cancer, does such protection against possible death count as a need that generates a right to a service for which others have a moral obligation to pay? Or is the nonprovision of such a service unfortunate, but not unfair? Or, if one's admission to a critical-care unit will convey a small chance of survival at a very high cost, does one have a need for health care that generates a right to the resources of others in order to purchase such critical care? Or is the nonavailability of such resources, save for the rich, simply unfortunate, not unfair?

There are, in addition, substantive disagreements regarding how to understand the relationship among individuals, communities, societies, and states. These disagreements are functions of different accounts of how one should characterize the communal, societal, and/or political space within which individuals find different kinds of morally authoritative structures. For example, should welfare, in the sense of group-provided insurance against losses in the natural and social lotteries,[7] be provided at the level of the state for all citizens, or instead at the level of particular communities and associations? One might envisage such provision occurring not just through companies, but also through religious and ideological groups. A number of these could transcend national boundaries, such as, perhaps, a worldwide Vaticare health-care welfare system for Roman Catholics, with the payment for care denominated in Vatican lira. Past history indicates that such approaches can succeed quite well even when they are unassociated with a particular religious or moral vision. In our contemporary postmodern world of deep disagreements regarding appropriate moral understandings of health care, such associations offer the opportunity

of maintaining moral and religious integrity within structures committed to a particular vision of health care. Under such an arrangement, one will need to tolerate others' doing evil within their own associations; yet when associations (rather than governments) are the social structures which embody content-full moralities, one can distance oneself as a citizen from such undertakings and avoid immediate collaboration with what one recognizes as wrong.

IV. HEALTH-CARE WELFARE PROVISION: WHY IT IS SO INTRUSIVE AND PROBLEMATIC

The provision of health care as a basic uniform civil right is more intrusive than any other element of the welfare state: health care dramatically touches all the important passages of life, from reproduction and birth to suffering and death. The commitment to a particular package of services brings with it a particular interpretation of the significance of reproduction, birth, health, suffering, death, and equality (e.g., it involves specific positions regarding artificial insemination by donors, prenatal diagnosis with the possibility of selective abortion, physician-assisted suicide, voluntary active euthanasia, and unequal access to better basic health care). A uniform welfare right to health care involves endorsing and establishing one among a number of competing concrete moralities of life, death, and equality. Because of this tie to morally controversial interventions, the establishment of uniform, universal health-care welfare rights directly or indirectly involves citizens, patients, physicians, nurses, and others in receiving or providing health care in a health-care system which they may find morally opprobrious.

Since all elements of personal behavior have some impact on the likelihood of disease, disability, and death, the establishment of a uniform, encompassing health-care welfare system involves the risk of medically politicizing all elements of personal conduct. For example, how should one regard a person who smokes heavily? Does a smoker irresponsibly expose the nation's health-care system to unnecessary costs? Or is such an individual a super-patriot, supporting the long-term fiscal solvency of the government? That is, should one consider such an individual a cost-saver, taking into account not only the costs of health care for smoking-related illnesses, but also the Social Security obligations (which would increase if the person were to live a more wholesome, longer life), possible long-term Medicare costs (which would be incurred if the individual adopted wholesome, nonsmoking behaviors, and thus lived to be eligible), and possible long-term Medicaid costs (which would rise if the individual adopted wholesome, nonsmoking behaviors, lived longer, and developed Alzheimer's, etc.)? Should one also consider the affluence and therefore increased life expectancies that may result from wealth generated from the tobacco industry? Who burdens whom, and under what circumstances, depends on who pays as well as on the freedom of individuals to agree to engage in certain behaviors and to accept the consequences involved.

An encompassing health-care welfare entitlement does not merely tend to impose a particular vision of morality, human flourishing, and responsible risk-taking; it also tends to constrain the free choice of those with disposable resources. The notion of a guaranteed basic benefit package can take on a coercive character, so that individuals are not allowed to purchase better basic care but may only purchase additional care which is not provided through the guaranteed benefit package. For example, after being compelled by state force to contribute to a Medicare system, so-called beneficiaries may not offer more money for a covered service in order to gain access to a premier physician. Current Medicare law forbids Medicare patients from rewarding their physicians and health-care providers for better basic service. Nor may they legally offer to pay more for a longer, more careful provision of the basic services covered under Medicare. Once covered by Medicare for physician services, for example, they may not volunteer to pay five times the reimbursement schedule (i.e., have Medicare pay its fee and they pay four times that in addition) for a house call by a distinguished internist. In short, their resources are devalued by a system to which they are compelled to contribute and which will then not allow them to benefit from their required contributions if they wish to purchase better basic care. Substantive, coercively imposed health-care policies come into tension with the free and peaceable choices of individuals (e.g., the patient who might wish to purchase better basic care from a willing physician, while still receiving Medicare benefits which that patient has been compelled to fund).

Health-care welfare rights are, for all these reasons, problematic. The framing of health-care policy requires (1) gambling with human life, (2) accepting unavoidable inequalities in morbidity and mortality, (3) recognizing multiple and competing notions of equality in health care, and (4) acknowledging the intrusiveness of health-care rights if they bring with them particular moral visions of reproduction, suffering, and death. It also requires (5) appreciating the dangers of imposing a particular medicalized view of lifestyles in the service of health policy, and (6) noting the temptation to restrict free choices in order to achieve what is taken to be, on some particular understanding, a suitable level of efficiency or equity, while (7) confronting the diversity of our moral visions.

V.   WHY THE MORAL DISPUTES WILL NOT GO AWAY, WHY WE ARE NOT ONE MORAL COMMUNITY WHEN IT COMES TO MATTERS OF HEALTH-CARE WELFARE PROVISION, AND WHY A PARTICULAR SUBSTANTIVE MORAL VISION OF FAIRNESS MAY NOT BE IMPOSED ON ALL

It is not merely a matter of fact or of sociological circumstance that we possess diverse understandings of the significance of reproduction, birth, disability, suffering, and death, as well as diverse understandings of how one ought to gamble in the face of finitude or how one ought to take account of our inequalities and disparate misfortunes with respect to death and suffering. The crucial point is that we do not possess the basis for resolving such controversies in terms of a content-full morality. The goal of demonstrating that we are one secular moral community—such that we ought to agree as a matter of justice, fairness, or moral probity regarding an all-encompassing health-care welfare system—is elusive. Rather than uniting citizens in a single moral community, the attempt to develop a uniform, encompassing health-care welfare right, as a matter of principle, and not only as a matter of fact, reveals our moral differences concerning the meaning and importance of equality, as well as our differences concerning the proper understanding of reproduction, suffering, and death.

The difficulty in resolving our moral controversies is foundational: one must already possess particular background moral premises, together with rules of moral evidence and inference, in order to resolve a moral controversy by sound rational argument. One needs a perspective from which one can make a morally authoritative choice among competing visions of the right and the good. An appeal to moral intuitions will not suffice. One's own moral intuitions will conflict with other moral intuitions. An appeal to ever-higher levels of moral intuition will not be decisive either, for further disagreements and appeals can in principle be extended indefinitely. Nor will an appeal to a consensus be any more successful. It will simply raise a number of questions: How does any particular consensus confer moral authority? How extensive must a consensus be to confer such authority? And from whom does such authority derive? (The appeal to consensus appears to invoke a secular version of a claim for the divine authority of majorities: *vox populi, vox Dei.*) In short, how much of a majority authorizes what use of force and why? In order to establish policy, one must know which substantive account of the right and/or the good is authoritative. However, the higher-level perspective from which one would make such a choice must itself be informed by an understanding of the right and/or the good.

Imagine that one agrees that a society—through public policy in general, and in health-care policy in particular—should attempt to maximize liberty, equality, prosperity, and security. To calculate and compare the consequences of alternative approaches, one must already know how to compare liberty, equality, prosperity, and security. The comparative consequences of competing approaches cannot be assessed simply by an appeal to consequences. One must already have an independent morality allowing one to compare the different kinds of outcomes at stake, namely, liberty consequences, equality consequences, prosperity consequences, and security consequences. Nor will attempting to maximize the preferences of citizens determine which health policy has the best consequences. One must first know how to compare impassioned versus rational preferences. One must know how, if at all, one is to revise or correct preferences. In addition, one will need to know God's discount rate for preference satisfaction over time; that is, one must have an absolute standard or must know whether each person's own standard should be used, whatever it might be, in the moment the person attempts the discounting. Nor will it do to appeal to a disinterested observer, a hypothetical chooser, or a set of hypothetical contractors. If such are truly disinterested, they will have no moral sense and will be unable to make a principled choice. To make a principled choice, they must already be informed by a particular moral sense or thin theory of the good. But of course, the choice of the correct moral sense or thin theory of the good is what is at stake. The same difficulty can be recapitulated for any account of moral rationality or of the decision-theoretic resolution of disputes. In order morally to assess behavior or policy, one must appeal to a standard. To use a standard, however, one must know which standard is morally canonical. The result is that a canonical content-full moral vision can be established as binding by sound rational argument only by begging the question. To choose with moral authority, one must already have authoritative normative guidance. The question is: "Which (and whose) guidance?"

Postmodernity as an epistemological predicament, not merely as a sociological fact, is the recognition that, outside of a revelation of a canonical standard, one cannot authoritatively choose among content-full understandings of moral probity, justice, or fairness without begging the question or engaging in an infinite regress. In order to show how a conclusion is warranted, one must always ask whose moral rationality, which sense of justice, is being invoked. At the same time, one must recognize that there are numerous competing moral accounts or narratives. As we have seen, there are numerous and competing understandings of the importance and significance of equality. In such a circumstance, if all do not listen to God, so as to find revealed to them the canonical content-full notion of moral probity, fairness, justice, and equality, and if all attempts by sound rational argument to establish the canonical content-full account of moral probity, justice, and fairness beg the question, then one can arrive at moral authority when individuals meet as moral strangers, not by drawing authority either from God or from reason, but only from the permission of those who participate. Moral authority will not be the authority of God or reason, but of consent, agreement, or permission. General secular moral authority is thus best construed as authorization.[8] The practice of deriving moral authority from permission makes possible a sparse practice of secular morality that does not presume any particular content-full view of the right or the good.

In such circumstances, permission or the authority it provides becomes the source of moral authority without any endorsement of permission as either good or bad. The securing of permission provides authority even when it does not provide motivation (permission does secure secular moral authority for the appropriate, albeit limited, use of state coercion, which can motivate compliance with the practice of deriving authority from permission). The point is that it is possible to secure a justification for state coercion and to determine which instances of coercion carry secular moral authority. The question is not "What will motivate moral action?" (though this issue is important), or "What level of moral disagreement makes governance difficult or impossible?" (or, for that matter, "What strategies by governments support public peace or effective governance?"). The question is, rather, "Under what circumstances can those ruling claim secular moral authority, so that those who disobey laws are not only at risk of being punished, but also at risk of being blameworthy?" Acting with permission offers a sparse, right-making condition for the collaboration of individuals who do not share a common understanding of what God demands or what moral rationality requires, but who claim an authority for their common endeavors.

Secular morality is procedural, and its legitimacy is limited by the consent of those who participate in common endeavors. Consequently, the paradigm moral activities of secular morality are the free market, contract formation, and the establishment of limited democracies.

In particular, democracies will have only that secular moral authority which can be derived either from the actual consent of all their members or from the practice of never using persons without their permission. The result will be that one will at most be able to justify the material equivalent of Robert Nozick's ultraminimal state. The point is that, in the absence of a canonical, content-full secular morality, (1) health-care policy must derive its authority from the consent of the governed, (2) not from a prior understanding of justice, fairness, or

equality, and (3) may not be all-encompassing, because the scope of its authority is limited by the limits of the consent of those involved. One will need to create policy instead of attempting to discover guidance in secular morality. One must proceed not by an appeal to a canonical, content-full understanding of the right or the good, but by an appeal to the permission of those involved. There will be no way to discover the correct balance among the various undertakings to which a community could direct its resources (e.g., how one should use common funds when faced with the claims of partisans of whooping cranes versus those of aged humans). As a consequence, limited democracies will be obliged to leave space so that individuals and communities can peaceably pursue their own visions of human flourishing and of appropriate health care. Still, if the state has legitimately acquired common resources, it is at liberty to create limited policy answers. One can explore many of the secular moral limits in health-care policy without attending to the general secular moral limits on state authority, by assuming that the state possesses legitimately acquired funds.[9]

VI.   TAKING MORAL DIVERSITY AND LIMITED DEMOCRACY SERIOUSLY

The concern to establish health-care welfare provision is encumbered by a cluster of moral difficulties tied to the inability to establish, by sound rational argument, a canonical morality regarding equality in access, not to mention regarding such important issues as third-party-assisted reproduction, abortion, physician-assisted suicide, and euthanasia. Though there is, on the part of many, a strong desire to establish an encompassing and equal right to health care, there are even stronger grounds for recognizing the morally problematic character of this desire. The substantial and significant differences in moral vision concerning matters of equality—and concerning the appropriate ways to regard reproduction, birth, suffering, and death—make any uniform, governmentally imposed right to health care highly morally problematic. Such an imposition would involve the secular equivalent of establishing a particular religious morality. If we do not share a common understanding of equality, fairness, and justice, and if there is in principle no way through sound rational argument to determine which understanding of justice, fairness, and equality should guide governmental undertakings, and if, in addition, health care is particularly intrusive and morally troubling when it brings with it a content-full moral understanding of reproduction, birth, suffering, and death, then the provision of any general protection against morbidity and mortality is best offered as a limited insurance against losses in the natural and social lotteries.

These considerations argue against any particular universally mandated set of health-care services and in favor of the equivalent of a voucher for the poor, which would allow the purchase of health care from various morally different health-care delivery networks. The limits of secular moral authority require acquiescing in the creation of health-care networks and associations providing morally different forms of basic health care. The only restrictions that may be imposed with secular moral authority will involve the guarantee that participants in the various health-care networks join freely in the particular medical moralities they choose.

In order to establish a limited welfare right to health care without going aground on diverse visions of moral probity and justice, secular health-care provision for the indigent may not be justified in terms of a particular account of equality, fairness, or justice, nor may it establish a particular medical morality regarding reproduction, suffering, and death. The use of vouchers could avoid much of this difficulty if such vouchers could be applied to different alternative, basic menus of service. Different communities or associations with different moral visions could then establish morally competing health-care systems into which individuals could enter for basic services using such vouchers. Better yet would be a policy that avoided even the necessity of establishing basic menus of service and instead allowed the use of health-care purchase accounts to which funds could be provided for the poor to use in purchasing basic medical services.

Under such circumstances, the government would provide basic health-care protection against morbidity and mortality for the indigent without imposing a content-full morality. Medical needs could be both defined and addressed in a range of significantly different terms. In a truly free and limited democracy,

competing health-care systems could come into existence to take advantage of the availability of the health-care vouchers (as well as the availability of payments from private insurers and direct payments from patients). For the sake of illustration, one could imagine two systems, one supported by Roman Catholics and another by New Age agnostics. The first would not offer artificial insemination by donors, prenatal diagnosis and abortion, or physician-assisted suicide and euthanasia. It would provide limitations on health-care expenditures in terms of religious understandings of the appropriate line between proportionate and disproportionate care, that is, between ordinary and extraordinary care. This line would vary with the social status of the individual (i.e., it would be *proportionem status*). In addition, religiously attentive hospice and comfort care would be offered to all.

In contrast, the system appealing to agnostic New-Agers would offer artificial insemination for unmarried women, prenatal diagnosis and selective abortion, and specially discounted treatment with an agreement to be euthanatized under certain conditions when health care is unlikely to provide a significant extension of life with an acceptable quality. Hospice care would be tied to effective and painless euthanasia. A voucher system or health-care purchase account that took moral diversity seriously would allow individuals to avoid interventions they recognized as morally inappropriate and to purchase in their stead those they saw as acceptable (or to select care so as to achieve a savings of funds). The result would be a policy that provided basic protection against health-care needs without establishing one view of equality and medical moral probity as dominant over the others.

The data indicate that such a basic welfare package would afford significant mortality protection. If individuals were left free to choose particular packages of basic health care (offered within particular medical moralities and constrained only by the free consent of the participants), then help could be provided for the poor while avoiding the significant moral costs of generally imposing one of the many secular medical moralities at the expense of the others. Such an approach to health-care policy would require accepting our finitude, including the limits of governmental moral authority, while acknowledging our moral diversity.

NOTES

1. The White House Domestic Policy Council, *The President's Health Security Plan* (New York: Times Books, 1993), presents a robustly egalitarian blueprint for health-care policy. In its "Ethical Foundations of Health Reform," the Clinton plan rejects a tiered system: "The system should avoid the creation of a tiered system providing care based only on differences of need, not individual or group characteristics" (p. 11). When the plan recommends that a new federal criminal statute be enacted prohibiting "the payment of bribes, gratuities or other inducements to administrators and employees of health plans, health alliances or state health care agencies" (p. 199), the goal is *inter alia* to proscribe payment to physicians for better basic care. The implications and the stated purpose of the plan are egalitarian.

2. I take it that the postmodern era is characterized by the circumstance, as a matter of sociological fact, (1) that all people do not share the same moral narrative or account, and (2) that this moral diversity is apparent and widely recognized. Moreover, as a matter of our epistemological condition, (3) there is no way to establish in purely secular terms the correct moral narrative or account without begging the question or engaging in an infinite regress, and (4) this is also widely recognized.

3. See also H. Tristram Engelhardt, Jr., *Bioethics and Secular Humanism: The Search for a Common Morality* (Philadelphia: Trinity Press International, 1991), esp. pp. 130–38.

4. One might interpret the so-called Oregon proposal as driven by an egalitarianism of altruism. Oregon proposed limiting the range of health-care resources available to Medicaid recipients so that all the poor could be covered. The proposal was that all the poor should be insured, although (1) Medicaid recipients would not receive the same level of health care as previously, and (2) the affluent would be able to purchase better basic care, as well as luxury care (i. e., there would be a tiered provision of health care with a limited package for the poor and with the affluent left free to purchase whatever they wished and could afford).

5. Schieber, Poullier, and Greenwald, "Health System Performance."

6. Norman Daniels provides a justification of an egalitarian approach to health care that, in the service of equality of opportunity, advances arguments for proscribing the purchase of better basic diagnostic and therapeutic interventions. See Norman Daniels, *Just Health Care* (New York: Cambridge University Press, 1985). Daniels was among the advisory members of the White House Task Force on National Health Reform, which developed President Clinton's 1993 health-care reform proposal.

7. The term "natural and social lotteries" identifies the natural and social forces that advantage and disadvantage individuals irrespective of their deserts: some live long and healthy lives, while others contract serious diseases and die young (examples of the natural lottery); some inherit fortunes, while others are born destitute (examples of the social lottery).

8. Moral constraints do exist within secular morality; they are derived from the right-making character of appeals to permission as the only source of authority in secular public policy. Even if all do not listen to God, and if reason cannot disclose a canonical content-full moral vision, one can still derive authority from common agreement, that is, from permission. See Engelhardt, *The Foundations of Bioethics*, 2nd ed. (New York: Oxford University Press, 1996), pp. 135–88.

9. I do not here explore the considerable difficulties faced in providing a general secular moral justification for taxation. Instead, attention is directed to how one ought to proceed in using common resources, presuming that they can be acquired legitimately. For my treatment of issues bearing on the legitimacy of taxation, see *The Foundations of Bioethics*, pp. 154–80.

SOCIAL DETERMINANTS OF HEALTH: THE SOLID FACTS

INTRODUCTION

Even in the most affluent countries, people who are less well off have substantially shorter life expectancies and more illnesses than the rich. Not only are these differences in health an important social injustice, they have also drawn scientific attention to some of the most powerful determinants of health standards in modern societies. They have led in particular to a growing understanding of the remarkable sensitivity of health to the social environment and to what have become known as the social determinants of health.

This publication outlines the most important parts of this new knowledge as it relates to areas of public policy. The ten topics covered include the lifelong importance of health determinants in early childhood, and the effects of poverty, drugs, working conditions, unemployment, social support, good food and transport policy. To provide the background, we start with a discussion of the social gradient in health, followed by an explanation of how psychological and social influences affect physical health and longevity.

In each case, the focus is on the role that public policy can play in shaping the social environment in ways conducive to better health: that focus is maintained whether we are looking at behavioural factors, such as the quality of parenting, nutrition, exercise and substance abuse, or at more structural issues such as unemployment, poverty and the experience of work.

. . .

The evidence on which this publication is based comes from very large numbers of research reports—many thousands in all. Some of the studies have used prospective methods, sometimes following tens of thousands of people over decades—sometimes

From *Social Determinants of Health: The Solid Facts*, 2nd ed., edited by Richard Wilkinson and Michael Marmot. Copenhagen: WHO Regional Office for Europe, 2003. Reprinted by permission of the World Health Organization.
Editors' note: Some text has been cut. Students who want to read the article in its entirety should consult the original.

from birth. Others have used cross-sectional methods and have studied individual, area, national or international data. Difficulties that have sometimes arisen (perhaps despite follow-up studies) in determining causality have been overcome by using evidence from intervention studies, from so-called natural experiments, and occasionally from studies of other primate species. Nevertheless, as both health and the major influences on it vary substantially according to levels of economic development, the reader should keep in mind that the bulk of the evidence on which this publication is based comes from rich developed countries and its relevance to less developed countries may be limited.

Our intention has been to ensure that policy at all levels—in government, public and private institutions, workplaces and the community—takes proper account of recent evidence suggesting a wider responsibility for creating healthy societies. But a publication as short as this cannot provide a comprehensive guide to determinants of public health. Several areas of health policy, such as the need to safeguard people from exposure to toxic materials at work, are left out because they are well known (though often not adequately enforced). As exhortations to individual behaviour change are also a well established approach to health promotion, and the evidence suggests they may sometimes have limited effect, there is little about what individuals can do to improve their own health. We do, however, emphasize the need to understand how behaviour is shaped by the environment and, consistent with approaching health through its social determinants, recommend environmental changes that would lead to healthier behaviour.

Given that this publication was put together from the contributions of acknowledged experts in each field, what is striking is the extent to which the sections converge on the need for a more just and caring society—both economically and socially. Combining economics, sociology and psychology with neurobiology and medicine, it looks as if much depends on understanding the interaction between material disadvantage and its social meanings. It is not simply that poor material circumstances are harmful to health; the social meaning of being, poor, unemployed, socially excluded, or otherwise stigmatized also matters. As social beings, we need not only good material conditions but, from early childhood onwards, we need to feel valued and appreciated. We need friends, we need more sociable societies, we need to feel useful, and we need to exercise a significant degree of control over meaningful work. Without these we become more prone to depression, drug use, anxiety, hostility and feelings of hopelessness, which all rebound on physical health.

We hope that by tackling some of the material and social injustices, policy will not only improve health and well-being, but may also reduce a range of other social problems that flourish alongside ill health and are rooted in some of the same socioeconomic processes.

1. THE SOCIAL GRADIENT

Life expectancy is shorter and most diseases are more common further down the social ladder in each society. Health policy must tackle the social and economic determinants of health.

What Is Known

Poor social and economic circumstances affect health throughout life. People further down the social ladder usually run at least twice the risk of serious illness and premature death as those near the top. Nor are the effects confined to the poor: the social gradient in health runs right across society, so that even among middle-class office workers, lower ranking staff suffer much more disease and earlier death than higher ranking staff (Fig. 1).

Both material and psychosocial causes contribute to these differences and their effects extend to most diseases and causes of death.

Disadvantage has many forms and may be absolute or relative. It can include having few family assets, having a poorer education during adolescence, having insecure employment, becoming stuck in a hazardous or dead-end job, living in poor housing, trying to bring up a family in difficult circumstances and living on an inadequate retirement pension.

These disadvantages tend to concentrate among the same people, and their effects on health accumulate during life. The longer people live in stressful

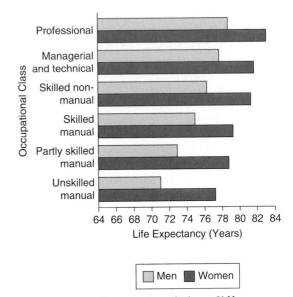

FIGURE 1   Occupational class differences in life expectancy, England and Wales, 1997–1999

Source: Donik A, Goldblatt P, Lynch K. Inequalities in life expectancy by social class 1972–1999. *Health Statistics Quarterly*, 2002, 15:5–15.

economic and social circumstances, the greater the physiological wear and tear they suffer, and the less likely they are to enjoy a healthy old age.

Policy Implications

If policy fails to address these facts, it not only ignores the most powerful determinants of health standards in modern societies, it also ignores one of the most important social justice issues facing modern societies.

- Life contains a series of critical transitions: emotional and material changes in early childhood, the move from primary to secondary education, starting work, leaving home and starting a family, changing jobs and facing possible redundancy, and eventually retirement. Each of these changes can affect health by pushing people onto a more or less advantaged path. Because people who have been disadvantaged in the past are at the greatest risk in each subsequent transition, welfare policies need to provide not only safety nets but also springboards to offset earlier disadvantage.

- Good health involves reducing levels of educational failure, reducing insecurity and unemployment and improving housing standards. Societies that enable all citizens to play a full and useful role in the social, economic and cultural life of their society will be healthier than those where people face insecurity, exclusion and deprivation.
- Other chapters of this publication cover specific policy areas and suggest ways of improving health that will also reduce the social gradient in health.

2. STRESS

Stressful circumstances, making people feel worried, anxious and unable to cope, are damaging to health and may lead to premature death.

What Is Known

Social and psychological circumstances can cause long-term stress. Continuing anxiety, insecurity, low self-esteem, social isolation and lack of control over work and home life, have powerful effects on health. Such psychosocial risks accumulate during life and increase the chances of poor mental health and premature death. Long periods of anxiety and insecurity and the lack of supportive friendships are damaging in whatever area of life they arise. The lower people are in the social hierarchy of industrialized countries, the more common these problems become.

Why do these psychosocial factors affect physical health? In emergencies, our hormones and nervous system prepare us to deal with an immediate physical threat by triggering the fight or flight response: raising the heart rate, mobilizing stored energy, diverting blood to muscles and increasing alertness. Although the stresses of modern urban life rarely demand strenuous or even moderate physical activity, turning on the stress response diverts energy and resources away from many physiological processes important to long-term health maintenance. Both the cardiovascular and immune systems are affected. For brief periods, this does not matter; but if people feel tense too often or the tension goes on for too long, they become more vulnerable to a wide range

of conditions including infections, diabetes, high blood pressure, heart attack, stroke, depression and aggression.

Policy Implications

Although a medical response to the biological changes that come with stress may be to try to control them with drugs, attention should be focused upstream, on reducing the major causes of chronic stress.

- In schools, workplaces and other institutions, the quality of the social environment and material security are often as important to health as the physical environment. Institutions that can give people a sense of belonging, participating and being valued are likely to be healthier places than those where people feel excluded, disregarded and used.
- Governments should recognize that welfare programmes need to address both psychosocial and material needs: both are sources of anxiety and insecurity. In particular, governments should support families with young children, encourage community activity, combat social isolation, reduce material and financial insecurity, and promote coping skills in education and rehabilitation.

3. EARLY LIFE

A good start in life means supporting mothers and young children: the health impact of early development and education lasts a lifetime.

What Is Known

Observational research and intervention studies show that the foundations of adult health are laid in early childhood and before birth. Slow growth and poor emotional support raise the lifetime risk of poor physical health and reduce physical, cognitive and emotional functioning in adulthood. Poor early experience and slow growth become embedded in biology during the processes of development, and form the basis of the individual's biological and human capital, which affects health throughout life.

Poor circumstances during pregnancy can lead to less than optimal fetal development via a chain that

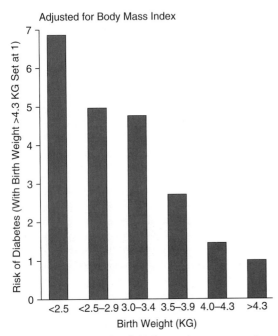

Adjusted for Body Mass Index

FIGURE 2   Risk of diabetes in men aged 64 years by birth weight

Source: Barker DJP. *Mothers, babies and disease in later life,* 2nd ed. Edinburgh, Churchill Livingstone, 1998.

may include deficiencies in nutrition during pregnancy, maternal stress, a greater likelihood of maternal smoking and misuse of drugs and alcohol, insufficient exercise and inadequate prenatal care. Poor fetal development is a risk for health in later life (Fig. 2).

Infant experience is important to later health because of the continued malleability of biological systems. As cognitive, emotional and sensory inputs programme the brain's responses, insecure emotional attachment and poor stimulation can lead to reduced readiness for school, low educational attainment, and problem behaviour, and the risk of social marginalization in adulthood. Good health-related habits, such as eating sensibly, exercising and not smoking, are associated with parental and peer group examples, and with good education. Slow or retarded physical growth in infancy is associated with reduced cardiovascular, respiratory, pancreatic and kidney development and function, which increase the risk of illness in adulthood.

Policy Implications

These risks to the developing child are significantly greater among those in poor socioeconomic circumstances, and they can best be reduced through improved preventive health care before the first pregnancy and for mothers and babies in pre- and postnatal, infant welfare and school clinics, and through improvements in the educational levels of parents and children. Such health and education programmes have direct benefits. They increase parents' awareness of their children's needs and their receptivity to information about health and development, and they increase parental confidence in their own effectiveness.

Policies for improving health in early life should aim to:

- increase the general level of education and provide equal opportunity of access to education, to improve the health of mothers and babies in the long run;
- provide good nutrition, health education, and health and preventive care facilities, and adequate social and economic resources, before first pregnancies, during pregnancy, and in infancy, to improve growth and development before birth and throughout infancy, and reduce the risk of disease and malnutrition in infancy; and
- ensure that parent–child relations are supported from birth, ideally through home visiting and the encouragement of good parental relations with schools, to increase parental knowledge of children's emotional and cognitive needs, to stimulate cognitive development and pro-social behaviour in the child, and to prevent child abuse.

4. SOCIAL EXCLUSION

Life is short where its quality is poor. By causing hardship and resentment, poverty, social exclusion and discrimination cost lives.

What Is Known

Poverty, relative deprivation and social exclusion have a major impact on health and premature death, and the chances of living in poverty are loaded heavily against some social groups.

Absolute poverty—a lack of the basic material necessities of life—continues to exist, even in the richest countries of Europe. The unemployed, many ethnic minority groups, guest workers, disabled people, refugees and homeless people are at particular risk. Those living on the streets suffer the highest rates of premature death.

Relative poverty means being much poorer than most people in society and is often defined as living on less than 60% of the national median income. It denies people access to decent housing, education, transport and other factors vital to full participation in life. Being excluded from the life of society and treated as less than equal leads to worse health and greater risks of premature death. The stresses of living in poverty are particularly harmful during pregnancy, to babies, children and old people. In some countries, as much as one quarter of the total population—and a higher proportion of children—live in relative poverty (Fig. 3).

Social exclusion also results from racism, discrimination, stigmatization, hostility and unemployment.

FIGURE 3 **Proportion of children living in poor households (below 50% of the national average income)**

Source: Bradshaw J. Child poverty in comparative perspective. In: Gordon D, Townsend P. *Breadline Europe: the measurement of poverty.* Bristol, The Policy Press, 2000.

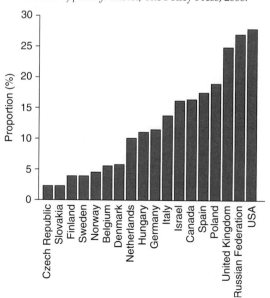

These processes prevent people from participating in education or training, and gaining access to services and citizenship activities. They are socially and psychologically damaging, materially costly, and harmful to health. People who live in, or have left, institutions, such as prisons, children's homes and psychiatric hospitals, are particularly vulnerable.

The greater the length of time that people live in disadvantaged circumstances, the more likely they are to suffer from a range of health problems, particularly cardiovascular disease. People move in and out of poverty during their lives, so the number of people who experience poverty and social exclusion during their lifetime is far higher than the current number of socially excluded people.

Poverty and social exclusion increase the risks of divorce and separation, disability, illness, addiction and social isolation and vice versa, forming vicious circles that deepen the predicament people face.

As well as the direct effects of being poor, health can also be compromised indirectly by living in neighbourhoods blighted by concentrations of deprivation, high unemployment, poor quality housing, limited access to services and a poor quality environment.

Policy Implications

Through policies on taxes, benefits, employment, education, economic management, and many other areas of activity, no government can avoid having a major impact on the distribution of income. The indisputable evidence of the effects of such policies on rates of death and disease imposes a public duty to eliminate absolute poverty and reduce material inequalities.

- All citizens should be protected by minimum income guarantees, minimum wages legislation and access to services.
- Interventions to reduce poverty and social exclusion are needed at both the individual and the neighbourhood levels.
- Legislation can help protect minority and vulnerable groups from discrimination and social exclusion.
- Public health policies should remove barriers to health care, social services and affordable housing.
- Labour market, education and family welfare policies should aim to reduce social stratification.

. . .

5. UNEMPLOYMENT

Job security increases health well-being and job satisfaction. Higher rates of unemployment cause more illness and premature death.

What Is Known

Unemployment puts health at risk, and the risk is higher in regions where unemployment is widespread. Evidence from a number of countries shows that, even after allowing for other factors, unemployed people and their families suffer a substantially increased risk of premature death. The health effects of unemployment are linked to both its psychological consequences and the financial problems it brings—especially debt.

The health effects start when people first feel their jobs are threatened, even before they actually become unemployed. This shows that anxiety about insecurity is also detrimental to health. Job insecurity has been shown to increase effects on mental health (particularly anxiety and depression), self-reported ill health, heart disease and risk factors for heart disease. Because very unsatisfactory or insecure jobs can be as harmful as unemployment, merely having a job will not always protect physical and mental health: job quality is also important (Fig. 4).

During the 1990s, changes in the economies and labour markets of many industrialized countries increased feelings of job insecurity. As job insecurity continues, it acts as a chronic stressor whose effects grow with the length of exposure; it increases sickness absence and health service use.

Policy Implications

Policy should have three goals: to prevent unemployment and job insecurity; to reduce the hardship suffered by the unemployed; and to restore people to secure jobs.

- Government management of the economy to reduce the highs and lows of the business cycle can make an important contribution to job security and the reduction of unemployment.
- Limitations on working hours may also be beneficial when pursued alongside job security and satisfaction.

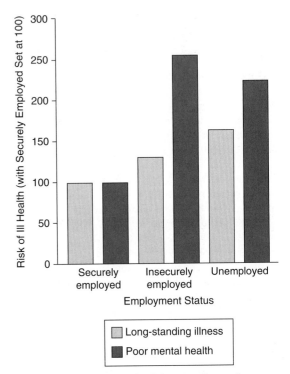

FIGURE 4   Effect of job insecurity and unemployment on health

Source: Ferrie JE et al. Employment status and health after privatisation in white collar civil servants: prospective cohort study. *British Medical Journal*, 2001, 322:647–651.

- To equip people for the work available, high standards of education and good retraining schemes are important.
- For those out of work, unemployment benefits set at a higher proportion of wages are likely to have a protective effect.
- Credit unions may be beneficial by reducing debts and increasing social networks.

6. SOCIAL SUPPORT

Friendship, good social relations and strong supportive networks improve health at home, at work and in the community.

What Is Known

Social support and good social relations make an important contribution to health. Social support helps give people the emotional and practical resources they need. Belonging to a social network of communication and mutual obligation makes people feel cared for, loved, esteemed and valued. This has a powerful protective effect on health. Supportive relationships may also encourage healthier behaviour patterns.

Support operates on the levels both of the individual and of society. Social isolation and exclusion are associated with increased rates of premature death and poorer chances of survival after a heart attack (Fig. 5). People who get less social and emotional support from others are more likely to experience less well-being, more depression, a greater risk of pregnancy complications and higher levels of disability from chronic diseases. In addition, bad close relationships can lead to poor mental and physical health.

The amount of emotional and practical social support people get varies by social and economic status. Poverty can contribute to social exclusion and isolation.

Social cohesion—defined as the quality of social relationships and the existence of trust, mutual obligations and respect in communities or in the wider society—helps to protect people and their health. Inequality is corrosive of good social relations. Societies with high levels of income inequality tend to have less social cohesion and more violent crime. High levels of mutual support will protect health while the breakdown of social relations, sometimes following greater inequality, reduces trust and increases levels of violence. A study of a community with initially high levels of social cohesion showed low rates of coronary heart disease. When social cohesion declined, heart disease rates rose.

Policy Implications

Experiments suggest that good social relations can reduce the physiological response to stress. Intervention studies have shown that providing social support can improve patient recovery rates from several different conditions. It can also improve pregnancy outcome in vulnerable groups of women.

- Reducing social and economic inequalities and reducing social exclusion can lead to greater social cohesiveness and better standards of health.

FIGURE 5 **Level of social integration and mortality in five prospective studies**
Source: House JS, Landis KR, Umberson D. Social relationships and health. *Science*, 1988, 241:540–545.

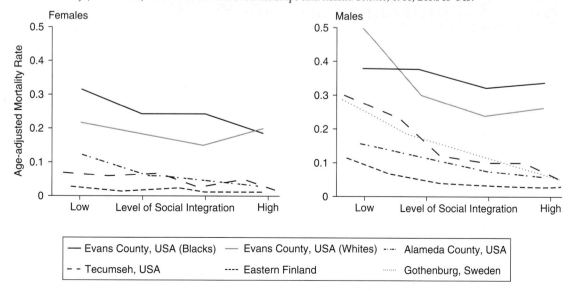

- Improving the social environment in schools, in the workplace and in the community more widely, will help people feel valued and supported in more areas of their lives and will contribute to their health, especially their mental health.
- Designing facilities to encourage meeting and social interaction in communities could improve mental health.
- In all areas of both personal and institutional life, practices that cast some as socially inferior or less valuable should be avoided because they are socially divisive.

7. ADDICTION

Individuals turn to alcohol, drugs and tobacco and suffer from their use, but use is influenced by the wider social setting.

What Is Known

Drug use is both a response to social breakdown and an important factor in worsening the resulting inequalities in health. It offers users a mirage of escape from adversity and stress, but only makes their problems worse.

Alcohol dependence, illicit drug use and cigarette smoking are all closely associated with markers of social and economic disadvantage (Fig. 6). In some of the transition economies of central and eastern Europe, for example, the past decade has been a time of great social upheaval. Consequently, deaths linked to alcohol use—such as accidents, violence, poisoning, injury and suicide—have risen sharply. Alcohol dependence is associated with violent death in other countries too.

The causal pathway probably runs both ways. People turn to alcohol to numb the pain of harsh economic and social conditions, and alcohol dependence leads to downward social mobility.

The irony is that, apart from a temporary release from reality, alcohol intensifies the factors that led to its use in the first place.

The same is true of tobacco. Social deprivation—whether measured by poor housing, low income, lone parenthood, unemployment or homelessness—is associated with high rates of smoking and very low rates of quitting. Smoking is a major drain on poor people's incomes and a huge cause of ill health

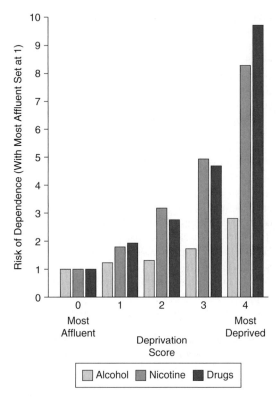

FIGURE 6   Socioeconomic deprivation and risk of dependence on alcohol, nicotine and drugs, Great Britain, 1993

Source: Wardle J et al., eds. Smoking, drinking, physical activity and screening uptake and health inequalities. In: Gordon D et al., eds. *Inequalities in health.* Bristol, The Policy Press, 1999:213–239.

and premature death. But nicotine offers no real relief from stress or improvement in mood.

The use of alcohol, tobacco and illicit drugs is fostered by aggressive marketing and promotion by major transnational companies and by organized crime. Their activities are a major barrier to policy initiatives to reduce use among young people; and their connivance with smuggling, especially in the case of tobacco, has hampered efforts by governments to use price mechanisms to limit consumption.

Policy Implications

- Work to deal with problems of both legal and illicit drug use needs not only to support and treat people who have developed addictive patterns of use, but also to address the patterns of social deprivation in which the problems are rooted.

- Policies need to regulate availability through pricing and licensing, and to inform people about less harmful forms of use, to use health education to reduce recruitment of young people and to provide effective treatment services for addicts.

- None of these will succeed if the social factors that breed drug use are left unchanged. Trying to shift the whole responsibility on to the user is clearly an inadequate response. This blames the victim, rather than addressing the complexities of the social circumstances that generate drug use. Effective drug policy must therefore be supported by the broad framework of social and economic policy.

8. FOOD

Because global market forces control the food supply, healthy food is a political issue.

What Is Known

A good diet and adequate food supply are central for promoting health and well-being. A shortage of food and lack of variety cause malnutrition and deficiency diseases. Excess intake (also a form of malnutrition) contributes to cardiovascular diseases, diabetes, cancer, degenerative eye diseases, obesity and dental caries. Food poverty exists side by side with food plenty. The important public health issue is the availability and cost of healthy, nutritious food (Fig. 7). Access to good, affordable food makes more difference to what people eat than health education.

Economic growth and improvements in housing and sanitation brought with them the epidemiological transition from infectious to chronic diseases—including heart disease, stroke and cancer. With it came a nutritional transition, when diets, particularly in western Europe, changed to overconsumption of energy-dense fats and sugars, producing more obesity. At the same time, obesity became more common among the poor than the rich.

World food trade is now big business. The General Agreement on Tariffs and Trade and the Common Agricultural Policy of the European Union allow

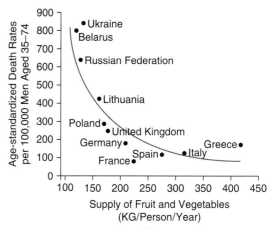

FIGURE 7 Mortality from coronary heart disease in relation to fruit and vegetable supply in selected European countries

Sources: FAOSTAT (Food balance sheets) [database online]. Rome, Food and Agriculture Organization of the United Nations, 25 September 2003.

WHO mortality database [database online]. Geneva, World Health Organization, 25 September 2003.

Health for all database [database online]. Copenhagen, WHO Regional Office for Europe, 25 September 2003.

global market forces to shape the food supply. International committees such as Codex Alimentarius, which determine food quality and safety standards, lack public health representatives, and food industry interests are strong. Local food production can be more sustainable, more accessible and support the local economy.

Social and economic conditions result in a social gradient in diet quality that contributes to health inequalities. The main dietary difference between social classes is the source of nutrients. In many countries, the poor tend to substitute cheaper processed foods for fresh food. High fat intakes often occur in all social groups. People on low incomes, such as young families, elderly people and the unemployed, are least able to eat well.

Dietary goals to prevent chronic diseases emphasize eating more fresh vegetables, fruits and pulses (legumes) and more minimally processed starchy foods, but less animal fat, refined sugars and salt. Over 100 expert committees have agreed on these dietary goals.

Policy Implications

Local, national and international government agencies, nongovernmental organizations and the food industry should ensure:

- the integration of public health perspectives into the food system to provide affordable and nutritious fresh food for all, especially the most vulnerable;
- democratic, transparent decision-making and accountability in all food regulation matters, with participation by all stakeholders, including consumers;

- support for sustainable agriculture and food production methods that conserve natural resources and the environment;
- a stronger food culture for health, especially through school education, to foster people's knowledge of food and nutrition, cooking skills, growing food and the social value of preparing food and eating together;
- the availability of useful information about food, diet and health, especially aimed at children;
- the use of scientifically based nutrient reference values and food-based dietary guidelines to facilitate the development and implementation of policies on food and nutrition.

WHY THE UNITED STATES IS NOT NUMBER ONE IN HEALTH

Ichiro Kawachi

Americans are quite accustomed to seeing their country rank at the very top of the medal chart at the Summer Olympic Games. Imagine our surprise, then, upon discovering that our health status ranks near the bottom among the 13 most economically advanced countries of the world. In the health Olympics, we rank twelfth overall on sixteen indicators of health status—behind Japan, Sweden, Canada, France, Australia, Spain, Finland, the Netherlands, the United Kingdom, Denmark, and Belgium. On specific indicators, we rank as follows:

- 13th (bottom) for percentage of low birth weight
- 13th for neonatal mortality and total infant mortality
- 13th for years of potential life lost
- 11th for life expectancy at age 1 for females, 12th for males

From *Healthy, Wealthy, and Fair: Health Care and the Good Society*, edited by James A. Morone and Lawrence R. Jacobs. New York: Oxford University Press, 2005. Reprinted by permission.

Editors' note: Some author's notes have been cut. Students who want to follow up on sources should consult the original article.

- 10th for life expectancy at age 15 for females, 12th for males
- 10th for life expectancy at age 40 for females, 9th for males
- 7th for life expectancy at age 65 for females, 7th for males

About the only health indicator for which we rank near the top of the medal chart is life expectancy, at age 80 (third for both females and males). If this were the sports Olympics, our Senate would order urgent public hearings to get to the bottom of our dismal performance and Congress would immediately pump millions of extra dollars into athletic programs to correct this source of national shame.

Why, then, do we not see a comparable level of outrage when it comes to our performance in the health Olympics? This chapter outlines three possible explanations for our curious complacency. First, the American public may be ignorant of its dismal health performance because the issue does not receive regular coverage on the nightly news in the way that our economic performance does. Second, even if we were aware of our health performance, some members of the public might not care about our relative rank compared to other rich nations, so long as average life expectancy continues to improve. Third, the public might ignore the problem because it is misinformed about the causes of our poor health performance and, hence, what can be done about it.

THE DOW JONES VERSUS THE DOUG JONES

It is quite understandable that most Americans mistakenly assume we rank first in the world on indicators of longevity and good health. After all, we are the wealthiest nation in the world, and everyone knows that a higher standard of living allows longer and healthier lives. We also spend by far the most of any nation on health care. We make up just 4% of the world's population, yet we expend about half of all the money spent on medical care across the globe. But contrary to most people's assumptions, even as far back as 1970, the United States ranked about fifteenth in the world in health indicators like life expectancy and infant mortality. Twenty years later, our position had slipped to about twenty-second, or near the bottom of the OECD (Organization of Economic Cooperation and Development) countries—behind almost all rich countries and even a few poorer ones. Japan, by contrast, started out near the bottom (twenty-third) of the health Olympics in 1960, but overtook the rest of the world by 1977.

If the American public was more generally aware of these kinds of comparisons, we might feel less smug about being the richest, most successful economy in the world. However, in contrast to the compulsive way in which we track the performance of our economy, Americans remain largely ignorant about the state of the nation's health, because there is no equivalent of the Dow Jones Industrial Average by which we can monitor our health performance. We are quite accustomed to following the ups and downs of the Dow Jones on a minute-by-minute basis. However, "in contrast to the tools, structures, and mechanisms of the economic sphere, the richness and variety of its indicators, and the regularity with which they are reported, our vision of the social sphere is far more obscure. Social data are collected once a year at best, rather than daily, weekly, monthly, or quarterly, as in economics."[1] Texas populist Jim Hightower has argued that our nation should develop an alternative to the Dow Jones index, one that better describes what is happening to

ordinary people. Such an index might track a combination of social indicators such as wages, unemployment, and benefits like health insurance. Hightower suggests calling it the "Doug Jones index," in honor of the working-class man. As it happens, the Miringoffs at the Fordham Institute for Innovation in Social Policy have developed exactly such an index, which they have dubbed the Index of Social Health. This index is made up of health indicators such as infant mortality, teenage suicide, homicides, health insurance coverage, drug abuse, rates of child abuse, and alcohol-related traffic fatalities, as well as broader social indicators such as children in poverty, high school dropouts, and affordable housing. When stacked up against our nation's market performance, the unavoidable conclusion is that our nation's health and social performance have stagnated, even as our economy has taken off.

In Figure 1, we see that our nation's Index of Social Health closely tracked the performance of the Dow Jones index up until the late 1970s. Since then, however, the two lines have diverged: our social health has slumped, while the Dow Jones currently

FIGURE 1   Index of Social Health and the Dow Jones Industrial Average, 1970–1993

Sources: Fordham Institute for Innovation in Social Policy; Statistical Abstract of United States; Survey of Current Business.

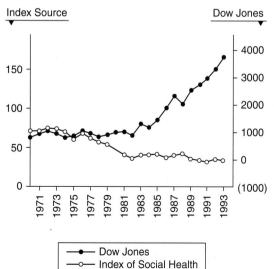

hovers around 10,000. The same pattern is repeated when we substitute a broader indicator of economic performance, such as growth in the per capita gross domestic product.

Granted, some indicators that comprise the Miringoffs' index have improved in recent years; for example, homicide rates. Even so, current rates of firearm homicide remain at levels above the rates that prevailed prior to the 1980s. Other health indicators not included in the Index of Social Health, such as rates of low birth weight, demonstrate little or no improvement over the past two decades. In fact, on a state-by-state basis, only New Hampshire did not record an increase in low birth-weight babies between 1985 and 1996. For the United States as a whole, rates increased by 9%, while in some midwestern states such as Minnesota, Iowa, and Indiana, rates rose by as much as 20%.

DIFFERENT YARDSTICKS: ABSOLUTE VERSUS RELATIVE HEALTH ACHIEVEMENTS

Even if Americans were made aware of our dismal health performance, some of us might argue that we need not be concerned about our relative ranking in the health Olympics, so long as, on average, everyone is living longer. In other words, our performance should be judged in terms of *absolute* gains in life expectancy and not with reference to our comparative performance vis-à-vis other rich countries. While this argument has superficial merit (we shouldn't envy the achievement of others), it falls down on the hard facts. Thus, while it is true that life expectancy for Americans has been improving *on average*, averages can obscure dramatic differences between groups. For African-Americans, life expectancy actually slid backward during the 1980s, even as the longevity for white Americans continued to rise (see Table 1).[2]

Even though the *average* life expectancy of Americans continues to improve, it is impossible to ignore the staggering disparities in longevity that have been documented across groups and regions of the United States. An African-American born in the District of Columbia can expect to live 57.9 years—lower than the life expectancy of the male citizens of Ghana (58.3 years), Bangladesh (58.1 years), or Bolivia (59.8 years). By contrast, an Asian-American woman born in Westchester County, New York, can expect to live on average for 90.3 years.[3] Regardless of one's

TABLE 1		
U.S. Life Expectancy at Birth, 1984–1992		
Year	White	Black
1984	75.3	69.5
1985	75.3	69.3
1986	75.4	69.1
1987	75.6	69.1
1988	75.6	68.9
1989	75.9	68.8
1990	76.1	69.1
1991	76.3	69.3
1992	76.5	69.6

Source: Williams, 2001, p. 74

views about how best to judge comparative health performance, the sheer magnitude of these disparities ought to cause alarm and concern.

MYTHS ABOUT LAGGING U.S. HEALTH PERFORMANCE

Supposing that the American public came to acknowledge our dismal health performance, there still remain some powerful myths about what can be done to improve our health status. These myths have attained the status of shibboleths. The first is that our poor health performance, especially with respect to racial disparities in health, reflects inherited differences in health stock. The second myth is that our poor health performance comes from poor people behaving badly. A third myth puts all the blame for our health status on the lack of universal access to health care. These myths warrant careful scrutiny.

Poor Health Equals Bad Genes

The "bad genes" line of argument will be familiar to readers who have followed the infamous "bell curve" controversy. According to this line of argument, our nation's lackluster health performance can be explained by the distribution of flawed genes in the population. For instance, the high incidence of obesity, hypertension, diabetes, and low birth weight can all be explained by a higher genetic predisposition within our communities (especially African-American communities) to develop these maladies. Although this unfortunate perception is still highly prevalent in our society (and we devote large sums of research dollars to pursue this hypothesis), the idea has been thoroughly discredited. In other words, while not denying the existence of an inherited predisposition to these diseases, we can reject the notion that our overall health performance can be blamed on the disproportionately high prevalence of individuals with such predispositions in our society.

We owe this insight to the work of researchers who have carefully compared the occurrence of these diseases across populations sharing the same genetic stock, but living in different societies. For instance, U.S.-born black women have twice the incidence of low birth-weight babies compared to white American women. However, when the birth weight patterns of *African-born* black women are compared to American black women, they much more closely resemble the distribution among U.S. *white* women than among U.S.-born black women. In other words, it is U.S.-born black women who exhibit a different pattern of birth weights compared to the other groups, even though African-born and U.S.-born black women presumably share the same genetic stock.[4] Similar findings have been reported for the distribution of blood pressure and hypertension among U.S.-born blacks compared to West African populations,[5] as well as the prevalence of diabetes.[6] These kinds of data refute the "bad genes" argument as an explanation for poor health status in our country.

Instead of blaming the flawed genes of our citizens, we ought to be searching for what it is about American society that is toxic to health. Even the longevous Japanese are not immune to the toxic influence of American society. According to the famous NiHonSan Study, which followed Japanese immigrants to the United States, the closer they settled to the American mainland, the higher their risk was of suffering a heart attack.[7] Death rates from heart attack were lowest among the Japanese who stayed behind, intermediate among those who settled in Honolulu, Hawaii, and highest among immigrants who moved to San Francisco.

Poor People Behaving Badly

The second, and in some ways most culturally ingrained, myth about our nation's health is that sick people—especially poor and uneducated people—bring poor health upon themselves through ill-informed or irresponsible risk-taking behaviors. This

line of reasoning owes its enduring appeal to other values that are held sacred in American culture, such as liberty, individualism, and moralism. According to this view, individuals are free to choose their "lifestyles," as long as they take responsibility for the consequences of their own choices and don't expect others to pay for them. Some would even assert that our poor health status is the price we pay for maintaining our values—but a worthwhile one for the liberty and opportunity guaranteed by the American way of life. If you don't like the American way, you can always defect to Cuba, where people live long (and, many would add, where life *feels* long).

The flaw in this logic is that people don't always *choose* to behave badly (by ignoring the doctor's advice to stop smoking, indulging in fast foods, or putting off regular exercise). Nobody denies that some "risky" behavior is freely chosen or that individuals should take some responsibility for their own actions. However, *how much* individual responsibility should be assigned to bad behaviors lies at the crux of the disagreement between those who say nothing can (or needs to) be done about our poor health status, versus those who see it as an avoidable blemish on our national record.

Adopting a life-course perspective often helps tease out the issues of individual freedom and responsibility from the claims of collective responsibility. For instance, in the case of cigarette smoking and its adverse health consequences, adult smokers are typically held accountable for their habits. But this ignores the reality that an overwhelming majority of adult smokers initiated their lifelong addiction as underage minors. Over 80% of smokers become addicted to nicotine before the legal age of purchase. Even staunch libertarians would concede that minors are not capable of making responsible decisions that may affect their future welfare. Yet American lawmakers (until very recently at least) routinely permitted tobacco manufacturers to peddle their products to children through the medium of cartoon characters, as well as advertising in youth-oriented magazines and public venues. The tobacco industry goes even further by systematically targeting its outdoor advertising to low-income and minority ethnic neighborhoods. In other words, the high prevalence of health-damaging behaviors (like smoking) among poor people is less a sign of their moral turpitude than a consequence of the workings of the not-so-invisible hand of the free market.

Similar arguments could be made about the deliberate decisions of fast food manufacturers to open their businesses near schools in low-income neighborhoods, or the lack of availability of healthy food choices where poor people shop. The ability to choose regular physical activity is also socially constrained. Parents may discourage their children from exercising outdoors in high-crime neighborhoods. Public exercise facilities, like playgrounds and bike paths, are more accessible, appealing, and safer in middle-class as opposed to impoverished neighborhoods. High-status employees have more flexible work schedules that permit them to take long lunch-hour workouts at the gym. Joining a health club requires membership fees that many low-income individuals cannot afford without sacrificing money needed for food, clothing, and other necessities. The long list of barriers to adopting a healthy lifestyle should give pause to those among us who would blame the poor health habits of fellow citizens on ignorance, sloth, or indifference.

Lack of Access to Health Care

A third persistent misconception about our lagging health performance is our lack of access to universal health care. The United States is unique among the world's rich countries in failing to assure universal access of citizens to medical care. And there can be no gainsaying that universal access to health care would improve the health of millions of Americans currently without coverage. Nor can there be denying that medical care makes a difference to the health status of sick individuals (sometimes dramatically so, as in fixing a broken limb).

However, the fallacy of ascribing our health performance to lack of universal coverage lies in the assumption that health care can account for variations in health status. It is the fallacy of confusing the cure with the cause of the illness—like blaming a patient's fever on a deficiency of aspirin.

Sometimes the (important) goal of achieving universal health care in this country is discussed as if it were an *alternative* to doing something about the non-medical determinants of health (and vice versa). This is a myth that ignores the fact that the two goals are, in fact, complementary. Inequality in access to medical care is, after all, just another manifestation of inequalities in access to broader resources (such as

wealth, credit, employment, and education), all of which contribute to our ability to lead healthy lives. Nor is inequality in access to medical care a simple yes/no phenomenon (you either have health insurance or you don't). Even in countries with a national health care system, such as Great Britain, there are lingering disparities in the quality of medical care, the geographic distribution of doctors and medical facilities, and so on. Additionally, what *type* of health care we get may matter. According to some analyses, lack of primary care accounts for a significant part of the dismal American health care performance. This implies a radical redirection of current efforts to reform health insurance, including restructuring medical care priorities in a system that is overwhelmingly focused on the delivery of specialist and hospital-based care.

IF IT'S NOT BAD GENES OR BAD BEHAVIORS, THEN WHAT IS IT?

If bad genes and bad behaviors can't explain America's dismal state of health, then what can? The answer lies in much more fundamental social causes. We now understand that the prerequisites for the health and well being of a population consist of fundamental social conditions, such as a fair distribution of resources as well as robust support for our self-respect. Translated into concrete terms, the social determinants of health include access to safe neighborhoods, productive employment, freedom from discrimination, and full participation in the life of communities. In turn, people's access to health-promoting social conditions is played out through the political process. Politics determine who gets what, how much, and when. As Rudolf Virchow famously asserted, "Medicine is a social science, and politics is nothing else but medicine on a grand scale."[8] To illustrate this point, consider the paradox identified at the beginning of this chapter, i.e., why, despite being the wealthiest country in the world, we are not the healthiest.

Economic Prosperity and Health

As it turns out, there is almost no correlation among the worlds' richest countries between their per capita wealth and life expectancy. A comparison of

TABLE 2

Comparison of Per Capita GNP in Selected Countries and Their Life Expectancies

Country	Per Capita GNP (U.S. $)	Average Life Expectancy (Years)
United States	29,080	76.7
Sweden	26,210	78.5
Netherlands	25,830	77.9
United Kingdom	20,870	77.2
France	26,300	78.1
Germany	28,280	77.2

Source: 1999 Human Development Report.

countries with roughly the same level of economic prosperity reveals dramatic differences in life expectancy (see Table 2).

Among rich countries, then, economic prosperity alone is no guarantee of stellar health performance. That is not to say that economic growth does not matter. Three-fifths of the world's people still live on less than $2 per day, and there is no denying that in poor countries, raising people's incomes, even by a small amount, would dramatically improve their life chances. That said, even among countries of middle economic development, we can find dramatic disconnects between the material standard of living and life expectancy. Amartya Sen has repeatedly pointed out the unexpected success of countries such as China, Sri Lanka, and the Kerala region of India, which have less than one-sixth the per capita gross national product of wealthier countries such as Brazil, Namibia, South Africa, and Gabon—but nonetheless record much higher performance on health indicators such as life expectancy.[9]

A major reason why the average income of a country is not correlated with its average health is because averages can hide deep divisions within society. For example, countries like Brazil and South Africa have much higher average incomes than Sri Lanka or China, but their wealth tends to be concentrated in the hands of the fortunate few. China and Sri Lanka, despite much lower average incomes, tend to spread their economic gains more evenly throughout the population, and economic growth is also plowed back into social spending that benefits all.

To turn to the United States, our spectacular economic growth in recent decades has not been equally shared across segments of the population. Beginning in the mid-1970s (incidentally, about the time that our Index of Social Health started to diverge from indicators of market performance—see Figure 1), the American economy began registering sharp increases in both earnings and income inequality. Over the past two and a half decades, the affluent sections of society have been pulling away sharply from the middle class and poor.[10] Between 1977 and 1999, the average after-tax incomes of the top fifth of American families rose by 43%. By contrast, the average incomes of the middle fifth of families rose by a meager 8% over the same 22-year period, or less than 0.5% per year. At the bottom, the incomes of poor families actually fell by 9%. Forty percent of American families are either no better off or worse off today in real terms than they were in 1977. But at the very top, the incomes of the wealthiest 1% of the population rose by a staggering 115% after adjusting for inflation.[11]

In other words, if you happened to have been born into the top fifth of the population (better still the top 1%) during the past 25 years, you probably lived the American dream. Conversely, if you happened to have been working class or poor, you would be justified in believing that life had not improved, or had possibly even gotten worse. Despite the sustained economic growth during recent years and the longest bull market in postwar history (which ended in 2001), America has scarcely made a dent on the number of households living in poverty. We may crow about our economic performance to the rest of the world, but our pattern of growth has been spectacularly lopsided.

Inequality, Poverty, and Health

Prosperity, by itself, cannot guarantee health. The Achilles' heel of the American economy is the high degree of economic inequality we tolerate in our society. A direct consequence of economic inequality is that people near the bottom of the income distribution are poorer than they otherwise would be. Poverty in America (and for that matter, anywhere else in the world) means that people lack the resources to purchase the necessary goods and services to maintain good health.

The mediocre performance of the economy for poor and working-class Americans might be sufficient to account for our dismal health performance as a nation. However, health research suggests that the deleterious consequences of economic inequality are not just confined to the officially poor. According to this new view, the unequal distribution of income and wealth—as distinct from the low absolute standard of living among the poor—exerts an independent, detrimental influence on population health. As it happens, the United States is one of the most unequal societies among developed countries. According to the Luxembourg Income Study, the distribution of incomes in this country is the most unequal of 22 industrialized countries that belong to the OECD—by quite a margin.[12] Wealthy Americans make considerably more money than their counterparts in other wealthy countries, while the bottom 10% of our households make considerably less than poor people in Europe or Japan. Consequently, the size of the gap between rich and poor is substantially wider in this country than in other societies.

An impression of the extent of inequality in this country can be swiftly, and vividly, gained by comparing the façade of public life in American cities compared to other countries. The visitor to any sizable American city is likely to be accosted by desperate panhandlers on the sidewalks and intersections. Homeless people are less noticeable in the major cities of other rich countries, or in the case of some places like Osaka, Japan, municipal authorities have gone to the extent of setting aside land in public parks to build temporary housing for itinerant populations. Americans drive around cities in hulking, gas-guzzling sport utility vehicles, while most Europeans, even wealthy ones, get by on more modest vehicles or take public transport.

The enormous gulf between the rich and poor in this country has led over time to what John Kenneth Galbraith once dubbed the paradox of private splendor amidst public squalor.[13] As private wealth becomes more concentrated, the quality of public life suffers.

Across the American states, researchers have found a striking association between the degree of household income inequality and mortality rates: The more inegalitarian the distribution of income, the more unhealthy people tend to be. Figure 2 shows the correlation between one measure of income inequality (aptly called the Robin Hood Index) and the mortality rate at the state level.[14] The Robin Hood Index is equivalent to the proportion of total income earned by all the households within a state that would need to be redistributed from the well-off to the less well-off in order to achieve income equality. Consequently, the higher the Robin Hood Index value, the more unequal the distribution of income in a given state.

As Figure 2 shows, the more unequal the distribution of income in a state, the higher the death rate. Other studies have shown that economic inequality is associated with higher rates of depression,[15] higher prevalence of hypertension and smoking,[16] and higher rates of teen pregnancy and birth,[17] as well as lower self-rated health (i.e., people reporting that their health is only fair or poor, as opposed to excellent or very good).[18]

FIGURE 2 The relationship of income inequality to mortality rates across the United States

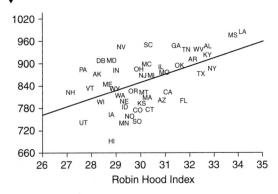

Why the United States Is Not Number One in Health
Age Adjusted Mortality

Correlations of this type do not prove causation, and so the evidence linking economic inequality to poor health status is not universally accepted.[19] In particular, many economists remain skeptical about such a link, primarily because other factors besides economic inequality (such as poverty or racial discrimination) might be driving the apparent association between income inequality and poor health status.[20] According to these views, the real culprit behind America's poor health performance is not economic inequality per se, but our persistent rate of poverty and/or history of strained race relations that have produced massive health disparities. These arguments are important and warrant scrutiny.

First of all, there is no contradiction in stating that persistent poverty, racism, and economic inequality are each, in and of themselves, important contributors to the poor health of Americans. There can be no gainsaying that the poorest Americans bear a disproportionately high burden of illness and premature mortality compared to the rest of society. However, the officially poor represent only 11% of the population, so we can't blame all of our lackluster health performance on that segment of the population. The health status of Americans is mediocre for the near poor, the working poor, and even middle-class Americans, especially if you happen to belong to a minority race/ethnic group, or if you happen to live in a deprived community. Living in an unequal society is toxic to just about everybody's health, and our poor ranking against other economically advanced countries can't simply be blamed on the misbehaving minority at the tail end of the bell curve.

More important, for the critics who assert that poverty is the real culprit behind our poor health achievement, not economic inequality, what they conveniently leave out is that income inequality is one of the major *mechanisms* by which a society ends up with a persistently high rate of poverty. Consider the case of Sweden and the United States, which look rather similar in terms of their family poverty rates prior to government intervention (20.7% and 23.2%, respectively). After redistributive taxes and transfer payments, the two countries look dramatically different. Compared to the United States, Sweden ends up with a more egalitarian distribution of income, a much lower rate of family poverty (3.8% compared to 18.9%), as well as a higher level of life expectancy.[21] In other words, if

our politicians are serious about tackling poverty, someone has to pay for the health care of low-income families, their prescription drug costs, their child care and children's education, and so forth. Leaving this to laissez-faire markets and trickle-down policies simply will not suffice. Tackling poverty and reducing income inequality are therefore complementary policy objectives; they are not mutually exclusive, as some critics appear to imply.

The question of reducing racial inequalities has also been posed as an alternative to tackling economic inequalities—to the detriment of both agendas. In the ongoing debate about whether economic inequality is harmful to health, some researchers have noted that the effects of income inequality on excess mortality are not robust after taking into account racial heterogeneity in the population.[22] In other words, it is America's racial heterogeneity (and presumably the resulting strained racial relations) that is to blame for our poor health achievement, not our degree of economic inequality. Once again, this is a false dichotomy. Racial heterogeneity and prejudice are surely part of the historical mechanism by which this country has ended up with, and continues to tolerate, high degrees of economic inequality. Racial heterogeneity is itself a marker for many kinds of inequality in access to resources, including not only wealth and income, but also education, health care, and residential quality. Furthermore, whereas government policy can alter the distribution of income, it can hardly influence the distribution of race (at least not democratically).

CONCLUSION

Considering all of the evidence, there is a good case to be made for implicating economic inequality as a major culprit behind America's mediocre health performance. Several lines of reasoning suggest why economic inequality is detrimental to our nation's health. In the realm of politics, income inequality translates into poor health via the polarized politics of rich and poor. That is, when the social distance widens between the rich and poor in society, governments tend to invest less in social infrastructure, such as public transport and amenities, public education, public health, and social welfare. In addition, our poor health performance reflects exposure to a variety of other adverse social circumstances as well, including residential segregation, racism, job insecurity, and the erosion of community bonds.

Health is an exquisitely sensitive mirror of our social conditions and political arrangements. It stands to reason, therefore, that improving our collective health requires investments to improve the circumstances of our families, communities, and workplaces.

NOTES

1. Marc Miringoff and Marque-Luisa Miringoff, *The Social Health of the Nation: How America Is Really Doing* (New York: Oxford University Press, 1999), 12.

2. David Williams, "Race and Health: Trends and Policy Implications," *Income, Socioeconomic Status, and Health: Exploring the Relationship,* ed. James A. Auerbach and Barbara Kimivae Krimgold (Washington, DC: National Policy Association and the Academy for Health Services Research and Health Policy, 2001), 74.

3. Christopher J. L. Murray, Catherine M. Michaud, M. T. McKenna, and James S. Marks, *U.S. Patterns of Mortality by County and Race, 1965–1994* (Cambridge, MA: Harvard Burden of Disease Unit, Harvard Center for Population and Development Studies, and the Centers for Disease Control and Prevention, 1998).

4. Richard J. David and James W. Collins, "Differing Birth Weight among Infants of U.S.-Born Blacks, African-Born Blacks, and U.S.-Born White Women," *New England Journal of Medicine* 337 (1997): 1209–1214.

5. Richard Cooper, C. N. Rotimi, S. Ataman, D. McGee, B. Osotimehin, S. Kadiri, W. Muna, S. Kingue, H. Fraser, T. Forrester, et al., "The Prevalence of Hypertension in Seven Populations of West African Origin," *American Journal of Public Health* 87 (1997): 160–168.

6. Richard Cooper, C. N. Rotimi, J. S. Kaufman, E. E. Owoaje, H. Fraser, T. Forrester, R. Wilks, L. K. Riste, and J. K. Cruickshank, "Prevalence of NIDDM among Populations of the African Diaspora," *Diabetes Care* 20 (1977): 343–348.

7. Michael Marmot and S. Leonard Syme, "Acculturation and Coronary Heart Disease in Japanese Americans," *American Journal of Epidemiology* 104 (1976): 225–247.

8. Anonymous, "Rudolf Virchow on Pathology Education," available at www.pathguy.com/lectures/virchow.htm.

9. Amartya Sen, *Development as Freedom* (New York: Alfred A. Knopf, 1999).

10. Lawrence Mishel, Jared Bernstein, and John Schmidt, *The State of Working America 1998–1999* (Washington, DC: Economic Policy Institute, 1999).

11. Figure 6, data from Mishel et al., *Working America.*

12. Timothy M. Smeeding, "U.S. Income Inequality in a Cross-National Perspective: Why Are We So Different?" *Inequality Paradox: Growth of Income Disparity,* ed. James A. Auerbach and Richard S. Belous (Washington, DC: National Policy Association, 1998), 194–217.

13. John Kenneth Galbraith, *The Affluent Society* (Boston: Houghton Mifflin, 1958).

14. Bruce P. Kennedy, Ichiro Kawachi, and Deborah Prothrow-Stith, "Income Distribution and Mortality: Cross-Sectional Ecological Study of the Robin Hood Index in the United States," *British Medical Journal* 312 (1996): 1004–1007. See also erratum, *British Medical Journal* 312 (1996): 1253.

15. Robert S, Kahn, Paul H. Wise, Bruce P. Kennedy, and Ichiro Kawachi, "State Income Inequality, Household Income, and Maternal Mental and Physical Health: Cross-sectional National Survey," *British Medical Journal* 321 (2000): 1311–1315.

16. Ana V. Diez-Roux, Bruce G. Link, and Mary E. Northridge, "A Multilevel Analysis of Income Inequality and Cardiovascular Disease Risk Factors," *Social Science & Medicine* 50 (2000): 673–687.

17. Rachel Gold, Ichiro Kawachi, Bruce P. Kennedy, John W. Lynch, and Frank A. Connell, "Ecological Analysis of Teen Birth Rates: Association with Community Income and Income Inequality," *Maternal and Child Health Journal* 5 (2001): 161–167.

18. Bruce P. Kennedy, Ichiro Kawachi, Roberta Glass, and Deborah Prothrow-Stith, "Income Distribution, Socioeconomic Status, and Self Rated Health in the United States: Multilevel Analysis," *British Medical Journal* 317 (1998): 917–921.

19. Christopher Jencks, "Does Inequality Matter?" *Daedalus* (Winter 2002): 49–65.

20. Jennifer Mellor and Jeffrey Milyo, "Re-examining the Evidence of an Ecological Association between Income Inequality and Health," *Journal of Health Politics, Policy and Law* 26 (2001): 487–522.

21. Clyde Hertzman, "The Case for an Early Childhood Development Strategy," *Isuma* 1 (2000): 1–19.

22. Angus Deaton and Darren Lubotsky, "Mortality, Inequality and Race in American Cities and States," *Social Science & Medicine* 56 (2001): 1139–1153.

JUSTICE, HEALTH, AND HEALTHCARE

Norman Daniels

A theory of justice for health and healthcare should help us answer three central questions. First, is healthcare special? Is it morally important in ways that justify (and explain) the fact that many societies distribute healthcare more equally than many other social goods? Second, when are health inequalities unjust? After all, many socially controllable factors besides access to healthcare affect the levels of population health and the degree of health inequalities in a population. Third, how can we meet competing healthcare needs fairly under reasonable resource constraints? General principles of justice that answer the first two questions do not, I argue, answer some important questions about rationing fairly. Is there instead a fair process for making rationing decisions?

About twenty years ago I answered the first question by claiming healthcare was special because of its impact on opportunity. Specifically, the central function of healthcare is to maintain normal functioning. Disease and disability, by impairing normal functioning, restrict the range of opportunities open to individuals. Healthcare thus makes a distinct but limited contribution to the protection of equality of opportunity. Though I construed healthcare broadly to include public health as well as individual preventive, acute, and chronic care, I ignored other factors that have a profound effect on population health. Unfortunately, focusing on just healthcare adds to the popular misconception that our vastly improved health in the last century is primarily the result of healthcare.

During the last twenty years, a major literature has emerged exploring the social determinants of health. We have long known that the richer people

are, the longer and healthier their lives. The powerful findings of the last couple of decades, however, have deepened our understanding of the factors at work producing these effects on population health and the distribution of health within populations. It is less tenable to think that it is simply poverty and true deprivation that diminishes the health of some people, for there is growing evidence that race and class effects operate across a broad range of inequalities. Since social policies—not laws of human nature or economic development—are responsible for the social and economic inequalities that produce these health effects, we are forced to look upstream from the point of medical delivery and ask about the fairness of the distribution of these goods. Rawls's theory of justice as fairness, quite serendipitously, contains principles that give a plausible account of the fair distribution of those determinants, thus providing an answer to the second question.

· · ·

WHICH HEALTH INEQUALITIES ARE UNJUST?

Universal access to appropriate healthcare—just healthcare—does not break the link between social status and health, a point driven home in studies of the effects on health inequality of the British National Health Service and confirmed by work in other countries as well. Our health is affected not simply by the ease with which we can see a doctor—though that surely matters—but also by our social position and the underlying inequality of our society. We cannot, of course, infer causation from these correlations between social inequality and health inequality (though later I explore some ideas about how the one might lead to the other). Suffice to say that, while the exact processes are not fully understood, the evidence suggests that there are social determinants of health.

If social factors play a large role in determining our health, then efforts to ensure greater justice in health outcomes should not focus simply on the traditional health sector. Health is produced not merely by having access to medical prevention and treatment, but also—to a measurably greater extent—by the cumulative experience of social conditions over the course of one's life. By the time a sixty-year-old heart attack victim arrives at the emergency room, bodily insults have accumulated over a lifetime. For such a person, medical care is, figuratively speaking, "the ambulance waiting at the bottom of the cliff." Much contemporary discussion about reducing health inequalities by increasing access to medical care misses this point. Of course, we still want that ambulance there, but we should be looking as well to improve social conditions that help to determine the health of societies.

As I noted earlier, Rawls's theory of justice as fairness was not designed to address issues of healthcare. He assumed a completely healthy population, and argued that a just society must assure people equal basic liberties, guarantee that the right of political participation has roughly equal value for all, provide a robust form of equal opportunity, and limit inequalities to those that benefit the least advantaged. When these requirements of justice are met, Rawls argued, we can have reasonable confidence that others are showing us the respect that is essential to our sense of self-worth. The fair terms of cooperation specified by these principles promote our social and political well-being.

The conjecture I explore is that by establishing equal liberties, robustly equal opportunity, a fair distribution of resources, and support for our self-respect—the basics of Rawlsian justice—we would go a long way toward eliminating the most important injustices in health outcomes. To be sure, social justice is valuable for reasons other than its effects on health (or Rawls could not have set aside issues of health when arguing for justice as fairness). And social reform in the direction of greater justice would not eliminate the need to think hard about fair allocation of resources within the healthcare system. Still, acting to promote social justice is a crucial step toward improving our health because there is this surprising convergence between what is needed for our social and political well-being and for our mental and physical health.

To see the basis for this conjecture about Rawlsian principles, let us review very briefly some of the central findings in the recent literature on the social determinants of health. If we look at cross-national studies, we see that a country's prosperity is related to its health, as measured, for example, by life expectancy: In richer countries, people tend to live longer. But the relationship between per capita gross domestic product (GDPpc) and life expectancy levels off at around $8,000 to $10,000; beyond this threshold, further economic advance buys virtually no further gains in life expectancy. This leveling effect is most apparent among the advanced industrial economies. Nevertheless, even within this relationship, there are telling variations. Though Cuba and Iraq are equally poor (each has a GDPpc of about $3,100), life expectancy in Cuba exceeds that in Iraq by 17.2 years. The poor state of Kerala in India, which invested heavily in education, especially female literacy, has health outcomes far superior to the rest of India and more comparable to those in much wealthier countries. The difference between the GDPpc for Costa Rica and the United States is enormous (about $21,000), yet Costa Rica's life expectancy exceeds that of the United States (76.6 to 76.4).

Taken together, these observations show that the health of nations depends, in part, on factors other than wealth. Culture, social organization, and government policies also help determine population health. Variations in these factors—not fixed laws of economic development—may explain many of the differences in health outcomes among nations.

One especially important factor in explaining the health of a society is the distribution of income: the health of a population depends not just on the size of the economic pie, but also on how the pie is shared. Differences in health outcomes among developed nations cannot be explained simply by the absolute deprivation associated with low economic development—lack of access to the basic material conditions necessary for health, such as clean water, adequate nutrition and housing, and general sanitary living conditions. The degree of relative deprivation within a society also matters.

Numerous studies support this *relative-income hypothesis,* which states, more precisely, that inequality is strongly associated with population mortality and life expectancy across nations. Rich countries vary in life expectancy, and that variation dovetails with income distribution. In particular, wealthier countries with more equal income distributions, such as Sweden and Japan, have higher life expectancies than the United States, despite having lower per capita GDP. Likewise, countries with low GDPpc but remarkably high life expectancy, such as Costa Rica, tend to have a more equitable distribution of income.

We find a similar pattern when we compare states within the United States. If we control for differences in state wealth, income inequality accounts for about 25% of the between-state variation in age-adjusted mortality rates. Furthermore, a recent study across U.S. metropolitan areas found that areas with high income inequality had an excess of death compared to areas with low inequality—a very large excess, equivalent in magnitude to all deaths due to heart disease. Longitudinal studies, which look at a single place over time and examine widening income differentials, support similar conclusions.

At the individual level we also find that inequality is important. Numerous studies have documented what has come to be known as the socioeconomic gradient: At each step along the economic ladder, we see improved health outcomes over the rung below (even in societies with universal health insurance). Differences in health outcomes are not confined to the extremes of rich and poor, but are observed across all levels of socioeconomic status.

The slope of the socioeconomic gradient varies substantially across societies. Some societies show a relatively shallow gradient in mortality rates: Being better off confers a health advantage, but not so large an advantage as elsewhere. Others, with comparable or even higher levels of economic development, show much steeper gradients. The slope of the gradient appears to be fixed by the level of income inequality in a society. The more unequal a society is in economic terms, the more unequal it is in health terms. Moreover, middle income groups in a country with high income inequality typically do worse in terms of health than comparable or even poorer groups in a society with less income inequality. We find the same pattern within the United States when we examine state and metropolitan area variations in inequality and health outcomes.

Earlier, I cautioned that correlations between inequality and health do not necessarily imply causation. Still, there are enough plausible and identifiable pathways through which social inequalities

appear to produce health inequalities to make a reasonable case for causation. In the United States the states with the most unequal income distributions invest less in public education, have larger uninsured populations, and spend less on social safety nets. Studies of educational spending and educational outcomes are especially striking. Controlling for median income, income inequality explains about 40% of the variation between states in the percentage of children in the fourth grade who are below the basic reading level. Similarly strong associations are seen for high school drop-out rates. It is evident from these data that educational opportunities for children in high income inequality states are quite different from those in states with more egalitarian distributions. These effects on education have an immediate impact on health, increasing the likelihood of premature death during childhood and adolescence (as evidenced by the much higher death rates for infants and children in the high inequality states). Later in life these effects appear in the socioeconomic gradient in health.

When we compare countries, we also find that differential investment in human capital—in particular, education—is a strong predictor of health. Indeed, one of the strongest predictors of life expectancy among developing countries is adult literacy, particularly the disparity between male and female adult literacy, which explains much of the variation in health achievement among these countries after accounting for GDPpc. For example, among the 125 developing countries with GDPpcs of less than $10,000, the difference between male and female literacy accounts for 40% of the variation in life expectancy (after factoring out the effect of GDPpc). In the United States differences among the states in women's status—measured in terms of economic autonomy and political participation—are strongly correlated with higher female mortality rates.

These societal mechanisms—for example, income inequality leading to educational inequality leading to health inequality—are tightly linked to the political processes that influence government policy. For example, income inequality appears to affect health by undermining civil society. Income inequality erodes social cohesion, as measured by higher levels of social mistrust and reduced participation in civic organizations. Lack of social cohesion leads to lower participation in political activity (such as voting, serving in local government, volunteering for political campaigns). And lower participation, in turn, undermines the responsiveness of government institutions in addressing the needs of the worst off. States with the highest income inequality, and thus lowest levels of social capital and political participation, are less likely to invest in human capital and provide far less generous social safety nets.

Rawls's principles of justice thus turn out to regulate the key social determinants of health. One principle assures equal basic liberties, and specifically provides for guaranteeing *effective* rights of political participation. The fair equality opportunity principle assures access to high quality public education, early childhood interventions (including day care) aimed at eliminating class or race disadvantages, and universal coverage for appropriate healthcare. Rawls's "Difference Principle" permits inequalities in income only if the inequalities work (e.g., through incentives) to make those who are worst off as well off as possible. This principle is not a simple "trickle down" principle that tolerates any inequality so long as there is some benefit that flows down the socioeconomic ladder; it requires a maximal flow downward. It would therefore flatten socioeconomic inequalities in a robust way, assuring far more than a "decent minimum." In addition, the assurances of the value of political participation and fair equality of opportunity would further constrain allowable income inequalities.

The conjecture is that a society complying with these principles of justice would probably flatten the socioeconomic gradient even more than we see in the most egalitarian welfare states of northern Europe. The implication is that we should view health inequalities that derive from social determinants as unjust unless the determinants are distributed in conformity with these robust principles. Because of the detailed attention Rawls's theory pays to the interaction of these terms of fair cooperation, it provides us—through the findings of social science—with an account of the just distribution of health.

The inequalities in the social determinants that are still permitted by this theory may produce a socioeconomic gradient, albeit a much flatter one than we see today. Should we view these residual health inequalities as unjust and demand further redistribution of the social determinants?

I believe the theory I have described does not give a clear answer. If the Rawlsian theory insists that protecting opportunity takes priority over other matters and cannot be traded for other gains (and Rawls generally adopts this view), then residual health inequalities may be unjust. If health can be traded for other goods—and all of us make such trades when we take chances with our health to pursue other goals—then the account may be more flexible. Still, Rawls's principles give us more specific guidance in thinking about the distribution of the social determinants than is given by the fair equality of opportunity account of just healthcare alone.

There is considerable convergence between the opportunity-based view I defend and A. K. Sen's appeal to a capabilities-based account (or freedom based account) of the target of justice. The convergence is even more pronounced when Sen discusses the ways in which health in developing countries is affected by different development strategies and emphasizes the importance of education and the growth of democratic culture and institutions. Rawls's focus on the "capabilities of free and equal citizens" suggests the convergence works in both directions. Both approaches allow us [to] talk informatively about justice and the distribution of health.

· · ·

OPPORTUNITY IS NOT THE KEY

Gopal Sreenivasan

Norman Daniels highlights and provides an overview of three strands in his seminal work on justice and healthcare. He associates each strand with a central question: Is healthcare special? When are health inequalities unjust? How can we meet competing healthcare needs fairly under reasonable resource constraints?

I suggest there is an inherent tension between the strands corresponding to the first two questions. More specifically, the empirical data on the social determinants of health, which motivate Daniels's second question, raise serious doubts about his answer to the first. These data indicate that healthcare is *not* special. Indeed, it seems to me, they fuel the suspicion that Daniels's fair equality of opportunity account is simply the wrong framework for thinking about what justice requires in the way of access to healthcare.

On Daniels's analysis, healthcare is special because *health* is special. Health, in turn, is special because it constitutes what Daniels calls "species-typical normal functioning," which is required to preserve an individual's *fair share* of the "normal range of opportunity" in his or her society. This share is defined and protected by a moral principle of fair equality of opportunity, which principle serves as the touchstone of Daniels's account.

Healthcare, then, derives its special status from its connection to a fair share of opportunity. However, this connection has not one, but *two* links in it. There is a link between health and a fair share of opportunity, and a further link between health and *healthcare*. Similarly, we need *two* steps to reach the

conclusion that fair equality of opportunity requires universal access to healthcare. One step takes us from a fair share of opportunity to a fair share of health. From a fair share of health, we still need a second step to get to a fair share of healthcare, which Daniels seems to interpret as requiring universal access.

In *Just Healthcare* (1985), Daniels concentrated on securing the link between health and a fair share of opportunity. He took the link between health and healthcare more or less completely for granted, as seems intuitively reasonable. More recently, Daniels has been in the forefront of drawing our attention to the so-called "social determinants" of health. Yet, while he concedes that social determinants have an impact on health that is "measurably greater" than that of access to medical prevention and treatment, Daniels continues to take the link between health and healthcare for granted.

I am sceptical that this link can be sustained. Let us take the distribution of income, the distribution of education, and the distribution of workplace control as examples of the social determinants of health. Here is a dramatic way of making the point: Suppose the introduction of a national health insurance scheme—full blown universal access—makes *no* difference to a particular society's social gradient in health status, so that the distribution of health outcomes across the society remains essentially unchanged. (Since this is more or less what happened in the U.K., the premise is hardly far-fetched). Suppose, further, that the very considerable cost of a national scheme would significantly reduce this society's social gradient in health, if it were applied instead to equalizing the distribution of income, education, or workplace control. In that case, the society can produce a better net distribution of health outcomes by minimizing people's chances of getting sick than it can produce by guaranteeing their chances of getting treatment once they get sick. Devoting the entire healthcare budget to ameliorating the social determinants of health, rather than to healthcare, would thus move citizens closer to their "fair share of health," however exactly this is defined.

Editors' note: The author's notes have been cut. A longer version of this article appears as "Health Care and Equal Opportunity," *Hastings Center Report* 37, no. 2 (2007): 2–12.

If a fair share of opportunity was the key, this society would be *required* not to spend anything on healthcare and, a fortiori, not to provide universal access. Variations in access to care would only matter insofar as they have an impact on opportunity; and they can do *that* only insofar as they have an impact on health. In the case described, failure to provide healthcare has no adverse impact on the distribution of health outcomes. So no complaint of justice could be raised. Daniels's account avoids this consequence only to the extent that the case itself is empirically unrealistic. But the evidence on social determinants that he himself adduces does not favor this escape hatch.

Nothing turns here on my dramatic assumption that the best allocation of a fixed health budget would allocate very little to personal medical services. This bears emphasis. Given any division of the total health budget, the issue arises of how to *distribute* whatever resources are allocated to personal medical services *across the citizenry*, and thereby to determine their access to healthcare more narrowly construed. Many different distributions of access to personal medical services, including radically unequal ones, will be compatible with the same resultant distribution of health outcomes across the society. All of these distributions have the same impact on health, and hence on opportunity. Daniels's fair equality of opportunity account is therefore committed to the verdict that they are all equally just.

Can it really be that universal access to medical services has no greater title to the mantle of justice than does radically unequal access? That is what Daniels's account tells us, once we digest the facts about the link between health and healthcare. Those who balk at this conclusion thus have good reason to question his account.

ALLOCATING SCARCE RESOURCES

BONE MARROW TRANSPLANTS FOR ADVANCED BREAST CANCER: THE STORY OF CHRISTINE DEMEURERS

Alex John London

It was a frightening discovery.[1] At 32, Christine deMeurers was an active woman with a husband, two children, and a new job as a school teacher. It was 1992 and in the heat of late August the deMeurers were unprepared for the turn their lives were about to take. Christine had been at her new job for less than two months when she found a small lump in her left breast. A visit to her physician and some tests revealed that her worst fears were true; Christine had breast cancer.

The reality of her situation hit like a thunderclap. The speed with which breast cancer is treated can mean the difference between life and death, and the deMeurers knew it. Moving as quickly as possible, Christine underwent a radical mastectomy, radiation therapy, and a course of chemotherapy which ended in March of 1993. By May it was clear that her cancer had spread and Christine was told she had Stage IV metastatic breast cancer.

Like many Americans, the deMeurers received their health insurance through their employer, and like a growing number of people in this country they were members of a managed care plan. Christine had recently been hired to teach at the same school in Elsinore, California, where her husband had been teaching since 1989, and they had each signed up for the least expensive of the three health plans their school offered, Health Net of Woodland Hills, California.

There is no reason to think that the deMeurers were unhappy with the treatment Christine had received from Health Net by the end of March 1993. Although it had not stopped the spread of her cancer, Christine had received prompt and aggressive treatment for a disease that affects 1 of every 9 American women and is the second leading cause of cancer deaths among women. At the end of these first months of 1993, Christine had exhausted the standard therapies that were available at the time, and it looked as though her cancer would soon overtake her.

Reprinted with permission from the author.

Yet Christine's oncologist, Dr. Mahesh Gupta, offered hope. He suggested that Christine might be a candidate for a new procedure known as high-dose chemotherapy with autologous bone marrow transplant, or HDC/ABMT. Although the use of this procedure on women with Stage IV breast cancer was new and its efficacy largely unknown, HDC/ABMT was already accepted as a successful treatment of many non-solid forms of cancer such as Hodgkins disease and leukemia. The theory behind the procedure is simple. There is a direct correlation between the dose of chemotherapy a patient receives and its effect on the targeted cancer. The problem, however, is that there is a natural limit to the amount of these toxic agents the body can endure. In HDC/ABMT physicians remove stem cells from a patient's bone marrow, purify them of cancer cells, and then freeze them for later use. Patients are then exposed to near lethal doses of chemotherapy, up to 10 times the normal level. In addition to killing cancer cells, however, such concentrated amounts of these potent chemicals inevitably kill much of the patient's remaining bone marrow. So after receiving this high dose of chemotherapy the harvested and purified stem cells are transplanted back into the patient. There was, nevertheless, very little information and certainly no consensus among experts as to the efficacy of this procedure on solid tumors like Christine's.

Nevertheless, Dr. Gupta assured Christine that there were still options available, and in a breach of Health Net policy he referred her directly to a colleague at the Scripps Clinic in nearby La Jolla. Dissatisfied with their reception there, the deMeurers flew to Denver where Christine was evaluated by Dr. Roy B. Jones at the University of Colorado. Unlike their reception at Scripps, the deMeurers found a welcome ally in Dr. Jones who examined Christine on June 8, 1993 and told her that she might benefit from the HDC/ABMT procedure. It was a ray of hope in a very dark period of their lives.

On the same day that Christine was being examined by Dr. Jones, however, Health Net formally decided not to pay for the procedure on the grounds that the treatment "is not uniformly accepted as proven and effective for the treatment of metastatic breast cancer." The treatment was excluded under the so-called "investigational clause" in the Health Net contract. The deMeurers were crushed, but undaunted. Together they decided to try to obtain the new procedure any way they could, and they began taking every step possible. Christine secured permission to see a new oncologist who agreed with Dr. Jones' assessment of her situation and agreed to refer her to UCLA medical center. At the same time they began trying to raise the $100,000 it would take to pay for the procedure, and they hired a lawyer to write a formal appeal to Health Net's decision on Christine's behalf.

On June 25, Christine met with Dr. John Glaspy at the UCLA medical center who spelled out the risks involved with the procedure itself, the three months it would take to recover from the severity of the chemotherapy, and the rather steep price tag it entailed. Dr. Glaspy was himself a cautious proponent of the use of HDC/ABMT on women with Stage IV breast cancer, even though a 1992 review article by the respected health policy expert Dr. David Eddy had concluded that there were no data to support the claim that this procedure was in any way superior to the standard dose of chemotherapy when treating women with metastatic breast cancer.[2] Cautious but optimistic, Dr. Glaspy said that he would perform the procedure if that was what they wanted. The deMeurers readily accepted.

What Dr. Glaspy did not know, what the deMeurers had purposefully made sure he would not know, was that Christine was a member of the Health Net plan. Wary of the influence that they suspected Health Net administrators had already exerted on the course of Christine's care, the deMeurers had decided to present themselves to Dr. Glaspy as paying customers rather than as members of a managed care plan. Ironically, this also prevented the deMeurers from finding out that Dr. Glaspy was a member of the Health Net committee which earlier that year had voted to deny coverage for bone marrow transplants to patients with Stage IV breast cancer.

Soon after their visit to UCLA, the deMeurers learned that Health Net had rejected their appeal. Preliminary tests at UCLA had shown that Christine's cancer had responded to initial doses of chemotherapy, but it was also quickly becoming clear that they would be unable to raise such a substantial amount of money on their own. So the deMeurers authorized their attorney to file for an injunction to force Health Net to pay for treatment and they enlisted Dr. Glaspy's help. The revelation that Christine was a member of Health Net put

Dr. Glaspy in a terrible position. As a member of Health Net's transplantation committee, he had advocated covering HDC/ABMT for metastatic breast cancer. But in the end he had agreed with the committee's consensus to exclude it from coverage. Committed to advocating for his patient's interests, on September 13 Dr. Glaspy wrote to Health Net in support of Christine's injunction, "As a physician representing Christine, I have a responsibility to represent her interests and to help her achieve her goals in her health care." Exactly one week later, however, at the request of Health Net lawyers, he submitted a second, much less sanguine statement to Health Net concluding "This procedure is of unproven efficacy in the treatment of metastatic breast cancer, and the results of clinical trials to date are not sufficient to establish beyond doubt that it is superior to standard dose chemotherapy."

The deMeurers felt betrayed and alone. The second letter from Dr. Glaspy only strengthened their resentment of Health Net and their distrust of its doctors. Dr. Glaspy was also painfully aware of the blow he had dealt to the deMeurer's trust. But he was also aware of the dissatisfaction his first letter had caused at Health Net, especially in light of the fact that he was a member of the committee that voted not to cover this procedure. Health Net was upset that a member of its own committee was actively trying to thwart the very regulations he had helped to design, and the phone calls of Health Net officials to Dr. Glaspy's boss, Dr. Dennis Slamon, revealed the depth of the company's dissatisfaction.

In an attempt to salvage as much of the medical center's relationship with the deMeurers and with Health Net as possible, Dr. Slamon arrived at a compromise. He decided that UCLA would absorb the costs of Christine's procedure, thus relieving Health Net of any obligation to pay and enabling Christine to receive the health care she so desperately wanted. On September 23, 1993 Christine was admitted to UCLA to begin the first phase of treatment. According to her husband, she experienced four disease-free months after recovering from the severe chemotherapy, but by the Spring of 1994 she was ill again and on March 10, 1995 Christine deMeurers succumbed to her cancer.

The story of Christine deMeurers is not typical of most people's experience with managed care, but because it is such an extreme case it casts some of the

most serious problems facing the American health care system into stark relief. It is the story of a family coping with a terrible disease and unifying around the common cause of exhausting every possible treatment option. It is also the story of a woman who must not only battle cancer, but must also struggle with her insurance company for the treatment she so desperately wants. Similarly, Christine's story illustrates the way physicians have found themselves trapped between two worlds of health care. In Dr. Glaspy we see the old fee-for-service system and the new medicine under managed care clashing in its most palpable form. In these ways, Christine's story is a miniature portrait of the way we think about health care in America and the problems we are facing as the cost of care outstrips our collective ability to pay for it.

After World War II, medical research in the United States flourished, and the marriage of increased research funding with top-flight science gave birth to a formidable array of new therapeutic drugs and devices that enabled physicians to conquer injuries and diseases in a way that would have been unthinkable only years earlier. As amazing as the feats such advances were making possible, however, was the price tag that came with them. The nation's health care expenditures began to climb sharply in the post-war years, and by 1976 General Motors announced that it was spending more money on the health care of its workers than on steel. As the decade drew to a close there was a collective recognition on the part of the corporate sector that something had to be done to keep the cost of health care from hemorrhaging out of control.[3]

Because most Americans receive their health insurance through their employers, the corporate sector was coming to see the high cost of their employees' benefits as a threat to their ability to remain competitive. The choice seemed terrible but unavoidable. How long before industry would have to choose between competitive viability and employee health care? It was in response to this dilemma that managed care companies like Health Net arose with the mandate of stemming the swiftly rising tide of health care costs.

In an important way, the rise of managed care and our reaction to the way it has tried to carry out its mandate illustrates the fundamentally paradoxical relationship that Americans have to medicine in general and to their health care providers in particular.

On the one hand, we embrace the values of frugality and fiscal sensibility which lead us to protest against the dizzying rate at which health care costs have been rising. At the same time, we will not tolerate receiving anything less than the latest, most sophisticated health care.[4] We don't want to see restrictions put on our liberty when it comes to being able to seek out and obtain the latest and most advanced medical procedures from the most well-trained providers, yet we also bristle at the restrictions on our liberty that come in the form of the higher taxes, product prices, or insurance premiums that inevitably result from the exercise of this freedom.

In the story of Christine deMeurers we have a concrete and powerful illustration of the way these conflicting values can intersect in the lives of the most vulnerable people. Christine represents the way we have come to look to the frontiers of medicine in the face of the ravages of sickness and disease. Here is a young, productive woman with a life of her own, a family, children, who is also dying from a terrible disease. When the standard modalities of treatment are exhausted, she looks to the frontiers of medical science and places her hopes in a relatively untested procedure of questionable therapeutic value for the chance to live out some portion of her remaining months free of disease. With no other medical options and without the resources to secure this chance for herself, she looks to a third party to cover the expenses and make it possible.

Debate over the benefit that receiving HDC/ABMT had for Christine deMeurers is still mixed. The officials at Health Net stick by their initial decision to deny coverage and Dr. Glaspy admits that Christine would probably have lived longer without the treatment. Clinical trials to test the efficacy of the procedure are under way in a number of cities across the country, but there is still no consensus on whether HDC/ABMT is more effective than standard chemotherapy for women with metastatic breast cancer. For Alan deMeurers, however, the procedure was worth it. It allowed his wife to live a better quality of life for a few short months and to spend one final Christmas with him and their two children. Even if Dr. Glaspy is right, it is the quality of the life Christine led for those four months that matters most to her husband, not simply the length of time she remained alive.

The public reaction to cases like Christine's has mostly been one of outrage. The media was critical of the influence Health Net officials exerted on the medical decisions of the program's physicians, and juries were eager to teach the plan's plutocratic administrators a lesson. In 1993 Health Net lost a lawsuit filed by Jim Fox, the husband of Nelene Fox, a Health Net subscriber who had been denied HDC/ABMT for her Stage IV breast cancer on the grounds that it was experimental and investigational. The jury awarded Nelene's estate $12 million in actual damages and $77 million in punitive damages, although Health Net later agreed to pay only $5 million in exchange for their right to appeal the verdict. Nevertheless, the members of the jury were eager to send a message to health care companies. "You cannot substitute profits for good-quality health care," one juror was quoted as saying.

The Fox verdict precipitated a rash of similar judgments on behalf of women who had been denied coverage for HDC/ABMT for advanced breast cancer, and in 1995 a California arbitration board awarded one million dollars to the estate of Christine deMeurers on the ground that phone calls which Health Net officials had placed to Christine's physicians at various stages in her treatment had exerted undue influence on the doctor-patient relationship. In addition to a fury of litigation, these cases have given rise to legislation in a number of states requiring insurers to pay for HDC/ABMT for women with metastatic breast cancer. The result of these suits and of state congressional action has been to free up patients' access to specialists and to procedures which their insurance providers would otherwise have excluded as investigational or experimental. Yet, amidst the lurid details of some of the questionable activities on the part of officers at Health Net and other HMOs, and in the rush to right what look like injustices that were being perpetrated against the women who were denied access to HDC/ABMT, we seem to have lost sight of the difficult but enduring questions at the very heart of this issue. Should we, should the government or insurance companies, pay for people's access to procedures of this nature? Should we pay for costly medical procedures of unknown therapeutic benefit when there are people struggling to get access to a host of genuinely effective therapies?

Are four disease-free months in the life of a terminally ill person worth the $100,000 to $200,000 it takes to secure them? Could this money be better spent somewhere else? If we do not draw the line on medical expenses in front of cases like this, then where do we draw it?

In the wake of cases like those of the deMeurers and the Foxes, we have struggled with these questions in a very piecemeal and largely inchoate way. On the one hand, the judiciary has consistently sided with plaintiffs in these cases, making it very clear that those with the resources to make themselves heard and with voices articulate enough to make their case compelling can receive access to these sorts of therapies while the less articulate and less well-off cannot. On the other hand, as of the end of 1995 at least seven states had mandated coverage for HDC/ABMT for breast cancer although such mandates do not necessarily apply to all forms of insurance providers, and it is rare that such mandates are formulated around a coherent set of health care goals.[5]

The patchwork of judicial and legislative decisions rendered in response to these cases amounts to a de facto way of answering the difficult questions posed a moment ago. But surely this is no way to deal with such important and fundamental issues of public policy. The system may provide greater access for some, but in a way that seems arbitrary at best and inequitable or unjust at worst. We may benefit from the psychological comforts of avoiding some very public, "tragic choices," but this is very likely the illusory comfort of the fine new garments the Emperor is wearing.[6] We have to ask ourselves whether we have responded to these cases in such a way as to make the system more just, or whether we haven't simply shifted the burden of injustice off of those who are most capable of defending themselves onto those who are least able to do so.

By acquiescing to the de facto practice that has emerged for dealing with these cases, we have done ourselves, our health care providers, and our third-party payers a terrible disservice. We have left unanswered important questions about which kinds of medical interventions we should be in the business of helping people obtain. We have left the insurance industry without substantive guidelines by which to determine the kinds of interventions they need to

cover and the kinds they may need to exclude. This in turn perpetuates a system of disclosure on the part of insurers which keeps subscribers largely in the dark as to the nature of excluded therapies, the methods used for making such determinations, and the process by which the subscriber can influence these guidelines or appeal such decisions. This may have provided litigious subscribers with the power to obtain exotic medical interventions, but the system in which this kind of arbitrary power exists seems to work against our common commitment to reducing health care costs and to spreading the burdens of doing so evenly among the members of society. To that extent, the maintenance of this piecemeal way of creating public policy works against many of our own explicit and publicly held commitments to fairness and fiscal responsibility.

This leaves subscribers with the unenviable feeling of being trapped in an unfriendly system that has been imposed on them from above. In the absence of some form of communal conversation about these difficult and enduring questions, we will make little headway against the antagonistic and largely adversarial relationship developing between patients, their insurance providers, and the health care workers who are increasingly asked to facilitate the very different aims of these two parties.[7] We need to ask ourselves why so many of these cases wound up in the judicial system. Would subscribers who were given a more active role in the creation of policy guidelines or in the decision-making process of their insurance provider feel the need to take their claims to court? How can we facilitate a more active role for subscribers? Similarly, are there ways we could improve the system so that subscribers whose claims have been denied can appeal their decision and feel that their needs are receiving legitimate and sincere consideration? Would subscribers be as eager to litigate if they felt their claims had received fair consideration in an equitable review process? Would lawsuits have as much merit if insurance companies could point to such a process of appeal?

By giving subscribers a more active role in the formation of the guidelines that govern their care, insurance providers will give their subscribers a stake in making sure such guidelines are both fair and effective. It will also reassure subscribers that they are being treated as ends in themselves and not as mere means. But in order to accomplish these goals we are going to have to improve the way that insurance providers disclose information to their subscribers, and this means that providers and subscribers alike are going to have to deliberate together on how to answer some very important questions. In the case of HDC/ABMT this means that we are going to have to ask whether women with advanced breast cancer should receive coverage for this procedure, and if not, why not.

Health Net, like most managed care companies, denied coverage for HDC/ABMT on the grounds that it was investigational or experimental. The rationale behind this move was simple. First, insurers could make a strong case that there is only an obligation to pay for therapies that are proven to have some therapeutic benefit. The case for this normative claim looks especially strong when we add the premise that there are not even enough resources to cover everyone's access to proven therapies. Second, with this argument on the table the claim that a drug or a procedure is experimental looks more like a straightforward descriptive claim than it does a controversial normative judgment. So excluding an intervention as experimental allowed the insurance provider to maintain the appearance of making coverage decisions without having to make delicate and controversial judgments about the monetary value of the length and quality of human life. Finally, this general attitude toward experimental treatments was perfectly consistent with the public's view of human experimentation in the wake of scandals such as Willowbrook, Tuskegee, and the Jewish Chronic Disease Hospital case.* That is, the denial of access to experimental drugs and procedures fit nicely with the public's view that such things were usually dangerous and to be avoided.

In the 1980s, however, social attitudes towards experimental treatments started to change as patients dying of AIDS began to clamor for access to the experimental drugs and devices which were being held up in what they came to view as a paternalistic system of federal oversight. In the 1980s experimental drugs and procedures came to be seen, not as dangerous things to which no one wanted to be subjected, but rather as the last desperate hope for dying patients. This shift in attitude put pressure on the normative claim that people should not receive access to experimental drugs, but it also brought into question the notion that labeling something as experimental was a purely descriptive and non-normative claim.

Time and again the insurance industry's claim that HDC/ABMT was experimental was challenged by lawyers and physicians. What makes a drug or procedure experimental? Is it the fact that it is not a part of the established medical practice? But medicine is a notoriously recalcitrant social practice and it can take some time for innovative and effective procedures to be widely adopted. This raises the question of whose medical practice we are talking about. Are we concerned with the standard practices of the larger medical community or only of the most knowledgeable experts? Lawyers had no problem finding expert oncologists to testify about the number of their colleagues who were performing HDC/ABMT on women with advanced breast cancer at some of the most prestigious medical institutions in the world. So if this was the criterion for something's being "experimental," HDC/ABMT didn't seem to fit the bill. Perhaps then something is experimental when it has not received FDA approval. But many of the drugs and procedures involved in HDC/ABMT had received FDA approval for other uses, and there are many drugs and procedures that are used effectively for purposes for which they were not initially approved. Also, FDA approval often requires that a procedure's efficacy be shown in a randomized clinical trial, but there are difficult moral problems associated with conducting this kind of trial on a procedure of this sort.

As a result, in case after case, judges and juries told managed care companies that the experimental exclusion clause in their subscriber contract did not apply to HDC/ABMT for advanced breast cancer. But these judgments were based on the inadequate definitions offered by the managed care companies. They should not be taken as speaking to the underlying question of whether this is the sort of treatment third parties should be financing. If policy holders and their providers are going to have an open and productive debate about this question, then they are going to have to ask frank questions about the kinds of health care goals they are willing to support and to what degree. Undoubtedly this is

---

*Editor's note: See Part 6, Section 1.

going to require each of us to look at the giant pink elephant standing in the middle of the room: How much money are we willing to spend to improve the quality of a terminally ill patient's life for a few months given the other kinds of health care needs our plan must meet?

The questions raised by cases like that of Christine deMeurers are often perceived as instances of the familiar and intractable conflict between consequentialist concerns about money and utility and deontic concerns for the dignity of persons. Although they can easily be understood along these lines, it is important to see that this is not the only or necessarily the best way to think about them. It is true that a careful look at the historical record will show that at the time, many of these cases may have in fact been about a straightforward conflict between money and autonomy. But this might simply be evidence for the inadequacy of this way of structuring the problem rather than for the claim that this is the only way to structure it.

One thing seems clear. To the extent that plan members are forced to submit to policies which they themselves have not either helped to shape or voluntarily chosen, people will continue to feel that someone else has put a price on the length and quality of their lives, and this will continue to foster feelings of antagonism and resentment.[8] To the extent that plan members can actively participate in shaping the policies which govern their treatment or choose their plan based on the policies that best reflect their conception of the value of health care, the restrictions placed on their care will represent an extension of their own autonomy. To that extent they will represent people's considered judgments about the way their needs should be met given the fact of fiscal scarcity and the need to distribute the benefits and burdens of health care fairly amongst the members of the plan. Considerations of costs and benefits may be important factors which shape these decisions, but in the end the moral legitimacy of these decisions will be based on the fact that the resulting policies are the product of the autonomous and considered judgments of the very people they are meant to cover.

In the end, the story of Christine deMeurers confronts us with two basic and interconnected problems. First, how should we answer the difficult questions with which this case confronts us? Second, how can we make sure that there are not more cases like this? How can we ensure that there are structures in place which will facilitate our ability to deliberate about these questions together, and which will reflect the conclusions that such deliberations reach? How can we shape the practices and procedures of our health care system in a way that will facilitate and accommodate this increased interaction between providers, subscribers, and health care workers? We should not shrink from making these difficult decisions together or from the recognition that some of these choices may be tragic, so long as we can maintain the conviction that the decisions we make are fair and that the system we create is more just than the one we have now.

NOTES

1. The details presented here about Christine deMeurers' battle with breast cancer and her HMO have been taken from published accounts by Erik Larson, "The Soul of an HMO," *Time Magazine* (January 22, 1996) and George Anders, *Health Against Wealth* (New York: Houghton Mifflin Company, 1996), chapter seven.
2. David Eddy, "High Dose Chemotherapy with Autologous Bone Marrow Transplantation for the Treatment of Metastatic Breast Cancer," *Journal of Clinical Oncology* 1992, 10(4):657–670.
3. For a more detailed account of the rise of managed care see E. Haavi Morreim, *Balancing Act: The New Medical Ethics of Medicine's New Economics* (Washington, D.C.: Georgetown University Press, 1995) pp. 8–17 and George Anders, *Health Against Wealth* op cit.
4. For a trenchant criticism of the conflicting views Americans have about health and health care see Daniel Callahan, *What Kind of Life* (Washington, D.C.: Georgetown University Press, 1994).
5. Reinhard Priester, Karen G. Gervais and Dorothy E. Vawter, *Improving Coverage for Unproven Health Care Interventions* (Minnesota Center for Health Care Ethics, August, 1996), p. 5.
6. For the view that we should avoid the appearance of making tragic choices, even when the choices themselves are unavoidable, see Guido Calabresi and Philip Bobbitt, *Tragic Choices* (New York: W. W. Norton and Company, 1978).
7. For an analysis of the way the interests of these three parties can conflict and some suggestions for managing these conflicts see my "Thrasymachus and Managed Care: How Not to Think About the Craft of Medicine" in Ronald Polansky and Mark Kuczewski, eds. *Bioethics: Ancient Themes in Contemporary Issues* (Cambridge: MIT Press, 2000).

8. For a view of the importance of subscriber consent within a managed care plan, see Paul T. Menzel, *Strong Medicine* (New York: Oxford University Press, 1990). For the importance of being able to select a plan that coheres with one's vision of the role of health care in one's life, see Ezekiel J. Emanuel, *The Ends of Human Life* (Cambridge: Harvard University Press, 1991).

JUSTICE AND THE HIGH COST OF HEALTH

Ronald Dworkin

I

Everyone agrees that the United States now spends too much on health care. Medical services accounted for 14 percent of our gross domestic product in 1991—France and Germany spent 9 percent and Japan and Britain 8 percent—and economists predict that without reform medical expenses will grow to 18 percent by the year 2000. But how much should a nation like ours spend on its citizens' health? How do we know that other nations are not spending too little, rather than that we are spending too much?

Most people also agree that health care is unjustly distributed in America. Forty million Americans have grossly inadequate medical coverage or none at all, and many who now have adequate insurance will lose it, because they will lose their jobs or develop a disease or condition that makes them uninsurable. In all, without reform, a quarter of all Americans will be without health insurance for some period during the next five years. But how much health care should a decent society make available for everyone? We can't provide everyone with the medical care that the richest among us can buy for themselves. How do we decide what lesser level of health care justice demands even the poorest should have?

Reprinted by permission of the publisher from *Sovereign Virtue* by Ronald Dworkin, pp. 307–319, Cambridge, Mass.: Harvard University Press, Copyright © 2000 by Ronald Dworkin. First appeared under another title in *New York Review of Books*, January 13, 1994.

Editors' note: Some author's notes have been cut. Students who want to follow up on sources should consult the original article.

The health-care plan that President Clinton presented to Congress in 1993, but was never adopted, would have instituted a form of health-care rationing. It provided a basic package of health care that would be guaranteed to almost everyone. The plan specified some components of this basic package in considerable detail: the package included, for example, a comprehensive schedule of immunization for infants and children, routine screening and physical examinations at different intervals for different age groups, and mammograms to detect breast cancer for women every two years starting at age fifty. The plan also specifically excluded some kinds of treatment from the basic package altogether—most cosmetic surgery, for example.

The plan's most important rationing provision, however, was not detailed but extremely abstract: it provided that medical treatment be part of the basic package only if it was "necessary and appropriate," and it would have created a National Health Board charged with the responsibility of determining what kinds of treatment were necessary and appropriate and in what circumstances. That board would have had to decide, for example, whether bone-marrow transplants or other experimental forms of treatment were necessary and appropriate for particular diseases; it would have had to determine whether most people could have such expensive procedures when doctors told them that was their only chance, slim though it might be.

How should an agency charged with such a responsibility make such decisions? When should expensive magnetic resonance imaging be provided to those who cannot afford it on their own? Should speculative bowel and liver transplants ever be provided? If so, to which patients suffering from which diseases? If a nation cannot buy all the tests and treatment that its citizens might want or need, how should it decide, as a nation, how much it should spend, collectively and on each citizen?

Some critics deny that any such rationing of health care is really necessary: they argue that if the waste and greed in the American health-care system were eliminated, we could save enough money to give men and women all the medical treatment that could benefit them. But though administrative expenses account for a significant part of hospital costs,[1] and American doctors' salaries are extremely large by other nations' standards,[2] the greatest contribution to the rise in medical costs in recent decades has been the availability of new, high-tech means of diagnosis like magnetic resonance imaging and new and very expensive techniques like organ transplants and, on the horizon, monoclonal-antibody treatment for cancer. America is not paying all that much more for the medicine it formerly bought more cheaply; rather, it now has so much more medicine to buy.

Many politicians and some doctors say that much of the new technology is "unnecessary" or "wasteful." They do not mean that it provides no benefit at all. They mean that its benefit is too limited to justify its cost, and this is an argument for rationing, not an argument that rationing is unnecessary. There is an emerging consensus among doctors that routine mammograms for women under fifty, which are expensive, do not save many women's lives. But they do save some. Heroic transplants that rarely work do work rarely. So we cannot defend the rationing decisions that any health-care plan would make as simply avoiding waste. We cannot avoid the question of justice: what is "appropriate" medical care depends on what it would be unfair to withhold on the grounds that it costs too much.

II

For millennia doctors have paid lip service, at least, to an ideal of justice in medicine which I shall call the rescue principle. It has two connected parts. The first holds that life and health are, as René Descartes put it, chief among all goods: everything else is of lesser importance and must be sacrificed for them. The second insists that health care must be distributed on grounds of equality: that even in a society in which wealth is very unequal and equality is

otherwise scorned, no one must be denied the medical care he needs just because he is too poor to afford it. These are understandable, even noble, ideals. They are grounded in a shared human understanding of the horror of pain, and, beyond that, of the indispensability of life and health to everything else we do. The rescue principle is so ancient, so intuitively attractive, and so widely supported in political rhetoric that it might easily be thought to supply the right standard for answering questions about rationing.

In fact, however, the rescue principle is almost wholly useless for that purpose, and the assumption that it sets the proper standard for health-care reform has done more harm than good. The principle does offer an answer to the question of how much America should spend on health care overall: it says we should spend all we can until the next dollar would buy no gain in health or life expectancy at all. No sane society would try to meet that standard, any more than a sane person would organize his life on that principle. In past centuries, however, there was not so huge a gap between the rhetoric of the rescue principle and what it was medically possible for a community to do. But now that science has created so many vastly expensive forms of medical care, it is preposterous that a community should treat longer life as a good that it must provide at any cost—even one that would make the longer lives of its people lives barely worth living.

So the rescue principle's answer to the question of how much a society should spend on health care overall must be rejected as incredible. Once that answer is rejected, the principle has no second-best or fallback level of advice: it simply is silent. That is worse than unhelpful, because it encourages the idea that justice has nothing to say about how much a society should spend on health care, as against other goods, like education or controlling crime or material prosperity or the arts.

The rescue principle does have something helpful, though negative, to say about the other question of justice, which is how health care should be distributed. It says that if rationing is necessary, it should not be done, as it now largely is in the United States, on the basis of money. But we need more positive advice: What should the basis of rationing be? The egalitarian impulse of the principle suggests that medical care should be distributed according to need. But what does that mean—how is need to be measured? Does someone "need" an operation that might save his life but is highly unlikely to do so? Is someone's need for life-saving treatment affected by the quality his life would have if the treatment were successful? Does the age of the patient matter—does someone need or deserve treatment less at seventy than at a younger age? Why? How should we balance the need of many people for relief from pain or incapacity against the need of fewer people for life-saving care? At one point the procedures of an Oregon commission appointed to establish medical priorities ranked tooth-capping ahead of appendectomy, because so many teeth can be capped for the price of one operation. Why was that so clearly a mistake?

We need a different, more helpful statement of ideal justice in health care, and we should start by noticing one problem that seems to make reform mandatory. Why does America spend so much—so much more than other nations—on medicine? In large part because individual decisions about how much health care to buy are made by patient and doctor but paid for by a third party, the insurance company, so that those who make the decisions have no direct incentive to save money. Insurance premiums are tax-deductible, moreover, and an employer's contribution is not treated as part of the employee's taxable income. So health insurance makes patients insensitive to cost at the moment of decision, and the real price of that insurance is subsidized by the nation. People would probably spend less on their own or their family's care if they had to pay the actual cost themselves, at the expense of other goods and opportunities they might also want or want their families to have.

Of course, in the long run most people do pay the true costs of their health care, but they do so indirectly and unwisely, because employer contributions and tax funds could be used to buy what they would choose to have if they made the choice themselves: better schools for their children, for example, or economic investments and programs that would improve America's competitiveness and give them greater job security. Our medical expenditures are therefore irrational: the system makes choices for people that they would not make for themselves, and the result is that our collective expenditures are

too high—measured, as they should be, by how much care we really want, taken together, at the price we really want to pay.

Conservative economists seize on this fact: they say we should create a free market in health care by removing all tax benefits and subsidies so that people can have only the care they can afford. While that is, of course, an unacceptable solution, it is important to see why. It is unacceptable for three reasons. First, wealth is so unfairly distributed in America that many people would be unable to buy any substantial health insurance at market rates. Second, most people have very inadequate information about health risks and medical technology; they do not know what the risk of breast cancer is before the age of fifty, for example, or how many years having routine mammography before that age would add to their life expectancy. Third, in an unregulated market, insurance companies would charge some people higher premium rates because they were greater health risks (as, indeed, many insurance companies now do) so that people with a poor health history, or who were members of ethnic groups particularly susceptible to certain diseases, or who lived in areas where the risk of violent injury was greater would be charged prohibitive rates.

This analysis points to a more satisfactory ideal of justice in health care—the "prudent insurance" ideal. We should allocate resources between health and other social needs, and between different patients who need treatment, by trying to imagine what health care would be like if it were left to a free and unsubsidized market, and if the three deficiencies I have just described were somehow corrected. So try to imagine that America is transformed in three ways. Suppose, first, that the distribution of wealth and income is as fair as it possibly can be. In my view, that means that the resources people can initially command, in making their decisions about education, work, and investment, are as nearly equal as possible; but you should imagine an economic distribution that is fair according to your own views, whatever these are. (I shall assume, however, that on your views, as on mine, the wealth of everyone in a fair society would be much closer to the average than is true in America now: the great extremes between rich and poor that mark our economic life now would have largely disappeared.)

Second, imagine that America has also changed so that all the information that might be called state-of-the-art knowledge about the value and cost and side effects of particular medical procedures—everything, in other words, that good doctors know—is generally known by the public at large as well. Third, imagine that no one—including insurance companies—has any information available about how likely any particular person is to contact any particular disease or to suffer any particular kind of accident. No one would be in a position to say, of himself or anyone else, that that person is more or less likely to contract sickle-cell anemia, or diabetes, or to be the victim of violence in the street, than anyone else.

The changes I am asking readers to imagine are very great, but they are not, I think, beyond the reach of the imagination. Now suppose that health-care decisions in the transformed community are left simply to individual market decisions in as free a market as we can imagine, so that doctors and hospitals and drug companies are free to charge whatever they wish. Medical care is not provided by the government for anyone, nor are medical expenses or health-insurance premiums tax deductible. There is no need to subsidize medical care in any such way, because people have enough resources to buy, for themselves the medical care they decide is appropriate. What kind of health-care institutions would actually develop in such a community? Would most people join health maintenance organizations that provided care by staff doctors at a relatively inexpensive rate? Would any substantial number choose more-expensive insurance arrangements that allowed more freedom of choice in doctors or hospitals? Would the average plan or policy provide coverage for routine medical examinations or diagnostic screenings? What kind, how often, and at what age? How many plans or policies would provide, at appropriately high rates or premiums, experimental or very expensive or high-risk or low-expected-benefit procedures of different kinds? How much of its aggregate resources would the community devote to medical care through these various individual decisions?

It is impossible to answer these questions with any precision. But we can nevertheless make two crucial claims about justice. First, whatever that transformed community actually spends on health care in the aggregate is the morally appropriate amount for it to spend: it could not be criticized, on grounds of justice, for spending either too much or too little. Second, however health care is distributed in that society is just for that society: justice would not require providing health care for anyone that he or his family had not purchased. These claims follow directly from an extremely appealing assumption: that a just distribution is one that well-informed people create for themselves by individual choices, provided that the economic system and the distribution of wealth in the community in which these choices are made are themselves just.[3]

These important conclusions help us to decide what health care we should aim to provide for everyone in our own, imperfect, and unjust community. We can speculate about what kind of medical care and insurance it would be prudent for most Americans to buy for themselves if the changes I imagined had really taken place; and we can use those speculations as guidelines in deciding what justice requires now—in deciding, for example, which medical tests and procedures the National Health Board should decide are "necessary and appropriate" if the Health Security Act is passed.

Consider a twenty-five-year-old with average wealth and prospects and state-of-the-art knowledge of medicine. Suppose he can choose from a wide variety of possible arrangements to provide for the health care be might want, under various contingencies, over the course of his life. What arrangements would it be prudent for him to make? He might be tempted, initially, to buy insurance providing every form of treatment or care that might conceivably be beneficial for him under any circumstance. But he would soon realize that the cost of such wildly ambitious insurance would be prohibitive—he would have nothing left for anything else—and decide that prudence required a much less comprehensive insurance program.

Of course, what is prudent for someone depends on that person's own individual needs, tastes, personality, and preferences, but we can nevertheless make some judgments with confidence that they would fit the needs and preferences of most contemporary Americans. We can be confident, for example, about what medical insurance it would not be prudent for most people to buy, because some insurance would be a mistake no matter what happened in the future, including the worst out-come. It would be irrational for almost any twenty-five-year-old to insure himself as to provide for life-sustaining treatment if he falls into a persistent vegetative state, for example. The substantial sum he would have to spend in insurance premiums, year by year, to provide that coverage would be much better used in other ways to enhance his actual, conscious life. Even someone who lived only a few months after purchasing the insurance before he fell into a vegetative state would have made, in retrospect, a mistake, giving up resources that could have made his short remaining conscious life better in order to buy a longer unconscious state.

We can enlarge this claim to include dementia as well as unconsciousness: it would not be prudent, for almost anyone, to purchase insurance provid-ing for expensive medical intervention, even of a life-saving character, after he entered the late stages of Alzheimer's disease or other form of irreversible dementia. The money spent on premiums for such insurance would have been better spent, no matter what happens, in making life before dementia more worthwhile. Of course, most prudent people would want to buy insurance to provide custodial care, in conditions of dignity and adequate com-fort, if they became demented; providing for such care would be much less expensive than providing for life-saving treatment—for example renal dialy-sis or an organ transplant—if it were needed.

Now consider a somewhat more controversial sug-gestion. In most developed countries, a major fraction of medical expense—over a quarter of Medicare pay-ments in the United States, for example—is spent on people in the last six months of their lives. Of course, doctors do not always know whether a particular patient will die within a few months no matter how much is spent on his care. But in many cases, sadly, they do know that he will. Most young people on reflecting would not think it prudent to buy insurance that could keep them alive, by expensive medical intervention, for four or five more months at the most if they had already lived into old age. They would think it wiser to spend what that insurance would cost on better health care earlier, or on education or training or investment that would provide greater benefit or more important security. Of course, most people would want to live those additional months if they did fall ill; most people want to remain alive as long as possible, provided they remain conscious and alert and the pain is not too great. But prudent people would nevertheless not want to guarantee those addi-tional months at the cost of sacrifices in their earlier, vigorous life, although, once again, they would cer-tainly want insurance to provide the much less expen-sive care that would keep them as comfortable and as free of pain as possible.

We can use these assumptions about what most people would think prudent for themselves, under fairer conditions than those we now have, as guides to the health care that justice demands everyone have now. If most prudent people would buy a cer-tain level of medical coverage in a free market if they had average means—if nearly everyone would buy insurance covering ordinary medical care, hospital-ization when necessary, prenatal and pediatric care, and regular checkups and other preventative medi-cine, for example—then the unfairness of our society is almost certainly the reason some people do not have such coverage now. A universal health-care system should make sure, in all justice, that every-one does have it.

On the other hand, if even under fair conditions very few prudent people would want to insure themselves to a much higher level of coverage—if, as I said, very few people would insure to provide life-saving care when demented, or heroic and expensive treatment that could prolong their lives only by a few months, for instance—then it is a dis-service to justice to force everyone to have such insurance through a mandatory scheme. Of course, any judgment about what most prudent people would do is subject to exceptions: some people have special preferences and would make very different decisions from those that many other people would. Some people might think, even on reflection, that guaranteeing a few extra months of life at the end was worth great sacrifice earlier, for example. But it seems fair to construct a mandatory coverage scheme on the basis of assumptions about what all but a small number of people would think appropri-ate, allowing those few who would be willing to spend more on special care to do so, if they can afford it, through supplemental insurance.

If we substituted the prudent insurance approach for the rescue principle as our abstract ideal of justice in health care, we would therefore accept certain limits on universal coverage, and we would accept these not as compromises with justice but as required by it. Expensive treatment for unconscious or demented or terminally ill patients would be relatively easy cases to decide if we adopted that approach. Other decisions would be more difficult to make, including, for example, heart-wrenching decisions about the care of babies born so deformed or diseased that they are unlikely to live more than a few weeks even with the most heroic and expensive medical intervention. A few years ago doctors in Philadelphia separated newborn Siamese twins who shared a single heart, though the operation would certainly kill one baby and give the other only a one-in-a-hundred chance of surviving for long, and though the total cost was estimated to be a million dollars. (The twins' parents had no medical insurance, but Indiana, where they lived, paid $1,000 a day toward the cost, and the Philadelphia hospital absorbed the rest.) The chief surgeon justified the procedure by appealing to the rescue principle: "There has been a unanimous consensus," he said, "that if it is possible to save one life, then it is worth doing this."

But the different standard I am defending would probably have recommended against the operation. Suppose people of average wealth, when they marry, are offered the opportunity to buy one of two insurance policies: the first provides that if any of their children is born with a life-threatening defect, neonatal treatment will be covered only if it offers a reasonable (say, 25 percent) chance of success, and the second—much more expensive—provides that such treatment will be guaranteed even if it offers only the barest hope. Most potential parents would decide, I believe, that it would be better for them and their families to buy the first policy, and to use the premiums they would save each year to benefit their healthy children in other ways—to provide better routine medical care, or better housing, or better education, for example—even though they would be giving up the chance for a desperate gamble to save a defective child if they ever had one.

Any public body charged with overseeing the distribution of health care would have to decide what medical procedures are "necessary and appropriate" and thus should be part of a comprehensive package of benefits everyone is guaranteed. Some of these decisions would be particularly difficult: deciding when very expensive diagnostic techniques or experimental organ transplants with a low chance of success are appropriate, for example. Such decisions must of course be based on the best and latest medical evidence, and must constantly be reviewed as that evidence changes. But they, too, should be guided by the standard of individual prudence: Would it make sense for someone to insure himself when young to guarantee a vastly expensive blood test which would improve the diagnosis of a heart attack by a very small percentage of accuracy if he should ever have doubtful symptoms of cardiac disease? Or to provide a risky, expensive, and probably ineffective bowel and liver transplant if doctors decided it would give him a small chance to live?

The rescue principle insists that society provide such treatment whenever there is any chance, however remote, that it will save a life. The prudent insurance principle balances the anticipated value of medical treatment against other goods and risks: it supposes that people might think they lead better lives overall when they invest less in doubtful medicine and more in making life successful or enjoyable, or in protecting themselves against other risks, including economic ones, that might also blight their lives. An agency might well decide that while prudent people would provide their family with the prenatal and well-child care that so many Americans lack, and would insure against serious medical risks at all stages of their lives by providing tested and reasonably effective treatment should they need it, they would forgo heroic treatment of improbable value if they needed it in return for more certain benefits like education, housing, and economic security. If so, then justice demands that a universal health scheme not provide such treatment.

In summary, the prudent insurance test helps to answer both questions of justice I mentioned at the beginning: How much should America spend overall on its health care, and how should that health care be distributed among its citizens? The test asks what people would decide to spend on their own medical care, as individuals, if they were buying insurance under fair free-market conditions, and it insists, first, that we as a nation should spend what individuals would spend, collectively, under those conditions; and, second, that we should use that aggregate expenditure to make sure that all have now, as individuals, what they would have then.

Of course some of the decisions I have been discussing would be made differently by different people trying to apply the prudent insurance test. It is very important that any agency charged with those decisions should be made up of representatives of different groups that might be expected to make such judgments differently; it should have doctors and health-care specialists, of course, but it should also have ordinary people of various ages drawn from different parts of the country and, if possible, different ways of life. Such an agency could draw on the experience of countries with "single-payer" government-run health services which have had systematically to ration health care.

In Britain, for example, doctors in the national health system have been forced to allocate scare resources like renal dialysis machines and organs for transplant, and they have worked out informal guidelines that take into account a potential recipient's age, general health, life quality, and prospects, as well as prospects for adequate care by family or friends. Though this supposed cost-benefit test is different from the prudent insurance test, the decisions doctors have made under the former presumably reflect their judgments, guided by experience, about the relative value of different kinds of treatment at different ages and in different circumstances, and these are also judgements that a prudent insurer would be required to make.

The prudent insurance test also makes plain why it is so important to consult public opinion before rationing decisions are made. Since rationing should reflect not just technical cost-benefit calculations but also the public's sense of priorities, consultation is essential. When Oregon sought to establish priorities in health care under Medicaid, it organized a series of "town meetings," and a "parliament" to discuss the matter, and though the meetings were criticized by some because they were attended by very few of the poor whose health care was being debated, the meetings were nevertheless valuable sources of information about what those who did participate thought would be prudent insurance decisions.

Still, no matter how much information an agency seeking to apply the prudent insurance test is able to gather, its results must be provisional, open to revision on the basis of further evidence of public preference as well as of medical technology and experience. Clinton's failed health-care plan would have allowed people covered by the plan to purchase supplemental health insurance at market prices, with no tax deduction or subsidy. That provision would have fitted the prudent insurance approach particularly well. If, after an agency has established a basic coverage package, a very substantial number of people of average income buy supplemental insurance, in spite of its expense, the basic package should be expanded. If most men of average wealth bought supplemental coverage providing yearly prostate examinations beginning at a younger age than the basic package specified, for example, the prudent insurer test would require that the age specified in the basic package be lowered.

III

Clinton's health-care plan failed, and conventional political wisdom now holds that no health-care reform even approaching the scope of that plan will be adopted in the United State for at least a generation. If that is true, our national disgrace will continue; it is disgraceful that so prosperous a nation cannot guarantee even a decent minimum of medical care to all those over whom it exercises dominion. Clinton's plan was, in retrospect, too complex, in some respects ill judged, and in any case artlessly presented. But some of the plan's most forceful opponents argued, not just that the scheme was wrong in detail or even in design, but that it was rooted in the unacceptable "socialistic" idea that government should watch over people from cradle to grave rather than allow them to take responsibility for themselves.

If the argument of this chapter—and indeed of this book as a whole—is sound, then this objection is wholly misguided. A community that is committed to equality of resources, so that people can make their own decisions about what lives are best for them, enforces rather than subverts proper principles of individual responsibility. It does accept that the intervention of government is sometimes necessary to provide the circumstances in which it is fair to ask all citizens to take responsibility for their own lives. But it respects the personal judgments of need and value that citizens have actually made, or would be likely to make under appropriate conditions, in the exercise of this responsibility. That goal is at the heart of the resource conception of equality, and of the hypothetical insurance strategy it recommends. A health-care scheme constructed to respect the decisions of citizens as prudent insurers is indeed egalitarian. But it is the very opposite of paternalistic.

NOTES

1. According to a *New England Journal of Medicine* study, administrative costs were 2 percent of hospital costs in 1990. See Erik Eckholm, "Study Links Paperwork to 25% of Hospital Costs," *New York Times,* August 5, 1993.

2. The average medical salary in the United States in 1992 was over $160,000. Salary varies dramatically by medical specialty: the average salary of a cardiovascular surgeon was $574,769, that of a family practitioner $119,186. See "Health Plan Would Hurt Most the Doctors Who Make the Most," *New York Times,* November 7, 1993, p. 1.

3. My claim needs minor qualification. Even in the imagined community, some paternalistic interference might be necessary to protect people from imprudent insurance decisions, particularly when they are young. And some constraints might be necessary to provide adequate resources for later generations.

IMPOSING PERSONAL RESPONSIBILITY FOR HEALTH

Robert Steinbrook

The concept of personal responsibility in health care is that if we follow healthy lifestyles (exercising, maintaining a healthy weight, and not smoking) and are good patients (keeping our appointments, heeding our physicians' advice, and using a hospital emergency department only for emergencies), we will be rewarded by feeling better and spending less money. The details of programs that emphasize personal responsibility, however, are often sketchy, and many difficult questions related to individual freedom and patients' autonomy remain unanswered. For instance, which well-meaning measures to promote responsible behavior actually make a difference, and which are primarily coercive and potentially counterproductive? Which measures may actually improve health or save money, and which may merely shift costs from government, private insurers, or employers to patients?

There are many examples of initiatives that are meant to promote personal responsibility. The World Health Organization will no longer hire persons who smoke, suck, chew, or snuff any tobacco product, although it will still recruit people "who do not have a healthy lifestyle." In the United

States, some employers target smokers, some even going so far as to fire workers who smoke when they are not at work. At some companies, health insurance may cost less for nonsmokers or for people who complete weight-loss programs, and employees may receive financial incentives to participate in health screenings, fitness programs, or tobacco-cessation programs. Wal-Mart has considered discouraging unhealthy people from applying for work by including some physical activity in all jobs. A national survey conducted in July 2006 estimated that 53 percent of Americans think it is "fair" to ask people with unhealthy lifestyles to pay higher insurance premiums and higher deductibles or copayments for their medical care than people with healthy lifestyles.[1] In November 2003, the comparable figure was about 37 percent. A healthy lifestyle was defined as not smoking, frequent exercising, and weight control.

Promoting personal responsibility for health and for obtaining health care is also part of the federal government's "Roadmap to Medicaid Reform." Under the Deficit Reduction Act of 2005, states have increased flexibility in designing and implementing their Medicaid programs, which are jointly financed with the federal government. For example, they can require cost sharing for certain medical services, such as the use of nonpreferred drugs and nonemergency care furnished in a hospital emergency

From *New England Journal of Medicine* 355, no. 8 (August 24, 2006): 753–756. Copyright © 2004 Massachusetts Medical Society. All rights reserved.

department, and can participate in a demonstration program to evaluate the potential effectiveness of Medicaid-funded personal health accounts, which are similar to health savings accounts.[2]

The redesign of the West Virginia Medicaid program has recently become a leading but controversial example of efforts to reward personal responsibility. West Virginia has a population of 1.8 million; as compared with the United States, it has a higher percentage of residents with Medicaid coverage and near-poor or poor incomes (see graphs). In May 2006, the federal government approved the state's plan to provide reduced basic benefits to most healthy children and adults who are eligible for Medicaid

because of low income while allowing them to qualify for enhanced benefits by signing and adhering to a "Medicaid Member Agreement" (see box).[3] The enhanced benefits include all mandatory services as well as additional age-appropriate services that focus on wellness. Examples include diabetes care beyond basic inpatient and outpatient services, cardiac rehabilitation, tobacco-cessation programs, education in nutrition, and chemical-dependency and mental health services. Under the basic plan, prescriptions are limited to four per month; under the enhanced plan, there is no monthly limit. According to Nancy Atkins, the commissioner of the Bureau for Medical Services in the West Virginia Department of Health

Health Insurance Coverage and Income in West Virginia and the United States

Source: Data are for 2003–2004 and are from the Kaiser Commission on Medicaid and the Uninsured.

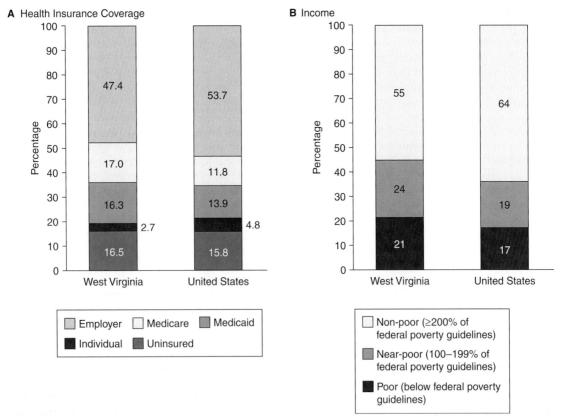

West Virginia Medicaid Member Agreement

This Agreement outlines your Rights and Responsibilities as a person in the West Virginia Medicaid Program. It also is about ways you can work with your doctor and other health care providers to become healthier.

Member Responsibilities

I will follow the requirements of the West Virginia Medicaid program.

I will do my best to stay healthy. I will go to health improvement programs as directed by my medical home.

I will read the booklets and papers my medical home gives me. If I have questions about them, I will ask for help.

I will go to my medical home when I am sick.

I will take my children to their medical home when they are sick.

I will go to my medical home for check-ups.

I will take my children to their medical home for check-ups.

I will take the medicines my health care provider prescribes for me.

I will show up on time when I have my appointments.

I will bring my children to their appointments on time.

I will call the medical home to let them know if I cannot keep my appointments or those for my children.

I will let my medical home know when there has been a change in my address or phone number for myself or my children.

I will use the hospital emergency room only for emergencies.

Member Rights

1. I have the right to pick my medical home. This is where I go for check-ups or when I am sick and where my health care records will be.
2. I have a right to decide things about my health care and the health care of my children. I have a right to see my medical records. I have the right to ask questions about my health care and the health care of my children.
3. I will be treated fairly and with respect. I will get the care and treatment I need as soon as possible. I will not be treated differently because I am in the Medicaid program.
4. I have a right to know about all laws and rules of the Medicaid Program.
5. I can contact Medicaid or my health plan with any question about my health care.
6. I have a right to be sent a written notice when West Virginia Medicaid decides to deny or limit my Medicaid eligibility. I have a right to appeal a decision about my eligibility.
7. I have a right to appeal a decision that says I have not kept the member responsibilities in this agreement.

Member Acknowledgement

The information in this paper has been explained to me and I agree to follow this Medicaid Member Agreement.

and Human Resources, the goals of the redesign are to streamline administration; tailor benefits to specific groups; coordinate care, especially for members with chronic conditions; and "provide members with the opportunity and incentive to maintain and improve their health."

To remain in the enhanced plan, members must keep their medical appointments, receive screenings, take their medications, and follow health improvement plans; West Virginia will monitor "successful compliance with these four responsibilities."[4] Members whose benefits are to be reduced because they have not met these criteria will receive advance notice and have the right to appeal. Those who meet their health goals will receive "credits" that will be placed in a "Healthy Rewards Account" to be used for purchasing services that are not covered by the Medicaid plan. Although details about how these accounts will work and what services will be eligible for purchase are forthcoming, the services might include fitness-club memberships for adults or vouchers for healthful foods for children. In July 2006, transition to the new plan began in three West Virginia counties; the program will eventually include about 160,000 people—or about half the state's Medicaid beneficiaries. Beneficiaries who are 65 years of age or older or who have disabilities will retain their current level of coverage, as will some others, such as children in foster care.

There have been no previous efforts to change Medicaid benefits in the way West Virginia intends to do, nor are there comparable examples among private health insurance programs. Thus, it is difficult to predict the effects, including those on costs, beneficiaries' health, and medical practice. Many specifics are uncertain, including the level of acceptance of the member agreement on the part of Medicaid enrollees and the criteria beneficiaries must meet to remain in the enhanced plan, as well as program regulations and implementation details. Although there is no limit on the number of eligible beneficiaries who can receive the enhanced benefits, the percentage who do receive them will not be known for several years. According to the Washington-based Center on Budget and Policy Priorities, which monitors policies and programs affecting low- and moderate-income Americans, West Virginia's assumption that Medicaid beneficiaries will change their behavior in such a way as to improve their health (and maintain their eligibility for enhanced benefits) as a result of signing a member agreement is "unproven and untested."[5]

There are many reasons why patients might not comply with medical recommendations. These include poor physician–patient communication; side effects of medication; advice that is impractical to follow for reasons that include job responsibilities and difficulties with transportation or child care, psychiatric illness, cost, the complexity of the recommendations, or the language in which they are communicated; and cultural barriers.[6] Patients who may benefit from additional services, such as diabetes care, education in nutrition, or chemical-dependency and mental health services, include many who might have difficulty with compliance, thus increasing the likelihood that they will not be eligible for these services under the West Virginia program. Moreover, as compared with elderly Medicaid beneficiaries and those with disabilities, healthy children and adults are inexpensive to cover. Any savings for these groups could be offset by the costs of administering the changes in Medicaid or by increased costs for mandatory services for patients who remain in the basic plan.[7]

Although personal responsibility for health and for obtaining health care may seem intuitively attractive, the design and implementation of specific insurance initiatives may be complicated. Before such plans are implemented, it would be best to evaluate them rigorously in a controlled trial conducted by an independent group. If they do not improve health or save money, or have unanticipated negative effects, they can be discarded or revised.

NOTES

1. Wall Street Journal Online/Harris Interactive Health-Care Poll. Many Americans back higher costs for people with unhealthy lifestyles. July 19, 2006. (Accessed August 2, 2006, at http://online.wsj.com/article_print/SB115324313567509976.html.)

2. Center for Medicare and Medicaid Services. Roadmap to Medicaid reform: new options to improve and expand insurance coverage for acute care needs. March 31. 2006. (Accessed August 2, 2006, at http://www.cms.hhs.gov/smdl/downloads/Rvacutecare.pdf.)

3. West Virginia's Medicaid State Plan Amendment (SPA) 06-02, approved by the Centers for Medicare & Medicaid Services, Department of Health and Human Services, May 3, 2006. (Accessed August 2, 2006, at http://www.wvdhhr.org/bms/.)

4. Ibid.

5. Solomon J. West Virginia's Medicaid changes unlikely to reduce state costs or improve beneficiaries' health. Washington, D.C.: Center on Budget and Policy Priorities, May 31, 2006. (Accessed August 2, 2006, at http://www.cbpp.org/5-31-06health.htm.)

6. Osterberg L., Blaschke T. Adherence to medication. N Engl J Med 2005; 353:487–97.

7. Solomon, West Virginia's Medicaid changes.

RESPONSIBILITY IN HEALTH CARE: A LIBERAL EGALITARIAN APPROACH

Alexander W. Cappelen and Ole Frithjof Norheim

People make different choices about how to live their lives. These choices also affect their health, the risks they face, and their need for medical treatment in the future. A key question is how considerations of individual responsibility should enter into the design of health care policies. Two issues are of particular importance in this context. First, if the same treatment is given to all patients the total cost of treatment will depend on how people behave. We then need to consider whether, and to what extent, the distribution of the costs of treatment should be related to a patient's behaviour. Secondly, in a situation where the budgets for health care are limited, it is necessary to ration treatment. Another important question is therefore whether the extent to which a disease is a result of individual choices should be allowed to affect the degree to which it is given priority.

Studies from WHO show that most of the leading risk factors contributing to the burden of disease in high income countries can be attributed to unhealthy life styles (table 1). WHO has also estimated that "in the developed countries of North America, Europe and the Asian Pacific, at least one-third of all disease burden is attributable to these five risk factors: tobacco, alcohol, blood pressure, cholesterol and obesity"[1] The idea that individuals must take responsibility for their own health is also an increasingly focused topic in the popular press. Articles on health, fitness, and self-help seem to comprise an increasing proportion of consumer directed feature articles in newspapers.

Holding individuals accountable for their choices in the context of health care is, however, controversial.

From *Journal of Medical Ethics* 31, no. 18 (2005): 476–480. Reproduced with permission from the BMJ Publishing Group Ltd.

Editors' note: Some authors' notes have been cut. Students who want to follow up on sources should consult the original article.

TABLE 1
Leading 10 selected risk factors as percentage causes of disease burden in developed countries measured in disability adjusted life years

Risk factor	% cause of disease burden
Tabacco	12.2
Blood pressure	10.9
Alcohol	9.2
Cholesterol	7.6
Overweight	7.4
Low fruit and vegetable intake	3.9
Physical inactivity	3.3
Illicit drugs	1.8
Unsafe sex	0.8
Iron deficiency	0.7

(*Source:* Modified from World Health Organization, 2002[1])

The aim of this article is to propose a plausible interpretation of liberal egalitarianism with respect to responsibility and health care, and assess it against reasonable counter-arguments.

TWO TYPES OF ARGUMENT FOR THE IMPORTANCE OF RESPONSIBILITY IN HEALTH CARE

What does it mean to hold somebody responsible in the context of health policy? We shall say that any health policy that links either the relative payment for treatment or the extent of treatment to factors that are under an individual's control holds that person responsible.

Generally there are two types of reason why we would want to link treatment or payment to individual behaviour. The first is backwards looking and related to the idea that the distribution of burdens and benefits should be linked to how different individuals contributed to the creation of these burdens and benefits. When applied to health policy this implies that, in order to determine how treatment or the cost of treatment should be distributed, we must ask how the need for treatment arose. More precisely it argues that the extent to which an individual contributed to the need for treatment might be a morally relevant factor. The basic intuition behind this view is that individuals are free to make certain choices about how to live their life and that they should be held responsible for such choices to the extent that they affect their need for treatment. For example, since smoking increases the risk for cancer and cardiovascular disease, people who freely decide to smoke should be held accountable for this choice.

The backward looking responsibility argument has been most important as a reason for not including certain types of treatment in public health care systems. Most people would, for example, agree that the cost of surgical removal of tattoos should be paid by the individual, not by the public. This intuition holds even if the subjective suffering is equal to that associated with disfiguring birthmarks, the removal of which is typically financed by the health service.

The second type of reason is consequentialist and forward looking. Consequentialist normative theories evaluate alternatives by comparing their consequences and the best alternative is simply the one that has the best consequences. Consequentialist arguments are not concerned with what individuals have done, but rather with how they will behave in the future. It links the distribution of costs or treatment to behaviour because it wants to affect future conduct in a certain way by creating incentives or disincentives to certain types of behaviour. Holding individuals responsible for their choices is seen simply as a means to an end.

Many prominent normative theories of distributive justice focus only on the second of these two reasons. For example, the quality of life years approach requires that limited resources are distributed between alternative treatments so as to maximize health outcomes in terms of quality adjusted

life years. Such consequentialist theories are forward looking and exclude all types of backward looking considerations.

The arguments for health promotion in the literature are also based on forward looking or consequentialist normative theories, such as utilitarianism. The idea is that in order to promote health people must face the right incentives. Holding people responsible for their choices with respect to unhealthy life-styles could be justified purely by incentive arguments. Incentive mechanisms are often implemented at population level. Taxes and laws governing conduct can discourage people from smoking and excessive drinking. Governments or insurance plans could cover in full screening programmes such as mammography, smoking cessation programmes, and vaccinations, as well as testing and treatment for sexually transmitted diseases in order to encourage appropriate behavior. Both negative and positive incentives can play a role in health promotion.

The disincentive argument has also been important in the design of effective treatment procedures. Many physicians, as well as national commissions on priorities, argue that patients should be held responsible for actions affecting the effectiveness of treatment. For example, continuous smoking will negatively affect the outcome of coronary bypass surgery as well as surgery for intermittent claudication. Continuous intravenous drug abuse could interfere with the effect of valve replacements because of re-infection. Excessive drinking reduces the chance of organ survival after liver transplantation. Consequently, many doctors argue that they are justified in requiring behavioural change if this is necessary for the treatment to be effective and that they should be allowed to refuse treatment if these requirements are not followed.

The implications of the forward looking and the backward looking perspectives often coincide. Clearly, one way of creating incentives is to link payment or treatment to past behaviour. However, even if the implications of the backward looking and the forward looking arguments sometimes coincide, this is far from always the case, and the difference in justification can hardly be exaggerated. This is easily seen by considering the situation in which there are no incentive effects—that is, where people's behaviour is unaffected by the incentive structure. In such a situation there is no forward looking reason for relating treatment or payment to past behaviour but a backward looking argument could still be relevant. To illustrate, consider a situation where smoking behaviour is unaffected by taxes on tobacco. In such a situation there would be no incentive reason for tobacco taxes, but it could still be argued that those who smoke should pay the expected cost of treatment.

Despite these powerful arguments, individual responsibility is, as we noted in the introduction, in general rejected as an important criterion in the distribution of resources in health care. We agree that there are forceful reasons why individual responsibility has been relegated to the background of political and theoretical arguments about distributive justice in health care. Below we consider two types of argument that justify this state of affairs.

TWO TYPES OF ARGUMENT AGAINST INDIVIDUAL RESPONSIBILITY

It is convenient to distinguish between normative and practical arguments against allowing individual responsibility for health to be an important factor in the distribution of health care. The latter are often as compelling as the former.

Normative Objections

We shall distinguish between three different normative objections to holding individuals accountable. The first is what we will call the 'humanitarian objection'. According to this, we have an obligation to help people who are in real need, regardless of why they are in such a situation, provided that helping is possible and would not impose unacceptable sacrifices on those who provide the help. Consider a man who is a long-term smoker who at age 60 develops coronary heart disease. He now suffers from angina pectoris and is at risk for myocardial infarction, or a stroke. The cardiologist makes further diagnostic tests and tells him he needs a percutaneous coronary intervention. Many think it would be a harsh judgement to deny him the procedure because the disease could be said to be self-inflicted. The humanitarian concern would be even stronger if we assume that the patient has already suffered a myocardial infarction, is in a great deal of pain and

at high risk of dying. Should treatment be denied him? Many would strongly object to this.

The 'liberal objection' is concerned with the collateral effects of denying a person treatment. Even if we could accept inequality in health, there are other types of inequality—for example, political inequality, which we would not accept. Some theorists within the liberal egalitarian tradition argue that giving weight to individual responsibility in the context of health care would violate the liberal principle of equal political and civil rights because persons cannot exercise these rights if their health condition is sufficiently bad. Haavi Morreim suggests that exclusion, or disenrolment, from health insurance plans could be a likely consequence of implementing responsibility. Such a result would be even worse than denial of treatment for a single condition, and would further undermine people's opportunity to exercise their political and civil rights.

Perhaps the most fundamental normative objection is what we could call the 'fairness objection'. This focuses on the fact that the actual consequences of a choice partly depend on factors outside the individual's control. Those who make the same choices may not have the same need for treatment. This could partly be due to different degrees of luck (for example, that the parachute did not open), or different genetic dispositions (for example, a disposition to develop cancer or cardiovascular diseases). If people are forced to pay for their own treatment when the need for it can be said to be self-inflicted, then we are holding individuals responsible for too much.

Practical Objections

The second type of objection holds that, even though individual responsibility for health may be important in principle, introducing such considerations into actual policy is difficult and will create new problems.

The 'informational objection' is concerned with two types of problem. The first is related to asymmetric information about a patient's past behaviour. Typically, the patient knows far more about his or her own past behaviour than the doctor. If this asymmetry is to be corrected there is a danger of jeopardising the physician–patient relationship. The physician providing treatment is the most likely person to enforce the necessary measures for holding patients responsible for the consequences of their actions and to gather information about their past behaviour. For example, denial of care based on this rationale can seriously undermine the physician's identity as caregiver and thus the physician–patient relationship itself. Moreover, the physician being assigned a controlling role might easily intrude on patients' privacy. A second informational problem is related to the fact that information about the relationship between behaviour and the need for treatment is often uncertain, even when information about patients' past behavior is readily available. Although much is known about the relationship between unhealthy life-styles and disease, this is strongly mediated by genetic and environmental factors. Establishing a causal relationship between behaviour and outcomes is difficult for most conditions and it is hard to establish with certainty that a particular type of behaviour is the sole cause of the disease in question.

The objection of "non-neutrality" is concerned with the possibility that only certain types of risky behaviour will be identified as of special concern. What kind of risky behaviour should be identified as of special concern? Why should smokers be "punished" while those who eat too much or exercise too little are not? One such important worry is the possibility of opening up for "moralism". How do we draw the line between "justified" inequalities and "moralistic" judgements about a person's choice or character? A liberal state should be neutral to the ways of life people choose. Identification of those types of behaviour for which people should be held responsible should be determined by the impact on health, but considering the high emotions aroused when tobacco, alcohol, and unsafe sex are debated, there is reason to fear that in practice it is difficult to draw this line.

A LIBERAL EGALITARIAN RESPONSE: HOLDING INDIVIDUALS RESPONSIBLE FOR THEIR CHOICE, NOT FOR THE CONSEQUENCES OF THEIR CHOICE

The arguments outlined above are compelling. However, most of them are aimed at what we believe is a wrong interpretation of what it means to hold people responsible for their choices, namely the view that it implies they should be held accountable for the actual consequences of their choices. Liberal egalitarian theories suggest an alternative interpretation of what it means to hold a person responsible that avoids most of the objections presented above. In order to show this, we give a brief presentation of the main features of liberal egalitarian theories of justice.

The revival of liberal egalitarian theories of justice, and the focus on responsibility in contemporary normative theory, can be traced back to the seminal work by John Rawls.[2] As noted by Thomas Nagel:

> [W]hat Rawls has done is to combine the very strong principles of social and economic equality associated with European socialism with the equally strong principles of pluralistic toleration and personal freedom associated with American liberalism, and he has done so in a theory that traces them to a common foundation. The result is closer in spirit to European social democracy than to any mainstream American political movement.[3]

The link between freedom and individual responsibility has evolved as a central topic in contemporary political theory. Rawls' early contribution—as a critique of what Amartya Sen later labeled welfarism—was to introduce individual responsibility, but only for preferences. Dworkin deepens the critique of welfarism and develops the theory of equality of resources. People are to be held responsible for their ambitions, but not the resources they receive in the social and natural "lottery".[4] Inequalities arising from brute luck in the social and natural lottery should be compensated. If resources are distributed equally, what people do with their resources is irrelevant for a theory of equality. Sen, in his way,[5] and Roemer,[6,7] Cohen,[8] and Arneson[9] have developed fine-tuned versions of the equal opportunity principle where the *equalisandum* is defined as capabilities, advantage, opportunity for welfare, etc.

Liberal egalitarian theories of distributive justice argue that a central goal of public policy should be to secure equal opportunities for all individuals. All equal opportunity approaches argue that society should eliminate inequalities that arise from some, but not all, factors. However, different versions of this approach disagree about which factors are legitimate sources of inequality and which are not.

One prominent position argues that equal opportunity requires that all inequalities that arise from factors outside the agent's control in the social and the natural lottery, such as a person's natural and genetic abilities, should be eliminated, but that inequalities or costs that arise from factors under the agent's control should be accepted.[10] Cohen refers to the factors outside the agent's control as "circumstances" and the factors that are within the person's control as "choice".[11] A liberal egalitarian approach can then be seen as consisting of two parts. First, the liberal principle that people should be held accountable for their choices, what we may call the principle of responsibility, and secondly the egalitarian principle that individuals who make the same choices should also have the same outcomes, what we may call the "principle of equalisation". Applied to the context of health care the principle of equalisation implies that all individuals who make the same choices should be treated as if they were identical with respect to all factors outside their own control—that is, as if they had the same disposition to become sick and faced the same health risks.

It is important to distinguish the liberal egalitarian theory from the liberalist theory. Both are concerned with the equalisation of opportunities, but while liberal egalitarian theories want to eliminate the effect of all factors outside individuals' control, the liberalists are primarily concerned with non-discrimination. Liberals who argue for equal opportunities are mostly concerned about eliminating formal and informal barriers. They are not supporting a substantial positive commitment to securing equal opportunities ("levelling the playing field"). In other words, the liberal argument is more focused on responsibility and only formally interested in equality.[12]

Having said this, we are now in a position to state a common misunderstanding of liberal egalitarianism. The most important misinterpretation is that these theories argue that individuals should be held responsible for the consequences of their choice. In the context of health care this would imply that individuals should be refused treatment (or collectively financed treatment) if they could have avoided the need for treatment by making different choices. However, the principle of responsibility states that individuals should be held responsible for their choices, not for the consequences of their

choices. It is only in the special case where the outcome depends solely on the individual's choices and not on any other factors that this principle implies that individuals should be held responsible for the consequences of their actions. To hold people responsible for the actual consequences of their choice would therefore be to hold them responsible for too much. Some people are lucky and some are unlucky when they engage in risky behaviour. It would be unfair to hold people responsible for differences in luck. Ideally we would therefore want to reward or tax the behaviour as such rather than the consequences of the action. This means that the correct place to introduce responsibility is not at the sick bed or beside the road accident victim.

This interpretation suggests ways in which individual responsibility can be introduced in health care without falling victim to the objections discussed above. Below we present one way of doing this, by levying taxes on certain types of behaviour, and argue that this way of holding individuals responsible would avoid most of the objections presented above.

HOLDING PEOPLE RESPONSIBLE FOR THEIR CHOICES THROUGH TAXES

To see the implications of this view it is useful to take an example. Consider a situation in which physicians and the health care system treat all individuals as equals, regardless of the choices they have made. That is, everyone is given the best available treatment. The question then becomes how we should distribute the costs of treatment between individuals in the economy. Assume furthermore that the need for treatment of a particular disease is proportionally related to the consumption of a particular good (for example, tobacco) and that this good can be taxed. In this situation the implication of the liberal egalitarian theory is straightforward. This theory would, in the absence of an efficient insurance market, want to tax tobacco in order to finance the costs of treatment rather than to require that patients pay for their own treatment. The theory does not determine uniquely how the level of taxes should be decided, but one plausible alternative would be to set the per-unit taxes on tobacco so that the total tax revenues are equal to the additional cost of treatment associated with smoking.

Another implication of the theory is that all smokers should pay the same tax rate independent of their genetic disposition and the expected cost of their treatment. To do otherwise would violate the principle that all individuals who make the same choice should also face the same costs.

Let us now examine how this way of introducing individual responsibility avoids the objections discussed above. The first point to note is that holding people responsible for choices through taxes will not violate humanitarian concerns. No patients would be denied diagnostics or treatment because of their choices. Of course the tax burden imposed on each person ex ante (at the point of choice) could be considered as inhumanitarian if it imposes an extremely high tax. However, the range of taxes implemented in most cases would probably not invoke such an objection. Secondly, this policy would avoid the liberal objection since everyone who becomes sick is treated and taxes on tobacco will not, unless excessively high, restrict the set of health related opportunities. Rather, it secures that other people's opportunity sets remain unrestricted by the smoker's choice.

Most importantly, the liberal egalitarian theory avoids the fairness objection since the whole point of the tax is to eliminate the effect of factors outside the control of the agent. Individuals with different luck or with a different disposition to become sick are given the same treatment and face the same taxes. The fairness objection is directed against the liberalist interpretation of responsibility that holds individuals responsible for the actual consequences of their choices.

The tax policy also avoids objections based on practice-ability. Tax policies will not, and this is important, undermine the physician–patient relationship. Physicians are not assigned the role of holding people responsible for their choices. Many (but not all) choices regarding life-style involve "consumption" of various types of goods, such as cigarettes, alcohol, food (including salt), organised sport, or exercise, etc. Taxes or tax deductions can easily be attached to the consumption of these goods and need not involve any active role for physicians or providers.

Furthermore, the rejection of responsibility based on the argument that we do not know whether there is a direct connection between a patient's condition

and his or her choice of life-style does not undermine the liberal egalitarian approach. Holding people responsible for their choices is justified if one can demonstrate that a particular choice is likely to impose a higher risk on that person when compared with another person who is equal in all other relevant aspects.

The use of the tax mechanism would not eliminate the problem of non-neutrality. It will still be possible to use the responsibility argument as a way of introducing "moralistic" judgement. However, it is likely to reduce this problem because tax policies will typically be decided through democratic procedures and not by individuals in the health care system.

DISCUSSION

Even if we believe that the liberal egalitarian response answers many of the objections, there are still problems with this approach. A fundamental— and remaining—issue is the informational problem of drawing the precise cut between those factors that are under a person's control and those that are outside it. New genetic knowledge might clarify which risk factors are attributable to choice and which are not. We therefore believe that as we obtain more genetic information on susceptibility, the understanding of individual responsibility within liberal egalitarianism could become increasingly more important.

Moreover, people have different probabilities of becoming a smoker or an alcoholic depending on family background, social class, etc. It is well documented that not only is unhealthy behaviour statistically more likely among people who are poor, but also that people with lower socioeconomic status on average have inferior health. This suggests that it can be misleading to view unhealthy behaviour as freely chosen (see Roemer for a good discussion on this point[13]).

Another unresolved issue is that not all types of behaviour can be associated with a taxable product. It is relatively easy to levy taxes on consumer goods, but how should we tax choices such as exercising too little or having unsafe sex? Although it is possible to assign tax exemptions to membership of fitness clubs, on condoms etc., we acknowledge the problem that not all unhealthy life-style choices can be handled in the same way.

In this article we have focused on the liberal egalitarian argument for holding individuals responsible for their choices. This must, of course, be combined with the incentive argument. We have ignored the incentive argument in most of our discussion in order to focus on the backward looking arguments for holding individuals responsible. Even if people's behaviour is totally unaffected by the existence of taxes, in which case there is no incentive argument for taxes, we still contend that justice requires that smokers or others who make risky choices should contribute more to the financing of health care.

REFERENCES

1. World Health organization. *The world health report: reducing risks, promoting healthy life*. Geneva: WHO, 2002.

2. Rawls J. *A theory of justice*. Cambridge, MA: Belknap Press of Harvard University Press, 1971.

3. Nagel T. *Concealment and exposure and other essays*. Cambridge, MA: Oxford University Press, 2002.

4. Dworkin R. What is equality? Part 2: Equality of resources. *Philosophy and Public Affairs* 1981; 10: 283–345.

5. Sen AK. *Inequality reexamined*. Oxford: Clarendon Press, 1992.

6. Roemer J. A pragmatic theory of responsibility for the egalitarian planner. *Philosophy and Public Affairs* 1993; 22: 146–66.

7. Roemer J. *Equality of opportunity*. Cambridge, MA: Harvard University Press, 1998.

8. Cohen GA. On the currency of egalitarian justice. *Ethics* 1989; 99: 906–44.

9. Arneson R. Equality and equal opportunity for welfare. *Philosophical Studies* 1989; 56: 159–94.

10. Buchanan A, Brock D, Daniels N, et al. *From chance to choice. Genetics and justice*. Cambridge, MA: Oxford University Press, 2002.

11. Cohen, On the currency of egalitarian justice.

12. Buchanan, Brock, Daniels, et al., *From chance to choice*.

13. Roemer, *Equality of opportunity*.

LAST-CHANCE THERAPIES AND MANAGED CARE: PLURALISM, FAIR PROCEDURES, AND LEGITIMACY

Norman Daniels and James Sabin

I. COVERAGE FOR UNPROVEN LAST-CHANCE THERAPIES

The most difficult and explosive responsibility for any health care system is deciding whether patients with life-threatening illnesses will receive insurance coverage for unproven treatments they believe may make the difference between life and death.

Potentially life-saving treatments with proven efficacy and safety (proven net benefit) and quack treatments for which there is no scientific rationale, rarely pose major problems about insurance coverage.

In a country as wealthy as the United States, effective last-chance treatments without alternatives generally are and should be covered virtually all the time. When shared resources from cooperative schemes are involved, as in public or private insurance, rather than individuals paying with their own resources, quack treatments will and should virtually never be covered, even if the patient or doctor passionately believe in the purported cure.

The difficult practical and ethical challenges come from promising but unproven last-chance treatments, for which we use high-dose chemotherapy with autologous bone marrow transplant (ABMT) for advanced breast cancer as our key example.[1] Not covering treatments that ultimately prove to be effective lets curable patients die prematurely, and even

From *Hastings Center Report* 28, no. 2 (1998): 27–41. Reprinted by permission of The Hastings Center.

if a treatment ultimately proves to be ineffective, not covering it may create the impression that critically ill patients are being abandoned in their moment of need. Covering treatments that ultimately prove to be ineffective or harmful reduces the quantity and quality of the patient's remaining life, wastes substantial resources, and undermines clinical research. These are the moral stakes in the decision.

There are also other costs and risks in these decisions. Denials of coverage for seriously ill people are highly visible. Even health plans that use impeccable science and patient-centered deliberation while trying to hold the traditional, contractually-specified line against unproven therapies risk horrendous publicity, expensive litigation, and legislative mandates requiring coverage.

We shall later see (in Section II) that there is room for reasonable people to disagree about how to weigh the conflicting values and principles in these cases. There is no convincing, principled argument or social consensus for determining the relative importance of (1) giving some (how much?) priority to meeting the *urgent claims* of patients in last-chance situations, (2) providing *stewardship* of collective resources, (3) producing the public good of *scientific knowledge* about the effectiveness of unproven therapies, and (4) respecting *patient autonomy* through collaborative decision making about risks and benefits.

We can try to gloss over the ethical uncertainties in these cases by pretending that terms like "investigational," "experimental," and "medical necessity" tell us what to do. These terms, however, explain little and dodge the genuine ethical dilemmas. Without extensive explanation of the reasoning process they will not—and should not—satisfy the public or the courts. The ethical challenges posed by unproven but promising last-chance technologies are not helped at all by the language of current medical insurance benefit contracts. They are also made harder to solve by the climate of distrust that surrounds insurers, including managed care organizations (MCOs) of all types. Why should the public accept as *legitimate* decisions made by MCOs that limit access to "unproven" last-chance therapies, especially if some responsible clinicians and their patients believe them to be effective?

In a three-year research project involving collaboration with a number of leading managed care organizations, we have been investigating, through a series of policy case studies, how insurers and health plans make coverage decisions about the adoption and application of new technologies.[2] In this policy discussion, we report on some very promising "exemplary practices" we have observed for managing last-chance therapies. We believe it would be premature to try to choose among these "exemplary practices." Because of the deep moral disagreement about the underlying issues, it would be wise for society to experiment with several promising strategies in order to learn more over time about how well they work and how morally acceptable they seem in light of actual practice.

Before describing the moral disagreement in more detail in Section III, we shall begin with some background about the scientific and societal context in which the practices we describe have been developed. In Section IV, we describe the "exemplary practices" in more detail, showing how the differences among them might be mapped onto different moral views about the weight we should assign various relevant considerations. In Section V, we return to the issue of the legitimacy of MCO decisions, suggesting how some of these practices could meet more general conditions for establishing legitimacy. In Section VI, we discuss a consequence of our view that we should experiment with a variety of fair procedures, namely that we may have to learn to tolerate what looks like violations of a formal requirement of justice. Finally, in the concluding section, we suggest ways in which the different "exemplary practices" can provide valuable lessons about coming to grips with limits in the domain of health care.

II.   A BRIEF SOCIAL HISTORY

By 1989, and definitely by 1990, patients with advanced breast cancer, with the support of some clinicians, began to seek coverage for admittedly experimental use of ABMT from MCOs, including our collaborating sites. Analogues to this treatment had proven effective for some lymphatic cancers, and there was some scientific rationale for extending the treatment to solid tumors. Despite the enthusiasm of the clinicians, and the desperate belief of the breast cancer patients, many of whom were well-organized and informed, there was at the time no hard clinical evidence, and especially no controlled trials, that showed an advantage to the risky treatment over standard treatments.

During this period in the early 1990s, technology assessment of the therapy was undertaken at a number of our collaborating MCOs and by the Medical Advisory Panel (MAP) of the Blue Cross/ Blue Shield (BC/BS) Technology Evaluation Center (TEC).[3] The National Cancer Institute authorized four randomized clinical trials for ABMT in advanced breast cancer in 1991 (with support from TEC), but these results would not be available for some time. There were no published controlled clinical trials until the Bezwoda et al. study in 1995.[4] Early evaluations of this technology had to be based on weaker forms of evidence. Between 1991 and 1994, several MCOs (as well as the Oregon Health Services Commission) decided that the technology was not ready for standard coverage, based on this early evidence regarding safety and efficacy. (As early as 1990, one of our collaborating sites, Health Partners, provided coverage under "alternative funding" for participation in clinical trials.) Similarly, early evaluations by the MAP found that there was inadequate evidence of efficacy or net benefit for ABMT for advanced breast cancer.

It was not until February 1996 that the BC/BS Medical Advisory Panel (MAP) finally decided that the therapy did meet its criteria for status as a non-investigational technology. At its February 1996 meeting, the MAP evaluated evidence from the only published study of a randomized clinical trial (Bezwoda et al. 1995), as well as evidence from ongoing studies. The discussion suggested that the published study could not support conclusions about the greater efficacy of the therapy over standard treatments used in the U.S., but the MAP voted that its criteria were met.[5] A consideration of the identical evidence in June 1996 by California State Blue Shield led to the decision that the MAP criteria were not yet satisfied.[6] Several MCOs that had undertaken similar technology assessments also continued to believe, as of mid-1996, that there was insufficient evidence to show that the therapy met reasonable criteria of safety and efficacy for advanced breast cancer in comparison to standard treatments—even if it had by then become nearly "standard" therapy.

Like HIV patients desperate to try "promising" drugs prior to full FDA testing, however, breast cancer patients in the early 1990s demanded that they be allowed to decide whether the risks were worth taking.[7] The "gatekeeper" here, however, was not the FDA, charged with keeping unsafe pharmaceuticals off the market, but insurers, who, by contract, had no obligation to provide coverage for "investigational" treatments. When some MCOs, with adequate, evidence-based reason on their side, insisted the therapy was still "investigational" and "unproven," and might even prove worse than standard therapies, patients pursued both litigation and legislation, and the media "exposed" the denials. As early as 1991, *60 Minutes* featured a story about Aetna declining coverage for ABMT for breast cancer. In California in 1993, the estate of Nelene Fox won an $89 million suit against Health Net, which had originally denied coverage, then provided it. The suit charged the delay cost Fox her life. This suit cast a pall over traditional procedures for assessing the status of last-chance therapies.

Throughout the early 1990s, many insurers were providing coverage for patients participating in approved clinical trials. Unfortunately, this coverage seemed "arbitrary and capricious" according to an important study in the *New England Journal of Medicine*, which said coverage was not correlated with pretreatment clinical characteristics of the patients, the design or phase of the study, or the response to induction therapy.[8] That study showed that as many as three out of four patients seeking coverage for participation in a trial were granted it, and another half of those who threatened legal action when initially denied also received coverage. Activism clearly paid off for patients seeking treatment.

Responding to well-organized and highly visible advocates for these women, some state legislatures mandated coverage as early as 1994 and 1995, despite protests, for example in Minnesota and Massachusetts, that the mandates would make it impossible to continue proper clinical trials aimed at finding out if the procedure was truly superior to standard therapy. In other states, though legislative mandates were not passed, lawsuits in effect compelled coverage, since large punitive damages were imposed where coverage was denied or delayed. The resulting legal climate made it too risky and costly to deny what was still an unproven therapy.

Some insurers responded earlier than others to the handwriting on the wall, reading the message that traditional efforts to manage last-chance therapies by "holding the line" against investigational treatments were not working. Following the *60 Minutes* expose in 1991, Aetna, under the initiative of William McGivney, introduced a procedure in which an independent panel would be invoked when patients wanted a last-chance treatment that internal review denied coverage for (see Section IV for more detailed discussion). The same approach was adopted by Kaiser of Northern California in 1993. Other approaches were introduced in the same period, including Oregon Blue Cross Blue Shield's (1994) use of a transplant coordinator to manage the coverage of clinical trials for unproven last-chance therapies. In 1996, Health Partners introduced a special process for evaluating "promising therapies" that fall in the space between clearly investigational and standard treatment. It is this "new wave" of approaches that is the focus of our discussion in subsequent sections.

Before turning to the details of these newer approaches, we want to make three points. First, the social climate—including well-organized women's groups, a crusading media, committed practitioners, suspicious courts, and opportunistic legislators—clearly made the standard "technology assessment" approach to holding the line against coverage for last-chance "investigational" therapies untenable. Second, the legal and political interventions also had the effect of making it more difficult to find out if high-dose chemotherapy with stem cell support actually worked for advanced breast cancer. Although some MCOs decided to provide coverage for clinical trials, others (for example Harvard Community Health Plan, in an evaluation just before the Massachusetts mandate in 1994) were ethically uneasy about insisting on participation in trials, where patients would not always get the experimental regimen. The effect of compelling coverage meant that enrollment in NIH sponsored clinical trials was slowed. The public intervention through the courts and legislatures thus had the effect of frustrating another publicly supported goal in health care, namely, to make the system more efficient by pushing it to adopt "outcomes-based" medicine.

Third, the challenge to limit-setting by MCOs has its international analogues in publicly administered and financed health care systems that offer universal coverage. Even where public agencies

might be thought to be a more "legitimate" locus for limit-setting decisions, a similar moral challenge is made. The suggestion is that "bureaucratic" decisions driven too much by "budget limitations" ignore the fact of urgent need in these cases, that is, that the moral priorities of decision makers are inappropriate. It would take us too far afield to discuss the similarities and differences between these cases (e.g., in England, Norway, and New Zealand) and those in the U.S., but it is important to see that the moral dimension of these issues arises across differences in institutional design, financing, national culture, and even incentives. We return to this issue briefly in Section V.

III.   MORAL DISAGREEMENT AND ACCESS TO LAST-CHANCE THERAPIES

Reasonable people disagree about the best way to manage access to last-chance therapies because they disagree about the relative importance of several values or principles that come into conflict in these cases. In a pluralist society, where the underlying disagreement may involve conflicts among more comprehensive and systematic moral views, this means there is no one way of managing last-chance therapies that all agree is morally superior. In effect, we may have to learn to live with alternative best practices, not agreement on one approach, even if, as we shall see in Section V, this raises a challenge to one aspect of our traditional thinking about fairness and justice.

The general and difficult moral problem that all health plans must solve is how to meet the diverse needs of the insured population under reasonable resource constraints. This problem involves balancing population-centered concerns against patient-centered ones. Promising but unproven last-chance treatments evoke the general problem especially sharply since so much is at stake for the individual patients while at the same time the proposed treatments are often quite costly.

The major population-centered concerns are the prudent use of shared resources ("stewardship") and the promotion of public goods, such as knowledge about safety and efficacy produced through clinical trials. Those who emphasize these concerns will prefer policies under which collective resources would only be used for last-chance treatments that meet a threshold of established net benefit, and unproven therapies, if paid for at all, would only be covered in the context of controlled clinical trials, including randomized controlled trials in which a patient might receive a placebo or the standard treatment.

The key patient-centered concerns include: giving proper attention to patient needs, especially urgent needs as in the last-chance situations; avoiding harm, including the psychological harm that can arise from adversarialism; and managing uncertainties and risks through collaborative treatment planning. Those who emphasize these concerns will prefer policies for last-chance treatments that create a much lower standard of evidence that must be met for a treatment to be offered to a patient and that allow patients and their clinicians more leeway in judging the relative weight of risks and benefits. They are less likely to promote policies that would require patients to enter controlled trials, since they have no assurance in those trials of receiving the desired treatment.

Reasonable people will differ, however, in the degree to which they want to trade population-centered values in favor of patient-centered ones because of the urgency of the situation. There is no higher-level agreement on how much weight to give to the competing values or principles. Careful deliberation may resolve some of the conflicts, for often our views are not systematically considered, but it is unlikely to eliminate all of them. In many cases, the disagreement about weights may reflect significant differences in comprehensive moral views that people hold. For example, some "communitarians" will give more weight to guardianship of collective resources and the maximization of health benefits for a community that is cooperating to share resources. Classic liberals will give more weight to respect for individual autonomy. "Communitarians" and "liberals" will recognize the relevance of the reasons to which the other gives priority, since in other contexts, these factors also count as reasons for them in their thinking about how to solve the general problem of meeting needs under resource constraints. But the disagreement about weights or priorities will probably persist.

This disagreement about weights will then lead people to have different views about the acceptability of different ways of managing last-chance therapies. In the next section, we draw on our empirical study of decision making about coverage in MCOs to describe in more detail a set of "exemplary practices" regarding promising but unproven last-chance therapies. Our point is to show how they can be thought to reflect these different judgments about how to weigh competing values. We do not try to show that any one is best, since we know of no persuasive argument to that conclusion. Rather, we present each as a reasonable, good-faith effort to solve the problem.

IV. SOME EXEMPLARY PRACTICES IN MANAGING LAST-CHANCE THERAPIES

We begin with the earliest approach to managing last-chance therapies, the terminal illness program William McGivney started at Aetna in 1991. This program, used primarily in an indemnity insurance context, served as Aetna's *modus operandi* until the end of 1996 after Aetna purchased and merged with U.S. Healthcare. It was later adapted for use in an MCO setting by Northern California Kaiser Permanente and eventually became the model for the 1996 Friedman-Knowles legislation in California.

In the Aetna program, when medical directors in the field received a request for an unproven but promising last-chance cancer treatment that was not covered under established company policy, they referred the request to the home office at Hartford, where a consulting oncologist reviewed the clinical situation. A key feature of the program was that the home-office oncologist was only empowered to *approve* requests. If the consulting oncologist believed the request did not represent reasonable clinical practice for the particular patient, the case was automatically referred outside the company for independent review by the Medical Care Ombudsman Program in Bethesda, Maryland.

The Ombudsman Program, which was founded by Grace Monaco in 1991, provides independent expert opinion about appropriate treatment in serious but ambiguous clinical situations. On a timetable which can be as short as 24 hours, the Ombudsman

Program will put together a panel of 2–3 experts with no affiliation to the insurer or the provider of the proposed treatment, to assess whether the proposed treatment has any scientific rationale for the particular patient. This is not a technology assessment of the new technology but an expert clinical assessment of the *potential value of the technology for a particular patient*. Typically, at least one of the experts is prepared to testify in court if the case should come to litigation.

Aetna did not restrict its own consulting oncologist from rendering negative coverage decisions because the consultant lacked competence. Any time that specialized technical expertise was needed, Aetna could have hired additional consultants at less cost to itself than using the Ombudsman Program. The problem Aetna was trying to solve with its terminal illness program was one of *trust*, not lack of technical expertise. The fact and appearance of "conflict of interest" was removed: if Aetna would say no only if an independent consultant said no, then the "no" should not be construed as a cost-driven decision. In circumstances of life-threatening illness and ambiguous information, the patient's trust in the decision-making process can be the difference between peace and outrage, or acceptance versus litigation.

In 1993, the Northern California region of Kaiser Permanente took the program that Aetna had developed in a primarily *indemnity* insurance context and adapted it for its own 3600 physician *prepaid group practice HMO*. Kaiser's experience helps us understand the mechanism through which Aetna's innovative way of addressing the patient's concern about the insurer's potential conflict of interest helps the decision-making process.[9]

Like Aetna, Northern California Kaiser Permanente decided to let patients in last-chance situations know that they could go outside of Kaiser for an independent opinion from the Ombudsman Program if they were not satisfied with the internal decision-making process. This was a controversial step for Kaiser to take. Some Kaiser doctors worried that allowing automatic appeal outside the HMO would diminish the group's ability to manage care rationally and feared that the program itself might be very costly.

What actually happened was exactly the opposite of what was feared. From 1994–1996, only 6 of the 2.5 million northern California members asked for referral to the Ombudsman program. When the patients' concerns about insurer trustworthiness and potential conflict of interest were addressed in advance by the option of going outside of Kaiser for independent consultation, patients and families were much readier to enter into a reflective dialogue with their Kaiser physicians about what treatment approach really made sense for them.

The Aetna-Kaiser "last-chance" policy might simply be dismissed as a cost-benefit calculation made by the MCO. Put cynically, it is better to pay for a few treatments than face lawsuits, any one of which would be more costly than a bunch of treatments. But it also can be defended—and is by some MCOs that adopt it—on more explicitly moral grounds that connect its adoption with our earlier discussion.

The policy can be defended morally in this way. It recognizes the fundamental importance in a medical system of "shared decision making" between patients and clinicians about risk taking. If an unproven last-chance therapy is viewed by some acknowledged experts as the most appropriate treatment for the patient, and if the patient understands the risks as presented by parties on all sides, then organizations have no better option than to rely on the informed decision of the patient and her clinician. This is not the same as saying that a patient can be granted just any last wish regarding treatment: there must be some basis in evidence and expert view that the therapy is not quackery. In the external review model, that expert view is provided by the independent panel. Under those conditions, simply refusing to provide coverage fails to acknowledge the obligation not to impose paternalistically a plan's own judgment about acceptable risks and benefits on the choices of desperately ill patients with few options. To be sure, the role of the MCO as a guardian of shared resources is reduced, but this is defensible in light of both the urgency of the patients' needs, and the special importance, in light of the uncertainty and the severity of need, of promoting a climate of shared decision making. Indeed, a proponent of this view might even say that the decision to hold to a hard-line denial is so likely to lead to a waste of resources in the legal and political climate that actually surrounds MCOs that the more efficient way to respect resources is to adopt the more lenient strategy toward last-chance therapies.

The Aetna-Kaiser approach has been embodied in new legislation. Under the Friedman-Knowles Experimental Treatment Act, passed by the California legislature in 1996, the kind of independent consultation process that Aetna and Kaiser Northern California have piloted will become mandatory for all California insurers starting July 1, 1998. The provisions of the bill are quite detailed, but the basic concept is simple. If a patient with a condition that has no effective therapy and is likely to cause death within two years is denied coverage for a new treatment that has some scientific promise, an independent expert review of the decision must be offered.

What is so important about the Friedman-Knowles bill is the effort to use legislation to influence the quality of the decision-making process without making any attempt to mandate what the decisions themselves should be. The bill does not mandate any specific treatments as so many states have done and continue to do. Rather, it mandates an organizational decision-making process designed to reduce fears about conflict of interest and increase deliberative reflection and clarity about the reasons for coverage decisions. (We note that in August 1997, the California Legislature considered legislation that takes a step backwards—toward mandating coverage for ABMT for breast cancer. Some proponents of the legislation say it eliminates "inequities" in coverage, since state employee benefits mandate ABMT but other insurers do not, an issue we return to in Section VI; critics say the state should not be making these disease-specific sorts of coverage decisions.)

Oregon Blue Cross Blue Shield has developed an approach to unproven bone marrow transplant regimens that reflects a slightly different moral framework. In 1993, in the aftermath of the *Fox* v. *Health Net* case, Oregon Blue Cross Blue Shield created a new, full-time role of transplant coordinator. The transplant coordinator is a clinically experienced nurse whose job is to work directly with patients and families, transplant programs, employers, and the Oregon Blue Cross Blue Shield benefit systems to create mutually satisfactory individualized treatment plans.

Whereas Aetna and Kaiser use the option for independent review outside of the organization to allay patient concerns about conflict of interest and promote collaboration, Oregon Blue Cross Blue Shield's distinctive approach is an unusually open and accountable process of deliberation and reason-giving and an especially strong emphasis on supporting scientific treatment evaluation. Instead of the infamous "gag rule," the Oregon program has developed what might be called a "let's talk it over openly and at great length rule!"

In ethics classes at medical, nursing, and business schools we try to teach students to identify the key facts and values in a situation and to develop options to advance the most important values that apply. This is what the Blue Cross transplant coordinator does every day, except she does it in circumstances of time pressure and high emotion, not in a classroom. When we interviewed her for our research project, we told her that her role seemed to be $1/3$ nurse clinician, $1/3$ nurse manager, and $1/3$ ethics professor.

Here are the kinds of things the transplant coordinator says in dealing with the multiple stakeholders in the decision-making process:

- To a confused and frightened patient: "Do you have this article about the treatment? Have you read this other one? I'm going to be at the library this afternoon—why don't you come and meet me there and we can go over the information together?"
- To explain the importance of consistency to a wealthy patient: "Just because you're a VIP who lives in the West Hills, you don't really want to make me treat you any differently than the person who comes to clean your house, do you?"
- To an employer who wants Blue Cross to cover an employee for a treatment that has no scientific justification: "But it's not based on sound science. Do you want to do the same thing for all the other women in your employee group? And even if you do, what will you tell their sisters who can't have the treatment? We want to be able to support scientific research that's going to answer the question."
- And, to a provider who is asking the insurer to cover an unproven treatment: "Then build your case to us, make your proposal so that when we make this decision, we can have sound rationale for a similar case on the next patient that you or someone else may send to us."

These comments illustrate the kind of deliberative dialogue that will have to happen hundreds of thousands and perhaps millions of times for doctors, patients, health plans, and society to move along a learning curve towards a more patient-centered, cost-effective, and ethical health care system.

The Oregon Blue Cross process, like the Aetna-Kaiser, places its ultimate emphasis on encouraging open deliberation between patient, clinician, and, in this case, coordinator. When we asked the coordinator how she was able to achieve trust with patients without the promise of an external, independent review, as in the Aetna-Kaiser approach, she said that she would view an instance of a patient going to external review as a failure on her part to have engaged the patient in the kind of deliberative give and take that her approach requires. The promise of external review, she feared, could lure patients away from the need to engage in deliberation with her.

Although deliberation and shared decision making were the key goals, Oregon Blue Cross Blue Shield has another priority as well—supporting clinically important research. If a promising but unproven last-chance treatment is available in a scientifically valid clinical trial, the plan will cover it. The coordinator claimed that as of our visit in June, 1996, no patients had resorted to litigation, and a significant number decided that the unproven treatments they initially requested were, after careful thinking, not really what they wanted.

In contrast to the Aetna-Kaiser approach, Oregon Blue Cross Blue Shield appears to put more emphasis on redirecting its stewardship responsibility toward supporting research. At the same time, since outright denial of unproven therapies was much less likely than in a traditional "hold the line" approach, it became possible to involve the patient in shared decision making.

In 1996, Health Partners, a prominent HMO in Minnesota, began to develop a special policy regarding "promising" but still unproven therapies. For selected "promising treatments," Health Partners will provide coverage even though the technology still falls into the category of "investigational" and would traditionally be excluded from coverage by contract language. The rationale for singling out the category of "promising treatments" is to introduce consistent policy about a particular technology, thereby avoiding case-by-case responses to individual requests.

Although this approach clearly relaxes the traditional hard line about stewardship, it keeps the health plan in control of what counts as "promising." Compared to the case-by-case decision-making by Aetna, Kaiser of Northern California, and Oregon Blue Cross Blue Shield, the Health Partners approach appears to place more emphasis on the organization's stewardship role. It remains to be seen whether the approach of offering greater consistency technology-by-technology at the cost of less flexibility in deciding individual cases leads to more or less conflict and litigation.

V.   LEGITIMACY AND FAIRNESS

MCOs operate in a social climate of distrust. The vigorous effort at cost containment initiated by large employers (and the government) has largely been invisible to the public. Instead, managed care organizations have taken the heat for cost containment and system change. In this climate of distrust, the issue of legitimacy arises in a sharp form: why should patients or clinicians who think they are being denied medically appropriate treatments, even unproven last-chance therapies, accept as legitimate the decisions of MCOs? More to the point, under what conditions should the public come to view these decisions as legitimate?

Elsewhere,[10] we have argued that if the following four conditions were met, MCOs would take a large step toward earning legitimacy, at least over time:

1. Decisions regarding coverage for new technologies (and other limit-setting decisions) and their rationales must be publicly accessible.
2. The rationales for coverage decisions should aim to provide a *reasonable* construal of how the organization should provide "value for money" in meeting the varied health needs of a defined population under reasonable resource constraints. Specifically, a construal will be "reasonable" if it appeals to reasons and principles that are accepted as relevant by people who are disposed to finding terms of cooperation that are mutually justifiable.
3. There is a mechanism for challenge and dispute resolution regarding limit-setting decisions, including the opportunity for revising decisions in light of further evidence or arguments.

4. There is either voluntary or public regulation of the process to ensure that conditions 1–3 are met.

These four conditions capture at least the central necessary elements of a solution to the legitimacy and fairness problems for coverage decisions about new treatments. Condition 1 requires openness or publicity, that is, clarity about the reasons for decisions. Condition 2 involves some constraints on the kinds of reasons that can play a role in the rationale: it recognizes the fundamental interest all parties have to finding a justification all can accept as reasonable. Conditions 3 and 4 provide mechanisms for connecting deliberation and decisions within MCOs to a broader deliberative process, that is, for making them accountable to the results of a wider deliberation about what fairness requires.[11]

The procedures for managing last-chance therapies discussed in the previous section can meet these conditions. The first point to note is that the rationale for a plan's adopting one procedure rather than another should itself be made public, as Condition 1 requires. In such a rationale, giving more weight to responsibility for stewardship (as perhaps in the "promising-therapy" strategy) than another strategy does is the type of reason that meets Condition 2; so does the opposite weighting. Our main point in the discussion in the previous section is that each of the exemplary strategies could be defended publicly with reasons that meet these legitimacy conditions. What varies among these procedures is not the appeal to inappropriate reasons but the different weights reasonable people might give to relevant reasons.

In their implementation, any of these procedures should meet the conditions as well. For example, in the procedure followed by Oregon Blue Cross Blue Shield in managing patients who may be left out of available clinical trials, there is an effort to engage the patient in reason-giving of exactly the sort required by Condition 2. Similarly, the results of previous deliberations about particular cases could be made publicly available (still respecting confidentiality), so they were accessible to other patients seeking to develop claims about coverage in their cases. In effect, a kind of case law should emerge that governs the operation of the MCO and is accessible to patients and clinicians. Similarly, the kind of deliberation engaged in by the external ombudsman

program used by Aetna and Kaiser, and now mandated by California law, could also meet the publicity conditions and the restrictions on types of reason-giving.

We noted earlier that the legitimacy problem in the U.S. has its analogue in publicly administered systems. In other countries, even where public commissions have been established to approve "principles" for priority-setting and limit-setting in those systems, the agencies that make actual decisions often keep their results quiet, perhaps implicit in quietly made budget decisions, and fail to meet the conditions we articulate. We believe compliance with these conditions would contribute to establishing greater legitimacy for hard choices made in those systems as well.

VI. FORMAL VS. PROCEDURAL JUSTICE

There may not be just one best or fairest way to manage last-chance therapies. At least, reasonable people may not agree on what the best procedure is, and in light of that disagreement, we should experiment with a family of "best practices," or so we have argued. There is a troubling implication of this view that some may view as a fatal objection. We see it not as a flaw in our approach but as a manifestation of an unavoidable moral uncertainty, which we must learn to respect and to live with.

Here is the problem. Suppose we have two patients, Groucho and Harpo, who are indistinguishable with regard to the relevant features of their cases. Both make the same claim that they need a particular high-dose chemotherapy with stem cell support for their advanced cancers. Let us suppose that this treatment has not yet been shown to provide a net benefit for the condition, which is in any case fatal on standard treatments. Groucho belongs to BestHealth and Harpo to GreatCare, two responsible MCOs that manage last-chance therapies in different ways. For the sake of specificity, suppose BestHealth uses a version of the external appeal procedure (like Aetna or Kaiser) and that GreatCare covers people in clinical trials if they meet the protocols or can make a reasonable case that they should be so covered (like Oregon Blue Cross Blue Shield). Suppose finally that Groucho is denied the transplant but that Harpo is given it. When Groucho hears about Harpo, should we agree if he complains that one of them has been treated unfairly?

Groucho claims that a fundamental principle of justice has been violated, the *formal* principle that like cases be treated similarly. If his case is just like Harpo's in all relevant ways, then they should either both get the treatment or neither should. The formal principle does not tell us how both should be treated, only that they should be treated similarly. Specifically, if there are *reasons* why Harpo should get the treatment, Groucho insists, then they apply equally to him, and he should receive it as well.

Groucho's complaint that a formal principle of justice is violated actually turns on there being a substantive reason or principle that grounds the decision to treat Harpo. To see this point, consider this variation on the case: in both MCOs, a coin is flipped about whether to give the treatment. Groucho loses and Harpo wins. When Groucho complains that like cases are being treated dissimilarly, we can now say to him, "The cases are unlike: there was a coin toss, and you lost and he won." There is no violation of the formal principle if there is a non-reason-based procedure used to distinguish the cases, as there is in the case of a coin toss. Alternatively, we can construe this as a case in which a principle is appealed to and uniformly applied, namely the principle that winners but not losers of coin-tosses (or other random processes) will get the treatment.

Neither BestHealth nor GreatCare flips coins, however. Within their different procedures, each encourages the giving of reasons and the deliberation about cases in light of reasons. We presuppose that the difference in their procedures for managing these cases rests on a difference in the ways the two organizations weight certain values, i.e., the values of urgency, stewardship, and shared decision-making with patients. Suppose further that we are right to claim there is no argument we all can accept that shows that one weighting (and thus one procedure) is clearly morally more justifiable than the other. That weighting, and thus the choice of fair procedure, is itself the focus of reasonable disagreement.

Generally, when there is a violation of the formal principle of justice, we are challenged to evaluate the weight attributed to a reason or principle that was applied in one case but not the other. We are asked to find a difference in the cases, that is, to show that they were not really similar in all relevant ways, or to affirm the uniform application of that reason or principle or of some alternative principle. But in the condition of moral pluralism we face, we have no candidate principle that purports to enjoy "our" endorsement independently of the fair procedure we are employing. A reason that may seem compelling or decisive in one process may not have that force in another. To be sure, we are not flipping coins in either case. We are deliberating carefully in a reason-driven and reason-giving way. But the weight given reasons in each setting is a reasonable reflection of other moral disagreements and moral uncertainty—the very uncertainty about what counts as a just outcome that compels us to adopt a procedural approach to fair outcomes. Groucho can be told this: Harpo was given the treatment because his plan reasoned about his case differently than your plan, and both ways of reasoning are relevant and arguably fair.

How tolerable would a system be if it produced situations in which a Groucho and Harpo were treated differently? We might think it makes a difference how centralized or decentralized a system is. In a decentralized system such as ours, for example, it may be difficult to require that insurance schemes use one rather than another procedurally fair way of deliberating about cases (though legislation such as the Friedman-Knowles Experimental Treatment Act imposes uniformity, at least at one stage of decision making). On what basis should the choice between procedures and weightings be made? Can we show a superior outcome to insisting on one such process rather than another? Without such a compelling regulatory reason, we might have trouble justifying public regulation requiring just one form of managing last-chance cases.

Despite the decentralization in our health care system, however, our courts arguably can impose a kind of unifying framework. Groucho might sue BestHealth, saying that not only does he want the treatment, and not only does some clinician he prefers say it is appropriate, but GreatCare has given the treatment to someone just like him. In practice, the courts could make unworkable an effort to experiment with different fair procedures to see what their advantages and disadvantages really are. On the other hand, what has often carried the day in actual suits on these matters is a demonstration of a lack of fair process and a kind of arbitrariness within an organization. If each of the fair procedures constitutes a reasonable defense against that sort of claim, then the courts might welcome an effort to rely more directly on fair procedures applied within plans. An analogy here would be the way in which the courts have welcomed decision making by ethics committees in hospitals as a preferable route to having these kinds of cases continuously adjudicated in the courts.

Would it be a compelling regulatory reason that we find differential treatment unacceptable and have to avoid it, if only by insisting on uniform process by convention? That might be true in a decentralized system, but it seems even more likely to be true in a national health care system. In the U.K., for example, it might seem more troubling that Groucho did not get his transplant in London but Harpo got his in Manchester. Here too, however, there might be disagreements among *meaningful political units,* the districts, about what constituted the "best" procedure. If that is true, then there might be even more reason to tolerate variation than there is in the U.S., where people are grouped into insurance schemes, not meaningful political units that have ways of selecting their procedures in a democratic fashion.

How acceptable differential treatment would be seems to depend, then, on whether a persuasive political rationale for uniformity can be developed. In a decentralized system, the political rationale would have to be sufficient to override the presumption that "private" insurers have the authority to select from among a set of comparably fair procedures. Of course, the political rationale might simply be that the legal system would not allow differential treatment; but that too remains to be seen.

In a national health care system, the political rationale for uniformity would have to show that differential treatment among districts was less acceptable than giving them the autonomy to select their own procedures. If meaningful political units, like districts, felt strongly enough about their choices of procedures, the costs of uniformity might be too high. For the problem we are facing, then, it remains unclear how unacceptable it would be for Harpo to get a last chance when Groucho does not.

VII. CONCLUSIONS

Making decisions and policies about payment for promising but unproven last-chance therapies presents the most difficult moral and clinical policy challenge a health care system can face. Important values, all of which command respect and attention, inevitably come into conflict in these difficult situations, especially (1) giving some (how much?) priority to meeting the *urgent claims* of patients in last-chance situations, (2) providing *stewardship* of collective resources, (3) producing the public good of *scientific knowledge* about the effectiveness of unproven therapies, and (4) respecting *patient autonomy* through collaborative decision making about risks and benefits.

General principles of distributive justice do not tell us how to weigh the relative claims of these competing considerations. Nevertheless, the insurers and MCOs whose programs we describe have developed procedures for making decisions and policies that can be defended on the basis of justifiable—although different—weights they give to the different values. In our decentralized, competitive system—largely in response to political and legal pressures patients and clinicians have focused on these plans—an important social experiment has emerged. Different procedural "solutions" to the problem of limit setting in the case of new technologies are being developed and honed in practice. What can we learn from the experiment?

If we as a society can tolerate the inevitable differences in decisions and policies that the different configurations of values will create, we will have an opportunity to learn from the dialectic between principles and practice. We will see more clearly through a legacy of specific decisions and their outcomes just what the moral and nonmoral benefits and costs of the different approaches are. What we learn will help us refine our notions of fair procedure and in turn help us produce better solutions to the general problem of limit-setting in health care that all societies are struggling with. In the last 20–30 years, we have learned much and seen important changes in how individual clinicians and patients negotiate the difficult issues of clinical planning in the context of threats to life itself. If we have enough societal fortitude, and a modicum of strong political leadership, close study of the experiences generated by the kinds of programs we have described can help us do the same at the level of social policy.

NOTES

1. We distinguish the case of promising but unproven last-chance therapies from the case of treatments that professionals decide are futile. In futility cases, the judgment of the professional is that there will be harm to the patient, or there is at least clear evidence that there will be no benefit. The patient or family might disagree, perhaps because they seek miracles or perhaps because they view mere physiological functioning as a benefit. Here there is a conflict between stewardship and the somewhat confusing notion of patient "autonomy." The conflict eases if we restrict the plausible core of patient autonomy to a (positive) right to participate in decisions about treatment and a (negative) right to refuse treatment, and we distinguish that core from an (implausible) "entitlement" to have whatever treatment one desires, which involves unrestricted claims on resources held by others. There is also a conflict between paternalism (in the form of a legitimate concern to avoid doing harm) and a patient's or family's judgment about what counts as a benefit. These are interesting issues, but this kind of case is marked by clear professional judgment rooted in considerable *certainty about the evidence*. In the last-chance cases we are concerned with, it is professional *uncertainty*, not certainty, that is key.

2. Case studies completed to date include Sabin, J., Daniels, N., 1997a. "How MCOs deliberated about coverage for lung volume reduction surgery: A Focal Case Study" (unpublished manuscript), and Wilkinson, S., Sabin, J., and Daniels, N. 1997. "How MCOs decided to cover pallidotomy for advanced Parkinson's Disease: A Focal Case Study" (unpublished manuscript). See also Daniels, N. and Sabin, J. 1997. "Limits to Health Care: Fair Procedures, Democratic Deliberation, and the Legitimacy Problem for Insurers," *Philosophy and Public Affairs* 26, no. 4 (Fall 1997): 303–350.

3. Other technology assessment centers not affiliated with MCOs, such as ECRI, also undertook evaluations.

4. Bezwoda, W.R., Seymour, L., Dansey, R.D., "High-dose Chemotherapy with Hematopoietic Rescue as Primary Treatment for Metastatic Breast Cancer: A Randomized Trial." 1995. *J Clin Oncol* 13:2483–89.

5. The MAP criteria are as follows:

   (1) The technology must have final approval from the appropriate government regulatory body.
   (2) The scientific evidence must permit conclusions concerning the effect of the technology on health outcomes.
   (3) The technology must improve the net health outcome.
   (4) The technology must be as beneficial as any established alternative.
   (5) The improvement must be attainable outside the investigational settings.

   The South African study used as its control a regimen of standard chemotherapy that was inferior in outcomes to the conventional therapy that would standardly be available in the U.S. and elsewhere. Showing that high-dose chemotherapy was superior to a conventional regimen that itself was far inferior to conventional therapy commonly in use should not persuade us of the superior efficacy of the high-dose regimen.

6. The California Blue Shield evaluation took place in a public setting, the only such open technology assessment process that we know of aside from Oregon Health Resources Commission. At its discussion, the panel seemed comfortable supporting its conclusion only after it was assured that no one actually wanting the high-dose chemotherapy was unable to get it, despite its investigational status.

7. See Norman Daniels, *Seeking Fair Treatment: From the AIDS Epidemic to National Health Care Reform*, New York: Oxford University Press, 1995, Chapter 6.

8. Peters, W.P., and Rogers, M.C. 1994. "Variation in Approval by Insurance Companies for Coverage of Autologous Bone Marrow Transplantion for Breast Cancer," *NEJM* 330:7:473–7.

9. Beebe, D.B., Rosenfeld, A.B., Collins, N.: "An Approach to Decisions about Coverage of Investigational Treatments." *HMO Practice* 11(2): 65–67, 1997 (June).

10. See Daniels and Sabin, "Limits to Health Care: Fair Procedures, Democratic Deliberation, and the Legitimacy Problem for Insurers," *Philosophy and Public Affairs* 26, no. 4 (Fall 1997): 303–350.

11. These conditions were developed independently but fit reasonably well with the principles of publicity, reciprocity, and accountability governing democratic deliberation cited by Amy Gutmann and Dennis Thompson, *Democracy and Disagreement* (Cambridge: Harvard University Press, 1996). For reservations about their account, see Norman Daniels, "Enabling Democratic Deliberation," Pacific Division of the American Philosophical Association, March 1997.

ILLEGAL IMMIGRANTS, HEALTH CARE, AND SOCIAL RESPONSIBILITY

James Dwyer

Illegal immigrants form a large and disputed group in many countries. Indeed, even the name is in dispute. People in this group are referred to as illegal immigrants, illegal aliens, irregular migrants, undocumented workers, or, in French, as *sans papiers*. Whatever they are called, their existence raises an important ethical question: Do societies have an ethical responsibility to provide health care for them and to promote their health?

This question often elicits two different answers. Some people—call them nationalists—say that the answer is obviously no. They argue that people who have no right to be in a country should not have rights to benefits in that country. Other people—call them humanists—say that the answer is obviously yes. They argue that all people should have access to health care. It's a basic human right.

I think both these answers are off the mark. The first focuses too narrowly on what we owe people based on legal rules and formal citizenship. The other answer focuses too broadly, on what we owe people qua human beings. We need a perspective that is in between, that adequately responds to the phenomenon of illegal immigration and adequately reflects the complexity of moral thought. There may be important ethical distinctions, for example, among the following groups: U.S. citizens who lack health insurance, undocumented workers who lack health insurance in spite of working full time, medical visitors who fly to the United States as tourists in order to obtain care at public hospitals, foreign citizens who work abroad for subcontractors of American firms, and foreign citizens who live in impoverished countries. I believe that we—U.S. citizens—have

ethical duties in all of these situations, but I see important differences in what these duties demand and how they are to be explained.

In this paper, I want to focus on the situation of illegal immigrants. I will discuss several different answers to the question about what ethical responsibility we have to provide health care to illegal immigrants. (I shall simply assume that societies have an ethical obligation to provide their own citizens with a reasonably comprehensive package of health benefits.) The answers that I shall discuss tend to conceptualize the ethical issues in terms of individual desert, professional ethics, or human rights. I want to discuss the limitations of each of these approaches and to offer an alternative. I shall approach the issues in terms of social responsibility and discuss the moral relevance of work. In doing so, I tend to pull bioethics in the direction of social ethics and political philosophy. That's the direction I think it should be heading. But before I begin the ethical discussion, I need to say more about the phenomenon of illegal immigration.

HUMAN MIGRATION

People have always moved around. They have moved for political, environmental, economic, and familial reasons. They have tried to escape war, persecution, discrimination, famine, environmental degradation, poverty, and a variety of other problems. They have tried to find places to build better lives, earn more money, and provide better support for their families. A strong sense of family responsibility has always been an important factor behind migration.

But while human migration is not new, *illegal* immigration is, since only recently have nation-states tried to control and regulate the flow of immigration. Societies have always tried to exclude people they viewed as undesirable: criminals, people unable to support themselves, people with contagious

From *Hastings Center Report* 34, no. 5 (January–February 2004): 34–41. Reprinted by permission of The Hastings Center.

Editors' note: Some author's notes have been cut. Students who want to follow up on sources should consult the original article.

diseases, and certain ethnic or racial groups. But only in the last hundred years or so have states tried in a systematic way to control the number and kinds of immigrants.

In contrast, what the Athenian polis tried to control was not immigration, but citizenship. Workers, merchants, and scholars came to Athens from all over the Mediterranean world. They were free to work, trade, and study in Athens, although they were excluded from the rich political life that citizens enjoyed. Today, political states try to control both citizenship and residency.

Modern attempts to control residency are not remarkably effective. There are illegal immigrants residing and working all over the globe. When people think about illegal immigrants, they tend to focus on Mexicans in the United States or North-Africans in France. But the phenomenon is really much more diverse and complex. Illegal immigrants come from hundreds of countries and go wherever they can get work. There are undocumented workers from Indonesia in Malaysia, undocumented workers from Haiti in the Dominican Republic, and undocumented workers from Myanmar in Thailand. Thailand is an interesting example because it is both a source of and a destination for undocumented workers: while many people from poorer countries have gone to work in Thailand, many Thais have gone to work in richer countries.

Since illegal activities are difficult to measure, and people are difficult to count, we do not know exactly how many people are illegal immigrants. The following estimates provide a rough idea. The total number of illegal immigrants in the U.S. is probably between five and eight million. About 30–40 percent of these people entered the country legally, but overstayed their visas. Of all the immigrants in Europe, about one third are probably illegal immigrants. A small country like Israel has about 125,000 foreign workers (not counting Palestinians). About 50,000 of these are in the country illegally.

I believe that a sound ethical response to the question of illegal immigration requires some understanding of the work that illegal immigrants do. Most undocumented workers do the jobs that citizens often eschew. They do difficult and disagreeable work at low wages for small firms in the informal sector of the economy. In general, they have the worst jobs and work in the worst conditions in such

sectors of the economy as agriculture, construction, manufacturing, and the food industry. They pick fruit, wash dishes, move dirt, sew clothes, clean toilets.

Japan is a good example of this. In the 1980s many foreign workers came to Japan from the Philippines, Thailand, China, and other countries. Yoshio Sugimoto summarizes the situation:

> The unprecedented flow of foreign workers into Japan stemmed from the situations in both the domestic and foreign labor markets. "Pull" factors within Japan included the ageing of the Japanese workforce and the accompanying shortage of labor in unskilled, manual, and physically demanding areas. In addition, the changing work ethic of Japanese youth has made it difficult for employers to recruit them for this type of work, which is described in terms of the three undesirable Ks (or Ds in English): kitanai (dirty), kitsui (difficult), and kiken (dangerous). Under these circumstances, a number of employers found illegal migrants, in particular from Asia, a remedy for their labor shortage.

The pattern is much the same in other countries.

In the global economy, in which a company can shift its manufacturing base with relative ease to a country with cheaper labor, illegal immigrants often perform work that cannot be shifted overseas. Toilets have to be cleaned, dishes have to be washed, and children have to be watched *locally*. This local demand may help to explain a relatively new trend: the feminization of migration. Migrants used to be predominantly young men, seeking work in areas such as agriculture and construction. But that pattern is changing. More and more women migrants are employed in the service sector as, for example, maids, nannies, and health care aides.

Women migrants are also employed as sex workers. The connection between commercial sex and illegal immigration is quite striking. As women in some societies have more money, choices, schooling, and power, they are unwilling to work as prostitutes. These societies seem to be supplying their demands for commercial sex by using undocumented workers from poorer countries. Before brothels were legalized in the Netherlands, about 40 to 75 percent of the prostitutes who worked in Amsterdam were undocumented workers. About 3,000 of the 7,000 prostitutes in Berlin are from Thailand. Japan has over 150,000 foreign prostitutes, most of them from Thailand, China, and the Philippines. Thailand has about 25,000 prostitutes from Myanmar.

Even when prostitution is voluntary, it is difficult and dangerous. Leah Platt notes that prostitution is

a job without overtime pay, health insurance, or sick leave—and usually without recourse against the abuses of one's employer, which can include being required to have sex without a condom and being forced to turn tricks in order to work off crushing debts.[1]

And for some illegal immigrants, prostitution is not a voluntary choice. Some are deceived and delivered into prostitution. Others are coerced, their lives controlled by pimps, criminal gangs, and human traffickers.

Some of the worst moral offenses occur in the trafficking of human beings, but even here it is important to see a continuum of activities. Sometimes traffickers simply provide transportation in exchange for payment. Sometimes, they recruit people with deceptive promises and false accounts of jobs, then transport them under horrible and dangerous conditions. If and when the immigrants arrive in the destination country, they are controlled by debt, threat, and force. Some become indentured servants, working without pay for a period of time. Others are controlled by physical threats or threats to expose their illegal status. A few are enslaved and held as property.

Not all illegal immigrants are victims, however, and an accurate account of illegal immigration, even if only sketched, must capture some of its complexity. My task is to consider how well different ethical frameworks deal with that complexity.

A MATTER OF DESERT

The abstract ethical question of whether societies have a responsibility to provide health care for illegal immigrants sometimes becomes a concrete political issue. Rising health care costs, budget reduction programs, and feelings of resentment sometimes transform the ethical question into a political debate. This has happened several times in the United States. In 1996, the Congress debated and passed the "Illegal Immigration Reform and Immigrant Responsibility Act." This law made all immigrants ineligible for Medicaid, although it did allow the federal government to reimburse states for emergency treatment of illegal immigrants.

In 1994, the citizens of California debated Proposition 187, an even more restrictive measure. This ballot initiative proposed to deny publicly funded health care, social services, and education to illegal immigrants. This law would have required publicly funded health care facilities to deny care, except in medical emergencies, to people who could not prove that they were U.S. citizens or legal residents.

This proposition was approved by 59 percent of the voters. It was never implemented because courts found that parts of it conflicted with other laws, but the deepest arguments for and against it remain very much alive. Because they will probably surface again, at a different time or in [a] different place, it is worthwhile evaluating the ethical frameworks that they assume.

The first argument put forward is that illegal aliens should be denied public benefits because they are in the country illegally. Although it is true that illegal aliens have violated a law by entering or remaining in the country, it is not clear what the moral implication of this point is. Nothing about access to health care follows from the mere fact that illegal aliens have violated a law. Many people break many different laws. Whether a violation of a law should disqualify people from public services probably depends on the nature and purpose of the services, the nature and gravity of the violation, and many other matters.

Consider one example of a violation of the law. People sometimes break tax laws by working off the books. They do certain jobs for cash in order to avoid paying taxes or losing benefits. Moreover, this practice is probably quite common. I recently asked students in two of my classes if they or anyone in their extended family had earned money that was not reported as taxable income. In one class, all but two students raised their hands. In the other class, every hand went up.

No one has suggested that health care facilities deny care to people suspected of working off the books. But undocumented work is also a violation of the law. Furthermore, it involves an issue of fairness because it shifts burdens onto others and diminishes funding for important purposes. Of course, working off the books and working without a visa are not alike in all respects. But without further argument, nothing much follows about whether it is right to deny benefits to people who have violated a law.

Proponents of restrictive measures also appeal to an argument that combines a particular conception of desert with the need to make trade-offs. Proponents of California's Proposition 187 stated that, "while our own citizens and legal residents go wanting, those who chose to enter our country ILLEGALLY get royal treatment at the expense of the California taxpayer."[2] Proponents noted that the legislature maintained programs that included free prenatal care for illegal aliens but increased the amount that senior citizens must pay for prescription drugs. They then asked, "Why should we give more comfort and consideration to illegal aliens than to *our* own needy American citizens?"

The rhetorical question is part of the argument. I would restate the argument in the following way: Given the limited public budget for health care, U.S. citizens and legal residents are more deserving of benefits than are illegal aliens. This argument frames the issue as a choice between competing goods in a situation of limited resources.

There is something right and something wrong about this way of framing the issue. What is right is the idea that in all of life, individual and political, we have to choose between competing goods. A society cannot have everything: comprehensive and universal health care, good public schools, extensive public parks and beaches, public services, and very low taxes. What is false is the idea that we have to choose between basic health care for illegal aliens and basic health care for citizens. Many other trade-offs are possible, including an increase in public funding.

The narrow framework of the debate pits poor citizens against illegal aliens in a battle for health care resources. Within this framework, the issue is posed as one of desert. Avoiding the idea of desert is impossible. After all, justice is a matter of giving people their due—giving them what they deserve. But a narrow conception of desert seems most at home in allocating particular goods that go beyond basic needs, in situations where the criteria of achievement and effort are very clear. For example, if we are asked to give an award for the best student in chemistry, a narrow notion of desert is appropriate and useful. But publicly funded health care is different and requires a broader view of desert.

The discussion of restrictive measures often focuses on desert, taxation, and benefits. Proponents tend to picture illegal immigrants as free riders who are taking advantage of public services without contributing to public funding. Opponents are quick to note that illegal immigrants do pay taxes. They pay sales tax, gas tax, and value-added tax. They often pay income tax and property tax. But do they pay enough tax to cover the cost of the services they use? Or more generally, are illegal immigrants a net economic gain or a net economic loss for society?

Instead of trying to answer the economic question, I want to point out a problem with the question itself. The question about taxation and benefits tends to portray society as a private business venture. On the business model, investors should benefit in proportion to the funds they put into the venture. This may be an appropriate model for some business ventures, but it is not an adequate model for all social institutions and benefits. The business model is not an adequate model for thinking about voting, legal defense, library services, minimum wages, occupational safety, and many other social benefits.

Consider my favorite social institution: the public library. The important question here is not whether some people use more library services than they pay for through taxation, which is obviously true. Some people pay relatively high taxes but never use the library, while others pay relatively low taxes but use the library quite often. In thinking about the public library, we should consider questions such as the following. What purposes does the library serve? Does it promote education, provide opportunity, and foster public life? Does it tend to ameliorate or exacerbate social injustice? Given the library's purposes, who should count as its constituents or members? And what are the rights and responsibilities of the library users? In the following sections, I shall consider analogous questions about illegal immigrants and the social institutions that promote health.

A MATTER OF PROFESSIONAL ETHICS

Some of the most vigorous responses to restrictive measures have come from those who consider the issue within the framework of professional ethics. Tal Ann Ziv and Bernard Lo, for example, argue that "cooperating with Proposition 187 would undermine professional ethics."[3] In particular, they argue that cooperating with this kind of restrictive measure is inconsistent with physicians' "ethical responsibilities to protect the public health, care for persons in medical need, and respect patient confidentiality."

Restrictive measures may indeed have adverse effects on the public health. For example, measures that deny care to illegal aliens, or make them afraid to seek care, could lead to an increase in tuberculosis. And physicians do have a professional obligation to oppose measures that would significantly harm the public health. But the public health argument has a serious failing, if taken by itself. It avoids the big issue of whether illegal immigrants should be considered part of the public and whether public institutions should serve their health needs. Instead of appealing to an inclusive notion of social justice, the argument suggests how the health of illegal immigrants may influence citizens' health, and then appeals to citizens' sense of prudence. The appeal to prudence is not wrong, but it avoids the larger ethical issues.

The second argument against Proposition 187 is that it restricts confidentiality in ways that are not justified. It requires health care facilities to report people suspected of being in the country illegally and to disclose additional information to authorities. Ziv and Lo argue that "Proposition 187 fails to provide the usual ethical justifications for overriding patient confidentiality." Reporting a patient's "immigration status serves no medical or public health purpose, involves no medical expertise, and is not a routine part of medical care." Thus this restriction on confidentiality is a serious violation of professional ethics.

But if restrictive measures work as designed, issues of confidentiality may not even arise. Illegal aliens will be deterred from seeking medical care or will be screened out before they see a doctor. Thus the issue of screening may be more important than the issue of confidentiality. First, if the screening is carried out, it should not be by physicians, because it is not their role to act as agents for the police or the immigration service. Professional ethics requires some separation of social roles, and terrible things have happened when physicians have become agents of political regimes. The bigger issue, though, is not who should do the screening, but whether it should be done at all.

Ziv and Lo note that "clerks will probably screen patients for their immigration status, just as they currently screen them for their insurance status." They object to this arrangement, and they argue that physicians bear some responsibility for arrangements that conflict with professional ethics. In their view, screening out illegal aliens conflicts with physicians' ethical responsibility to "care for persons in medical need."

This claim is important, but ambiguous. It could mean simply that physicians have an obligation to attend to anyone who presents to them in need of emergency care. That seems right. It would be wrong not to stabilize and save someone in a medical emergency. It would be inhumane, even morally absurd, to let someone die because her visa had expired. But a claim that physicians have an enduring obligation to provide emergency care is consistent with measures like Proposition 187 and the 1996 federal law.

The claim might also mean that the selection of patients should be based only on medical need, never on such factors as nationality, residency, immigration status, or ability to pay. This is a very strong claim. It means that all private practice is morally wrong. It means that most national health care systems are too restrictive. It means that transplant lists for organs donated in a particular country should be open to everyone in the world. It might even mean that physicians have an ethical responsibility to relocate to places where the medical need is the greatest. I shall say more about the strong claim in the next section. Here I just want to note one point. This claim goes well beyond professional ethics. It is an ethical claim that seems to be based on a belief about the nature of human needs and human rights.

Finally, Ziv and Lo's claim about physicians' responsibility to care for people in medical need might be stronger than the claim about emergency care but weaker than the universal claim. Perhaps we should interpret it to mean that it is wrong to turn patients away when society has no other provisions and institutions to provide them with basic care. The idea then is that society should provide all members with basic health care and that physicians have some responsibility to work to realize this idea.

There is something appealing and plausible about this interpretation, but it too goes beyond professional ethics. It has more to do with the nature of social justice and social institutions than with the nature of medical practice. It makes an ethical claim based on a belief about social responsibility and an assumption that illegal aliens are to be counted as members of society. I shall try to elaborate this belief and assumption later.

Let me sum up my main points so far. Political measures that restrict medical care for illegal immigrants often involve violations of professional ethics, and health care professionals should oppose such measures. But the framework of professional ethics is not adequate for thinking about the larger ethical issues. It fails to illuminate the obligation to provide medical care. Furthermore, it fails to consider factors such as work and housing that may have a profound impact on health. In the next two sections I shall consider broader frameworks and discourses.

A MATTER OF HUMAN RIGHTS

To deal with the issue of health care and illegal immigrants, some adopt a humanistic framework and employ a discourse of human rights. They tend to emphasize the right of all human beings to medical treatment, as well as the common humanity of aliens and citizens, pointing to the arbitrary nature of national borders.

National borders can seem arbitrary. Distinctions based on national borders seem even more arbitrary when one studies how borders were established and the disparities in wealth and health that exist between countries. Since it doesn't seem just that some people should be disadvantaged by arbitrary boundaries, it may also seem that people should have the right to emigrate from wherever they are and to immigrate to wherever they wish. But does this follow from the fact that national borders can be seen as arbitrary?

John Rawls thinks not. He writes:

> It does not follow from the fact that boundaries are historically arbitrary that their role in the Law of Peoples cannot be justified. On the contrary, to fix on their arbitrariness is to fix on the wrong thing. In the absence of a world state, there *must* be boundaries of some kind, which when viewed in isolation will seem arbitrary, and depend to some degree on historical circumstances.[4]

Even if boundaries depend on historical circumstances, a defined territory may allow a people to form a government that acts as their agent in a fair and effective way. A defined territory may allow a people to form a government that enables them to take responsibility for the natural environment, promote the well-being of the human population, deal with social problems, and cultivate just political institutions.

From functions like these, governments derive a qualified right to regulate immigration. This right is not an unlimited right of communal self-determination. Societies do not have a right to protect institutions and ways of life that are deeply unjust. Furthermore, even when a society has a right to regulate immigration, there are ethical questions about whether and how the society should exercise that right. And there are ethical questions about how immigrants should be treated in that society.

The committed humanist, who begins with reflections on the arbitrary nature of national boundaries, sometimes reaches the same conclusion as the global capitalist: that all restrictions on labor mobility are unjustified. In their different ways, both the humanist and the capitalist devalue distinctions based on political community. To be sure, there is much to criticize about existing political communities, but we need to be cautious about some of the alternatives. Michael Walzer warns us about two possibilities. He says that to "tear down the walls of the state is not . . . to create a world without walls, but rather to create a thousand petty fortresses."[5] Without state regulation of immigration, local communities may become more exclusionary, parochial, and xenophobic. Walzer also notes another possibility: "The fortresses, too, could be torn down: all that is necessary is a global state sufficiently powerful to overwhelm the local communities. Then the result would be . . . a world of radically deracinated men and women."

Of course, the humanist need not be committed to an abstract position about open borders. The humanist might accept that states have a qualified right to regulate immigration, but insist that all states must respect the human rights of all immigrants—legal and illegal. That idea makes a lot of sense, although much depends on how we specify the content of human rights.

The idea that all human beings should have equal access to all beneficial health care is often used to critique both national and international arrangements. In an editorial in the *New England*

Journal of Medicine, Paul Farmer reflects on the number of people who go untreated for diseases such as tuberculosis and HIV. He writes:

> Prevention is, of course, always preferable to treatment. But epidemics of treatable infectious diseases should remind us that although science has revolutionized medicine, we still need a plan for ensuring equal access to care. As study after study shows the power of effective therapies to alter the course of infectious disease, we should be increasingly reluctant to reserve these therapies for the affluent, low-incidence regions of the world where most medical resources are concentrated. Excellence without equity looms as the chief human-rights dilemma of health care in the 21st century.[6]

I too am critical of the gross inequalities in health within countries and between countries, but here I only want to make explicit the framework and discourse of Farmer's critique. His critique appeals to two ideas: that there is a lack of proportion between the medical resources and the burden of disease and that there is a human right to equal access.

What is wrong with the claim that equal access to health care is a human right? First, to claim something as a right is more of a conclusion than an argument. Such claims function more to summarize a position than to further moral discussion. A quick and simple appeal to a comprehensive right avoids all the hard questions about duties and priorities. When faced with grave injustices and huge inequalities, claiming that all human beings have a right to health care is easy. Specifying the kind of care to which people are entitled is harder. Specifying duties is harder yet. And getting those duties institutionalized is hardest of all.

In addition to the general problems with claims about rights, a problem more specific to the issue of illegal immigration exists. Since a claim based on a human right is a claim based on people's common humanity, it tends to collapse distinctions between people. Yet for certain purposes, it may be important to make distinctions and emphasize different responsibilities. We may owe different things to, for example, the poor undocumented worker in our country, the middle-class visitor who needs dialysis, the prince who wants a transplant, people enmeshed in the global economy, and the most marginalized people in poor countries.

Rather than claiming an essentially limitless right, it makes more sense to recognize a modest core of human rights and to supplement those rights with a robust account of social responsibility, social justice, and international justice. I do not know if there is a principled way to delineate exactly what should be included in the core of human rights. But even a short list of circumscribed rights would have important consequences if societies took responsibility for trying to protect everyone from violations of these rights. Illegal immigrants are sometimes killed in transport, physically or sexually abused, held as slaves, kept in indentured servitude, forced to work in occupations, and denied personal property. These are clear violations of what should be recognized as human rights. But this core of recognized rights should be supplemented with an account of social justice and responsibility.

A MATTER OF SOCIAL RESPONSIBILITY

Framing the issue in terms of social responsibility helps to highlight one of the most striking features of illegal immigration: the employment pattern within society. As I noted before, illegal immigrants often perform the worst work for the lowest wages. Illegal immigrants are part of a pattern that is older and deeper than the recent globalization of the economy. Societies have often used the most powerless and marginalized people to do the most disagreeable and difficult work. Societies have used slaves, indentured servants, castes, minorities, orphans, poor children, internal migrants, and foreign migrants. Of course, the pattern is not exactly the same in every society, nor even in every industry within a society, but the similarities are striking.

I see the use of illegal immigrants as the contemporary form of the old pattern. But it is not a natural phenomenon beyond human control. It is the result of laws, norms, institutions, habits, and conditions in society, and of the conditions in the world at large. It is a social construction that we could try to reconstruct.

Some might object that no one forces illegal immigrants to take unsavory jobs and that they can return home if they wish. This objection is too simple. Although most undocumented workers made a voluntary choice to go to another country, they often had inadequate information and dismal alternatives, and voluntary return is not an attractive option when they have substantial debts and poor earning potential at home. More importantly, even a fully informed and voluntary choice does not settle the question of social justice and responsibility. We have gone through this debate before. As the industrial revolution developed, many people agreed to work under horrible conditions in shops, factories, and mines. Yet most societies eventually saw that freedom of contract was a limited part of a larger social ethic. They accepted a responsibility to address conditions of work and to empower workers, at least in basic ways. Decent societies now try to regulate child labor, workplace safety, minimum rates of pay, workers' rights to unionize, background conditions, and much more. But because of their illegal status, undocumented workers are often unable to challenge or report employers who violate even the basic standards of a decent society.

We need to take responsibility for preventing the old pattern from continuing, and the key idea is that of "taking responsibility." It is not the same as legal accountability, which leads one to think about determining causation, proving intention or negligence, examining excuses, apportioning blame, and assigning costs. Taking responsibility is more about seeing patterns and problems, examining background conditions, not passing the buck, and responding in appropriate ways. A society need not bear full causal responsibility in order to assume social responsibility.

Why should society take responsibility for people it tried to keep out of its territory, for people who are not social members? Because in many respects illegal immigrants are social members. Although they are not citizens or legal residents, they may be diligent workers, good neighbors, concerned parents, and active participants in community life. They are workers, involved in complex schemes of social co-operation. Many of the most exploited workers in the industrial revolution—children, women, men without property—were also not full citizens, but they were vulnerable people, doing often undesirable work, for whom society needed to take some responsibility. Undocumented workers' similar role in society is one reason that the social responsibility to care for them is different from the responsibility to care for medical visitors.

If a given society had the ethical conviction and political will, it could develop practical measures to

transform the worst aspects of some work, empower the most disadvantaged workers, and shape the background conditions in which the labor market operates. The interests of the worst-off citizens and the interests of illegal immigrants need not be opposed. Practical measures may raise labor costs and increase the price of goods and services, as they should. We should not rely on undocumented workers to keep down prices on everything from strawberries to sex.

I can already hear the objection. "What you propose is a perfect recipe for increasing illegal immigration. All the practical measures that you suggest would encourage more illegal immigration." Whether improving the situation of the worst-off workers will increase illegal immigration is a complex empirical question. The answer probably depends on many factors. But even if transforming the worst work and empowering the worst-off workers leads to an increase in illegal immigration, countries should take those steps. Although we have a right to regulate immigration, considerations of justice constrain the ways we can pursue that aim. A society might also decrease illegal immigration by decriminalizing the killing of illegal immigrants, but no one thinks that would be a reasonable and ethical social policy. Nor do I think that the old pattern of using marginalized people is a reasonable and ethical way to regulate immigration.

I have left out of my account the very point with which I began, namely, health and health care, and I ended up talking about work and social responsibility. Surely work and social responsibility are at the heart of the matter. Where then does health care fit in?

Good health care can, among other things, prevent death and suffering, promote health and well-being, respond to basic needs and vulnerabilities, express care and solidarity, contribute to equality of opportunity, monitor social problems (such as child abuse or pesticide exposure), and accomplish other important aims. But health care is just one means, and not always the most effective means, to these ends. To focus on access to and payment of health care is to focus our ethical concern too narrowly.

I believe that societies that attract illegal immigrants should pursue policies and practices that (1) improve the pay for and conditions of the worst forms of work; (2) structure and organize work so as to give workers more voice, power, and opportunity to develop their capacities; and (3) connect labor to unions, associations, and communities in ways that increase social respect for all workers. I cannot justify these claims in this paper, but I want to note how they are connected to health care. Providing health care for all workers and their families is a very good way to improve the benefit that workers receive for the worst forms of work, to render workers less vulnerable, and to express social and communal respect for them. These are good reasons for providing health care for all workers, documented and undocumented alike. And they express ethical concerns that are not captured by talking about human rights, public health, or the rights of citizens.

THE RIGHT DISCUSSION

I have examined the frameworks that are employed in discussions about illegal immigrants and health care. I argued against conceptualizing the issues in terms of desert, professional ethics, or even human rights. Although all of these concepts highlight something important, they tend to be too narrow or too broad. And because they provide the wrong

perspective, they fail to focus attention on the crux of the matter.

I have suggested that the issues should be framed in terms of social justice and social responsibility. I realize that I did not fully justify my view, and that other people may give a different account of what social justice requires. But I had a different aim. I did not want to convince everyone of the rectitude of my account, but to shift the discussion into the realm of social justice and responsibility.

REFERENCES

1. L. Platt, "Regulating the Global Brothel," *The American Prospect*, Special Supplement, Summer 2001: 11.
2. This and the following quotations are from the California Ballot Pamphlet, 1994, available at http://www.holmes.uchastings.edu/cgibin/starfinder/5640/calprop/txt, accessed September 30, 2002.
3. T.A. Ziv and B. Lo, "Denial of Care to Illegal Immigrants," *NEJM* 332 (1995): 1095–1098.
4. J. Rawls, *The Law of Peoples* (Cambridge, Mass.: Harvard University Press, 1999), 39.
5. M. Walzer, *Spheres of Justice* (New York: Basic Books, 1983), 39.
6. P. Farmer, "The Major Infectious Diseases in the World—To Treat or Not to Treat?" *NEJM* 345 (2001): 208–210.

RATIONING VACCINE DURING AN AVIAN INFLUENZA PANDEMIC: WHY IT WON'T BE EASY

John D. Arras

The specter of an avian influenza pandemic poses enormous technical and logistical challenges. For example, how can such a looming catastrophe be avoided? If we cannot prevent it, how can we best

Reprinted by permission of *Yale Journal of Biology and Medicine*.

Editors' note: Some author's notes have been cut. Students who want to follow up on sources should consult the original article.

mobilize our medical and social resources to effectively blunt its impact? How can we quickly mobilize production of sufficient quantities of effective vaccines and antiviral agents to either prevent infection or mitigate the burden of illness in the infected? While we hope and trust that our scientists and public health officials will do their best to prevent a pandemic, it would be fool-hardy to assume they will succeed against such a formidable foe, especially when many of our most distinguished and knowledgeable influenza experts warn that the operative question isn't whether, but rather when, a pandemic will strike. And while virologists in both the public and private sectors are no doubt searching feverishly for new ways to hasten production of effective vaccines, a full-blown pandemic will most likely overwhelm their best efforts. Thus, in addition to posing scientific, technical, and logistical problems, the threat of an avian influenza pandemic poses equally important ethical problems, the most vexing of which is the age-old question, "Who shall live when not all can live?" In short, how should influenza vaccine and antivirals be rationed in the context of a global pandemic?

In the absence of revolutionary breakthroughs in the design and production of influenza vaccines, we can expect acute shortages of vaccine in the early months of a pandemic. Given current egg-based methods of producing vaccines, experts anticipate a ramp-up period of roughly six months before large quantities of drug will be ready for distribution. Since pandemic influenza strains achieve their global reach by virtue of their novelty and our corresponding lack of immunological defenses against them, it takes time to identify the new strain and design a tailor-made vaccine against it. Thus, during the first six months of a pandemic, there is likely to be little or no carefully tailored vaccine available to combat the first wave of influenza. (There may, however, be stocks of generic vaccine on hand, such as the H5N1 vaccine currently being developed at the National Institutes of Health. Just how effective such a generic vaccine will be against a specific, newly mutated influenza strain remains to be seen. Preliminary studies indicate that the generic vaccine is effective but only at extremely high doses—a result that does not bode well for widespread distribution during a pandemic.) One authoritative source estimates that, during the following six months, worldwide vaccine production would most likely be limited to roughly 1 billion doses. Since we won't have any built-up immunity to this particular strain of influenza, as we do against garden variety influenza strains that circulate among us from year to year, it will most likely require two doses of this vaccine to effectively protect each recipient. This means that only roughly 500 million people, or 14 percent of the world's population,

could be effectively immunized during the second half of the pandemic's first year. Other authorities estimate that current production capacity in the United States would only yield enough drug in one year to effectively vaccinate about half of the American population. A realistic approach to the threat of pandemic influenza must, therefore, assume that there will be significant shortfalls in vaccine availability, which, in turn, will force us to choose, especially in the early stages of an epidemic, who will live and who will die. We will have to decide not only who gets scarce vaccines, but also who gets (less) scarce antiviral medications, hospital beds, and ventilators. In this paper, I will limit the ambit of my attention to the problem of justice in vaccine distribution. Because such awesome choices are fraught with ethical and political ramifications, it is imperative that we begin drafting and publicly justifying our selection criteria now, well before a pandemic is upon us. The stakes are so high, and the issue so volatile, that the public must come to understand and accept, if only somewhat passively, the rationale for distribution well before an epidemic strikes that will inevitably stir up social chaos in its wake.

In this paper, I shall argue that the ethical principles governing the distribution of vaccine during the so-called "interpandemic" influenza seasons will be inadequate to deal with the medical, social, and ethical challenges of a genuine avian flu pandemic. Our criteria for just distribution will have to expand to include protection of key personnel and social infrastructures. I shall also argue, however, that once we have articulated these additional criteria, we will have to acknowledge that we lack rational grounds or a social consensus on how to set priorities among them. This conclusion will lead to the further claim that when rational priority-setting among distributional criteria founders in this way, efforts to legitimize rationing during a pandemic should focus on the development of a transparent and democratic process for making such decisions. Even when such a legitimizing process has been deployed, however, rationing will still be difficult due to ubiquitous empirical uncertainties. In short, I shall argue that even though rationing during an avian flu pandemic is potentially legitimate and ethically justifiable, it won't be easy.

I.   RATIONING DURING INTERPANDEMIC FLU SHORTAGES

We already occasionally experience manufacturing disruptions that lead to shortages in vaccine supply during normal, "interpandemic" influenza seasons—the most recent occurring in the fall of 2004—and the United States and other countries have by now settled upon criteria for vaccine rationing during such periods. One might well ask why we should not simply deploy these same criteria during a genuine influenza pandemic. A comparison of the phenomena of interpandemic and pandemic influenza shows why this would be a bad idea.

Although vaccine shortages during interpandemic influenza seasons pose a serious threat to thousands of vulnerable individuals, such "crises" are not generally regarded as a threat to the functioning of society at large. Consequently, rationing strategy during such periods tends to focus rather narrowly on protecting those most at risk for influenza-associated mortality and hospitalization. This approach thus gives highest priority to people over 65 with co-morbid conditions, elderly residents of long-term care facilities, those under 65 with co-morbid conditions, children aged 6 to 23 months, and pregnant women. The CDC's recently published priority ranking also lists health care personnel and the household contacts of children under the age of 6 months. (Direct vaccination of children in this category is not recommended.)

A solid social consensus exists with regard to this narrowly focused rationing scheme. There is general agreement that during interpandemic shortages, scarce life-saving medical resources should go to those most in need. No consideration is given here to maintaining the smooth functioning of important social institutions, such as schools, prisons, the courts, or legislatures. Indeed, when the news media report that high-ranking politicians or sports teams have jumped the queue, this behavior tends to be roundly criticized. Although health-care providers are included in the CDC's list, the justification for their inclusion had nothing to do with maintaining the smooth functioning of our medical infrastructure. Given the likely impact of a normal influenza season upon unvaccinated health-care workers, officials at the CDC were not worried about the ability of the health care system to con-

tinue to function. Their primary concern with health-care providers is helpfully telegraphed by this group's proximity on the list to household contacts and out-of-home caretakers of children under 6 years. All three of these groups were given priority because they are potential vectors of influenza transmission to the populations most at risk for influenza-related illness and death. (Imagine the potential impact of a single infected physician or nurse upon the frail, immune-compromised residents of a nursing home.) Thus, the one item on the list that might appear to suggest a social objective, rather than a narrowly medical focus, turns out to represent merely an indirect means of achieving the single goal of protecting the neediest and most vulnerable individuals.

This consensus on the correct rationing principle for interpandemic shortages has important implications for policy. First, agreement on a single rationing principle tends to obviate the need for much attention to the development of fair and/or elaborate procedures for the distribution of scarce resources. If we agree in principle on who should get scarce vaccine, and if our sole criterion is based upon medical considerations, then, assuming serious scarcity, the major procedural question will be how to ensure as far as possible that *only* the most vulnerable persons actually end up receiving the vaccine. So we will need screening mechanisms carefully designed by medical professionals to exclude younger and healthier persons (e.g., politicians) from receiving priority. Inevitably, some unscrupulous, relatively healthy people will slip through the screen, but those doing the screening will at least know exactly what they are looking for. The philosopher John Rawls called this an example of "imperfect procedural justice"—i.e., a case in which there exists an independent criterion for the correct outcome, but there is no feasible procedure guaranteed to yield it.

Interestingly, given this interpandemic emphasis upon a single agreed-upon criterion of selection—and a corresponding de-emphasis upon the elaboration of some sort of "fair procedure"—those political units (e.g., towns, counties, states) that resort to non-medical decision procedures in order to achieve a perceived measure of "fairness" might actually be judged as acting in an unprincipled, unjust manner. During fall 2004, for example, the media published accounts of municipalities that responded to the impending shortfall in vaccine supplies by instituting lotteries or first-come, first-served policies at public health clinics. Apparently flummoxed by the magnitude of the shortfall, the intensity of demand from all quarters, and lack of clear guidance from the CDC at that time, some political leaders adopted a seemingly fair procedure that would at least give everyone a fair shot at obtaining an injection. Notice, however, that if we really do have consensus upon a rationing principle—such as: "protect those most likely to suffer illness or death due to influenza"— then resort to other kinds of procedures like lotteries or town meetings will be either unjust or unnecessary. Since they already agree on the correct principle, and since the fairest process will be predicated upon medical judgments, those attending a town meeting would have nothing to discuss. A lottery, on the other hand, would give equal consideration or an equal chance not only to those who are most vulnerable (e.g., sick nursing home residents) but also to those who are merely somewhat vulnerable (e.g., healthy adults over 65), which would defeat the point of the principle.

Consensus on a rationing principle during interpandemic vaccine shortages also has implications for the locus of decision making. During the 2004 season, a controversy arose regarding the relative desirability of national versus local decision making. After it became apparent that only half the usual doses would be available due to a manufacturing snafu at Chiron Corporation, local health departments looked to the federal government, and in particular to the CDC, for guidance in allocating their scarce remaining stocks. For its part, the CDC had not yet developed an authoritative priority list and pondered the wisdom of hastily publishing recommendations without a firm factual basis or much time to deliberate carefully. Some CDC officials worried that publishing a priority list in the midst of that flu season, after many local health officials had already made tough but unavoidable choices in distributing vaccine, might have the unintended effect of undercutting local health departments and possibly subjecting them to lawsuits from irate citizens who had been denied vaccination. Abstracting from the crisis atmosphere of that period, we can now ask at our leisure whether centralized federal or diffuse local decision making, or perhaps some

complex mix of the two, should govern such rationing choices during interpandemic shortages.

Supposing that we have a well-founded consensus on a rationing principle exclusively focused on the prevention of morbidity and mortality in the most vulnerable categories of people, the case for local decision-making is greatly attenuated. In many circumstances, policy makers rightly favor localized decision making. Conditions may vary from place to place. The residents of different geographical locations might have different value rankings, and, especially when information concerning particulars is at a premium, only local actors might possess a sufficiently nuanced appreciation of the facts on the ground to make sound decisions. Such is the case, for example, regarding decisions to forgo life-sustaining treatments, which most thoughtful observers believe are best delegated to the involved parties and perhaps local hospital ethics committees rather than to members of the U.S. Senate. During interpandemic flu seasons, however, none of these conditions prevail, so the national government via the CDC seems to be the locus of proper decision making. To be sure, local public health officers and other officials will require discretion in carrying out the recommendations of federal agencies—for example, regarding the number and placement of screening and vaccination sites—but they require no discretion in identifying the proper policy objectives.

Finally, note that vaccine shortages during interpandemic flu seasons are at least somewhat compatible with a private market in vaccines. During ordinary flu seasons, it is at least somewhat "business as usual" in that various health care providers (e.g., hospitals, nursing homes, managed care organizations, local public health agencies, etc.) already will have contracted for their standing orders of vaccine long before a crisis emerges. When a serious shortage looms, such institutions rightly expect their prior contractual agreements to be honored. The problem, of course, is that many other institutions—ranging from corporations to professional sports teams—have also placed standing orders, but few (if any) of their members might satisfy the criteria set forth in the CDC's priority ranking list. In situations such as this, government agencies can wheedle, cajole, and perhaps even threaten such private institutions to cede their stocks of vaccine to those who are truly needy, such as the residents of nursing homes that had the bad luck to have contracted with a defaulting supplier. In cases such as this, the market is a notoriously bad mechanism for achieving just or tolerably fair results. Notwithstanding much urgent talk about the need for fair and equitable dissemination of scarce vaccine stocks in fall 2004, the brute fact was that preexisting market transactions had already precluded fair and equitable distribution for many highly vulnerable citizens. For rationing to be both equitable and efficient, those doing the rationing (e.g., legislators, public health officials, etc.) must effectively control the resources to be distributed; otherwise, they have no leverage in bringing about desired results. Fortunately, that flu season turned out not to be as devastating as originally predicted, and many virtuous citizens who regularly get flu shots decided to forgo them. So an impending medical and moral crisis was averted, but this close call served to highlight the limits of unfettered markets in the distribution of vaccine.

II.　RATIONING DURING PANDEMICS

When we move from rationing during interpandemic periods to full-scale pandemic rationing, the situation is entirely different. In the first place, there will be much less room for the workings of the free market if or when the United States is engulfed by waves of avian flu. Given the predicted extent of shortages and their implications for large-scale devastation of the population, it will be imperative for the federal government to control all available stocks of avian flu vaccine from the beginning. Naturally, the government will have to purchase these stocks from the private companies that produce them, but we cannot repeat during a pandemic the unfocused, ad hoc, and socially blind workings of the market seen during the last interpandemic crisis, a process that delivered vaccines to the members of Congress and, one suspects, to high-ranking officials of large corporations. This does not mean, however, that the government should control the chain of distribution along its entire length and breadth. There may well be a powerful case for distributing avian flu vaccine not only through public

health clinics, but also through private hospitals, managed care organizations, and other private enterprises. The key point is that such decisions must be made by a single entity that controls all available vaccine. They must, moreover, conform to the strictly defined objectives of the vaccination program, and not according to people's willingness and ability to pay.

Another crucial difference between interpandemic and pandemic rationing situations is that the latter may exhibit several (possibly competing) policy goals, whereas the former only featured the single goal of reducing mortality and morbidity within the most vulnerable categories of citizens. The latter policy objective might certainly continue to play a role in the thinking and planning of public health officials during a pandemic, in which case distribution would continue to favor the most medically needy and vulnerable—e.g., the elderly and children with co-morbid conditions, such as acute asthma, nursing home residents, and the people (including physicians and family members) who care for them. But this is only one possibility. During the crunch of a genuine flu pandemic, other important objectives for social policy beckon. Before we enumerate and discuss these additional policy goals, some of which supplement a narrow medical focus with a concern for the continued functioning of crucial social institutions, we need to confront an important threshold question: viz, is it ever morally permissible to weigh the social value of various possible recipients and uses of scarce medical resources?

This question was posed at the birth of the modern bioethics movement by Dr. Belding Scribner's development of an arterio-venous shunt for dialysis patients in end-stage kidney failure: viz, who would live when not all could live? According to many observers at the time, one key factor that should count either for or against any given candidate for this scarce, life-saving resource was his or her value to society. It seemed axiomatic to these commentators that if not all could be saved, then the cancer researcher or the church-going mother of four should receive ongoing dialysis rather than the bachelor street sweeper with a drinking problem. From this angle, the best solution to this problem was the formation of a committee with diverse membership, whose job it would be to tote up the potential net social contributions of the various candidates. If there wasn't enough to go around, we should bestow our scarce societal resources upon those most likely to give us maximal "return on investment." Clearly, this position was animated by an unapologetic and unvarnished version of utilitarianism, according to which resources should be distributed so as to maximize social value (e.g., happiness, welfare, the satisfaction of desires, etc.). According to this view, everyone's gains or losses in welfare would be counted, but the prize would go to those who had the most social value on offer.

Notwithstanding its intuitive plausibility to many observers, the social value criterion was subjected to withering criticism at the time of the Seattle allocation experiment, and it was subsequently abandoned by both clinicians and social policy experts in the area of organ transplantation. According to the influential Protestant moral theologian Paul Ramsey, deciding who should live or die according to judgments of social worth necessarily violates the equal intrinsic worth of every human being.[1] To say that the cancer researcher or the banker is more valuable to society than a disabled single man on welfare, and thus that the former should live while the latter should die, is, argued Ramsey, "to presume to make a (nearly) total estimate of a man's life,"[2] and thus to make a repugnant and indefensible judgment. Repugnant because such a judgment denies what most religions and liberal political philosophies steadfastly insist upon: viz, that each of us is, respectively, either a child of God morally equal in God's eyes, or a citizen of a democratic polity deserving of equal concern and respect. Indefensible, because we lack the epistemological resources to know who is more socially worthy than whom. What if the single man on welfare devotes himself to the well-being of his neighbors, while the banker turns out to be a selfish tyrant, ruining the lives of his workers and family? Ramsey concluded that, in the ordinary run of such tragic choices, the only way to acknowledge our equal worth as human beings was to decide who would live on the basis of a random decision procedure, such as a lottery.

Ramsey conceded, however, that there might be some highly unusual social circumstances in which judgments of social worth could be morally permissible. In two of Ramsey's examples, war and catastrophic triage situations, human beings are reduced to a state of affairs in which a single overarching social goal—e.g., defeating the enemy or saving those who can be most easily saved following a natural catastrophe—effectively eclipses all other concerns. Thus, during World War II, it was decided that the scarce stocks of the newly developed "magic bullet," penicillin, would go first to soldiers "wounded in brothels" rather than on the battlefield. During the North African campaign of 1943, the myriad values and goals ordinarily littering the social landscape were reduced to a single imperative: Get as many troops into battle as soon as possible in order to defeat the German army. Here the great plurality of social values and criteria for selection boil down to a "focused" concern "where objectives were closely defined."[3] In such desperate straits, social worthiness can and should, Ramsey conceded, be both effectively measured and deployed as a decisive criterion for life and death decisions. He maintained, however, that dire straits of this severity were a rare social occurrence and continued to advocate his principle of random selection for the vast majority of "tragic choice" situations, including the rationing of dialysis machines and transplantable organs.

Although they routinely claim many thousands of lives each year, bringing untold grief to those left behind, interpandemic flu seasons do not bring society to its knees; they do not count as exceptions to Ramsey's general rule against the deployment of social worth criteria. Although many die, life goes on for the vast majority of citizens, and the variegated infrastructure of society remains intact. Our field of vision thus remains highly pluralistic rather than "focused" upon a single overarching social imperative, and so it makes sense to avoid social value criteria. But the specter of a genuine avian flu pandemic may well provide us with yet another example of a catastrophic situation so drastic and so threatening to the fabric of society as to legitimate the limited use of social value criteria.

Consider in this connection the havoc wreaked by the infamous "Spanish flu" pandemic of 1918. This was an exceptionally lethal virus that killed with frightening speed and efficiency. Young adults, a category usually spared by most interpandemic flu viruses, were singled out for particularly harsh treatment. It is estimated that as many as 8 to 10 percent of all young adults then living in the world were felled by this virus. Five hundred thousand Americans and as many as 50 million deaths worldwide have been attributed to the Spanish flu. As the historian John M. Barry, puts it, this flu killed more people than any other outbreak in human history. It "killed more people in a year than the Black Death of the Middle Ages killed in a century; it killed more people in twenty-four weeks than AIDS has killed in twenty-four years."[4] Military bases with their cramped, fetid quarters provided ideal growth conditions for the virus and were quickly decimated. In the city of Philadelphia, it took only 10 days for the epidemic to explode from one or two deaths per day to hundreds of thousands ill and hundreds dropping dead. Federal, city, and state courts closed down, and all public meetings were banned. Swaths of black crepe, indicating a death in the house, hung everywhere in every neighborhood. "People were dying like flies," one observer noted, "every other house had crepe over the door."[5] There were not nearly enough doctors and nurses to attend to the ill, as if their paltry defenses at the time would have made any difference against that virus, nor were there enough undertakers to bury the mounting toll of dead.

A flu pandemic threatening anything resembling the devastation of 1918 would no doubt qualify as an exception to Paul Ramsey's rejection of social value criteria. In the United States alone, hundreds of thousands would perish, key social institutions (e.g., the courts, prisons, legislatures) would be crippled, and commerce would grind to a halt in many cities. Air travel, a primary medium for the spread of such viruses, would be suspended for weeks, if not months, thereby throwing the whole industry into a financial tail spin. Confronted by the looming threat of such a pandemic, our usual commitment to the equal moral worth of each citizen would predictably and justifiably yield to a social value perspective narrowly focused on survival and the minimization of social disruption. At such a perilous juncture, it would be reasonable for those in charge of the national welfare to consider the following possible goals:

(1) Protection of the most vulnerable

For example, children and the elderly, those with co-morbid conditions, their caregivers, etc. As we have seen, this goal, which focuses attention on the medically worst off group, constitutes the sole objective of current government policy during periods of interpandemic flu. During an epidemic of pandemic flu, however, this important goal may well have to be weighed and balanced against other values and social priorities. Thus, in addition to upholding the value of social equality and the equal worth of every person, society may have to engage in trade-offs with some of the following social goals.

(2) Protection of key personnel in health care, public health and safety, and crisis response infrastructures

Whereas current government interpandemic rationing policy does include health care workers providing direct support to infected or highly vulnerable persons, the rationale for their inclusion, as we saw above, rested exclusively on their role as potential vectors of the disease to vulnerable populations. During a pandemic, however, both the categories of key workers and the rationale for their inclusion would expand to encompass explicitly social goals, such as the maintenance of crucial health-related infrastructures. Thus, in addition to those health care workers directly caring for patients, our priority list would also include vaccine manufacturers and key public health personnel on both the national and local levels, as well as front-line crisis responders, including personnel from the Department of Homeland Security. This list could be expanded to include key elected officials with administrative responsibilities for managing social crises, such as the U.S. president, key cabinet officers, state governors, etc.

(3) The protection of key social functions—including transportation, fire and police departments, food production, utilities, and undertakers

Some key sectors of the economy, such as trucking, obviously play a role in the distribution of crucial medical supplies such as vaccines and anti-viral drugs. Clearly, these sectors would have priority during a flu pandemic. Nevertheless, many crucial, non-health related social functions would be threatened during a pandemic. As we saw during hurricane Katrina, natural catastrophes can overwhelm the usual bulwarks of law and public order. Police and fire personnel, as well as members of the National Guard, might thus be high on our priority list. Depending on the mortality rate of a given pandemic flu virus, even undertakers might be singled out for preferential treatment under a vaccine rationing plan. The plausibility of such a scenario is graphically underscored in Barry's account of the 1918 outbreak in Philadelphia: "But the most terrifying aspect of the epidemic was the piling up of bodies. Undertakers, themselves sick, were overwhelmed. They had no place to put the bodies. . . . The city morgue had room for thirty-six bodies. Two hundred were stacked there. The stench was terrible. . . . No more bodies could fit. Bodies lay in homes where they died, as they died, often with bloody liquid seeping from the nostrils or mouths. . . . Corpses were wrapped in sheets, pushed into corners, left there sometimes for days, the horror of it sinking in deeper each hour. . ."[6]

(4) Maximization of economic benefits
Supposing that one were inclined to maximize the economic benefits flowing from the deployment of vaccines and anti-virals, and supposing that the greatest economic cost exacted by a flu pandemic would be attributable to massive loss of life in the healthy working population, then planners might reasonably target vaccines at a broad swath (e.g., 40 to 60 percent) of healthy workers in the general adult population. While traditional criteria for vaccine priority tend to be explicitly "Hippocratic" in nature, this ordering of priorities would be dictated entirely by cost-benefit analysis—more specifically, by an analysis of the costs associated with a catastrophic shutdown of major industries, such as air travel, telecommunications, food production and distribution, tourism and entertainment, and so on.

(5) "Fair innings"
Another controversial rationing principle with a credible claim to justification is rationing by age. According to this view, those who have already reached old age and thus enjoyed their "fair innings" should receive lower priority for vaccines and other scarce resources than those who have yet to live a full life. Thus, even though relatively healthy persons over the age of 65 might be at greater risk for influenza-related morbidity and mortality than healthy children, teens, and young adults, the fair innings principle would give priority to these latter groups. Although this principle reaches many of the same conclusions as rationing according to social value, its rationale is very different. While some appeals to age-based rationing, like the economic maximization scheme described directly above, are

grounded in utilitarian calculations of the likely social benefits of immunizing various competing age cohorts, the fair innings argument, focusing as it does on securing for everyone an equal opportunity to live a full life, is actually grounded in a concern for fairness and justice.

III. WHY PANDEMIC RATIONING WILL BE SO DIFFICULT

In a pandemic flu situation, the four policy goals enumerated above—i.e., protection of the most vulnerable individuals, of key health-related personnel, of important societal infrastructures, and, finally, the achievement of maximal social utility—would all be on the table as possible options for key decision makers. But not all of these goals are mutually compatible. The protection of the most vulnerable would obviously allot highest priority to the elderly debilitated residents of nursing homes. Living in close proximity to scores or hundreds of other patients, most with already compromised immune systems, these residents are clearly at highest risk for infection and death. On the other hand, because they are no longer working, their deaths would not exact great economic costs. In addition, precisely because their immune systems are already often severely compromised, giving nursing home residents first priority will not amount to an efficient use of scarce vaccine stocks. So a policy focused upon the protection of the most vulnerable would inevitably threaten at least two other worthy goals—viz., maximizing both economic value and the purely medical effectiveness of the vaccine.

   While most of these goals individually represent plausible policy options, as would various permutations and combinations among them, it is highly unlikely that any one value or any single combination of values will emerge as uniquely and obviously correct. Part of the problem stems from our epistemological limitations. We will often not have sufficient information to choose among various key players representing health care, the public health system, government, or the economic infrastructure. Who among them is truly "indispensable"? Which will have the greatest impact on stemming the rising tide of the pandemic or maintaining social stability? In all likelihood, we just won't have complete answers to such empirical questions, although we can be quite confident about the crucial importance of some groups, such as front-line emergency medical and public health personnel.

But this epistemological embarrassment won't be the worst of our problems. In addition, there's the equally embarrassing fact that we apparently lack a canonical value ordering that would allow us to prioritize, weigh, and balance the available policy goals and values already on the table before us. How, for example, should we weigh and balance the competing goals of protecting the most vulnerable and safeguarding our key health and security infrastructures? In the value ordering of many people, protecting the most vulnerable should have top priority, especially when compared with, say, the maximization of economic efficiency, but at what cost? The vulnerable certainly won't be protected if our public health infrastructure collapses.

Here's a related problem: How should we weigh and balance the competing goals of protecting the most vulnerable and achieving the best results in terms of lives saved per dose of vaccine? We all might agree that the debilitated elderly in nursing homes deserve protection, but what if the very fact of their immunological debilitation means that they will be extremely inefficient hosts for the vaccine? What if focusing our attention on the debilitated elderly means that we won't be able to save thousands more younger and healthier people whose bodies could put the vaccine to better use and who perhaps have a stronger claim based upon the fair innings principle? Should we then abandon the elderly completely, giving them no chance at the vaccine, or should we rather allot them a major (or minor) portion of the vaccine, fully realizing that our commitment to protecting this vulnerable population will have serious costs in terms of other lives lost? Questions of this sort go to the heart of the rationing problem, yet we lack both a rational decision procedure and a clear political consensus on how best to answer them. (For a worthy initial attempt at grappling with these difficult problems, see the suggested priority schemes of two federal committees advising the Department of Health and Human Services at www.hhs.gov/pandemicflu/plan/appendixd.html. Additional information concerning the U.S. government's preparations for an avian flu pandemic, see the National Strategy for Pandemic Influenza: Implementation Plan, available at http://www.whitehouse.gov/homeland/nspi_implementation.pdf).

Norman Daniels and James Sabin have acknowledged in their recent work the baffling nature of such fundamental questions at the very heart of the health care rationing project. They have concluded that, in the absence of canonical answers to them, the legitimacy of political decision-making about scarce life-saving resources depends upon the fairness of the processes through which they are made. In contrast to the sort of rationing problem posed by interpandemic flu, a situation in which we share a solid consensus on the correct principle, pandemic flu confronts us with multiple values, goals, and principles, all of which are to some extent plausible, but none of which (or no combination of which) is obviously rationally correct. For Daniels and Sabin, this failure of reason leads directly to an emphasis on fair procedures for settling on public policies. Although this is no place for a full examination of their theory of fair process, these authors stress the importance, inter alia, of publicity (rationales must be publicly accessible), of broadly intelligible and acceptable reasons (rather than sectarian appeals), and of mechanisms for challenge and dispute resolution. If such fair procedures are not followed, Daniels and Sabin contend, political choices may well be reasonable and sound, but they will not be viewed as legitimate by the people subject to them. This is, I would argue, a crucial consideration for medical and public health leaders who would suggest rationing principles favoring members of their own professions. Although a highly plausible case can be made for vaccinating front-line doctors, nurses, and public health officials in a context of pandemic flu, we must keep in mind that such a rationing principle does override or violate (even if justifiably) Paul Ramsey's principle of equal moral worth. In the absence of a well-planned process of sharing information, deliberation and consensus building with the public, such a recommendation may well strike many people as a case of well off medical types helping themselves to the lion's share of a scarce life-saving resource. In this connection, it appears that the Canadians, who have already deployed an ambitious consensus-building project on pandemic flu preparations, are already well ahead of the U.S.

Another important difference between interpandemic and pandemic flu follows from this discussion. We saw above how consensus on a moral principle for rationing in the context of interpandemic flu rendered otiose much of the debate over the locus of decision making. If we all (or most of us) agree on a single principle of distribution, then our usual preference for local decision making over the ruminations of distant government bureaucrats loses most of its force. In a context of reasonable disagreement over a host of plausible principles and their various permutations in combination, however, local differences in approaching these intractable questions may well come to the fore. In theory, at least, officials in Maine and California may have a different take on how such goals as protecting the vulnerable, securing the best medical results, safeguarding infrastructures, and achieving maximal economic benefit should be ranked and combined with other goals. So in order for such decisions to acquire legitimacy in the eyes of the public, it may well take more than an edict from the federal government coming out of Atlanta. On the other hand, such political theoretic considerations will have to be balanced against the real world demands of efficiency in the context of an emerging flu pandemic. Since it would only take weeks or even days for a virulent avian flu virus to begin to wreak havoc across the globe, this would not be the time for leisurely democratic deliberation in uncoordinated town meetings. Such rationing decisions will either have to be made long before a pandemic strikes, or they will have to be left to centralized government actors and agencies in the thick of the battle. The former course is obviously preferable to the latter, but does our society have the will to confront well ahead of time such potentially harsh but uncertain realities? Recent events in New Orleans indicate otherwise.

In addition to our epistemological limitations and our lack of consensus on key values, pandemic rationing decisions will be hampered by much uncertainty. An avian flu pandemic may come in the near future, but then again it may not. How much of our national treasure should we devote to hedging against this possibility? Advance planning will also be stymied by uncertainty about the virus itself and its effects. Until an avian viral strain breaks out into the human population, we won't know exactly how virulent it is. The Spanish flu strain of 1918 killed

roughly 2.5 percent of its victims, which doesn't sound like much until you recall that it struck one-fifth of the world's population. Garden-variety flu viruses, by contrast, only kill one-tenth of 1 percent during a normal influenza season. A great deal obviously hangs on where a new strain of avian flu would fall on this continuum between worldwide catastrophe and business-as-usual. Planning for pandemic rationing will also be hampered by uncertainty about the virus' age-specific fatality rate. Even if we have decided well ahead of time through legitimate processes of democratic deliberation to devote a certain percentage of vaccine stocks to protecting the most vulnerable members of society, we won't know exactly who the most vulnerable are until the virus strikes. Ordinarily, the elderly and small children are most at risk from flu viruses, but the 1918 flu primarily targeted young adults. Since pandemics by definition are driven by new viral strains against which we have no built up immunity, we won't know how bad they are going to be or who is going to be hardest hit until the epidemic is well under way.

These uncertainties will pose serious problems for any rationing scheme we could possibly devise. Because we cannot predict either a strain's virulence or its affinity for certain age groups, public health officials will have to be exceedingly attentive to its patterns of infectivity and mortality and be willing to alter pre-established rationing strategies in the middle of the crisis. This will be especially problematic with regard to the threshold question of whether any given epidemic merits the overriding of our standard concerns about equal moral worth and subsequent deployment of social value criteria. Suppose a strain of avian flu does break out into the human population but is comparatively weak, resembling more the strain of Hong Kong flu in 1968 than the Spanish flu of 1918. How bad will it have to be before we jettison our governing norms of equality and start giving preference to health care professionals, politicians, and truck drivers bearing stocks of vaccine? Just because we agree that social value criteria can legitimately be invoked in a genuine social crisis doesn't mean that we will unerringly know when one is upon us. A false positive judgment here would lead to the unnecessary and morally problematic abandonment of a crucially important social norm bearing on the moral equality of all citizens. A false-negative judgment, on the other hand, would lead to misplaced complacency and social chaos.

I close this review of moral difficulties attendant upon pandemic rationing schemes with two additional related considerations. First, any ethical rationing scheme for pandemic influenza must plan effectively to counterbalance our society's well-documented tendency to give short shrift to minorities and the poor. As hurricane Katrina amply demonstrated, in our society the rich and well-placed command resources and the high ground, while the poor suffer, die, and are swept away. We saw this pattern repeated during the last interpandemic rationing crisis in Fall 2004. In spite of all the urgent talk of distributing scarce vaccine equitably among the most vulnerable, the wealthy and powerful unerringly found their way to the vaccine through the medium of the market and the power of political office. Crisis planners would thus do well to keep the somber lessons of Katrina firmly in mind as they devise distribution strategies for vaccine and anti-virals during a flu pandemic.

Finally, in addition to the problem of the poor at home, there is the problem of global poverty and lack of access to medical resources in developing countries. Notwithstanding the urgency of problems on the domestic front, we nevertheless must consider what obligations we (and other advanced industrialized nations) have toward the distant needy. Numerous principles of moral and political philosophy converge on the moral necessity of doing more, much more, than we currently do to help those suffering from starvation, malnutrition, and stunted lives abroad. Whether the analysis focuses on the utilitarian-inspired principles of beneficence and common decency, a strong principle of global distributive justice, considerations of rectification for past and ongoing wrongs, or a relatively weak principle of assistance to burdened societies derived from John Rawls' last work, the conclusion is the same: our current efforts to stem the tide of poverty, malnutrition, and premature death in the developing world are pitifully lame. If this conclusion encompasses an obligation to provide the world's poor with drugs to combat HIV, why would it not also include an obligation to make flu vaccine available to those who cannot afford it? Clearly, this is not a burden that the U.S. can or

should bear alone. Other technologically advanced and wealthy nations must join forces to create vastly expanded capacity to manufacture vaccines. This moral imperative will be extremely difficult, if not impossible, to carry out if we follow the usual pattern of waiting for the epidemic to happen before kicking our pharmaceutical machinery into high gear. Now that a generic vaccine for the H5N1 avian flu virus has been successfully developed, however, we will not have to wait that long, even though this vaccine might not be as effective as one tailor made for an emerging pandemic.

CONCLUSION

I have argued in this paper that the ethical challenges posed by a possible pandemic of avian flu are nearly as formidable as the scientific and public health challenges. Assuming a high degree of mortality associated with the viral strain, a genuine pandemic would claim millions of lives worldwide and threaten the integrity of key medical, public health, social, and political infrastructures. A pandemic on such a scale would justify the temporary abandonment of our traditional commitment to the principle of equal moral worth and the concomitant embrace of social value criteria for health care rationing. But no sooner do we admit the justifiability of such criteria than we realize that we lack a canonical rank ordering of them and their many possible permutations. In the absence of social consensus on priorities, adhering to fair processes becomes critical for the public legitimation of rationing scarce life-saving resources, especially when health care providers and public health officials play a major role in allotting flu vaccines and anti-viral medications to themselves. Whatever rationing principles are ultimately forged within a context of public democratic deliberation, we will still be faced with the difficulty of deploying them under conditions of debilitating factual uncertainty. Finally, the rationing principles we develop must remain vigilant against the ever-present temptation to discriminate against the poor and dispossessed, whether here at home or in the far reaches of the developing world.

REFERENCES

1. Ramsey P. *The Patient as Person*. New Haven, Connecticut: Yale University Press; 1970, 253.
2. Ibid., 259.
3. Ibid., 257.

4. Barry JM. *The Great Influenza*. New York: Viking; 2004, 4–5.
5. Ibid., 223.
6. Ibid., 223–24.

WHO SHOULD GET INFLUENZA VACCINE WHEN NOT ALL CAN?

Ezekiel J. Emanuel and Alan Wertheimer

The potential threat of pandemic influenza is staggering: 1.9 million deaths, 90 million people sick, and nearly 10 million people hospitalized, with almost 1.5 million requiring intensive-care units (ICUs) in the United States.[1] The National Vaccine Advisory Committee (NVAC) and the Advisory Committee on Immunization Policy (ACIP) have jointly recommended a prioritization scheme that places vaccine workers, health-care providers, and the ill elderly at the top, and healthy people aged 2 to 64 at the very bottom even under embalmers[2] (see table). The primary goal informing the recommendation was to "decrease health impacts including severe morbidity and death"; a secondary goal was minimizing societal and economic impacts.[3] As the NVAC and ACIP acknowledge, such important policy decisions require broad national discussion. In this spirit, we believe an alternative ethical framework should be considered.

THE INESCAPABILITY OF RATIONING

Because of current uncertainty of its value, only "a limited amount of avian influenza A (H5N1) vaccine is being stockpiled."[4] Furthermore, it will take at least 4 months from identification of a candidate

Reprinted from *Science* 312 (May 12, 2006): 854–855. Reprinted by permission.

Editors' note: Some authors' notes have been cut. Students who want to follow up on sources should consult the original article.

vaccine strain until production of the very first vaccine.[5] At present, there are few production facilities worldwide that make influenza vaccine, and only one completely in the USA. Global capacity for influenza vaccine production is just 425 million doses per annum, if all available factories would run at full capacity after a vaccine was developed. Under currently existing capabilities for manufacturing vaccine, it is likely that more than 90% of the U.S. population will not be vaccinated in the first year.[6] Distributing the limited supply will require determining priority groups.

Who will be at highest risk? Our experience with three influenza pandemics presents a complex picture. The mortality profile of a future pandemic could be U-shaped, as it was in the mild-to-moderate pandemics of 1957 and 1968 and interpandemic influenza seasons, in which the very young and the old are at highest risk. Or, the mortality profile could be an attenuated W shape, as it was during the devastating 1918 pandemic, in which the highest risk occurred among people between 20 and 40 years of age, while the elderly were not at high excess risk. Even during pandemics, the elderly appear to be at no higher risk than during interpandemic influenza seasons.

Clear ethical justification for vaccine priorities is essential to the acceptability of the priority ranking and any modifications during the pandemic. With limited vaccine supply, uncertainty over who will be at highest risk of infection and complications, and questions about which historic pandemic experience is most applicable, society faces a fundamental ethical dilemma: Who should get the vaccine first?

THE NVAC AND ACIP PRIORITY RANKINGS

Many potential ethical principles for rationing health care have been proposed. "Save the most lives" is commonly used in emergencies, such as burning buildings, although "women and children first" played a role on the Titanic. "First come, first served" operates in other emergencies and in ICUs when admitted patients retain beds despite the presentation of another patient who is equally or even more sick; "Save the most quality life years" is central to cost-effectiveness rationing. "Save the worst-off" plays a role in allocating organs for transplantation. "Reciprocity"—giving priority to people willing to donate their own organs—has been proposed. "Save those most likely to fully recover" guided priorities for giving penicillin to soldiers with syphilis in World War II. Save those "instrumental in making society flourish" through economic productivity or by "contributing to the well-being of others" has been proposed by Murray and others.

The save-the-most-lives principle was invoked by NVAC and ACIP. It justifies giving top priority to workers engaged in vaccine production and distribution and health-care workers. They get higher priority not because they are intrinsically more valuable people or of greater "social worth," but because giving them first priority ensures that maximal life-saving vaccine is produced and so that health care is provided to the sick. Consequently, it values all human life equally, giving every person equal consideration in who gets priority regardless of age, disability, social class, or employment. After these groups, the save-the-most-lives principle justifies priority for those predicted to be at highest risk of hospitalization and dying. We disagree with this prioritization.

LIFE-CYCLE PRINCIPLE

The save-the-most-lives principle may be justified in some emergencies when decision urgency makes it infeasible to deliberate about priority rankings and impractical to categorize individuals into priority groups. We believe that a life-cycle allocation principle (see table), based on the idea that each person should have an opportunity to live through all the stages of life is more appropriate for a pandemic. There is great value in being able to pass through each life stage—to be a child, a young adult, and to then develop a career and family, and to grow old—and to enjoy a wide range of the opportunities during each stage.

Multiple considerations and intuitions support this ethical principle. Most people endorse this principle for themselves. We would prioritize our own resources to ensure we could live past the illnesses of childhood and young adulthood and would allocate fewer resources to living ever longer once we reached old age. People strongly prefer maximizing the chance of living until a ripe old age, rather than being struck down as a young person.

Death seems more tragic when a child or young adult dies than an elderly person—not because the lives of older people are less valuable, but because the younger person has not had the opportunity to live and develop through all stages of life. Although the life-cycle principle favors some ages, it is also intrinsically egalitarian. Unlike being productive or contributing to others' well-being, every person will live to be older unless their life is cut short.

THE INVESTMENT REFINEMENT

A pure version of the life-cycle principle would grant priority to 6-month-olds over 1-year-olds who have priority over 2-year-olds, and on. An alternative, the investment refinement, emphasizes gradations within a life span. It gives priority to people between early adolescence and middle age on the basis of the amount the person invested in his or her life balanced by the amount left to live. Within this framework, 20-year-olds are valued more than 1-year-olds because the older individuals have more developed interests, hopes, and plans but have not had an opportunity to realize them. Although these groupings could be modified, they indicate ethically defensible distinctions among groups that can inform rationing priorities.

One other ethical principle relevant for priority ranking of influenza vaccine during a pandemic is public order. It focuses on the value of ensuring safety and the provision of necessities, such as food and fuel. We believe the investment refinement combined with the public-order principle (IRPOP) should be the ultimate objective of all pandemic response measures, including priority ranking for vaccines and interventions to limit the course of the

Priorities for Distribution of Influenza Vaccine

Tier*	NVAC and ACIP recommendations (subtier)†	Life-cycle principle (LCP)	Investment refinement of LCP including public order
1	Vaccine production and distribution workers	Vaccine production and distribution workers	Vaccine production and distribution workers
	Frontline health-care workers	Frontline health-care workers	Frontline health-care workers
	People 6 months to 64 years old with ≥2 high-risk conditions or history of hospitalization for pneumonia or influenza		
	Pregnant women		
	Household contacts of severely immunocompromised people		
	Household contacts of children ≤6 months of age		
	Public health and emergency response workers		
	Key government leaders		
2	Healthy people ≥65 years old	Healthy 6-month-olds	People 13 to 40 years old with <2 high-risk conditions, with priority to key government leaders; public health, military, police, and fire workers; utility and transportation workers; telecommunications and IT workers; funeral directors
	People 6 months to 64 years old with 1 or more high-risk conditions	Healthy 1-year-olds	People 7 to 12 years old and 41 to 50 years old with <2 high-risk conditions with priority as above
	Healthy children 6 months to 23 months old	Healthy 2-year-olds	People 6 months to 6 years old and 51 to 64 years old with <2 high-risk conditions, with priority as above‡
	Other public health workers, emergency responders, public safety workers (police and fire), utility workers, transportation workers, telecommunications and IT workers	Healthy 3-year-olds etc.	People ≥65 years old with <2 high-risk conditions
3	Other health decision-makers in government	People with life-limiting morbidities or disabilities, prioritized according to expected life years	People 6 months to 64 years old with ≥2 high-risk conditions
	Funeral directors		
4	Healthy people 2 to 64 years old		People ≥65 years old with ≥2 high-risk conditions

*Tiers determine priority ranking for the distribution of vaccine if limited in supply.

†Children 6 months to <13 years would not receive vaccine if they can be effectively confined to home or otherwise isolated.

pandemic, such as closing schools and confining people to homes. These two principles should inform decisions at the start of an epidemic when the shape of the risk curves for morbidity and mortality are largely uncertain.

Like the NVAC and ACIP ranking, the IRPOP ranking would give high priority to vaccine production and distribution workers, as well as healthcare and public health workers with direct patient contact. However, contrary to the NVAC and ACIP prioritization for the sick elderly and infants, IRPOP emphasize people between 13 and 40 years of age. The NVAC and ACIP priority ranking comports well with those groups at risk during the mild-to-moderate 1957 and 1968 pandemics. IRPOP prioritizes those age cohorts at highest risk during the devastating 1918 pandemic. Depending on patterns of flu spread, some mathematical models suggest that following IRPOP priority ranking could save the most lives overall.[7]

CONCLUSIONS

The life-cycle ranking is meant to apply to the situation in the United States. During a global pandemic, there will be fundamental questions about sharing vaccines and other interventions with other countries. This raises fundamental issues of global rationing that are too complex to address here.

Fortunately, even though we are worried about an influenza pandemic, it is not upon us. Indeed, the current H5N1 avian flu may never develop into a human pandemic. This gives us time both to build vaccine production capacity to minimize the need for rationing and to rationally assess policy and ethical issues about the distribution of vaccines.

REFERENCES AND NOTES

1. U.S. Department of Health and Human Services (HHS), *HHS Pandemic Influenza Plan* (HHS, Washington, DC, 2005), supplement E at (www.hhs.gov/pandemicflu/plan/) (accessed 29 March 2006).
2. Ibid.
3. Ibid.
4. Ibid.
5. Ibid.
6. Ibid.
7. M. E. Halloran, I. M. Longini Jr., *Science* 311, 615 (2006).

ORGAN TRANSPLANTATION: GIFTS VERSUS MARKETS

THE CASE FOR ALLOWING KIDNEY SALES

Janet Radcliffe-Richards, Abdallah S. Daar, Ronald D. Guttmann, Raymond Hoffenberg, Ian Kennedy, Margaret Lock, Robert A. Sells, Nicholas L. Tilney, International Forum for Transplant Ethics

When the practice of buying kidneys from live vendors first came to light some years ago, it aroused such horror that all professional associations denounced it and nearly all countries have now made it illegal. Such political and professional unanimity may seem to leave no room for further debate, but we nevertheless think it important to reopen the discussion.

The well-known shortage of kidneys for transplantation causes much suffering and death. Dialysis

is a wretched experience for most patients, and is anyway rationed in most places and simply unavailable to the majority of patients in most developing countries. Since most potential kidney vendors will never become unpaid donors, either during life or posthumously, the prohibition of sales must be presumed to exclude kidneys that would otherwise be available. It is therefore essential to make sure that there is adequate justification for the resulting harm.

Most people will recognise in themselves the feelings of outrage and disgust that led to an outright ban on kidney sales, and such feelings typically have a force that seems to their possessors to need no further justification. Nevertheless, if we are to deny treatment to the suffering and dying we need better reasons than our own feelings of disgust.

In this paper we outline our reasons for thinking that the arguments commonly offered for prohibiting organ sales do not work, and therefore that the

Reprinted from *The Lancet*, Vol. 351, J. Radcliffe-Richards, A. S. Daar, R. D. Guttmann, R. Hoffenberg, I. Kennedy, M. Lock, R. A. Sells, N. Tilney, for the International Forum for Transplant Ethics, "The Case for Allowing Kidney Sales," pp. 1950–2. Copyright © 1998, with permission from Elsevier.

Editors' note: All authors' notes have been cut. Students who want to follow up on sources should consult the original article.

debate should be reopened. Here we consider only the selling of kidneys by living vendors, but our arguments have wider implications.

The commonest objection to kidney selling is expressed on behalf of the vendors: the exploited poor, who need to be protected against the greedy rich. However, the vendors are themselves anxious to sell, and see this practice as the best option open to them. The worse we think the selling of a kidney, therefore, the worse should seem the position of the vendors when that option is removed. Unless this appearance is illusory, the prohibition of sales does even more harm than first seemed, in harming vendors as well as recipients. To this argument it is replied that the vendors' apparent choice is not genuine. It is said that they are likely to be too uneducated to understand the risks, and that this precludes informed consent. It is also claimed that, since they are coerced by their economic circumstances, their consent cannot count as genuine.

Although both these arguments appeal to the importance of autonomous choice, they are quite different. The first claim is that the vendors are not competent to make a genuine choice within a given range of options. The second, by contrast, is that poverty has so restricted the range of options that organ selling has become the best, and therefore, in effect, that the range is too small. Once this distinction is drawn, it can be seen that neither argument works as a justification of prohibition.

If our ground for concern is that the range of choices is too small, we cannot improve matters by removing the best option that poverty has left, and making the range smaller still. To do so is to make subsequent choices, by this criterion, even less autonomous. The only way to improve matters is to lessen the poverty until organ selling no longer seems the best option; and if that could be achieved, prohibition would be irrelevant because nobody would want to sell.

The other line of argument may seem more promising, since ignorance does preclude informed consent. However, the likely ignorance of the subjects is not a reason for banning altogether a procedure for which consent is required. In other contexts, the value we place on autonomy leads us to insist on information and counseling, and that is what it should suggest in the case of organ selling as well. It may be said that this approach is impracticable,

because the educational level of potential vendors is too limited to make explanation feasible, or because no system could reliably counteract the misinformation of nefarious middlemen and profiteering clinics. But even if we accepted that no possible vendor could be competent to consent, that would justify only putting the decision in the hands of competent guardians. To justify total prohibition it would also be necessary to show that organ selling must always be against the interests of potential vendors, and it is most unlikely that this would be done.

The risk involved in nephrectomy is not in itself high, and most people regard it as acceptable for living related donors. Since the procedure is, in principle, the same for vendors as for unpaid donors, any systematic difference between the worthwhileness of the risk for vendors and donors presumably lies on the other side of the calculation, in the expected benefit. Nevertheless the exchange of money cannot in itself turn an acceptable risk into an unacceptable one from the vendor's point of view. It depends entirely on what the money is wanted for.

In general, furthermore, the poorer a potential vendor, the more likely it is that the sale of a kidney will be worth whatever risk there is. If the rich are free to engage in dangerous sports for pleasure, or dangerous jobs for high pay, it is difficult to see why the poor who take the lesser risk of kidney selling for greater rewards—perhaps saving relatives' lives, or extricating themselves from poverty and debt—should be thought so misguided as to need saving from themselves.

It will be said that this does not take account of the reality of the vendors' circumstances: that risks are likely to be greater than for unpaid donors because poverty is detrimental to health, and vendors are often not given proper care. They may also be underpaid or cheated, or may waste their money through inexperience. However, once again, these arguments apply far more strongly to many other activities by which the poor try to earn money, and which we do not forbid. The best way to address such problems would be by regulation and perhaps a central purchasing system, to provide screening, counselling, reliable payment, insurance, and financial advice.

To this it will be replied that no system of screening and control could be complete, and that both vendors and recipients would always be at risk of exploitation and poor treatment. But all the evidence we have shows that there is much more scope for exploitation and abuse when a supply of desperately wanted goods is made illegal. It is, furthermore, not clear why it should be thought harder to police a legal trade than the present complete ban.

Furthermore, even if vendors and recipients would always be at risk of exploitation, that does not alter the fact that if they choose this option, all alternatives must seem worse to them. Trying to end exploitation by prohibition is rather like ending slum dwelling by bulldozing slums: it ends the evil in that form, but only by making things worse for the victims. If we want to protect the exploited, we can do it only by removing the poverty that makes them vulnerable, or, failing that, by controlling the trade.

Another familiar objection is that it is unfair for the rich to have privileges not available to the poor. This argument, however, is irrelevant to the issue of organ selling as such. If organ selling is wrong for this reason, so are all benefits available to the rich, including all private medicine, and, for that matter, all public provision of medicine in rich countries (including transplantation of donated organs) that is unavailable in poor ones. Furthermore, all purchasing could be done by a central organisation responsible for fair distribution.

It is frequently asserted that organ donation must be altruistic to be acceptable, and that this rules out payment. However, there are two problems with this claim. First, altruism does not distinguish donors from vendors. If a father who saves his daughter's life by giving her a kidney is altruistic, it is difficult to see why his selling a kidney to pay for some other operation to save her life should be thought less so. Second, nobody believes in general that unless some useful action is altruistic it is better to forbid it altogether.

It is said that the practice would undermine confidence in the medical profession, because of the association of doctors with money-making practices. That, however, would be a reason for objecting to all private practice; and in this case the objection could easily be met by the separation of purchasing and treatment. There could, for instance, be independent trusts to fix charges and handle accounts, as well as to ensure fair play and

high standards. It is alleged that allowing the trade would lessen the supply of donated cadaveric kidneys. But although some possible donors might decide to sell instead, their organs would be available, so there would be no loss in the total. And in the meantime, many people will agree to sell who would not otherwise donate.

It is said that in parts of the world where women and children are essentially chattels there would be a danger of their being coerced into becoming vendors. This argument, however, would work as strongly against unpaid living kidney donation, and even more strongly against many far more harmful practices which do not attract calls for their prohibition. Again, regulation would provide the most reliable means of protection.

It is said that selling kidneys would set us on a slippery slope to selling vital organs such as hearts. But that argument would apply equally to the case of the unpaid kidney donation, and nobody is afraid that that will result in the donation of hearts. It is entirely feasible to have laws and professional practices that allow the giving or selling only of non-vital organs. Another objection is that allowing organ sales is impossible because it would outrage public opinion. But this claim is about western public opinion: in many potential vendor communities, organ selling is more acceptable than cadaveric donation, and this argument amounts to a claim that other people should follow western cultural preferences rather than their own. There is, anyway, evidence that the western public is far less opposed to the idea, than are medical and political professionals.

It must be stressed that we are not arguing for the positive conclusion that organ sales must always be acceptable, let alone that there should be an unfettered market. Our claim is only that none of the familiar arguments against organ selling works, and this allows for the possibility that better arguments may yet be found.

Nevertheless, we claim that the burden of proof remains against the defenders of prohibition, and that until good arguments appear, the presumption must be that the trade should be regulated rather than banned altogether. Furthermore, even when there are good objections at particular times or in particular places, that should be regarded as a reason for trying to remove the objections, rather than as an excuse for permanent prohibition.

The weakness of the familiar arguments suggests that they are attempts to justify the deep feelings of repugnance which are the real driving force of prohibition, and feelings of repugnance among the rich and healthy, no matter how strongly felt, cannot justify removing the only hope of the destitute and dying. This is why we conclude that the issue should be considered again, and with scrupulous impartiality.

AN ETHICAL MARKET IN HUMAN ORGANS

Charles A. Erin and John Harris

While people's lives continue to be put at risk by the dearth of organs available for transplantation, we must give urgent consideration to any option that may make up the shortfall. A market in organs from living donors is one such option. The market should be ethically supportable, and have built into it, for example, safeguards against wrongful exploitation. This can be accomplished by establishing a single purchaser system within a confined marketplace.

Statistics can be dehumanising. The following numbers, however, have more impact than most: as of 24th November, during 2002 in the United Kingdom, 667 people have donated organs, 2055 people have received transplants, and *5615 people are still awaiting transplants.* It is difficult to estimate how many people die prematurely for want of donor organs. "In the world as a whole there are an estimated 700 000 patients on dialysis. . . . In India alone 100 000 new patients present with kidney failure each year" (few if any of whom are on dialysis and only 3000 of whom will receive transplants). Almost "three million Americans suffer from congestive heart failure . . . deaths related to this condition are estimated at 250 000 each year . . . 27 000 patients die annually from liver disease. . . . In Western Europe as a whole 40 000 patients await a kidney but only . . . 10 000 kidneys" become available. Nobody knows how many people fail to make it onto the waiting lists and so disappear from the statistics. It is clear that loss of life, due in large measure to shortage of donor organs, is a major crisis, and a major scandal.

At its annual meeting in 1999, the British Medical Association voted overwhelmingly in favour of the UK moving to a system of presumed consent for organ donation, a proposed change in policy that the UK government immediately rejected. What else might we do to increase the supply of donor organs? At its annual meeting in 2002, the American Medical Association voted to encourage studies to determine whether financial incentives could increase the supply of organs from cadavers. In 1998, the International Forum for Transplant Ethics concluded that trade in organs should be regulated rather than banned. In 1994, we made a proposal in which we outlined possibly the only circumstances in which a market in donor organs could be achieved ethically, in a way that minimises the dangers normally envisaged for such a scheme. Now may be an appropriate time to revisit the idea of a market in donor organs. Our focus then, as now, is organs obtained from the living since creating a market in cadaver organs is uneconomic and is more likely to reduce supply than increase it and the chief reason for considering sale of organs is to improve availability.

To meet legitimate ethical and regulatory concerns, any commercial scheme must have built into it safeguards against wrongful exploitation and show concern for the vulnerable, as well as taking into account considerations of justice and equity.

There is a lot of hypocrisy about the ethics of buying and selling organs and indeed other body products and services—for example, surrogacy and gametes. What it usually means is that everyone is paid but the donor. The surgeons and medical team are paid, the transplant coordinator does not go

From *Journal of Medical Ethics* 29 (2003): 137–138. Reproduced with permission from the BMJ Publishing Group Ltd. *Editors' note:* All authors' notes have been cut. Students who want to follow up on sources should consult the original article.

unremunerated, and the recipient receives an important benefit in kind. Only the unfortunate and heroic donor is supposed to put up with the insult of no reward, to add to the injury of the operation.

We would therefore propose a strictly regulated and highly ethical market in live donor organs and tissue. We should note that the risks of live donation are relatively low: "The approximate risks to the donor . . . are a short term morbidity of 20% and mortality, of 0.03%. . . . The long term risks of developing renal failure are less well documented but appear to be no greater than for the normal population." And recent evidence suggests that living donor organ transplantation has an excellent prognosis, better than cadaver organ transplantation. Intuitively, the advantage also seems clear: the donor is very fit and healthy, while cadaver donors may well have been unfit and unhealthy, although this will not be true of many accident victims.

The bare bones of an ethical market would look like this: the market would be confined to a self governing geopolitical area such as a nation state or indeed the European Union. Only citizens resident within the union or state could sell into the system and they and their families would be equally eligible to receive organs. Thus organ vendors would know they were contributing to a system which would benefit them and their families and friends since their chances of receiving an organ in case of need would be increased by the existence of the market. (If this were not the case the main justification for the market would be defeated.) There would be only one purchaser, an agency like the National Health Service (NHS), which would buy all organs and distribute according to some fair conception of medical priority. There would be no direct sales or purchases, no exploitation of low income countries and their populations (no buying in Turkey or India to sell in Harley Street). The organs would be tested for HIV, etc, their provenance known, and there would be strict controls and penalties to prevent abuse.

Prices would have to be high enough to attract people into the marketplace but dialysis, and other alternative care, does not come cheap. Sellers of organs would know they had saved a life and would be reasonably compensated for their risk, time, and altruism, which would be undiminished by sale. We do not after all regard medicine as any the less a caring profession because doctors are paid. So long as thousands continue to die for want of donor organs we must urgently consider and implement ways of increasing the supply. A market of the sort outlined above is surely one method worthy of active and urgent consideration.

BODY VALUES: THE CASE AGAINST COMPENSATING FOR TRANSPLANT ORGANS

Donald Joralemon and Phil Cox

The issue of financial compensation for organ donation is back on center stage as a result of legislative proposals in Congress and recommendations adopted by the American Medical Association, the United Network for Organ Sharing, and the American Society of

From *Hastings Center Report* 33, no. 1 (January–February 2003): 27–33. Reprinted by permission of The Hastings Center. *Editors' note:* Most authors' notes have been cut. Students who want to follow up on sources should consult the original article.

Transplant Surgeons. Recently introduced Congressional bills relating to organ donation include two that would authorize tax credits for cadaveric donations. Another bill, by some readings, would grant authority to the Secretary of Health and Human Services to override the prohibition against donor compensation in the National Organ Transplantation Act of 1984 so as to support pilot studies assessing the impact of moderate incentives (such as funeral benefits) on donor rates.

The AMA's House of Delegates, at its Annual Meeting in June 2002, approved a recommendation

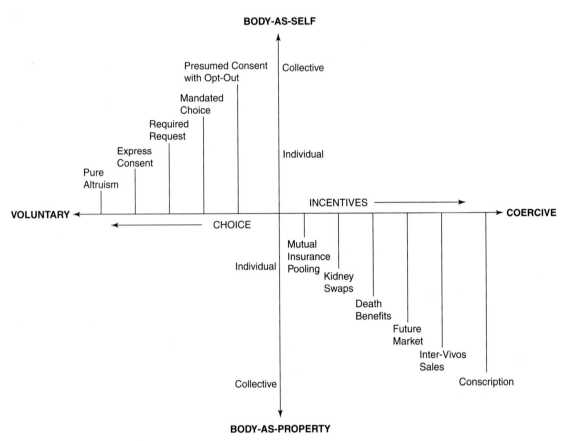

FIGURE 1   Body, Self, and Organ Acquisition

The Major Alternatives for Acquiring Organs

The horizontal axis distinguishes plans based on "choice" from those that assume "incentives" are required to get persons to give up their organs, or those of their deceased relatives. The axis is meant to indicate a continuum between two extremes. The vertical axis distinguishes plans that view the physical body as integral to the self from plans that view the body as property. Both conceptions of the body's relationship to the self range from individualistic to collectivist conceptions of personal identity.

"Pure altruism" characterizes the present system, in which a person's organs may be taken only if prior consent had been expressed or if the relatives agree after the person's death. In a system that relied on "express consent," the next of kin would not be able to override a deceased's documented wish to donate. "Required request," also already in effect in the United States, requires doctors to request organ donation in every suitable case. In a "mandated choice" system, all persons would be required to indicate on some common official document (such as a driver's license) whether they wished to donate. If we adopted "presumed consent with opt-out," agreement to donate would be a default assumption, but individuals could express disagreement.

Six proposed plans involve incentives to varying degrees. In "mutual insurance pooling," individuals who had signed an organ donor card while healthy would be given preference when they need an organ. In "kidney swaps," if a relative of someone on a waiting list for a kidney donates a kidney to another patient, the person on the waiting list is given a higher status. Kidney swaps may be employed if the relative and the person on the waiting list are not histocompatible.

Incentives would shift from quid pro quos to cash if "death benefits"—payments to defray funeral costs—were made to relatives who agree to donation. In a "futures market," contracts for organs would be written for healthy persons, to be activated should that person die in a fashion that makes the organs useful for transplantation. The contracts could be sold and purchased on a secondary market, and the owner of the contract would then sell the organs to people in need of them. Kidneys are available in some countries through inter-vivos sales. In a system that relied on conscription, incentives give way altogether; the state assumes ownership of bodies after death and does not have to solicit consent to salvage organs.

from the organization's Council on Ethical and Judicial Affairs to encourage pilot studies of compensation for cadaveric donations. The studies would have to include consultations with the population affected, their methods would have to pass scientific muster and be approved by oversight bodies, and they could use only "incentives of moderate value and at the lowest level that can be reasonably expected to increase organ donation."[1] The studies would involve only cadaveric donations, not donations from live donors, and they would not sidestep the present organ allocation system (as governed by UNOS). UNOS and ASTS quickly responded to the AMA action with supporting resolutions.

The AMA proposal is based on a utilitarian ethic that is especially clear in the following passage: "Whether or not [incentives] are ethical depends upon the balance of benefits and harms that result from them."[2] A number of opponents agreed with past AMA President Lonnie Bristow when she said, "Please do not be seduced by the idea that the ends justify the means."[3] Rex Greene, an oncologist and a delegate to the AMA's House of Delegates from California, made a similar point when he said, "I would state that, no matter what the outcomes of these studies, it does not answer ethical questions."[4] Despite this strong opposition and in the face of a negative recommendation from the Reference Committee on Amendments to Constitution and Bylaws, the proposal passed.

These are only the most recent episodes in a two-decade-long discussion about whether organs and money can ethically be mixed. The combination of legislative proposals and aggressive support from medical societies indicates that proponents of incentives believe the time is right to move the discussion from the pages of bioethics journals to the public arena. In doing so, they seek to inoculate their proposals against attack by claiming the moral high ground—they ostensibly seek only to advance the interests of desperate patients on waiting lists—and by minimizing the scope of the actions proposed—they propose "incentives," not payments, and only "pilot studies," not policy changes.

This paper responds to the most frequent criticisms of the present altruism-based system, and elaborates on the case for keeping the cash out of transplantation. The arguments canvassed here refer variously both to the cadaveric organ acquisition addressed by the AMA proposal and to the use of live donors—or vendors—which is known as "inter vivos" donation. Although the AMA proposal is only for cadaveric organ acquisition, a natural next step is to consider employing financial incentives for inter vivos donation.

The major alternative schemes proposed for organ acquisition range from fully voluntary to coercive, where "coercive" plans are those that attempt to encourage or force people to do something that they would not otherwise be inclined to do. (See the accompanying figure.) Plans also vary in terms of what they posit about the relationship between physical bodies and the 'self' or 'person.' Some treat the 'person' as having a necessarily embodied existence. In these, 'I' am not distinct from my physical being; body is understood *as* the self. Others treat the body as property, as something distinct from the self that is "owned" by a disembodied (or at least anatomically localized) self. Both of these conceptions range from individualistic to collectivist understandings of identity. For example, the property conception can justify an individual's rights to dispose of his or her body parts ("I own my own body"), or it can be generalized to legitimate disposal by some collective entity ("The State owns my body"). Likewise, "embodiment" can be seen in purely individualistic terms or in reference to a shared identity with some larger social group.

COMMODIFICATION

Proponents of incentives have repeatedly advanced several critiques of the current altruism-based approach to organ procurement. Three critiques seem to be especially significant: (1) that compensating for organs is no different from many other permissible forms of body commodification; (2) that it is hypocritical to prohibit an activity that you would wish to engage in were you in a similar situation; and (3) that it is unethical not to do everything possible to increase donation because so many die for the lack of an adequate supply of organs.

The worry about commodification is that the buying and selling of human organs would lead to an increasing objectification of the human body. Commerce in organs would encourage people to view individual human beings as saleable commodities and would to that extent compromise and denature human dignity, so the argument goes. Other forms of this concern are voiced in discussions of surrogate motherhood, cloning, genetic testing and therapy, and some other topics in biotechnology and medical research.

Yet commercialization advocates have a ready rejoinder: Selling an organ is not different in kind from selling one's labor in other, often quite legal, ways—commercial surrogate motherhood, choosing to work a very risky job, and in some jurisdictions, the sexual service industry. Physical risk, exploitation, or commodification are arguably a matter of degree rather than of kind, and one cannot consistently deny the "choice" of engaging in these other activities while exceptionalizing organ commerce.

However, admitting the similarities (or even ethical identities) between, say, the presumed exploitation of prostitution and the exploitation of organ selling should not be taken as an argument for legally, socially, or ethically embracing all kinds of exploitation. Working as a diamond miner in South Africa is demonstrably dangerous to life and limb; selling the right lobe of one's liver, or a lung, is also demonstrably dangerous. Both force a devil's bargain on the economically desperate of trading life and limb for sustenance. Yet admitting the exploitative and hence ethically objectionable nature of highly dangerous working conditions is not an argument for *expanding* the range of dangerous occupations or risky labor-body exchanges. Rather, objecting to such kinds of exploitation or to the selling of one's labor or physical well-being should be taken as a reason for working to *reduce* the kinds of work or exchange that are so risky.

The concern about commodification takes on additional considerations in the context of cadaveric donation—the sort of donation that the AMA proposal addresses. Most commentators agree that as a matter of law and common morality, inter vivos donations should rely on noncoercive, voluntary organ acquisition plans that endorse what we refer to as the "body-as-self" view. When cadaveric donations are considered, however, commentators differ. Some still prefer voluntary, body-as-self organ acquisition, but some argue for using incentives to encourage donation, and they favor the "body-as-property" view of the organ. The key point of contention, in courts of law as well as at the

bedside of patients, is whether death immediately ends the body-as-self connection and opens the door to the application of property concerns and the logic of commodities—since the 'person' is no longer there, who owns the material body and how much may they profit from its disposition? Even scholars sensitive to the significance of body-self integrity seem prepared to accept that death means instant disembodiment of the person and transformation of the body to property, or at least a circumscription of the continuing right of the deceased to have his or her wishes honored in respect to the treatment of the corpse.

We know from a massive ethnographic record that the cessation of biological functions is rarely seen as being commensurate with the separation of the self from the body. The distinction made by social scientists between social and biological death captures the undeniable fact that a person's identity is commonly thought to remain with the body for some time after physical death has occurred. The cultural work achieved by mourning rituals is to complete the disconnection that biological death initiates. This is not, as Margaret Radin would have it, an example of fetishism—a superstitious belief that rational thought ought to banish. Rather, it is a basic human recognition that our 'self', our identity, exists in the space of social relations, and that the ongoing flow of social life necessitates a gradual disaggregation of the deceased from the ties to the living that constituted the social self.

These observations help explain the moral intuition some feel that the commodification of cadavers is abhorrent. It is this intuition that causes medical staff to hesitate when called upon to request a donation, that explains the fear felt by kin that their loved one's body would be mutilated during organ removal, and that makes understandable the reservations felt around the world to declaring a person dead at brain death and permitting cadaveric organ transplantation. The claim that dead bodies "are no longer inextricably intertwined with a person," and are therefore only protected as property, may capture the direction of recent legal interpretations, but it is badly out of sync with the real world and the way families actually respond to the death of relatives. It would be wise to assess plans for acquiring organs against a real world standard, rather than by legal or philosophical reasoning alone.

Reason and Rescue

Inter vivos sales have also been promoted by what could be called the "reasoned ideal" argument. In response to anti-incentive critics, some ask, "But what would *you* do if your child's life depended on your selling one of your kidneys? How can you deny to others a choice that you yourself might make if you were in their circumstances?" This claim often invokes an example of a parent in the developing world who has already lost some of her children to malnutrition or preventable disease. The sale of a kidney can generate the equivalent of ten years' wages for, say, an itinerant Indian worker (although the promised financial gain often fails to materialize, and serious long-term health problems are common). Isn't this just the kind of sacrifice that we generally applaud in developed countries, when a loving parent gives up a kidney to save a child with a life threatening kidney disease?

There is often something to this charge of hypocrisy. However, philosophers who make this charge should take more care to distinguish the arguments that might incline one to sell an organ—such as Kantian notions of a duty to family—from the utilitarian argument that enfranchising the practice would lead to the greater social acceptance of similar transactions. By way of analogy, consistency does not require that entertaining the proposition, "A parent may save the life of her child by cutting off a leg or selling herself into slavery," commits one to accept an effort to legalize, let alone facilitate, dismemberment or slavery. Two different questions are being asked here: What actions are morally understandable under conditions of desperation, and what social institutions or policies might be ethically justified to accommodate "choices" made under such desperate circumstances.

Another objection to philosophical arguments concerns what might be called the "rescue obligation." Proponents of incentives—whether arguing for inter-vivos sales or for cash rewards for cadaveric organs (including tax rebates and funeral "stipends" as well as cash paid outright for each organ taken)—frequently argue that the number of persons who die before an organ is available for them presents a compelling moral case for shifting the burden of argument back onto those who support the preservation of the current altruism-based system. Recitations of the statistics on the ever-increasing gap between those awaiting organs and the number of organs available typically preface rhetorical charges of avoidable tragedies, of life-saving body parts being left for the worms, and even of criminal liability for refusals to donate. A letter to the *British Medical Journal* puts the underlying claim clearly: "We all have a moral duty to do everything we can to give the living the best possible quality of life."

What's wrong with this claim? First, there is precious little legal or custom-based support for an obligation to rescue those whose organs have failed. Courts in the United States, for example, have repeatedly found that there is no duty to aid a person in need: "The common law has consistently held to a rule which provides that one human being is under no legal compulsion to give aid or rescue or to take action to save another. . . . The rule is founded upon the very essence of our free society."[5] This rule has traditionally been applied to living persons, but the mandate that organs may be removed for transplantation only with consent—expressed or presumed—would indicate that even after death the default assumption is that there is no presumptive obligation to rescue.

Indeed, it is precisely the absence of an obligation to rescue that gives the decision to donate organs its positive moral weight. If this presumption were reversed, say by conscripting cadavers for their organs regardless of dissent, then no moral value would attach to the persons from whom organs are extracted, or from their next of kin. This would introduce a crass instrumentality into organ transplantation that is directly at odds with its long-standing ethos.

The claim that society as a whole has a positive duty to rescue those on transplant waiting lists is actually weakened by utilitarian calculation: there are immense numbers of other persons whose lives could more easily be improved or saved with the financial resources required for organ replacement. Even as strong a defender of organ transplantation as Richard Evans must admit that "from a public health perspective, more harm than good has already been done [by organ transplantation]"; in the United States "nearly $6 billion is spent [annually] on a handful of solid organ transplant recipients."[6] We might contrast this expenditure, for example, to the $0.26 per vaccine to immunize against measles, which kills 900,000 children around the world. In a world of finite resources for health care, it is hard to argue that the extraordinary expenditure associated with organ transplantation constitutes the best possible way to serve the needs of the living.

A third problem with the rescue claim is that organ transplantation is not the medical miracle it claims to be. Given the severity of the diseases from which transplant candidates suffer and the stubborn reality of organ rejection, many of those who die before receiving an organ might very well have died within several years even with a replacement organ. Survival rates vary significantly by the organ replaced, but the average 20 percent loss of life at the one-year point increases significantly after five years. Furthermore, the profession of transplant medicine has consistently overstated recipients' quality of life and understated the long-term toll of powerful anti-rejection medications.

A final problem with the "rescue obligation" is that high technology medicine is, more often than not, unavailable to persons whose bank accounts or insurance status are inadequate to the expense. In all of Africa, between 1978–1994, only 163 transplant surgeries were performed; during the same period, over 124,000 transplants were performed in the United States alone. Even within developed countries, the "green screen" determines who gets to the waiting list for organs and who can afford the medications after surgery. If society has a moral duty to rescue, the obligation surely is not limited to rescuing those of means.

SCIENCE AND SUPERSTITION

Many medical professionals believe that the body-as-self conception—especially when it is extended to include the recently dead—is a superstition that must eventually disappear as "scientific" understandings of the body penetrate ever more deeply into the general culture. They point to the growing number of body fluids and parts that are openly marketed—from gametes to skin and corneas—as evidence that, at least in the United States, we are witnessing a shift toward property conceptions of the body and an acceptance of bodily commodification. If this is the case, then one could predict an

inevitable trend toward incentives in organ procurement, first for cadaveric and then for living "donations." Indeed, advocates of commerce frequently claim that incentives would cross no new or substantially relevant threshold, since other body parts are already treated as commodities.

But this modernist view of how medical science influences the general culture may be out of step. Physicians and other health professionals come to a disembodied view of the self—if they do—only after the desensitizing socialization of medical school, where the curriculum promotes a Cartesian distinction between mind and body that accords well with the objectification of organ systems. Rather than treating this way of thinking as the inevitable endpoint of a progressive culture, it would be just as reasonable to see it as a clinically useful but culturally aberrant view.

This alternative interpretation is supported by evidence that even those most fully immersed in the world view of modern medicine appear to have difficulty reconciling their scientific understandings of the body with their intuitive responses. How else can one explain why physicians often do not sign organ donor cards, or the ambivalent responses by health care staff to persons declared brain dead or in a persistent vegetative state. The strong dissent voiced at the AMA over the incentive proposal might be taken as additional evidence that even doctors are yet to be fully persuaded by the body-as-property view.

There are other indications that the corpse continues to be treated as integral to the self. Consider the extraordinary investment of time and money in the recovery of the smallest of body parts from the ruins of the World Trade Center, or the public horror occasioned by news of bodies left uncremated at a Georgia facility. Persistent accounts of organ recipients who express concern about the identity and character of the donor, and of donor kin who believe that the deceased lives on in the recipient, also show how firmly rooted in common intuition is the idea that a person's identity is embodied.

Clearly, the AMA's proposal entails much more than an innocent experiment. Rather than doing ethics by pilot study, it would be better to reflect more deeply on where the "is" and the "ought" of incentives line up. There is more at stake than encouraging donation.

REFERENCES

1. CEJA Report 1:A-02, "Cadaveric Organ Donation: Encouraging the Study of Motivation," presented at the 2002 American Medical Association House of Delegates Annual Meeting, Chicago. Ill., June 15–20, 2002.
2. CEJA Report 1:A-02.
3. Quoted in A. Robeznieks, "Boosting Organ Donations Ultimate Focus of Initiative," Amednews.com, 8/15 July 2002.
4. Robeznieks, "Boosting Organ Donations Ultimate Focus of Initiative."
5. J. Rutherford-McClure, "To Donate or Not to Donate Your Organs: Texas Can Decide for You When You Cannot Decide for Yourself," *Texas Wesleyan Law Review* 6 (2000): 241. While U.S. common law has not given rise to any establishment of a "duty to rescue," most European countries have passed such laws. In the United States, five states have legislatively enacted related statutes, though in four of them "duty to rescue" simply means "duty to report a crime," if such can be done without risk to the reporter. Only in Vermont is a person obligated to provide "reasonable assistance" when another person "is exposed to grave physical harm," but again only if such can be done without danger or peril to self or others. See E. Volokh, "Duties to Rescue and the Anticooperative Effects of Law," *Georgetown Law Journal* 88 (1999): 105–14.
6. R.W. Evans, "How Dangerous Are Financial Incentives to Obtain Organs?" *Transplantation Proceedings* 31 (1999): 1337–41.

POVERTY, HEALTH, AND JUSTICE BEYOND NATIONAL BORDERS

RESPONSIBILITIES FOR POVERTY-RELATED ILLNESS

Thomas W. Pogge

My view on justice in regard to health is distinctive in two ways. First, I hold that the strength of our moral reasons to prevent or to mitigate particular medical conditions does not depend only on what one might call distributional factors, such as how badly off the people affected by these conditions are in absolute and relative terms, how costly prevention or treatment would be, and how much patients would benefit from given treatment. Rather, it depends also on relational factors, that is, on how we are related to the medical conditions they suffer. This point is widely accepted in regard to conduct. You have, for instance, stronger moral reason to make sure that people are not harmed through your negligence than you have to ensure that they are not harmed through causes outside your control (others' negligence or their own, say, or bad weather). And your moral reason to help an accident victim is stronger if you were materially involved in causing her accident.

I assert an analogous point also in regard to any social institutions that agents are materially involved in upholding: in shaping an institutional order, we should be more concerned, morally, that it not contribute substantially to the incidence of medical conditions than we should be that it prevent medical conditions caused by other factors. Thus, we should design any institutional order so that it prioritizes the alleviation of those medical conditions it substantially contributes to. In institutional contexts as well, what is important to moral assessment is not merely the distribution of health

Thomas W. Pogge, "Responsibilities for Poverty-Related Ill Health," *Ethics & International Affairs* 19, no. 1 (March 2005): 9–18.

Editors' note: This article is a revised version of the original article from Thomas W. Pogge, "Responsibilities for Poverty-Related Ill Health," *Ethics & International Affairs,* Blackwell Publishers.

outcomes as such, but also whether and how social factors contribute to their incidence. The latter consideration is needed to distinguish different degrees of responsibility for medical conditions and for their prevention and mitigation.

My second thesis builds on the first. It is generally believed that one's moral reason to help prevent and mitigate others' medical conditions is stronger when these others are compatriots than when they are foreigners. I reject this belief in regard to medical conditions in whose incidence one is materially involved. People can be so involved through their ordinary conduct or through their role in upholding an institutional order. In the case of ordinary interpersonal relations, for example, one's moral reasons to drive carefully and to help victims of any accident one has caused do not weaken when traveling abroad. And in institutional contexts, we ought especially to ensure that any institutional order we help impose avoids causing adverse medical conditions and makes the alleviation of any medical conditions it does cause a priority. Here my second thesis holds that this responsibility is not sensitive to whether the medical conditions at stake are suffered by foreigners or by compatriots.

Putting both theses together, I hold then that foreigners' medical conditions in whose incidence we are materially involved have greater moral weight for us than compatriots' medical conditions in whose incidence we are not materially involved. In interpersonal contexts, this combined thesis is not likely to be very controversial. Suppose two children have been injured by speeding drivers and money is needed to pay for an expensive medical treatment necessary to restore their health and appearance completely. In one case, the child is a foreigner and you were the driver. In the other case, the child is a compatriot and someone else was the driver. My view entails that in a situation like this you have (other things being equal) stronger moral reason to buy the expensive treatment for the foreign child, and most would probably agree.

In institutional contexts, by contrast, my view is likely to be quite controversial. It might be stated as follows: Foreigners' medical conditions, if social institutions we are materially involved in upholding substantially contribute to their incidence, have greater moral weight for us than compatriots'

medical conditions in whose causation we are not materially involved. This combined thesis is radical if social institutions we are materially involved in upholding do substantially contribute to the incidence of medical conditions abroad. Is this the case?

SOCIAL INSTITUTIONS, POVERTY, AND HEALTH

Many kinds of social institutions can substantially contribute to the incidence of medical conditions. Of these, economic institutions—the basic rules governing ownership, production, use, and exchange of natural resources, goods, and services—have the greatest impact on health. This impact is mediated, for the most part, through poverty. By avoidably engendering severe poverty, economic institutions substantially contribute to the incidence of many medical conditions. And persons materially involved in upholding such economic institutions are then materially involved in the causation of such medical conditions.

In our world, poverty is highly relevant to human health. In fact, poverty is far and away the most important factor in explaining existing health deficits. Because they are poor, 830 million persons are malnourished, 1.1 billion lack access to safe water, 2.6 billion lack access to basic sanitation,[1] about 2 billion lack access to essential drugs (www.fic.nih.gov/about/plan/exec_summary.htm), approximately 1 billion have no adequate shelter and 2 billion no electricity.[2] Some 250 million children between 5 and 14 do wage work outside their household—often under harsh or cruel conditions: as soldiers, prostitutes, or domestic servants, or in agriculture, construction, textile or carpet production.[3] About one third of all human deaths, 18 million annually, are due to poverty-related causes,[4] including 10.6 million deaths each year of children under 5.[5] Females, children, and people of color are heavily overrepresented in all these figures.

This massive poverty is not due to overall scarcity. At market exchange rates, the World Bank's higher ("$2/day") international poverty line corresponds today to about $280 per person per year in a typical poor country (and to $1,120 in the more expensive U.S.). The 2.7 billion persons living below this line, 42 percent below it on average,[6] thus have aggregate annual income of roughly $440 billion and a $320 billion collective shortfall from the $2/day poverty line. By contrast, the aggregate gross national incomes (GNIs) of the "high-income countries" with 1 billion citizens amount to over $35,000 billion. However daunting the figure of 2.7 billion poor people may sound, global inequality is now so enormous that eradicating world poverty solely at the expense of the high-income countries would barely be felt in the latter.[7]

It cannot be denied that the distribution of income and wealth is heavily influenced by economic institutions, which regulate the distribution of a jointly generated social product. What can be said, and is said quite often, is that the economic institutions that substantially contribute to extreme poverty in the less developed countries are *local* economic institutions in whose imposition we, citizens of the developed countries, are not materially involved. Economists tirelessly celebrate the success stories of the Asian tigers or of Kerala (a state in India), leading us to believe that those who remain hungry have only their own institutions and governments (and hence themselves and their own compatriots) to blame. Even the philosopher Rawls feels called upon to reiterate that poverty has local explanations: "The causes of the wealth of a people and the forms it takes lie in their political culture and in the religious, philosophical, and moral traditions that support the basic structure, as well as in the industriousness and cooperative talents of its members, all supported by their political virtues. . . . Crucial also is the country's population policy."[8]

It is quite true, of course, that local economic institutions, and local factors more generally, play an important role in the reproduction of extreme poverty in many less developed countries. But this fact does not show that social institutions we are materially involved in upholding play no substantial role. That the effects of flawed domestic institutions are as bad as they are is often due to global institutions: National borders allow affluent populations to prevent the poor from migrating to where their work could earn a decent living, for example. And health systems in poor countries fail to cope in good part because, under the TRIPS Agreement, pharmaceutical innovations must be rewarded through monopoly pricing

powers, which exclude the poor from advanced medicines for the sake of incentivizing solutions to the health problems of the affluent. There are straightforward alternative ways of incentivizing pharmaceutical innovation that would not exclude the poor from its benefits.[9]

Global institutions also have a profound impact on the indigenous institutional schemes of less developed countries. Such institutions recognize anyone holding effective power in a country—regardless of how they acquired or exercise it and to how they are regarded by the population—as entitled to sell the country's resources and to dispose of the proceeds of such sales, to borrow in the country's name and thereby to impose debt service obligations upon it, to sign treaties on the country's behalf and thus to bind its present and future population, and to use state revenues to buy the means of internal repression. By assigning such powers to any de-facto rulers, we support, reward, and encourage the undemocratic acquisition and repressive exercise of political power especially in the resource-rich poorer countries.

The national institutional schemes of developed countries, too, can have a profound influence on the national institutional schemes of poorer countries. An obvious example is that, until recently, most affluent countries (though not, after 1977, the United States) have allowed their firms to pay bribes to officials of poor countries, and even to deduct such bribes from their taxable revenues. Such authorization and moral support for bribery have greatly contributed to the now deeply entrenched culture of corruption in many less developed countries.

If the social institutions of the developed countries and the global institutional order these countries uphold contribute substantially to the reproduction of poverty, then it is hard to deny that we citizens of developed countries are therefore materially involved in it as well. It is true of course that these institutions are shaped by our politicians. But we live in reasonably democratic states where we can choose politicians and political programs from a wide range of alternatives, where we can participate in shaping political programs and debates, and where politicians and political parties must cater to the popular will if they are to be elected and reelected. If we really wanted our domestic and international institutions to be shaped so as to avoid reproducing extreme poverty, politicians committed to that goal would emerge and be successful. But the vast majority of citizens of the developed countries want national and global institutions to be shaped in the service of their own interests and therefore support politicians willing so to shape them. At least the citizens in this large majority can then be said to be materially involved in the reproduction of poverty and the associated health deficits. And they, at least, have then stronger moral reason to discontinue their support, and to help the foreign victims of current institutions, than to help fund most services provided under ordinary health programs (such as Medicare) for the benefit of their compatriots—or so the view I have outlined would suggest.

Superficially similar conclusions are sometimes defended on cost/benefit grounds, by reference to how thousands of children in poor countries can be saved from their trivial diseases at the cost of terminal care for a single person in a developed country. My view, by contrast, turns on the different ways in which we are related to the medical conditions of others and thus may tell us to favor foreigners even if costs and benefits are equal.

This summary of my larger view on health equity was meant to be introductory, not conclusive. Seeing what is at stake, I would expect even the most commonsensical of my remarks about the explanation of global poverty to be vigorously disputed; and I certainly do not believe that this brief outline can lay such controversies to rest.[10]

RELATIONAL RESPONSIBILITIES

Let me expand on my first thesis by sketching how a conception of social justice might weight the impact that social institutions have on relevant quality of life according to how they have this impact. Let me illustrate by distinguishing, in a preliminary fashion, six basic ways in which an institutional order may have an impact on the medical conditions persons suffer under it. This illustration distinguishes scenarios in which some particular medical condition suffered by certain innocent persons can be traced to the fact that they, due to the arrangement of social institutions, avoidably lack some vital nutrients V (the vitamins contained in fresh fruit, perhaps, which are essential to good health). The six scenarios are arranged in order of

their moral weight, according to my intuitive, pre-reflective judgment:

- In scenario 1, the nutritional deficit is *officially mandated*, paradigmatically by the law: legal restrictions bar certain persons from buying foodstuffs containing V.
- In scenario 2, the nutritional deficit results from *legally authorized* conduct of private persons: sellers of foodstuffs containing V lawfully refuse to sell to certain persons.
- In scenario 3, social institutions *foreseeably and avoidably engender* (but do not specifically require or authorize) the nutritional deficit through conduct they stimulate: certain persons, suffering severe poverty within an ill-conceived economic order, cannot afford to buy foodstuffs containing V.
- In scenario 4, the nutritional deficit arises from private conduct that is *legally prohibited but barely deterred*: sellers of foodstuffs containing V illegally refuse to sell to certain persons, but enforcement is lax and penalties are mild.
- In scenario 5, the nutritional deficit arises from social institutions *avoidably leaving unmitigated the effects of a natural defect*: certain persons are unable to metabolize V due to a treatable genetic defect, but they avoidably lack access to the treatment that would correct their handicap.
- In scenario 6, finally, the nutritional deficit arises from social institutions *avoidably leaving unmitigated the effects of a self-caused defect*: certain persons are unable to metabolize V due to a treatable self-caused disease—brought on, perhaps, by their maintaining a long-term smoking habit in full knowledge of the medical dangers associated with it—and avoidably lack access to the treatment that would correct their ailment.

This differentiation of six ways in which social institutions may be related to the goods and ills persons encounter is preliminary in that it fails to isolate the morally significant factors that account for the descending moral weight of the relevant medical conditions. Lacking the space to do this here, let me merely venture the hypothesis that what matters is not merely the *causal* role of social institutions, how they figure in a complete causal explanation of the nutritional deficit in question, but also (what one might call) the implicit *attitude* of social institutions toward this deficit.[11]

My preliminary classification is surely still too simple. In some cases one will have to take account of other, perhaps underlying causes; and one may also need to recognize interdependencies among causal influences and fluid transitions between the classes.[12] Bypassing these complications here, let me emphasize once more the decisive point missed by the usual accounts of justice: to be morally plausible, a criterion of social justice must take account of—and its application thus requires information about—the particular relation between social institutions and human quality of life, which may determine whether some institutionally avoidable deficit is an injustice at all and, if so, how great an injustice it is. Such a criterion must take into account, that is, not merely the comparative impact a social order has on the distribution of quality of life, but also *how* it exerts this influence. If this is right, then it is no more true of social rules than of persons and conduct that they are just if and insofar as they promote a good overall distribution. Appraising overall distributions of goods and ills (or of quality of life) may be an engaging academic and theological pastime, but it fails to give plausible moral guidance where guidance is needed: for the assessment and reform of social rules as well as of persons and their conduct.

IN CONCLUSION

An institutional order can be said to contribute substantially to medical conditions if and only if it contributes to their genesis through scenarios 1, 2, and 3. Supposing that at least the more privileged adult citizens of affluent and reasonably democratic countries are materially involved in upholding not only the economic order of their own society but also the global economic order, we can say two things about such citizens: pursuant to my second thesis, they have equally strong moral reason to prevent and mitigate *compatriots'* medical conditions due to avoidable poverty engendered by *domestic* economic institutions as they have to prevent and mitigate *foreigners'* medical conditions due to avoidable poverty engendered by *global* economic institutions. And pursuant to my combined thesis, they have stronger moral reason to prevent and mitigate foreigners' medical conditions due to

avoidable poverty engendered by global economic institutions than to prevent and mitigate compatriots' medical conditions that are not due to mandated, authorized, or engendered deficits.

In the United States, some 50 million mostly poor citizens avoidably lack adequate medical insurance. Due to their lack of coverage, many of these people, at any given time, suffer medical conditions that could be cured or mitigated by treatment not in fact accessible to them. This situation is often criticized as manifesting an injustice in the country's social order. Now imagine that the poverty of the 50 million were so severe that it not only rendered them unable to gain access to the medical care they need (scenarios 5 and 6), but also exposed them to various medical conditions owing specifically to poverty-related causes (scenario 3). This additional feature, which plays a substantial role for some fraction of the 50 million, considerably aggravates the injustice. And it is central to the plight of the world's poorest populations. The global poor generally lack access to adequate care for the medical conditions they suffer, of course. But the main effect of an extra $50 or $100 of annual income for them would not be more medical care, but much less need for such care. If they were not so severely impoverished, they would not suffer in the first place most of the medical conditions for which, as things are, they also cannot obtain adequate treatment.

I have tried to lend some initial plausibility to the view that such poverty-induced medical conditions among the global poor are, for us, morally on a par with poverty-induced medical conditions among the domestic poor and of greater moral weight than not-socially-induced medical conditions among poor compatriots. In the first two cases, but not in the third, we are materially involved in upholding social institutions that contribute substantially to the incidence of medical conditions and of the countless premature deaths resulting from them.

NOTES

1. United Nations Development Programme (UNDP), *Human Development Report 2006* (Houndsmills: Palgrave Macmillan 2006), pp. 174 and 33. These figures compare to a world population of about 6.5 billion.
2. UNDP, *Human Development Report 1998* (Oxford: Oxford University Press 1998), p. 49.

3. See www.ilo.org/public/english/standards/ipec/ simpoc/stats/4stt.htm and International Labour Organisation, *A Future Without Child Labour* (Geneva: ILO 2002), pp. 9, 11, and 18.

4. World Health Organization (WHO), *The World Health Report 2004* (Geneva: WHO Publications 2004), pp. 120–25. Also at www.who.int/whr/2004.

5. UNICEF (United Nations Children's Fund), *The State of the World's Children 2005* (New York: UNICEF). Also at www.unicef.org/publications/files/SOWC_2005_ (English).pdf.

6. Chen, Shaohua and Martin Ravallion, "How Have the World's Poorest Fared since the Early 1980s?," *World Bank Research Observer,* 19 (2004): 141–69.

7. In fact, these countries spend some $18 billion (0.05 percent of their collective GNIs) on poverty eradication: about $11 billion through their governments in official development assistance for "basic social services" (www.oecd.org) and another $7 billion through private giving to international non-governmental organizations.

8. John Rawls, *The Law of Peoples* (Cambridge MA: Harvard University Press 1999), p. 108.

9. See Thomas Pogge: "Human Rights and Global Health" in Christian Barry and Thomas Pogge, eds.: *Global Institutions and Responsibilities* (Oxford: Blackwell 2005), for a fuller discussion of how pharmaceutical innovation could be incentivized without excluding the poor from its benefits.

10. For more detail, see my *World Poverty and Human Rights* (Cambridge: Polity Press 2002).

11. This implicit attitude of social institutions is independent of the attitudes or intentions of the persons shaping and upholding these institutions: Only the former makes a difference to how just the institutions are— the latter only make a difference to how blameworthy persons are for their role in imposing them.

12. The case of smoking, for instance, may exemplify a fluid transition between scenarios 2 and 6 insofar as private agents (cigarette companies) are legally permitted to try to render persons addicted to nicotine.

DO WE OWE THE GLOBAL POOR ASSISTANCE OR RECTIFICATION?

Mathias Risse

A central theme throughout Thomas Pogge's path-breaking *World Poverty and Human Rights* is that the global political and economic order *harms* people in developing countries, and that our duty toward the global poor is therefore not to *assist* them but to *rectify injustice*. But does the global order *harm* the poor? I argue elsewhere that there is a sense in which this is indeed so, at least if a certain empirical thesis is accepted. In this essay, however, I seek to

Mathias Risse, "Do We Owe the Global Poor Assistance or Rectification?" *Ethics & International Affairs,* 16, no. 2 (September 2002): 71–79, Blackwell Publishers.

Editors' note: Some text and author's notes have been cut. Students who want to read the article in its entirety should consult the original.

show that the global order not only does not harm the poor but can plausibly be credited with the considerable improvements in human well-being that have been achieved over the last 200 years. Much of what Pogge says about our duties toward developing countries is therefore false.

Let me begin by clarifying what I mean by "the global political and economic order" ("the global order"). For the first time in history, there is one continuous global society based on territorial sovereignty. This system has emerged from the spread of European control since the fifteenth century and the formation of new states through wars of independence and decolonization. Even systems that escaped Western imperialism had to follow legal and diplomatic practices imposed by Europeans.

This state system is governed by rules, the most important of which are embodied in the UN Charter. The Bretton Woods institutions (the World Bank, IMF, and later the GATT/WTO) were founded as a framework for economic cooperation that would prevent disasters like the Great Depression of the 1930s. These institutions, together with economically powerful states acting alone or in concert, shape the economic order. Although this order is neither monolithic nor harmonious, it makes sense to talk about a global order that includes but is not reducible to the actions of states.

In what follows, then, I argue that this global order does not harm the poor according to the benchmarks of comparison used by Pogge, but that on the contrary, according to those benchmarks, this order has caused amazing improvements over the state of misery that has characterized human life throughout the ages. The global order is not fundamentally unjust; instead, it is *incompletely* just, and it should be credited with the great advances it has brought.

BENCHMARKS FOR HARM: HISTORICAL REFERENCES

One might think the present extents of poverty and inequality by themselves reveal the injustice of the global order.[1] But they do not. While indeed 1.2 billion people in 1998 lived below the poverty line of $1.08 PPP (Purchasing Power Parities) 1993 per day, it is also true that there is now less misery than ever before, at least as measured in terms of any standard development indicator. The progress made over the last 200 years is miraculous. In 1820, 75 percent of the world population lived on less than $1 a day (appropriately adjusted). Today, in Europe, almost nobody does; in China, less than 20 percent do; in South Asia, around 40 percent do; and globally, slightly more than 20 percent do. The share of people living on less than $1 a day fell from 42 percent in 1950 to 17 percent in 1992. Historically *almost everybody* was poor, but that is no longer true.

It is true that the high-income economies include 15 percent of the population but receive 80 percent of the income. Around 1820, per capita incomes were similar worldwide, and low, ranging from around $500 in China and South Asia to $1,000–$1,500 in some European countries. So the gap between rich and poor was 3 to 1, whereas, according to UNDP

statistics, in 1960 it was 60 to 1, and in 1997, 74 to 1. But it is also true that, between 1960 and 2000, real per capita income in developing countries grew on average 2.3 percent (doubling living standards within thirty years). Britain's GDP grew an average of 1.3 percent during its nineteenth-century economic supremacy. For developing countries, things have been better recently than they were for countries at the height of their power during any other period in history. The average income per capita in 1950 worldwide was $2,114, while in 1999 it was $5,709 (in 1990 dollars PPP); for developing countries income per capita increased from $1,093 to $3,100 (in 1990 dollars PPP) during this period. Similar improvements were achieved in life expectancy, which rose from forty-nine years to sixty-six years worldwide, and from forty-four years to sixty-four years in developing countries, and thus has increased more in the last fifty years than in the preceding 5,000 years. Literacy rose from 54 percent in 1950 to 79 percent in 1999. Infant mortality fell from 156 to 54 per 1,000 live births worldwide. Furthermore, while the UNDP inequality statistics quoted above used international exchange rates, things look different if one uses the Purchasing-Power-Parity standard. According to such calculations, which account for what money buys in different countries, inequality had risen by 1960 to 7 to 1 and has since fallen to about 6 to 1 because of higher growth in the developing world.

Development aid, which has often been given for strategic reasons, has declined since the end of the Cold War, and currently makes up a tiny percentage of donor countries' GDP.[2] Nevertheless, the resources transferred are substantial for those who receive them. In 1993, sub-Saharan countries received on average 11.5 percent of *their* GNP as aid (Zambia, 23.6 percent; Tanzania, 40 percent).[3] The Marshall Plan, hailed as the greatest aid program ever, has been estimated to have given its recipients on average 2.1 percent of GNP annually.[4]

WTO negotiations have not yet done as much for the poor as one might have hoped, and negotiators representing rich countries possess more bargaining power and often also more expertise than those of poor countries. Indeed, the WTO has so far opened markets too little. But it is also true that the WTO, by and large, represents a significant improvement over the GATT, and, for that matter, any previous system (for example, ad hoc bilateral treaties or no clear rules at all) of regulating international trade. The GATT mostly aimed to reduce tariffs in OECD countries and in sectors that mattered to them, while developing countries, through "special and preferential treatment," had a second-class status: in virtue of their "special and preferential" treatment they were free riders on GATT treaties, but their concerns were not on the agenda. That agriculture and textiles became part of WTO negotiations was a tremendous change for countries with a comparative advantage in such goods. Progress has been made in both areas. While the final results of the Doha Round of WTO negotiations with regard to agriculture are not settled (as of February 2005), the WTO is committed to eliminating export subsidies and to restricting other forms of export support in agriculture. Moreover, the quota system that has governed the textile sector since the 1960s is being phased out, and, as of January 1, 2005, all quotas have been eliminated. Things are changing slowly, but despite setbacks (such as the agreement on Trade-Related Aspects of Intellectual Property Rights [TRIPs], which will probably lead to a net redistribution to developed countries), great progress has arguably been made here too. Historically, negotiations exploring mutually acceptable solutions for worldwide problems are an anomaly. We are making progress.

What conclusion such statistics warrant depends on the time horizon considered (sub-Saharan Africa has made progress over a 200-year horizon, but not for the last 20 years), whether one looks at absolute or relative quantities (the number of abysmally poor has remained unchanged for 15 years, but their share of the world population decreased), and whether one looks at individuals or countries (the median developing country has experienced zero growth over the last 20 years; still, inequality between any two randomly chosen individuals has fallen, because of growth in India and China). Still, what is remarkable is not that so many now live in poverty, but that so many do not; not that so many die young, but that so many do not; not that so many are illiterate, but that so many are not. By and large, if one looks at the last 200, 100, or 50 years, things have improved dramati-

cally for the poor. The 200-year and the 50-year horizon (roughly speaking) are especially significant. The former captures the period in which the industrial revolution has perfected the system of the division of labor, which has in turn led to technological advancements (originating largely in what are nowadays industrialized countries) that have benefited everyone. The 50-year horizon captures the period in which a network of international organizations characterizing the global order has come into its own—a network whose absence would harm its weakest members the most. Historically speaking, the global order seems to have greatly benefited the poor.

OTHER BENCHMARKS FOR HARM: COUNTERFACTUAL AND FAIRNESS

My argument so far may seem philosophically naive. For while these data may be useful to get some sense of the status quo and its historical background, it may be argued (in agreement with Pogge) that such data is useless *as a benchmark of whether harm has been done*. Surely, one may say, developing countries are better off now than 200 years ago—but so were African Americans under Jim Crow vis-à-vis the antebellum days. Even 200 years ago "we" and "they" belonged to a single global system, and "they" were already on a trajectory toward their current disadvantaged status. So it may seem cynical to say that developing countries are not being harmed because they are better off than at an earlier stage of an ongoing oppressive relationship. Should we not assess whether harm has been done by asking what things would have been like had European supremacists never invaded the rest of the globe?

The trouble with this benchmark is that it is impossible to say anything about it. It is conceivable, for example, that political structures would have emerged in Africa that would have allowed indigenous peoples to exploit the natural resource wealth of their continent, enabling them to build a culturally sophisticated and economically prosperous civilization. But it is equally conceivable that wars would have thwarted such efforts. The point is not that a certain threshold of reasonable certainty cannot be met, but that we must plead complete ignorance. The uncertainty of what people who, as it happened, were never born, would have done across centuries, how events would have turned out that, as it happened, never occurred, how lives would have been changed by innovations that, as it happened, were never made—such factors make it impossible to say what things would be like had the past been different. If we evaluate counterfactuals, we normally first assess what the world would be like were the antecedent true and then resort to cases where some claim similar to the antecedent in fact was true to evaluate whether the consequent of the counterfactual will be true in a world in which the antecedent is. Assessing the relevant counterfactuals here is impossible, especially since much turns on exercises of the will of merely possible people.

Researchers in comparative politics do engage heavily in counterfactual reasoning since causal claims depend on such speculation: they try to reduce the speculative part by *comparing*; that is, holding other factors constant, they compare countries in the WTO with similarly situated ones outside it; or they compare a country's period of not belonging to the WTO with its period of belonging. However, when assessing the global order as such, we cannot apply this technique of holding other factors constant and judge what the world would be like had the current global order not developed. We have only this one world to work with. So while we can make sense of claims about what the development of Poland would have been had it not joined the European Union, we cannot make sense of claims of what the world would now be like had the global order not developed.

Yet, *surely*, one may say, developing countries would be better off had they been left alone! While those counterfactuals may be difficult to assess conclusively, they are *plausible*, and worrying about their verifiability violates Aristotle's advice to adjust accuracy standards to the subject matter. However, I suspect one may find this position obvious because one compares developing countries to industrialized countries, observes that the latter did not face similar interference, and concludes that without such interference Africa, for example, would have prospered. We must resist such reasoning, since the reasons why such regions fell to con-

querors may be the same reasons why they would have been unable to prosper without external interference. The political scientist Jeffrey Herbst has emphasized, for example, that facts of physical geography in Africa made it difficult for powerful states to emerge, and this by itself makes for a big difference to Europe. And the historian Bernard Lewis has argued that the decline of Islamic societies was due to internal developments rather than interference. While these are topics on which I cannot take a stance, we cannot simply assume that other parts of the world would have done better had they been left alone, and it is easy to see why we incline to do so.

Maybe we get guidance to assessing the claim that "they" would be better off had "we" never invaded them by considering more empirically tractable claims, such as that developed countries are rich because they have oppressed developing countries, and that colonialism has inflicted lasting harm. The first view was defended prominently by dependency theorists. Dependency theory comes in different versions, the strongest claiming that the development of "the North" entailed the underdevelopment of "the South" and a weaker version claiming that there is some other dependency of the South on the North—for instance, that the terms of trade weakened for "the South" as its natural resources became cheaper over time relative to manufactured goods from "the North." Yet dependency theory and related theories have become incredible to all but "a dwindling group of Marxist historians." Such views have not withstood scrutiny, and even some of their strongest erstwhile defenders, like Brazil's former president Fernando Henrique Cardoso, have abandoned them. The exploitation, theft, and murder they brought upon other parts of the world notwithstanding, developed countries became rich because they industrialized, thereby benefiting from an ever more refined division of labor.

It is tempting to say that the global order must be unjust because colonialism has created disadvantaged countries. Yet this is not obvious. While it happened, colonialism disrupted people's lives, killing, mutilating, or enslaving many. But past injustice does not make the present order unjust, any more than past kindness makes it kind. We need arguments that there is persisting injustice rooted in colonialism. Historians tend to come to differentiated assessments of the colonial heritage. For instance, Fernand Braudel writes:

> Education and a certain level of technology, of hygiene, of medicine and of public administration: these were the greatest benefits left by the colonists, and some measure of compensation for the destruction which contact with Europe brought to old tribal, family, and social customs. . . . It will never be possible to gauge the full results of such novelties as employment for wages, a money economy, writing and individual ownership of land. Each was undoubtedly a blow to the former social regime. Yet these blows were surely a necessary part of the evolution taking place today. On the other hand, colonization had the real disadvantage of dividing Africa into a series of territories—French, English, German, Belgian, and Portuguese—whose fragmentation has been perpetuated today in too large a cluster of independent states, which are sometimes said to have "Balkanized" Africa.[5]

Most historians find colonial rule to have been inadequate while it lasted, but that does not mean that its legacy, all things considered, continues to impose harm that outweighs technological advances in infrastructure, medicine, and other areas that it brought. One does not need to be callous to think that, no matter how bad it was, one should not take for granted that colonialism created a world where the essence of the relationship between developed and developing countries is that the former *harm* the latter.

There is yet another way of articulating that developing countries are being harmed by the global order: a benchmark of fairness, where the reference point is a state of nature in which resources are distributed fairly. "Worldwide 34,000 children under age five die daily from hunger and preventable diseases.' Try to conceive a state of nature that can match this amazing feat of our globalized civilization!" writes Pogge.[6] However, no such state-of-nature references can help in this context. They cannot distinguish between the view that *the global order* harms developing societies (Pogge's view), and any other view explaining how the present magnitude of global poverty could have arisen. Such references can only show that things are not as they should be, which does not reveal who is to blame for it.

To conclude: the historical benchmark is the only benchmark among the three considered that we can make sense of, and in relation to that benchmark the global order has brought tremendous advances. Moreover, advances in medicine and food production are largely due to countries that have shaped that order. So, *as far as we can tell*, the global order has benefited the poor.

Let me briefly return to the scenario of African Americans under Jim Crow: that, as some might argue, African Americans were better off under Jim Crow vis-à-vis the antebellum days. About this scenario we can say more than that things were better in 1950 than in 1850. We can say that some participants in a single society sharing economic and political institutions were relegated to an inferior status. This evil can also be attributed to a group of perpetrators. By contrast, we have not yet been able to identify an ongoing evil for which the global order is responsible that is comparable to the way in which Southern whites were responsible for the plight of African Americans long after the abolition of slavery. My reasoning does not therefore entail that Jim Crow should have inspired gratitude.

. . .

Pogge suggests that one goal of macro-explanations transcending national factors is to explain why so many countries are poor and so few are rich (as opposed to explaining the economic status of this or that country). Yet we must be careful in looking for this explanation. If one considers suicide rates in specific countries, micro-explanations at the level of individual suicides will not capture the full story: societal factors have to be considered. There are two senses in which we can inquire about such factors. First, we may ask a noncomparative question about which societal factors matter; and second, we may ask a comparative question about why some particular country has a different suicide rate than similar countries. These two approaches are related (assessing the comparative claim is a way of ensuring that the noncomparative explanation is complete; assessing the noncomparative claim identifies those countries to which one should draw comparisons), but they respond to different inquiries.

Now consider the question, "Why are so many countries poor and so few rich?" This question can only be asked noncomparatively: we have no sense of "what is to be expected" in the same way we do when other countries with certain characteristics have a lower suicide rate than the country we are considering. It is plausible to say that the country with a higher suicide rate "than expected" has good reason to identify and try to change the relevant factors because something is obviously going wrong in that society that does not go wrong in similarly situated societies. But this sort of reasoning does not apply if we have no clear sense of "what is to be expected," as is the case with the question, "Why are so many countries poor and so few rich?" Whatever is wrong with the fact that "so many countries are poor and so few are rich," it is not that there is an obvious gap between "what is to be expected" and what is the case. The perception that there is such a gap may contribute to the intuition that evils like poverty and starvation must be attributable to some entity that can be regarded as "doing the harming." This perception rests on a mistake.

NOTES

1. Unless otherwise noted, data are from World Bank, *World Development Report 2000/2001: Attacking Poverty* (Washington, D.C.: World Bank, 2000); available at web.worldbank.org/WBSITE/EXTERNAL/TOPICS/EXTPOVERTY/o,,contentMDK:20195989~pagePK:148956~piPK:216618~theSitePK:336992,00.html; United Nations, "Report of the High-Level Panel on Financing for Development" ("Zedillo Report"); available at www.un.org/reports/ financing/full_report.pdf; "World Development Indicators 2002"; available at www .worldbank. org/data/wdi2002/cdrom; and Angus Maddison, *The World Economy: A Millennial Perspective* (Paris: OECD Development Center, 2001), table B 22, p. 265. See also Bjorn Lomborg, *The Skeptical Environmentalist: Measuring the Real State of the World* (Cambridge: Cambridge University Press, 2001), esp. Part II for the different approaches to measuring inequality.

2. Alberto Alesina and David Dollar, "Who Gives Foreign Aid to Whom and Why?" *Journal of Economic Growth* 5 (2000), pp. 33–64. According to the Zedillo Report, official development aid in 2000 was $53.1 billion, down from $60.9 billion in 1992; in 1998, $12.1 billion went to the least developed countries; official development aid in 1992 averaged 0.33% of *donors'* GNP, down to 0.22% in 2000, contrasted with the 0.7% of GNP that is widely agreed upon.

3. Nicolas Van de Walle and Timothy Johnston, *Improving Aid to Africa* (Washington, D.C.: Johns Hopkins University Press for the Overseas Development Council, 1996), p. 20.

4. Herbert Giersch, Karl-Heinz Paqué, and Holger Schmieding, *The Fading Miracle: Four Decades of Market Economy in Germany* (Cambridge: Cambridge University Press, 1992), p. 98.

5. Fernand Braudel, *A History of Civilizations* (New York: Penguin, 1987), p. 134.

6. Thomas W. Pogge, "'Assisting' the Global Poor," in Deen K. Chatterjee, ed., *The Ethics of Assistance: Morality and the Distant Needy* (Cambridge: Cambridge University Press, 2004), pp. 260–89.

RECOMMENDED SUPPLEMENTARY READING

GENERAL WORKS

Abraham, Laurie K. *Mama Might Be Better Off Dead: The Failure of Health Care in Urban America*. Chicago: University of Chicago Press, 1993.

Agich, George J., and Charles E., Begley, eds. *The Price of Health*. Boston: D. Reidel, 1986.

Annas, George J. *Standard of Care: The Law of American Bioethics*. Oxford: Oxford University Press, 1993.

Beauchamp, Dan E. *The Health of the Republic: Epidemics, Medicine, and Moralism as Challenges to Democracy*. Philadelphia. Temple University Press, 1988.

Brock, Dan W. *Life and Death: Philosophical Essays in Biomedical Ethics*. New York: Cambridge University Press, 1993.

Cates, Diana Fritz, and Paul Lauritzen. *Medicine and the Ethics of Care*. Washington, DC: Georgetown University Press, 2001.

Daniels, Norman. *Just Health Care.* Cambridge: Cambridge University Press, 1985.

———. *Seeking Fair Treatment: From the AIDS Epidemic to National Health Care Reform.* New York: Oxford University Press, 1995.

Daniels, Norman, Donald W. Light, and Ronald L. Caplan. *Benchmarks of Fairness for Health Care Reform.* New York: Oxford University Press, 1996.

Dougherty, Charles. *Back to Reform: Values, Markets, and the Health Care System.* New York: Oxford University Press, 1996.

Emanuel, Ezekiel. *The Ends of Human Life: Medical Ethics in a Liberal Polity.* Cambridge, MA: Harvard University Press, 1991.

Hall, Mark A. *Making Medical Spending Decisions: The Law, Ethics, and Economics of Rationing Mechanisms.* New York: Oxford University Press, 1996.

Light, Donald, and David Hughes. *Sociological Perspectives on Health Care Rationing.* Oxford: Basil Blackwell, 2001.

Loewy, Erich H., and Roberta Springer Loewy, eds. *Changing Health Care Systems from Ethical, Economic, and Cross Cultural Perspectives.* New York: Kluwer Academic, 2001.

Mechanic, David. "Disadvantage, Inequality, and Social Policy." *Health Affairs,* 21, no. 2 (2002): 48–59.

Morreim, E. Haavi. *Balancing Act: The New Medical Ethics of Medicine's New Economics.* Washington, DC: Georgetown University Press, 1995.

President's Commission for the Study of Ethical Problems in Medicine and Biomedical and Behavioral Research. *Securing Access to Health Care.* Washington, DC: U.S. Government Printing Office, 1983.

Whitehead, Margaret. "The Concepts and Principles of Equity and Health." *International Journal of Health Services* 22 (1992): 429–445.

Zoloth, Laurie. *Health Care and the Ethics of Encounter: A Jewish Discussion of Social Justice.* Chapel Hill: University of North Carolina Press, 1999.

JUSTICE, HEALTH, AND HEALTH CARE

Arras, John. "Retreat from the Right to Health Care: The President's Commission and Access to Health Care." *Cardozo Law Review* 6 (1984): 321–345.

Bayer, Ronald. "Ethics, Politics, and Access to Health Care: A Critical Analysis of the President's Commission." *Cardozo Law Review* 6 (1984): 303–320.

Brock, Dan, Allen Buchanan, Norman Daniels, and Daniel Wikler. *From Chance to Choice: Genetics and Justice.* New York: Cambridge University Press, 2000.

Brody, Baruch. "Why the Right to Health Care Is Not a Useful Concept for Policy Debates." In *Rights to Health Care,* edited by T. J. Bole III and W. B. Bondeson. Netherlands: Kluwer Academic, 1991.

Buchanan, Allen. "Equal Opportunity and Genetic Intervention." *Social Philosophy and Policy* 12, no. 2 (Summer 1995): 105–135.

Callahan, Daniel. *What Kind of Life: The Limits of Medical Progress.* New York: Simon and Schuster, 1990.

Daniels, Norman. *Seeking Fair Treatment: The Lesson of AIDS for National Health Care.* New York: Oxford University Press, 1995.

Daniels, Norman, Bruce Kennedy, and Ichiro Kawachi. *Is Inequality Bad for Our Health?* Boston: Beacon Press, 2000.

Daniels, Norman, and James E. Sabin. *Setting Limits Fairly: Can We Learn to Share Medical Resources?* New York: Oxford University Press, 2002.

Evans, Robert G. "Health Care as a Threat to Health: Defense, Opulence, and the Social Environment." *Daedalus* 123, no. 4 (Fall 1994): 21–43.

Evans, Timothy, Margaret Whitehead, Finn Diderichsen, Abbas Bhuiya, and Meg Wirth, eds. *Challenging Inequities in Health: From Ethics to Action.* New York: Oxford University Press, 2001.

Gutmann, Amy. "For and Against Equal Access to Health Care." *Milbank Quarterly* 59 (Fall 1981): 542–560.

Hofrichter, Richard, ed. *Health and Social Justice: Politics, Ideology, and Inequity in the Distribution of Disease.* Hoboken, NJ: Jossey-Bass, 2003.

LaVeist, Thomas, ed. *Race, Ethnicity, and Health: A Public Health Reader.* Hoboken, NJ: Jossey-Bass, 2002.

Marmot, M. G., and Richard G. Wilkinson, eds. *Social Determinants of Health.* New York: Oxford University Press, 1999.

Marmot, Michael. *The Status Syndrome: How Social Standing Affects Our Health and Longevity.* New York: Times Books/Henry Holt, 2004.

Morreim, E. Haavi. *Holding Health Care Accountable: Law and the New Medical Marketplace.* New York: Oxford University Press, 2001.

Murphy, Timothy F., and Marc A. Lappé, eds. *Justice and the Human Genome Project.* Berkeley: University of California Press, 1994.

Rosenbaum, Sara. "Racial and Ethnic Disparities in Healthcare: Issues in the Design, Structure, and Administration of Federal Healthcare Financing Programs Supported through Direct Public Funding." *Unequal Treatment: Confronting Racial and Ethnic Disparities in Healthcare.* Washington, DC: National Academies Press, 2003: 664–698.

Trivedi, A. N. et al. "Trends in the Quality of Care and Racial Disparities in Medicare Managed Care." *New England Journal of Medicine* 353, no. 7 (August 18, 2005): 692–700.

van Ryn, Michelle, and Jane Burke. "The Effect of Patient Race and Socioeconomic Status on Physicians' Perceptions of Patients." *Social Science and Medicine* 50 (2000): 813–828.

Veatch, Robert M. *The Foundations of Justice: Why the Retarded and the Rest of Us Have Claims to Equality.* New York: Oxford University Press, 1986.

Walzer, Michael. *Spheres of Justice: A Defense of Pluralism and Equality.* New York: Basic Books, 1983.

ALLOCATING SCARCE RESOURCES

Aaron, Henry J., and William B. Schwartz. *The Painful Prescription: Rationing Health Care.* Washington, DC: Brookings Institution, 1984.

Anand, Sudhir, Fabienne Peter, and Amartya Sen, eds. *Public Health, Ethics, and Equity.* Oxford: Oxford University Press, 2004: 201–219.

Axtell-Thompson, L. M. "Consumer Directed Health Care: Ethical Limits to Choice and Responsibility." *Journal of Medical Philosophy* 30, no. 2 (April 2005): 207–226.

Blank, Robert H. *The Price of Life: The Future of American Health Care.* New York: Columbia University Press, 1997.

Churchill, Larry R. *Rationing Health Care in America: Perceptions and Principles of Justice.* Notre Dame, IN: University of Notre Dame Press, 1987.

Daniels, Norman. "Rationing Fairly: Programmatic Considerations." *Bioethics* 7, nos. 2–3 (1993): 224–233.

Daniels, Norman et al. "Meeting the Challenges of Justice and Rationing." *Hastings Center Report* 24, no. 4 (July–August 1994): 27–42.

Daniels, Norman, and James Sabin. "Limits to Health Care: Fair Procedures, Democratic Deliberation, and the Legitimacy Problem for Insurers." *Philosophy and Public Affairs* 26, no. 4 (Fall 1997): 303–350.

Denier, Yvonne. *Efficiency, Justice and Care: Philosophical Reflections on Scarcity in Health Care (International Library of Ethics, Law, and the New Medicine).* New York: Springer, 2007.

Eddy, David M. *Clinical Decision Making: From Theory to Practice.* Sudbury, MA: Jones and Bartlett, 1996.

———. "High-Dose Chemotherapy with Autologous Bone Marrow Transplantation for the Treatment of Metastatic Breast Cancer." *Journal of Clinical Oncology* 10, no. 4 (1992): 657–670.

Hall, Mark A. *Making Medical Spending Decisions: The Law, Ethics, and Economics of Rationing Mechanisms.* New York: Oxford University Press, 1997.

Kamm, Frances M. *Morality, Mortality: Death and Whom to Save From It.* Oxford: Oxford University Press, 1993.

"The Law and Policy of Health Care Rationing: Models and Accountability." *University of Pennsylvania Law Review* 140, no. 5 (May 1992): 1505–1998.

Light, Donald, and David Hughes, eds. *Sociological Perspectives on Health Care Rationing.* Oxford: Basil Blackwell, 2001.

"Managed Care Systems: Emerging Health Issues from an Ethics Perspective." *Journal of Law, Medicine and Ethics* 23, no. 3 (symposium, 1995).

Mann, Jonathan M. *Health and Human Rights: A Reader.* New York: Routledge, 1999.

Menzel, Paul T. *Medical Costs, Moral Choices.* New Haven, CT: Yale University Press, 1983.

———. *Strong Medicine: The Ethical Rationimg Medical Care.* New York: Oxford University Press, 1990.

Nelson, James Lindemann. "Measured Fairness, Situated Justice: Feminist Reflections on Health Care Rationing." *Kennedy Institute of Ethics Journal* 6 (1996): 53–68.

Nord, Erik. *Cost-Value Analysis in Health Care: Making Sense Out of QALYs.* New York: Cambridge University Press, 1999.

Pongrace, Paul Earl III. "HDC/ABMT Experimental Treatment or Cure All? (Ask the Insurance Companies)." *The Journal of Pharmacy & Law* 2, no. 2 (1994): 329–356.

Priester, Reinhard, Karen G. Gervais, and Dorothy E. Vawter. *Improving Coverage for Unproven Health Care Interventions.* Minneapolis: Minnesota Center for Health Care Ethics, 1996.

Schut, F. T., and W. P. Van de Ven. "Rationing and Competition in the Dutch Health-Care System." *Health Economics* 14 suppl. 1 (September 2005): S59–S74.

Tauber, A. I. "A Philosophical Approach to Rationing." *Medical Journal of Australia* 178, no. 9 (May 5, 2003): 454–456.

Tengs, T. O. "An Evaluation of Oregon's Medicaid Rationing Algorithms." *Health Economics* 5, no. 3 (May–June 1996): 171–181.

Ubel, Peter A. *Pricing Life: Why It's Time for Health Care Rationing.* Cambridge, MA: MIT Press, 1999.

Wikler, Daniel. "Ethics and Rationing: 'Whether,' 'How,' or 'How Much'?" *Journal of the American Geriatrics Society* 40, no. 4 (1992): 398–403.

Wong, Kenman L. *Medicine and the Marketplace: The Moral Dimensions of Managed Care.* Notre Dame, IN: University of Notre Dame Press, 1998.

ORGAN TRANSPLANTATION: GIFTS VERSUS MARKETS

Burrows, L. "Selling Organs for Transplantation." *Mount Sinai Journal of Medicine* 71, no. 4 (September 2004): 251–254.

Cherry, Mark J. *Kidney for Sale by Owner: Human Organs, Transplantation, and the Market.* Washington DC: Georgetown University Press, 2005.

Cohen, I. Glenn. "The Price of Everything. The Value of Nothing. Reframing the Commodification Debate." *Harvard Law Review* 117 (2003): 689–710.

Crowley-Matoka M., and R. M. Arnold. "The Dead Donor Rule: How Much Does the Public Care . . . and How

Much Should We Care?" *Kennedy Institute of Ethics Journal* 14, no. 3 (September 2004): 319–332.

Delmonico, F. L., R. Arnold, N. Scheper-Hughes, L. A. Siminoff, J. Kahn, and S. J. Youngner. "Ethical Incentives—Not Payment—for Organ Donation." *New England Journal of Medicine* 346, no. 25 (June 20, 2002): 2002–2005.

Goodwin, Michele. *Black Markets: The Supply and Demand of Body Parts.* Cambridge: Cambridge University Press, 2006.

Goyal, M., R. L. Mehta, L. J. Schneiderman, and A. R. Sehgal. "Economic and Health Consequences of Selling a Kidney in India." *Journal of the American Medical Association* 288, no. 13 (October 2002): 1589–1593.

Taylor, James Stacy. *Stakes and Kidneys: Why Markets in Human Body Parts Are Morally Imperative (Live Questions in Ethics and Moral Philosophy).* London: Ashgate, 2005.

POVERTY, HEALTH, AND JUSTICE BEYOND NATIONAL BORDERS

Farmer, Paul. *Pathologies of Power: Health, Human Rights, and the New War on the Poor (California Series in Public Anthropology, 4).* Berkeley: University of California Press, 2004.

Leon, David A., and Gill Walt, eds. *Poverty, Inequality and Health: An International Perspective.* New York: Oxford University Press, 2001.

Nagel, T. "The Problem of Global Justice." *Philosophy & Public Affairs* 33, no. 2 (2005): 113–147.

Pogge, T. "Severe Poverty as a Violation of Negative Duties." *Ethics and International Affairs* 19, no. 1 (2005): 55–83.

PART THREE

DEFINING DEATH, FORGOING LIFE-SUSTAINING TREATMENT, AND EUTHANASIA

Death remains as inevitable as always, yet somehow today it seems harder to achieve. In the past, diseases such as pneumonia, formerly called "the old man's friend," led to a speedy and fairly gentle death. Today such infections can be treated, and many of the more rapid causes of death can be staved off. Thus, the benefits of medical advances bring with them burdens, and here the burden is the possibility of a lingering death, surrounded not by loved ones in the home, but by medical hardware in an intensive care unit.

Indeed, it is now possible to sustain individuals for years in a "persistent vegetative state" (PVS), a state in which they do not feel, think, or have any awareness of their surroundings. Some would argue that someone who lacks a capacity for *any* conscious activity is not, in any meaningful ethical sense, alive. This raises the first issue of this chapter: How do we define death?

THE DEFINITION OF DEATH

Most scholars accept that to analyze the concept of "death," you first need to agree on its definition, then formulate a measurable criterion to show that the definition has been fulfilled, and finally develop a series of clinical tests to show that the criterion has been satisfied. The definition of "death" might seem straightforward, since "death" is a nontechnical word that is used widely and correctly. Someone is dead when he or she is no longer living; death is the end and absence of life. However, developments in medical technology over the last few decades, as well as reflective scholarship on those developments, have called into question not only the clinical tests for determining when an individual has died, but also what the tests should measure (the criterion of death) and even our understanding of what death is (its definition).

Before the development of high-technology forms of life support—in particular, the respirator—death was pretty straightforward. People were dead when they stopped breathing and their hearts stopped beating. The traditional criterion of death, then, is the cessation of heart–lung, or cardiopulmonary, function. And the clinical test for determining the cessation of cardiopulmonary function might be as simple as putting a mirror in front of the patient's mouth to see if he or she was still breathing, or listening for a heartbeat. Today, however, people whose respiration and heartbeat have ceased can be resuscitated, and their breathing can be artificially maintained; and when this is done, the heart can continue to beat even in the absence of any input from the brain. Hence, a patient with an intact heart can be maintained on a respirator even when his or her brain functions have ceased entirely.

This new state of affairs created the need for rethinking death. In 1968, an ad hoc committee of the Harvard Medical School, chaired by Henry K. Beecher,* issued a report recommending that patients on life support, whose brain function had completely and irreversibly ceased, be declared dead and then removed from the respirator. Beecher favored brain-based, or neurological, criteria for diagnosing death, not primarily to resolve conceptual uncertainties about the meaning of death, but to solve several practical problems stemming from new technologies, including organ transplantation and the prevention of waste of medical resources (Pernick 1999). Organs that remain in a patient's dead body quickly deteriorate and become unusable. Transplant surgeons needed to remove organs quickly without risking accusations of murder. In addition, Beecher wanted to end the futile waste of scarce and expensive medical resources, such as respirators, on patients who could no longer benefit from them.

By the late 1970s, the issue of providing futile care and prolonging dying, epitomized by the case of Karen Quinlan (see Section 3, "Advance Directives"), gave further impetus to the shift to neurological criteria for diagnosing death. Quinlan herself did not meet the criteria of whole-brain death, recommended by the Harvard committee, since her brain stem continued to function. She was not brain dead, but rather alive in a PVS, a state in which the capacity for thought and feeling, or for conscious awareness of any kind, has been permanently lost. Nevertheless, in the case of both PVS and brain-dead patients, the continued use of life support appeared futile and wasteful to many people, and emphasized the need for a shift to neurological criteria for diagnosing death.

Two main schools of thought have emerged regarding neurological criteria of death. One is the whole-brain criterion, advocated by the Harvard report. The Harvard criteria specified that death

required the termination of all functions of the whole brain, both conscious and reflexive activities. The other approach is the higher-brain criterion. It maintains that death occurs when there is the permanent loss of consciousness. Since consciousness has its seat in the cerebral cortex, the individual is dead when the cortex or higher brain irreversibly loses function, even if there is brain stem activity.

The whole-brain criterion was adopted by the influential President's Commission for the Study of Ethical Problems in Medicine and Biomedical and Behavioral Research. A selection from the Commission's 1981 report *Defining Death* is the first reading in Section 1. Unlike the Harvard Committee, the President's Commission explicitly grounds its whole-brain criterion in a rejection of a "higher-brain" definition of death, which it regards as too radical, too far from the ordinary conception of death. In rejecting the "neocortical death" or "higher-brain death" proposal, the Commission argues that whole-brain death is not, as one might think, a wholly new concept of death. Rather, the Commission suggests, it is simply that artificial ventilation has made the traditional cardiopulmonary indicators of death invalid for a set of patients, and brain death substitutes new diagnostic measures for them.

According to the Commission, then, the *concept* of death remains the same, whatever the *criteria* for determining death are taken to be. If this is right, then even the term "brain dead" is misleading: after all, we do not say that someone diagnosed as dead according to traditional cardiopulmonary criteria is "heart dead" or "lung dead." Moreover, if someone who is brain dead is really dead, it is a mistake to say (as newspapers sometimes do) that the patient was declared brain dead on a certain day and "died" on a subsequent day. But is the confusion that exists among medical specialists and bioethicists as much as among laypeople merely verbal confusion as we adjust to new criteria for death? Or is brain death something distinct from death as it is commonly understood?

It might seem that the definition of "death" is a matter for science, in particular, biology. Certainly, science has a role to play in our understanding of death, for example, in determining the most reliable criteria of death. However, the issue is not simply which criteria most reliably mark the irreversible

---

Editors' note: Beecher, a respected anesthesiologist, is the author of a 1966 article in the *New England Journal of Medicine* that called attention to a number of experimental studies that had put patients at risk and were done without informed consent. See Part 6, "Experimentation on Human Subjects."

loss of life. Rather, our understanding of what constitutes human death depends on our understanding of what it is to be a human being. As one commentator has put it, "The ensuing controversy between advocates of whole-brain and higher-brain criteria for diagnosing brain death often reflected a conceptual contest over whether mental activity or bodily integration constitute the essence of human life" (Pernick 1999). This conceptual contest is primarily a philosophical, not a scientific, question. If we think of the human being primarily as an *organism,* and if we take the brain to be the organ that coordinates and unifies the organism's biological functioning, then the whole-brain theory might provide the best account of death, for the organism dies when the entire brain permanently ceases functioning. But if we think of the human being primarily as a *person,* and if we think that the person is gone when the capacities for awareness, thought, and social interaction are permanently lost, then the higher-brain criterion might be considered the better view. Thus, the concept of death, while undoubtedly partly biological, is also metaphysical and evaluative. Moreover, death traditionally has had medical, social, and legal consequences. It marks the point at which medical treatment can be unilaterally withdrawn (that is, without consent), organs harvested (with appropriate consent), property disposed of, the body buried or cremated, the surviving spouse can remarry, and so forth. If death is an ethically and legally significant boundary, after which it is permissible to do things that it is not permissible to do before, then we need a moral argument for where this boundary should be drawn.

James L. Bernat attempts to provide such an argument in "The Whole-Brain Concept of Death Remains Optimum Public Policy." Pointing out that the determination of death using brain-death tests has become worldwide over the past several decades, Bernat argues that "despite admitted shortcomings, the classical formulation of whole-brain death remains both conceptually coherent and forms a solid foundation for public policy surrounding human death determination and organ transplantation."

What are these admitted shortcomings? Some have argued that it is time to abandon brain death on the ground that the whole-brain criterion of death has become obsolete. Even when the brain is permanently nonfunctioning, isolated brain cells can continue to live, and small amounts of electrical activity can be recorded on an electroencephalogram. For this reason, no one really believes anymore that literally all functions of the whole brain must be irreversibly lost for an individual to be dead. However, Bernat maintains that the whole-brain approach does not require the loss of all neuronal activity. Rather, death occurs when all clinical functions of the brain are irreversibly lost. This raises the question of what "irreversible" means and how irreversibility is to be determined, in light of reports of patients who were diagnosed as brain dead but whose circulation and visceral organ functioning were successfully maintained for months or longer. Bernat suggests that the mere assertion of irreversibility may no longer be sufficient to diagnose brain death and that further tests to show cessation of all intracranial blood flow should be mandatory, "at least if there is any question about the diagnosis or if the examiner is inexperienced."

Another objection to brain death focuses on the rationale for according a special role to brain function. Alan Shewmon argues that the brain performs no qualitatively different forms of integration than the spinal cord, and therefore should have no special status in death determination. Furthermore, fetuses have continued to live and grow inside the bodies of brain-dead women, making the very concept of brain death inherently counterintuitive. Moreover, since an explicit rationale for the adoption of neurological, or brain-based, criteria for diagnosing death was to facilitate organ transplantation, some, like Robert Taylor, have concluded that brain death is nothing more than a legal fiction: Those "we declare 'brain dead' are not truly dead, but we consider them dead for the socially beneficial goal of organ procurement."

Bernat acknowledges that the whole-brain formulation is not perfect, but he thinks it is the best approach to determining death in the real world, where compromises are necessary to achieve acceptable practices and laws. Jeff McMahan, in "An Alternative to Brain Death," disagrees, in part because he think that critics of neurological criteria are correct in maintaining that the brain is not necessary for the integrated functioning of an organism. Indeed, early embryos do not have brains, and they seem to be living human organisms. But McMahan wishes to make a deeper philosophical point, which is to reject the underlying assumption that we are essentially organisms. Instead, McMahan argues, we are essentially embodied minds. When the capacity for consciousness is irreversibly lost, *we* cease to exist, even if our organisms continue to be biologically alive, as in PVS. Like others, such as Robert Veatch, McMahan adopts a higher-brain criterion of death, but does not apply this criterion to human organisms. Thus, his view avoids the "embarrassing implication" that an organism with spontaneous respiration and heartbeat is dead. The organism is not dead, though the person whose organism it was no longer exists. For McMahan, then, the question of organ donation turns not on when the death of the organism occurs, but rather on whether taking organs from someone in PVS, causing the death of the organism, is morally permissible. To this question he answers, "if the person had consented in advance, there would be no moral objection to killing the unoccupied organism in order to use its organs to save the lives of others."

One of the fundamental challenges for bioethics today is to decide when to terminate treatment for patients who are, by present definitions, alive. Competent patients have a well-established, common-law right to refuse even life-sustaining medical treatment. As articulated by the eminent judge Benjamin Cardozo in a rightly celebrated formulation, "Every adult human being of adult years and sound mind has a right to determine what shall be done with his own body." But what exactly do we mean by a "sound mind," and how are we to distinguish sound minds from unsound minds?

DECISIONAL CAPACITY AND THE RIGHT TO REFUSE TREATMENT

Although most patients either clearly possess or clearly lack the capacity for autonomous decision making, a significant portion fall into a troublesome gray area between competence and incompetence.* In Section 2, the factual and conceptual difficulties

involved in determining competency are well illustrated in the case of Mary Northern, a stubborn 72-year-old woman suffering from gangrene of both feet. Although Ms. Northern's physicians insisted that surgical amputation of her feet was required to save her life, she adamantly refused to grant them permission to operate. Contrary to the opinion of her physicians, she maintained that her feet were improving and that surgery was thus unnecessary. While her physicians characterized her refusal as irrational, a court-appointed guardian remarked on her good memory and overall coherence and intelligence. Her physicians found her to be "psychotic" with regard to discussions about her feet, but her guardian concluded that she was of "sound mind." Mary Northern's own testimony, delivered from her bed in an intensive care unit, supported both conclusions. Who was right? More important, what do we mean by "competency," and what standards of decision-making capacity should be imposed on patients like Mary Northern?

According to Allen Buchanan and Dan W. Brock in "Deciding for Others: Competency," competency ought to be understood not as a global attribute, but rather as a "decision-relative" concept. In other words, persons should be thought of as competent to do this or that, or to make this or that decision. Obviously, the same patient might thus be competent to refuse an easily explainable procedure but incompetent to manage her own complex finances. In addition, Buchanan and Brock argue that our concept of competency encompasses not merely an assessment of the patient's actual psychological capacities, but also a complex societal weighting of the values of well-being and autonomy. Noting that our task is to avoid two diametrically opposed kinds of error—stripping capable patients of the autonomy or allowing impaired patients to make foolish and self-destructive decisions—Buchanan and Brock contend that our standard of competency must be *decided* rather than merely *discovered*. Contrary to those who argue for some minimal standard of competency in every case or judge a patient's choice according to some objective canon of normalcy, Buchanan and Brock focus our attention on the quality of the patient's process of reasoning and on the risks and benefits posed by the decision. In Mary Northern's case, for example, a situation involving a life-or-death decision by a woman of questionable

---

Editors' note: Strictly speaking, "competence" is a legal term. Thus understood, only judges have the authority to declare a patient "incompetent." In the less formal context of this book, however, we define "competency" as the capacity for autonomous decision making.

competence, they would have insisted that the patient meet a high standard of decision-making capacity. We leave it to readers to decide whether this "sliding-scale" approach masks ethically problematic, paternalistic judgments as objective medical or psychiatric competency determinations; or whether it correctly avoids attributing autonomy to all conscious patients, regardless of cognitive impairment, whose decisions may be manifestly against their own best interests.

Some refusals of treatment cause consternation among physicians not because there is genuine doubt about the ability of the patient to understand his or her condition, treatment alternatives, possible outcomes, and the like, but rather because the patient's refusal seems patently irrational. Must all treatment refusals be honored, or only those that meet certain standards of rationality, legal competence, or professional medical ethics? Must doctors honor the refusal of any legally competent patient, no matter how irrational the choice might seem? What if sound medical practice offers a high probability of curing an otherwise fatal condition—should our medical ethic condone such self-destructive treatment refusals? Is the paternalistic imposition of therapy against the patient's will ever justified?

These questions converge in this section's case study. A freak accident left Don Cowart with severe burns on over 65 percent of his body. Despite the severity of his injuries, he was clearly competent, and he repeatedly asked to be allowed to die. Don's doctor at first dismissed his patient's pleas to stop treatment as the typical response of burn victims to the pain of their wounds and treatment. In time, however, he discussed Don's wish to die with Don, his mother, and his lawyer. Should Don have been allowed to discontinue his painful daily treatments in order to go home and die? Should his mother and lawyer have been able to block his treatment refusal? And is the ultimate outcome of Don's life—completing a law degree, passing the bar, and setting up a small practice—relevant to whether he should have been allowed to die?

ADVANCE DIRECTIVES

Advance directives are documents created by competent individuals to express their preferences regarding treatment, should they become incompetent.

The best known form of advance directive is the "living will." The nation's first living-will statute was enacted in California in 1976, prompted by the case of Karen Ann Quinlan, who slipped into a coma in April 1975. When it became clear that she was in a persistent vegetative state (PVS), her parents sought to have her respirator removed. Her doctors refused, and her parents took the case to court. The court found that Karen, were she competent, would have had a right to refuse treatment, and held that Karen's guardian could assert that right on Karen's behalf, provided that she would have wanted it exercised in such circumstances. The problem was that Karen had never specified what she would want done—she was, after all, a healthy 21-year-old prior to her sudden loss of consciousness. Despite this lack of evidence for implementing the standard that has come to be known as "the substituted judgment test," the court favored the right of Karen's family to make the decision to refuse her treatment. It stated that if *their* decision was that Karen would have wanted treatment stopped, they could exercise Karen's right of privacy. The court found such a choice permissible based on the medical prognosis—Karen had lost all chance of returning to a sapient, cognitive existence—and suggested that hospitals set up "ethics committees" to oversee such decisions and, in particular, confirm the prognoses.

The *Quinlan* case prompted the enactment of the nation's first living-will statute, California's Natural Death Act, in 1976. A living will is a document executed by a competent adult that directs medical treatment in the event of his or her future incapacitation. The California statute is very narrow. It allows the removal of life-sustaining treatment only after the patient has been diagnosed with a terminal illness that will cause death imminently. "Thus," as George J. Annas notes in "The Health Care Proxy and the Living Will," "even though this statute was inspired by her story, it would not have helped Quinlan, because she was not terminally ill." Indeed, she continued to live for another ten years after being taken off the respirator.

A second landmark case involved another young woman, Nancy Cruzan, who entered a PVS, in this case, as a result of a car accident in 1983. Like Karen Quinlan, Nancy Cruzan did not die when removed from the respirator, but continued to breathe on her own and was placed on a feeding tube. After four years, when it became apparent that her condition would not change, her father attempted to have the feeding tube removed so that she could die. Nancy's parents were granted permission by a Missouri trial court to terminate her artificial nutrition and hydration, but the Missouri Supreme Court reversed the decision on the grounds that there was not "clear and convincing evidence" that she would have wanted the feeding tube removed. On June 25, 1990, the U.S. Supreme Court upheld, by a 5–4 decision, the judgment of the Missouri Supreme Court. This was the first so-called right-to-die case to reach the U.S. Supreme Court.

The Court made two notable claims in *Cruzan.* First, it rejected the view that there is a moral or legal difference between taking someone off a respirator and removing a feeding tube. The Court said that in this context they are both forms of medical treatment, and both can be rejected. Second, the Court upheld Missouri's right to use the most stringent standard—the clear and convincing evidence standard—in determining whether life-prolonging treatment may be removed from incompetents. The Court did not say that this standard *must* be used, only that there is nothing in the Constitution that prevents a state from applying this test.

At this point, other people came forward who had known Nancy Cruzan by her married name of Davis and so did not connect her with the case until they heard the details from the media. They had worked with her in a program for children with disabilities, where she had stated repeatedly that she would not want to be force fed or kept alive on a machine. The Cruzans returned to court with this testimony in October 1990, and this time Missouri's attorney general and Ms. Cruzan's court-appointed guardian ad litem did not object to the Cruzans' request. The judge who had originally said that the tube could be removed repeated his findings of three years before. The tube was removed and, twelve days later, on December 26, 1990, Nancy Cruzan died.

Living wills are intended to provide "clear and convincing" evidence of what the person "would have wanted," thus providing a basis for proxy decision making. However, relatively few people (roughly 18 percent of Americans) make living wills. Moreover, according to Annas, virtually all living-will statutes suffer from four major shortcomings: They are applicable only to those who are "terminally ill" (thus inapplicable to PVS patients who can survive for years); they limit the types of treatment that can be refused, usually allowing refusal only of "artificial" or "extraordinary" therapies; they make no provision for the designation of a decision maker to act on the person's behalf; and there is no penalty if health care providers do not honor these documents. Another problem with living wills is that it is extremely difficult to foresee every medical problem and possible treatment that might arise. Living wills also require physicians to make treatment decisions based on their interpretation of the document, rather than on a discussion of the treatment options with a person acting on the patient's behalf.

In "Enough: The Failure of the Living Will," Angela Fagerlin and Carl E. Schneider add another reason that living wills fail: Patients often do not have enough information to give informed consent for even contemporaneous decisions, much less prospective ones. Moreover, patients' preferences often are not stable. In particular, healthy people are likely to discount the strength of their desire to live when ill and misjudge their own end-of-life preferences. Even if they knew their own desires, it is unlikely they would be able to articulate them clearly, largely because of the uncertainty and range of medical choices. The inevitable imprecision of living wills makes it difficult to apply them to specific clinical situations, which in turn leads physicians either to disregard them or to read them in light of their own preferences. Thus, having a living will is unlikely to change the treatment a patient receives. Fagerlin and Schneider conclude that while living wills may have some use for some individuals, getting everyone to have one is not a wise public policy.

A solution to the problems of foresight and interpretation is to replace living wills with durable-power-of-attorney forms, which would name a "health care proxy" or "surrogate" empowered to make medical decisions for the incapacitated person. Every state already has a durable-power-of-attorney law; however, the current trend is for states to enact additional proxy laws that deal specifically with health care. These laws authorize a proxy to make any decisions that the patient would have made if he or she were still competent. These decisions must prove consistent with the wishes of the patient, if known, or they must prove otherwise consistent with the patient's best interests.

Many people find the "clear and convincing" standard imposed in *Cruzan* and other cases far too stringent, especially in the case of individuals who are permanently and irreversibly unconscious. Such critics may ask whether life is of any benefit or value to someone who cannot hear, feel, think, or be aware of anything. A much more difficult decision arises in the case of minimally conscious patients, for they may get some benefit out of their lives, severely limited though they are. Some argue that a family, based on its intimate knowledge of the person over a lifetime, should have the right to terminate life support for a severely demented relative. However, in many cases it is extremely difficult even for family members to know what the patient would have wanted.

Even if it is possible to ascertain what the patient would have wanted when he or she was competent, should this be the deciding factor? That is, should treatment decisions be made on the basis of the preferences and values of the once-competent individual, or on the basis of the interests of the patient as he or she is now? This issue is sharply highlighted in the scenarios by Norman L. Cantor ("Testing the Limits of Prospective Autonomy: Five Scenarios") and in Section 4, "Choosing for Once-Competent Patients."

CHOOSING FOR ONCE-COMPETENT PATIENTS

In February 1990, Theresa Schiavo, aged 26, collapsed in her home. Doctors believe a potassium imbalance, probably due to an eating disorder, caused her heart to temporarily stop, cutting off oxygen to her brain. Soon afterward, she went into a coma that became a PVS. Like Karen Quinlan and Nancy Cruzan before her, Theresa was able to be weaned from a respirator and began to breathe on her own. The *Schiavo* case raised the question, raised earlier in *Cruzan*, of whether a feeding tube may be removed from a PVS patient. Seemingly, that issue had been settled (see the preceding section, "Advance Directives"). The removal of a feeding tube from a PVS patient was—or so it seemed—no longer a live issue in bioethics or in law. Yet the

Schiavo case created a political firestorm and media circus. It went through every level of the Florida judicial system and several federal courts. The U.S. Congress and even the president became involved. The interesting question is, why?

In part, the answer has to do with abortion politics. Having lost—at least for the time being—the battle to make abortion illegal, many in the pro-life movement are turning to end-of-life issues, to fight against both assisted suicide and the termination of treatment for incapacitated patients. In this they have been joined by many members of the disability community who argue that brain damage—even damage resulting in permanent unconsciousness—should not influence treatment decisions. In part, *Schiavo* was different from previous cases and raised different questions. One important difference is that this case involved a battle within a family. Whereas the Quinlan and the Cruzan families had to fight the hospital or the state for the right to remove the respirator or feeding tube keeping their daughters alive, the court battle in this case was between Theresa's husband, Michael Schiavo, and her parents, Robert and Mary Schindler, a battle that is sympathetically described by Jay Wolfson, Theresa's guardian ad litem, in "Erring on the Side of Theresa Schiavo: Reflections of the Special Guardian ad Litem," the first essay in this section. The Schindlers maintained that Theresa was not in a PVS and that, with adequate care, her condition could improve. For a long time Michael Schiavo also clung to the belief that his wife could recover, taking her from doctor to doctor, trying various kinds of experimental treatments, and stays in rehabilitation centers. Eventually, however, he accepted the diagnosis of PVS, which led to his petition to have her feeding tube removed in 1998. As he said in a statement in 2003, "After more than seven years of desperately searching for a cure for Terri, the death of my own mother helped me realize that I was fooling myself. More important, I was hiding behind my hope, and selfishly ignoring Terri's wishes. I wanted my wife to be with me so much that I denied her true condition."

In addition to denying the diagnosis of PVS, the Schindlers also argued that Michael should not be allowed to make medical decisions for their daughter because he did not have Theresa's best interest at heart. Rather, they said, he wanted Theresa dead so that he could remarry and inherit her estate. (He had begun living with another woman during the fifteen years that his wife was unconscious, and they had two children together.) These allegations (and others, including the suggestion that Michael had physically abused his wife) were found to be baseless by the court. The Schindlers' attempt to have Michael removed as his wife's guardian failed.

From 2000 to 2005, the feeding tube was ordered removed, replaced, and removed several times, as Michael Schiavo and the Schindlers fought each other in court. On October 20, 2003, the Florida House of Represenatatives passed a bill called Terri's Law that allowed the governor to issue a "one-time stay in certain cases." After passing the Florida Senate, Gov. Jeb Bush issued an executive order directing reinsertion of the percutaneous endoscopic gastrostomy (PEG) tube. Dr. Jay Wolfson, a public health professor at the University of South Florida, who holds both medical and law degrees, was appointed her (third) guardian ad litem, to represent her "best interest" although not to make medical decisions for her. On December 1, 2003, Dr. Wolfson submitted his report concluding that Theresa Schiavo was in a persistent vegetative state with no chance of improvement.

In May 2004, a circuit judge ruled that Terri's Law was unconstitutional. This ruling was upheld by the Florida Supreme Court in September. In January 2005 the U.S. Supreme Court refused to hear the appeal brought by the governor's attorneys. The trial court judge, Judge George Greer, issued one last emergency stay blocking removal of Theresa Schiavo's feeding tube, saying he needed time to decide whether her parents should be allowed to pursue other legal and medical options. Finally, on February 25, 2005, Judge Greer gave Michael Schiavo permission to order the removal of the feeding tube at 1 p.m. on March 18.

Meanwhile, on March 8, U.S. Rep. David Weldon (R-FL) introduced in the U.S. House of Representatives a bill that would permit a federal court to review the Schiavo matter through a habeas corpus lawsuit. A compromise bill was passed by the House and the Senate, and signed into law by President George W. Bush on March 21. He had cut short his vacation on his ranch in Texas—the first time he had ever done so—to return to Washington to sign this legislation.

On March 22, federal district court judge James D. Whittemore refused to order the reinsertion of the PEG tube. The Schindlers appealed to the Eleventh Circuit Court of Appeals, which dismissed their appeal. On March 24, the U.S. Supreme Court refused to hear the case. On March 31, 2005, Theresa Schiavo died. The diagnosis of PVS was confirmed by her autopsy in June 2005. According to the autopsy report, "The brain weighed 615 grams, roughly half of the expected weight of a human brain. . . . This damage was irreversible, and no amount of therapy or treatment would have regenerated the massive loss of neurons."

For many people, the fact that the autopsy proved that Theresa Schiavo was indeed in a persistent vegetative state would settle the moral and legal issues: Why would anyone want to be kept alive indefinitely in a state of permanent and irreversible unconsciousness? But some argue that even PVS patients should receive medical treatment and have their lives sustained. In "'Human Non-Person': Terri Schiavo, Bioethics, and Our Future," Wesley J. Smith worries about a slippery slope in which we go from disconnecting the feeding tubes of patients with "profound cognitive disabilities" to harvesting the organs of still-living, terminally ill patients. Groups like Not Dead Yet, which picketed in front of the hospital, regard the issues in the *Schiavo* case as fundamentally disability rights issues—"issues which affect tens of thousands of people with disabilities who, like Ms. Schindler-Schiavo, cannot currently articulate their views and so must rely on others as substitute decision-makers" (Not Dead Yet 2005). However, it can be argued that it is a mistake to characterize PVS as a disability, on the ground that there is a real distinction between those whose cognitive abilities are impaired and those who are permanently unconscious and therefore do not have any cognitive abilities at all.

One of the difficult questions raised by the *Schiavo* case was determining what Theresa Schiavo would have wanted. To answer that question, we may look to explicit statements made by the patient, or to the implicit values expressed in the kind of life she made. However, the question of whether life-sustaining treatment should be continued is made more complicated when the patient is not permanently unconscious. In that case, in addition to the patient's prior wishes, we have to consider her present interests, however attenuated these may be.

In the Matter of Claire C. Conroy posed this question, which was decided by the same court that decided *In re Quinlan*. *Conroy* held that when it is not clear what the patient *would have wanted* (the subjective test), a patient's family can still terminate treatment if they meet an objective test: If they can prove that the burdens of the patient's life "clearly and markedly" outweigh the benefits, where both burdens and benefits are measured in terms of physical pain and suffering. In his partial dissent, Justice Handler rejected the notion that benefits and burdens should be understood in purely physical terms, arguing that notions like personal privacy, dignity, and bodily integrity should be considered as well.

In "The Severely Demented, Minimally Functional Patient: An Ethical Analysis," John D. Arras reiterates the difficulties of determining what a previously competent, now incompetent patient like Claire Conroy (Mrs. Smith, in his article) "would have wanted." Does the fact that she repeatedly pulls out her feeding tube signify a desire to die—or only a desire to have the irritation caused by the tube stop? Previous independence and avoidance may or may not mean that the patient would prefer death to being sustained by feeding tubes. (Fagerlin and Schneider make precisely this point in Section 3 when they discuss the malleability of patient preferences.) So should we eschew a subjective standard in favor of an objective best-interests standard? In the case of PVS patients, it is far from clear that such a standard makes any sense: Does a permanently and irreversibly unconscious individual even have interests or a welfare in the ordinary sense of these terms? A best-interests standard would require that treatment always continue, given the very slight possibility of recovery or misdiagnosis and the absence of pain or other burdens—a result Arras terms "paradoxical," since if anyone's life need not be maintained, surely PVS patients are at the top of the list. If, as Arras maintains, PVS patients cannot be benefited or burdened, then the rationale for nontreatment is not that continuing to be tube fed is bad for the patient. Rather, it is that the *person* has ceased to exist, even though her body continues to live. As Michael Schiavo expressed it in his 2003 statement: "The reality is that Terri left us 13 years ago, and none of us can bring her back."

Decision making is very different for marginally or moderately functional individuals who can think,

feel, and relate to others. Even if such patients are incapable of rational decision making, they nevertheless are clearly persons with interests that can be either advanced or frustrated by their caregivers. These patients are, Arras says, entitled to a "patient-centered best-interests" medical analysis. However, applying a best-interests analysis to minimally functional patients, such as Arras's Mrs. Smith, is problematic. It is difficult to determine either the benefits or the burdens of continued existence in her condition. Nevertheless, Arras maintains that it is highly doubtful that the burdens of Mrs. Smith's life "clearly and markedly" outweigh the benefits; thus, a literal application of the *Conroy* formula would lead to the conclusion that the G-tube should be surgically implanted. The trouble with this conclusion is that it appears to leave out something important: namely, the patient's probable feelings about privacy, dependency, dignity, and bodily integrity. To focus solely on physical pain is to reduce Mrs. Smith "from the full-fledged person that she once was to a mere physical repository of pleasures and pains."

Considerations of this sort led Justice Handler to his eloquent dissent in *Conroy*. Arras notes, however, that Handler's dissent is also problematic. If we consider only Mrs. Smith's *present interests*, then these are indeed reduced to sensations of pleasure and pain. In her present state, she is not bothered by a lack of dignity or bodily integrity. If we consider the interests of the formerly competent Mrs. Smith, it is possible that she would have been appalled at being kept alive in her present condition. The trouble is that we cannot know this, since she left behind neither an advance directive nor a pattern of analogous choices that clearly demonstrate what she would have wanted under her present circumstances. Thus, the ambiguities of substituted judgment lead to the adoption of an objective best-interests standard, while the deficiencies of the objective standard—with its narrow focus on pain to the exclusion of other important values—send us back to the substituted judgment test. To get us out of this dilemma, Arras opts for a procedural solution, one that allows families or other trustworthy surrogates to make treatment decisions—including removing feeding tubes—for severely demented patients as they see fit, unless their decisions clearly violate the patient's best interests.

Opposed to Arras's "quality of life" approach is the statement from the U.S. Bishops' Pro-Life

Committee titled "Nutrition and Hydration: Moral and Pastoral Reflections." It enumerates some basic principles of the Catholic moral tradition that apply to decisions about medically assisted nutrition and hydration. In a careful and nuanced discussion, the bishops affirm their opposition to the deliberate taking of life, even permanently unconscious life, while at the same time they express support for the view that one is not obliged to prolong the life of a dying person by every possible means.

The *Conroy* case and the five case studies presented by Cantor raise the question of whether treatment decisions should be made on the basis of the interests the patient had when she was previously competent, or only on the basis of the interests she has now, as someone who is no longer competent. In other words, is it the "then-self" or the "now-self" that matters?

Rebecca S. Dresser and John A. Robertson opt for basing treatment decisions on the actual interests of the incompetent patient in "Quality of Life and Non-Treatment Decisions for Incompetent Patients: A Critique of the Orthodox Approach." They criticize "the orthodox judicial approach," as enunciated in *Quinlan*, as both conceptually flawed and dangerous. In the orthodox approach, incompetent patients have the same right to refuse treatment as do competent ones, a right that may be exercised on their behalf by surrogates, or proxies. The proxy is to determine what the incompetent patient would have chosen, either by relying on advance directives or by using substituted judgment. The orthodox approach ostensibly promotes patient self-determination, protects individuals from overtreatment, recognizes a central role for family discretion, and avoids troublesome quality-of-life determinations. However, Dresser and Robertson fault the orthodox approach on all these counts. The first issue, the autonomy of incompetent patients, cannot be respected because autonomy is literally a characteristic that belongs only to patients capable of making their own choices. Also, it is wrong to assume that the incompetent patient's prior preferences indicate the patient's current interests. Competent individuals have interests in work, family, friendships, and hobbies. They may feel that life without the possibility of pursuing these interests would be no longer worth living. However, severely demented individuals no longer have these interests. A life that may

seem demeaning to a competent individual may still be of value to the incompetent patient. Why should the values and preferences of the person, while competent, prevail over the interests of the incompetent person? This is unlike the situation of a person making an ordinary will, since the testator no longer has interests after he or she is dead. By contrast, the maker of a living will may be authorizing decisions that are contrary to his or her own best interests.

The orthodox approach is dangerous, according to Dresser and Robertson, because it is likely to lead to undertreatment. They discuss several cases, including *Spring* and *Hier,* in which courts authorized nontreatment for elderly incompetent patients based on substituted judgment. Use of this standard "opens the door to nontreatment of nursing home residents and other severely debilitated persons" based on what others think they would have wanted. Instead, Dresser and Robertson recommend that such decisions be based on the patients' actual interests. Such an approach requires a forthright consideration of quality of life. If the patient is permanently unconscious, then treatment is not warranted because, in their view, some capacity to interact with the environment must be present for life to be of value to an individual. Moreover, when the patient has no interest in continued existence, then the family's burdens and financial costs may be taken into account. Treatment might also be withheld from barely conscious patients on the grounds that their lives are not of value to them. Like Arras, Dresser and Robertson would allow families to request nontreatment for minimally conscious individuals, not because the patient would prefer nontreatment, but rather on the grounds that such life does not clearly confer a genuine benefit. However, people can differ dramatically on what kinds of life constitute a benefit. Wesley J. Smith would argue that letting minimally conscious or even permanently unconscious individuals die because others view their lives as having little worth violates the right to life. For those who maintain that continued existence is always in patients' best interests, a current interests approach that allows for the removal of life-prolonging treatment is no more likely to prevent undertreatment for nursing home residents and other severely debilitated persons than a substituted judgment approach.

Nancy K. Rhoden attempts to answer the question posed by Dresser and Robertson in "The Limits of Legal Objectivity": Why should the values and preferences of the once-competent person take precedence over the interests of the incompetent person? Her answer is that respect for persons requires us to adhere to the express and implicit wishes of individuals when they were competent. She says, "It is at least one, if not an overriding, component of treating persons with respect that we view them as they view themselves. If we are to do this, we must not ignore their prior choices and values." Applying this approach to the *Conroy* case, Rhoden suggests that the objective test strips the individual of his or her uniqueness and personality. She reminds us that Claire Conroy was not "just anyone; she was a specific human being—Aunt Claire." While we can, and should, make quality-of-life assessments from a present-oriented perspective for individuals who were never competent (infants and severely retarded people), something is wrong, Rhoden argues, when we treat formerly competent patients as if they were never competent. She acknowledges that paying attention to advance directives and prior values does give primacy to the competent person, but this is not inexplicable or unjustifiable: "[I]t is, after all, competent persons who have the considered moral values, life plans, and treatment preferences that underlie our respect."

Rhoden also argues that the objective test endangers all of our choices, because any of us could become suddenly incapacitated. In the objective current interests approach, a competent patient's "right" to refuse treatment will be upheld only for the time he remains competent. If he has a stroke that renders him incompetent, treatment decisions will be made on the basis of his present interests. Rhoden says, "Taken to an extreme, this could mean that a Jehovah's Witness could refuse a blood transfusion until he 'bled out,' after which he could be transfused."

CHOOSING FOR NEVER-COMPETENT PATIENTS

The tension between a subjective standard based on the patient's wishes and an objective best-interests standard is not relevant in the case of never-competent patients, such as infants or those with profound cognitive disabilities. It is not possible to consider what the patient would want, because without the ability to consider treatment options, or whether life "like that" is preferable to death, never-competent patients do not have preferences or wishes to consult. However, such cases raise their own difficulties, both substantive and procedural. How do we determine what is in the never-competent patient's best interests? Should decisions to terminate treatment be made by the parents, and if so, on what ground? Clearly, the claim that families are in a better position to know the wishes of once-competent patients is not relevant in the case of never-competent persons.

"Termination of Life-Support for a Never-Competent Patient: The Case of Sheila Pouliot," presented by law professor Alicia R. Ouellette, illustrates how wrong laws intended to protect individuals with disabilities can go. Despite the agreement of Pouliot's entire family and all of her doctors, New York's law would not allow the removal of nutrition and hydration from a patient without clear and convincing evidence that this is what the patient would have wanted—something that is clearly impossible to prove in the case of someone who has never had the mental ability to consider the issue. After Pouliot died in 2000, New York passed a very narrow law permitting the termination of life-sustaining treatment by a surrogate for individuals with mental retardation. However, the law does not apply to formerly competent individuals where there is not clear and convincing evidence of their wishes, nor does it apply to infants or young children.

The Texas case *Miller* v. *HCA* raises the question of the right of parents to withhold life-sustaining treatment from an extremely premature newborn. After the infamous Baby Doe case in 1981, and the subsequent passage of the federal Child Abuse Amendments (CAA) of 1984, the question of treating infants with genetic and chromosomal abnormalities has been largely settled. Not only have there been significant improvements in medical care, but in addition disability advocates have helped increase public awareness that individuals with disabilities, even serious ones, have the potential to lead happy and fulfilling lives. Therefore, the practice—once fairly common—of withholding life-sustaining treatment from babies with Down syndrome or spina bifida has generally ceased. The cases of very premature and low-birth-weight infants are often more difficult precisely because of the uncertainty of prognosis. With intensive care and aggressive medical treatment, a very premature baby may survive and go on to become a healthy child and adult. But there is also the risk of mortality (50 percent or higher with babies younger than 25 weeks' gestation or weighing less than 750 grams) and the even greater chance of significant disability.

Two questions arise in cases of infants on the threshold of viability: Who should make medical decisions for them, their parents or their doctors? And on what basis should the decisions be made? In "Extreme Prematurity and Parental Rights After Baby Doe," John A. Robertson supports the decision of the Texas Supreme Court on the ground that the withholding of life-sustaining treatment on the basis of expected disability can be seen as discriminatory. He acknowledges the importance of parental autonomy, but insists that "it is not so robust that parents have the right to deny a disabled child the medical resources necessary for life regardless of the child's interests in living or ability to interact with others." John J. Paris, Michael D. Schreiber, and Alun C. Elias-Jones, on the other hand, regard the court's decision as a regrettable departure from present standards of good neonatal practice. In "Resuscitation of the Preterm Infant against Parental Wishes" they agree that the appropriate standard is the best interest of the child, but they deny that this necessarily implies lifesaving measures in all cases. Mechanical ventilation that causes the infant to suffer and merely prolongs life for weeks or months "might be judged an even greater tragedy than death." They argue that the determination of whether the risks and benefits warrant the use of aggressive technology is not a medical assessment, and therefore there is no reason to substitute the physician's values for those of the parents when the parties disagree. Moreover, since it is the parents who, along with the infant, will bear the burden of a decision to resuscitate, the decision properly belongs to them.

PHYSICIAN-ASSISTED DEATH

Whether life is always worthwhile, or whether there are times when death is preferable to life, is an issue that has become more pressing in recent years. One reason for the growing importance of this issue is the ability of modern medicine to keep people alive who would have died in earlier medical eras. The elongation of dying through modern medical technology has raised the issue of euthanasia even more persistently than in the past. "Euthanasia" (literally, a "beautiful death") means an easy or painless death, but has come to stand for deliberately bringing about such a death through action or inaction. On the one hand, euthanasia would appear to be antithetical to all that medical practice stands for (indeed, the Hippocratic oath specifically enjoins inducing death, even if the patient requests it). On the other hand, if the purpose of medicine is not simply to prevent death but to alleviate suffering, then perhaps euthanasia is not entirely foreign to good, ethical medical practice. Indeed, it has been practiced openly by physicians for a number of years in the Netherlands, with the acceptance of the country's highest court and a broad majority of physicians and the populace. In 2001, euthanasia became fully legal in the Netherlands, provided specific guidelines are met.

Another reason for the recent attention to euthanasia, suicide, and physician-assisted suicide (PAS) is the AIDS epidemic. Many people with AIDS want the solace of knowing that they will be able to end their lives before either the pain becomes unbearable or they become demented. However, suicide is not always easily accomplished. According to a New York doctor with a large AIDS practice, "the reality is that most people with AIDS have very strong cardiovascular systems. Taking overdoses of most common prescription pills is not going to kill you" (*New York Times* 1994). Also, people can develop a tolerance for morphine. A botched suicide attempt may leave a person alive, but without any brain function. When doctors are involved, things are less likely to go wrong. For this reason, many doctors say they favor changing laws that currently prohibit them from legally assisting in suicides of people with terminal illnesses; other doctors, however, still say they have qualms about assisted suicide, even in the case of AIDS.

There are two distinctions of fundamental importance to the moral assessment of euthanasia. The first is between active euthanasia (deliberately *bringing about death* through some action, such as administering a lethal injection) and passive euthanasia (deliberately *allowing death to occur* through some form of inaction, such as refraining from performing corrective surgery). Often this distinction has been characterized as the difference between "killing" and "letting die." A second distinction is made between voluntary euthanasia (actively requested by the patient) and nonvoluntary euthanasia, in which the patient (for example, a PVS patient) lacks the capacity to consent. Writers on the topic disagree as to whether all forms of euthanasia are permissible, or only some forms. Most people would agree that the voluntary/nonvoluntary distinction is at least relevant to, if not decisive in determining, the permissibility of euthanasia; some still maintain, however, that the distinction between active and passive euthanasia—if it can be coherently drawn at all—has no moral relevance (Steinbock and Norcross 1994).

Legally, nevertheless, there is an important difference between actively causing someone's death and allowing him or her—even deliberately—to die. Liability for allowing to die depends on the relation between the "victim" and the one who allows him or her to die. A doctor who stops treatment at the request of a patient is unlikely to be liable for the patient's death, as long as the doctor acts within the bounds of accepted medical practice. Indeed, a doctor who continues treating a competent patient who has refused treatment is theoretically liable for battery (although few, if any, doctors have ever been successfully sued for treating without consent). Killing a patient, even at his or her request, is quite another matter. Assisting a suicide is a crime in most jurisdictions. In recent years, California and Washington have attempted initiatives to legalize doctor-assisted suicide; neither state succeeded. In 1994, Oregon became the only state to legalize PAS. Under the state's Death with Dignity Act, a terminally ill patient may be given a prescription for lethal drugs if two doctors agree the person has less than six months to live and is mentally competent to make the decision to end his or her life. Opponents sought to repeal the act, but this attempt was rejected by the voters, with a greater margin than had passed the original act, in November 1997. In the first four years of legalization, about 90 people have died after ingesting medications received under the act. Many more have obtained lethal prescriptions but have died of natural causes before taking the drugs.

One of the few jurisdictions where there was no law, until recently, against assisting a suicide was Michigan. For this reason, the controversial Dr. Jack Kevorkian chose Michigan as the place to perform several "medicides," as he calls them, using the "suicide machine" he invented for the purpose. Michigan quickly moved to pass a statute making assisted suicide a crime so that Dr. Kevorkian could be charged the next time he helped someone die. However, on May 2, 1994, a Detroit jury acquitted Dr. Kevorkian of charges that he had violated Michigan's law barring assisted suicide. Comments from jurors made it clear that the jury regarded Dr. Kevorkian as justified in helping terminally ill patients die. However, he was convicted of second-degree murder in 1999 and served eight years of a 10- to 25-year sentence before being released on June 1, 2007.

Dr. Timothy E. Quill, the first author in Section 6 ("Death and Dignity: A Case of Individualized Decision Making"), prescribed barbiturates for his long-time patient Diane, who requested them to kill herself in order to avoid a lingering, painful (or drugged) death from leukemia. Many commentators have contrasted Dr. Quill with Dr. Kevorkian. Dr. Kevorkian is a retired pathologist; Dr. Quill a practicing internist. Dr. Kevorkian has helped about 100 people die; Dr. Quill only 1. Dr. Kevorkian does not know the individuals he helps die, neither the details of their medical conditions nor their psychological states. Dr. Quill knew Diane very well, and met regularly with her over several months after she requested the barbiturates. Clearly, Dr. Quill is a conscientious, compassionate physician who had the deepest concern for his patient's well-being and the deepest respect for her choices. Having said that, did Dr. Quill do the right thing? And should such behavior be sanctioned by law?

During 1996, two federal appeals courts held that state laws criminalizing assisted suicide violated the Fourteenth Amendment to the United States Constitution. In June 1997, the Supreme Court reversed the decisions in both *Washington* v. *Glucksberg* and *Vacco* v. *Quill*, holding that there is no constitutional right to physician-assisted suicide. This has settled (for the time being) the constitutional question. However, the moral and legal debate over whether one has a right to die is far from over. The Court decision, most legal commentators said, simply returns the question to the states. However, the ability of states to make their own decisions regarding PAS has been challenged. On November 6, 2001, Attorney General John Ashcroft, declaring that assisted suicide is *not* a "legitimate medical purpose" for prescribing or dispensing medication, authorized federal drug agents to revoke the license of any doctor who prescribes lethal drugs, even one acting within all terms of the Oregon law. Ashcroft's action illustrates a tension between the constitutional doctrine of federal supremacy and the principle of states' rights. Although conservatives generally support the rights of states to make their own decisions on most policy matters, social and religious conservatives have long sought to undermine or even abolish the Oregon law, holding that any official sanction of suicide is immoral. Oregon officials said they would go to court to try to block the order, and "even those who said they were personally opposed to physician-assisted suicide, generally responded with outrage to an action in the nation's capital that so clearly undercut the expressed will of the states' voters" (Verhovek 2001). A temporary restraining order, blocking Ashcroft's move, was granted by a federal judge in November 2001, enabling doctors to continue prescribing lethal medication under the terms of the law. On April 17, 2002, federal district court judge Robert R. Jones confirmed the temporary restraining order. In a decision sharply critical of Ashcroft, Judge Jones called his directive an attempt by opponents of Oregon's law "to get through the administrative door what they could not get through the Congressional door" and said that there is no indication in any federal statute, including the drug law, "that Congress delegated to federal prosecutors the authority to define what constitutes legitimate *medical* practices" (Liptak 2002).

The case in favor of assisted suicide is made by six well-known moral philosophers in "The Philosophers' Brief," the third article in Section 6. The basis of their position is the general moral principle that every competent person has the right to make momentous personal decisions about life's value, including decisions about when life ceases to be worth living. At the same time, the authors acknowledge that people may make such momentous decisions impulsively or out of depression, and that the state has the right to adopt safeguards to ensure that a patient's decision for suicide is informed, competent, and free. The philosophers address the risk that legalizing PAS might jeopardize vulnerable patients, and they conclude that such patients might be better, rather than less, well

protected if assisted suicide were legalized with appropriate safeguards.

In "Physician-Assisted Suicide: A Tragic View," John D. Arras lays out the pros and cons of legalizing PAS. Although Arras is "deeply sympathetic to the central values motivating the push for PAS and euthanasia," he ultimately concludes that the social risks of legalization outweigh the benefits. While there may be individual cases in which assisted suicide is the best choice, it does not follow that legalizing PAS is the wisest social policy. A better approach would be to improve radically the palliative care terminally ill patients receive. "At the end of this long and arduous process," Arras writes, "when we finally have an equitable, effective, and compassionate health care system in place . . . , then we might well want to reopen the discussion of PAS and active euthanasia."

Margaret P. Battin has updated her article "Euthansia: The Way We Do It, The Way They Do It," providing a cross-cultural comparison of assistance in dying in the Netherlands, Germany, and the United States, as well as in countries whose policies are to some extent patterned after them: Belgium, Switzerland, Australia, Canada, and the United Kingdom. In the Netherlands, voluntary active euthanasia, while until recently prohibited by statute, has nevertheless been legally tolerated, provided the physician meets a rigorous set of guidelines. Euthanasia and assisted suicide are infrequently chosen, but are a "conspicuous option in terminal illness."

The painful history of Nazism in Germany, and the killing of mentally and physically disabled patients (which led eventually to the Holocaust), has resulted in Germany's rejection of physician participation in causing death. "Euthanasia is viewed as always wrong, and the Germans view the Dutch as stepping out on a dangerously slippery slope," writes Battin. At the same time, assisted suicide is not a violation of the law, and the German Society for Humane Dying publishes a booklet listing drugs available by prescription, together with the specific dosages necessary for producing a certain, painless death. However, the removal of physicians from participating in assisted suicide means that decisions for suicide are not necessarily medically evaluated, either to confirm the patient's diagnosis or prognosis, or to rule out treatable depression as the motivating factor.

The United States differs from both the Netherlands and Germany in significant ways. Unlike all the countries discussed here—not only the Netherlands and Germany, but also Belgium, Switzerland, Canada, Australia, and the United Kingdom—we have no national health insurance, and cost increasingly plays a role in health care decisions. Battin, who generally supports physician aid-in-dying for the reasons given in "The Philosophers' Brief," briefly examines the ways in which some safeguards function in different societies and concludes that PAS is a better alternative in the United States than euthanasia, given our cultural context, because PAS grants physicians a measure of control while it leaves the fundamental decision up to the patients themselves.

Nearly fifty years ago, in an influential article criticizing proposed "mercy-killing" legislation, Yale Kamisar warned against giving the choice of euthanasia to gravely ill patients, saying:

> Will we not sweep up, in the process, some who are not really tired of life, but think others are tired of them; some who do not really want to die, but who feel they should not live on, because to do so when there looms the legal alternative of euthanasia is to do a selfish or a cowardly act? Will not some feel an obligation to have themselves "eliminated" in order that funds allocated for their terminal care might be better used by their families or, financial worries aside, in order to relieve their families of the emotional strain involved? (Kamisar 1958)

Most defenders of PAS try to argue that, with proper safeguards, Kamisar's fears will not materialize. By contrast, in what may be the most provocative article in this collection ("Is There a Duty to Die?"), John Hardwig suggests that there can be a moral obligation (not merely a right) to choose death. The basis of this obligation is the burden imposed on family members who care for sick and dying patients. It might seem that Hardwig is using a consequentialist analysis to derive a duty to die. In fact, his reasoning owes at least as much to Kantian ethics as to utilitarianism, for he says, "To think that my loved ones must bear whatever burdens my illness, debility, or dying process might impose upon them is to reduce them to means to my well-being. And that would be immoral." We leave it to the reader to decide whether Hardwig's claim of a duty to die is a moral advance, or, as Felicia Nimue Ackerman argues in "'For Now I Have My Death': The 'Duty to Die' versus the Duty to Help the Ill Stay Alive," a reflection of "our society's bias against and systematic devaluation of the old and ill."

REFERENCES

1. Kamisar, Yale. 1958. Some non-religious views against proposed "mercy-killing" legislation. *Minnesota Law Review* 42:969–1042.
2. Liptak, Adam. 2002. Judge blocks U.S. bid to ban suicide law. *New York Times*, April 18:A16.
3. *New York Times*. 1994. AIDS patients seek solace in suicide but many find pain and uncertainty. June 14:C6.
4. Not Dead Yet. 2005, March 20. Schiavo case is about disability rights [press statement]. Not Dead Yet Web site, http://www.notdeadyet.org/docs/schiavostatement032005.html.
5. Pernick, Martin S. 1999. Brain death in a cultural context: The reconstruction of death, 1967–1981. In *The definition of death: Contemporary controversies*, eds. Stuart J. Youngner, Robert M. Arnold, and Renie Schapiro. Baltimore: Johns Hopkins University Press.
6. Steinbock, Bonnie, and Alastair Norcross, eds. 1994. *Killing and letting die*. 2nd ed. New York: Fordham University Press.
7. Verhovek, Sam Howe. 2001. Federal agents are directed to stop physicians who assist suicides. *New York Times*, November 7:A20.

THE DEFINITION OF DEATH

DEFINING DEATH

President's Commission for the Study of Ethical Problems in Medicine and Biomedical and Behavioral Research

WHY UPDATE DEATH?

For most of the past several centuries, the medical determination of death was very close to the popular one. If a person fell unconscious or was found so, someone (often but not always a physician) would feel for the pulse, listen for breathing, hold a mirror before the nose to test for condensation, and look to see if the pupils were fixed. Although these criteria have been used to determine death since antiquity, they have not always been universally accepted.

From the President's Commission for the Study of Ethical Problems in Medicine and Biomedical and Behavioral Research, *Defining Death: A Report on the Medical, Legal and Ethical Issues in the Determination of Death*, Washington, DC: U.S. Government Printing Office, 1981:12–20, 31–43.

Editors' note: Some text and the notes have been cut. Students who want to read the article in its entirety should consult the original.

Developing Confidence in the Heart-Lung Criteria

In the eighteenth century, macabre tales of "corpses" reviving during funerals and exhumed skeletons found to have clawed at coffin lids led to widespread fear of premature burial. Coffins were developed with elaborate escape mechanisms and speaking tubes to the world above . . . , mortuaries employed guards to monitor the newly dead for signs of life, and legislatures passed laws requiring a delay before burial.

The medical press also paid a great deal of attention to the matter. In *The Uncertainty of the Signs of Death and the Danger of Precipitate Interments* in 1740, Jean-Jacques Winslow advanced the thesis that putrefaction was the only sure sign of death. In the years following, many physicians published articles agreeing with him. This position had, however, notable logistic and public health disadvantages. It also disparaged, sometimes with unfair vigor, the skills of physicians as diagnosticians of death.

In reply, the French surgeon Louis published in 1752 his influential *Letters on the Certainty of the Signs of Death*. The debate dissipated in the nineteenth century because of the gradual improvement in the competence of physicians and a concomitant increase in the public's confidence in them.

Physicians actively sought to develop this competence. They even held contests encouraging the search for a cluster of signs—rather than a single infallible sign—for the diagnosis of death. One sign did, however, achieve prominence. The invention of the stethoscope in the mid–nineteenth century enabled physicians to detect heartbeat with heightened sensitivity. The use of this instrument by a well-trained physician, together with other clinical measures, laid to rest public fears of premature burial. The twentieth century brought even more sophisticated technological means to determine death, particularly the electrocardiograph (EKG), which is more sensitive than the stethoscope in detecting cardiac functioning.

The Interrelationships of Brain, Heart, and Lung Functions

The brain has three general anatomic divisions: the cerebrum, with its outer shell called the cortex; the cerebellum; and the brainstem, composed of the midbrain, the pons, and the medulla oblongata. . . . Traditionally, the cerebrum has been referred to as the "higher brain" because it has primary control of consciousness, thought, memory, and feeling. The brainstem has been called the "lower brain," since it controls spontaneous, vegetative functions such as swallowing, yawning, and sleep-wake cycles. It is important to note that these generalizations are not entirely accurate. Neuroscientists generally agree that such "higher brain" functions as cognition or consciousness probably are not mediated strictly by the cerebral cortex; rather, they probably result from complex interrelations between brainstem and cortex.

Respiration is controlled in the brainstem, particularly the medulla. . . . Neural impulses originating in the respiratory centers of the medulla stimulate the diaphragm and intercostal muscles, which cause the lungs to fill with air. Ordinarily, these respiratory centers adjust the rate of breathing to maintain the correct levels of carbon dioxide and oxygen. In certain circumstances, such as heavy exercise, sighing, coughing, or sneezing, other areas of the brain modulate the activities of the respiratory centers or even briefly take direct control of respiration.

Destruction of the brain's respiratory center stops respiration, which in turn deprives the heart of needed oxygen, causing it too to cease functioning. The traditional signs of life—respiration and heartbeat—disappear: the person is dead. The "vital signs" traditionally used in diagnosing death thus reflect the direct interdependence of respiration, circulation, and the brain.

The artificial respirator and concomitant life-support systems have changed this simple picture. Normally, respiration ceases when the functions of the diaphragm and intercostal muscles are impaired. This results from direct injury to the muscles or (more commonly) because the neural impulses between the brain and these muscles are interrupted. However, an artificial respirator (also called a ventilator) can be used to compensate for the inability of the thoracic muscles to fill the lungs with air. Some of these machines use negative pressure to expand the chest wall (in which case they are called "iron lungs"); others use positive pressure to push air into the lungs. The respirators are equipped with devices to regulate the rate and depth of "breathing," which are normally controlled by the respiratory centers in the medulla. The machines cannot compensate entirely for the defective neural connections since they cannot regulate blood gas levels precisely. But, provided that the lungs themselves have not been extensively damaged, gas exchange can continue and appropriate levels of oxygen and carbon dioxide can be maintained in the circulating blood.

Unlike the respiratory system, which depends on the neural impulses from the brain, the heart can pump blood without external control. Impulses from brain centers modulate the inherent rate and force of the heartbeat but are not required for the heart to contract at a level of function that is ordinarily adequate. Thus, when artificial respiration provides adequate oxygenation and associated medical treatments regulate essential plasma components and blood pressure, an intact heart will continue to beat, despite loss of brain functions.

At present, however, no machine can take over the functions of the heart except for a very limited time and in limited circumstances (e.g., a heart-lung machine used during surgery). Therefore, when a severe injury to the heart or major blood vessels prevents the circulation of the crucial blood supply to the brain, the loss of brain functioning is inevitable because no oxygen reaches the brain.

Loss of Various Brain Functions

The most frequent causes of irreversible loss of functions of the whole brain are (1) direct trauma to the head, such as from a motor vehicle accident or a gunshot wound, (2) massive spontaneous hemorrhage into the brain as a result of ruptured aneurysm or complications of high blood pressure, and (3) anoxic damage from cardiac or respiratory arrest or severely reduced blood pressure.

Many of these severe injuries to the brain cause an accumulation of fluid and swelling in the brain tissue, a condition called cerebral edema. In severe cases of edema, the pressure within the closed cavity increases until it exceeds the systolic blood pressure, resulting in a total loss of blood flow to both the upper and lower portions of the brain. If deprived of blood flow for at least 10 to 15 minutes, the brain, including the brainstem, will completely cease functioning. Other pathophysiologic mechanisms also result in a progressive and, ultimately, complete cessation of intracranial circulation.

Once deprived of adequate supplies of oxygen and glucose, brain neurons will irreversibly lose all activity and ability to function. In adults, oxygen and/or glucose deprivation for more than a few minutes causes some neuron loss. Thus, even in the absence of direct trauma and edema, brain functions can be lost if circulation to the brain is impaired. If blood flow is cut off, brain tissues completely self-digest (autolyze) over the ensuing days.

When the brain lacks all functions, consciousness is, of course, lost. While some spinal reflexes often persist in such bodies (since circulation to the spine is separate from that of the brain), all reflexes controlled by the brainstem as well as cognitive, affective, and integrating functions are absent. Respiration and circulation in these bodies may be generated by a ventilator together with intensive medical management. In adults who have experienced irreversible cessation of the functions of the entire brain, this mechanically generated functioning can continue only a limited time because the heart usually stops beating within two to ten days. (An infant or small child who has lost all brain functions will typically suffer cardiac arrest within several weeks, although respiration and heartbeat can sometimes be maintained even longer.)

Less severe injury to the brain can cause mild to profound damage to the cortex, lower cerebral structures, cerebellum, brainstem, or some combination thereof. The cerebrum, especially the cerebral cortex, is more easily injured by loss of blood flow or oxygen than is the brainstem. A 4 to 6 minute loss of blood flow—caused by, for example, cardiac arrest—typically damages the cerebral cortex permanently, while the relatively more resistant brainstem may continue to function.

When brainstem functions remain, but the major components of the cerebrum are irreversibly destroyed, the patient is in what is usually called a "persistent vegetative state" or "persistent noncognitive state." Such persons may exhibit spontaneous, involuntary movements such as yawns or facial grimaces, their eyes may be open, and they may be capable of breathing without assistance. Without higher brain functions, however, any apparent wakefulness does not represent awareness of self or environment (thus, the condition is often described as "awake but unaware"). The case of Karen Ann Quinlan has made this condition familiar to the general public. With necessary medical and nursing care—including feeding through intravenous or nasogastric tubes, and antibiotics for recurrent pulmonary infections—such patients can survive months or years, often without a respirator. (The longest survival exceeded 37 years.)

Conclusion: The Need for Reliable Policy

Medical interventions can often provide great benefit in avoiding irreversible harm to a patient's injured heart, lungs, or brain by carrying a patient through a period of acute need. These techniques have, however, thrown new light on the interrelationship of these crucial organ systems. This has created complex issues for public policy as well.

For medical and legal purposes, partial brain impairment must be distinguished from complete and irreversible loss of brain functions or "whole brain death." The President's Commission regards the cessation of the vital functions of the entire brain—and not merely portions thereof, such as those responsible for cognitive functions—as the only proper neurologic basis for declaring death. This conclusion accords with the overwhelming consensus of medical and legal experts and the public.

Present attention to the "definition" of death is part of a process of development in social attitudes and legal rules stimulated by the unfolding of biomedical knowledge. In the nineteenth century increasing knowledge and practical skill made the public confident that death could be diagnosed reliably using cardiopulmonary criteria. The question now is whether, when medical intervention may be responsible for a patient's respiration and circulation, there are other equally reliable ways to diagnose death.

The Commission recognizes that it is often difficult to determine the severity of a patient's injuries, especially in the first few days of intensive care following a cardiac arrest, head trauma, or other similar event. Responsible public policy in this area requires that physicians be able to distinguish reliably those patients who have died from those whose injuries are less severe or are reversible. . . .

Understanding the "Meaning" of Death

It now seems clear that a medical consensus about clinical practices and their scientific basis has emerged: certain states of brain activity and inactivity, together with their neurophysiological consequences, can be reliably detected and used to diagnose death. To the medical community, a sound basis exists for declaring death even in the presence of mechanically assisted "vital signs." Yet before recommending that public policy reflect this medical consensus, the Commission wished to know whether the scientific viewpoint was consistent with the concepts of "being dead" or "death" as they are commonly understood in our society. These questions have been addressed by philosophers and theologians, who have provided several formulations.

The Commission believes that its policy conclusions . . . including the [Uniform Determination of Death Act] must accurately reflect the social meaning of death and not constitute a mere legal fiction. The Commission has not found it necessary to resolve all of the differences among the leading concepts of death because these views all yield interpretations consistent with the recommended statute.

Three major formulations of the meaning of death were presented to the Commission: one focused upon the functions of the whole brain, one upon the functions of the cerebral hemispheres, and one upon non-brain functions. Each of these formulations (and its variants) is presented and evaluated.

The "Whole Brain" Formulations

One characteristic of living things which is absent in the dead is the body's capacity to organize and regulate itself. In animals, the neural apparatus is the dominant locus of these functions. In higher animals and man, regulation of both maintenance of the internal environment (homeostasis) and interaction with the external environment occurs primarily within the cranium.

External threats, such as heat or infection, or internal ones, such as liver failure or endogenous lung disease, can stress the body enough to overwhelm its ability to maintain organization and regulation. If the stress passes a certain level, the organism as a whole is defeated and death occurs.

This process and its denouement are understood in two major ways. Although they are sometimes stated as alternative formulations of a "whole brain definition" of death, they are actually mirror images of each other. The Commission has found them to be complementary; together they enrich one's understanding of the "definition." The first focuses on the integrated functioning of the body's major organ systems, while recognizing the centrality of the whole brain, since it is neither revivable nor replaceable. The other identifies the functioning of the whole brain as the hallmark of life because the brain is the regulator of the body's integration. The two conceptions are subject to similar criticisms and have similar implications for policy.

The Concepts   The functioning of many organs—such as the liver, kidneys, and skin—and their integration is "vital" to individual health in the sense that if any one ceases and that function is not restored or artificially replaced, the organism as a whole cannot long survive. All elements in the system are mutually interdependent, so that the loss of any part leads to the breakdown of the whole, and eventually, to the cessation of functions in every part.

Three organs—the heart, lungs, and brain—assume special significance, however, because their interrelationship is very close and the irreversible cessation of any one very quickly stops the other two and consequently halts the integrated functioning of the organism as a whole. Because they were easily measured, circulation and respiration were traditionally the basic "vital signs." But breathing and heartbeat are not life itself. They are simply used as signs—as one window for viewing a deeper and more complex reality: a triangle of interrelated systems with the brain at its apex. As the biomedical scientists who appeared before the Commission made clear, the traditional means of diagnosing death actually detected an irreversible cessation of integrated functioning among the interdependent bodily systems. When artificial means of support mask this loss of integration as measured by the old methods, brain-oriented criteria and tests provide a new window on the same phenomenon.

On this view, death is that moment at which the body's physiological system ceases to constitute an integrated whole. Even if life continues in individual cells or organs, life of the organism as a whole requires complex integration, and without the latter, a person cannot properly be regarded as alive.

This distinction between systemic, integrated functioning and physiological activity in cells or individual organs is important for two reasons. First, a person is considered dead under this concept even if oxygenation and metabolism persist in some cells or organs. There would be no need to wait until all metabolism had ceased in every body part before recognizing that death has occurred.

More importantly, this concept would reduce the significance of continued respiration and heartbeat for the definition of death. This view holds that continued breathing and circulation are not in themselves tantamount to life. Since life is a matter of integrating the functioning of major organ systems, breathing and circulation are necessary but not sufficient to establish that an individual is alive. When an individual's breathing and circulation lack neurologic integration, he or she is dead.

The alternative "whole brain" explanation of death differs from the one just described primarily in the vigor of its insistence that the traditional "vital signs" of heartbeat and respiration were merely surrogate signs with no significance in themselves. On this view, the heart and lungs are not important as basic prerequisites to continued life but rather because the irreversible cessation of their functions shows that the brain had ceased functioning. Other signs customarily employed by physicians in diagnosing death, such as unresponsiveness and absence of pupillary light response, are also indicative of loss of the functions of the whole brain.

This view gives the brain primacy not merely as the sponsor of consciousness (since even unconscious persons may be alive), but also as the complex organizer and regulator of bodily functions. (Indeed, the "regulatory" role of the brain in the organism can be understood in terms of thermodynamics and information theory.) Only the brain can direct the entire organism. Artificial support for the heart and lungs, which is required only when the brain can no longer control them, cannot maintain the usual synchronized integration of the body. Now that other traditional indicators of cessation of brain functions (i.e., absence of breathing) can be obscured by medical interventions, one needs, according to this view, some new standards for determining death—that is, more reliable tests for the complete cessation of brain functions.

Critique Both of these "whole brain" formulations—the "integrated functions" and the "primary organ" views—are subject to several criticisms. Since both of these conceptions of death give an important place to the integrating or regulating capacity of the whole brain, it can be asked whether that characteristic is as distinctive as they would suggest. Other organ systems are also required for life to continue—for example, the skin to conserve fluid, the liver to detoxify the blood.

The view that the brain's functions are more central to "life" than those of the skin, the liver, and so on, is admittedly arbitrary in the sense of representing a choice. The view is not, however, arbitrary in the sense of lacking reasons. As discussed previously, the centrality accorded the brain reflects both its overarching role as "regulator" or "integrator" of other bodily systems and the immediate and devastating consequences of its loss for the organism as a whole. Furthermore, the Commission believes that this choice overwhelmingly reflects the views of experts and the lay public alike.

A more significant criticism shares the view that life consists of the coordinated functioning of the various bodily systems, in which process the whole brain plays a crucial role. At the same time, it notes that in some adult patients lacking all brain functions it is possible through intensive support to achieve constant temperature, metabolism, waste disposal, blood pressure, and other conditions typical of living organisms and not found in dead ones. Even with extraordinary medical care, these functions cannot be sustained indefinitely—typically, no longer than several days—but it is argued that this shows only that patients with nonfunctional brains are dying, not that they are dead. In this view, the respirator, drugs, and other resources of the modern intensive-care unit collectively substitute for the lower brain, just as a pump used in cardiac surgery takes over the heart's function.

The criticism rests, however, on a premise about the role of artificial support vis-à-vis the brainstem which the Commission believes is mistaken or at best incomplete. While the respirator and its associated medical techniques do substitute for the functions of the intercostal muscles and the diaphragm, which without neuronal stimulation from the brain cannot function spontaneously, they cannot replace the myriad functions of the brainstem or of the rest of the brain. The startling contrast between bodies lacking *all* brain functions and patients with intact brainstems (despite severe neocortical damage) manifests this. The former lie with fixed pupils, motionless except for the chest movements produced by their respirators. The latter cannot only breathe, metabolize, maintain temperature and blood pressure, and so forth, *on their own* but also sigh, yawn, track light with their eyes, and react to pain or reflex stimulation.

It is not easy to discern precisely what it is about patients in this latter group that makes them alive while those in the other category are not. It is in part that in the case of the first category (*i.e.*, absence of all brain functions) when the mask created by the artificial medical support is stripped away what remains is not an integrated organism but "merely a group of artificially maintained subsystems." Sometimes, of course, an artificial substitute can forge the link that restores the organism as a whole to unified functioning. Heart or kidney transplants, kidney dialysis, or an iron lung used to replace physically impaired breathing ability in a polio victim, for example, restore the integrated functioning of the organism as they replace the failed function of a part. Contrast such situations, however, with the hypothetical of a decapitated body treated so as to prevent the outpouring of blood and to generate respiration: continuation of bodily functions in that case would not have restored the requisites of human life.

The living differ from the dead in many ways. The dead do not think, interact, autoregulate, or maintain organic identity through time, for example. Not all the living can always do *all* of these activities, however; nor is there one single characteristic (*e.g.*, breathing, yawning, etc.) the loss of which signifies death. Rather, what is missing in the dead is a cluster of attributes, all of which form part of an organism's responsiveness to its internal and external environment.

While it is valuable to test public policies against basic conceptions of death, philosophical refinement beyond a certain point may not be necessary. The task undertaken in this Report is to provide and defend a statutory standard for determining that a human being has died. In setting forth the standards recommended in this Report, the Commission has used "whole brain" terms to clarify the understanding of death that enjoys near-universal acceptance in our society. The Commission finds that the "whole brain" formulations give resonance and depth to the biomedical and epidemiological data presented in [a part of the study not reproduced here]. Further effort to search for a conceptual "definition" of death is not required for the purpose of public policy because, separately or together, the "whole brain" formulations provide a theory that is sufficiently precise, concise, and widely acceptable.

Policy Consequences   Those holding to the "whole brain" view—and this view seems at least implicit in most of the testimony and writing reviewed by the Commission—believe that when respirators are in use, respiration and circulation lose significance for the diagnosis of death. In a body without a functioning brain, these two functions, it is argued, become mere artifacts of the mechanical life supports.

The lungs breathe and the heart circulates blood only because the respirator (and attendant medical interventions) cause them to do so, not because of any comprehensive integrated functioning. This is "breathing" and "circulation" only in an analogous sense: the function and its results are similar, but the source, cause, and purpose are different between those individuals with and those without functioning brains.

For patients who are not artificially maintained, breathing and heartbeat were, and are, reliable signs either of systemic integration and/or of continued brain functioning (depending on which approach one takes to the "whole brain" concept). To regard breathing and respiration as having diagnostic significance when the brain of a respirator-supported patient has ceased functioning, however, is to forget the basic reasoning behind their use in individuals who are not artificially maintained.

Although similar in most respects, the two approaches to "whole brain death" could have slightly different policy consequences. The "primary organ" view would be satisfied with a statute that contained only a single standard—the irreversible cessation of all functions of the entire brain. Nevertheless, as a practical matter, the view is also compatible with a statute establishing irreversible cessation of respiration and circulation as an alternative standard, since it is inherent in this view that the loss of spontaneous breathing and heartbeat are surrogates for the loss of brain functions.

The "integrated functions" view would lead one to a "definition" of death recognizing that collapse of the organism as a whole can be diagnosed through the loss of brain functions as well as through loss of cardiopulmonary functions. The latter functions would remain an explicit part of the policy statement because their irreversible loss will continue to provide an independent and wholly reliable basis for determining that death has occurred when respirators and related means of support are *not* employed.

The two "whole brain" formulations thus differ only modestly. And even conceptual disagreements have a context; the context of the present one is the need to clarify and update the "definition" of death in order to allow principled decisions to be made about the status of comatose respirator-supported patients. The explicit recognition of both standards—cardiopulmonary and whole brain—solves that problem fully. In addition, since it requires only a modest reformulation of the generally accepted view, it accounts for the importance traditionally accorded to heartbeat and respiration, the "vital signs" which will continue to be the grounds for determining death in the overwhelming majority of cases for the foreseeable future. Hence the Commission, drawing on the aspects that the two formulations share and on the ways in which they each add to an understanding of the "meaning" of death, concludes that public policy should recognize both cardiopulmonary and brain-based standards for declaring death.

The "Higher Brain" Formulations

When all brain processes cease, the patient loses two important sets of functions. One set encompasses the integrating and coordinating functions, carried out principally but not exclusively by the cerebellum and brainstem. The other set includes the psychological functions which make consciousness, thought, and feeling possible. These latter functions are located primarily but not exclusively in the cerebrum, especially the neocortex. The two "higher brain" formulations of brain-oriented definitions of death discussed here are premised on the fact that loss of cerebral functions strips the patient of his psychological capacities and properties.

A patient whose brain has permanently stopped functioning will, by definition, have lost those brain functions which sponsor consciousness, feeling, and thought. Thus the higher brain rationales support classifying as dead bodies which meet "whole brain" standards, as discussed in the preceding section. The converse is not true, however. If there are parts of the brain which have no role in sponsoring consciousness, the higher brain formulation would regard their continued functioning as compatible with death.

The Concepts Philosophers and theologians have attempted to describe the attributes a living being must have to be a person. "Personhood" consists of the complex of activities (or of capacities to engage in them) such as thinking, reasoning, feeling, and human intercourse which make the human different from, or superior to, animals or things.

One higher brain formulation would define death as the loss of what is essential to a person. Those advocating the personhood definition often relate these characteristics to brain functioning. Without brain activity, people are incapable of these essential activities. A breathing body, the argument goes, is not in itself a person; and, without functioning brains, patients are merely breathing bodies. Hence personhood ends when the brain suffers irreversible loss of function.

For other philosophers, a certain concept of "personal identity" supports a brain-oriented definition of death. According to this argument, a patient literally ceases to exist as an individual when his or her brain ceases functioning, even if the patient's body is biologically alive. Actual decapitation creates a similar situation: the body might continue to function for a short time, but it would no longer be the "same" person. The persistent identity of a person as an individual from one moment to the next is taken to be dependent on the continuation of certain mental processes which arise from brain functioning. When the brain processes cease (whether due to decapitation or to "brain death") the person's identity also lapses. The mere continuation of biological activity in the body is irrelevant to the determination of death, it is argued, because after the brain has ceased functioning the body is no longer identical with the person.

Critique   Theoretical and practical objections to these arguments led the Commission to rely on them only as confirmatory of other views in formulating a definition of death. First, crucial to the personhood argument is acceptance of one particular concept of those things that are essential to being a person, while there is no general agreement on this very fundamental point among philosophers, much less physicians or the general public. Opinions about what is essential to personhood vary greatly from person to person in our society—to say nothing of intercultural variations.

The argument from personal identity does not rely on any particular conception of personhood, but it does require assent to a single solution to the philosophical problem of identity. Again, this problem has persisted for centuries despite the best attempts by philosophers to solve it. Regardless of the scholarly merits of the various philosophical

solutions, their abstract technicality makes them less useful to public policy.

Further, applying either of these arguments in practice would give rise to additional important problems. Severely senile patients, for example, might not clearly be persons, let alone ones with continuing personal identities; the same might be true of the severely retarded. Any argument that classified these individuals as dead would not meet with public acceptance.

Equally problematic for the "higher brain" formulations, patients in whom only the neocortex or subcortical areas have been damaged may retain or regain spontaneous respiration and circulation. Karen Quinlan is a well-known example of a person who apparently suffered permanent damage to the higher centers of the brain but whose lower brain continues to function. Five years after being removed from the respirator that supported her breathing for nearly a year, she remains in a persistent vegetative state but with heart and lungs that function without mechanical assistance.* Yet the implication of the personhood and personal identity arguments is that Karen Quinlan, who retains brainstem function and breathes spontaneously, is just as dead as a corpse in the traditional sense. The Commission rejects this conclusion and the further implication that such patients could be buried or otherwise treated as dead persons.

Policy Consequences   In order to be incorporated in public policy, a conceptual formulation of death has to be amenable to clear articulation. At present, neither basic neurophysiology nor medical technique suffices to translate the "higher brain" formulation into policy. First, as was discussed in [a part of the study not reproduced here], it is not known which portions of the brain are responsible for cognition and consciousness; what little is known points to substantial interconnections among the brainstem, subcortical structures, and the neocortex. Thus, the "higher brain" may well exist only as a metaphorical concept, not in reality. Second, even when the sites of certain aspects of consciousness can be found, their cessation often cannot be assessed

_____

Editors' note: Karen Quinlan died on June 11, 1985.

with the certainty that would be required in applying a statutory definition.

Even were these difficulties to be overcome, the adoption of a higher brain "definition" would depart radically from the traditional standards. As already observed, the new standard would assign no significance to spontaneous breathing and heartbeat. Indeed, it would imply that the existing cardiopulmonary definition had been in error all along, even before the advent of respirators and other life-sustaining technology.

In contrast to this, the position taken by the Commission is deliberately conservative. The statutory proposal presented in [the Uniform Determination of Death Act] offers legal recognition for new diagnostic measures of death, but does not ask for acceptance of a wholly new concept of death. On a matter so fundamental to a society's sense of itself—touching deeply held personal and religious beliefs—and so final for the individuals involved, one would desire much greater consensus than now exists before taking the major step of radically revising the concept of death.

Finally, patients declared dead pursuant to the statute recommended by the Commission would be also considered dead by those who believe that a body without higher brain functions is dead. Thus, all the arguments reviewed thus far are in agreement that irreversible cessation of *all* brain functioning is sufficient to determine death of the organism.

The Non-Brain Formulations

The Concepts   The various physiological concepts of death so far discussed rely in some fashion on brain functioning. By contrast, a literal reading of the traditional cardiopulmonary criteria would require cessation of the flow of bodily "fluids," including air and blood, for death to be declared. This standard is meant to apply whether or not these flows coincide with any other bodily processes, neurological or otherwise. Its support derives from interpretations of religious literature and cultural practices of certain religious and ethnic groups, including some Orthodox Jews and Native Americans.

Another theological formulation of death is, by contrast, not necessarily related to any physiologic phenomenon. The view is traditional in many faiths that death occurs the moment the soul leaves the body. Whether this happens when the patient loses psychological capacities, loses all brain functions, or at some other point, varies according to the teachings of each faith and according to particular interpretations of the scriptures recognized as authoritative.

Critique   The conclusions of the "bodily fluids" view lack a physiologic basis in modern biomedicine. While this view accords with the traditional criteria of death, as noted above, it does not necessarily carry over to the new conditions of the intensive care unit—which are what prompt the reexamination of the definition of death. The flow of bodily fluids could conceivably be maintained by machines in the absence of almost all other life processes; the result would be viewed by most as a perfused corpse, totally unresponsive to its environment.

Although the argument concerning the soul could be interpreted as providing a standard for secular action, those who adhere to the concept today apparently acknowledge the need for a more public and verifiable standard of death. Indeed, a statute incorporating a brain-based standard is accepted by theologians of all backgrounds.

Policy Consequences   The Commission does not regard itself as a competent or appropriate forum for theological interpretation. Nevertheless, it has sought to propose policies consistent with as many as possible of the diverse religious tenets and practices in our society.

The statute set forth in the UDDA [Uniform Determination of Death Act] does not appear to conflict with the view that the soul leaves the body at death. It provides standards by which death can be determined to have occurred, but it does not prevent a person from believing on religious grounds that the soul leaves the body at a point other than that established as marking death for legal and medical purposes.

The concept of death based upon the flow of bodily fluids cannot be completely reconciled with the proposed statute. The statute is partially consistent with the "fluids" formulation in that both would regard as dead a body with no respiration and circulation. As noted previously, the overwhelming majority of patients, now and for the foreseeable future, will be diagnosed on such basis. Under the statute, however, physicians would declare dead those bodies in which respiration and circulation continued *solely* as a result of artificial maintenance, in the absence of all brain functions. Nonetheless, people who believe that the continued flow of fluids in such patients means they are alive would not be forced by the statute to abandon those beliefs nor to change their religious conduct. While the recommended statute may cause changes in medical and legal behavior, the Commission urges those acting under the statute to apply it with sensitivity to the emotional and religious needs of those for whom the new standards mark a departure from traditional practice. Determinations of death must be made in a consistent and evenhanded fashion, but the statute does not preclude flexibility in responding to individual circumstances after determination has been made.

THE WHOLE-BRAIN CONCEPT OF DEATH REMAINS OPTIMUM PUBLIC POLICY

James L. Bernat

The definition of death is one of the oldest and most enduring problems in biophilosophy and bioethics. Serious controversies over formally defining death began with the invention of the positive-pressure mechanical ventilator in the 1950s. For the first time, physicians could maintain ventilation and, hence, circulation on patients who had sustained what had been previously lethal brain damage. Prior to the development of mechanical ventilators, brain injuries severe enough to induce apnea quickly progressed to cardiac arrest from hypoxemia. Before the 1950s, the loss of spontaneous breathing and heartbeat ("vital functions") were perfect predictors of death because the functioning of the brain and of all other organs ceased rapidly and nearly simultaneously thereafter, producing a unitary death phenomenon. In the pretechnological era, physicians and philosophers did not have to consider whether a human being who had lost certain "vital functions" but had retained others was alive, because such cases were technically impossible.

From *Journal of Law, Medicine & Ethics* 34, no. 1 (Spring 2006): 35–43. Reprinted by Permission of the American Society of Law, Medicine & Ethics, Copyright © 2006, all rights reserved.

Editors' note: Some author's notes have been cut. Students who want to follow up on sources should consult the original article.

With the advent of mechanical support of ventilation (permitting maintenance of circulation) the previous unitary determination of death became ambiguous. Now patients were encountered in whom some vital organ functions (brain) had ceased totally and irreversibly, while other vital organ functions (such as ventilation and circulation) could be maintained, albeit mechanically. Their life status was ambiguous and debatable because they had features of both dead and living patients. They resembled dead patients in that they could not move or breathe, were utterly unresponsive to any stimuli, and had lost brain stem reflex activity. But they also resembled living patients in that they had maintained heartbeat, circulation and intact visceral organ functioning. Were these unfortunate patients in fact alive or dead?

In a series of scientific articles addressing this unprecedented state, several authors made the bold claim that patients who had totally and irreversibly lost brain functions were dead, despite their continued heartbeat and circulation. In the 1960s, they popularized the concept they called "brain death" to acknowledge this idea. The intuitive attractiveness of the concept of "brain death" led to its rapid acceptance by the medical and scientific community, and to legislators expeditiously drafting public laws permitting physicians to determine death on the basis of loss of brain functioning. Interestingly, largely by virtue of its intuitive appeal, the academy, medical practitioners, governments, and the public accepted the validity of brain death prior to the development of a rigorous biophilosophical proof that brain dead patients were truly dead. Medical historians have emphasized utilitarian factors in this rapid acceptance, because a determination of brain death permitted the desired societal goals of cessation of medical treatment and organ procurement.

The practice of determining human death using brain death tests has become worldwide over the past several decades. The practice is enshrined in law in all 50 states in the United States and in approximately 80 other countries, including nearly all of the developed world and much of the undeveloped world. A 1995 conference on the definition of death sponsored by the Institute of Medicine concluded that, despite certain theoretical and practical shortcomings, the practice of diagnosing brain death was so successful and so well accepted by the medical profession and the public that no major public policy changes seemed desirable.

Yet despite this consensus, from its beginning, a persistent group of critics have attacked the concept and practice of brain death as being conceptually invalid or a violation of religious beliefs. Recently, through the intellectual leadership of Alan Shewmon, additional critics have concluded that the concept of brain death is incoherent, anachronistic, unnecessary, a legal fiction, and should be abandoned. In this essay I show that, despite admitted shortcomings, the classical formulation of whole-brain death remains both conceptually coherent and forms a solid foundation for public policy surrounding human death determination and organ transplantation.

AN ANALYSIS OF DEATH

Defining death is a formidable task. In their rigorous, thoughtful, and highly influential book *Defining Death,* the President's Commission for the Study of Ethical Problems in Medicine and Biomedical and Behavioral Research chose as their conceptual foundation the analysis of death that I published with my Dartmouth colleagues Charles Culver and Bernard Gert.[1] Our analysis was conducted in three sequential phases: (1) the philosophical task of determining the definition of death by making explicit

the consensual concept of death that has been confounded by technology; (2) the philosophical and medical task of determining the best criterion of death, a measurable condition that shows that the definition has been fulfilled by being both necessary and sufficient for death; and (3) the medical-scientific task of determining the tests of death for physicians to employ at the patient's bedside to demonstrate that the criterion of death has been fulfilled with no false positive and minimal false negative determinations. Most subsequent scholars have accepted this method of analysis, if not our conclusions, with two recent exceptions.

Following a series of published critiques and rebuttals of our position over the past two decades, I concluded that much of the disagreement over our account of death resulted from the lack of acceptance by dissenting scholars of the "paradigm of death." By "paradigm of death" I refer specifically to a set of conditions and assumptions that frame the discussion of the topic of death by identifying the nature of the topic, the class of phenomena to which it belongs, how it should be discussed, and its conceptual boundaries. Accepting a paradigm of death permits scholars to rationally analyze and discuss death without falling victim to the fallacy of category noncongruence and consequently talking past each other. But the paradigm remains useful even if scholars do not agree on all its elements, because it can help clarify the root of their disagreement.

My paradigm of death comprises seven sequential elements. First, the word "death" is a common, nontechnical word that we all use correctly to refer to the cessation of a human being's life. The philosophical task of defining death seeks not to redefine it by contriving a new meaning, but rather to divine and make explicit the implicit meaning of death that we all accept but that has been made ambiguous by technological advances. Some scholars have gone astray by not attempting to capture our consensual concept of death and instead redefining death for ideological purposes or by overanalyzing death to a metaphysical level of abstraction—thereby rendering it devoid of its ordinary meaning.

Second, death is fundamentally a biological phenomenon. We all agree that life is a biological entity; thus also should be its cessation. Accepting that death is a biological phenomenon neither denigrates the richness and beauty of various cultural and religious practices surrounding death and dying, nor denies societies their proper authority to govern practices and establish laws regulating the determination and time of death. But death is an immutable and objective biological fact and not fundamentally a social contrivance. For the definition and criterion of death, the paradigm thus exclusively considers the ontology of death and ignores its normative aspects.

Third, we restrict our analysis to the death of higher vertebrate species for which death is univocal. That is, we mean the same phenomenon of "death" when we say our cousin died as we do when we say our dog died. Although individual cells within organisms and single celled organisms also die, our analysis of defining human death is simplified by restricting our purview to the death of related higher vertebrate species. Determining the death of cells, organs, protozoa, or bacteria are valid biophilosophical tasks but are not the task at hand here.

Fourth, the term "death" can be applied directly and categorically only to organisms. All living organisms must die and only living organisms can die. Our use of language may seem to confuse this point, for example, when we say "a person died." But by this usage we are referring directly to the death of the living organism that embodied the person, not to a living organism ceasing to be a person. Personhood is a psychosocial construct that can be lost but cannot die, except metaphorically. Similarly, other uses of the term "death" such as "the death of a culture" clearly are metaphorical and fall outside the paradigm.

Fifth, a higher vertebrate organism can reside in only one of two states, alive or dead: no organism can be in both states or in neither. Based on the theory of fuzzy sets, the concept that the world does not easily divide itself into sets and their complements, Amir Halevy and Baruch Brody proposed that an organism may reside in a transitional state between alive and dead that shares features of both states.[2] This claim appears plausible when considering cases of gradual, protracted dying, in which it may be difficult and even appear arbitrary to identify the precise moment of death. But this claim ignores the important distinction between our ability to identify an organism's biological state and the nature of that state. Simply because we currently lack the technical ability to always accurately identify an organism's

state does not necessitate postulating an in-between state. Using the terminology of fuzzy set theory as a guide, the paradigm requires us to view alive and dead as mutually exclusive (non-overlapping) and jointly exhaustive (no other) sets.

Sixth, and inevitably following from the preceding premise, death must be an event and not a process. If there are only two exclusive underlying states of an organism, the transition from one state to the other, at least in theory, must be sudden and instantaneous, because of the absence of an intervening state. Disagreement on this point, highlighted since the original debate over 30 years ago in *Science* by Robert Morison and Leon Kass,[3] centers on the difference between our ability to accurately measure the presence of a biological state and the nature of that biological state. To an observer, it may appear that death is an ineluctable process within which it is arbitrary to stipulate the moment of death, but such an observation simply underscores our current technical limitations. For technical reasons, the event of death may be determinable with confidence only in retrospect. As my colleagues and I first observed in 1981, death is best conceptualized not as a process but as the event separating the biological processes of dying and bodily disintegration.

Seventh and finally, death is irreversible. By its nature, if the event of death were reversible it would not be death but rather part of the process of dying that was interrupted and reversed. Advances in technology permit physicians to interrupt the dying process in some cases and postpone the event of death. So-called "near-death experiences," reported by some critically ill patients who subsequently recovered, do not indicate returning from the dead but are rather recalled experiences that result from alterations in brain physiology during incipient dying that was reversed in a timely manner.

THE DEFINITION OF DEATH

Given the set of assumptions and conditions comprising the paradigm of death, we can now explore the definition, criterion, and tests of death. Defining death is the conceptual task of making explicit our understanding of it. It poses an essential question: what does it mean for an organism to die, particularly in our contemporary circumstance in which technology can compensate for the failure of certain vital organs?

We all agree that by "death" we do not require the cessation of functioning of every cell in the body, because some integument cells that require little oxygen or blood flow continue to function temporarily after death is customarily declared. We also do not simply mean the cessation of heartbeat and respiration, though this circumstance will lead to death if untreated. Although some religious believers assert that the soul departs the body at the moment of death, this is not an adequate definition of death because it is not what religious believers fundamentally mean by "death."

Beginning early in the brain-death debate, Robert Veatch advocated a position that became known as the "higher-brain formulation of death."[4] He claimed that death should be defined formally as "the irreversible loss of that which is considered to be essentially significant to the nature of man." He expressly rejected the idea that death should be related to an organism's "loss of the capacity to integrate bodily function" asserting that "man is, after all, something more than a sophisticated computer. His project attempted not to reject brain death, but to refine the intuitive thinking underlying the brain death concept by emphasizing that it was the cerebral cortex that counted in a brain death concept and not the more primitive integrating brain structures.

Irrespective of the attractiveness of this idea (it has spawned a loyal following) the higher-brain formulation contains a fatal flaw as a candidate for a definition of death: it is not what we mean when we say "death." Its logical criterion of death would be the irreversible loss of consciousness and cognition, such as that which occurs in patients in an irreversible persistent vegetative state (PVS). Thus a higher-brain formulation of death would count PVS patients as dead. However, despite their profound and tragic disability, all societies, cultures, and laws consider PVS patients as alive. Thus, despite its potential merits, the higher-brain formulation fails the first condition of the paradigm: to make explicit our underlying consensual concept of death and not to contrive a new definition of death.

In 1981, my colleagues and I strove to capture the essence of the concept of human death that formed the intuitive foundation of the brain-based criterion of death. We defined death as "the cessation of functioning of the organism as a whole." This definition utilized a biological concept proposed by Jacques Loeb in 1916.[5] Loeb explained that organisms are not simply composites of cells, tissues, and organs, but possess overarching functions that regulate and integrate all systems to maintain the unity and interrelatedness of the organism to promote its optimal functioning and health. The organism as a whole comprises that set of functions that are greater than the mere sum of the organism's parts.

More recently, biophilosophers have advanced the concept of "emergent functions" to explain this type of phenomenon with greater conceptual clarity. An emergent function is a property of a whole that is not possessed by any of its component parts, and that cannot be reduced to one or more of its component parts. The physiological correlate of the organism as a whole is the set of emergent functions of the organism. The irretrievable loss of the organism's emergent functions produces loss of the critical functioning of the organism as a whole and therefore is the death of the organism.

In early writings on brain death, a few scholars proposed similar ideas. Most noteworthy was Julius Korein who asserted that the brain was the "critical system" of the organism whose loss indicated the organism's death.[6] Using thermodynamics theory, Korein argued that once the critical system was irretrievably lost (death), an irreversible and unstoppable process ensued of increasing entropy that constituted the process of bodily disintegration. The concept of the demise of the organism's critical system relies on concepts analogous to the cessation of functions of the organism as a whole.

Examples of critical functions of the organism as a whole include: (1) consciousness, which is necessary for the organism to respond to requirements for hydration and nutrition; (2) control of circulation, respiration, and temperature control, which are necessary for all cellular metabolism; and (3) integrating and control systems involving chemoreceptors, baroreceptors, and neuroendocrine feedback loops to maintain homeostasis. Death is the irreversible and permanent loss of the critical functions of the organism as a whole.

THE CRITERION OF DEATH

The next task is to identify the criterion of death, the general measurable condition that satisfies the definition of death by being both necessary and sufficient for death. There are several plausible candidates for a criterion of death. Among brain death advocates, three separate criteria have been proposed: (1) the whole-brain formulation, the criterion recommended by the Harvard Committee and the President's Commission, and accepted throughout the United States and in most parts of the world; (2) the higher-brain formulation, popular in the academy but accepted in no jurisdictions anywhere; and (3) the brain stem formulation accepted in the United Kingdom.

The whole-brain criterion requires cessation of all brain clinical functions including those of the cerebral hemispheres, diencephalon (thalamus and hypothalamus), and brain stem. Whole-brain theorists require widespread cessation of neuronal functions because each part of the brain serves the critical functions of the organism as a whole. The brain stem initiates and controls breathing, regulates circulation, and serves as the generator of conscious awareness through the ascending reticular activating system. The diencephalon provides the center for bodily homeostasis, regulating and coordinating numerous neuroendocrine control systems such as those regulating body temperature, salt and water regulation, feeding behavior, and memory. The cerebral hemispheres have an indispensable role in awareness that provides the conditions for all conscious behavior that serves the health and survival of the organism.

Clinical functions are those that are measurable at the bedside. The distinction between the brain's clinical functions and brain activities, recordable electrically or through other laboratory means, was made by the President's Commission in *Defining Death* though, for the sake of brevity, it did not appear in the Uniform Determination of Death Act proposed by the Commission. All clinical brain functions measurable at the bedside must be lost and the absence must be shown to be irreversible. But the whole-brain criterion does not require the loss of all neuronal activities. Some neurons may survive and contribute to recordable brain activities (by an electroencephalogram, for example) but not to clinical functions.[7] The precise number, location,

and configuration of the minimum number of critical neuron arrays remain unknown.

Despite the fact that the whole-brain criterion does not require the cessation of functioning of every brain neuron, it does rely on a pathophysiological process known as brain herniation to assure widespread destruction of the neuron systems responsible for the brain's clinical functions. When the brain is injured diffusely by trauma, hypoxicischemic damage during cardiorespiratory arrest or asphyxia, meningoencephalitis, or enlarging intracranial mass lesions such as neoplasms, brain edema causes intracranial pressure to rise to levels exceeding mean arterial blood pressure. At this point, intracranial circulation ceases and nearly all brain neurons that were not destroyed by the initial brain injury are secondarily destroyed by lack of intracranial circulation. Thus the whole-brain formulation provides a failsafe mechanism to eliminate false-positive brain death determinations and assure the loss of the critical functions of the organism as a whole. Showing the absence of all intracranial circulation is sufficient to prove widespread destruction of all critical neuronal systems. Similarly, it satisfies Korein's requirement for the loss of the irreplaceable critical system of the organism.

The higher-brain formulation fails to provide an adequate criterion of death because its conditions are insufficient for the loss of the critical functions of the organism as a whole. Its criterion is the irreversible loss of consciousness and cognition. The most common clinical manifestation of this condition is the PVS, caused by diffuse damage to the cerebral hemispheres, thalami, or disconnections between those structures. In most cases of PVS, brain stem neurons and their functions remain intact, so PVS patients, although unaware, have retained wakefulness and sleep-wake cycles (through the function of the intact ascending reticular activating system), have continued control of respiration and circulation by the intact medulla, and retain other brain stem mediated regulatory functions. The higher-brain formulation, thus, serves as neither an adequate definition nor criterion of death.

The criterion of the brain stem formulation is the loss of consciousness and the capacity for breathing. Diffuse damage to the brain stem that is sufficient to destroy the ascending reticular activating system and the medullary breathing center satisfies this criterion. But the brain stem formulation does not require commensurate damage to the diencephalon or cerebral hemispheres. It therefore leaves open the possibility of misdiagnosis of death because of a pathological process that appears to destroy brain stem activities but that permits some form of residual conscious awareness that cannot be easily detected. It thus lacks the fail-safe feature of whole-brain death to test for and guarantee the irreversible loss of these critical systems.

As a criterion of death, the circulation formulation fails for precisely the opposite reason of the higher-brain and brain stem formulations. Whereas the higher-brain and brain stem criteria both fail because they are necessary but not sufficient for death, the circulation criterion fails because it is sufficient but not necessary for death. The loss of all systemic circulation produces the destruction of all bodily organs and tissues so it is clearly a sufficient condition for death. But it is unnecessary to require the cessation of functions of organs that do not serve the critical functions of the organism as a whole.

THE TESTS OF DEATH

Brain death tests must be used to determine death only in the unusual case in which a patient's ventilation is being supported. If positive-pressure ventilation is neither employed nor entertained, the traditional tests of death—prolonged absence of breathing and heartbeat—can be used successfully. These traditional tests are absolutely predictive that the brain will be rapidly destroyed by lack of blood flow and oxygen, at which time death will have occurred. Traditional examinations for death, in addition to testing for heartbeat and breathing, always included tests for responsiveness and pupillary reflexes that directly measure brain function.

The bedside tests satisfying the whole-brain criterion of death have been designed with a sufficiently high degree of concordance to permit the drafting of widely accepted clinical practice guidelines on the determination of brain death. The tests require demonstrating the loss of all clinical brain functions, irreversibility, and a known structural process sufficient to produce the clinical findings. Laboratory tests showing the absence of intracranial blood flow or the absence of electrical activity in the

hemispheres and brain stem can be used to confirm the clinical diagnosis to expedite the determination.

Irreversibility is an indispensable requirement for brain death. There is general belief that irreversibility can be adequately demonstrated by conducting serial neurological examinations, excluding potentially reversible factors, and demonstrating a structural cause that is sufficient to account for the clinical signs. But, while highly plausible, these conditions have never been proved to assure irreversibility. Two recent factors prompted me to reassess my previous position that irreversibility could be proved solely by clinical factors and to suggest that a laboratory test showing cessation of all intracranial blood flow should become mandatory in brain death determination.

There are several published studies documenting the alarming frequency of physician variations and errors in performing brain death tests, despite clear guidelines for performing and recording the tests. Patients with "chronic brain death" have been reported who were diagnosed as brain dead but whose circulation and visceral organ functioning were successfully physiologically maintained for months or longer. Eelco Wijdicks and I questioned whether all of the reported patients were correctly diagnosed, and if some brain-damaged but not brain dead patients were included because of inadequate examinations and resultant incorrect brain death determinations.[8] Reacting to both these findings, I proposed that the mere assertion of irreversibility may no longer be sufficient to diagnose brain death and that a test showing cessation of all intracranial blood flow, such as transcranial Doppler ultrasonography, radionuclide angiography, or computed tomographic angiography, should become mandatory, at least if there is any question about the diagnosis or if the examiner is inexperienced.

PUBLIC POLICY ON DEATH

Brain death is widely regarded as the prime example of a formerly contentious bioethical and biophilosophical issue that has been resolved to the point of widespread public consensus. Evidence for this consensus is the enactment of effective and well-accepted brain death laws and policies throughout the world. In the United States, the Uniform Determination of

Death Act, recommended by the President's Commission and the National Conference of Commissioners on Uniform State Laws, has been enacted in most states, and others have enacted statutes with similar language. Contemporaneously, the Law Reform Commission of Canada produced a similar statute.

But an observer unaware of this consensus and public acceptance, who relied solely on reading the output of scholarly articles and university conferences on brain death, would reach a far different conclusion. The publication of anti-brain death articles has never been greater than during the past decade. Yet, despite those arguments, the 1995 Institute of Medicine conference on brain death recommended no changes in public laws in the United States, no jurisdiction has abandoned its brain death statute, and there is evidence that many additional countries have embraced the practice of determining brain death during the past decade of scholarly dissention. What accounts for the mismatch between public acceptance and scholarly agitation?

Higher-brain proponents continue to accept brain death but argue that the criterion of death should be changed to the higher-brain formulation. Brain stem death proponents also accept the conceptual validity of brain death but hold that the criterion of death should be the brain stem formulation. Religious authorities continue a debate that has raged for 40 years about whether brain death is compatible with the doctrines of the world's principal religious traditions. Protestantism, including fundamentalism, has accepted brain death. The debate in Roman Catholicism was largely settled by Pope John Paul's 2000 pronouncement embracing brain death as consistent with Catholic teachings. In Judaism, brain death is accepted by Reform and Conservative authorities, but an Orthodox rabbinic debate continues between those who declare brain death compatible with Jewish law and those who do not.[9] Brain death determination is also practiced in several Islamic societies, Hindi societies, and in Confucian-Shinto Japan.

The principal active opponents within the academy are those who reject the concept of brain death outright and promote the concept that a human being is not dead until the systemic circulation ceases and all organs are destroyed. The circulation proponents see no special role for brain functions in a determination of death. Alan Shewmon, the intellectual leader of the circulationists, has written eloquently on the conceptual problems inherent within the whole-brain (or any brain criterion) formulation. He cites evidence that the brain performs no qualitatively different forms of integration than the spinal cord and argues that therefore it should enjoy no special status above other organs in death determination. He claims further that his cases of "chronic brain death" show that the concept of brain death is inherently counterintuitive, for how could a dead body gestate infants or grow?

Another critic, Robert Taylor, has called the brain death concept a "legal fiction" that is accepted by society in a manner analogous to the concept of legal blindness. Taylor explains that legal blindness is a concept invented by society to permit people who are functionally blind from severe visual impairment to receive the same social benefits as those enjoyed by people who are totally blind. We all know that most people who are declared legally blind are not truly blind. But we employ a legal fiction and use the term "blindness" in a biologically incorrect way for its socially beneficial purpose. Taylor argues that, by analogy, we know that people we declare "brain dead" are not truly dead, but we consider them dead for the socially beneficial goal of organ procurement.[10]

As a longstanding proponent of whole-brain death, I acknowledge that the whole-brain formulation, although coherent, is imperfect, and that my attempts to defend it have not adequately addressed all valid criticisms. But my inadequacies must be viewed within the larger context of the relationship of biology to public policy. Our attempts to conceptualize, understand, and define the complex and subtle natural concepts of life and death remain far from perfect. Perhaps we will never be able to achieve uniform definitions of life and death that everyone accepts and that no one criticizes for conceptual or practical shortcomings.

In the real world of public policy on biological issues, we must frequently make compromises or approximations to achieve acceptable practices and laws. For these compromises to be tolerable, generally they should be minor and not affect outcomes. For example, in the current practice of organ donation after cardiac death (formerly known as non-heart-beating organ donation), I and others raised the question of whether the organ donor patients were truly dead after only five minutes of asystole.

The five-minute rule was accepted by the Institute of Medicine as the point at which death could be declared and the organs procured. Ours was a biologically valid criticism because, at least in theory, some such patients could be resuscitated after five minutes of asystole and still retain measurable brain function. If that was true, they were not yet dead at that point so their death declaration was premature.

But thereafter I changed my position to support programs of organ donation after cardiac death. I decided that it was justified to accept a compromise on this biological point when I realized that donor patients, if not already dead at five minutes of asystole, were incipiently and irreversibly dying because they could not auto-resuscitate and no one would attempt their resuscitation. Because their loss of circulatory and respiratory functions was permanent if not yet irreversible, there would be no difference whatsoever in their outcomes if their death were declared after five minutes of asystole or after 60 minutes of asystole. I concluded that, from a public policy perspective, accepting the permanent loss of circulatory and respiratory functions rather than requiring their irreversible loss was justified. The good accruing to the organ recipient, the donor patient, and the donor family resulting from organ donation justified overlooking the biological shortcoming because, although the difference in the death criteria was real, it was inconsequential.

Of course Alan Shewmon is correct that not all bodily system integration and functions of the organism as a whole are conducted by the brain (though most are) and that the spinal cord and other structures serve relevant roles. And Robert Taylor is correct that many people view brain death as a legal fiction and regard such patients "as good as dead" but not biologically dead. But despite its shortcomings, the whole-brain formulation remains coherent on the grounds of the critical functions of the organism as a whole and on the additional grounds of Korein's critical system theory. The whole-brain death formulation comprises a concept and public policy that make intuitive and practical sense and have been well accepted by the public throughout many societies. Therefore, while I am willing to acknowledge that whole-brain death formulation remains imperfect, I continue to support it because on the public policy level its shortcomings are relatively inconsequential.

Those scholars attacking the established whole-brain death formulation have a duty to show that their proposed alternative formulations not only more accurately represent biological reality, but also can be translated into successful public policy that is intuitively acceptable and maintains public confidence in physicians' accuracy in death determination and in the integrity of the organ procurement enterprise. Although I acknowledge certain weakness of the whole-brain death formulation, I hold that it most accurately maps our consensual implicit concept of death in a technological age and, as a consequence, it has been accepted by societies throughout the world.

REFERENCES

1. J. L. Bernat, C. M. Culver and B. Gert, "On the Definition and Criterion of Death," *Annals of Internal Medicine* 94 (1981): 389–394.
2. A. Halevy and B. Brody, "Brain Death: Reconciling Definitions, Criteria, and Tests," *Annals of Internal Medicine* 119 (1993): 519–525.
3. R. S. Morison, "Death: Process or Event?" *Science* 173 (1971): 694–698 and L. Kass, "Death as an Event: A Commentary on Robert Morison," *Science* 173 (1971): 698–702.
4. R. M. Veatch, "The Whole Brain-Oriented Concept of Death: An Outmoded Philosophical Formulation," *Journal of Thanatology* 3 (1975): 13–30; R. M. Veatch, "Brain Death and Slippery Slopes," *Journal of Clinical Ethics* 3 (1992): 181–187; and R. M. Veatch, "The Impending Collapse of the Whole-Brain Definition of Death," *Hastings Center Report* 23, no. 4 (1993): 18–24.
5. J. Loeb, *The Organism as a Whole* (New York: G. P. Putnam's Sons, 1916).
6. J. Korein, "The Problem of Brain Death: Development and History," *Annals of the New York Academy of Sciences* 315 (1978): 19–38. For the most recent refinement of Korein's argument, see J. Korein and C. Machado, "Brain Death: Updating a Valid Concept for 2004," *Advances in Experimental Medicine and Biology* 550 (2004): 1–14.
7. Residual EEG activity seen on unequivocally brain dead patients has been described by M. M. Grigg, M. A. Kelly, G. G. Celesia, M. W. Ghobrial, and E. R. Ross, "Electroencephalographic Activity after Brain Death," *Archives of Neurology* 44 (1987): 948–954.
8. E. F. M. Wijdicks and J. L. Bernat, "Chronic 'Brain Death': Metaanalysis and Conceptual Consequences" (letter to the editor), *Neurology* 53 (1999): 1639–1640.

9. The rabbinic debate is explained in F. Rosner, "The Definition of Death in Jewish Law," in S. J. Youngner, R. M. Arnold, and R. Schapiro, eds., *The Definition of Death: Contemporary Controversies* (Baltimore: Johns Hopkins University Press, 1999): 210–221.

10. R. M. Taylor, "Re-examining the Definition and Criterion of Death," *Seminars in Neurology* 17 (1997): 265–270.

AN ALTERNATIVE TO BRAIN DEATH

Jeff McMahan

SOME COMMON BUT MISTAKEN ASSUMPTIONS ABOUT DEATH

Most contributors to the debate about brain death, including Dr. James Bernat, share certain assumptions. They believe that the concept of death is univocal, that death is a biological phenomenon, that it is necessarily irreversible, that it is paradigmatically something that happens to *organisms,* that we are human organisms, and therefore that our deaths will be deaths of organisms. These claims are supposed to have moral significance. It is, for example, only when a person dies that it is permissible to extract her organs for transplantation.

It is also commonly held that our univocal notion of death is the permanent cessation of integrated functioning in an organism and that the criterion for determining when this has occurred in animals with brains is the death of the brain as a whole—that is, brain death. The reason most commonly given for this is that the brain is the irreplaceable master control of the organism's integration.

Before presenting my own view, let me say something about a couple of these assumptions and about the case for brain death. It is, perhaps, a measure of the heretical cast of my mind that I reject *all* of these widely shared assumptions.

I do not think the concept of death is univocal. When Jesus says that "whosoever liveth and believeth in me shall never die," he does not mean that some human organisms will remain functionally integrated forever. He means that believers will never cease to exist. (Admittedly, Jesus did not use the English word "die." But this seemed an intelligible use of the word to the translators.)

But "death" also has a biological meaning. It makes sense to say that when a unicellular organism, such as an ameba, undergoes binary fission, it ceases to exist; but in the biological sense it does not *die.* There is no cessation of functioning that turns this once-living organism into a corpse. So death as a biological phenomenon is different from the ceasing to exist of a living being and may or may not involve an entity's ceasing to exist. It is intelligible, for example, to say that when an animal organism dies, it does not cease to exist. Rather, it simply becomes a corpse. The living animal becomes a dead animal—but nothing ceases to exist until the animal organism disintegrates.

I also do not think our concept of death makes it a necessary truth that death is irreversible. If that were true, the claim that Lazarus was raised from the dead, or that Jesus was resurrected, would be incoherent. I think these claims are false; but if it were a conceptual truth that death is irreversible, they would not be false, but nonsensical.

I do think, however, that there is something true and important in the idea that death as a biological phenomenon is irreversible. It may well be a conceptual truth that an organism can be revived from death only by a violation of the laws of nature—that is, only by a literal miracle of the sort that Jesus is

From *Journal of Law, Medicine &Ethics* 34, no. 1 (Spring 2006): 44–48. Reprinted by Permission of the American Society of Law, Medicine &Ethics, Copyright © 2006, all rights reserved.

thought by some to have performed. For in cases not involving miracles, if an organism that was thought to be dead is restored to integrated functioning, our tendency is to conclude that we were mistaken in assuming that it was dead. (Subsequent references to irreversibility should be understood as having the implicit qualification "except by miracle.")

Some people, of course, will say that the organism was dead but was non-miraculously restored to life. To make this claim acceptable, they will need to offer good reasons for thinking the organism was dead, given that it is now alive. For reasons that I will give later, I think that nothing of importance depends on this. It is just a question of how we use certain words. But for those who believe that we are organisms and that we always have special value or sanctity while we are alive, this is a very important issue indeed.

While we are considering whether death is necessarily irreversible, I should mention that I am puzzled that Bernat and others define death as the permanent cessation of functioning—or of the critical functions—of an organism as a whole.[1] Surely what they should say is that it is the irreversible cessation of functioning. (By "irreversible" I mean irreversible in principle, not in practice.) If an organism stops functioning but its functioning could be recovered by means of a device that we do not in fact possess, it is not dead. There are, however, metaphysically determined constraints on what kind of device this could be. It would, for example, have to restore the same life, not create a new one.

Let me explain why the notion of irreversibility is preferable to that of permanence. Suppose there is an organism in which integrated functioning has ceased but could be revived. If it is up to you whether to revive the functioning, your decision now will determine whether the organism was dead a moment ago. For if you decide to revive the functioning, the cessation will not have been permanent and the organism will have been alive a moment ago. But if you decide not to revive it, you thereby make permanent the cessation of functioning that occurred in the past. But whether the organism was dead a moment ago is a matter of its intrinsic state at the time; it cannot be determined retroactively by what you do now. (Bernat, I should note, urges a similar point in his cogent objections to the proposal for non-heart-beating organ donation.[2])

BRAIN DEATH AND THE CESSATION OF INTEGRATED FUNCTIONING

Turn now to the central contention of the defenders of brain death, which is that at least certain critical functions of the brain are necessary for integrated functioning in the organism. (I put aside the interesting question whether they are also sufficient.) This claim raises two related questions. First, what counts as the right sort of integration? Second, is the claim empirical or conceptual?

There are several ways in which the functions of the various organs and subsystems of an organism might be integrated so as to maintain homeostasis and resist entropy. It might be, for example, that integration occurs via a central integrator, a master control that receives signals from the various organs and subsystems, processes them, and then sends return signals that coordinate the functions of the organism's many parts. The defenders of brain death typically claim that the only possible central integrator is the brain. They say that the brain is irreplaceable, that nothing else could possibly carry out its regulative functions.

Critics of brain death, by contrast, often speculate that a mechanical brain—or to be more precise, a mechanical substitute for the brain stem—could adequately replicate the regulative functions of the brain and hence could be the central integrator of a living human organism. Some, indeed, have claimed that the resources of the modern intensive care unit (ICU) already constitute an external and multifaceted substitute for the regulatory functions of the brain stem.[3]

In defending the irreplaceability of the brain, Bernat writes that, "although some of the brain's regulatory functions may be replaced mechanically, the brain's functions of awareness, sentience, sapience, and its capacities to experience and communicate cannot be reproduced or simulated by any machine."[4] Let us grant that this is true. The problem is that these are not somatic regulatory functions.[5]

A second way in which the functions of an organism's various organs and subsystems might be integrated is through decentralized interaction, in which these parts achieve coordination by sending, receiving, and processing signals among themselves. In a series of papers, Alan Shewmon has argued that this sort of decentralized integration of functioning can and sometimes does occur among the parts of an organism without any input from the brain at all.[6] He cites numerous actual cases involving high cervical transaction, functional isolation of the brain in Guillain-Barré Syndrome, or even brain death with artificially induced respiration in which there is a high degree of functional integration in the absence of regulation by the brain—and, indeed, without any central integrator at all. He notes, for example, that some brain dead organisms have the same range of functions as certain uncontroversially living patients in an ICU, and yet maintain these functions with *fewer* sources of external support.

If the familiar claims about the necessary role of the brain in integrating the functions of an organism are empirical claims, I think that Shewmon's cases and arguments force the defender of brain death to admit defeat. But it is possible for the defender of brain death to respond to Shewmon's challenge by interpreting the claim that the brain is necessary for integrated functioning as a conceptual rather than empirical claim.

The defender of brain death can, in other words, retreat to the claim that while certain forms of integrated functioning can be sustained via an artificial central regulator or via decentralized interaction, these forms of integration are not the kind of integration that is necessary for life in a human organism. Only the brain as central regulator can provide that. This may be a reasonable interpretation of Bernat's claim that "the brain is the critical system of the organism without which the remaining organs may continue to function independently but cannot together comprise an organism as a whole."[7] He might be saying that, even if all the organs are alive and doing their job, they cannot together constitute a living organism without the mediation of the brain.

There are various responses to such a view. One is to ask how much the brain must contribute to the integration of functioning among the parts of the organism in order for the organism to be alive. Clearly it need not regulate *every* aspect of functioning. Indeed, it seems that those who would defend the idea that somatic regulation by the brain is a conceptually necessary condition for life in a human organism must accept something like the following. First we have to identify a range of "critical" regulatory functions. As long as the brain continues to carry out any single one of these functions, that is sufficient for life in the organism. For if we were to

insist on the necessity of the brain's carrying out more than one, then an organism in which the brain carried out only one critical regulatory function would be dead—but it would not be brain dead.

But now imagine a case in which only one critical regulatory function is being carried out by the brain. All others are being carried out by external life support. Suppose that right at the moment the brain is about to lose the capacity to carry out this one remaining critical function, a mechanical replacement takes over for it with perfect efficiency. Could *this* be the difference between life and death? Note that, because the mechanical replacement would carry out the regulatory functions in exactly the same way the brain did, the state of the organism would be unchanged apart from this one small change in the brain itself. It is very hard to believe that such a change could make the difference between life and death in an organism, either as a matter of fact or, especially, as a matter of conceptual necessity.

If presented only with information about the loss of supposed critical functions in the brain and information about the unchanged but externally supported functioning of the various organs and subsystems within the organism, most people, I suspect, would not know what to say about whether such an organism was alive or dead. Our concept of death simply fails to deliver an immediately intuitive verdict that the organism is dead. This strongly suggests that the loss by the brain of critical regulatory functions is no part of our *concept* of death.

Another response is simply to point to the case of human embryos, which seem to be living human organisms whose somatic functions are not regulated or integrated by the brain. If this is a correct description, it cannot be a necessary truth that the kind of integrated functioning necessary for life must be regulated to some degree by the brain.

There are a great many other problems with the notion of brain death but I will not rehearse them here.[8] Instead I will conclude by sketching an alternative view.

AN ALTERNATIVE UNDERSTANDING OF DEATH

I accept that it is largely correct to say that a human organism dies when it irreversibly loses the capacity for integrated functioning among its various major organs and subsystems. But the death of a human organism will necessarily be *my* death only if I am an organism. The view that we are organisms is the most important of the widely shared assumptions that I noted at the outset. But, as I mentioned, I think it is mistaken.

The question whether we are organisms is not a biological question, or even a scientific question—just as it is not a scientific question whether a statue and the lump of bronze of which it is composed are one and the same thing or distinct substances. Whether we are organisms is also, and more obviously, not an ethical question. It is a metaphysical question.

There are two arguments that convince me that the answer to this question is "no." One appeals to the hypothetical case of brain transplantation—or, better yet, cerebrum transplantation. If my cerebrum were successfully grafted onto the brain stem of my identical twin brother (whose own cerebrum had been excised), I would then exist in association with what was once his organism. What was formerly my organism would have an intact brain stem and might, therefore, be idling nicely in a persistent vegetative state without even mechanical ventilation. Since I can thus in principle exist separately from the organism that is now mine, I cannot be identical with it.

The second argument appeals not to a science fiction scenario but to an actual phenomenon: dicephalus. Certain instances of dicephalic twinning, in which two heads sprout from a single torso, seem to be clear cases in which a single organism supports the existence of two distinct people. The transitivity of identity prevents us from saying that *both* these people *are* that organism; for that implies that the people are identical, that is, that there are not really two people but only one. And because each twin's relation to the organism is the same as the other's, it cannot be that one twin but not the other is the organism. The best thing to say, therefore, is that neither of them is identical to the organism. Since we are essentially the same kind of thing they are, we cannot be organisms either.

If I am right that we are not organisms, what are we? The most widely held alternative view is that each of us is essentially a cartesian soul—that is, a nonmaterial conscious entity that in life is linked with a particular brain and body but at death continues to exist and indeed remains conscious and is psychologically continuous with the person prior to death. Because the soul, so conceived, is nonphysical, it can be individuated only by reference to a single

field of consciousness. Thus, any conscious state that is not accessible in my field of consciousness must belong to a different person, or soul. This conception of the soul is, however, undermined by what we know about the results of hemispheric commissurotomy—a procedure in which the tissues connecting a patient's cerebral hemispheres are surgically severed. This procedure gives rise, at least in certain experimental settings, to two separate centers of consciousness in a single human organism. If persons were cartesian souls, we would have to conclude that the procedure creates two persons where formerly there was only one. Since this is clearly not what happens, we cannot be cartesian souls.[9]

How should we think about the problem of determining what kind of thing we essentially are? Here is a quick thought-experiment. Imagine that you were facing the prospect of progressive dementia. At what point would you cease to exist? To most of us it seems clear that you would persist at least as long as the brain in your body retained the capacity for consciousness. For there would be somebody there, and who might it be, if not you? But would you still survive if your brain irreversibly lost the capacity for consciousness? It seems that the only thing there that might qualify as you would be a living human organism. But if I am right that you are not a human organism and there would be nothing else there for you to be, it seems that you must have ceased to exist when your brain lost the capacity for consciousness. I infer from this that you are in fact a mind, a mind that is necessarily embodied.

Recall now my earlier claim that the concept of death is not univocal. The term "death" can refer to our ceasing to exist (as in the earlier quotation from Jesus) or it can refer to a biological event in the history of an organism. This makes things easy; for we already have the two concepts of death that we require if I am right that we are not organisms.

An organism dies in the biological sense when it loses the capacity for integrated functioning. The best criterion for when this happens is probably a circulatory-respiratory criterion. There is bound to be considerable indeterminacy about how much functional integration is required for life in an organism. But if we are not organisms, this is of little consequence.

What it is important to be able to determine is when we die in the nonbiological sense—that is, when we cease to exist. If we are embodied minds, we die or cease to exist when we irreversibly lose the capacity for consciousness—or, to be more precise, when there is irreversible loss of function in those areas of the brain in which consciousness is realized. The best criterion for when this happens is a higher-brain criterion—for example, what is called "cerebral death." But I do not pretend to any expertise here.

Note that when I say the right criterion of our death is a higher-brain criterion, I am not claiming that a human organism in a persistent vegetative state is dead. If persistent vegetative state involves the loss of the capacity for consciousness, then neither you nor I could ever exist in a persistent vegetative state. But you could be survived by your organism, which could remain biologically alive in a persistent vegetative state even though you were dead (that is, had ceased to exist). My view thus avoids the embarrassing implication of most proposals for a higher-brain criterion of death that an organism with spontaneous respiration and heartbeat might be dead.

From an ethical point of view, what matters is not whether an organism remains alive, but whether one of us continues to exist. Of course, we cannot survive unless our organisms remain alive (though this might change if brain transplantation were to become possible). Indeed, although brain death is not sufficient for the biological death of a human organism, it is sufficient for the death or ceasing to exist of a person.

The problematic cases are those in which a person has ceased to exist but her organism remains alive. Might it be permissible to remove the organs from such an organism for transplantation? I believe that it would be, provided that this would not be against the expressed will of the person whose organism it was. But if the person had consented in advance, there would be no moral objection to killing the unoccupied organism in order to use its organs to save the lives of others.

The organism itself cannot be harmed in the relevant sense, it has no rights, and it is not an appropriate object of respect in the Kantian sense. I believe that the treatment of a living but unoccupied human organism is governed morally by principles similar to those that govern the treatment of a corpse. The latter also cannot be harmed or possess rights. But respect for the person who once animated a corpse dictates that there are certain things that must not be done to it. Taking its organs for transplantation with the person's prior consent is not one of these.

REFERENCES

1. J. L. Bernat, "A Defense of the Whole-Brain Concept of Death," *Hastings Center Report* 28, no. 2 (1998): 14–23, at 17.
2. See J. L. Bernat, "Defending Challenges to the Concept of 'Brain Death,'" *at* <http://www.lahey.org/NewsPubs/Publications/Ethics/Journal Fall1998/Journal_Fall1998_Feature.asp> (last visited December 5, 2005); and M. A. DeVita and R. M. Arnold, "The Concept of Brain Death," *at* <http://www.lahey.org/NewsPubs/Publications/Ethics/JournalWinter1999/Journal_Winter1999_Dialogue.asp> (last visited December 5, 2005).
3. For an early suggestion of this sort, see M. B. Green and D. Wikler, "Brain Death and Personal Identity," *Philosophy and Public Affairs* 9 (1980): 105–33, at 113.
4. Bernat, *supra* note 1, at 19.
5. Bernat also claims that "consciousness, which is required for the organism to respond to requirements for hydration, nutrition, and protection, among other needs," is therefore among the "critical functions of the organism as a whole." *Ibid.*, at 17. But this still does not make it a somatic regulatory function of the brain.
6. See, for example, A. Shewmon, "Recovery from 'Brain Death': A Neurologist's Apologia," *Linacre Quarterly* 64 (1997): 30–96; A. Shewmon, "Chronic 'Brain Death,'" *Neurology* 51 (1998): 1538–45; and A. Shewmon, "The Disintegration of Somatic Integrative Unity: Demise of the Orthodox but Physiologically Untenable Physiological Rationale for 'Brain Death,'" manuscript on file with the author.
7. Bernat, *supra* note 2.
8. See J. McMahan, *The Ethics of Killing: Problems at the Margins of Life* (New York: Oxford University Press: 2002): chapter 5, section 1.2.
9. For further argument, see McMahan, *supra* note 8, at 7–24.

DECISIONAL CAPACITY AND THE RIGHT TO REFUSE TREATMENT

STATE OF TENNESSEE DEPARTMENT OF HUMAN SERVICES V. MARY C. NORTHERN

Court of Appeals of Tennessee, Middle Section, Feb. 7, 1978

On January 24, 1978, the Tennessee Department of Human Services filed this suit alleging that Mary C. Northern was 72 years old, with no available help from relatives; that Miss Northern resided alone under unsatisfactory conditions as a result of which she had been admitted to and was a patient in Nashville General Hospital; that the patient suffered from gangrene of both feet which required the removal of her feet to save her life; that the patient lacked the capacity to appreciate her condition or to consent to necessary surgery.

Attached to the complaint are identical letters from Drs. Amos D. Tackett and R. Benton Adkins, which read as follows:

Mrs. Mary Northern is a patient under our care at Nashville General Hospital. She has gangrene of both feet probably secondary to frostbite and then thermal burning of the feet. She has developed infection along with the gangrene of her feet. This is placing her life in danger. Mrs. Northern does not understand the severity or consequences of her disease process and does not appear to understand that failure to amputate the feet at this time would probably result in her death. It is our recommendation as the physicians in charge of her case, that she undergo amputation of both feet as soon as possible.

On January 24, 1978, the Chancellor appointed a guardian ad litem to defend the cause and to receive service of process pursuant to Rule 4.04(2) T.R.C.P. On January 25, 1978, the guardian ad litem answered as follows:

The Respondent, by and through her guardian ad litem, states as follows:

1. She is 72 years of age and a resident of Davidson County, Tennessee.

Editors' note: The suit was filed under the state Protective Services for the Elderly Act, which permits a court to appoint a guardian for the purposes of consent to medical treatment if an elderly person is in imminent danger of death without treatment and lacks capacity to consent to it. Some text has been cut. Students who want to read the article in its entirety should consult the original.

2. She is presently in the intensive care unit of General Hospital, Nashville, Tennessee, because of gangrenous condition in her two feet.
3. She feels very strongly that her present physical condition is improving, and that she will recover without the necessity of surgery.
4. She is in possession of a good memory and recall, responds accurately to questions asked her, is coherent and intelligent in her conversation, and is of sound mind.
5. She is aware that the Tennessee Department of Human Services has filed this complaint, knows the nature of the complaint, and does not wish for her feet to be amputated.

.   .   .

On January 26, 1978, there was filed in this cause a letter from Dr. John J. Griffin, reporting that he found the patient to be generally lucid and sane, but concluding:

> Nonetheless, I believe that she is functioning on a psychotic level with respect to ideas concerning her gangrenous feet. She tends to believe that her feet are black because of soot or dirt. She does not believe her physicians about the serious infection. There is an adamant belief that her feet will heal without surgery, and she refused to even consider the possibility that amputation is necessary to save her life. There is no desire to die, yet her judgment concerning recovery is markedly impaired. If she appreciated the seriousness of her condition, heard her physicians' opinions, and concluded against an operation, then I would believe she understood and could decide for herself. But my impression is that she does not appreciate the dangers to her life. I conclude that she is incompetent to decide this issue. A corollary to this denial is seen in her unwillingness to consider any future plans. Here again I believe she was utilizing a psychotic mechanism of denial.
>
> This is a schizoid woman who has been urged by everyone to have surgery. Having been self-sufficient previously (albeit a marginal adjustment), she is continuing to decide alone. The risks with surgery are great and her lifestyle has been permanently disrupted. If she has surgery there is a tremendous danger for physical and psychological complications. The chances for a post-operative psychosis are immense, yet the surgeons believe an operation is necessary to save her life. I would advise delaying surgery (if feasible) for a few days in order to attempt some work for strengthening her psychologically. Even if she does not consent to the operation after that time, however, I believe she is incompetent to make the decision.

On January 28, 1978, this Court entered an order reciting the following:

From all of the above the Court finds:

1. That the respondent is not now in 'imminent danger of death' in the extreme sense of the words, but that her present condition is such that 'imminent danger of death' may reasonably be expected during her continued hospitalization.
2. That both feet of respondent are severely necrotic and affected by wet gangrene, an infection which probably will result in death unless properly treated by amputation of the feet.
3. That the probability of respondent's survival without amputation is from 5 percent to 10 percent and the probability of survival after amputation is about 50 percent, with possible severe psychotic results.
4. That, with or without amputation, the prognosis of respondent's condition is poor.
5. That respondent is an intelligent, lucid, communicative, and articulate individual who does not accept the fact of the serious condition of her feet and is unwilling to discuss the seriousness of such condition or its fatal potentiality.
6. That, because of her inability or unwillingness to recognize the actual condition of her feet which is clearly observable by her, she is incompetent to make a rational decision as to the amputation of her feet.
7. That respondent has no wish to die, but is unable or unwilling to recognize an obvious condition which will probably result in her death if untreated.

This Court is therefore of the opinion that a responsible individual should be named with authority to consent to amputation of respondent's feet when urgently recommended in writing by respondent's physicians because of the development of (symptoms) indicating an emergency and severe imminence of death.

.   .   .

[Appellant's first assignment of error states:]

Such actions by the Court were injurious to the appellant because they deprived her of her right to make her own decisions—regardless as to whether death might be a probable consequence—as to whether she was willing to surrender control of her own person and life.

This controversy arises from the fact that Miss Northern's attending physicians have determined that all of the soft tissue of her feet has been killed by frostbite, that said dead tissue has become infected with gangrene, and that the feet must be removed to prevent loss of life from spreading of gangrene and its effects to the entire body. Miss Northern has refused to consent to the surgery.

The physicians have determined, and the Chancellor and this Court have found, that Miss Northern's life is critically endangered; that she is mentally incapable of comprehending the facts which constitute that danger; and that she is, to that extent, incompetent, thereby justifying State action to preserve her life.

As will be observed from the bill of exceptions, a member of this Court asked Miss Northern if she would prefer to die rather than lose her feet, and her answer was "possibly." This is the most definitive expression of her desires in this record.

The patient has *not* expressed a desire to die. She evidences a strong desire to live and an equally strong desire to keep her dead feet. She refuses to make a choice.

If the patient would assume and exercise her rightful control over her own destiny by stating that she prefers death to the loss of her feet, her wish would be respected. The doctors so testified; this Court so informed her; and this Court now reiterates its commitment to this principle.

The appellant has filed three supplemental assignments of error, of which the first is:

1. The statute, T.C.A. §§ 14-2301, *et seq.*, is impermissibly vague; and, therefore, void and unconstitutional. The two phrases used in the statute, 'imminent danger of death' and 'capacity to consent' have not been defined in the statute nor is the Court given any assistance to determine when either standard has been met in the legal context, rather than a medical context.

In the judgment of this Court, the words "imminent danger of death" are no more vague than is consistent with the nature of the subject matter.

. . .

The words, "imminent danger of death" mean conditions calculated to and capable of producing within a short period of time a reasonably strong probability of resultant cessation of life if such conditions are not removed or alleviated. Such is undoubtedly the legislative intent of the words.

"Imminent danger of death" should be reasonably interpreted to carry out the purposes of the statute. For an authorization to mildly encroach upon the freedom of the individual, a relatively mild imminence or danger of death may suffice. On the other hand, the authorization of a drastic encroachment upon personal freedom and bodily integrity would require a correspondingly severe imminence of death.

In the present case, the Chancellor was not called upon to act until the imminence of death was moderately severe. By the time of the hearing before this Court, the imminence of death had lessened somewhat but remained real and appreciable. Accordingly this Court, recognizing a present real and appreciable imminence of death, made provision for drastic emergency measures to be taken only in event of severe and urgent imminence of death.

Appellant also complains of vagueness of the meaning of "capacity to consent." Capacity means mental ability to make a rational decision, which includes the ability to perceive, to appreciate all relevant facts, and to reach a rational judgment upon such facts.

Capacity is not necessarily synonymous with sanity. A blind person may be perfectly capable of observing the shape of small articles by handling them, but not capable of observing the shape of a cloud in the sky.

A person may have "capacity" as to some matters and may lack "capacity" as to others.

In 44 C.J.S. Insane Persons § 2, pp. 17, 18, partial insanity is defined as follows:

Partial insanity. Although it is hard to define the invisible line that divides perfect and partial insanity, the law recognizes a state of mind called 'partial insanity,' that is, insanity on a particular subject only, sometimes denominating it 'insane delusion' or 'monomania.' The use of the term, however, has been criticized. Partial insanity has been said to be the derangement of one or more of the faculties of the mind, which prevents freedom of action. Ordinarily it is confined to a particular subject, the person being sane on every other. The degree of insanity, as partial or total, is to be measured by the extent and number of the delusions existing in the mind of the person in question. . . .

In the present case, this Court has found the patient to be lucid and apparently of sound mind generally. However, on the subjects of death and amputation of her feet, her comprehension is blocked, blinded, or dimmed to the extent that she is incapable of recognizing facts which would be obvious to a person of normal perception.

For example, in the presence of this Court, the patient looked at her feet and refused to recognize the obvious fact that the flesh was dead, black, shriveled, rotting, and stinking.

The record also discloses that the patient refuses to consider the eventuality of death which is, or ought to be, obvious in the face of such dire bodily deterioration.

As described by the doctors and observed by this Court, the patient wants to live and keep her dead feet, too, and refuses to consider the impossibility of such a desire. In order to avoid the unpleasant experience of facing death and/or loss of feet, her mind or emotions have resorted to the device of denying the unpleasant reality so that, to the patient, the unpleasant reality does not exist. This is the "delusion" which renders the patient incapable of making a rational decision as to whether to undergo surgery to save her life or to forgo surgery and forfeit her life.

The physicians speak of probabilities of death without amputation as 90 to 95 percent and the probability of death with surgery as 50–50 (1 in 2). Such probabilities are not facts, but the existence and expression of such opinions are facts which the patient is unwilling or unable to recognize or discuss.

If, as repeatedly stated, this patient could and would give evidence of a comprehension of the facts of her condition and could and would express her unequivocal desire in the face of such comprehended facts, then her decision, however unreasonable to others, would be accepted and honored by the Courts and by her doctors. The difficulty is that she cannot or will not comprehend the facts.

The first supplemental assignment of error is respectfully overruled.

The second supplemental assignment of error is as follows:

> 2. The Chancellor erred by denying the Appellant her rights to substantive and procedural due process. The entire legal proceedings involved in this case and on appeal are unprecedented; the order of the Chancellor granting the appeal but refusing the automatic stay of thirty days allowed by the Rules is one example of the procedural wrongs which was not in accordance

with the established legal practice, and contrary to the expected procedure to be followed. The proposed amputation will not only permanently deprive the Appellant of her two limbs, but most likely will significantly and irreparably alter her personality for the worse, and make her mentally and physically dependent upon the State.

Whatever the propriety or impropriety of the action of the Chancellor in attempting to effectuate his action in spite of the appeal, the error, if any, has been rendered harmless by the action of this Court, after appeal, in reviewing and modifying his actions.

This Court does not recognize that it has been guilty of any improper deviation from correct procedure. The gravity of the condition of the patient and the resultant emergency in time required the unusual action of the Court under § 27-327 T.C.A. and the unusual acceleration of hearings and actions taken.

This Court is painfully and acutely aware of the possible tragic results of amputation. According to the doctors, the patient has only a 50 percent chance of surviving the surgery; and, if she survives, she will never be able to walk and may suffer severe mental and emotional problems.

On the other hand, the doctors testified, and this Court finds, that the patient's chances of survival without amputation are from 5 percent to 10 percent—a rather remote and fragile chance. Moreover, as testified by the doctors and found by this Court, even if the patient should survive without amputation, she will never walk because the dead flesh will fall off the bones of her feet leaving only bare bones.

IT IS, THEREFORE, ORDERED, ADJUDGED AND DECREED that

1. Mary C. Northern is in imminent danger of death if she does not receive surgical amputation of her lower extremities and she lacks the capacity to consent or refuse consent for such surgery.
2. That Honorable Horace Bass, Commissioner of Human Services of the State of Tennessee or his successor in office is hereby designated and authorized to act for and on behalf of said Mary C. Northern in consenting to surgical amputation of her lower extremities and of exercising such custodial supervision as is necessarily incident thereto at any time that Drs. Amos D. Tackett and R. Benton Adkins

join in signing a written certificate that Mary C. Northern's condition has developed to such a critical stage as to demand immediate amputation to save her life. The previous order of this Court is likewise so modified.

As modified, the order of the Chancellor is affirmed. The cause is remanded for further appropriate proceedings.

.   .   .

Modified, Affirmed, and Remanded.*

_____

*On May 1, 1978, Mary Northern died in a Nashville hospital as a result of a clot from the gangrenous tissue migrating through the bloodstream to a vital organ. Because of complications rendering surgery more dangerous, the proposed surgery was never performed.

TRANSCRIPT OF PROCEEDINGS: TESTIMONY OF MARY C. NORTHERN
January 28, 1978

Testimony of Mary Northern: [The following interview took place at the bedside of Mary Northern in the Intensive Care Unit of the Nashville General Hospital. Present were Judge Todd, Judge Drowota, and the Reverend Palmer Sorrow, a friend and frequent visitor of the patient. Eds.]

Judge Todd: Now, Mrs. Mary, you know that there have been some proceedings in court about you, and that's the reason why the judges are here. And we wanted to see you and talk to you.

Miss Northern: Yes.

Judge Todd: And give you a chance to talk to us.

Miss Northern: Yeah.

Judge Todd: I understand that you had a little problem of getting too cold out there at your house.

Miss Northern: Yes.

Judge Todd: That's right.

Miss Northern: Yes. Well, now, it's a point of this, the swelling of my foot was—was very dangerous looking.

Judge Todd: Yes ma'am.

Miss Northern: And so that's what caused most of the trouble, and the—it's starting to go down. Give it a chance, it is starting to go down, and it's almost . . . Well, these—these ankles and the—along on these legs have gone down wonderfully.

Judge Todd: Yes, now, Mrs. Mary, these doctors have been talking to us at great length about the condition of your feet.

Mr. Sorrow: I think it's okay.

Miss Northern: Okay.

Judge Todd: —and they tell us this about your feet. Now, mind you . . . we don't know whether it's so or not, but I want you to know what they have told us. . . . They tell us that your feet have been frostbitten before, and that they got well.

Miss Northern: Yes.

Judge Todd: What they tell us, that your feet were frostbitten a great deal worse this time than they were . . . before.

Miss Northern: Yes.

Judge Todd: And they tell us this,—now I am going to say some things to you that might be a little uncomfortable, but I want—I don't believe these doctors have told it to you just like they told it to us.

Miss Northern: Yeah.

Judge Todd: So I want to give it to you just like they have given it to us. They tell us that this time every bit of the flesh on your two feet is completely dead.

Miss Northern: I know—No, it isn't, it will revive.

Judge Todd: I understand.

Miss Northern: Four or five days ago it started to go down.

Judge Todd: All right. Now they tell us this, that when you came in . . . here that your feet were swollen. . . . And they tell us that the swelling has gone down.

Miss Northern: Yes.

Judge Todd: But they tell us that your feet are shriveling up like a dead person's feet—

Miss Northern: Unh-unh.

Judge Todd:—rather than a live person's feet.

Miss Northern: No, no. . . . I can get and walk all the way down to the shopping places.

Judge Todd: Now they tell us—We questioned them very, very thoroughly about this thing, and they tell us that you can move your toes. And then I asked them how could a person move his toes if his foot was dead? You see? And here's what they tell us. They tell us that the ligaments that move the toes . . . are dead, but they are still just like strings,—

Miss Northern: Yeah.

Judge Todd: —and that the muscles that move the toes are up here where they are still alive, and therefore a dead foot can move its toes.

Miss Northern: Well, they are not going to—they are not going to take my legs away. They are not going to take my legs away from me, you understand this?

Judge Todd: Yes, ma'am.

Miss Northern: And they are not going to—I think it's rather silly, because they all—all of em have gotten viable.

Judge Todd: Yes, ma'am. Yes, ma'am. Now here is the thing that disturbs us. The doctors tell us that you have a very heavy infection which they are keeping in control by antibiotics, but that your temperature has started to rise, that you have a hundred and one temperature . . . which indicates that the infection is increasing. And we questioned them very closely now, we have been a long time—

Miss Northern: You understand they are going to do it. Now, does this have something to do with the Metropolitan Government, has it not? Well, the Metropolitan Government can't take anything—do me this way, you know?

Judge Todd: Yes, sir. Now, here is what I want to present to you. You are a very intelligent woman for your age. I want to compliment you on that, you really are. I said you were like my mother, but you do circles around my mother as far as talking and thinking.

Now, you are educated, and you know this business of "if," and I want to ask you an "if" question. If your feet, the flesh of your feet, really is dead, and if you have one chance in ten of living without surgery, that it is, if—if the feet are left on, that nine

chances to one that you will not live, it will kill you,—

Miss Northern: I am not going to have—

Judge Todd: —would you still say, "I want that one chance?"

Miss Northern: Well, of course,—

Judge Todd: Ma'am?

Miss Northern: —this is not going to do anything like this. All—All of these thing,—

Judge Todd: Yes, ma'am.

Miss Northern: —and my feet have gone down.

Judge Todd: Yes, ma'am.

Miss Northern: My ankles are—

Judge Todd: Yes, ma'am. Now, let me ask you one more question.

Miss Northern: I am not going to—Let me tell you something. I am not going to argue any more with you, because I know you have a multiple of opinions.

Judge Todd: No, I haven't formed any opinions, that's the reason I came up to talk to you. I haven't decided.

Miss Northern: It's an opinion you formed, and I am not going to let you tell me—

Judge Todd: I am just telling you what they told me. Now let me ask you one more little thing.

If the time comes that this infection gets so bad that you are practically unconscious and can't talk to anybody, would you then be willing for the doctors to go ahead and do what they think should be done? . . .

Mr. Sorrow: That's an "if"—That's an "if" question.

Judge Todd: "If."

Miss Northern: I think that's an understandable idea.

Judge Todd: Yes, ma'am.

Miss Northern: An amongst your—your own opinion former—opinion former.

Judge Todd: Yes. Now, if the time comes that you are so sick that you can't make the decision, are you willing for the doctors to make the decision for you then?

Miss Northern: Well, I think that that's an unreasonable way to look at it because you want an opinion.

Judge Todd: Yes, ma'am.

Miss Northern: And you see, that's—that—Groundhog Day and the—all the weather and everything else, now, it's an opinion.

Judge Todd: Judge, is there anything you would like to ask?

Judge Drowota: Well, I have the same questions, though, with the "if." And as Reverend Sorrow has said, if in fact at some day there is a feeling that—and you are unconscious and we can't ask you—

Mr. Sorrow: It's a question of whether to let you die.

Judge Drowota: —should we let you die, or would you rather live your life without your feet?

Miss Northern: I am giving my feet a chance to get well.

Mr. Sorrow: Right, right. Okay. Let's say we have given it a chance to get well, and if the infection didn't get out of your system and you became unconscious, he is saying, would you rather—

Miss Northern: I am not making any further . . . statement.

Judge Todd: In other words, you are not willing to admit that you might get unconscious?

Miss Northern: No.

Judge Todd: I see. All right.

Miss Northern: You are pretty handsome; it's rather nice to have all you handsome men come at you this morning.

Mr. Sorrow: Can they look at your feet?

Miss Northern: No, no. Can you see me?

Judge Todd: I think maybe you better see your feet.

Miss Northern: You know where they are? . . . They are there.

Judge Todd: I need to ask you this, Miss Mary. . . . When have you seen your feet?

Mr. Sorrow: Have you seen them recently? Have they let you see your feet real close?

Miss Northern: They let me see my feet. I can see my feet.

Judge Todd: When did you see them, do you remember?

Miss Northern: I seen them two or three times. Don't look at the feet. Let's don't look at the feet.

Judge Todd: I tell you what let's do.

Miss Northern: Don't look at the feet.

Judge Todd: Let's don't look at the feet. I tell you what let's do. . . . Let's you and I look at them together at the same time and see what we can.

Miss Northern: They are down there.

Judge Todd: I want you to look at them with me. Would you do it?

Miss Northern: Isn't—I just don't understand, it's sadism about it. I can't understand it.

A Nurse: Let's all look at your feet.

Miss Northern: Okay. All right, General.

A Nurse: All of us together. Let's get your gown down. There we go. Now—

Miss Northern: That's all peeling off of that. It's all getting well. It's all going down.

Judge Drowota: Do you have feeling in your feet?

Miss Northern: Oh, yes, they were knocking all around, and they're banging up against this thing and everything.

Mr. Sorrow: Can you feel it when you do that?

Miss Northern: Yeah.

Mr. Sorrow: Is there feeling?

Miss Northern: Yeah. . . .

Judge Todd: —Would you—would you just bear with us just for one more thing?

Miss Northern: You want to establish your point.

Judge Todd: No, we don't. I am asking you—

Miss Northern: You got your points all in writing and established it, according to your own—

Judge Todd: Yes, ma'am. If the time comes that you have to choose between losing your feet and dying, would you rather just go ahead and die than lose your feet? If that time comes?

Miss Northern: It's possible—It's possible only if I—Just forget it. I—You are making me sick talking.

Judge Todd: I know. I know. And I am sorry. Would you be willing to say to me that you just don't want to live if you can't have your feet? Is that the way you feel?

Miss Northern: I don't understand why it's so important to you people, why it's so important. . . .

Judge Todd: Mrs. Mary, you see a judge has to see both sides of the thing, and these people have come and told us something, and now we want you to tell us what you want to tell us so we can decide.

Miss Northern: A billion of you have been here.

Judge Todd: I understand. And that's the reason we came out to see you, so we could let you—

Miss Northern: I don't want to discuss it any more. I made my point.

Judge Todd: I believe, Mrs. Mary, that you have made your point that you would rather—that you don't want to live if you can't have your feet; isn't that about it?

Miss Northern: That's possible. . . . It's possible to see it that way, to have that opinion. I don't want you all to change your opinion.

Judge Todd: No. I want you to tell me if you really feel that way. Tell me because I want to know it. I want to consider how you feel.

Judge Drowota: Or if you would rather live and have your feet. I mean, without your feet. See, you have got me confused, Miss Mary.

Judge Todd: She wants to live and have her feet.

Mr. Sorrow: That's exactly what she wants.

Miss Northern: This is ridiculous. I am tired. And ridiculous, you know it is.

Mr. Sorrow: I think they are trying to look at your side of it and understand how you feel, and, of course, somebody else in your position, we don't know what we would do, and so I guess they are saying so many people have told these judges so much they want to see Miss Mary and say, "How do you feel, how do you feel?"

Miss Northern: It's gotten a little roll.

Mr. Sorrow: Like a snowball.

Miss Northern: This is—Let's leave it alone. Let's leave it alone. And you keep your opinions. I am through with it.

Judge Todd: I wish I could be through with it. Let me leave you with a little thought, Miss Mary.

Miss Northern: All right. . . .

Judge Todd: Did you ever read the Sermon on the Mount?

Miss Northern: Yes.

Judge Todd: You remember one thing the Good Lord said?

Miss Northern: What?

Judge Todd: If thy eye offend thee,—

Miss Northern: Oh, yes, take the eye out.

Judge Todd: —cast it out. If thy hand offend you, cut it off. Now, if and when your feet begin to offend you, maybe, maybe, you will remember that little verse.

Miss Northern: I thank you.

DECIDING FOR OTHERS: COMPETENCY

Allen Buchanan and Dan W. Brock

COMPETENCE AND INCOMPETENCE

Discussions of competence have often been hampered by a failure to distinguish carefully among the following questions:

- What is the appropriate *concept* of competence?
- Given an analysis of the appropriate concept of competence, what *standard* (or standards) of competence must be met if an individual is to be judged to be competent?
- What are the most reliable *operational measures* for ascertaining whether a given standard of competence is met?

From Allen Buchanan and Dan W. Brock, "Deciding for Others: Competency," *Milbank Quarterly* 64, no. 2 (1986): 67–80, Blackwell Publishers.

Editors' note: Authors' notes have been cut. Students who want to follow up on sources should consult the original article.

- *Who* ought to make a determination of competence?
- What *sorts of institutional arrangements* are needed to assure that determinations of competence are made in an accurate and responsible way?

Each of these questions will be addressed separately. This section—which is concerned with the theoretical underpinnings of determinations of competence—will concentrate on the first three questions. The last two, which raise more practical and concrete concerns, can only be addressed in detail after the ethical framework has been laid out and the realities of current practices have been described.

THE CONCEPT OF COMPETENCE

Competence as Decision-Relative

The statement that a particular individual is (or is not) competent is incomplete. Competence is always competence *for some task*—competence *to do something.*

The concern here is with competence to perform the task of making a decision. Hence, competence is to be understood as *decision-making capacity.* But the notion of decision-making capacity is itself incomplete until the nature of the choice as well as the conditions under which it is to be made are specified. Thus competence is decision-relative, not global. A person may be competent to make a particular decision at a particular time, under certain circumstances, but incompetent to make another decision, or even the same decision under different conditions. A competency determination, then, is a determination of a particular person's capacity to perform a particular decision-making task at a particular time and under specified conditions.

Any individual may be competent to perform some tasks (e.g., drive a car), but not others (e.g., solve differential equations). The tasks relevant to this article vary substantially, and include making decisions about medical treatment, entering into contracts, deciding whether to continue to live on one's own in an unsupervised setting, and so forth. It is true, of course, that for some individuals, decision-making capacity is entirely lacking (for instance, when the individual is permanently unconscious), but these are the unproblematic cases.

Decision-making tasks vary substantially in the capacities they require for performance at an appropriate level of adequacy. For example, even restricted to medical treatment decisions, there is substantial variation in the complexity of information that is relevant to a particular treatment decision and that, consequently, must be understood by the decision maker. There is, therefore, variation in what might be called the *objective demands* of the task in question—here, the level of abilities to understand, reason, and decide about the options in question. But there is also variation of several sorts in a subject's ability to meet the demands of a particular decision. Many factors that diminish or eliminate competence altogether vary over time in their presence or severity in a particular person. For example, the effects of dementia on a person's cognitive capacities is at some stages commonly not constant, particularly in cases of borderline competence. Instead, mental confusion may come and go; periods of great confusion are sometimes followed by comparative lucidity.

In other cases, the environment and the behavior of others may affect the relative level of decision-making competence. For example, side effects of medications often impair competence, but a change of medication may reduce those effects. Behavior of others may create stresses for a person that diminish decision-making capacities, but that behavior can often be altered, or the situations in which it occurs can be avoided. Further, cognitive functioning can sometimes be enhanced by familiar surroundings and diminished by unfamiliar ones. A person may be competent to make a decision about whether to have an elective surgical procedure if the choice is presented in the familiar surroundings of home by someone known and trusted, but may be incompetent to make that same choice in what is found to be the intimidating, confusing, and unfamiliar environment of a hospital.

Factors such as these mean that even for a given decision, a person's competence may vary over time, and so be intermittent. The values that support the right of the competent person to participate in health care decisions also require that caretakers utilize periods of lucidity when they occur. Sometimes the emergency nature of the situation will not permit this, but it is no doubt possible to involve intermittently competent persons in decision making substantially more than is done at present. Sometimes, with opportune timing or other appropriate measures (such as medications), the intermittently competent person may be able to be involved in decision making at a time when he or she is clearly competent. Often, however, the person either consistently remains in, or can only be brought to, a state of borderline competence for the decision at hand. These borderline cases of questionable competence require more careful analysis of and clarity about the nature of the competency determination. They also illustrate the need for greater sophistication on the part of medical care providers and others about physical and mental problems that frequently affect the elderly.

Capacities Needed for Competence

What capacities are necessary for a person competently to decide about such matters as health care, living arrangements, financial affairs, and so forth? As already noted, the demands of these different decisions will vary, but it is nevertheless possible to generalize about the necessary abilities. Two may be distinguished: the capacity for communication and understanding, and the capacity for reasoning and deliberation. Although these capacities are not entirely distinct, significant deficiencies in any of them can result in diminished decision-making competence. A third important element of competence is that the individual must have a set of values or conception of the good.

Under *communication and understanding* are included the various capacities that allow a person to take part in the process of becoming informed on and expressing a choice about a given decision. These include the ability to communicate and the possession of various linguistic, conceptual, and cognitive abilities necessary for an understanding of the particular information relevant to the decision at hand. The relevant cognitive abilities, in particular, are often impaired by disease processes to which the elderly are especially subject, including most obviously various forms of dementia, but also aphasia due to stroke and, in some cases, reduced intellectual performance associated with depression (pseudodementia). Even where cognitive function is only minimally impaired, ability to express desires and beliefs may be greatly diminished or absent (as in some patients with amyotrophic lateral sclerosis).

Understanding also requires the ability to appreciate the nature and meaning of potential alternatives—what it would be and "feel" like to be in possible future states and to undergo various experiences. In young children this is often prevented by the lack of sufficient life experience. In the case of elderly persons facing diseases with progressive and extremely debilitating deterioration, it is hindered by people's generally limited ability to understand a kind of experience radically different from their own and by the inability of severely impaired individuals to communicate the character of their own experience to others. Major psychological blocks—such as fear, denial, and depression—can also significantly impair the appreciation of information about an unwanted or dreaded alternative. In general, communication and understanding require the capacities to receive, process, and make available for use the information relevant to particular decisions.

Competence also requires *capacities for reasoning and deliberation*. These include capacities to draw inferences about the consequences of making a certain choice and to compare alternative outcomes based on how they further one's good or promote one's ends. Some capacity to employ rudimentary probabilistic reasoning about uncertain outcomes will commonly be necessary, as well as the capacity to give due consideration to potential future outcomes in a present decision. Reasoning and deliberation obviously make use of both capacities mentioned earlier: understanding the information and applying the decision maker's values.

Finally, a competent decision maker also requires *a set of values or conception of what is good* that is reasonably consistent and stable. This is needed in order to be able to evaluate particular outcomes as benefits or harms, goods or evils, and to assign different relative weight or importance to them. Often what will be needed is the capacity to decide on the import and relative weight to be accorded different values, since that may not have been fully determined before a particular choice must be made. Competence does not require a fully consistent set of goals, much less a detailed "life plan" to cover all contingencies. Sufficient internal consistency and stability over time in the values relative to a particular decision, however, are needed to yield a decision outcome. Although values change over time and although ambivalence is inevitable in the difficult choices faced by many persons of questionable competence concerning their medical care, living arrangements, and personal affairs, sufficient value stability is needed to permit, at the very least, a decision that can be stated and adhered to over the course of its discussion, initiation, and implementation.

Competence as a Threshold Concept, Not a Comparative One

Decision-making competence, and the skills and capacities necessary to it, is one of the three components in standard analyses of the requirements for informed consent in health care decision making. The informed-consent doctrine requires the free and informed consent of a competent patient to medical procedures that are to be performed. The idea underlying this doctrine is that of a patient deciding, in consultation with a physician, what health care, if any, will best serve the patient's aims and needs. If the decision is not voluntary, but instead coerced or manipulated, it will likely serve another's ends or another's view of the patient's good, not the patient's own view, and will, in a significant sense, originate with another and not the patient. If the appropriate information is not provided to the individual in a form the patient can understand, the patient will not be able to ascertain how available alternatives might serve his or her aims. Finally, if the patient is not competent, either the individual will be unable to decide at all or the decision-making process will be seriously flawed.

Sometimes incompetence will be uncontroversially complete, as with patients who are in a persistent vegetative state or who are in a very advanced state of dementia, unable to communicate coherently at all. Often, however, defects in the capacities and skills noted above as necessary to competence will be partial and a matter of degree, just as whether a patient's decision is voluntary or involuntary, informed or uninformed, is also often a matter of degree. Does this mean that competence itself should be thought of as sometimes partial and possessed in different degrees? It is certainly the case that persons are commonly thought of and said to be more or less competent to perform many tasks, not just decision making. Nevertheless, because of the role competency determinations play in health care generally, and in the legal process in particular, it is important to resist the notion that persons can be determined to be more or less competent, or competent to some degree. The difficulty with taking literally the notion that competence is a matter of degree can be seen clearly by looking at the function of the competency determination within the practice of informed consent for health care, or within other areas of the law in which it plays a role, such as conservatorship or guardianship for financial affairs.

That function is, first and foremost, to sort persons into two classes: (1) those whose voluntary decisions (about their health care, financial affairs, and so on) must be respected by others and accepted as binding, and (2) those whose decisions, even if uncoerced, will be set aside and for whom others will be designated as surrogate decision makers. The function of the competency determination, then, is to make an "all or nothing" classification of persons

with regard to their competence to make particular decisions, not to make "matter of degree" findings about their decision-making capacities and skills. Persons are judged, both in the law and more informally in health care settings, to be either competent or incompetent to make a particular decision—even though the underlying capacities and skills forming the basis of that judgment are possessed in different degrees. Competence, then, is in this sense a threshold concept, not a comparative one.

The foregoing makes clear that the crucial question in the competency determination is *how* defective an individual's capacities and skills to make a particular decision must be for the individual to be found incompetent to make that decision, so that a surrogate decision maker becomes necessary. In keeping with the primary objective of this article, the analysis of that question focuses on medical decisions. Here, the familiar doctrine of informed consent provides considerable guidance.

The central purpose of assessing competence is to determine whether a patient may assert his or her right to decide to accept or refuse a particular medical procedure, or whether that right shall be transferred to a surrogate. We must, therefore, ask what values are at stake in whether people are allowed to make such decisions for themselves. The informed-consent doctrine assigns the decision-making right to patients themselves; but what fundamental values are served by the practice of informed consent? In the literature dealing with informed consent, many different answers—and ways of formulating answers—to that question have been proposed, but we believe the most important values at stake are: (1) promoting and protecting the patient's well-being, and (2) respecting the patient's self-determination. It is in examining the effect of these two values that the answer to the proper standard of decision-making competence will be found.

STANDARDS OF COMPETENCE: UNDERLYING VALUES

Promotion of Individual Well-Being

There is a long tradition in medicine that the physician's first and most important commitment should be to serve the well-being of the patient. The more recent doctrine of informed consent is consistent with that tradition, if it is assumed that, at least in general, competent individuals are better judges of their own good than others are. The doctrine recognizes that while the physician commonly brings to the physician-patient encounter medical training that the patient lacks, the patient brings knowedge that the physician lacks: knowledge of particular subjective aims and values that are likely to be affected by whatever decision is made.

As medicine's arsenal of possible interventions has dramatically expanded in recent decades, alternative treatments (and the alternative of no treatment) now routinely promise different mixes of benefits and risks to the patient. Moreover, since health is only one value among many, and is assigned different importance by different persons, there is commonly no one single intervention for a particular condition that is best for everyone. Which, if any, intervention best serves a particular patient's well-being will depend in part on that patient's aims and values. Health care decision making thus usually ought to be a joint undertaking between physician and patient, since each brings knowledge and experience that the other lacks, yet that is necessary for decisions that will best serve the patient's well-being.

In the exercise of their right to give informed consent, then, patients often decide in ways that they believe will best promote their own well-being as they conceive it. As is well known, and as physicians are frequently quick to point out, however, the complexity of many treatment decisions—together with the stresses of illness with its attendant fear, anxiety, dependency, and regression, not to mention the physical effects of illness itself—means that a patient's ordinary decision-making abilities are often significantly diminished. Thus, a patient's treatment choices may fail to serve his or her good or well-being, even as that person conceives it. Although one important value requiring patient participation in their own health care decision making is the promotion of patient well-being, that same value sometimes also requires persons to be protected from the harmful consequences to them of their own choices.

Respect for Individual Self-Determination

The other principal value underlying the informed-consent doctrine is respect for a patient's self-determination, understood here as a person's interest in making important decisions about his or her own life. Although often conceived in the law under the right to privacy, the leading legal decisions in the informed-consent tradition appeal fundamentally to the right of individual self-determination. No attempt will be made here to analyze the complex of ideas giving context to the concept of individual self-determination, nor of the various values that support its importance. But it is essential to underline that many persons commonly want to make important decisions about their life for themselves, and that desire is in part independent of whether they believe that they are always in a position to make the best choice. Even when we believe that others may be able to decide for us better than we ourselves can, we sometimes prefer to decide for ourselves so as to be in charge of and responsible for our lives.

The interest in self-determination should not be overstated, however. People often wish to make such decisions for themselves simply because they believe that, at least in most cases, they are in a better position to decide what is best for themselves than others are. Thus, when in a particular case others are demonstrably in a better position to decide for us than we ourselves are, a part, but not all, of our interest in deciding for ourselves is absent.

Conflict Between the Values of Self-Determination and Well-Being

Because people's interest in making important decisions for themselves is not based solely on their concern for their own well-being, these two values of patient well-being and self-determination can sometimes conflict. Some people may appear to decide in ways that are contrary to their own best interests or well-being, even as determined by their own settled conception of their good, and others may be unable to convince them of their mistake. In other cases, others may know little of a person's own settled values, and the person may simply be deciding in a manner sharply in conflict with how most reasonable persons would decide. It may be difficult or even impossible to determine, however, whether this conflict is simply the result of a difference in values between this individual and most reasonable persons (for example, a difference in the weights assigned to various goods), or whether it results from some failure of the patient to assess correctly what will best serve his or her own interests or good.

In the conflict between the values of self-determination and patient well-being, a tradeoff between avoiding two kinds of errors should be sought. The first error is that of failing to protect a person from the harmful consequences of his or her decision when the decision is the result of serious defects in the capacity to decide. The second error is failing to permit someone to make a decision and turning the decision over to another, when the patient is able to make the decision him or herself. With a stricter or higher standard for competence, more people will be found incompetent, and the first error will be minimized at the cost of increasing the second sort of error. With a looser or more minimal standard for competence, fewer persons will be found incompetent, and the second sort of error is more likely to be minimized at the cost of increasing the first.

Evidence regarding a person's competence to make a particular decision is often uncertain, incomplete, and conflicting. Thus, no conceivable set of procedures and standards for judging competence could guarantee the elimination of all error. Instead, the challenge is to strike the appropriate balance and thereby minimize the incidence of either of the errors noted above. No set of procedures will guarantee that all and only the incompetent are judged to be incompetent.

But procedures and standards for competence are not merely inevitably imperfect. They are inevitably *controversial* as well. In the determination of competence, there is disagreement not only about which procedures will minimize errors, but also about the proper standard that the procedures should be designed to approximate. The core of the controversy derives from the different values that different persons assign to protecting individuals' well-being as against respecting their self-determination. We believe there is no uniquely "correct" answer to the relative weight that should be assigned to these two values, and in any event it is simply a fact that different persons do assign them different weight.

DECIDING ON STANDARDS OF COMPETENCE

Focusing only on the two values of patient well-being and self-determination is an oversimplification. Because other values are at stake, room for controversy about the proper standard of competence increases. For example, also important to the appropriate standard of competence is the value of maintaining public confidence in the integrity of the medical profession, so as to protect and foster the trust necessary to physician-patient relationships that function well.

The standard of competence, then, cannot be discovered. There is no reason to believe that there is one and only one optimal tradeoff to be struck between the competing values of well-being and self-determination, nor, hence, any one uniquely correct level of capacity at which to set the threshold of competence—even for a particular decision under specified circumstances. In this sense, setting a standard for competence is a value choice, not a scientific or factual matter. Nevertheless, the choice need not be and should not be arbitrary. Instead, it should be grounded in (1) a reflective appreciation of the values in question, (2) a clear understanding of the goals that the determination of competence is to serve, and (3) an accurate prediction of the practical consequences of setting the threshold at this level rather than elsewhere.

People may disagree on exactly where the threshold should be set not only because they assign different weights to the values of self-determination and well-being, but also because they make different estimates of the probability that others will err in trying to promote a person's interests. Unanimous agreement on an optimal standard is not necessary, however, for workable social arrangements for determining competence, any more than it is for determining who may vote or who may drive an automobile.

Different Standards of Competence

A number of different standards of competence have been identified and supported in the literature, though statutory and case law provide little help in articulating precise standards. It is not feasible to discuss here all the alternatives that have been proposed. Instead, the range of alternatives will be delineated and the difficulties of the main standards will be examined.

No single standard is adequate for all medical treatment decisions, much less so for decisions about living arrangements, financial affairs, participation in research, and so forth. It was argued above that a standard of competence must set a balance between the two principal values at stake in health care decision making: promoting and protecting the patient's well-being while respecting the patient's self-determination.

An example of a minimal standard of competence is that the patient merely be able to express a preference. This standard respects every expressed choice of a patient, and so is not, in fact, a criterion of *competent* choice at all. It entirely disregards whether defects or mistakes are present in the reasoning process leading to the choice, whether the choice is in accord with the patient's conception of his or her good, and whether the choice would be harmful to the patient. It thus fails to provide any protection for patient well-being, and it is insensitive to the way the value of self-determination itself varies with differences in people's capacities to choose in accordance with their conceptions of their own good.

At the other extreme are standards that look to the *content* or *outcome* of the decision, for example, the standard that the choice be a reasonable one, or be what other reasonable or rational persons would choose. On this view, failure of the patient's choice to match some such allegedly objective standard of choice entails that it is an incompetent choice. Such a standard maximally protects patient well-being—according to the standard's conception of well-being—but fails adequately to respect patient self-determination.

At bottom, a person's interest in self-determination is his or her interest in defining, revising over time, and pursuing his or her own particular conception of the good life. There are serious risks associated with any purportedly objective standard for the correct decision—the standard may ignore the patient's own distinctive conception of the good and may involve the substitution of another's conception of what is best for the patient. Moreover, even such a standard's claim to protect maximally a patient's well-being is only as strong as the objective account of a person's well-being on which the standard rests.

The issue is theoretically complex and controversial, but any standard of individual well-being that does not ultimately rest on an individual's own informed preferences is both problematic in theory and subject to intolerable abuse in practice. Thus, a standard that judges competence by comparing the content of a patient's decision to some objective standard for the correct decision may fail even to protect appropriately a patient's well-being. An adequate standard of competence will focus primarily not on the content of the patient's decision, but on the *process* of reasoning that leads up to that decision.

While an adequate competency evaluation and standard focuses on the patient's understanding and reasoning, rather than upon the particular decision that issues from them, the key issue remains. What level of reasoning is required for the patient to be competent? In other words, how well must the patient understand and reason to be competent? How much can understanding be limited or reasoning be defective and still be compatible with competence? It is important to emphasize another question faced by those evaluating competence. How certain must those persons evaluating competence be about how well the patient has understood and reasoned in coming to a decision? This last question is important because it is common in cases of marginal or questionable competence for there to be a significant degree of uncertainty about the patient's decision-making process that can never be eliminated.

Relation of the Standard of Competence to Expected Harms and Benefits

Because the competency evaluation requires setting a balance between the two values of respecting patients' rights to decide for themselves and protecting them from the harmful consequences of their own choices, it should be clear that no single standard of competence—no single answer to the questions above—can be adequate. That is simply because the degree of expected harm from choices made at a given level of understanding and reasoning can vary from virtually none to the most serious, including major disability or death.

There is an important implication of this view that the standard of competence ought to vary with the expected harms or benefits to the patient of acting in accordance with a choice—namely, that just because a patient is competent to consent to a treatment, it does not follow that the patient is competent to refuse it, and vice versa. For example, consent to a low-risk life-saving procedure by an otherwise healthy individual should require a minimal level of competence, but refusal of that same procedure by such an individual should require the highest level of competence.

Because the appropriate level of competence properly required for a particular decision must be adjusted to the consequences of acting on that decision, no single standard of decision-making competence is adequate. Instead, the level of competence appropriately required for decision making varies along a full range from low/minimal to high/maximal. Table 1 illustrates this variation.

The presumed net balance of expected benefits and risks of patient choice in comparison with other alternatives refers to the physician's assessment of the expected effects in achieving the goals of prolonging life, preventing injury and disability, and relieving suffering from a particular treatment option as against its risks of harm. The table indicates that the relevant comparison is with other available alternatives, and the degree to which the net benefit/risk balance of the alternative chosen is better or worse than that for other treatment options. It should be noted that a choice might properly require only low/minimal competence, although its expected risks

exceeded its expected benefits, because all other available alternatives had substantially worse expected risk/benefit ratios.

Table 1 also indicates, for each level of competence, the grounds for believing that a patient's own choice best promotes his or her well-being. This brings out an important point. For all patient choices, other people responsible for deciding whether those choices should be respected should have grounds for believing that the choice, if it is to be honored, is reasonably in accord with the patient's good and does reasonably protect or promote the patient's well-being (though the choice need not, of course, *maximize* the patient's interests). When the patient's level of decision-making competence is only at the low/minimal level, the grounds derive only minimally from the fact that the patient has chosen the option in question; they principally stem from others' positive assessment of the choice's expected effects for life and health.

At the other extreme, when the expected effects of the patient's choice for life and health appear to be substantially worse than available alternatives, the requirement of a high/maximal level of competence provides grounds for relying on the patient's decision

---

TABLE 1

Decision-Making Competence and Patient Well-Being

Presumed net balance of expected benefits and risks of patient choice in comparison with other alternatives	Level of decision-making competence required	Grounds for believing patient's choice best promotes/protects own well-being
Net balance substantially better than for possible alternatives.	Low/minimal	Principally the benefit/risk assessment made by others.
Net balance roughly comparable to that of other alternatives.	Moderate/median	Roughly equally from the benefit/risk assessment made by others and from the patient's decision that the chosen alternative best fits patient's conception of own good.
Net balance substantially worse than for another alternative or alternatives.	High/maximal	Principally from patient's decision that the chosen alternative best fits own conception of own good.

as itself establishing that the choice best fits the patient's good (his or her own particular aims and ends). That highest level of competence is required to rebut the presumption that if the choice seems not best to promote life and health, then that choice is not, in fact, reasonably related to the patient's interests.

When the expected effects for life and health of the patient's choice are approximately comparable to those of alternatives, a moderate/median level of competence is sufficient to provide reasonable grounds that the choice promotes the patient's good and that his or her well-being is adequately protected. It is also reasonable to assume that as the level of competence increases (from minimal to maximal), the value or importance of respecting the patient's self-determination increases as well, since a part of the value of self-determination rests on the assumption that persons will secure their good when they choose for themselves. As competence increases, the likelihood of this happening increases.

Thus, according to the concept of competence endorsed here, a particular individual's decision-making capacity at a given time may be sufficient for making a decision to refuse a diagnostic procedure when forgoing the procedure does not carry a significant risk, although it would not necessarily be sufficient for refusing a surgical procedure that would correct a life-threatening condition. The greater the risk—where risk is a function of the severity of the expected harm and the probability of its occurrence—the greater the level of communication, understanding, and reasoning skills required for competence to make that decision. It is not always true, however, that if a person is competent to make one decision, then he or she is competent to make another decision so long as it involves equal risk. Even if this risk is the same, one decision may be more complex, and hence require a higher level of capacity for understanding options and reasoning about consequences.

Relation of Refusal of Treatment to Determination of Incompetence

A common criticism of the way physicians actually practice is that patients' competence is rarely questioned until they refuse to consent to a physician's recommendation for treatment. It is no doubt true

that patients' competence when they accept physicians' treatment recommendations should be questioned more often than it now is, because consent without understanding provides little basis for believing the choice is best for the patient, and because the physician's judgment about what is medically best is fallible. Nevertheless, treatment refusal does reasonably raise the question of a patient's competence in a way that acceptance of recommended treatment does not. It is a reasonable assumption that physicians' treatment recommendations are more often than not in the interests of their patients. Consequently, it is a reasonable presumption—though rebuttable in any particular instance—that a treatment refusal is contrary to the patient's interest. Exploration of the reasons for the patient's response, including determination of whether the decision was a competent one, are appropriate—though reassessment of the recommendation is often appropriate as well.

It is essential to distinguish here, however, between grounds for calling a patient's competence into question and grounds for a finding of incompetence. Treatment refusal does reasonably serve to trigger a competency evaluation. On the other hand, a disagreement with the physician's recommendation or refusal of a treatment recommendation is no basis whatsoever for a finding of incompetence. This conclusion follows from the premise noted earlier that the competency evaluation, as well as evidence in support of a finding of incompetence, should address the *process* of understanding and reasoning of the patient, *not* the *content* of a decision.

Another essential distinction is between two quite different types of treatment refusal: a refusal of all the treatment options offered, and refusing the one treatment that the physician believes to be best while accepting an alternative treatment that lies within the range of medically sound options. If there is more than one medically sound treatment option—in the sense that competent medical judgment is divided as to which of two or more treatments would be optimal—then the patient's refusal to accept the option that the physician believes is optimal should not even raise the question of the patient's competence, much less entail a finding of incompetence, at least so long as the option the patient chooses lies within the range of medically sound options.

CONTRAST WITH FIXED MINIMUM THRESHOLD CONCEPTION OF COMPETENCE

Before elaborating the implications of this analysis for operational measurements of competence, it will be useful to contrast it with a widely held alternative conception that has been implicitly rejected here. According to this other conception—which may be called the "fixed minimal capacity" view—competence is *not* decision-relative. The simplest version of this view holds that a person is competent if he or she possesses the relevant decision-making capacities at some specified level, regardless of whether the decision to be made is risky or nonrisky, and regardless of whether the information to be understood or the consequences to be reasoned through are simple or complex. This concept of competence might also be called the "minimal threshold status concept," since the idea is that if a person's decision-making capacities meet or exceed the specified threshold, then the status of being a *competent individual* is to be ascribed to that person. According to this view, competence is an attribute of persons dependent solely on the level of decision-making capacities they possess (though these may vary, of course, from day to day or even from hour to hour, depending upon the effects of disease, medications, emotional states, and so on).

In contrast, according to the conception of competence espoused here, competence is a *relational* property. Whether a person is competent to make a given decision depends not only upon that person's own capacities but also upon certain features of the decision—including risk and information requirements. There are at least five points in favor of this approach.

First, a concept that allows a raising or lowering of the standard for decision-making capacities depending upon the risks of the decision in question is clearly more consonant with the way people actually make informal competency determinations in areas of judgment in which they have the greatest confidence and in which there is the most consensus. For example, you may decide that your 5-year-old child is competent to choose between a hamburger and a hotdog for lunch, but you would not think the child competent to make a decision about how to invest a large sum of money. This is because the risk

in the latter case is greater, and the information required for reasoning about the relevant consequences of the options is much more complex. It is worth emphasizing that incompetence due to developmental immaturity, as in the case of a child, is in many respects quite different from the increasing incompetence due to a degenerative disease such as Alzheimer's. These and other cases of incompetence do have in common, however, the relevance of the degree of risk for determining the appropriate level of competence.

Second, the decision-relative concept of competence also receives indirect support from the doctrine of informed consent. The more risky the decision a patient must make, and the more complex the array of possible benefits and burdens, the greater the amount of information that must be provided and the higher the standard of understanding required on the part of the patient. For extremely low-risk procedures, with a clear and substantial benefit and an extremely small probability of significant harm, the information that must be provided to the patient is correspondingly less.

Third, perhaps the most important reason for preferring the decision-relative concept of competence is that it better coheres with our basic legal framework in two distinct respects. First, in its treatment of minors, the law has already tacitly adopted the decision-relative concept and rejected the minimum threshold concept. The courts as well as legislatures now recognize that a child can be competent to make some decisions but not others—that competence is not an all-or-nothing status—and that features of the decision itself (including risk) are relevant factors in determining whether the child is competent to make that decision. This approach is increasingly popular, and is utilized in, for example, "limited conservatorships," where some decision-making authority is expressly left with the conservatee.

In addition, the law in this country has, in general, steadfastly refused to recognize a right to interfere with a *competent* patient's voluntary choice on purely paternalistic grounds—that is, solely to prevent harms or to secure benefits for the competent patient him or herself. Instead, the law makes a finding of incompetence a necessary condition for justified paternalism. According to the decision-relative concept of competence, the greater the potential harm to the individual, the higher the standard of competence.

From this it follows that a finding of incompetence is more likely in precisely those instances in which the case for paternalism is strongest—cases in which great harm can be easily avoided by taking the decision out of the individual's hands. Thus, the concept of competence favored here allows paternalism in situations in which the case for paternalism seems strongest, while at the same time preserving the law's fundamental tenet that, in general, people may be treated paternalistically only when they are incompetent to make their own decisions.

The fourth reason for preferring the decision-relative concept of competence is that it allows a finding of incompetence for a particular decision to be limited to that decision, and so it is not equivalent to a change in the person's overall status as a decision maker. Consequently, the decision-relative concept of competence contains a built-in safeguard to allay the fear that paternalism—even if justified in a particular case considered in isolation—is likely to spill over into other areas, eventually robbing the individual of all sovereignty over his or her own life. Further, any finding of incompetence is likely to evoke strong psychological reactions from some patients because to be labeled as "an incompetent" is to be returned to a childlike status. By making it clear that incompetence is decision-relative and hence may be limited to certain areas, the concept of competence used here can at least minimize the potentially devastating assault on self-esteem that a finding of incompetence represents to some individuals.

Finally, the decision-relative concept of competence has another clear advantage over the minimum threshold concept: It allows a better balance between the competing values of self-determination and well-being that are to be served by a determination of competence. The alternative concept, on its most plausible interpretation, also represents a balancing of these fundamental values, but in a cruder fashion. Setting a minimal threshold of decision-making capacities represents a choice about the proper balance of tradeoff between respect for self-determination and concern for well-being, but it does so on the basis of an extremely sweeping, unqualified generalization—about the probability that unacceptable levels of harm will occur if individuals are left free to choose—over an indefinitely large number of highly diverse potential decisions.

But as indicated earlier, decisions can vary enormously in their information requirements, in the reasoning ability needed to draw inferences about relevant consequences, and in the magnitude of risk involved. Hence, any such sweeping generalization will be very precarious. If the generalization errs in one direction—by underestimating the overall harm that would befall individuals if the threshold for competence were set at one level—then the minimal threshold of decision-making capacities will be set so low that many people who are judged competent will make disastrous choices. If the generalization errs in the other direction—by overestimating the harm that would result if the threshold were set at a particular level—then many people will be interfered with for no good reason. Thus, regardless of where the minimal threshold is set, it seems likely that it will provide either too much protection or too little. The decision-relative concept of competence avoids relying upon such crude generalizations about harm and permits a finer balance to be struck between the goods of protecting well-being and respecting self-determination.

A CHRONICLE: DAX'S CASE AS IT HAPPENED

Keith Burton

. . . *The story of Don Cowart is remarkable in some ways but commonplace in others. A man's wish to die is rather extraordinary in and of itself; but the pattern of events that shapes such a wish often is woven of the fabric of life's everyday occurrences. Such is the case with Cowart.*

Ray and Ada Cowart moved their family from the Rio Grande Valley to the small East Texas town of Henderson in the sixties. Ray prospered over the years as a rancher and real estate agent. Ada became a teacher in the Henderson school district. Their three children—Don, Jim, and Beth—were no different from other kids reared in a close-knit community. In fact, they were ordinary people living ordinary lives.

"Donny Boy," as he came to be called by his father, was popular in school and excelled in athletics. He was captain of his high school football team and performed in rodeos. He liked to take risks, a trait that often dismayed his mother. It was risk taking that would later lure him to skydiving, surfing, and other sports of chance.

Don Cowart left Henderson in 1966 to attend the University of Texas at Austin. He had planned to return home at his graduation three years later to join his father in business; however, when notified of his military draft selection, Cowart instead elected to join the U.S. Air Force. He became a pilot and served in Vietnam. He married a high school sweetheart in 1972, but they divorced eight months later. In May 1973 he was discharged from active duty and returned to Henderson, where he began working with his father in real estate.

July 23, 1973, seemed no different to Cowart from any other Wednesday. It was hot and sultry as the afternoon sun slipped low along the pine trees in the countryside near Henderson. Ray and Don had driven out to a ranch to look over some property being offered for sale by the owner. They parked their car on a bridge over a dry creek and took off by foot. They talked and laughed together as they surveyed points of interest on the land. Their business completed, the Cowarts then returned to their car to go home for dinner.

The accident happened with no warning. The Cowart men had returned to their car but had not been able to start the engine. Ray had lifted the hood and removed the air cleaner from the engine. He primed the carburetor by hand and instructed Don to try the ignition. Several tries failed. It seemed to Don that the battery was near exhaustion. A final attempt proved fateful, however, as a blue flame shot from the carburetor and ignited a terrible explosion and fire.

Ray Cowart was hurled into heavy underbrush by the force of the explosion. The blast rocked the car and showered window glass over Don's body. Around them, the fireball spread quickly, consuming pine trees and the scrub vegetation in the area. Don reacted quickly. He climbed from the burning car and began running toward the woods. But he was forced to stop by a fear that he would become entangled in the underbrush and slowly burn to death.

Don wheeled about and decided to chance the dirt road on which they had driven in. He ran through three walls of fire, emerged into a clearing, then fell to the ground and rolled his body to extinguish the flames. He got back to his feet and resumed running in search of help for his father.

It all seemed dreamlike. Don noticed his vision was blurred as though swimming under water. His eyes had been badly burned. Now the pain was coming in waves, and he knew it was real. He kept running.

Loud voices filtered through the woods. Don collapsed at the roadside as help arrived. He heard the footsteps of a man and then the exclamation, "Oh, my God!" when a farmer found him. Don sent the man after his father and lay wondering how badly he was burned. When the man returned, Don asked him to bring a gun—a gun he would use to kill himself. The farmer refused.

In shock, Don assumed he and his father had caused the explosion by igniting gasoline from the car's engine. Later he would learn that the explosion actually had been caused by a leaking propane gas transmission line in the area where they had parked. It was a freak event.

From *Dax's Case: Essays in Medical Ethics and Human Meaning,* edited by Lonnie D. Kliever, Southern Methodist University Press, 1989. Reprinted with permission.

Editors' note: Some text has been cut. Students who want to read the article in its entirety should consult the original.

A pocket of propane gas had formed in the dry creek bed. When the carburetor flamed up, it had ignited the gas.

Rescuers took the Cowart men to a hospital in nearby Kilgore. There, a decision was made to transport them by ambulance to a special burn unit at Dallas's Parkland Hospital. Ray Cowart died en route to Dallas. Don Cowart remembers incredible pain, his begging for pain medication, and the paramedic's refusal to administer drugs prior to their arrival in Dallas. By this time, Ada Cowart, too, was on her way to Dallas. She had returned home first to pack several changes of clothes. The radio had said the men were badly hurt. She didn't expect to return to Henderson any time soon.

Even as the ambulance sped the 140 miles from Kilgore to Dallas, Don Cowart's treatment regimen had begun. By telephone, Dr. Charles Baxter, head of Parkland's burn unit, had directed fluid therapies to help in preventing shock to vital organs. On examination in Dallas, Baxter found Cowart had severe burns over 65 percent of his body. His face suffered third-degree burns and both eyes were severely damaged. His ears and hands were also deeply burned. Fluid therapies continued and were aided by several other measures: the insertion of an intertracheal tube to control the airway, catheters placed in every body opening, treatment with antibiotics, cleansing the wounds with antibacterial drugs, and tetanus prophylaxis. Heavy doses of narcotics were given for the pain.

In the early days of Don's 232-day hospitalization at Parkland, doctors could not predict whether he would survive. It was touch and go for many weeks. Ada Cowart felt helpless; she could do little more than sit in the waiting area outside the intensive care unit with relatives of other burn victims, where she prayed and hoped for the best. Doctors permitted only short visits with her son. Don had given his mother power of attorney in the Parkland emergency room, and she in turn deferred to the medical professionals on treatment decisions.

For Cowart, there were countless whirlpool tankings in solutions to cleanse his wounds, procedures to remove dead tissue, grafts to protect living tissue, the amputation of badly charred fingers from both hands and the removal of his right eye. The damaged left eye was sewn shut. And there was terrible pain.

Through it all, Don had remained constant in his view that he did not want to live. His demands to die had started with the farmer at the accident site. They had continued at the Kilgore hospital, in the ambulance, and now at Parkland. He didn't want treatment that would extend his misery and he made this known to his mother and

family, Dr. Charles Baxter, a nurse named Leslie Kerr, longtime friend Art Rousseau, attorney Rex Houston, and many others.

Baxter remained undaunted by Don's pleas to stop treatment, dismissing them at first as the typical response of burn victims to the pain of their wounds and treatment. In time, however, he openly discussed Cowart's wish to die with Don, his mother, and his lawyer, considering all the medical and legal ramifications. Failing to get Ada Cowart's and Rex Houston's consent to the withdrawal of treatment, Baxter continued to deliver it.

For her part, Ada Cowart understood her son's pain and anguish. She was haunted, nonetheless, by these thoughts: What if treatment were ceased and Don changed his mind in a near-death state? Would it be too late? Furthermore, her religious beliefs simply made mercy killing or suicide deplorable options. These religious constraints were reinforced by her fear that her son had not yet made his "peace with God."

Rex Houston also had mixed feelings about Don's wishes. On the one hand, he sympathized with Cowart's condition—being unable to so much as take medication to end his life without the assistance of others. On the other hand, it was Houston's duty to reach a favorable resolution of a lawsuit filed against the pipeline owners for Ray Cowart's death and for Don Cowart's disability. With regard to the latter, he needed a living plaintiff to achieve the best damage award for the Cowart family. Moreover, Houston believed that such an award would provide the financial means necessary for Don Cowart's ultimate rehabilitation. He therefore encouraged Cowart to see the legal proceedings through.

In February 1974, the lawsuit was settled out of court—one day prior to trial. Almost immediately, Don's demands to die quickened. There had been talk before with Art Rousseau of getting a gun. Don had asked Leslie Kerr if she would help him by injecting an overdose of medication. Now Cowart even talked with Houston about helping him get to a window of his sixth-floor hospital room, where presumably he would leap to his death. All listened but none agreed to help.

On March 12, 1974, Don was discharged from Parkland. He, his family, and his doctors agreed that his condition had improved sufficiently to warrant his transfer to the Texas Institute for Research and Rehabilitation in Houston. Nine months removed from his medical residency, Dr. Robert Meier of TIRR found Cowart to be a passive recipient of medical care, although the philosophy of treatment in this rehabilitation center encouraged patient involvement in treatment decisions. Previously Don had no say in his care; now he would be offered choices in his own treatment.

All seemed to go well during the first three weeks of his stay, until Cowart realized the pain he had endured might continue indefinitely, thanks to a careless comment by a resident plastic surgeon that his treatment would be years in completion. Faced with that prospect, Cowart refused treatment for his open burn areas and stopped taking food and water. In a matter of days, Cowart's medical condition deteriorated rapidly. Finding his patient in serious condition, Dr. Meier was deeply perplexed about what to do next. He believed it his duty to help Cowart achieve the highest measure of rehabilitation, but he was not inclined to force upon the patient care he did not wish to receive. Faced with this dilemma, he called for a meeting with Ada Cowart and Rex Houston to discuss with Don the future course of his treatment.

Ada Cowart was outraged by Don's condition. She had been discouraged from staying with her son at TIRR, and in her absence his burns had worsened. He was again near death, due to his refusal of whirlpool tankings and dressing changes. It was agreed in the meeting that Cowart would be transferred to the burn unit of John Sealy Hospital of the University of Texas Medical Branch in Galveston, where his injuries could again be treated by burn specialists.

On April 15, 1974, Don was admitted to the Galveston hospital, in chronic distress from infected wounds, poor nutrition, and severe depression. His right elbow and right wrist were locked tight. The stubs of his fingers on both hands were encased in grotesque skin "mittens." There was practically no skin on his legs. His right eye socket and closed left eye oozed infection. And excruciating pain remained his constant nemesis.

Active wound care was initiated immediately and further skin grafts were advised by Dr. Duane Larson to heal the open wounds on Cowart's chest, legs, and arms. But Cowart bitterly protested the daily tankings and refused to consent to surgery. One night he even crawled out of bed, hoping to throw himself through the window to his death, but he was discovered on the floor and returned to bed.

Frustrated by Cowart's behavior, Dr. Larson consulted Dr. Robert White of psychiatric services for an evaluation of Don's mental competency. White remembers being puzzled by Cowart: Was he a man who tolerated discomfort poorly or perhaps was profoundly depressed? Or was this an extraordinary man who had undergone such an incredible ordeal that he was frustrated beyond normal limits? White concluded, and a colleague confirmed, that Cowart was certainly not mentally incompetent. In fact, he was so impressed with the clarity of Cowart's expressed wish to die that he asked permission to do a videotape interview for classroom use in presenting the medical, ethical, and legal problems surrounding such cases. That filmed interview, which White entitled Please Let Me Die, eventually became a classic on patient rights in the field of medical ethics.

Having been declared mentally competent, Cowart still found it difficult to gain control over his treatment. He and his mother argued constantly over treatment procedures. Rex Houston helped get changes in his wound care but turned a deaf ear to Cowart's plea to go home to die from his wounds or to take his own life. In desperation, Cowart turned to other family members for assistance in securing legal representation, but without success. Finally, with White's help, Cowart reached an attorney who had represented Jehovah's Witnesses attempting to refuse medical treatment, but he was not optimistic that a lawsuit would free him from the hospital.

Rebuffed on every hand, Cowart reluctantly became more cooperative. White secured changes in Don's pain medication before and after the daily tankings, making treatments more bearable. Psychotherapy and medication helped improve his overall outlook by relieving his depression and improving his sleep. Encouraged that he might still regain sight in his left eye, Don more or less accepted his daily wound care and even agreed to surgical skin grafts early in June 1974. By July 15, his physical condition had improved enough to allow him to transfer out of the burn unit of the John Sealy Hospital to the psychiatric unit of the Jennie Sealy Hospital in the University of Texas Medical Branch under White's direct care while his wounds continued to heal.

Amid these changes there were still periodic conflicts between Cowart and those around him over his confinement in the hospital. There were reiterated demands to die and protests against treatment. A particularly explosive encounter between Cowart and Larson occurred on the day preceding his second and last major surgical procedure in the Galveston hospital. Cowart had agreed to undergo surgery to free up his hands, but the night before he changed his mind. The next morning, Larson angrily confronted Cowart with the challenge that, if he really wanted to die, he would agree to the surgery that would enable him to leave the hospital and go home where he could take his own life if he wished. Anxious to do exactly *that, Cowart consented to the surgery, which was performed on July 31.*

Don Cowart's stormy stay at Galveston finally ended on September 19, 1974. He had been hospitalized for a total of fourteen months, but at last he was going home. His prognosis upon dismissal was listed simply as "guarded."

Cowart was glad to be back in Henderson. The little things counted the most—sleeping in his own bed, listening to music, visiting with friends. But it was different for him than before the accident. He was totally blind, his left eye having failed to recover. His hands and arms remained useless. He was badly scarred. A dropped foot now required that someone assist him in walking. Some of his burn sites still were not healed.

Everything he did required the help of others. Someone had to feed him, bathe him, and help with personal functions. The days seemed endless. He tried to find peace in sleep, but even this dark release was impossible without drugs. While he couldn't see himself, Don knew his appearance drew whispers and stares in restaurants.

He had his tapes, talking books, television, and CB radio. He could use his sense of hearing, though not as well as before due to the explosion and burns. And he could think. For a while, he could see in his mind's eye the memories of earlier times. Then the memories started to fade.

Ada Cowart had lost much, but she never lost her religious faith. There had been times when even she had admitted that maybe it would have been best if Don had died with her husband. She reconciled her doubt with the thought that no mother can give up the life of a son. Ada never gave up hope that Don could find new faith in God.

Homecoming brought peace for a time. As Don's early excitement for returning home gave way to deep depression and despair, however, conflict returned to their lives. They argued about how he could occupy himself, how he dressed, his personal habits, and his future. Frustration led to a veiled suicide attempt, Don stealing away from the house during the night to try throwing himself in the path of trucks hauling clay to a brick plant. The police found him and brought him home quietly.

For the next five years, Cowart lived in a shadow world of painful rehabilitation, chronic boredom, and failed relationships. His difficulties were not for want of trying. With Rex Houston's encouragement and assistance he tried pursuing a law degree. Fortunately, his legal settlement with the pipeline company provided the financial means for the nursing care and tutorial assistance which would be required because of his massive handicaps.

Cowart tested out his abilities as a blind student in two undergraduate courses at the University of Texas in Austin during the fall of 1975. He spent the spring at home in Henderson preparing for the tests that were required for admission to law school. In the summer of 1976, he enrolled for a part-time course load in Baylor University's School of Law.

Don handled his studies at Baylor in fine fashion despite his handicaps, but the strain was tremendous. He was forced to live with other people, his independence was limited, and his sleep problems persisted. When a special relationship with a woman ended abruptly in the spring of 1977, his life caved in. He tried to commit suicide by taking an overdose of pain and sleep medications, but he was discovered in time to have his stomach pumped at the hospital emergency room. He had trouble picking up his studies again, so he dropped out before the spring quarter was completed.

Cowart returned home defeated and discouraged, living with his mother for the next half year. He resumed his studies at Baylor in the spring of 1978, only to drop out again before he had completed the third quarter in the fall of 1979. He again retreated to his mother's home, filled with doubts that he would ever be able to pass the bar. By the spring of 1980, he was ready for another try at schooling, this time in a graduate program in building construction of Texas A&M University. Once again, the old patterns of sleepless nights and boring days got the best of him and he made a half hearted effort at slashing his wrists with a razor blade.

Looking back, Cowart saw his futile efforts to take his own life as a bitter human comedy. The doctors in Galveston had encouraged him to accept treatment that would free him of hospitalization and permit him to end his life, if that was his wish. But he found it difficult to find a way of killing himself without bringing further misery on himself—brain damage or further hospitalization. Ironically, he realized that he was no more successful in ending his life than in making his life work.

As a last resort, Cowart contacted White for help and was voluntarily readmitted under White's care to the Jennie Sealy Hospital on April 12, 1980. During his month-long stay, he met with White for psychotherapy treatments daily. Even more important, his sleep problems were finally resolved by weaning him away from the heavy sleep medications that he had taken for years. Cowart describes that experience as being like "coming out of a fog." For the first time since his harrowing burn treatment ordeal, his sleep became normal and his depression lifted.

It was during this stay that I met Don Cowart and we began early discussions of a film that would eventually come to be known as Dax's Case. *I still call him Don because that is how I know him, but he legally changed his name to Dax in the summer of 1982. Some commentators on the film speculate that this change of name reflects some personal metamorphosis that Cowart went through during his lengthy rehabilitation period. But Cowart offers a simpler explanation. As a blind man with impaired hearing, he often found himself responding to comments addressed to others bearing the name of Don. I accepted his reasons for changing his name but asked him not to think the poorer of me for persisting in calling him Don.*

It would be easy to believe that Dax's Case, *more than five years in the making, served as a crucible for Don Cowart's rehabilitation. During this time, new hope and independence came into his life. He started a mail-order specialty foods business in Henderson using his creative powers. He moved into his own house. He became an articulate spokesperson for "the right to die" under auspices of Concern for Dying. And he married a former high school classmate in February 1983.*

There is always another chapter, however. Even now, Don's life continues to shift. His first venture in business did not succeed financially. His second marriage ended unhappily. Amid failure has also come achievement. He returned to law school at Texas Tech University in Lubbock, where he completed his law degree in May and passed the bar in the summer of 1986. He set up a small law practice in Henderson and has recently taken in his first partner. He continues to represent his views on patient rights at educational symposiums and public forums. In time, he hopes to become a specialist in personal injury cases.

COMMENTARY

Robert B. White

Donald's wish seemed in great measure logical and rational; as my psychiatric duties brought me to know him well, I could not escape the thought that if I were in his position I would feel as he did. I asked two other psychiatric colleagues to see the patient, and they came to the same conclusion. *Should his demand to die be respected?* I found myself in sympathy with his wish to put an end to his pathetic plight. On the other hand, the burden on his mother would be unthinkable if he left the hospital, and none of us who were responsible for his care could bring ourselves to say, "You're discharged; go home and die."

Another question occurred to me as I watched this blind, maimed, and totally helpless man defy and baffle everyone: could his adamant stand be the only way available for him to regain his independence after such a prolonged period of helplessness and total dependence?

Consequently, I decided to assist him in the one area where he did want help—obtaining legal assistance. He obviously had the right to legal recourse, and I told him I would help him obtain it. I also told him that I and the other doctors involved could not accede immediately to his demand to leave; we could not participate in his suicide. Furthermore, he was, I said, in no condition to leave unless his mother took him home, and that was an unfair burden to place on her. I urged him to have the surgery; then, when he was able to be up and about, he could take his own life if he wished without forcing others to arrange his death.

But Donald remained adamant, and the patient, his attorney, and I had several conferences. Finally, the attorney reluctantly agreed to represent the patient in court. The patient and I agreed that if the court ruled that he had the right to refuse further treatment, the life-sustaining daily trips to the Hubbard tank and all his other life-sustaining treatment would be stopped. If he wished, he could remain in the hospital in order to be kept as free of pain as possible until he died.

From the *Hastings Center Report*, July 1975:9–10. Reprinted by permission of The Hastings Center.

Had Donald been burned a few years ago, before our increasingly exquisite medical and surgical technology became available, none of the moral, humanitarian, medical, or legal questions his case raised would have had time to occur; he would simply have died. But Donald lived, and never lost his courage or tenacity. He has imposed upon us the responsibility to explore the questions he has asked. On one occasion Donald put the matter very bluntly: "What gives a physician the right to keep alive a patient who wants to die?"

As we increase our ability to sustain life in a wrecked body we must find ways to assess the wishes of the person in that body as accurately as we assess the viability of his organs. We can no longer blindly hold to our instinctive tendency to regard death as an adversary to be defeated at any price. Nor must we accept immediately and at face value a patient's demand to be allowed to die. That demand may often be his only way to assert his will in the face of our unyielding determination to defeat death. The problem is relatively simple when brain death has occurred or when a patient refuses surgery for cancer. But what of the patient who

has entered willingly on a prolonged and difficult course of treatment, and then, at the point at which he will obviously survive if the treatment is continued, decides that he does not want further treatment because he cannot tolerate the kind of future life that his injuries or illness will impose upon him?

The outcome of Donald's case does not resolve these questions but it should add to the depth of our reflections. Having won his point, having asserted his will, having thus found a way to counteract his months of total helplessness, Donald suddenly agreed to continue the treatment and to have the surgery on his hands. He remained in the hospital for five more months until medically ready to return home. In the six months since he left, Donald has regained a considerable measure of self-sufficiency. Although still blind, he will soon have surgery on his eye, and it is hoped some degree of useful vision will be restored. He feeds himself, can walk as far as half a mile, and has become an enthusiastic operator of a citizen's band radio. When I told him of my wish to publish this case report, he agreed, and stated that he had been thinking of writing a paper about his remarkable experiences.

COMMENTARY

H. Tristram Engelhardt, Jr.

This case raises a fundamental moral issue: how can one treat another person as free while still looking out for his best interests (even over his objections)? The issue is one of the bounds and legitimacy of paternalism. Paternalistic interventions are fairly commonplace in society: motorcyclists are required to wear helmets, no one may sell himself into slavery,

From *Hastings Center Report*, June 1975:9–10. Reprinted by permission of The Hastings Center.
Author's note: This article explores the sparse secular morality that can bind moral strangers, not the thick morality that should guide all persons in their choices regarding dying and death. The first is not adequate for a good death.

etc. In such cases society chooses to intervene to maintain the moral agency of individuals so that their agency will not be terminated in death or in slavery. Society chooses in the purported best interest (i.e., to preserve the condition of self-determination itself—freedom) of the would-be reckless motorcyclist or slave. Or, in the paradigmatic case of paternalism, the choice by parents for their children is justifiable in that at a future time as adults, the children will say that their parents chose in their best interests (as opposed to the parents simply using their children for their own interests). That is, the paternalism involved in surrogate consent can be justified if the individual himself cannot choose, and one chooses in that individual's best interests so that if that person were (or is in the future) able to choose, he or she would (will) agree with the choice that has been made in his or her behalf.

Thus, one can justify treating a burned patient when first admitted even if that person protested: one might argue that the individual was not able to choose freely because of the pain and serious impact of the circumstances, and that by treating initially one gave the individual a reasonable chance to choose freely in the future. One would interpret the patient to be temporarily incompetent and have someone decide in his behalf. But once that initial time has passed, and once the patient is reasonably able to choose, should one respect a patient's request to refuse lifesaving therapy even if one has good reason to believe that later the patient might change his or her mind? This is the problem that this case presents.

Yet, what are the alternatives which are morally open: (1) to compel treatment, (2) at once to cease treatment, or (3) to convince the patient to persist, but if the patient does not agree, then to stop therapy. Simply to compel treatment is not to acknowledge the patient as a free agent (i.e., to vitiate the concept of *consent* itself), and simply to stop therapy at once may abandon the patient to the exigencies of unjustified despair. The third alternative recognizes the two values to be preserved in this situation: the freedom of the patient and the physician's commitment to preserve the life of persons.

But in the end, individuals, when able, must be allowed to decide their own destiny, even that of death. When the patient decides that the future quality of life open to him is not worth the investment of pain and suffering to attain that future quality of life, that is a decision proper to the patient. Such is the case *even if* one had good reasons to believe that once the patient attained that future state he would be content to live; one would have unjustifiably forced an invest-

ment of pain that was not agreed to. Of course, there are no easy answers. Physicians should not abandon patients when momentary pain overwhelms them; physicians should seek to gain consent for therapy. But when the patient who is able to give free consent does not, the moral issue is over. A society that will allow persons to climb dangerous mountains or do dare-devil stunts with cars has no consistent grounds for paternalistic intervention here. Further, unlike the case of the motorcyclist or the would-be slave, in this case one would force unchosen pain and suffering on another in the name of their best interests, but in circumstances where their best interests are far from clear. That is, even if such paternalistic intervention may be justifiable in some cases (an issue which is different from the paternalism of surrogate decision-making, and which I will not contest at this point), it is dubious here, for the patient's choice is not a capricious risking on the basis of free action, but a deliberate choice to avoid considerable hardship. Further, it is a uniquely intimate choice concerning the quality of life: the amount of pain which is worth suffering for a goal. Moreover, it is, unlike the would-be slave's choice, a choice which affirms freedom on a substantial point—the quality of one's life.

In short, one must be willing, as a price for recognizing the freedom of others, to live with the consequences of that freedom: some persons will make choices that they would regret were they to live longer. But humans are not only free beings, but temporal beings, and the freedom that is actual is that of the present. Competent adults should be allowed to make tragic decisions, if nowhere else, at least concerning what quality of life justifies the pain and suffering of continued living. It is not medicine's responsibility to prevent tragedies by denying freedom, for that would be the greater tragedy.

ADVANCE DIRECTIVES

THE HEALTH CARE PROXY AND THE LIVING WILL

George J. Annas

American medicine is awash in forms: insurance forms, disability forms, informed-consent forms, and forms for various examinations, to name just a few. Forms can help make the practice of medicine more efficient, but they can also make it more routinized, impersonal, and bureaucratic. Congress and the President have decreed that beginning December 1, 1991, all hospitals, nursing facilities, hospice programs, and health maintenance organizations that serve Medicare or Medicaid patients must provide all their new adult patients with written information describing the patients' rights under state law to make decisions about medical care, including their right to execute a living will or durable power of attorney. New forms will be routinely added to the

practice of medicine. Their purpose is to help implement a right that has been universally recognized: the right to refuse any and all medical interventions, even life-sustaining interventions. The challenge is to use these forms to foster communication between doctor and patient, as well as respect for the patient's autonomy.

HISTORICAL CONTEXT

The term "living will" was coined by Luis Kutner in 1969 to describe a document in which a competent adult sets forth directions regarding medical treatment in the event of his or her future incapacitation. The document is a will in the sense that it spells out the person's directions. It is "living" because it takes effect before death. Public interest in this document has always been high, and a national organization, Concern for Dying, has devoted most of its resources for the past 20 years to educating the public and professionals about the living will. A sister organization, Society for the Right to Die (which has merged with Concern for Dying to form the National Council for

From *New England Journal of Medicine* 324, no. 17 (April 25, 1991): 1210–1213. Copyright © 1991, Massachusetts Medical Society. All rights reserved. Reprinted with permission.
Editors' note: Author's notes have been cut. Students who want to follow up on sources should consult the original article.

Death and Dying), simultaneously devoted its primary efforts to encouraging states to pass legislation giving formal legal recognition to the living will.

In 1976 the country's attention focused on the case of Karen Ann Quinlan, a young woman in a persistent vegetative state, and her parents' attempts to have her ventilator removed so she could die a natural death. The New Jersey Supreme Court granted the parents' petition and held that an "ethics committee" could grant all parties concerned legal immunity for their actions. The court did this because it believed that it was the fear of legal liability that prevented Quinlan's physicians from honoring her parents' request. Her story prompted the enactment of the nation's first living-will statute, California's Natural Death Act, in 1976. The California statute is very narrow. A legally enforceable declaration can be executed only 14 days or more after a person is diagnosed as having a terminal illness, defined as one that will cause the patient's death "imminently," whether or not life-sustaining procedures are continued. Thus, even though this statute was inspired by her story, it would not have helped Quinlan, because she was not terminally ill.

By 1991, more than 40 states had enacted living-will statutes. All these laws provide immunity to physicians and other health care professionals who follow the patient's wishes as expressed in a living will. Virtually all of them also suffer from four major shortcomings, however: they are applicable only to those who are "terminally ill"; they limit the types of treatment that can be refused, usually to "artificial" or "extraordinary" therapies; they make no provision for the person to designate another person to make decisions on his or her behalf, or set forth the criteria for such decisions; and there is no penalty if health care providers do not honor these documents.

ADDRESSING THE LIMITATIONS OF THE LIVING WILL

These problems led to calls for second-generation legislation on the living will. Other shortcomings were also noted. Living wills require a person to predict accurately his or her final illness or injury and what medical interventions might be available to postpone death, and living wills require physicians to make decisions on the basis of their interpretation of a document, rather than a discussion of the treatment options with a person acting on behalf of the patient. The proposed solution to these problems was not to modify the living will but to replace it with another form, one assigning a durable power of attorney to a designated person (known, in this context, as appointing a health care proxy). The person named in the document (also called the health care proxy) is variously known as the attorney, the agent, the surrogate, or the proxy—four terms that are synonyms in this context.

Every state has a durable-power-of-attorney law that permits persons to designate someone to make decisions for them if they become incapacitated. Although these statutes were enacted primarily to permit the agent to make financial decisions, no court has ever invalidated a durable power of attorney specifically designed to enable the designated person to make health care decisions. In the recent *Cruzan* case—in which Nancy Cruzan's parents, basing their attempt on their daughter's previous statements, sought to have her tube feeding discontinued after she had been left in a persistent vegetative state by an automobile accident—Justice Sandra Day O'Connor advised citizens to employ this device. In her concurring opinion, O'Connor observed that the decision in *Cruzan* "does not preclude a future determination that the Constitution requires the States to implement the decisions of a duly appointed surrogate." The *Cruzan* case itself, which involved facts essentially identical to those in *Quinlan*, gave impetus to the concept of a health care proxy, just as the *Quinlan* case had previously increased interest in the living will. Physicians are legally and ethically bound to respect the directions of a patient set forth in a living will, but living wills are limited because no one can accurately foretell the future, and interpretation may be difficult. Attempts to make the living will less ambiguous by developing comprehensive checklists with alternative scenarios may be too confusing and abstract to be useful to either patients or heath care providers, although opinions on this differ.

THE MOVE TO DESIGNATE HEALTH CARE PROXIES

Although new laws are not necessary in any state (because of existing laws regarding the assignment of a durable power of attorney), the current trend in the United States is for states to enact additional proxy laws that specifically deal with health care.

Such laws generally specify the information that must be included in the proxy form and the standards on which treatment decisions must be based and grant good-faith immunity for all involved in carrying out the treatment decision. Two of the best-written proxy laws have recently become effective in New York (in January 1991) and Massachusetts (in December 1990). The New York law is based on a recommendation of the New York State Task Force on Life and the Law, and that group's statement of its rationale is still the best introduction to the concept of the health care proxy. The Massachusetts proxy law is largely modeled on the New York law.

The heart of both laws (and all proxy laws) is the same: to enable a competent adult (the "principal") to choose another person (the "proxy" or "agent") to make treatment decisions for him or her if he or she becomes incompetent to make them. The agent has the same authority to make decisions that the patient would have if he or she were still competent. Instead of having to decipher a document, the physician is able to discuss treatment options with a person who has the legal authority to grant or withhold consent on behalf of the patient. The manner in which the agent must exercise this authority is also crucial. The agent must make decisions that are consistent with the wishes of the patient, if these are known, and otherwise that are consistent with the patient's best interests.

Proxy laws also permit the principal to limit the authority of the agent in the document (for example, by not granting authority to refuse cardiopulmonary resuscitation or tube feeding), but the more limitations the principal puts on the agent, the more the document appointing a health care proxy resembles a living will. In addition, because every limitation is subject to interpretation, the likelihood that a dispute will arise about the meaning of the document is increased. One compromise is to give the agent blanket authority to make decisions and to detail one's values and wishes with as much precision as possible in a private letter to the agent. The agent could use this letter when it was relevant to the actual decision and keep it private when it was not relevant.

IMPLEMENTING LAWS REGARDING HEALTH CARE PROXIES

The goal of appointing a proxy is to simplify the process of making decisions and to make it more likely that the patient's wishes will be followed—not to complicate existing problems. If hospitals and hospital lawyers cooperate, this goal will be attained, because the vast majority of physicians will welcome the ability to discuss treatment options with a person, chosen by the patient, who has the legal authority to give or withhold consent. Hospitals can help their patients by making a simple proxy form available, by educating their medical, nursing, and social-service staffs about the laws governing health care proxies, and by supporting decisions made by the agents. Hospitals can impede the process of making good decisions, however, if they concentrate on the paperwork rather than on the way in which decisions are made. Some Massachusetts attorneys, for example, have already drafted a 13-page, singlespaced proxy form that is all but unintelligible to nonlawyers. Others have begun to explore and to catalogue all the reasons why physicians and hospitals might want to seek judicial review before honoring the decision of a health care agent. Neither of these strategies is constructive. The use of complex forms and obstructive strategies makes it likely that treatment decisions will actually be made by the hospital's lawyers and the agent's lawyers, not by the agent and the physician. If this happens, the trend to designating a health care agent will be frustratingly counterproductive, since, instead of encouraging a focus on the patient and the patient's wishes, where it belongs, the new proxy forms will add another layer of bureaucracy and another outsider to the decision process.

The most useful form for both patients and providers is a simple one-page document that sets forth all necessary information in easily comprehensible language. [A] one-page form, which is easily understood and meets all the requirements of the new Massachusetts proxy law (as well as those of the New York law) was developed by a broad-based task force made up of representatives of all the major health care organizations in the state, including the Massachusetts Medical Society, the Massachusetts Hospital Association, the Massachusetts Nurses Association, the Massachusetts Federation of Nursing Homes, and also the Massachusetts Department of Public Health, as well as the Massachusetts Executive Office of Elder Affairs and the Massachusetts Bar Association. This model form (available in bulk from Massachusetts Health Decisions, 101 Tremont St., No. 600, Boston, MA 02108), which also includes instructions and spaces for the optional signatures of the agent and an alternate (naming an alternate is not required), will be distributed across the state. The degree of cooperation in its development was virtually unprecedented and may provide a model for future efforts.

ADDING TO THE DOCUMENT DESIGNATING A PROXY

Perhaps out of concern for efficiency, some commentators have advocated combining an organ-donor form with the form designating a health care proxy. This is a serious error for at least two reasons. First, much effort has been expended over the past 20 years to separate the issues of organ donation and treatment decisions in the public's mind, since the main reason people do not sign organ-donor cards is that they believe doctors might "do something to me before I'm really dead." Tying organ donation to treatment refusals that might lead to death only heightens this concern and is likely to lead people to use neither form. Second, the proxy form takes effect when the patient becomes incompetent; in contrast, the organ-donor form takes effect only on the patient's death. The health care agent can have nothing to say about organ donation, because the agent can make only treatment decisions, an authority that dies with the patient. Organ donation is laudable, but it is not related to the designation of a health care agent, and the principal should authorize donation on a separate form designed for that purpose. Organ-donor forms may teach another lesson as well. No physician in the United States will honor an organ-donor form over the objections of the patient's family. Similarly, physicians have difficulty honoring a patient's living will over the family's objections. Because it identifies a person with legal authority to talk with the physician, the health care proxy is likely to be a more effective mechanism to implement the patient's wishes.

It should be stressed that forms naming a health care proxy do not substantively change existing law; they merely make it procedurally easier for a person to designate an agent who is authorized to make whatever health care decisions the person could legally make if competent, and they give health care providers legal immunity for honoring such decisions. The patient can, for example, give

the agent the authority to refuse any and all medical care, but the agent has no more legal authority than the principal to insist on assisted suicide or to demand a lethal injection. The naming of an agent also solves the problem of a dispute among family members concerning treatment, since the agent has the legal and ethical right and responsibility to make the decision. When a long-lost relative arrives and demands that "everything be done or I'll sue," the physician can refer that person to the agent, rather than try to achieve a consensus.

LIMITS OF THE CONCEPT OF THE HEALTH CARE PROXY

Only competent adults who actually execute a document can name a health care agent. Since fewer than 10 percent of Americans have either living wills or organ-donor cards, few may use this mechanism. It has no application to children, the mentally retarded, or others unable to appreciate the nature and consequences of their decisions. Treatment decisions for these groups will continue to be governed by the vague "best interests" standard, which is the functional equivalent of "reasonable medical care," "appropriate medical care," or "indicated medical care." The document will also be of limited use in the emergency department, although in rare cases the health care agent may arrive with the principal and there may be time for consultation and informed consent before a specific intervention is tried. Nor will the document solve problems of futility. Physicians will retain the right not to offer treatment that is contraindicated, useless, or futile.

THE RESPONSIBILITY OF PHYSICIANS

I have encouraged members of both the Boston Bar Association and the Massachusetts Bar Association to make health care–proxy forms available to the public and their clients free of charge as a public service. Many have agreed. It will also be useful to the public if physicians make such forms available to their patients and encourage them to fill them out. Physicians may also be more comfortable about relying on the decisions of the designated agent if patients are willing to discuss their choice of agent with the physician, although this is not a requirement. Any form that is used must be written in language that both patients and health care providers can easily understand; the form need not be written by a lawyer and should not require a lawyer to interpret.

Like soldiers in past wars, Americans serving in the Persian Gulf wrote their wills. This time, however, many also wrote living wills or executed durable powers of attorney. As one reporter observed, "In the process, the soldiers had to clarify ambiguous personal relationships, chart out their children's lives, and, in some cases, confront their own mortality for the first time." Designating a health care agent gives us all the opportunity to confront our mortality and to determine who among our friends and relatives we want to make treatment decisions on our behalf when we are unable to make them ourselves. A clear focus on these substantive issues, rather than on forms or formalities, could help patients feel more secure that their wishes regarding medical treatment will be respected, and could help health care professionals be more secure that the treatment decisions made for incompetent patients actually reflect the patients' wishes. These are certainly worthy goals.

ENOUGH: THE FAILURE OF THE LIVING WILL

Angela Fagerlin and Carl E. Schneider

By their fruits ye shall know them.

Enough. The living will has failed, and it is time to say so.

We should have known it would fail: A notable but neglected psychological literature always provided arresting reasons to expect the policy of living wills to misfire. Given their alluring potential, perhaps they were worth trying. But a crescendoing empirical literature and persistent clinical disappointments reveal that the rewards of the campaign to promote living wills do not justify its costs. Nor can any degree of tinkering ever make the living will an effective instrument of social policy.

As the evidence of failure has mounted, living wills have lost some of their friends. We offer systematic support for their change of heart. But living wills are still widely and confidently urged on patients, and they retain the allegiance of many bioethicists, doctors, nurses, social workers, and patients. For these loyal advocates, we offer systematic proof that such persistence in error is but the triumph of dogma over inquiry and hope over experience.

A note about the scope of our contentions: First, we reject only living wills, not durable powers of attorney. Second, there are excellent reasons to be skeptical of living wills on principle. For example, perhaps former selves should not be able to bind latter selves in the ways living wills contemplate. And many people do and perhaps should reject the view of patients, their families, and their communities that informs living wills. But we accept for the sake of argument that living wills desirably serve a strong version of patients' autonomy. We contend, nevertheless, that living wills do not and cannot achieve that goal.

And a stipulation: We do not propose the elimination of living wills. We can imagine recommending them to patients whose medical situation is plain, whose crisis is imminent, whose preferences are specific, strong, and delineable, and who have special reasons to prescribe their care. We argue on

From *Hastings Center Report*, 34, no. 2 (March–April 2004): 30–42. Reprinted by permission of The Hastings Center.

Editors' note: Some authors' notes have been cut. Students who want to follow up on sources should consult the original article.

the level of public policy: In an attempt to extend patients' exercise of autonomy beyond their span of competence, resources have been lavished to make living wills routine and even universal. This policy has not produced results that recompense its costs, and it should therefore be renounced.

Living wills are a bioethical idea that has passed from controversy to conventional wisdom, from the counsel of academic journals to the commands of law books, from professors' proposal to professional practice. Advance directives generally are embodied in federal policy by the Patient Self-Determination Act, which requires medical institutions to give patients information about their state's advance directives. In turn, the law of every state provides for advance directives, almost all states provide for living wills, and most states "have at least two statutes, one establishing a living will type directive, the other establishing a proxy or durable power of attorney for health care."[1] Not only are all these statutes very much in effect, but new legislative activity is constant. Senators Rockefeller, Collins, and Specter have introduced bills to "strengthen" the PSDA and living wills,"[2] and state legislatures continue to amend living will statutes and to enact new ones.

Courts and administrative agencies too have become advocates of living wills. The Veterans Administration has proposed a rule to encourage the use of advance directives, including living wills. Where legislatures have not granted living wills legal status, some courts have done so as a matter of common law, and where legislatures have granted them legal status, courts have cooperated with eager enthusiasm. Living wills have assumed special importance in states that prohibit terminating treatment in the absence of strong evidence of the patient's wishes. One supreme court summarized a common theme: "[A] written directive would provide the most concrete evidence of the patient's decisions, and we strongly urge all persons to create such a directive."[3]

The grandees of law and medicine also give their benediction to the living will. The AMA's Council on Ethical and Judicial Affairs proclaims: "Physicians should encourage their patients to document their treatment preferences or to appoint a health care proxy with whom they can discuss their values regarding health care and treatment."[4] The elite National Conference of Commissioners on Uniform

State Laws continues to promulgate the Uniform Health-Care Decisions Act, a prestigious model statute that has been put into law in a still-growing number of states. Medical journals regularly admonish doctors and nurses to see that patients have advance directives, including living wills. Bar journals regularly admonish lawyers that their clients—*all* their clients—need advance directives, including living wills. Researchers demonstrate their conviction that living wills are important by the persistence of their studies of patients' attitudes toward living wills and ways of inveigling patients to sign them.

Not only do legislatures, courts, administrative agencies, and professional associations promote the living will, but other groups unite with them. The Web abounds in sites advocating the living will to patients. The web site for our university's hospital plugs advance directives and suggests that it "is probably better to have written instructions because then everyone can read them and understand your wishes."[5]

Our own experience in presenting this paper is that its thesis provokes some bioethicists to disbelief and indignation. It is as though they simply cannot bear to believe that living wills might not work. How can anything so intuitively right be proved so infuriatingly wrong? And indeed, bioethicists continue to investigate ways the living will might be extended (to deal with problems of the mentally ill and of minors, for example) and developed for other countries.

Although some sophisticated observers have long doubted the wisdom of living wills, proponents have tended to respond in one of three ways, all of which preserve an important role for living wills. First, proponents have supposed that the principal problem with living wills is that people just won't sign them. These proponents have persevered in the struggle to find ways of getting more people to sign up.

Second, proponents have reasserted the usefulness of the living wills. For example, Norman Cantor, distinguished advocate of living wills, acknowledges that "[s]ome commentators doubt the utility or efficacy of advance directives" (by which he means the living will), but he concludes that "these objections don't obviate the importance of advance directives."[6] Other proponents are daunted by the criticisms of living wills but offer new justifications for them.

Linda Emanuel, another eminent exponent of living wills, writes that "living wills can help doctors and patients talk about dying" and can thereby "open the door to a positive, caring approach to death."[7]

Third, some proponents concede the weaknesses of the living will and the advantages of the durable power of attorney and then propose a durable power of attorney that incorporates a living will. That is, the forms they propose for establishing a durable power of attorney invite their authors to provide the kinds of instructions formerly confined to living wills.

None of these responses fully grapples with the whole range of difficulties that confound the policy promoting living wills. In fairness, this is partly because the case against that policy has been made piecemeal and not in a full-fledged and full-throated analysis of the empirical literature on living wills.

In sum, the law has embraced the principle of living wills and cheerfully continues to this moment to expound and expand that principle. Doctors, nurses, hospitals, and lawyers are daily urged to convince their patients and clients to adopt living wills, and patients hear their virtues from many other sources besides. Some advocates of living wills have shifted the grounds for their support of living wills, but they persist in believing that they are useful. The time has come to investigate those policies and those hopes systematically. That is what this article attempts.

We ask an obvious but unasked question: What would it take for a regime of living wills to function as their advocates hope? First, people must have living wills. Second, they must decide what treatment they would want if incompetent. Third, they must accurately and lucidly state that preference. Fourth, their living wills must be available to people making decisions for a patient. Fifth, those people must grasp and heed the living will's instructions. These conditions are unmet and largely unmeetable.

DO PEOPLE HAVE LIVING WILLS?

At the level of principle, living wills have triumphed among the public as among the princes of medicine. People widely say they want a living will, and living wills have so much become conventional medical wisdom "that involvement in the process is being portrayed as a duty to physicians and others."[8]

Despite this, and despite decades of urging, most Americans lack them. While most of us who need one have a property will, roughly 18 percent have living wills."[9] The chronically or terminally ill are likelier to prepare living wills than the healthy, but even they do so fitfully. In one study of dialysis patients, for instance, only 35 percent had a living will, even though all of them thought living wills a "good idea."[10]

Why do people flout the conventional wisdom? The flouters advance many explanations. They don't know enough about living wills, they think living wills hard to execute, they procrastinate, they hesitate to broach the topic to their doctors (as their doctors likewise hesitate). Some patients doubt they need a living will. Some think living wills are for the elderly or infirm and count themselves in neither group. Others suspect that living wills do not change the treatment people receive; 91 percent of the veterans in one study shared that suspicion. Many patients are content or even anxious to delegate decisions to their families, often because they care less what decisions are made than that they are made by people they trust. Some patients find living wills incompatible with their cultural traditions. Thus in the large SUPPORT and HELP studies, most patients preferred to leave final resuscitation decisions to their family and physician instead of having their own preferences expressly followed (70.8% in HELP and 78.0% in SUPPORT). This result is so striking that it is worth restating: not even a third of the HELP patients and hardly more than a fifth of the SUPPORT patients "would want their own preferences followed."[11]

If people lacked living wills only because of ignorance, living wills might proliferate with education. But studies seem not to "support the speculations found in the literature that the low level of advance directives use is due primarily to a lack of information and encouragement from health care professionals and family members." Rather, there is considerable evidence "that the elderly's action of delaying execution of advance directives and deferring to others is a deliberate, if not an explicit, refusal to participate in the advance directives process."[12]

The federal government has sought to propagate living wills through the Patient Self-Determination Act, which essentially requires medical institutions to inform patients about advance directives. However, "empirical studies demonstrate that: the PSDA has generally failed to foster a significant increase in advance directives use; it is being implemented by medical institutions and their personnel in a passive manner; and the involvement of physicians in its implementation is lacking."[13] One commentator even thinks "the PSDA's legal requirements have become a ceiling instead of a floor."[14]

In short, people have reasons, often substantial and estimable reasons, for eschewing living wills, reasons unlikely to be overcome by persuasion. Indeed, persuasion seems quickly to find its limits. Numerous studies indicate that without considerable intervention, approximately 20 percent of us complete living wills, but programs to propagate wills have mixed results.[15] Some have achieved significant if still limited increases in the completion of living wills, while others have quite failed to do so.

Thus we must ask: If after so much propaganda so few of us have living wills, do we really want them, or are we just saying what we think we ought to think and what investigators want to hear?

DO PEOPLE KNOW WHAT THEY WILL WANT?

Suppose, counterfactually, that people executed living wills. For those documents to work, people would have to predict their preferences accurately. This is an ambitious demand. Even patients making contemporary decisions about contemporary illnesses are regularly daunted by the decisions' difficulty. They are human. We humans falter in gathering information, misunderstand and ignore what we gather, lack well-considered preferences to guide decisions, and rush headlong to choice. How much harder, then, is it to conjure up preferences for an unspecifiable future confronted with unidentifiable maladies with unpredictable treatments?

For example, people often misapprehend crucial background facts about their medical choices. Oregon has made medical policy in fresh and controversial ways, has recently had two referenda on assisted suicide, and alone has legalized it. Presumably, then, its citizens are especially knowledgeable. But only 46 percent of them knew that patients may legally withdraw life-sustaining treatment. Even experience is a poor teacher: "Personal experience with illness . . . and authoring an advance directive . . . were not significantly associated with better knowledge about options."[16]

Nor do people reliably know enough about illnesses and treatments to make prospective life-or-death decisions about them. To take one example from many, people grossly overestimate the effectiveness of CPR and in fact hardly know what it is. For such information, people must rely on doctors. But doctors convey that information wretchedly even to competent patients making contemporaneous decisions. Living wills can be executed without even consulting a doctor, and when doctors are consulted, the conversations are ordinarily short, vague, and tendentious. In the Tulsky study, for example, doctors only described either "dire scenarios . . . in which few people, terminally ill or otherwise, would want treatment" or "situations in which patients could recover with proper treatment."[17]

Let us put the point differently. The conventional—legal and ethical—wisdom insists that candidates for even a flu shot give "informed consent." And that wisdom has increasingly raised the standards for disclosure. If we applied those standards to the information patients have before making the astonishing catalog of momentous choices living wills can embody, the conventional wisdom would be left shivering with indignation.

Not only do people regularly know too little when they sign a living will, but often (again, we're human) they analyze their choices only superficially before placing them in the time capsule. An ocean of evidence affirms that answers are shaped by the way questions are asked. Preferences about treatments are influenced by factors like whether success or failure rates are used, the level of detail employed, and whether long- or short-term consequences are explained first. Thus in one study, "201 elderly subjects opted for the intervention 12% of the time when it was presented negatively, 18% of the time when it was phrased as in an advance directive already in use, and 30% of the time when it was phrased positively. Seventy-seven percent of the subjects changed their minds at least once when given the same case scenario but a different description of the intervention."[18]

If patients have trouble with contemporaneous decisions, how much more trouble must they have with prospective ones. For such decisions to be "true," patients' preferences must be reasonably stable. Surprisingly often, they are not. A famous study of eighteen women in a "natural childbirth" class found that preferences about anesthesia and avoiding pain were relatively stable before childbirth, but at "the beginning of active labor (4–5 cm dilation) there was a shift in the preference toward avoiding labor pains. . . . During the transition phase of labor (8–10 cm) the values remained relatively stable, but then . . . the mothers' preferences shifted again at postpartum toward avoiding the use of anesthesia during the delivery of her next child."[19] And not only are preferences surprisingly labile, but people have trouble recognizing that their views have changed. This makes it less likely they will amend their living wills as their opinions develop and more likely that their living wills will treasonously misrepresent their wishes.

Instability matters. The healthy may incautiously prefer death to disability. Once stricken, competent patients can test and reject that preference. They often do. Thus Wilfrid Sheed "quickly learned [that] cancer, even more than polio, has a disarming way of bargaining downward, beginning with your whole estate and then letting you keep the game warden's cottage or badminton court; and by the time it has tried to frighten you to death and threatened to take away your very existence, you'd be amazed at how little you're willing to settle for."[20]

At least sixteen studies have investigated the stability of people's preferences for life-sustaining treatment. A meta-analysis of eleven of these studies found that the stability of patients' preferences was 71 percent (the range was 57 percent to 89 percent).[21] Although stability depended on numerous factors (including the illness, the treatment, and demographic variables), the bottom line is that, over periods as short as two years, almost one-third of preferences for life-sustaining medical treatment changed. More particularly, illness and hospitalization change people's preferences for life-sustaining treatments. In a prospective study, the desire for life-sustaining treatment declined significantly after hospitalization but returned almost to its original level three to six months later. Another study concluded that the "will to live is highly unstable among terminally ill cancer patients."[22] The authors thought their findings "perhaps not surprising, given that only 10–14% of individuals who survive a suicide attempt

commit suicide during the next 10 years, which suggests that a desire to die is inherently changeable."

The consistent finding that interest in life-sustaining treatment shifts over time and across contexts coincides tellingly with research charting people's struggles to predict their own tastes, behavior, and emotions even over short periods and under familiar circumstances. People mispredict what poster they will like, how much they will buy at the grocery store, how sublimely they will enjoy an ice cream, and how they will adjust to tenure decisions. And people "miswant" for numerous reasons. They imagine a different event from the one that actually occurs, nurture inaccurate theories about what gives them pleasure, forget they might outwit misery, concentrate on salient negative events and ignore offsetting happier ones, and misgauge the effect of physiological sensations like pain. Given this rich stew of research on people's missteps in predicting their tastes generally, we should expect misapprehensions about end-of-life preferences. Indeed, those preferences should be especially volatile, since people lack experience deciding to die.

CAN PEOPLE ARTICULATE WHAT THEY WANT?

Suppose, *arguendo*, that patients regularly made sound choices about future treatments and write living wills. Can they articulate their choices accurately? This question is crucially unrealistic, of course, because the assumption is false. People have trouble reaching well-considered decisions, and you cannot state clearly on paper what is muddled in your mind. And indeed people do, for instance, issue mutually inconsistent instructions in living wills.

But assume this difficulty away and the problem of articulation persists. In one sense, the best way to divine patients' preferences is to have them write their own living wills to give surrogates the patient's gloriously unmediated voice. This is not a practical policy. Too many people are functionally illiterate, and most of the literate cannot express themselves clearly in writing. It's hard, even for the expert writer. Furthermore, most people know too little about their choices to cover all the relevant subjects. Hence living wills are generally forms that demand little writing. But the forms have failed. For example, "several studies suggest that even those patients who have completed AD forms . . . may not fully understand the function of the form or its language." Living wills routinely baffle patients with their

> syntactic complexity, concept density, abstractness, organization, coherence, sequence of ideas, page format, length of line of print, length of paragraph, punctuation, illustrations, color, and reader interest. Unfortunately, most advance directive forms . . . often have neither a reasonable scope nor depth. They do not ask all the right questions and they do not ask those questions in a manner that elicits clear responses.[23]

Doctors and lawyers who believe their clients are all above average should ask them what their living will says. One of us (CES) has tried the experiment. The modal answer is, in its entirety: "It says I don't want to be a vegetable."

No doubt the forms could be improved, but not enough to matter. The world abounds in dreadfully drafted forms because writing complex instructions for the future is crushingly difficult. Statutes read horribly because their authors are struggling to (1) work out exactly what rule they want, (2) imagine all the circumstances in which it might apply, and (3) find language to specify all those but only those circumstances. Each task is ultimately impossible, which is why statutes explicitly or implicitly confide their enforcers with some discretion and why courts must interpret—rewrite?—statutes. However, these skills and resources are not available to physicians or surrogates.

One might retort that property wills work and that living wills are not that far removed from property wills. But wills work as well as they do to distribute property because their scope is—compared to living wills—narrow and routinized. Most people have little property to distribute and few plausible heirs. As property accumulates and ambitions swell, problems proliferate. Many of them are resolvable because experts—lawyers—exclusively draft and interpret wills. Lawyers have been experimenting for centuries with testamentary language in a process which has produced standard formulas with predictable meanings and standard ways of distributing property into which testators are channeled. Finally, if testators didn't say it clearly enough in the right words and following the right procedures, courts coolly ignore their wishes and substitute default rules.

The lamentable history of the living will demonstrates just how recalcitrant these problems are. There have been, essentially, three generations of living wills. At first, they stated fatuously general desires in absurdly general terms. As the vacuity of over-generality became clear, advocates of living wills did the obvious: Were living wills too general? Make them specific. Were they "one size fits all"? Make them elaborate questionnaires. Were they uncritically signed? "Require" probing discussions between doctor and patient. However, the demand for specificity forced patients to address more questions than they could comprehend. So, generalities were insufficiently specific and insufficiently considered. Specifics were insufficiently general and perhaps still insufficiently considered. What was a doctor—or lawyer—to do? Behold the "values history," a disquisition on the patient's supposed overarching beliefs from which to infer answers to specific questions. That patients can be induced to trek through these interminable and imponderable documents is unproved and unlikely. That useful conclusions can be drawn from the platitudes they evoke is false. As Justice Holmes knew, "General propositions do not decide concrete cases."[24]

The lessons of this story are that drafting instructions is harder than proponents of living wills seem to believe and that when you move toward one blessing in structuring these documents, you walk away from another. The failure to devise workable forms is not a failure of effort or intelligence. It is a consequence of attempting the impossible.

WHERE IS THE LIVING WILL?

Suppose that, *mirabile dictu*, people executed living wills, knew what they will want, and could say it. That will not matter unless the living will reaches the people responsible for the incompetent patient. Often, it does not. This should be no surprise, for long can be the road from the drafteer's chair to the ICU bed.

First, the living will may be signed years before it is used, and its existence and location may vanish in the mists of time. Roughly half of all living wills are drawn up by lawyers and must somehow reach the hospital, and 62 percent of patients do not give their living will to their physician.[25] On admission to the hospital, patients can be too assailed and anxious to recall and mention their advance directives. Admission clerks can be harried, neglectful, and loath to ask patients awkward questions.

Thus when a team of researchers reviewed the charts of 182 patients who had completed a living will before being hospitalized, they found that only 26 percent of the charts accurately recorded information about those directives,[26] and only 16 percent of the charts contained the form. And in another study only 35 percent of the nursing home patients who were transferred to the hospital had their living wills with them.[27]

WILL PROXIES READ IT ACCURATELY?

Suppose, *per impossibile*, that patients wrote living wills, correctly anticipated their preferences, articulated their desires lucidly, and conveyed their document to its interpreters. How acutely will the interpreters analyze their instructions? Living wills are not self-executing: someone must decide whether the patient is incompetent, whether a medical situation described in the living will has arisen, and what the living will then commands.

Usually, the patient's intimates will be central among a living will's interpreters. We might hope that intimates already know the patient's mind, so that only modest demands need be made on their interpreting skills. But many studies have asked such surrogates to predict what treatment the patient would choose. Across these studies, approximately 70 percent of the predictions were correct—not inspiring success for life and death decisions.

Do living wills help? We know of only one study that addresses that question. In a randomized trial, researchers asked elderly patients to complete a disease- and treatment-based or a value-based living will. A control group of elderly patients completed no living will. The surrogates were generally spouses or children who had known the patient for decades. Surrogates who were not able to consult their loved one's living will predicted patients' preferences about 70 percent of the time. Strikingly, surrogates who consulted the living will did no better than surrogates denied it. Nor were surrogates more successful when they discussed living wills with patients just before their prediction.

What is more, a similar study found that primary care physicians' predictions were similarly unimproved by providing them with patients' advance directives. On the other hand, emergency room doctors (complete strangers) given a living will more accurately predicted patients' preferences than ER doctors without one.

DO LIVING WILLS ALTER PATIENT CARE?

Our survey of the mounting empirical evidence shows that none of the five requisites to making living wills successful social policy is met now or is likely to be. The program has failed, and indeed is impossible.

That impossibility is confirmed by studies of how living wills are implemented, which show that living wills seem not to affect patients' treatments. For instance, one study concluded that living wills "do not influence the level of medical care overall. This finding was manifested in the quantitatively equal use of diagnostic testing, operations, and invasive hemodynamic monitoring among patients with and without advance directives. Hospital and ICU lengths of stay, as well as health care costs, were also similar for patients with and without advance directive statements."[28] Another study found that in thirty of thirty-nine cases in which a patient was incompetent and the living will was in the patient's medical record, the surrogate decisionmaker was not the person the patient had appointed.[29] In yet a third study, a quarter of the patients received care that was inconsistent with their living will.[30]

But all this is normal. Harry Truman rightly predicted that his successor would "sit here, and he'll say, 'Do this! Do that!' And nothing will happen. Poor Ike—it won't be a bit like the army. He'll find it very frustrating." (Of course, the army isn't like the army either, as Captain Truman surely knew.) Indeed, the whole law of bioethics often seems a whited sepulchre for slaughtered hopes, for its policies have repeatedly fallen woefully short of their purposes. Informed consent is a "fairytale." Programs to increase organ donation have persistently disappointed. Laws regulating DNR orders are hardly better. Legal definitions of brain death are misunderstood by astonishing numbers of doctors and nurses. And so on.

But why don't living wills affect care? Joan Teno and colleagues saw no evidence "that a physician unilaterally decided to ignore or disregard an AD." Rather, there was "a complex interaction of . . . three themes." First (as we have emphasized), "the contents of ADs were vague and difficult to apply to current clinical situations." The imprecision of living wills not only stymies interpreters, it exacerbates their natural tendency to read documents in light of their own preferences. Thus "[e]ven with the therapy-specific AD accompanied by designation of a proxy and prior patient-physician discussion, the proportion of physicians who were willing to withhold therapies was quite variable: cardiopulmonary resuscitation, 100%; administration of artificial nutrition and hydration, 82%; administration of antibiotics, 80%; simple tests, 70%; and administration of pain medication, 13%."[31]

Second, the Teno team found that "patients were not seen as 'absolutely, hopelessly ill,' and thus, it was never considered the time to invoke the AD." Living wills typically operate when patients become terminally ill, but neither doctors nor families lightly conclude patients are dying, especially when that means ending treatment. And understandably. For instance, "on the day before death, the median prognosis for patients with heart failure is still a 50% chance to live 6 more months because patients with heart failure typically die quickly from an unpredictable complication like arrhythmia or infection."[32] So by the time doctors and families finally conclude the patient is dying, the patient's condition is already so dire that treatment looks pointless quite apart from any living will. "In all cases in which life-sustaining treatment was withheld or withdrawn, this decision was made after a trial of life-sustaining treatment and at a time when the patient was seen as 'absolutely, hopelessly ill' or 'actively dying.' Until patients crossed this threshold, ADs were not seen as applicable." Thus "it is not surprising that our previous research has shown that those with ADs did not differ in timing of DNR orders or patterns of resource utilization from those without ADs."[33]

Third, "family members or the surrogate designated in a [durable power of attorney] were not available, were ineffectual, or were overwhelmed with their own concerns and did not effectively advocate for the patient." Family members are crucial surrogates because they should be: patients commonly want them to be; they commonly want to be; they specially cherish the patient's interests. Doctors ordinarily assume families know the patient's situation and preferences and may not relish responsibility for life-and-death decisions, and doctors intent on avoiding litigation may realize that the only plausible plaintiffs are families. The family, however, may not direct attention to the advance directive and may not insist on its enforcement. In fact, surrogates may be guided by either their own treatment preferences or an urgent desire to keep their beloved alive.[34]

In sum, not only are we awash in evidence that the prerequisites for a successful living wills policy are unachievable, but there is direct evidence that living wills regularly fail to have their intended effect. That failure is confirmed by the numerous convincing explanations for it. And if living wills do not affect treatment, they do not work.

DO LIVING WILLS HAVE BENEFICIAL SIDE EFFECTS?

Even if living wills do not effectively promote patients' autonomy, they might have other benefits that justify their costs. There are three promising candidates.

First, living wills might stimulate conversation between doctor and patient about terminal treatment. However, at least one study finds little association between patients' reports of executing an advance directive and their reports of such conversations. Nor do these conversations, when they occur, appear satisfactory. James Tulsky and colleagues asked experienced clinicians who had relationships with patients who were over sixty-five or seriously ill to "discuss advance directives in whatever way you think is appropriate" with them. Although the doctors knew they were being taped, the conversations were impressively short and one-sided: The median discussion "lasted 5.6 minutes (range, 0.9 to 15.0 minutes). Physicians spoke for a median of 3.9 minutes (range, 0.6 to 10.9 minutes), and patients spoke for the remaining 1.7 minutes (range, 0.3 to 9.6 minutes). . . . Usually, the conversation ended without any specific follow-up plan."

The "[p]atients' personal values, goals for care, and reasons for treatment preferences were discussed in 71% of cases and were explicitly elicited by 34% of physicians." But doctors commonly "did not explore the reasons for patient's preferences and merely determined whether they wanted specific interventions."[35]

Nor were the conversations conspicuously informative: "Physicians used vague language to describe scenarios, asking what patients would want if they became 'very, very sick' or 'had something that was very serious.' . . ." Further, "[v]arious qualitative terms were used loosely to describe outcome probabilities." In addition, these brief conversations considered almost exclusively the two ends of the continuum—the most hopeless and the most hopeful cases. Conversations tended to ignore "the more common, less clear-cut predicaments surrounding end-of-life care." True, the patients all thought "their physicians 'did a good job talking about the issues,'" but this only suggests that patients did not understand how little they were told.

The second candidate for beneficial side effect arises from evidence that living wills may comfort patients and surrogates. People with a living will apparently gain confidence that their surrogates will understand their preferences and will implement them comfortably, and the surrogates concur. Improved satisfaction with decisions was also a rare positive effect of the SUPPORT study (which devoted enormous resources to improving end of life decisions and care but made dismayingly little difference). In another study, living wills reduced the stress and unhappiness of family members who had recently withdrawn life support from a relative. But even if living wills make patients and surrogates more confident and comfortable, those qualities are apparently unrelated to the accuracy of surrogates' decisions. Thus we are left with the irony that one of the best arguments for a tool for enhancing people's autonomy is that it deceives them into confidence.

Third, because living wills generally constrain treatment, they might reduce the onerous costs of terminal illness. Although several studies associated living wills with small decreases in those costs, several studies have reached the opposite conclusion. The old Scotch verdict, "not proven," seems apt.

THE COSTS

There is no free living will, and the better (or at least more thorough and careful) the living will, the more it costs. Living wills consume patient's time and energy. When doctors or lawyers help, costs soar. On a broader view, Jeremy Sugarman and colleagues estimated that the Patient Self-Determination Act imposed on all hospitals a start-up cost of $101,569,922 and imposed on one hospital (Johns Hopkins) initial costs of $114,528.[36] These figures omit the expenses, paid even as we write and you read, of administering the program. And this money has bought only *pro forma* compliance.

These are real costs incurred when over 40 million people lack health insurance and when we are spending more of our gross domestic product on health care than comparable countries without buying commensurately better health. If programs to promote and provide living wills showed signs of achieving the goals cherished for them, we would have to decide whether their valuable but incalculable rewards exceeded their diffuse but daunting costs. However, since those programs have failed, their costs plainly outweigh their benefits.

WHAT IS TO BE DONE?

Living wills attempt what undertakers like to call "pre-need planning," and on inspection they are as otiose as the mortuary version. Critically, empiricists cannot show that advance directives affect care. This is damning, but were it our only evidence, perhaps we might not be weary in well doing: for in due season we might reap, if we faint not. However, our survey of the evidence suggests that living wills fail not for want of effort, or education, or intelligence, or good will, but because of stubborn traits of human psychology and persistent features of social organization.

Thus when we reviewed the five conditions for a successful program of living wills, we encountered evidence that not one condition has been achieved or, we think, can be. First, despite the millions of dollars lavished on propaganda, most people do not have living wills. And they often have considered and considerable reasons for their choice. Second, people who sign living wills have generally not thought through its instructions in a way we should want for life-and-death decisions. Nor can we expect people to make thoughtful and stable decisions about so complex a question so far in the future. Third, drafters of living wills have failed to offer people the means to articulate their preferences accurately. And the fault lies primarily not with the drafters; it lies with the inherent impossibility of living wills' task. Fourth, living wills too often do not reach the people actually making decisions for incompetent patients. This is the most remediable of the five problems, but it is remediable only with unsustainable effort and unjustifiable expense. Fifth, living wills seem not to increase the accuracy with which surrogates identify patients' preferences. And the reasons we surveyed when we explained why living wills do not affect patients' care suggest that these problems are insurmountable.

The cost-benefit analysis here is simple: If living wills lack detectable benefits, they cannot justify any cost, much less the considerable costs they now exact. Any attempt to increase their incidence and their availability to surrogates must be expensive. And the evidence suggests that broader use of living wills can actually disserve rather than promote patients' autonomy: If, as we have argued, patients sign living wills without adequate reflection, lack necessary information, and have fluctuating preferences anyway, then living wills will not lead surrogates to make the choices patients would have wanted. Thus, as Pope suggests, the "PSDA, rather than promoting autonomy has 'done a disservice to most real patients and their families and caregivers.' It has promoted the execution of uninformed and under-informed advance directives, and has undermined, not protected, self-determination."[37]

If living wills have failed, we must say so. We must say so to patients. If we believe our declamations about truth-telling, we should frankly warn patients how faint is the chance that living wills can have their intended effect. More broadly, we should abjure programs intended to cajole everyone into signing living wills. We should also repeal the PSDA, which was passed with arrant and arrogant indifference to its effectiveness and its costs and which today imposes accumulating paperwork and administrative expense for paltry rewards.

Of course we recognize the problems presented by the decisions that must be made for incompetent patients, and our counsel is not wholly negative. Patients anxious to control future medical decisions should be told about durable powers of attorney. These surely do not guarantee patients that their wishes will blossom into fact, but nothing does. What matters is that powers of attorney have advantages over living wills. First, the choices that powers of attorney demand of patients are relatively few, familiar, and simple. Second, a regime of powers of attorney requires little change from current practice, in which family members ordinarily act informally for incompetent patients. Third, powers of attorney probably improve decisions for patients, since surrogates know more at the time of the decision than patients can know in advance. Fourth, powers of attorney are cheap; they require only a simple form easily filled out with little advice. Fifth, powers of attorney can be supplemented by legislation (already in force in some states) akin to statutes of intestacy. These statutes specify who is to act for incompetent patients who have not specified a surrogate. In short, durable powers of attorney are—as these things go—simple, direct, modest, straightforward, and thrifty.

In social policy as in medicine, plausible notions can turn out to be bad ideas. Bad ideas should be renounced. Bloodletting once seemed plausible, but when it demonstrably failed, the course of wisdom was to abandon it, not to insist on its virtues and to scrounge for alternative justifications for it. Living wills were praised and peddled before they were fully developed, much less studied. They have now failed repeated tests of practice. It is time to say, "enough."

REFERENCES

1. C.P. Sabatino, "End-of-Life Legal Trends," *ABA Commission on Legal Problems of the Elderly* 2 (2000).
2. Health Care Assurance of 2001. S. 26. 107th Congress ed; 2001; The Advance Planning and Compassionate Care Act of 1999. S. 628. 106th Congress ed; 1999.
3. In re Martin. 538 NW2d 399; Mich 1995.
4. Council on Ethical and Judicial Affairs of the American Medical Association, *Surrogate Decision Making* E8.081. http://www.ama-assn.org
5. Available at www.med.umich.edu/1libr/aha/umlegal04.htm
6. N.L. Cantor, "Twenty-five Years after Quinlan: A Review of the Jurisprudence of Death and Dying," *Journal of Law, Medicine & Ethics* 29 (2001): 182–96.

7. L. Emanuel, "Living Wills Can Help Doctors and Patients Talk about Dying," *Western Journal of Medicine* 173 (2000): 368.

8. D.M. High, "Why Are Elderly People Not Using Advance Directives?" *Journal of Aging and Health* 5, no. 4 (1993): 497–515.

9. Emanuel, "Advance Directives for Medical Care; Reply."

10. Holley et al., "Factors Influencing Dialysis Patients' Completion of Advance Directives."

11. C.M. Puchalski et al., Patients Who Want their Family and Physician to Make Resuscitation Decisions for Them: Observations from SUPPORT and HELP; *JAGS* 48 (2000): S84.

12. High, "Why Are Elderly People Not Using Advance Directives?"

13. J.L. Yates and H.R. Glick, "The Failed Patient Self-Determination Act and Policy Alternatives for the Right to Die," *Journal of Aging and Social Policy* 29 (1997): 29, 31.

14. M.T. Pope, "The Maladaptation of Miranda to Advance Directives: A Critique of the Implementation of the Patient Self-Determination Act," *Health Matrix* 9 (1999): 139.

15. Cox and Sachs, "Advance Directives and the Patient Self-Determinaction Act."

16. M.J. Silveira et al., "Patient's Knowledge of Options at the End of Life: Ignorance in the Face of Death," *JAMA* 284 (2000): 2483, 2486–87.

17. J.A. Tulsky et al., "Opening the Black Box: How Do Physicians Communicate about Advance Directives?" *Annals of Internal Medicine* 129 (1998): 441, 444.

18. Ott, "Advance Directives." pp. 514, 517.

19. J.J. Christensen-Szalanski, "Discount Functions and the Measurement of Patients' Values: Women's Decisions during Childbirth," *Medical Decision Making* 4, no. 1 (1984): 47–58.

20. W. Sheed, *In Love with Daylight: A Memoir of Recovery* (New York: Simon and Schuster, 1995): 14.

21. Coppola et al., "Are Life-Sustaining Treatment Preferences Stable over Time?"

22. H.M. Chochinov et al., "Will to Live in the Terminally Ill," *Lancet* 354 (1999): 816, 818.

23. Pope, "The Maladaptation of Miranda to Advance Directives." pp. 139, 165–66.

24. Lochner v. New York N. 198 U.S. 45: Supreme Court of the United States; 1905.

25. Roe et al., "Durable Power of Attorney for Health Care."

26. R.S. Morrison et al., "The Inaccessibility of Advance Directives on Transfer from Ambulatory to Acute Care Settings," *JAMA* 274 (1995): 478–82.

27. M. Danis et al., "A Prospective Study of the Impact of Patient Preferences on Life-Sustaining Treatment and Hospital Cost," *Critical Care Medicine* 24, 11 (1996): 1811–17.

28. M.D. Goodman, M. Tarnoff, and G.J. Slotman, "Effect of Advance Directives on the Management of Elderly Critically Ill Patients," *Critical Care Medicine* 26, no. 4 (1998): 701–704.

29. Morrison et al., "The Inaccessibility of Advance Directives."

30. M. Danis and J.M. Garrett, "Advance Directives for Medical Care: Reply," *NEJM* 325 (1991): PP NO?.

31. W.R. Mower and L.J. Baraff, "Advance Directives: Effect of Type of Directive on Physicians' Therapeutic Decision," *Archives of Internal Medicine* 153 (1993): 375, 378.

32. J. Lynn, "Learning to Care for People with Chronic Illness Facing the End of Life," *JAMA* 284 (2000): 2508–09.

33. J. Teno et al., "The Illusion of End-of-Life Resource Savings with Advance Directives. SUPPORT Investigators. Study to Understand Prognoses and Preferences for Outcomes and Risks of Treatment," *Journal of the American Geriatrics Society* 45, no. 4 (1997): 513–18.

34. A. Fagerlin et al., "Projection in Surrogate Decisions about Life-Sustaining Medical Treatments," *Health Psychology* 20, no. 3(2001): 166–75.

35. Tulsky et al., "Opening the Black Box." pp. 441, 445.

36. J. Sugarman et al., "The Cost of Ethics Legislation: A Look at the Patient Self-Determination Act," *Kennedy Institute of Ethics Journal* 3, no. 4 (1993): 387–99.

37. Pope, "The Maladaptation of Miranda to Advance Directives." pp. 139, 167.

TESTING THE LIMITS OF PROSPECTIVE AUTONOMY: FIVE SCENARIOS

Norman L. Cantor

Several examples will help crystallize the potential tension between an advance directive and the contemporaneous interests of an incompetent patient. In the following scenarios, assume that all patients were fifty years old at the time of making an advance directive and that the critical medical decisions are confronted five years later. Assume also that no evidence exists that the patient changed his or her mind or wavered in resolve between preparation of the advance directive and losing competence.

Scenario 1: Person A, a Jehovah's Witness, prescribes in an advance directive that blood transfusions should not be administered regardless of the life-saving potential of such medical intervention. She is aware of the life and death implications of this religiously motivated instruction. Later, A becomes prematurely senile and incompetent. Still later, the senile patient develops bleeding ulcers which demand blood transfusions. With a blood transfusion, she will survive and continue to live as a "pleasantly senile" person for a number of years. The senile A no longer has recollection of, or interest in, religion; however, she remained an avid Jehovah's Witness up until the time of incompetency. Should the attending physician administer a life-saving blood transfusion?

Scenario 2: Person B believes both that life should be preserved to the maximum extent possible and that suffering is preordained and carries redemptive value in an afterlife. B prepares an advance directive in which all possible life-extending medical intervention is requested and all pain relief is rejected. At the time of the preparation of the directive, B has a conversation with a physician in which the physician explicitly warns B that many terminal illnesses entail excruciating pain. Despite that admonition,

B directs that all means to preserve life be utilized and that analgesics be omitted. Subsequently, B suffers from cancer, which both affects his brain, rendering him incompetent, and causes him to suffer excruciating pain. Further medical treatment such as radiation or chemotherapy will extend B's life, but will not itself relieve the pain or cause any remission in which competence would return. Should the attending physician sedate the patient, or cease the life-prolonging medical intervention, or both?

Scenario 3: Person C is an individual with chronic heart problems. Physicians have informed C that at some stage he will need a heart transplant in order to survive. C prepares an advance directive stating that if he becomes incompetent and survival becomes dependent on a heart transplant, then such a transplant should be rejected because of its expense. C prefers to leave a substantial monetary legacy to his children. Later, C becomes prematurely senile and incompetent. Still later, C's heart deteriorates and a heart transplant becomes necessary to preserve C's life. With the transplant, C will very likely continue to live for three to five years. Without it, C will die within a few months. The transplant will cost $100,000 and is not covered by any insurance or government benefit program. C's estate totals $100,000. Should a life-extending heart transplant be performed?

Scenario 4: Person D is a health-care professional sensitive to society's needs for organ and tissue donations. In her advance directive, D provides that if she should become incompetent but remain physically healthy, then she wishes to donate a kidney and bone marrow to needy recipients. Later, D is afflicted with Alzheimer's disease and reaches a point of profound dementia. Needy recipients for kidney and bone marrow transplants have been located. The prospective transplant operations will pose only a slight risk to D and entail only mild pain. At the same time, the now incompetent D has no recollection of her prior instruction and no appreciation of

From *Advance Directives and the Pursuit of Death with Dignity* by Norman L. Cantor, Indiana University Press, 1993. Reprinted with permission from the publisher.

the altruism involved in donating an organ or tissue. She will derive no contemporaneous gain from the contemplated operations. Should the transplants be performed in accord with D's advance directive?

Scenario 5: Person E is a sociology professor known for her intellectual sharpness. E takes enormous pride in that intellectual acuity. E drafts an advance directive prescribing that if she should become mentally impaired and incompetent to the point where she can no longer read and comprehend a sociology text, then all life-preserving medical intervention should be withheld. When reminded by her spouse about the potential for happiness in an incompetent state, E replies that she deems significant mental dysfunction to be degrading and personally distasteful. For her, such a debilitated existence is a fate worse than death. Later, E suffers a serious stroke which renders her permanently incompetent and incapable of reading or performing intellectual tasks. E is also unable to swallow and is therefore dependent on artificial nutrition. At the same time, E does not appear to be in any pain and seems to derive some pleasure from listening to music. Should the life-preserving nasogastric tube be continued?

In each of the above situations, people have issued advance directives which effectuate their personal values and concepts of dignity. Yet implementation of those prior instructions conflict in some measure with the contemporaneous interests or well-being of the incompetent persona. Can the advance directive prevail? Does prospective autonomy encompass the prerogative to impact negatively on the incompetent persona?

CHOOSING FOR ONCE-COMPETENT PATIENTS

ERRING ON THE SIDE OF THERESA SCHIAVO: REFLECTIONS OF THE SPECIAL GUARDIAN AD LITEM

Jay Wolfson

For Theresa Marie Schiavo, good science, good medicine, and the careful application of the law were not enough. Her loving parents begged the world to save the life of their brain-damaged daughter, while her devoted husband sought removal of a feeding tube to fulfill what he believed were his wife's wishes not to be maintained in a diagnosed vegetative state. As the whole world watched, legal and political armamentaria were mightily assembled and deployed. The life and death conflict ended Easter week, 2005—some asserted from painful starvation and dehydration, others said from a peaceful, natural shutting down of her systems.

In October 2003, I was appointed Ms. Schiavo's guardian ad litem and was afforded thirty days to complete a report to the courts and the governor of

From *Hastings Center Report* 35, no. 3 (2005): 16–19. Reprinted by permission of The Hastings Center.

Florida. I was charged with preparing a comprehensive medical and legal summary of her care and with making recommendations about the feasibility of conducting additional swallowing tests, which the governor of Florida considered a benchmark for assessing her condition. During that time I met with Theresa, her parents, siblings, husband, hospice staff, attorneys, and the governor, and engaged the nearly fourteen years and thirty thousand pages of legal and medical records in her case. My goal was to maintain balance and seek to represent exclusively Theresa's interests. To do this, acquiring the trust and active input of all parties was essential. There had never been a permanent guardian ad litem appointed for Theresa, even though the dispute over her guardianship had lasted more than a decade.

Theresa suffered a cardiac arrest in February of 1990, possibly because of an eating disorder that may have caused the profound electrolyte imbalance diagnosed upon her admission to the hospital.

Over the course of more than six previous years, she had dropped from nearly 250 pounds to 110. Subsequent to her arrest, she remained anoxic, or without oxygen, for about eleven minutes, some five to seven minutes longer than most medical experts believe is possible without suffering profound, irreversible brain damage. At the insistence of her husband, Michael, she was intubated, given a tracheotomy so she could breathe, and placed on a respirator.

Had Theresa not been resuscitated and placed on a respirator, she would have died, as many do after such an event. But instead, she was caused to live, in a coma for the first two months and then in what was repeatedly diagnosed as a persistent vegetative state (PVS). She was removed from the respirator and able to breathe and swallow her saliva—reflexive behaviors—but she was unable to drink or eat food, which is characteristic of the vegetative state. She was kept functioning with an artificial feeding and hydration tube in her stomach.

Throughout this period, there was no challenge to either the diagnosis of PVS or to the appointment of Michael as her guardian. For three and a half years, her husband and parents struggled together to maintain her.

Within four years of her cardiac arrest, a long-shot lawsuit against a fertility doctor who had failed to detect her electrolyte imbalance resulted in a judgment of $300,000 to Michael for loss of consortium, and some $700,000 to be placed in a court-managed trust account to maintain and provide care for Theresa. Thereafter, what is for millions of Americans a profoundly private matter catapulted a close, loving family into an internationally watched blood feud. The end product was a most public death for a very private individual. Snippets of Theresa's partially clad body and manifestly disabled state were broadcast everywhere. It was like *The Truman Show*, the movie of a man whose daily life was watched, unbeknownst to him, by millions of viewers as part of an internationally broadcast television show, except that it was defined by anecdote, stuffed with third party hearsay, and fueled by a naturally voyeuristic media, fabulous amounts of clinical and legal misinformation, political opportunism of unprecedented scope and flavor, and vitriol that poisoned the already imploded family relationships beyond any hope of repair. Theresa was by all accounts a very shy, fun loving, and

sweet woman who loved her husband and her parents very much. The family breach and public circus would have been anathema to her.

The courts deemed that the competent medical and legal evidence produced in the records offered clear and convincing proof that Theresa had been correctly diagnosed as being in a persistent vegetative state, and that her husband had appropriately reflected her intentions and her best interests by requesting that she not be kept alive by artificial means, including nutrition and hydration. My findings concurred with the courts'. The guide for this determination was the express provisions of the Florida Rules of Civil Procedure, the Florida Rules of Evidence, and the Florida Guardianship Statute, which was crafted over fifteen years through bipartisan political and religious efforts. There was no quickly sewn-together panoply of rules used in this matter. Further, the laws included express provisions for PVS as an end of life condition, and tubal nutrition and hydration as artificial life supports for which a person may request termination.

But this was a difficult case, and it is said that difficult cases make for bad law. In October of 2003, following a second, court-ordered removal of Theresa's feeding tube, the Florida legislature passed what became known as "Terri's Law," which gave the Florida governor the prerogative of reinserting it and required the appointment of a special guardian ad litem to review her case. Although I completed the duties of the special guardian, Terri's Law was later deemed unconstitutional by the Florida Supreme Court, and the U.S. Supreme Court refused to overturn that decision. During the last week of Theresa's life, the U.S. Congress interposed with legislation to move the case from the Florida state court system to the federal courts. But the federal district court in Florida issued a lengthy opinion concluding that the evidence submitted by the Schindlers was insufficient to create a new trial or review, as did the 11th Circuit Court of Appeals in Atlanta in their subsequent opinion. The U.S. Supreme Court then refused to review the findings of the lower federal courts.

PVS is characterized by sleeping and waking cycles, unlike a coma. Waking periods include eye movement and the making of noises, which may sound like moans, laughter, or crying. But there is no evidence of consistent, responsive behaviors. The behaviors are reflexive, derived from brain stem and forebrain activities—not those of the cerebral cortex, which in Theresa's case had been reduced to liquid. PVS is further characterized by a lack of evidence that the patient is aware of or interacts with the environment. Observed behaviors are random, not consistent or responsive.

The evidence in Theresa's case supported these clinical characteristics. During the thirty days of my report preparation, I spent about twenty with Theresa. I stayed with her for as long as four hours at a time, sometimes several times a day. I also spent time with her parents and siblings, with her husband, and with the governor, to whom I was reporting. My time with Theresa was emotional and intense. I sat with her, stood by her side, held her hand, stroked her hair, cradled her head in my hands, and looked deeply and closely into her eyes. I implored, cajoled, begged, and sought to find a consistent response, any response—anything other than reflex.

Five physicians testified and provided documentation about Theresa's medical state during trial. Two were appointed by Michael Schiavo, two by the Schindlers, and one by the court. Michael Schiavo's physicians and the one appointed by the court were board-certified neurologists, all with strong academic bases. The Schindlers' physicians included one well-trained, board-certified neurologist and one radiologist who also practiced bariatric medicine. Neither had academic records of publication and research on PVS. Three of the physicians—those appointed by Michael Schiavo and the court—determined, following examination of the record and the patient, that Theresa was in a persistent vegetative state and that she would not improve. They relied on their own well-published research, current medical and scientific literature, and case studies of which they had personal experience and knowledge.

The Schindlers' two physicians stated that they believed Theresa was not in PVS, that they had successfully treated brain damaged persons, and that they would and could successfully treat Theresa. The court sought to validate these claims through data, publications, or case studies, but the

Schindlers' appointees offered their statements as medical and personal opinions and could produce no objective, scientific, peer-reviewed, or case-relevant data. (Late in the day they were joined by other physicians who claimed that Theresa was not suffering from PVS and that treatments could bring her back, but only one of these physicians had seen, much less examined, her.)

The Schindlers argued that Theresa was, as the moniker of the activist disabilities group has it, "not dead yet." Further, since she had never executed a living will, and since there was disagreement over the express intentions of their daughter, there was ambiguity about what to do that should weigh in favor of life. Michael Schiavo and others testified that, at two separate funerals of family members, each on artificial life support before they died, Theresa commented that she would never want to be kept alive in this way.

The court sided with Descartes, deducing that without evidence of cognition, Theresa *was not*. Lacking a cerebral cortex, and with only reflexive capacities, Theresa could not, according to the clear and convincing medical evidence, consciously interact with her environment or engage in responsive behaviors. (I suggested additional swallowing tests, but only if the parties agreed in advance as to how these would be used, and technical legal issues prevented that from happening.) The court also determined, on the grounds of clear and convincing legal evidence, that Theresa had expressed an intention never to be kept alive in that circumstance, even though she had not signed a living will. The process and substance conformed to the guidelines of Florida law.

Throughout much of the public discussion of this case, there were occasional allegations that Michael Schiavo had physically abused his wife prior to or perhaps even leading to her collapse. Some of these allegations were shared directly with me, but they were also shared with the state attorney's office long before I had been called to the case. During the last weeks of Theresa's life, they were also introduced in motions intended to create criminal culpability that could be investigated by the Florida Department of Children and Families. In addition, there were persistent claims that Michael Schiavo stood to gain economically from his wife's death.

But there was no evidence in the record of physical abuse or of any opportunity for his monetary gain. The evidence presented to me was beyond hearsay and third party claims. Early in the dispute with his in-laws, he had offered to abdicate any claims to residual trust fund monies if Theresa were to die before the fund was depleted. In April, the Florida Department of Children and Family Services, part of the executive branch of the state government that sought unsuccessfully to intervene in the case during the last weeks of Theresa's life, publicly announced the findings of their review of the allegations of abuse. It concluded that the allegations were wholly unfounded, and that there was no evidence of abuse whatsoever.

Nonetheless, the Schindlers were convinced that he was acting out of self-interest. Claiming that they would better uphold her interests, they repeatedly sought to gain custody of their daughter. During the extensive court battle, however, Michael Schiavo's attorney, George Felos, disemboweled their claim when he elicited testimony that they would, if it were medically necessary to save her life, amputate all of her limbs and subject her to additional surgery thereafter. The Schindlers also stated that even if Theresa had executed a formal, written living will, they would have fought to have it voided because they did not believe it was consistent with their and her beliefs. Finally, they allowed that just having their daughter alive produced "joy" for them. Based upon my discussions with the Schindlers and with Michael Schiavo, it was apparent that these statements hardened Michael Schiavo's intentions. He resolved not to allow the woman he loved to be subjected to treatment he believed she would have abhorred.

The resolution of the malpractice case, four years after Theresa's collapse, was a watershed event. Following years of being told there was no hope, Michael Schiavo had the opportunity to reassess the facts. His in-laws had encouraged him to meet other women and to get on with his life. They had even entertained his dates at their home. As he began to step away from the past, he came to understand that the consistent medical message he and the Schindlers had been given for years was correct. It was at this point that he and the Schindlers began to part ways.

But the Schindlers' position can also be understood. Bob and Mary Schindler are warm, caring, and loving—normal, decent people who found themselves in an extraordinary circumstance. The child they raised and loved was suddenly profoundly incapacitated, and they were told in no uncertain terms that there was no hope of recovery. For an adult parent, the prospect of a child predeceasing them goes against all they know to be right. The hope of parents is literally embodied in their children. And when they become adults, children may grow in many tangible ways still closer to their parents. The death of an adult child cannot be easily fathomed. It is a direct challenge to one's mortality and a deep blow to an essential part of one's reason for being here at all. For a parent to give up hope on a child can be the most extraordinary admission of defeat.

As parents try to maintain their hope, they are bound to find strength and solace from the tenets of their faith. Here, traditional Roman Catholic roots provided the Schindlers with the foundation and will to believe in something more than what was. Years before the Schindlers were joined by national Christian fundamentalist figures, they held fast to a personal belief that Theresa should not die.

I believe that the Schindlers and Michael Schiavo were honestly motivated by what they perceived as being right and in Theresa's interests. But both sides got so caught up in the legal process and in their positions that it became increasingly difficult for them to reconcile. Once third parties and the press became involved, the mold was set and there was no desire or capacity among the parties to seek compromise.

The evening before Theresa died, I left the capitol building in Tallahassee through a back door and encountered an orthodox rabbi who, though it was spring, was standing next to a pile of winter clothes. My greeting was met with a call for help; he had arrived earlier that afternoon from New York with the express purpose of saving Terri's life. Life, he pleaded, is more precious than anything. It must be assured and maintained. One life reflects the hope and essence of all life.

For some, hope as manifest in the life of one highly visible figure can become transformational.

With Theresa Schiavo, the transformational element reached a fever pitch. Theresa's last days coincided with the Easter season and what were obviously the last days of Pope John Paul II, creating an almost surreal landscape on which the polemics and legal acrobatics played out. But doubting and challenging the intentions of the zealous does not produce a platform for understanding or dialogue. Indeed, it darkened the lines of irreconcilability and impasse. Hearts were hardened—as when Michael Schiavo insisted on cremating Theresa's remains and refused to allow her to be buried in a Schindler site. He did, however, agree to allow an autopsy, which the Schindlers had requested as one of their many pleadings before the state judge. He had long refused to perform one, and so his reversal was a welcome surprise, though the Schindlers will likely not accept conclusions that are not consistent with their beliefs and contentions.

There could be no good outcome in this drama, at least for the family, though for Michael Schiavo, there may be some comfort in fulfilling what he seems to genuinely believe were his wife's wishes. For Theresa, we hope, there is peace. For the rest of us, the case may have been a special call to action, sincerely articulated on both sides of the Schiavo debate—if the white noise of the political opportunists and the fringe interests can be turned down. The ultimate sanctity of life and the prerogatives of the individual provide the boundaries for what National Public Radio commentator Daniel Schorr suggested was Ms. Schiavo's "unconscious" contribution to a badly needed, renewed national discussion of death, dying, and end of life decisions.

"HUMAN NON-PERSON": TERRI SCHIAVO, BIOETHICS, AND OUR FUTURE

Wesley J. Smith

My *debate* about Terri Schiavo's case with Florida bioethicist Bill Allen on Court TV Online eventually got down to the nitty-gritty:

Wesley Smith: Bill, do you think Terri is a person?
Bill Allen: No, I do not. I think having awareness is an essential criterion for personhood. Even minimal awareness would support some criterion of personhood, but I don't think complete absence of awareness does.

If you want to know how it became acceptable to remove tube-supplied food and water from people with profound cognitive disabilities, this exchange brings you to the nub of the Schiavo case—the "first principle," if you will. Bluntly stated, most bioethicists do not believe that membership in the human species accords any of us intrinsic moral worth. Rather, what matters is whether "a being" or "an organism," or even a machine, is a "person," a status achieved by having sufficient cognitive capacities. Those who don't measure up are denigrated as "non-persons."

Allen's perspective is in fact relatively conservative within the mainstream bioethics movement. He is apparently willing to accept that "minimal awareness would support some criterion of personhood"—although he doesn't say that awareness is determinative. Most of his colleagues are not so reticent. To them, it isn't sentience per se that matters but rather demonstrable rationality. Thus Peter Singer of Princeton argues that unless an organism is self-aware over time, the entity in question is a non-person. The British academic John Harris, the Sir David Alliance professor of bioethics of the University of Manchester, England, has defined a person as "a creature capable of valuing its own existence." Other bioethicists argue that the basic threshold of personhood should include the capacity to experience desire. James Hughes, who is more explicitly radical than many bioethicists (or perhaps, just more candid), has gone so far as to assert that people like Terri are "sentient property."

So who are the so-called human non-persons? All embryos and fetuses, to be sure. But many bioethicists also categorize newborn infants as human non-persons (although some bioethicists refer to healthy newborns as "potential persons"). So too are those with profound cognitive impairments such as Terri Schiavo and President Ronald Reagan during the latter stages of his Alzheimer's disease.

Personhood theory would reduce some of us into killable and harvestable people. Harris wrote explicitly that killing human non-persons would be fine because "Non-persons or potential persons cannot be wronged" by being killed "because death does not deprive them of something they can value. If they cannot wish to live, they cannot have that wish frustrated by being killed."

And killing isn't the half of it. Some of the same bioethicists who have been telling us how right and moral it is to dehydrate Terri Schiavo have also urged that people like Terri—that is, human non-persons—be harvested or otherwise used as mere instrumentalities. Bioethicist big-wig Tom Beauchamp of Georgetown University has suggested that "because many humans lack properties of personhood or are less than full persons, they . . . might be aggressively used as human research subjects or sources of organs."

Such thinking is not fringe in bioethics, a field in which the idea of killing for organs is fast becoming mainstream. In 1997, several doctors writing for the International Forum for Transplant Ethics opined in *The Lancet* that people (like Terri) diagnosed as being in a persistent vegetative state should be redefined as dead for purposes of organ procurement:

> If the legal definition of death were to be changed to include comprehensive irreversible loss of higher brain function, it would be possible to take the life of a patient (or more accurately to stop the heart, since the patient would be defined as dead) by a lethal injection, and then to remove the organs needed for transplantation subject to the usual criteria for consent.

Knowing that this kind of thinking predominates in contemporary bioethics, I decided to bring up the matter in my Court TV debate with Bill Allen.

Wesley Smith: If Terri is not a person, should her organs be procured with consent?
Bill Allen: . . . Yes, I think there should be consent to harvest her organs, just as we allow people to say what they want done with their assets.

Put that in your hat and ponder it for a moment: If organ harvesting from the cognitively devastated were legal today—thank goodness, it isn't— Michael Schiavo would be the one, no doubt sanctioned by Judge Greer, who could consent to doctors' "stopping" Terri's heart and harvesting her organs.

Think that's a horrid thought? Well, ponder this: More than ten years ago, transplant-medicine ethicists Robert M. Arnold and Stuart J. Youngner painted a disturbing picture of the kind of society that the bioethics movement is leading us toward: literally a culture in which organ procurement is a routine part of end-of-life care and "planned deaths." The ethicists predicted that in the not-too-distant future:

> Machine dependent patients could give consent for organ removal before they are dead. For example, a ventilator-dependent ALS patient could request that life support be removed at 5:00 P.M., but that at 9:00 A.M. the same day he be taken to the operating room, put under general anesthesia, and his kidneys, liver and pancreas removed. . . . The patient's heart would not be removed and would continue to beat throughout surgery, perfusing the other organs with warm, oxygen-and-nutrient-rich blood until they were removed. The heart would stop, and the patient would be pronounced dead only after the ventilator was removed at 5:00 P.M., according to plan, and long before the patient could die from renal, hepatic, or pancreatic failure.

Know this: There is a direct line from the Terri Schiavo dehydration to the potential for this stunning human strip-mining scenario's becoming a reality. Indeed, as Arnold and Youngner put it so well, "If a look into such a future hurts our eyes (or turns our stomachs), is our discomfort any different from what we would have experienced 30 years ago by looking into the future that is today?"

IN THE MATTER OF CLAIRE C. CONROY
Supreme Court of New Jersey. 98 N.J. 321, 486 A. 2d 1209, decided Jan. 17, 1985

SCHREIBER, J.

At issue here are the circumstances under which life-sustaining treatment may be withheld or withdrawn from incompetent, institutionalized, elderly patients suffering from severe and permanent mental and physical impairments and a limited life expectancy.

Plaintiff, Thomas C. Whittemore, nephew and guardian of Claire Conroy, an incompetent, sought permission to remove a nasogastric feeding tube, the primary conduit for nutrients, from his ward, an eighty-four-year-old bedridden woman with serious and irreversible physical and mental impairments, who resided in a nursing home. John J. Delaney, Jr., Conroy's guardian *ad litem*, opposed the guardian's petition. The trial court granted the guardian permission to remove the tube, and the Appellate Division reversed. . . .

At the time of trial, Ms. Conroy was no longer ambulatory and was confined to bed, unable to move from a semi-fetal position. She suffered from arteriosclerotic heart disease, hypertension, and diabetes mellitus; her left leg was gangrenous to her knee; she had several necrotic decubitus ulcers (bed sores) on her left foot, leg, and hip; an eye problem required irrigation; she had a urinary catheter in place and could not control her bowels; she could not speak; and her ability to swallow was very limited. On the other hand, she interacted with her environment in some limited ways: she could move her head, neck, hands, and arms to a minor extent; she was able to scratch herself, and had pulled at her bandages, tube, and catheter; she moaned occasionally when moved or fed through the tube, or when her bandages were changed; her eyes sometimes followed individuals in the room; her facial expressions were different when she was awake from when she was asleep; and she smiled on

occasion when her hair was combed, or when she received a comforting rub.

Dr. Kazemi and Dr. Davidoff, a specialist in internal medicine who observed Ms. Conroy before testifying as an expert on behalf of the guardian, testified that Ms. Conroy was not brain dead, comatose, or in a chronic vegetative state. They stated, however, that her intellectual capacity was very limited, and that her mental condition probably would never improve. Dr. Davidoff characterized her as awake, but said that she was severely demented, was unable to respond to verbal stimuli, and, as far as he could tell, had no higher functioning or consciousness. Dr. Kazemi, in contrast, said that although she was confused and unaware, "she responds somehow."

The medical testimony was inconclusive as to whether, or to what extent, Ms. Conroy was capable of experiencing pain. Dr. Kazemi thought that Ms. Conroy might have experienced some degree of pain from her severely contracted limbs, or that the contractures were a reaction to pain, but that she did not necessarily suffer pain from the sores on her legs. According to Dr. Davidoff, it was unclear whether Ms. Conroy's feeding tube caused her pain, and it was "an open question whether she [felt] pain" at all; however, it was possible that she was experiencing a great deal of pain. Dr. Davidoff further testified that she responded to noxious or painful stimuli by moaning. The trial court determined that the testimony of a neurologist who had examined Ms. Conroy would not be necessary, since it believed that it had sufficient evidence about her medical condition on which to base a decision.

Both doctors testified that if the nasogastric tube were removed, Ms. Conroy would die of dehydration in about a week. Dr. Davidoff believed that the resulting thirst could be painful but that Ms. Conroy would become unconscious long before she died. Dr. Kazemi concurred that such a death would be painful. . . .

Ms. Conroy's only surviving blood relative was her nephew, the guardian, Thomas Whittemore. He

---

Editors' note: Some text and most legal references have been cut.

had known her for over fifty years, had visited her approximately once a week for four or five years prior to her commitment to the nursing home, and had continued to visit her regularly at the nursing home for some time. The record contained additional evidence about the nephew's and aunt's financial situations and the history of their relationship. Based on the details of that record, there was no question that the nephew had good intentions and had no real conflict of interest due to possible inheritance when he sought permission to remove the tube.

Mr. Whittemore testified that Ms. Conroy feared and avoided doctors and that, to the best of his knowledge, she had never visited a doctor until she became incompetent in 1979. He said that on the couple of occasions that Ms. Conroy had pneumonia, "[y]ou couldn't bring a doctor in," and his wife, a registered nurse, would "try to get her through whatever she had." He added that once, when his wife took Ms. Conroy to the hospital emergency room, "as foggy as she was she snapped out of it, she would not sign herself in, and she would have signed herself out immediately." According to the nephew, "[a]ll [Ms. Conroy and her sisters] wanted was to . . . have their bills paid and die in their own house." He also stated that he had refused to consent to the amputation of her gangrenous leg in 1982 and that he now sought removal of the nasogastric tube because, in his opinion, she would have refused the amputation and "would not have allowed [the nasogastric tube] to be inserted in the first place."

. . .

The trial court decided to permit removal of the tube. It reasoned that the focus of inquiry should be whether life has become impossibly and permanently burdensome to the patient. If so, the court held, prolonging life becomes pointless and perhaps cruel. It determined that removal of the tube would lead to death by starvation and dehydration within a few days, and that the death might be painful. Nevertheless, it found that Ms. Conroy's intellectual functioning had been permanently reduced to a very primitive level, that her life had become impossibly and permanently burdensome, and that removal of the feeding tube should therefore be permitted.

The guardian *ad litem* appealed. While the appeal was pending, Ms. Conroy died with the nasogastric tube intact. Nevertheless, the Appellate Division decided to resolve the meritorious issues, finding that they were of significant public importance and that this type of case was capable of repetition but would evade review because the patients involved frequently die during litigation.

. . .

The Appellate Division . . . held that the right to terminate life-sustaining treatment based on a guardian's judgment was limited to incurable and terminally ill patients who are brain dead, irreversibly comatose, or vegetative, and who would gain no medical benefit from continued treatment. As an alternative ground for its decision, it held that a guardian's decision may never be used to withhold nourishment, as opposed to the treatment or attempted curing of a disease, from an incompetent patient who is not comatose, brain dead, or vegetative, and whose death is not irreversibly imminent. Depriving a patient of a basic necessity of life, such as food, under those circumstances, the court stated, would hasten death rather than simply allow the illness to take its natural course. The court concluded that withdrawal of Ms. Conroy's nasogastric tube would be tantamount to killing her— not simply letting her die—and that such active euthanasia was ethically impermissible. The Appellate Division therefore reversed the trial court's judgment.

We granted the guardian's petition for certification, despite Ms. Conroy's death, since we agree with the Appellate Division that the matter is of substantial importance and is capable of repetition but evades review. . . .

I

This case requires us to determine the circumstances under which life-sustaining treatment may be withheld or withdrawn from an elderly nursing-home resident who is suffering from serious and permanent mental and physical impairments, who will probably die within approximately one year even with the treatment, and who, though formerly competent, is now incompetent to make decisions about her life-sustaining treatment and is unlikely to regain such competence. . . .

The *Quinlan* decision dealt with a special category of patients: those in a chronic, persistent vegetative or comatose state. In a footnote, the opinion left open the question whether the principles it enunciated might be applicable to incompetent patients in "other types of terminal medical situations . . . , not necessarily involving the hopeless loss of cognitive or sapient life." We now are faced with one such situation: that of elderly, formerly competent nursing-home residents who, unlike Karen Quinlan, are awake and conscious and can interact with their environment to a limited extent, but whose mental and physical functioning is severely and permanently impaired and whose life expectancy, even with the treatment, is relatively short. The capacities of such people, while significantly diminished, are not as limited as those of irreversibly comatose persons, and their deaths, while no longer distant, may not be imminent. Large numbers of aged, chronically ill, institutionalized persons fall within this general category.

Such people (like newborns, mentally retarded persons, permanently comatose individuals, and members of other groups with which this case does not deal) are unable to speak for themselves on life-and-death issues concerning their medical care. This does not mean, however, that they lack a right to self-determination. The right of an adult who, like Claire Conroy, was once competent, to determine the course of her medical treatment remains intact even when she is no longer able to assert that right or to appreciate its effectuation. As one commentator has noted:

> Even if the patient becomes too insensate to appreciate the honoring of his or her choice, self-determination is important. After all, law respects testamentary dispositions even if the testator never views his gift being bestowed. [Cantor, 30 *Rutgers L.Rev.* at 259.] . . .
>
> Any other view would permit obliteration of an incompetent's panoply of rights merely because the patient could no longer sense the violation of those rights. [*Id.* at 252.]

Since the condition of an incompetent patient makes it impossible to ascertain definitively his present desires, a third party acting on the patient's behalf often cannot say with confidence that his treatment decision for the patient will further rather than frustrate the patient's right to control his body. Nevertheless, the goal of decision-making for incompetent patients should be to determine and effectuate, insofar as possible, the decision that the patient would have made if competent. Ideally, both aspects of the patient's right to bodily integrity—the right to consent to medical intervention and the right to refuse it—should be respected.

In light of these rights and concerns, we hold that life-sustaining treatment may be withheld or withdrawn from an incompetent patient when it is clear that the particular patient would have refused the treatment under the circumstances involved. The standard we are enunciating is a subjective one, consistent with the notion that the right that we are seeking to effectuate is a very personal right to control one's own life. The question is not what a reasonable or average person would have chosen to do under the circumstances but what the particular patient would have done if able to choose for himself.

The patient may have expressed, in one or more ways, an intent not to have life-sustaining medical intervention. Such an intent might be embodied in a written document, or "living will," stating the person's desire not to have certain types of life-sustaining treatment administered under certain circumstances. It might also be evidenced in an oral directive that the patient gave to a family member, friend, or health care provider. It might consist of a durable power of attorney or appointment of a proxy authorizing a particular person to make the decisions on the patient's behalf if he is no longer capable of making them for himself. It might take the form of reactions that the patient voiced regarding medical treatment administered to others. *See, e.g., Storar,* 52 N.Y.2d 363, 420 N.E.2d 64, 438 N.Y.S.2d 266 (withdrawal of respirator was justified as an effectuation of patient's stated wishes when patient, as member of Catholic religious order, had stated more than once in formal discussions concerning the moral implications of the *Quinlan* case, most recently two months before he suffered cardiac arrest that left him in an irreversible coma, that he would not want extraordinary means used to keep him alive under similar circumstances). It might also be deduced from a person's religious beliefs and the tenets of that religion, or from the patient's consistent pattern of conduct with respect to prior decisions about his own medical care. Of course, dealing with the matter in advance in some sort of thoughtful and explicit way is best for all concerned.

Any of the above types of evidence, and any other information bearing on the person's intent, may be appropriate aids in determining what course of treatment the patient would have wished to pursue. In this respect, we now believe that we were in error in *Quinlan*, to disregard evidence of statements that Ms. Quinlan made to friends concerning artificial prolongation of the lives of others who were terminally ill. Such evidence is certainly relevant to shed light on whether the patient would have consented to the treatment if competent to make the decision.

Although all evidence tending to demonstrate a person's intent with respect to medical treatment should properly be considered by either surrogate decision-makers, or by a court in the event of any judicial proceedings, the probative value of such evidence may vary depending on the remoteness, consistency, and thoughtfulness of the prior statements or actions and the maturity of the person at the time of the statements or acts. Thus, for example, an offhand remark about not wanting to live under certain circumstances made by a person when young and in the peak of health would not in itself constitute clear proof twenty years later that he would want life-sustaining treatment withheld under those circumstances. In contrast, a carefully considered position, especially if written, that a person had maintained over a number of years or that he had acted upon in comparable circumstances might be clear evidence of his intent.

Another factor that would affect the probative value of a person's prior statements of intent would be their specificity. Of course, no one can predict with accuracy the precise circumstances with which he ultimately might be faced. Nevertheless, any details about the level of impaired functioning and the forms of medical treatment that one would find tolerable should be incorporated into advance directives to enhance their later usefulness as evidence.

Medical evidence bearing on the patient's condition, treatment, and prognosis, like evidence of the patient's wishes, is an essential prerequisite to decision-making under the subjective test. The medical evidence must establish that the patient fits within the Claire Conroy pattern: an elderly, incompetent nursing-home resident with severe and permanent mental and physical impairments and a life expectancy of approximately one year or less. In addition, since the goal is to effectuate the patient's right of informed consent, the surrogate decision-maker must have at least as much medical information upon which to base his decision about what the patient would have chosen as one would expect a competent patient to have before consenting to or rejecting treatment. Such information might include evidence about the patient's present level of physical, sensory, emotional, and cognitive functioning; the degree of physical pain resulting from the medical condition, treatment, and termination of treatment, respectively; the degree of humiliation, dependence, and loss of dignity probably resulting from the condition and treatment; the life expectancy and prognosis for recovery with and without treatment; the various treatment options; and the risks, side effects, and benefits of each of those options. Particular care should be taken not to base a decision on a premature diagnosis or prognosis.

We recognize that for some incompetent patients it might be impossible to be clearly satisfied as to the patient's intent either to accept or reject the life-sustaining treatment. Many people may have spoken of their desires in general or casual terms, or, indeed, never considered or resolved the issue at all. In such cases, a surrogate decision-maker cannot presume that treatment decisions made by a third party on the patient's behalf will further the patient's right to self-determination, since effectuating another person's right to self-determination presupposes that the substitute decision-maker knows what the person would have wanted. Thus, in the absence of adequate proof of the patient's wishes, it is naive to pretend that the right to self-determination serves as the basis for substituted decision-making.

We hesitate, however, to foreclose the possibility of humane actions, which may involve termination of life-sustaining treatment, for persons who never clearly expressed their desires about life-sustaining treatment but who are now suffering a prolonged and painful death. An incompetent, like a minor child, is a ward of the state, and the state's *parens patriae* power supports the authority of its courts to allow decisions to be made for an incompetent that serve the incompetent's best interests, even if the person's wishes cannot be clearly established. This authority permits the state to authorize guardians to withhold or withdraw life-sustaining treatment from an incompetent patient if it is manifest that such action would further the patient's best interests in a narrow sense of the phrase, even though the subjective test that we articulated above may not be satisfied. We therefore hold that life-sustaining treatment may also be withheld or withdrawn from a patient in Claire Conroy's situation if either of two "best interests" tests—a limited-objective or a pure-objective test—is satisfied.

Under the limited-objective test, life-sustaining treatment may be withheld or withdrawn from a patient in Claire Conroy's situation when there is some trustworthy evidence that the patient would have refused the treatment, and the decision-maker is satisfied that it is clear that the burdens of the patient's continued life with the treatment outweigh the benefits of that life for him. By this we mean that the patient is suffering, and will continue to suffer throughout the expected duration of his life, unavoidable pain, and that the net burdens of his prolonged life (the pain and suffering of his life with the treatment less the amount and duration of pain that the patient would likely experience if the treatment were withdrawn) markedly outweigh any physical pleasure, emotional enjoyment, or intellectual satisfaction that the patient may still be able to derive from life. This limited-objective standard permits the termination of treatment for a patient who had not unequivocally expressed his desires before becoming incompetent, when it is clear that the treatment in question would merely prolong the patient's suffering.

Medical evidence will be essential to establish that the burdens of the treatment to the patient in terms of pain and suffering outweigh the benefits that the patient is experiencing. The medical evidence should make it clear that the treatment would merely prolong the patient's suffering and not provide him with any net benefit. Information is particularly important with respect to the degree, expected duration, and constancy of pain with and without treatment, and the possibility that the pain could be reduced by drugs or other means short of

terminating the life-sustaining treatment. The same types of medical evidence that are relevant to the subjective analysis, such as the patient's life expectancy, prognosis, level of functioning, degree of humiliation and dependency, and treatment options, should also be considered.

This limited-objective test also requires some trustworthy evidence that the patient would have wanted the treatment terminated. This evidence could take any one or more of the various forms appropriate to prove the patient's intent under the subjective test. Evidence that, taken as a whole, would be too vague, casual, or remote to constitute the clear proof of the patient's subjective intent that is necessary to satisfy the subjective test—for example, informally expressed reactions to other people's medical conditions and treatment—might be sufficient to satisfy this prong of the limited-objective test.

In the absence of trustworthy evidence, or indeed any evidence at all, that the patient would have declined the treatment, life-sustaining treatment may still be withheld or withdrawn from a formerly competent person like Claire Conroy if a third, pure-objective test is satisfied. Under that test, as under the limited-objective test, the net burdens of the patient's life with the treatment should clearly and markedly outweigh the benefits that the patient derives from life. Further, the recurring, unavoidable, and severe pain of the patient's life with the treatment should be such that the effect of administering life-sustaining treatment would be inhumane. Subjective evidence that the patient would not have wanted the treatment is not necessary under this pure-objective standard. Nevertheless, even in the context of severe pain, life-sustaining treatment should not be withdrawn from an incompetent patient who had previously expressed a wish to be kept alive in spite of any pain that he might experience.

Although we are condoning a restricted evaluation of the nature of a patient's life in terms of pain, suffering, and possible enjoyment under the limited-objective and pure-objective tests, we expressly decline to authorize decision-making based on assessments of the personal worth or social utility of another's life, or the value of that life to others. We do not believe that it would be appropriate for a court to designate a person with the authority to determine that someone else's life is not worth living simply because, to that person, the patient's "quality of life" or value to society seems negligible. The mere fact that a patient's functioning is limited or his prognosis dim does not mean that he is not enjoying what remains of his life or that it is in his best interests to die. But see *President's Commission Report*, at 135 (endorsing termination of treatment whenever the surrogate decision-maker in his discretion believes it is in the patient's best interests, defined broadly to "take into account such factors as the relief of suffering, the preservation or restoration of functioning, and the quality as well as the extent of life sustained"). More wide-ranging powers to make decisions about other people's lives, in our view, would create an intolerable risk for socially isolated and defenseless people suffering from physical or mental handicaps.

We are aware that it will frequently be difficult to conclude that the evidence is sufficient to justify termination of treatment under either of the "best interests" tests that we have described. Often, it is unclear whether and to what extent a patient such as Claire Conroy is capable of, or is in fact, experiencing pain. Similarly, medical experts are often unable to determine with any degree of certainty the extent of a nonverbal person's intellectual functioning or the depth of his emotional life. When the evidence is insufficient to satisfy either the limited-objective or pure-objective standard, however, we cannot justify the termination of life-sustaining treatment as clearly furthering the best interests of a patient like Ms. Conroy.

The surrogate decision-maker should exercise extreme caution in determining the patient's intent and in evaluating medical evidence of the patient's pain and possible enjoyment, and should not approve withholding or withdrawing life-sustaining treatment unless he is manifestly satisfied that one of the three tests that we have outlined has been met. When evidence of a person's wishes or physical or mental condition is equivocal, it is best to err, if at all, in favor of preserving life. . . .

II

We emphasize that in making decisions whether to administer life-sustaining treatment to patients such as Claire Conroy, the primary focus should be the patient's desires and experience of pain and enjoyment—not the type of treatment involved. Thus, we reject the distinction that some have made between actively hastening death by terminating treatment and passively allowing a person to die of a disease as one of limited use in a legal analysis of such a decision-making situation.

Characterizing conduct as active or passive is often an elusive notion, even outside the context of medical decision-making.

> Saint Anselm of Canterbury was fond of citing the trickiness of the distinction between "to do" (*facere*) and "not to do" (*non facere*). In answer to the question "What's he doing?" we say "He's just sitting there" (positive), really meaning something negative: "He's not doing anything at all." [*D. Walton*, at 234 (footnote omitted).]

The distinction is particularly nebulous, however, in the context of decisions whether to withhold or withdraw life-sustaining treatment. In a case like that of Claire Conroy, for example, would a physician who discontinued nasogastric feeding be actively causing her death by removing her primary source of nutrients, or would he merely be omitting to continue the artificial form of treatment, thus passively allowing her medical condition, which includes her inability to swallow, to take its natural course? The ambiguity inherent in this distinction is further heightened when one performs an act within an overall plan of nonintervention, such as when a doctor writes an order not to resuscitate a patient.

> Consequently, merely determining whether what was done involved a fatal act or omission does not establish whether it was morally acceptable. . . . [In fact, a]ctive steps to terminate life-sustaining interventions may be permitted, indeed required, by the patient's authority to forego therapy even when such steps lead to death. [*President's Commission Report*, at 67, 72.]

For a similar reason, we also reject any distinction between withholding and withdrawing life-sustaining treatment. Some commentators have suggested that discontinuing life-sustaining treatment once it has been commenced is morally more problematic than merely failing to begin the treatment. Discontinuing life-sustaining treatment, to some, is an "active" taking of life, as opposed to the more "passive" act of omitting the treatment in the first instance. In the words of one writer, "[T]he difference between taking away that which one has come to count on as normal support for life and not instituting therapy when a new crisis begins . . . fits nicely a basic moral distinction throughout life—we are not morally obligated to help another person, but we are morally obligated not to interfere with his life-sustaining routines."

This distinction is more psychologically compelling than logically sound. As mentioned above, the line between active and passive conduct in the context of medical decisions is far too nebulous to constitute a principled basis for decision-making. Whether necessary treatment is withheld at the outset or withdrawn later on, the consequence—the patient's death—is the same. Moreover, from a policy standpoint, it might well be unwise to forbid persons from discontinuing a treatment under circumstances in which the treatment could permissibly be withheld. Such a rule could discourage families and doctors from even attempting certain types of care and could thereby force them into hasty and premature decisions to allow a patient to die.

Some commentators, as indeed did the Appellate Division here, have made yet a fourth distinction, between the termination of artificial feedings and the termination of other forms of life-sustaining medical treatment. According to the Appellate Division:

> If, as here, the patient is not comatose and does not face imminent and inevitable death, nourishment accomplishes the substantial benefit of sustaining life until the illness takes its natural course. Under such circumstances nourishment always will be an essential element of ordinary care which physicians are ethically obligated to provide. [190 *N.J.Super.* at 473, 464, A.2d 303.]

Certainly, feeding has an emotional significance. As infants we could breathe without assistance, but we were dependent on others for our lifeline of nourishment. Even more, feeding is an expression of nurturing and caring, certainly for infants and children, and in many cases for adults as well.

Once one enters the realm of complex, high-technology medical care, it is hard to shed the "emotional symbolism" of food. However, artificial feedings such as nasogastric tubes, gastrostomies, and intravenous infusions are significantly different from bottle-feeding or spoon-feeding—they are

medical procedures with inherent risks and possible side effects, instituted by skilled health-care providers to compensate for impaired physical functioning. Analytically, artificial feeding by means of a nasogastric tube or intravenous infusion can be seen as equivalent to artificial breathing by means of a respirator. Both prolong life through mechanical means when the body is no longer able to perform a vital bodily function on its own.

Furthermore, while nasogastric feeding and other medical procedures to ensure nutrition and hydration are usually well tolerated, they are not free from risks or burdens; they have complications that are sometimes serious and distressing to the patient.

Nasogastric tubes may lead to pneumonia, cause irritation and discomfort, and require arm restraints for an incompetent patient. The volume of fluid needed to carry nutrients itself is sometimes harmful.

Finally, dehydration may well not be distressing or painful to a dying patient. For patients who are unable to sense hunger and thirst, withholding of feeding devices such as nasogastric tubes may not result in more pain than the termination of any other medical treatment. Indeed, it has been observed that patients near death who are not receiving nourishment may be more comfortable than patients in comparable conditions who are being fed and hydrated artificially. Thus, it cannot be assumed that it will always be beneficial for an incompetent patient to receive artificial feeding or harmful for him not to receive it.

Under the analysis articulated above, withdrawal or withholding of artificial feeding, like any other medical treatment, would be permissible if there is sufficient proof to satisfy the subjective, limited-objective, or pure-objective test. A competent patient has the right to decline any medical treatment, including artificial feeding, and should retain that right when and if he becomes incompetent. In addition, in the case of an incompetent patient who has given little or no trustworthy indication of an intent to decline treatment and for whom it becomes necessary to engage in balancing under the limited-objective or pure-objective test, the pain and invasiveness of an artificial feeding device, and the pain of withdrawing that device, should be treated just like the results of administering or withholding any other medical treatment.

III

The decision-making procedure for comatose, vegetative patients suggested in *Quinlan*, namely, the concurrence of the guardian, family, attending physician, and hospital prognosis committee, is not entirely appropriate for patients such as Claire Conroy, who are confined to nursing homes. . . .

Because of the special vulnerability of mentally and physically impaired, elderly persons in nursing homes and the potential for abuse with unsupervised institutional decision-making in such homes, life-sustaining treatment should not be withdrawn or withheld from a nursing-home resident like Claire Conroy in the absence of a guardian's decision, made in accordance with the procedure outlined below, that the elements of the subjective, limited-objective, or pure-objective test have been satisfied. A necessary prerequisite to surrogate decision-making is a judicial determination that the patient is incompetent to make the decision for himself and designation of a guardian for the incompetent patient if he does not already have one.

As noted above, the guardian will resolve the issues in these matters and make the ultimate decision with such concurrences as we have required. Ordinarily, court involvement will be limited to the determination of incompetency, and the appointment of a guardian unless a personal guardian has been previously appointed, who will determine whether the standards we have prescribed have been satisfied. The record in this case did not satisfy those standards. The evidence that Claire Conroy would have refused the treatment, although sufficient to meet the lower showing of intent required under the limited-objective test, was certainly not the "clear" showing of intent contemplated under the subjective test. More information should, if possible, have been obtained by the guardian with respect to Ms. Conroy's intent. What were her ethical, moral, and religious beliefs? She did try to refuse initial hospitalization, and indeed had "scorned medicine." However, she allowed her nephew's wife, a registered nurse, to care for her during several illnesses. It was not clear whether Ms. Conroy permitted the niece to administer any drugs or other forms of medical treatment to her during these illnesses. Although it may often prove difficult, and at times impossible, to ascertain a person's wishes, the Conroy case illustrates the sources to which the guardian might turn. For example, in more than eight decades of life in the same house, it is possible that she revealed to persons other than her nephew her feelings regarding medical treatment, other values, and her goals in life. Some promising avenues for such an inquiry about her personal values included her response to the illnesses and deaths of her sisters and others, and her statements with respect to not wanting to be in a nursing home.

Moreover, there was insufficient information concerning the benefits and burdens of Ms. Conroy's life to satisfy either the limited-objective or pure-objective test. Although the treating doctor and the guardian's expert testified as to Claire Conroy's condition, neither testified conclusively as to whether she was in pain or was capable of experiencing pain or thirst. There was medical agreement that removal of the tube would have caused pain during the period of approximately one week that would have elapsed before her death, or at least until she were to lapse into a coma. On the other hand, there was little, if any, evidence of the discomfort, suffering, and pain she would endure if she continued to be fed and medicated through the tube during her remaining life—contemplated to be up to one year. Apparently her feedings sometimes occasioned moaning, but it remains unclear whether these were reflex responses or expressions of discomfort. Moreover, although she tried to remove the tube, it is not clear that this was intentional, and there was little evidence that she was in distress. Her treating physician also offered contradictory views as to whether the contractures of her legs caused pain or whether, indeed, they might be the result of pain, without offering any evidence on that issue. The trial court rejected as superfluous the offer to present as an expert witness a neurologist, who might have been able to explain what Ms. Conroy's reactions to the environment indicated about her perception of pain.

The evidence was also unclear with respect to Ms. Conroy's capacity to feel pleasure, another issue as to which the information supplied by a neurologist might have been helpful. What was known of her awareness of the world? Although Ms. Conroy had some ability to smile and scratch, the relationship of these activities to external stimuli apparently was quite variable.

The trial transcript reveals no exploration of the discomfort and risks that attend nasogastric feedings. A casual mention by the nurse/administrator of the need to restrain the patient to prevent the removal of the tube was not followed by an assessment of the detrimental impact, if any, of those restraints. Alternative modalities, including gastrostomies, intravenous feeding, subcutaneous or intramuscular hydration, or some combination, were not investigated. Neither of the expert witnesses presented empirical evidence regarding the treatment options for such a patient.

It can be seen that the evidence at trial was inadequate to satisfy the subjective, the limited-objective, or the pure-objective standard that we have set forth. Were Claire Conroy still alive, the guardian would have been required to explore these issues prior to reaching any decision. Guardians—and courts, if they are involved—should act cautiously and deliberately in deciding these cases. The consequences are most serious—life or death. . . .

The judgment of the Appellate Division is reversed. In light of Ms. Conroy's death, we do not remand the matter for further proceedings.

HANDLER, J., concurring in part and dissenting in part. . . .

In my opinion, the Court's objective tests too narrowly define the interests of people like Miss Conroy. While the basic standard purports to account for several concerns, it ultimately focuses on pain as the critical factor. The presence of significant pain in effect becomes the sole measure of such a person's best interests. "Pain" thus eclipses a whole cluster of other human values that have a proper place in the subtle weighing that will ultimately determine how life should end.

The Court's concentration on pain as the exclusive criterion in reaching the life-or-death decision in reality transmutes the best-interests determination into an exercise of avoidance and nullification rather than confrontation and fulfillment. In most cases the pain criterion will dictate that the decision be one not to withdraw life-prolonging treatment and not to allow death to occur naturally. First, pain will not be an operative factor in a great many cases. "[P]resently available drugs and techniques allow pain to be reduced to a level acceptable to virtually every patient, usually without unacceptable sedation." *President's Commission Report*, at 50–51. *See id.* at 19 n. 19 *citing* Saunders, "Current Views on Pain Relief and Terminal Care," in *The Therapy of Pain* 215 (Swerdlow, ed. 1981) (a hospice reports complete control of pain in over 99% of its dying patients). Further, as was true in Miss Conroy's case, health care providers frequently encounter difficulty in evaluating the degree of pain experienced by a patient. Finally, "[o]nly a minority of patients—fewer than half of those with malignancies, for example—have substantial problems with pain. . . ." *President's Commission Report*, at 278. Thus, in a great many cases, the pain test will become an absolute bar to the withdrawal of life-support therapy.

The pain requirement, as applied by the Court in its objective tests, effectively negates other highly relevant considerations that should appropriately bear on the decision to maintain or to withdraw life-prolonging treatment. The pain standard may dictate the decision to prolong life despite the presence of other factors that reasonably militate in favor of the termination of such procedures to allow a natural death. The exclusive pain criterion denies relief to that class of people who, at the very end of life, might strongly disapprove of an artificially extended existence in spite of the absence of pain. Thus, some people abhor dependence on others as much, or more, than they fear pain. Other individuals value personal privacy and dignity, and prize independence from others when their personal needs and bodily functions are involved. Finally, the ideal of bodily integrity may become more important than simply prolonging life at its most rudimentary level. Persons, like Miss Conroy, "may well have wished to avoid . . . '[t]he ultimate horror [not of] death but the possibility of being maintained in limbo, in a sterile room, by machines controlled by strangers.'" *In re Torres*, 357 N.W.2d at 340, quoting Steel, "The Right to Die: New Options in California," 93 *Christian Century* [July–Dec. 1976].

Clearly, a decision to focus exclusively on pain as the single criterion ignores and devalues other important ideals regarding life and death. Consequently, a pain standard cannot serve as an indirect proxy for additional and significant concerns that may bear on the decision to forgo life-prolonging treatments. . . .

I would therefore have the Court adopt a test that does not rely exclusively on pain as the ultimately determinative criterion. Rather, the standard should consist of an array of factors to be medically established and then evaluated by the decision-maker both singly and collectively to reach a balance that will justify the determination to withdraw or to continue life-prolonging treatment. The withdrawal of life-prolonging treatment from an unconscious or comatose, terminally ill individual near death, whose personal views concerning life-ending treatment cannot be ascertained, should be governed by such a standard.

Several important criteria bear on this critical determination. The person should be terminally ill and facing imminent death. There should also be present the permanent loss of conscious thought processes in the form of a comatose state or profound unconsciousness. Further, there should be the irreparable failure of at least one major and essential bodily organ or system. Obviously the presence or absence of significant pain is highly relevant.

In addition, the person's general physical condition must be of great concern. Progressive, irreversible, extensive, and extreme physical deterioration, such as ulcers, lesions, gangrene, infection, incontinence, and the like, which frequently afflict the bedridden, terminally ill, should be considered in the formulation of an appropriate standard. The medical and nursing treatment of individuals in *extremis* and

suffering from these conditions entails the constant and extensive handling and manipulation of the body. At some point, such a course of treatment upon the insensate patient is bound to touch the sensibilities of even the most detached observer. Eventually, pervasive bodily intrusions, even for the best motives, will arouse feelings akin to humiliation and mortification for the helpless patient. When cherished values of human dignity and personal privacy, which belong to every person living or dying, are sufficiently transgressed by what is being done to the individual, we should be ready to say: enough.

In my view, our understanding as to how life should end must be infused with the fundamental human moral values that serve us while we live. As we have faced life, so should we be able to face death. When an individual's personal philosophy or moral values cannot otherwise be brought to bear to resolve the dilemma of whether to live or die, then factors that generally and normally shape basic human moral values should be taken into account. These factors should be assessed reasonably and fairly from the patient's perspective. They should be weighed and balanced by an appropriate, responsible surrogate decision-maker in reaching the final awesome decision whether to withdraw life-prolonging treatment from the unfortunate and hapless patient. I believe that a decision informed by these considerations would be conducive to the humane, dignified, and decent ending of life.

THE SEVERELY DEMENTED, MINIMALLY FUNCTIONAL PATIENT: AN ETHICAL ANALYSIS

John D. Arras

Mrs. Smith, an 85-year-old resident of a nursing home, was transferred to the hospital for treatment of pneumonia. Although she has responded well to

From *Journal of the American Geriatrics Society* 36 (1988): 938–944. Reprinted with permission.

antibiotic therapy, her overall condition and prognosis remain grim. For the past 3 years her mental state has been steadily deteriorating due to a series of strokes which have finally rendered her severely demented. She is now nonambulatory, incapable of sitting up in bed, and uncommunicative most of the time. When she does talk, her speech is completely incoherent and repetitive. Mrs. Smith shows no signs of recognizing or remembering her family and primary caregivers. The nurses in charge of her care assert that she appears to experience pleasure only when her hair is combed or her back rubbed.

During her recovery from the pneumonia, Mrs. Smith began to have problems with swallowing food. Following a precipitous decline in her caloric intake, her son and daughter (the only involved family members) consented to the placement of a nasogastric tube. Mrs. Smith continually pulled out the tube, however, and continues to resist efforts to reinsert it.

The health care team faces difficult choices regarding Mrs. Smith's care. Foremost among them is whether her physicians should surgically insert a gastrostomy tube in spite of her aversive behavior. Mrs. Smith has neither left behind a living will nor has she indicated to family or friends at the nursing home what her preferences would be regarding life-sustaining care in this sort of circumstance. Both her son and daughter have stated that she would nevertheless not have wanted a gastrostomy tube inserted and would, if she could presently decide, prefer an earlier death to being sustained indefinitely in the twilight of her minimally functional condition. In defense of this claim, they note that she has always been a very active, independent person who avoided doctors whenever possible.

PROBING THE PATIENT'S SUBJECTIVITY

The first order of business in deciding for incompetent patients is to inquire, whenever possible, what the patient would want were she presently able to communicate. In the absence of a designated proxy or living will that speaks with rare precision about which modes of treatment are to be forgone under which circumstances, this task is more difficult than many commentators and jurists would have us think. The case before us yields two distinct sources of revelation bearing on the patient's putative subjective wishes regarding the present decision. As we shall see, neither provides evidence sufficiently compelling for us to conclude with moral certitude that she would not allow the insertion of a G-tube.

Extrapolating from the Patient's Prior Values

First, we have the testimony of family members who claim that the patient's character traits of independence and aloofness from physicians point to the conclusion that she would not want to be sustained by a G-tube. Although this claim may well be *plausible* and at least *consistent* with Mrs. Smith's previously held attitudes and behaviors, it would require a great leap of both faith and logic to conclude that evidence of this sort *entails* a negative decision on life-sustaining treatment. As several commentators have pointed out, there is a great difference between the degree of respect owed to a patient's *actual choices*, even choices made prior to the advent of incompetency, and to his or her preferences or tastes.[1-4] It is one thing to have negative attitudes toward aggressive life support, but it is quite another to actually refuse it in your own case. By doing so, a person *commits* himself or herself to a particular course of action and it is this commitment, rather than mere attitudes or generalized preferences abstracted from the particular details of choosing situations, that commands especially stringent respect.

Even if someone's generalized views about life, dependency, and doctors deserve the status of right claims, which they do not, they usually do not yield unequivocal answers to treatment dilemmas. Supposing that Mrs. Smith was indeed fiercely independent and skeptical of the medical profession, does this necessarily mean that she would prefer death to her present "twilight state" sustained by tube feedings? Conversely, if Mrs. Smith were an exceptionally dependent sort of person who actively sought and followed the advice of physicians, would that mean that she would presently prefer an indefinite extension of her barely conscious existence to an early death? Although such character traits indisputably have *some* evidentiary value, they appear to be compatible with a range of possible responses.[5] In Mrs. Smith's case, it is certainly *plausible* that she would decline the insertion of a G-tube, but that is not the only plausible interpretation. For all we know, she might have been content, were she miraculously lucid and communicative for an instant, to accede to the operation rather than go peacefully into that dark night. The question for Mrs. Smith's caregivers, then—and we shall explore this point more fully later on—is not whether her loved ones have provided a uniquely correct extrapolation of her previous values to her present situation, for in most cases that will simply be an unattainable goal; rather, the question is whether their plausible invocations of her values and character traits should be given the benefit of the doubt.

The Evidentiary Value of Aversive Behavior

Mrs. Smith has been constantly pulling out her nasogastric tube and waving off the attentions of her caregivers. What are we to make of this behavior? In contrast to the patient's previous preferences and attitudes, which are ill-matched in their generality to the concreteness of the present situation, Mrs. Smith's aversive behavior at least has the advantage of being contemporaneous. She is extubating herself right here and now. According to Daniel Callahan,[6] a philosopher who generally sees no justification for terminating food and fluids in severely demented patients, such behavior constitutes a "clear signal" mandating withdrawal of the tube.

But a clear signal of what? It is crucial to remember at this juncture that Mrs. Smith is severely demented and completely incompetent. Even though her aversive behavior occurs in the present, it is the behavior of a woman who has completely lost her rational capacity. She cannot even recognize her family, let alone engage in sophisticated deliberations bearing on the respective benefits and burdens of continued tube feeding in her minimally functional state versus an earlier death. Aphasic but otherwise competent patients might be able to send clear signals under such circumstances, but not Mrs. Smith, whose behavior appears to be freighted with a variety of possible meanings.

It is possible that her tube-pulling represents a firm and fixed present desire to forgo aggressive life-sustaining treatments in favor of an early death. It is also possible that it signals some kind of deeply sedimented personal desire manifested in spite of her present incompetence. But it is equally possible that her aversive behavior is nothing more than an elemental reflex signaling only her transient irritation from the tube. Nasogastric tubes *are* bothersome and sometimes painful intrusions, and one need not entertain sophisticated benefit-burden calculations to wish merely to be rid of such noxious stimuli. Thus, the interpretive options range from deeply intentional options for death in the face of minimally functional existence to reflexes of an almost exclusively physiological nature.

Mrs. Smith's "signal" is thus anything but clear, and this is a significant fact for her caregivers to ponder. While aversive behavior expressive of deeply sedimented personal values should be accorded the same degree of respect allotted to general character traits and attitudes, aversive reflexes to unpleasant stimuli should command little, if any, deference from surrogate decision-makers. Small children extubate themselves all the time, but no one would view such actions as a "clear signal" of a wish to die. The real problem facing Mrs. Smith's physicians is that they have no reliable way of discerning the "real meaning" behind her ongoing resistance to feeding tubes. It would certainly help if Mrs. Smith had been known to shun tube feeding even while she was competent, for that would at least provide some plausible evidence connecting her presently aversive behavior to sedimented preferences. But in the absence of such a record, the meaning of her "rejection" remains profoundly unclear.

Given the inconclusiveness of this inquiry into the patient's previous attitudes and present behavior, her caregivers might reasonably shift their focus of attention away from the patient's elusive subjectivity and toward a more objective assessment of her "best interests."

THE BEST-INTERESTS STANDARD

In the absence of reliable indicators of the patient's actual or hypothetical preferences, courts and commentators recommend an inquiry into the best interests of the patient.[7,8] What course of action (or inaction) will bring about the best overall result for the patient? Rather than finding this "objective" path an easier route to the correct decision, caregivers attempting to apply such a test to the case of a severely demented, minimally functional patient such as Mrs. Smith will immediately confront a series of equally perplexing questions. What will be the actual impact of placing a G-tube on Mrs. Smith's well-being? What definition of the good will ground their assessments of her best interests? And, given her low level of functioning, is it quite accurate even to describe Mrs. Smith as a full-fledged "person" with actual, discernable interests? Since these exceedingly difficult questions lack intuitively obvious answers, perhaps the best way to proceed is to examine categories of patients on either side of Mrs. Smith on the continuum of incompetency, categories that do yield fairly firm moral intuitions, and then attempt to locate a proper response to her case by means of "moral triangulation." Needless to say, the clarity and distinctness of these idealized categories often become somewhat blurred in real clinical situations, but there is still considerable theoretical value in discussing our responses to clear-cut cases.

Patients in Persistent Vegetative States

What if, instead of being minimally functional, Mrs. Smith were completely nonfunctional? (We shall call this hypothetical patient Mrs. Jones.) What if, instead of slowly declining into a twilight of consciousness, she were to have experienced a protracted period of anoxia that consigned her to a persistently vegetative condition? Although still alive, Mrs. Jones would subsist on brain-stem activity alone, her neocortex—the physical substratum of her capacity for consciousness—having been completely destroyed. She would thus persist in countless sleep-wake cycles, unable to connect with the world and with her past through conscious awareness, unable to plan or hope for better circumstances, unable even to perceive pleasure or pain. What rights, if any, would Mrs. Jones have, and what duties would be owed her by caregivers? If we were to apply straightforwardly the best-interests test to the case of Mrs. Jones, we would be hard-pressed to discover actual interests that could be meaningfully imputed to her. Lacking consciousness, she lacks a conception of herself as a moral agent with real interests in continued life and in the pursuit of her own vision of the good. Lacking the ability to experience pleasure and pain, she cannot be physically benefited or harmed.[9] Indeed, as

several commentators have pointed out, her only remaining interest in staying alive is based on the miniscule possibility that she has been misdiagnosed and could possibly regain some degree of consciousness in the future.[10] Apart from that slimmest of chances, she has no interests that might be assessed through a best-interests test.

If we seek a solution to the problem of Mrs. Jones in an examination of her best interests, we discover the paradoxical result that her best interests will probably be served by further treatment. True, except for the possibility of misdiagnosis, she cannot be benefited in any way by continued existence, but her lack of capacity for conscious experience renders her equally incapable of being harmed by further treatments and the extension of her life. Thus, we cannot say, as the best-interests test would appear to require, that Mrs. Jones is being excessively burdened by her treatments or that she would be "better-off dead." This result is indeed paradoxical, because if anyone's life need not be maintained, one would think that patients in persistently vegetative conditions must be at the top of the list.

Given the vanishingly small likelihood of misdiagnosis, especially after the passage of several weeks, I would argue that it is ethically appropriate to treat all PVS patients as though they had no interests either for or against treatment. Since continued medical interventions cannot realistically be thought to benefit them in any way, since caregivers cannot realistically be thought to have duties toward patients who cannot be helped or harmed, and since such treatments entail considerable costs—including the expenditure of huge sums of money, the time and energy of caregivers, and emotional strains on survivors—they may be ethically forgone.

The important lesson here is that although a rigorously patient-centered best-interests test might be ethically appropriate in most cases involving incompetent patients, it cannot be meaningfully applied when the patient under consideration lacks all fundamentally human capacities. In cases such as this, a judgment in favor of nontreatment must be based not on an objective weighing of benefits and burdens to the patient—for such patients are capable of neither benefit nor burden—but rather upon a judgment that the patient has ceased to be a "person" in any meaningful moral sense. Once this determination has been made, it is then ethically permissible to consider the financial and emotional impact of continued treatment upon other interested parties.[11] Certainly some families will, for religious or other personal reasons, continue to request life-sustaining treatments for their persistently vegetative relations; but others would be acting ethically to request the termination of all medical care, including artificially administered food and fluids.

Marginally Functional Patients

On the other side of Mrs. Smith are those patients who might usefully be described as "marginally functional." Mr. Black, for example, is a 90-year-old man presenting with rectal bleeding and suspected colon cancer who refuses a laparotomy to confirm the diagnosis. "I have lived a good life," he says, "and I don't want any surgery." His daughter, to whom he appears very close, concurs with his decision. Although Mr. Black appears on the surface to be sufficiently competent to make this decision, subsequent examinations by liaison psychiatrists reveal a glaring absence of short-term memory and significant confusion about his medical diagnosis and surroundings. He is described as "pleasantly demented."

Although patients like Mr. Black are strictly speaking incapable of rational decision-making most or all of the time, they differ from Mrs. Jones in their ability to reason, albeit rather poorly, in their ability to relate to other persons, and in their capacities to experience emotions, pain, and pleasure. Notwithstanding their inability to make most health care decisions, these patients are clearly "persons" with a multitude of interests that can be advanced or frustrated by their caregivers. In spite of their deficits and relatively low quality of life, such moderately functional patients have every right to a patient-centered best-interests analysis. While invasive, painful, and risky surgery may or may not eventually be deemed to be in Mr. Black's best interests, his capacities for experiencing the world are sufficiently intact to rule out any thought of forgoing other sorts of life-sustaining therapies, such as artificial nutrition and hydration.

The Minimally Functional Patient

Returning now to the example of Mrs. Smith, we find her to fall squarely between the permanently vegetative and moderately functional patient. Like the totally nonfunctional, vegetative patient, she is so demented that she lacks most of the criteria of "moral personhood."[12] Unfortunately, she appears to have been reduced to a mere shell of her former self. She can no longer reason, communicate (except in the most rudimentary, reflexive manner), relate to her family, or experience manifestations of love. Indeed, it is doubtful that she can be accurately described as a self-conscious, moral agent whose identity through time is cemented by the bonds of memory. There is, in cases such as this where the psychological glue of memory has given out, simply no enduring "self" there.[13] Formerly a self-conscious moral agent with a well-defined idea of the good, hopes and plans for the future, Mrs. Smith has been reduced to a mere locus of transient sensations. As philosopher James Rachels[14] puts it, she continues to have biological life, but her *biographical* life has come to an end.

On the other hand, Mrs. Smith resembles Mr. Black at least in her possession of some conscious life, albeit on a very low level, and in her ability to experience pleasure, pain, and perhaps some rudimentary emotions. Although she is not a "person" in the strict sense, she does have some interests. Insofar as she is open to pleasure and pain, she has a definite interest in experiencing the former and avoiding the latter. How might a "best-interests" test be applied to someone like Mrs. Smith?

Better-Off Dead?   In order to justify the termination of food and fluids under a best-interests test, decision-makers would have to show that the burdens of a patient's life with the proposed treatment would clearly and markedly outweigh whatever benefits she might derive from continued life.[15] In other words, they would have to show that the patient would be "better-off dead."

The most influential formulation of this best-interests test, the majority opinion in the Conroy case, requires not merely that the burdens of life clearly outweigh the benefits, but also that further treatment would be inhumane due to the presence of severe and uncontrollable pain.[16] The court's motivation in establishing such a strict standard is not hard to grasp. While people might disagree about the desirability of persisting in a minimally functional condition, severe and intractable pain is presumably something that just about everyone would prefer to avoid. It is this nearly universal sentiment that death would be preferable to a life of unmitigated pain and suffering that gives this test an air of "objectivity," as opposed to the subjectivity of tests based upon the patient's past preferences.

How then would this strict formula apply to Mrs. Smith? As we have seen, there isn't much to place in the "benefits" column. No longer able to take food by mouth or to interact meaningfully with her family and caregivers, it appears that Mrs. Smith experiences few pleasures apart from an occasional rub or combing. The only possible benefit to be derived from further treatment would appear to be the indefinite continuation of this twilight existence. And although the patient might conceivably derive some pleasure merely from lying in bed and dwelling in her alien world, it is highly doubtful that such a patient—bereft of memory, a sense of continuing selfhood, hopes, and plans—could possibly have an interest in, or be benefitted by, *continued* existence.

Given Mrs. Smith's low level of existence, it is equally difficult to discern the burdens of continued treatment. To be sure, she will experience some degree of pain and discomfort from the surgical insertion of a G-tube, but this pain will not approximate the kind of prolonged, severe, and intractable pain required by the Conroy best-interests formula.

Another possible source of pain and suffering would be the forcible imposition of medical treatment against the wishes of the incompetent patient. Even incompetent patients can have strong preferences for or against treatment or diagnostic procedures, and even if these preferences are not well grounded in medical reality or in the patient's previously authentic value system, forcible treatment will often be experienced as a painful and humiliating violation. Although this kind of coercion need not be thought of as a violation of the patient's autonomy, which may have already been destroyed by dementia, the pain, humiliation, distrust, and hostility it engenders must nevertheless be counted in any best-interests calculation. In some cases, Mr. Black's for example, the negative consequences of forcing treatment may not be worth the gains.

In Mrs. Smith's case, however, the side effects of coercive treatment are likely to be nonexistent. As we have already seen, her aversive reaction to NG tube feeding could just as easily be ascribed to immediate physical discomfort as to some deep-seated desire to die through the refusal of life-sustaining treatment. Mrs. Smith is probably too demented at this point to have preferences about tube feedings or to acknowledge the forcible imposition of surgery over against her aversive behavior. It is highly unlikely, then, that she would experience the insertion of a G-tube as a violation of her wishes (no matter how distorted) or as a painful humiliation.

In the absence of any persistent and severe pain underlying her condition, it would appear highly doubtful that the burdens of Mrs. Smith's continued existence clearly and markedly outweigh the benefits, even when the benefits approach zero. A literal reading and application of the Conroy formula would thus lead to the conclusion that the G-tube should be surgically implanted and that she should be maintained indefinitely with artificial nutrition and hydration.

Limitations of the Best-Interests Standard Not everyone will be satisfied with this result. Those who believe that quality of life should never affect treatment decisions will no doubt applaud this conclusion, but others might well think that something important has been left out of our deliberations. Judge Handler,[17] the lone dissenter in *Conroy*, identifies this missing factor as a legitimate concern for the patient's probable feelings about broader issues, such as privacy, dependency, dignity, and bodily integrity. By focusing the entire best-interests discussion upon the narrow issue of pain, we tend to reduce the patient from the full-fledged person that she once was to the status of a mere physical repository of pleasures and pains. Is this crudely hedonistic notion of the good an adequate or desirable measure of humane treatment decisions for minimally functional patients? Should we simply ignore the patient's probable responses to such abject dependency and daily violations of dignity?

Although Judge Handler's dissent eloquently pinpoints a major shortcoming of the *Conroy* best-interests formula, it is problematical in its own right. Specifically, it is unclear how Judge Handler's concerns for these larger issues of privacy and dignity might be grafted onto the *Conroy* best-interests formula. That test, let us recall, attempts to ascertain the *present* best interests of patients; it asks about the present and future benefits and burdens likely to be experienced by the patient. The obvious problem for Judge Handler's proposed enlargement of this formula is that severely demented, minimally functional patients like Mrs. Smith are presently incapable of experiencing what more functional patients would describe as insults to their privacy, dignity, and physical integrity. Although it is quite possible that the formerly competent Mrs. Smith would have been appalled at the loss of dignity entailed by her present situation, the present Mrs. Smith knows nothing of dignitary insults or violations of privacy. She is so demented that she cannot be affected, one way or the other, by solicitude for her present responses to these larger, humanistic issues.

In order to vindicate Judge Handler's concerns, we will have to reintroduce them at the stage of our inquiry into the patient's prior preferences (i.e., the substituted judgment test). Under that test, we would have to show that Mrs. Smith would have clearly viewed continued treatment under these circumstances as an indignity, and that she would have preferred an early death to the insertion of a G-tube. The problem with this move is that, as we have already seen, Mrs. Smith left behind neither a precise advance directive nor a pattern of analogous choices that clearly demonstrate what she would have wanted under present circumstances. Indeed, our earlier failure to provide this sort of clear evidence mandated our present effort to find a solution in terms of Mrs. Smith's best interests.

So we have come full circle. Our inability to satisfy a rigorous substituted judgment test required us to search for a solution in terms of Mrs. Smith's best interests. But the best-interests test, at least as articulated in *Conroy*, led to an unacceptably narrow focus on pain that excluded important values. Mrs. Smith's present lack of capacity to appreciate such values finally led us back again to the substituted judgment test. Clearly, something has gone wrong here.

A PROCEDURAL SOLUTION

According to lawyer-bioethicist Nancy Rhoden,[18] the problem lies not in our inability to come up with better evidence of a patient's wishes or level of pain and suffering, but rather in the questions we are asking. She argues convincingly that both the substituted judgment and best-interests tests set the standard of evidence far too high. By requiring *clear and convincing* evidence either that a patient's prior values would dictate the withdrawal of life-sustaining treatment or that the burdens of a patient's life outweigh the benefits, these tests establish a standard that cannot realistically be met by the kinds of evidence we are likely to have at our disposal. As we have seen, in the absence of a carefully drafted living will, a durable power of attorney, or severe and intractable pain, it will rarely be *clear* either that a patient would have refused treatment or that death is in her best interests. Given the usual evidentiary materials at hand, in most cases the best we can do is conclude that forgoing treatment is *probably* what the patient would have wanted, or that death is *likely* to be in the patient's best interests, although we will never know for sure in either case.

To be sure, there are some easy cases where a patient's best interests are clearly and perceptibly being violated. For example, greedy relatives might request the termination of treatment that could realistically return the patient to a good quality of life; or guilt-ridden relatives might press for full resuscitative measures on a moribund patient riddled with metastatic cancer. But apart from such clear-cut cases of unmistakable undertreatment and overtreatment, most of the truly problematical cases (like Mrs. Smith's) fall into a vast gray area between these extremes where the patient's best interests will remain unclear and largely inscrutable. Our problem, then, is that we have been asking questions for which there exist, in most of the hard cases at least, no clearly correct answers.

Rhoden's solution, in which I concur, is to bypass this substantive impasse with a procedural solution. Taking her cue from the President's Commission report[19] addressed to the problem of severely impaired newborns, she argues that when a proposed course of action falls into the gray area of uncertainty, involved and well-intentioned family members should have discretion to decide as they see fit. Presumably, they will invoke precisely the same kinds of evidence bearing on the patient's value system, religious affiliation, quality of life, and the potential benefits and burdens of treatment, but they would not be held to a standard of evidence requiring that their choice be uniquely correct.

To be sure, many caring and well-meaning family members will also want to weigh the impact of continued treatment upon themselves and the family unit. Sometimes the ongoing provision of care and treatment to severely demented patients like Mrs. Smith can impose great burdens, both financial and emotional, upon families. I believe that such concerns are for the most part inevitable and that they often subtly color treatment decisions even when officially banished under the auspices of the usual ethical-legal standards. This is to be expected and should not give us grounds for concern so long as the case originally falls within the gray area of ethical ambiguity, and so long as the interests of family do not *clearly* violate the best interests of the patient.

The correct question for us, then, is not whether forgoing treatment is clearly the right answer, but rather whether Mrs. Smith's case falls into the problematical gray area. If it does, then the decision of a trustworthy surrogate should prevail over objections from caregivers, unless the latter can show a clear violation of best interests. Since a case must exhibit considerable ethical ambiguity to fall into this gray zone in the first place, we should expect that well-meaning and ethically sensitive people will reach different conclusions about the care of such patients. The opinions of trustworthy surrogates should be given priority simply because they are usually in the best position to assess the prior wishes and best interests of incompetent patients, and because their familial and emotional bonding to patients usually gives them a greater claim than members of the health care team.[20]

What, then, are the boundaries of the gray area? When is a case sufficiently ambiguous to warrant our trust in surrogate decision-making? We can begin with a reassertion of the *Conroy* case's best-interests formula. If a patient's capacity for benefitting from continued life appears to be eclipsed by the constant presence of severe and intractable pain,

then the case falls either in the gray area or the clear-cut zone of nontreatment. I would add that this imbalance of burdens over benefits need not be conclusively proven by clear and convincing evidence. It should be sufficient merely for the surrogate to make a strong case that the burdens are disproportionate to the benefits. In Mrs. Smith's case, however, no such claim can be made.

In the absence of severe pain, we must ask whether the patient is genuinely capable of benefitting from continued existence. Does she recognize and interact with other persons, including her family and caregivers? Does she have a sufficiently intact self to conceive of the future and to care about what happens in it? If the answers to these questions are negative, even if the patient is capable of some rudimentary physical pleasures, I would argue that the patient has no real interest in either continued life or the administration of life-sustaining treatments and thus falls squarely into the gray area.

Mrs. Smith fits this profile. She is so demented that she cannot recognize family or caregivers. Her memory is so depleted, and her sense of self so fractured, that she cannot be said to have genuinely human interests.

Since the boundaries of this morally ambiguous zone will inevitably correspond to the limits of societal toleration, it will often be helpful to ask what most reasonable people would want for themselves in this circumstance. Although this question is generally not allowed in more patient-centered inquiries into the patient's prior preferences or best interests, it should be allowable here, where we are merely trying to determine whether a case is sufficiently morally problematic to fit into the gray zone. If we ask the question with regard to Mrs. Smith, I think that the overwhelming majority of persons would say that they would rather die than continue to live in such a physically, emotionally, and socially impoverished state.

Another useful clue is to ask how we would have responded to Mrs. Smith's death from lack of adequate nutrition had it occurred prior to the advent of artificial feeding. No doubt there would have been the inevitable sadness associated with the death of any human being, but there would have been no shock, no outrage, no sense of tragedy, nor even any feeling that death had deprived her of any real benefits. The predominant response to such a death would most likely have been relief, both for the sake of the patient and for her loved ones.

In such cases, the only apparent rationale for the imposition of life-sustaining technologies is that since they exist, they must be used. And the more they are used, the more pervasive their presence in hospital and long-term care facilities, the more their expanded use assumes the necessity of a moral imperative. But it is precisely here, in cases such as Mrs. Smith's, that we must pause to ask about the proper uses of such technologies. If they do nothing to further the real interests of patients, if all they do is to prolong the biological existence of patients whose biographical lives have long since come to an end, then biomedical technologies assume the status of idols—i.e., inanimate objects worshipped by the human beings who created them, objects that return to dominate us rather than serving our purposes.

NOTES

1. Dworkin R: Autonomy and the Demented Self. *Milbank Quarterly* 64: supp. 2, 4–16, 1986.
2. Buchanan A, Brock DW: Deciding for Others. *Milbank Quarterly* 64: supp. 2, 71, 1986.
3. Dresser R: Life, Death, and Incompetent Patients: Conceptual Infirmities and Hidden Values in the Law. *Arizona Law Review* 28: 376–379, 1986.
4. Rhoden NK: Litigating Life and Death. *Harvard Law Review* 102: 2, 375–446, Dec. 1988.
5. Ibid.
6. Callahan D: *Setting Limits: Medical Goals in an Aging Society*. New York, Simon & Schuster, 1987, p. 192.
7. President's Commission for the Study of Ethical Problems in Medicine and Biomedical and Behavioral Research: Deciding to Forego Life Sustaining Treatment. Washington, D.C., U.S. Government Printing Office, 1983, p. 134 ff.
8. In re Conroy, 98 N.J. 321, 486 A.2d 1209 (1985).
9. Cranford RE: The Persistent Vegetative State: The Medical Reality (Getting the Facts Straight). *Hastings Cent Rep* 18:27–32, Feb./Mar. 1988.
10. Feinberg J: The Rights of Animals and Unborn Generations, in *Rights, Justice, and the Bounds of Liberty*. Princeton, Princeton University Press, 1980, pp. 176–177.
11. Arras JD: Quality of Life in Neonatal Ethics: Beyond Denial and Evasion, in Weil WB, Benjamin M, (eds): *Ethical Issues at the Outset of Life*. Boston, Blackwell, 1987, pp. 151–186.
12. Engelhardt HT: *The Foundations of Bioethics*. New York, Oxford University Press, 1986.
13. Brock DW: Justice and the Severely Demented Elderly. *J Med Philos* 13:1, 73–99, Feb. 1988.
14. Rachels J: *The End of Life*. New York, Oxford University Press, 1986.
15. In re Conroy.
16. Ibid.
17. Ibid.
18. Rhoden, Litigating Life and Death.
19. President's Commission.
20. Ibid.

NUTRITION AND HYDRATION: MORAL AND PASTORAL REFLECTIONS

U.S. Bishops' Pro-Life Committee

INTRODUCTION

Modern medical technology seems to confront us with many questions not faced even a decade ago. Corresponding changes in medical practice have benefited many, but have also prompted fears by some that they will be aggressively treated against their will or denied the kind of care that is their due as human persons with inherent dignity. Current debates about life-sustaining treatment suggest that our society's moral reflection is having difficulty keeping pace with its technological progress.

A religious view of life has an important contribution to make to these modern debates. Our Catholic tradition has developed a rich body of thought on these questions, which affirms a duty to preserve human life but recognizes limits to that duty.

Our first goal in making this statement is to reaffirm some basic principles of our moral tradition, to assist Catholics and others in making treatment decisions in accord with respect for God's gift of life.

These principles do not provide clear and final answers to all moral questions that arise as individuals make difficult decisions. Catholic theologians may differ on how best to apply moral principles to some questions not explicitly resolved by the church's teaching authority. Likewise, we understand that those who must make serious healthcare decisions for themselves or for others face a complexity of issues, circumstances, thoughts and emotions in each unique case.

This is the case with some questions involving the medically assisted provision of nutrition and hydration to helpless patients—those who are seriously ill, disabled or persistently unconscious. These questions have been made more urgent by widely publicized court cases and the public debate to which they have given rise.

Our second purpose in issuing this statement, then, is to provide some clarification of the moral issues involved in decisions about medically assisted nutrition and hydration. We are fully aware that such guidance is not necessarily final, because there are many unresolved medical and ethical questions related to these issues and the continuing development of medical technology will necessitate ongoing reflection. But these decisions already confront patients, families and health-care personnel every day. They arise whenever competent patients make decisions about medically assisted nutrition and hydration for their own present situation, when they consider signing an advance directive such as a "living will" or health-care proxy document, and when families or other proxy decision-makers make decisions about those entrusted to their care. We offer guidance to those who, facing these issues, might be confused by opinions that at times threaten to deny the inherent dignity of human life. We therefore address our reflections first to those who share our Judeo-Christian traditions, and secondly to others concerned about the dignity and value of human life who seek guidance in making their own moral decisions.

MORAL PRINCIPLES

The Judeo-Christian moral tradition celebrates life as the gift of a loving God and respects the life of each human being because each is made in the image and likeness of God. As Christians we also believe we are redeemed by Christ and called to share eternal life with him. From these roots the

Catholic tradition has developed a distinctive approach to fostering and sustaining human life. Our church views life as a sacred trust, a gift over which we are given stewardship and not absolute dominion. The church thus opposes all direct attacks on innocent life. As conscientious stewards we have a duty to preserve life, while recognizing certain limits to that duty:

(1) Because human life is the foundation for all other human goods, it has a special value and significance. Life is "the first right of the human person" and "the condition of all the others."

(2) All crimes against life, including "euthanasia or willful suicide," must be opposed. Euthanasia is "an action or an omission which of itself or by intention causes death, in order that all suffering may in this way be eliminated." Its terms of reference are to be found "in the intention of the will and in the methods used." Thus defined, euthanasia is an attack on life which no one has a right to make or request, and which no government or other human authority can legitimately recommend or permit. Although individual guilt may be reduced or absent because of suffering or emotional factors that cloud the conscience, this does not change the objective wrongfulness of the act. It should also be recognized that an apparent plea for death may really be a plea for help and love.

(3) Suffering is a fact of human life, and has special significance for the Christian as an opportunity to share in Christ's redemptive suffering. Nevertheless there is nothing wrong in trying to relieve someone's suffering; in fact it is a positive good to do so, as long as one does not intentionally cause death or interfere with other moral and religious duties.

(4) Everyone has the duty to care for his or her own life and health and to seek necessary medical care from others, but this does not mean that all possible remedies must be used in all circumstances. One is not obliged to use either "extraordinary" means or "disproportionate" means of preserving life—that is, means which are understood as offering no reasonable hope of benefit or as involving excessive burdens. Decisions regarding such means are complex, and should ordinarily be made by the patient in consultation with his or her family chaplain or pastor and physician when that is possible.

(5) In the final stage of dying one is not obliged to prolong the life of a patient by every possible means: "When inevitable death is imminent in spite of the means used, it is permitted in conscience to take the decision to refuse forms of treatment that would only secure a precarious and burdensome prolongation of life, so long as the normal care due to the sick person in similar cases is not interrupted."

(6) While affirming life as a gift of God, the church recognizes that death is unavoidable and that it can open the door to eternal life. Thus, "without in any way hastening the hour of death," the dying person should accept its reality and prepare for it emotionally and spiritually.

(7) Decisions regarding human life must respect the demands of justice, viewing each human being as our neighbor and avoiding all discrimination based on age or dependency. A human being has "a unique dignity and an independent value, from the moment of conception and in every stage of development, whatever his or her physical condition." In particular, "the disabled person (whether the disability be the result of a congenital handicap, chronic illness or accident, or from mental or physical deficiency, and whatever the severity of the disability) is a fully human subject, with the corresponding innate, sacred and inviolable rights." First among these is "the fundamental and inalienable right to life."

(8) The dignity and value of the human person, which lie at the foundation of the church's teaching on the right to life, also provide a basis for any just social order. Not only to become more Christian, but to become more truly human, society should protect the right to life through its laws and other policies.

While these principles grow out of a specific religious tradition, they appeal to a common respect for the dignity of the human person. We commend them to all people of good will.

QUESTIONS ABOUT MEDICALLY ASSISTED NUTRITION AND HYDRATION

In what follows we apply these well-established moral principles to the difficult issue of providing medically assisted nutrition and hydration to persons who are seriously ill, disabled or persistently unconscious. We recognize the complexity involved in applying these principles to individual cases and acknowledge that, at this time and on this particular issue, our applications do not have the same authority as the principles themselves.

1. IS THE WITHHOLDING OR WITHDRAWING OF MEDICALLY ASSISTED NUTRITION AND HYDRATION ALWAYS A DIRECT KILLING?

In answering this question one should avoid two extremes.

First, it is wrong to say that this could not be a matter of killing simply because it involves an omission rather than a positive action. In fact a deliberate omission may be an effective and certain way to kill, especially to kill someone weakened by illness. Catholic teaching condemns as euthanasia "an action or an omission which of itself or by intention causes death, in order that all suffering may in this way be eliminated." Thus "euthanasia includes not only active mercy killing but also the omission of treatment when the purpose of the omission is to kill the patient."

Second, we should not assume that all or most decisions to withhold or withdraw medically assisted nutrition and hydration are attempts to cause death. To be sure, any patient will die if all nutrition and hydration are withheld. But sometimes other causes are at work—for example, the patient may be imminently dying, whether feeding takes place or not, from an already existing terminal condition. At other times, although the shortening of the patient's life is one foreseeable result of an omission, the real purpose of the omission was to relieve the patient of a particular procedure that was of limited usefulness to the patient or unreasonably burdensome for the patient and the patient's family or caregivers. This kind of decision should not be equated with a decision to kill or with suicide.

The harsh reality is that some who propose withdrawal of nutrition and hydration from certain patients do directly intend to bring about a patient's death and would even prefer a change in the law to allow for what they see as more "quick and painless" means to cause death. In other words, nutrition and hydration (whether orally administered or medically assisted) are sometimes withdrawn not because a patient is dying, but precisely because a patient is not dying (or not dying quickly) and someone believes it would be better if he or she did, generally because the patient is perceived as having an unacceptably low "quality of life" or as imposing burdens on others.

When deciding whether to withhold or withdraw medically assisted nutrition and hydration, or other forms of life support, we are called by our moral tradition to ask ourselves: What will my decision do for this patient? And what am I trying to achieve by doing it? We must be sure that it is not our intent to cause the patient's death—either for its own sake or as a means to achieving some other goal such as the relief of suffering.

2. IS MEDICALLY ASSISTED NUTRITION AND HYDRATION A FORM OF "TREATMENT" OR "CARE"?

Catholic teaching provides that a person in the final stages of dying need not accept "forms of treatment that would only secure a precarious and burdensome prolongation of life," but should still receive "the normal care due to the sick person in similar cases." . . . But the teaching of the church has not resolved the question whether medically assisted nutrition and hydration should always be seen as a form of normal care.

Almost everyone agrees that oral feeding, when it can be accepted and assimilated by a patient, is a form of care owed to all helpless people. . . . But our obligations become less clear when adequate nutrition and hydration require the skills of trained medical personnel and the use of technologies that may be perceived as very burdensome—that is, as intrusive, painful or repugnant. Such factors vary from one type of feeding procedure to another, and from one patient to another, making it difficult to classify all feeding procedures as either "care" or "treatment."

Perhaps this dilemma should be viewed in a broader context. Even medical "treatments" are morally obligatory when they are "ordinary" means—that is, if they provide a reasonable hope of benefit and do not involve excessive burdens. Therefore we believe people should make decisions in light of a simple and fundamental insight: Out of respect for the dignity of the human person we are obliged to preserve our own lives and help others preserve theirs, by the use of means that have a reasonable hope of sustaining life without imposing unreasonable burdens on those we seek to help, that is, on the patient and his or her family and community.

We must therefore address the question of benefits and burdens next, recognizing that a full moral analysis is only possible when one knows the effects of a given procedure on a particular patient.

3. WHAT ARE THE BENEFITS OF MEDICALLY ASSISTED NUTRITION AND HYDRATION?

. . .

Nutrition and hydration, whether provided in the usual way or with medical assistance . . . benefit patients in several ways. First, for all patients who can assimilate them, suitable food and fluids sustain life, and providing them normally expresses loving concern and solidarity with the helpless. Second, for patients being treated with the hope of a cure, appropriate food and fluids are an important element of sound health care. Third, even for patients who are imminently dying and incurable, food and fluids can prevent the suffering that may arise from dehydration, hunger and thirst.

. . . But sometimes even food and fluids are no longer effective in providing this benefit because a patient has entered the final stage of a terminal condition. At such times we should make the dying person as comfortable as possible and provide nursing care and proper hygiene as well as companionship and appropriate spiritual aid. Such a person may lose all desire for food and drink and even be unable to ingest them. Initiating medically assisted feeding or intravenous fluids in this case may increase the patient's discomfort while providing no real benefit; ice chips or sips of water may instead be appropriate to provide comfort and counteract the adverse effects of dehydration. Even in the case of the imminently dying patient, of course, any action or omission that of itself or by intention causes death is to be absolutely rejected. . . .

4. WHAT ARE THE BURDENS OF MEDICALLY ASSISTED NUTRITION AND HYDRATION?

. . .

The risks and objective complications of medically assisted nutrition and hydration will depend on the procedure used and the condition of the patient. In a given case a feeding procedure may become harmful or even life-threatening. . . .

If the risks and burdens of a particular feeding procedure are deemed serious enough to warrant withdrawing it, we should not automatically deprive the patient of all nutrition and hydration but should ask whether another procedure is feasible that would be less burdensome. We say this because some helpless patients, including some in a "persistent vegetative state," receive tube feedings not because they cannot swallow food at all but because tube feeding is less costly and difficult for health-care personnel. . . .

Many people see feeding tubes as frightening or even as bodily violations. Assessments of such burdens are necessarily subjective; they should not be dismissed on that account, but we offer some practical cautions to help prevent abuse.

First, in keeping with our moral teaching against the intentional causing of death by omission, one should distinguish between repugnance to a particular procedure and repugnance to life itself. The latter may occur when a patient views a life of helplessness and dependency on others as itself a heavy burden, leading him or her to wish or even to pray for death. Especially in our achievement-oriented society, the burden of living in such a condition may seem to outweigh any possible benefit of medical treatment and even lead a person to despair. But we should not assume that the burdens in such a case always outweigh the benefits; for the sufferer, given good counseling and spiritual support, may be brought again to appreciate the precious gift of life.

Second, our tradition recognizes that when treatment decisions are made, "account will have to be taken of the reasonable wishes of the patient and the patient's family, as also of the advice of the doctors who are specially competent in the matter." . . .

Third, we should not assume that a feeding procedure is inherently repugnant to all patients without specific evidence. In contrast to Americans' general distaste for the idea of being supported by "tubes and machines," some studies indicate surprisingly favorable views of medically assisted nutrition and hydration among patients and families with actual experience of such procedures. . . .

While some balk at the idea, in principle cost can be a valid factor in decisions about life support. For example, money spent on expensive treatment for one family member may be money otherwise needed for food, housing and other necessities for the rest of the family. Here, also, we offer some cautions. . . . Even for altruistic reasons a patient should not directly intend his or her own death by malnutrition or dehydration, but may accept an earlier death as a consequence of his or her refusal of an unreasonably expensive treatment.

. . . Individual decisions about medically assisted nutrition and hydration should [not] be determined by macroeconomic concerns such as national budget priorities and the high cost of health care. These social problems are serious, but it is by no means established that they require depriving chronically ill and helpless patients of effective and easily tolerated measures that they need to survive.

Third, tube feeding alone is generally not very expensive and may cost no more than oral feeding. What is seen by many as a grave financial and emotional burden on caregivers is the total long-term care of severely debilitated patients, who may survive for many years with no life support except medically assisted nutrition and hydration and nursing care. . . .

In the context of official church teaching, it is not yet clear to what extent we may assess the burden of a patient's total care rather than the burden of a particular treatment when we seek to refuse "burdensome" life support. On a practical level, those seeking to make good decisions might assure themselves of their own intentions by asking: Does my decision aim at relieving the patient of a particularly grave burden imposed by medically

assisted nutrition and hydration? Or does it aim to avoid the total burden of caring for the patient? If so, does it achieve this aim by deliberately bringing about his or her death?

Rather than leaving families to confront such dilemmas alone, society and government should improve their assistance to families whose financial and emotional resources are strained by long-term care of loved ones.

5. WHAT ROLE SHOULD "QUALITY OF LIFE" PLAY IN OUR DECISIONS?

Financial and emotional burdens are willingly endured by most families to raise their children or to care for mentally aware but weak and elderly family members. It is sometimes argued that we need not endure comparable burdens to feed and care for persons with severe mental and physical disabilities, because their low "quality of life" makes it unnecessary or pointless to preserve their lives.

But this argument—even when it seems motivated by a humanitarian concern to reduce suffering and hardship—ignores the equal dignity and sanctity of all human life. Its key assumption—that people with disabilities necessarily enjoy life less than others or lack the potential to lead meaningful lives—is also mistaken. Where suffering does exist, society's response should not be to neglect or eliminate the lives of people with disabilities, but to help correct their inadequate living conditions. Very often the worst threat to a good "quality of life" for these people is not the disability itself, but the prejudicial attitudes of others—attitudes based on the idea that a life with serious disabilities is not worth living.

This being said, our moral tradition allows for three ways in which the "quality of life" of a seriously ill patient is relevant to treatment decisions:

(1) Consistent with respect for the inherent sanctity of life, we should relieve needless suffering and support morally acceptable ways of improving each patient's quality of life.

(2) One may legitimately refuse a treatment because it would itself create an impairment imposing new serious burdens or risks on the patient. This decision to avoid the new burdens or risks created by a treatment is not the same as directly intending to end life in

order to avoid the burden of living in a disabled state.

(3) Sometimes a disabling condition may directly influence the benefits and burdens of a specific treatment for a particular patient. For example, a confused or demented patient may find medically assisted nutrition and hydration more frightening and burdensome than other patients do because he or she cannot understand what it is. The patient may even repeatedly pull out feeding tubes, requiring burdensome physical restraints if this form of feeding is to be continued. In such cases, ways of alleviating such special burdens should be explored before concluding that they justify withholding all food and fluids needed to sustain life.

These humane considerations are quite different from a "quality of life" ethic that would judge individuals with disabilities or limited potential as not worthy of care or respect. It is one thing to withhold a procedure because it would impose new disabilities on a patient, and quite another thing to say that patients who already have such disabilities should not have their lives preserved. A means considered ordinary or proportionate for other patients should not be considered extraordinary or disproportionate for severely impaired patients solely because of a judgment that their lives are not worth living.

In short, while considerations regarding a person's quality of life have some validity in weighing the burdens and benefits of medical treatment, at the present time in our society judgments about the quality of life are sometimes used to promote euthanasia. The church must emphasize the sanctity of life of each person as a fundamental principle in all moral decision-making.

6. DO PERSISTENTLY UNCONSCIOUS PATIENTS REPRESENT A SPECIAL CASE?

Even Catholics who accept the same basic moral principles may strongly disagree on how to apply them to patients who appear to be persistently unconscious—that is, those who are in a permanent coma or a "persistent vegetative state" (PVS). Some moral questions in this area have not been explicitly resolved by the church's teaching authority.

On some points there is wide agreement among Catholic theologians:

(1) An unconscious patient must be treated as a living human person with inherent dignity and value. Direct killing of such a patient is as morally reprehensible as the direct killing of anyone else. Even the medical terminology used to describe these patients as "vegetative" unfortunately tends to obscure this vitally important point, inviting speculation that a patient in this state is a "vegetable" or a subhuman animal.

(2) The area of legitimate controversy does not concern patients with conditions like mental retardation, senility, dementia or even temporary unconsciousness. Where serious disagreement begins is with the patient who has been diagnosed as completely and permanently unconscious after careful testing over a period of weeks or months.

Some moral theologians argue that a particular form of care or treatment is morally obligatory only when its benefits outweigh its burdens to a patient or the care providers. In weighing burdens, they say, the total burden of a procedure and the consequent requirements of care must be taken into account. If no benefit can be demonstrated, the procedure, whatever its burdens, cannot be obligatory. These moralists also hold that the chief criterion to determine the benefit of a procedure cannot be merely that it prolongs physical life, since physical life is not an absolute good but is relative to the spiritual good of the person. They assert that the spiritual good of the person is union with God, which can be advanced only by human acts, i.e., conscious, free acts. Since the best current medical opinion holds that persons in the persistent vegetative state (PVS) are incapable now or in the future of conscious, free human acts, these moralists conclude that, when careful diagnosis verifies this condition, it is not obligatory to prolong life by such interventions as a respirator, antibiotics or medically assisted hydration and nutrition. To decide to omit non-obligatory care, therefore, is not to intend the patient's death, but only to avoid the burden of the procedure. Hence, though foreseen, the patient's death is to be attributed to the patient's pathological condition and not to the omission of care. Therefore, these theologians conclude, while it is always wrong directly to intend or cause the death of such patients, the natural dying process which would have occurred without these interventions may be permitted to proceed.

While this rationale is convincing to some, it is not theologically conclusive and we are not persuaded by it. In fact, other theologians argue cogently that theological inquiry could lead one to a more carefully limited conclusion.

These moral theologians argue that while particular treatments can be judged useless or burdensome, it is morally questionable and would create a dangerous precedent to imply that any human life is not a positive good or "benefit." They emphasize that while life is not the highest good, it is always and everywhere a basic good of the human person and not merely a means to other goods. They further assert that if the "burden" one is trying to relieve by discontinuing medically assisted nutrition and hydration is the burden of remaining alive in the allegedly undignified condition of PVS, such a decision is unacceptable because one's intent is only achieved by deliberately ensuring the patient's death from malnutrition or dehydration. Finally, these moralists suggest that PVS is best seen as an extreme form of mental and physical disability—one whose causes, nature and prognosis are as yet imperfectly understood—and not as a terminal illness or fatal pathology from which patients should generally be allowed to die. Because the patient's life can often be sustained indefinitely by medically assisted nutrition and hydration that is not unreasonably risky or burdensome for that patient, they say, we are not dealing here with a case where "inevitable death is imminent in spite of the means used." Rather, because the patient will die in a few days if medically assisted nutrition and hydration are discontinued, but can often live a long time if they are provided, the inherent dignity and worth of the human person obligates us to provide this patient with care and support.

Further complicating this debate is a disagreement over what responsible Catholics should do in the absence of a final resolution of this question. Some point to our moral tradition of probabilism, which would allow individuals to follow the appropriate moral analysis that they find persuasive. Others point to the principle that in cases where one might risk unjustly depriving someone of life, we should take the safer course.

In the face of the uncertainties and unresolved medical and theological issues, it is important to defend and preserve important values. On the one hand, there is a concern that patients and families should not be subjected to unnecessary burdens, ineffective treatments and indignities when death is approaching. On the other hand, it is important to ensure that the inherent dignity of human persons, even those who are persistently unconscious, is respected and that no one is deprived of nutrition and hydration with the intent of bringing on his or her death.

It is not easy to arrive at a single answer to some of the real and personal dilemmas involved in this issue. In study, prayer and compassion we continue to reflect on this issue and hope to discover additional information that will lead to its ultimate resolution.

In the meantime, at a practical level we are concerned that withdrawal of all life support, including nutrition and hydration, not be viewed as appropriate or automatically indicated for the entire class of PVS patients simply because of a judgment that they are beyond the reach of medical treatment that would restore consciousness. We note the current absence of conclusive scientific data on the causes and implications of different degrees of brain damage, on the PVS patient's ability to experience pain and on the reliability of prognoses for many such patients. We do know that many of these patients have a good prognosis for long-term survival when given medically assisted nutrition and hydration, and a certain prognosis for death otherwise—and we know that many in our society view such an early death as a positive good for a patient in this condition. Therefore we are gravely concerned about current attitudes and policy trends in our society that would too easily dismiss patients without apparent mental faculties as non-persons or as undeserving of human care and concern. In this climate, even legitimate moral arguments intended to have a careful and limited application can easily be misinterpreted, broadened and abused by others to erode respect for the lives of some of our society's most helpless members. . . .

QUALITY OF LIFE AND NON-TREATMENT DECISIONS FOR INCOMPETENT PATIENTS: A CRITIQUE OF THE ORTHODOX APPROACH

Rebecca S. Dresser and John A. Robertson

Since the Quinlan decision in 1976, courts and legislatures have made substantial progress in defining rules to govern non-treatment of dying and debilitated patients. For example, the right of the competent patient to refuse necessary care is now widely established, and the legality of withdrawing respirators and even nutrition and hydration from permanently unconscious patients is increasingly recognized.

More difficult questions arise, however, when the patient is neither competent nor permanently unconscious, but instead is in a conscious, severely demented and debilitated state, with experiences that appear quite limited. Thousands of patients in this condition are cared for in private homes, hospitals, and nursing homes, the victims of stroke, senility, Alzheimer's disease, and other illnesses. Even though they usually require only low-tech, minimally supportive care, such patients can impose great stress on their families and high financial costs on the health care system.

As the population of frail elderly and demented patients grows, determining the limits of family and societal obligations to sustain them has become a major ethical, legal, and policy issue. Its resolution requires balancing the importance of life in such compromised conditions against the social and familial burdens that prolonging such lives entails. A conflict between a patient-centered and other-directed approach inevitably arises, testing the scope of society's respect for vulnerable and debilitated persons.

Unfortunately, the orthodox judicial approach to non-treatment decisions is not an adequate guide to resolution of these issues. Judicial analysis is too focused on the model of a competent person refusing treatment, even when the case involves a person who is incompetent and unable to choose. Although many of the decided cases have produced defensible results, the courts' efforts to fit incompetent patients to the model of a competent decision-maker are seriously flawed and ultimately threaten harm to many incompetent patients.

Courts, legislators, and physicians would do better to focus directly on the interests of the incompetent patient before them. Competing interests, such as family distress and financial costs, may then be directly evaluated and their role in such decisions properly assigned. Such an approach has the best chance of respecting incompetent persons, while giving due regard to the interests of families and society.

THE ORTHODOX APPROACH: ADVANCE DIRECTIVES AND SUBSTITUTED JUDGMENT

Starting with *In re Quinlan*, and continuing with such cases as *Superintendent of Belchertown* v. *Saikewicz, Eichner* v. *Dillon, Barber* v. *Superior Court, In re Conroy, Brophy* v. *New England Sinai Hospital, Inc.*, and *In re Jobes*, the courts have found that life-sustaining treatment may be withheld or withdrawn from incompetent patients in certain circumstances.

The cases adopt the same general pattern of reasoning. Adopting a patient-centered approach, they require that patient choices concerning their medical care be respected. The basic legal premise, derived from common law and constitutional rights to self-determination and privacy, is that competent

From Rebecca S. Dresser and John A. Robertson, "Quality of Life and Non-Treatment Decisions for Incompetent Patients," *Law, Medicine & Health Care* 17, no. 3 (Fall 1989): 234–244. Reprinted by permission of Professors Dresser and Robertson and the American Society of Law, Medicine & Ethics.

Editors' note: Notes have been cut. Students who want to follow up on sources should consult the original article.

patients have a right to refuse necessary medical care when they face intrusive treatment or life in a compromised state. Countervailing state interests in preserving life, preventing suicide, and upholding the integrity of the medical profession are then found insufficient to override the patient's objection to treatment.

What, however, if the patient is incompetent and cannot make a choice about treatment? Here the courts in most jurisdictions make a conceptual move that determines the structure of subsequent analysis. They assume that respect for incompetent patients requires according such patients the same right to refuse treatment accorded competent patients. This assumption requires that the incompetent patient be viewed as a choosing individual and leads the courts to find or construct a competent person as decision-maker to determine the incompetent patient's choice.

Determining what the fictional competent person in the incompetent patient's situation would choose entails further moves. An incompetent patient's prior oral or written directive concerning treatment when incompetent is given great weight in determining that hypothetical choice. If no directive exists, courts typically adopt the substituted judgment doctrine and allow the family or other proxy to choose as they think the patients would have chosen when or if competent.

This approach to decision-making for incompetent patients was first enunciated in the landmark New Jersey Supreme Court case, *In re Quinlan*, when the court stated that the patient's guardian and family should determine whether she would herself choose non-treatment in her present circumstances: ". . . the only practical way to prevent destruction of the right [of privacy] is to permit the guardian and family of Karen to render their best judgment . . . as to whether she would exercise it in these circumstances."

This approach has shaped the reasoning and analysis in every subsequent non-treatment case involving incompetent patients. Indeed, eleven years later the New Jersey Supreme Court forcefully reiterated the accepted view in *Jobes*:

> . . . the patient's right to self-determination is the guiding principle in determining whether to continue or withdraw life-sustaining treatment; . . . therefore the goal of a surrogate decision-maker for an incompetent patient must be to determine and effectuate what that patient, if competent, would want.

The strategy of relying on prior expressed wishes or proxy inferred competent treatment preferences to determine treatment choices for incompetent patients has wide currency in ethical and policy analysis involving incompetent patients. Authoritative bodies such as the President's Commission for the Study of Ethical Problems in Medicine and the Hastings Center have also endorsed it. Living-will and durable-power-of-attorney legislation embodies a further acceptance of the theme. Health professionals and ethicists hail it as the best solution to the difficult problem of deciding when treatment should be withheld from incompetent patients. It has also been extended to govern medical treatment for patients who never were competent, psychiatric treatment for civilly committed persons, sterilization of retarded persons, and organ donation by incompetent persons.

THE ALLURE OF THE ORTHODOX APPROACH

The orthodox judicial approach of relying on the patient's prior directive or choice inferred by a proxy's substituted judgment has a strong allure for several reasons. One is the appearance of consistency with widely shared values of personal autonomy. When we look to what incompetent patients formerly wanted, or what we infer they would desire, if known, the patient as competent appears to be deciding. This position purportedly extends the freedom and autonomy of competent persons to situations of incompetency.

A second attraction is that the orthodox approach has generally operated to protect incompetent patients from overzealous medical interventions. Until recently, applications of the test in most jurisdictions have found that patients would have refused treatment if they were competent, and have thus permitted intrusive, expensive treatments to be forgone. Also, by ostensibly treating incompetent patients as choice-makers who control whether treatment occurs, the orthodox approach denies others the power, at least explicitly, to override the incompetent patient's interests for the sake of others.

The orthodox approach also attracts because it recognizes a central role for family discretion in treatment decisions for incompetent patients. Since families are so directly involved in the illness of loved ones, an approach that reposes authority in the family seems to respect present social mores. Although this discretion is couched in terms of ascertaining what the patient would choose if competent, or what the patient in fact once said, the family is usually the source of this information and hence is in a position to control it. Close scrutiny of the family's assessment of these questions is frequently omitted, thus giving them ultimate discretion to decide the matter.

Finally, the orthodox approach is attractive because it is comfortable. It enables decision-makers to finesse the dilemmas or tragic choices that make decisions for incompetent patients so difficult. By shifting the inquiry to what the patient when competent had or would have decided, it absolves decision-makers of the need to confront directly the value of debilitated life versus the burdens such life places on families, physicians, and society. It enables the courts to say, as they do in *Saikewicz* and *Brophy*, that they are not making quality of life choices or privileging other-directed interests but simply honoring what the patient has or would have chosen.

With these advantages, it is no surprise that the orthodox approach of treating the incompetent patient as a competent decision-maker so dominates legal and ethical thinking in this area. But its conceptual flaws and contradictions emerge when it is applied to the conscious, demented, and debilitated patients who now claim judicial and policy attention. When extended to this diverse group of individuals, the orthodox approach risks giving excessive and unexamined power to family and cost considerations in the guise of respecting patient autonomy.

THE ERRORS OF THE ORTHODOX APPROACH

Despite its allure and wide acceptance, the orthodox approach to non-treatment decisions for incompetent patients is conceptually confused and threatens to harm conscious incompetent patients.

The problems arise from its concept of the incompetent patient, which excludes the patient's current needs, and from its implementation method, which allows family and other interests to take control. To demonstrate these points, we examine three erroneous assumptions of the orthodox approach.

1. Incompetent Persons Must Be Treated as Autonomous Choice-Makers.

A major error in the orthodox approach is the assumption that equal respect for incompetent patients requires that they be treated as competent patients—that is, as choice-making actors. Equal respect for incompetent patients requires that their interests be protected and that they not be abused simply because they are incompetent. However, it does not follow that they must be treated as if they were exercising autonomy.

Choice is irrelevant if one lacks the capacity to choose, and incompetent persons are by definition incapable of exercising choice or self-determination. Rather than engage in the fiction of asking what they would choose, we should determine what interests, if any, they currently have in receiving life-sustaining treatment. As we will show, the interests of incompetent patients are not respected by an approach that analyzes their situations as if they were competent individuals exercising choice about treatment and continued life.

2. Expressed or Inferred Prior Choices Are an Accurate Indicator of Incompetent Persons' Current Interests.

A second conceptual error implicit in the orthodox approach is the assumption that the incompetent patient's own treatment choice, if known, would incorporate the preferences the patient had as a competent person. It is wrong to assume that the incompetent patient's prior competent preferences are the best indicator of the patient's current interests. If we could determine the choice that these patients would make if suddenly able to speak—if they could tell us what their interests in their compromised states are—such choices would reflect their current and future interests as incompetent individuals, not their past preferences.

Linking incompetent patients' past competent treatment preferences to their existing welfare is highly problematic. The desires competent persons have concerning their future medical care reflect the activities and goals that make life worthwhile for them as competent, choosing individuals. To most competent persons, work, family, friendships, exercise, hobbies, and related pursuits seem integral to a life worth living. Self-determination, bodily integrity, and personal privacy are also matters of deep concern. Many competent persons would refuse life-sustaining treatment that severely compromised those interests.

When people become incompetent and seriously ill, however, their interests may radically change. With their reduced mental and physical capacities, what was once of extreme importance to them no longer matters, while things that were previously of little moment assume much greater significance. An existence that seems demeaning and unacceptable to the competent person may still be of value to the incompetent patient, whose abilities, desires, and interests have so greatly narrowed.

It is difficult, if not impossible, for competent individuals to predict their interests in future treatment situations when they are incompetent because their needs and interests will have so radically changed. As a result, the directives they issue for future situations of incompetency, though they reflect their current needs and interests, may have little relevance to their needs and interests once they become incompetent. Indeed, their advance directives may even be detrimental to their interests once in that state.

Philosophical concepts of personal identity are relevant to this analysis. One contemporary theory, which is articulated most clearly by the British philosopher Derek Parfit, holds that a person's life can be a series of successive selves, with a new self emerging as the individual undergoes significant changes in beliefs, desires, memories, and intentions. According to this theory, advance directives for non-treatment could be issued by a different person than the subsequently incompetent individual. In such a situation, the former self's preferences would have no particular authority to govern the incompetent patient's treatment.

Yet our analysis does not depend on acceptance of Parfit's theory of personal identity, which could have radical implications for contract, criminal, and other rules of law. According to an alternate widely held view of personal identity, an essential core of

the individual persists over time. Persons retain a unitary identity during their entire lives, even though a person's interests may change dramatically as new personal situations arise. The position that a person's interests may change drastically once incompetency develops is consistent with this theory of a more unitary personal identity, and argues against taking the prior directive as an indication of the patient's current interests.

3. Personal Autonomy Includes the Right to Control the Future by Advance Directives.

Some persons might argue that the orthodox approach, especially in its reliance on advance directives, follows from the generally recognized right of autonomous persons to order their future in various ways. The advance directive against medical treatment is simply another way to exert control over one's fate, by minimizing the risk that one will be kept alive unnecessarily. If persons control their future by contract, will, and other self-binding arrangements, should they not also have the right to control their medical future by advance directives against life-prolonging treatment?

At the outset it should be noted that the argument from autonomy only partially supports the orthodox approach to non-treatment decisions regarding incompetent patients. Even if accepted, it would apply only to situations in which the person had issued an explicit directive concerning future conditions that have come to exist. This argument gives no support to the substituted judgment approach to decision-making for incompetent patients, for the proxy decision-maker is not then relying on an explicit directive issued by a person trying to exercise autonomy over her future. Instead, the proxy infers from general statements and behavior what the incompetent patient would have chosen if she had made a decision when competent or could now express a competent preference.

Even with this proviso, it is not clear why a person's directions concerning situations that arise when incompetent should be followed. Such directives are very different from ordering the future by contract or will. For example, unlike contracts, advance treatment directives are not promises on which other parties rely, in return for their own promise of performance or other consideration.

Other persons may have their own interests in enforcement of an advance directive, but they have no contractual right to enforcement, since they have not promised performance in return. Thus, an obligation to honor advance directives does not follow from the obligation to enforce contracts.

The advance directive is also dissimilar to a devise by will. At the time that a will takes effect the testator is dead and no longer has interests that can be harmed by a decision to honor the prior instructions. By contrast, honoring the advance directive occurs at a time when the maker is still alive and can very much be harmed by adherence to its provisions. Failing to honor a "living will" is, therefore, not inconsistent with honoring a "property will."

The argument from autonomy in effect represents a normative judgment that it is more important to give persons the advance certainty that they will not be overtreated than to prevent mistakes of undertreatment which their directives may cause. The security gained in empowering persons to control their medical future in this way is not cost-free. The cost—too often overlooked—is that adherence to the directive will lead to the death of incompetent patients who retain significant interests in continued life. Because interests change over time and the person executing the directive may not be assessing the situation from the perspective of the future incompetent patient, the interests of the competent person contemplating a hypothetical future and the interests of the incompetent person once that future occurs, may diverge. A policy favoring advance directives is not justified unless it recognizes and chooses to run this risk.

A recent New York case, *Evans* v. *Bellevue Hospital*, shows that this concern is more than theoretical. In *Evans*, an incompetent patient diagnosed with AIDS-related complex had when competent executed a document stating that life-sustaining treatment should be forgone if he suffered from "illness, disease or injury or experienced extreme mental deterioration, such that there is no reasonable expectation of recovering or regaining a meaningful quality of life." He also had executed a power of attorney authorizing another individual to make all medical decisions on his behalf.

The court case arose after physicians observed that the patient had multiple brain lesions, which they attributed to toxoplasmosis, a type of infection.

The patient's proxy decision-maker asked physicians to withhold antibiotic treatment for the infection. They refused, arguing that the treatment was expected to produce recovery from toxoplasmosis and restore the patient's ability to communicate. The court authorized the treatment, on grounds that the document's reference to "meaningful quality of life" was too ambiguous to sanction non-treatment in this case. The judge noted, however, that if the document had specified conditions that clearly applied to the patient's situation, the proxy would have been permitted to decline the treatment.

Evans sheds light on several major problems with the advance treatment directive. First is the document's imprecision. Living wills and other non-treatment directives tend to consist of broad statements that may supply little guidance on specific treatment questions. In fact they may have no binding effect at all simply because they are too vague or general to be construed to authorize nontreatment in a variety of circumstances never explicitly contemplated by the maker.

A second problem is the strong possibility that individuals who execute directives are unaware that they may be authorizing actions or omissions that conflict with their subsequent well-being. The argument for enforcing a prior directive even when it conflicts with the incompetent patient's interests is hardly compelling if the person, when competent, had not been made aware that his future interests may radically change, and thus be in conflict with what he judged—through the eyes of his previously competent self—to be in his interest.

The *Evans* decision also raises the more serious policy issue of whether to honor advance directives that appear clearly to conflict with the incompetent patient's existing interests. (Of course, many competent patients' advance directives will represent the patients' current interests as well, but in those cases there is no real need for an advance directive to justify forgoing treatment.) Although there is insufficient information to determine if a conflict between past wishes and present interests existed in the *Evans* case, the scenario illustrates the need for courts and legislatures to address this issue.

Avoiding unnecessary, nonbeneficial treatment is clearly a valid individual, family, and policy concern. Patients should not be treated unnecessarily whether or not they have issued a prior directive against such treatment. Withholding treatment in those cases is thus not dependent on issuing an advance directive. As we discuss below, the need to treat should be assessed independently in each case regardless of a directive. Since the directive is unnecessary to this end and may in other situations threaten the welfare of incompetent patients, the policy judgment in its favor is open to serious question. Respect for autonomy thus does not automatically include an obligation to adopt the orthodox approach on prior directives.

THE DANGERS OF THE ORTHODOX APPROACH: UNDERTREATMENT AND INAPPROPRIATE ATTENTION TO COSTS AND FAMILY DISTRESS

The orthodox approach threatens incompetent patients with undertreatment, because it overlooks the interests they may have in continued life in their diminished state. Prior directives made when patients were competent, as well as choices proxy decision-makers infer patients would make under substituted judgment, may conflict with patients' current interests, thus leading to non-treatment decisions that harm incompetent patients.

The potential for conflict with patient interests is heightened under the substituted judgment doctrine. This standard will affect many more people than the advance directive approach, given that few people issue explicit treatment directives. In most applications of substituted judgment, there is no express evidence speaking to the situation at hand. Instead, the family is asked what the formerly competent person would have wanted, if confronted with a choice about this situation. The patient's relatives are seen as having an "intimate understanding of the patient's medical attitudes and general world view." But in answering the treatment question, strong pressures may also move the family to focus on considerations other than the needs of the patient before them.

First, the question itself shifts attention to the patient at another time—to the preferences and needs the patient had as a competent person. As we noted previously, these can differ from the incompetent patient's existing interests. Second, families often have their own interests in being relieved of

the distress of seeing their loved ones in a chronic debilitated state. Although not conscious or directly influential, such distress may push the family to determine that the patient "would certainly have wanted treatment forgone." After all, they themselves would not want to be treated in those circumstances. Is it not reasonable to assume that the patient as a competent person would have wanted the same?

When the treatment decision is made, however, the patient is no longer competent, and thus, in most cases, lacks interests in privacy, dignity, and other values that presuppose some conscious appreciation of those concerns. Assigning these factors weight when they are no longer relevant to the patient actually gives priority to family interests and to generally held values of competent persons. Indeed, the real offense in maintaining debilitated patients is to competent observers, whose own concepts of what constitutes dignified and respectful medical treatment for seriously compromised human beings have been violated. Perhaps, as Justice Handler argued in his *Conroy* and *Jobes* opinions, these interests should be influential in the treatment setting. The orthodox approach, however, formally proclaims that they have no role while simultaneously permitting them *sub silentio* to shape non-treatment decisions that may conflict with the patient's current welfare.

The possibility of conflict between patients' interests and the outcomes permitted under the substituted judgment standard is not merely theoretical. Although the proxy's assumptions about the incompetent patient's choices "if competent" may coincide with the incompetent patient's current interests, they may also diverge in crucial ways. A key difference between the approaches emerges when the patient's current interests would seem to require treatment, contrary to the patient's inferred competent wishes.

This difficulty is evident in *Spring* and *Hier*, two Massachusetts cases that permitted life-sustaining care to be withheld from conscious incompetent patients. These cases illustrate how courts applying the substituted judgment approach have failed to examine and protect the actual interests of the individual incompetent patients before them. Both these opinions gave the patients' interests as incompetent individuals short shrift, focusing instead on their alleged interests in privacy and dignity, interests they appeared incapable of possessing at the time due to their incapacity. Moreover, the decisions are vulnerable to charges that family distress and cost considerations influenced the substituted judgment inquiry.

In re Spring concerned a 78-year-old senile but fully conscious nursing-home resident whose end-stage renal disease was being treated with dialysis. He sometimes resisted the procedure and required sedation during its administration. His family asked the court to authorize cessation of the dialysis. The court applied the substituted judgment test and, relying on the family's claim that if Spring were competent he would have refused treatment, held that the dialysis could be discontinued.

The judgment that Spring's competent decision would be to refuse dialysis ignored the possibility that in his incompetent state he obtained sufficient countervailing pleasure and satisfaction to make the benefits of continued life outweigh the discomforts of the dialysis necessary to preserve that life. Nor was there any examination of whether the burdens of dialysis could be reduced by less drastic means, such as behavior modification techniques. The court accepted with little scrutiny the family's view that the patient would have wanted treatment withheld because he had previously been an active outdoorsman.

While Spring's family might have been sincere in their assessment, they were really focusing on what some (certainly not all) competent persons in Spring's situation might choose, and not on what would serve the interests of a person who no longer was competent. The court also failed to consider the possibility that the family's own distress and expense in such a situation influenced their assessment of what the patient would have wanted. The opinion dispenses with any need to assess these possibilities by simply assuming that they would not influence the wishes of a family faced with chronic nursing-home care of a senile husband and father.

Similar conceptual weaknesses characterize the opinion in *In re Hier*, a case involving a 92-year-old nonterminally ill incompetent patient who required feeding by gastrostomy tube. When she pulled out the tube and resisted its reinsertion, the hospital sought judicial guidance. The Court refused to order the minor surgery necessary to replace the tube, stressing the procedure's risk and interpreting Hier's behavior as a "plea for privacy and personal dignity for a 92-year-old person who is seriously ill and for whom life has little left to offer."

The determination that Hier's resistance to feeding manifested a desire for privacy and personal dignity attributed the concerns of a competent individual to an incompetent patient who was probably expressing a simple response, such as irritation with the feeding apparatus or a demand for attention. As in *Spring*, the major deficiencies in this opinion are its omission of a systematic analysis of the patient's current capacities and experiences, and its failure to weigh and balance these elements in determining whether the patient had significant contemporaneous interests in continued life.

Particularly troubling is the *Hier* court's neglect of the pain and distress a conscious patient could experience if she were denied nourishment, as well as its omission of any inquiry into the possibility that she obtained pleasure and enjoyment from her restricted life. There also was evidence that one physician who testified against performing the surgery did so because Hier had already consumed "enough" health care resources. (After the appellate court decision, Hier's legal representative returned to the trial court, presented additional medical testimony, and convinced the lower court to order the surgery.)

These cases illustrate how the court's application of the substituted judgment standard opens the door to non-treatment of nursing-home residents and other severely debilitated persons based on what competent persons believe they would want in those situations, or on what meets the needs of their families and others, rather than on what serves the needs of the incompetent patients themselves. The more recent *Brophy* case reinforces this possibility. Although *Brophy* involved a patient who was irreversibly comatose, the court formulated the substituted judgment doctrine in broad terms that could affect all incompetent patients. The result is that respirators, antibiotics, nutrition, or any other treatment could be withheld from conscious incompetent patients whenever the family asserts that the incompetent patients would have found their current lives "degrading and without human dignity" when they were competent. Since many competent persons might so view such a diminished existence,

Brophy opens the door legally to withdrawing treatment from any conscious, incompetent nursing-home resident.

THE ORTHODOX APPROACH AND THE RISKS OF OVERTREATMENT

Although the orthodox approach has been generally favorable to family requests for non-treatment, sometimes granting such requests even when unjustified, it could as easily be interpreted to deny proxy requests for non-treatment that should be granted. *In re O'Connor*, decided last year by New York's highest court, exemplifies this problem. Ms. O'Connor was an elderly woman who had suffered a series of strokes that left her paralyzed and bedridden. The court described her as "severely demented" and "profoundly incapacitated," able to respond to some simple commands, but with severe, irreparable neurological damage. Yet the court ruled against removal of a nasogastric tube because the evidence of her past preferences was insufficient to establish that she would have opted against such treatment if she were competent. Similarly, in *Cruzan v. Harmon*, the Missouri Supreme Court recently prohibited cessation of tube feeding for a permanently unconscious patient, emphasizing the lack of evidence that she had expressed desires to avoid such treatment.

As in *Spring* and *Hier*, these courts failed to inquire systematically into the patients' current interests in continued life. Instead, they sought to apply the orthodox approach, but took a stricter approach to what counted as sufficient evidence of the patients' competent wishes. Since it is difficult to know what an incompetent patient "if competent" would have wanted, the standard of proof applied to answering that question will control the outcome. Unlike the *Spring* and *Hier* judges, the courts in *O'Connor* and *Cruzan* applied a higher standard of proof to answering that question, finding insufficient evidence that they would have chosen non-treatment.

These cases illustrate the ultimate indeterminacy of the fiction of treating the incompetent patient as a self-determining individual. While the predominant danger of the orthodox approach is undertreatment, it also poses a risk that unjustified overtreatment

will occur whenever the courts impose a strict standard for inferring the patient's choice if competent. In that case, medical zeal and rigid concern with right to life values may override patient and other interests. In either case, by focusing on the wrong question—the wishes of a past or hypothetical competent person—the interests of the incompetent patient as they now exist are ignored.

TOWARD A NEW LEGAL STANDARD: THE INCOMPETENT PATIENT'S CURRENT INTERESTS

The orthodox approach to non-treatment decisions for incompetent patients is seriously flawed and should be scrapped. It mistakenly assumes that incompetent patients should be regarded as choice-makers when they are incapable of decision, and then constructs a hypothetical competent decision-maker that confuses past or inferred preferences of patients with their current interests. By overlooking the conflict between past directives and current interests, it allows concerns with family stress and costs to override the real needs of incompetent patients, without an adequate evaluation of each. Alternatively, the test can be manipulated to require such a high standard of proof for inferring competent choice, that treatment can seldom be withheld, no matter how justified in terms of the patient's current interests.

An alternative approach that is more likely to protect conscious incompetent patients and to give factors external to patient welfare their proper role is to ask whether treatment actually serves the incompetent patient's existing interests. If treatment cannot succeed in supplying patients with an acceptable quality of life, then external considerations should be permitted to affect the decision. If treatment would serve patient interests but would impose heavy burdens on family or society, the conflict can be faced openly. Society's commitment to a patient-centered position can be reaffirmed or modified on the merits, not in the guise of determining what the incompetent patient would have chosen if competent.

To develop defensible standards governing the care of incompetent patients, legal decision-makers must directly assess the value to patients of their diminished or marginalized lives. The most appropriate method is to adopt a variation of the "best interests" standard and to ask whether treatment will advance the current and future welfare of the patient. This approach requires a systematic evaluation of the incompetent patient's personal contemporaneous interests, rather than the interests competent persons might have in those situations. Assessing these interests requires observers to evaluate, from the incompetent patient's perspective, indications of the patient's subjective state, and ultimately, to judge whether this state of existence is a sufficient good to justify further treatment of the patient. The question is not how a competent person would feel in such states, but whether these experiences are of value to a person in the incompetent person's situation. The important question is whether patients who cannot experience the richness of normal life still have experiences that make continued existence from their own perspective better than no life at all.

Such an approach has several advantages that recommend its adoption for all decision-making regarding incompetent patients. First, it is respectful of the individual whose treatment is at issue. The ethical commitment to a patient-centered approach requires a focus on the patient as she now is, and not on the desires that she previously had when her interests were quite different. This approach will better protect a debilitated patient's existing interests in continued life.

Second, it will permit non-treatment to occur when justified, e.g., when the patient cannot reasonably be said to have any continued interest in living because her level of awareness is so minimal that the patient is unable to appreciate being alive. For life to be of value to an individual, some capacity to interact with the environment must be present. Thus, incompetent patients with minimal "relational capacity," such as Nancy Cruzan, Claire Conroy, or Mary O'Connor, lack significant interests in having their lives maintained, and might have further treatment withheld under this test.

Third, the current-interests approach acknowledges the role of costs, family stress, and similar concerns, thus preventing them from influencing non-treatment decisions in an uncontrolled or unprincipled way. By focusing on the incompetent patient's current interests, room is given for these competing concerns when no significant patient interests are affected. Thus, for example, in cases involving permanently unconscious and barely conscious individuals, the family's burdens and financial costs may be taken into account because no interests of the patient are directly affected.

Fourth, a focus on current interests of the incompetent patient sharpens the conflict between a patient-centered and other-directed approach, thus requiring explicit consideration of the normative judgments supporting either approach. The desire to relieve family stress and reduce costs may operate at some level in treatment decisions affecting many severely debilitated patients. Unless these factors are candidly confronted, they risk influencing treatment decisions in an unprincipled fashion, potentially overriding the significant interests some incompetent patients have in obtaining life-sustaining treatment. While such directness may be discomforting, facing the question openly will keep other-directed concerns from operating subterraneously and hold them in check.

Finally, a current-interests approach still permits the family to be the initial or primary decision-maker—an important ingredient of any public policy. The family or other proxy will, in effect, be asked to determine whether the patient's life is so diminished that the patient has no further interests in living, not whether continued living is what the patient would have chosen. Doctors, courts, and others reviewing family decisions, however, will then explicitly apply a current-interests test to the proxy's choice. Ultimately a societal judgment about what states of diminished life are worth protecting will be brought to bear on those decisions.

Such an approach is not as radical a departure as it might initially sound, and is inevitable once the inability of the orthodox approach to handle more difficult cases becomes clear. Indeed, variations on this approach have already appeared. In *Saikewicz*, for example, the court purportedly applied the substituted judgment standard, couching its decision in terms of the patient's privacy and self-determination rights. In reality it performed a best interests analysis and concluded that in light of the patient's capacity to understand the pain that would be imposed to gain a few extra months of living, a decision against treatment would best serve his interests. Similarly, although its decision to require treatment might be questioned, the New York Court of Appeals in *Storar* based its decision on an individualized assessment of the burdens and benefits of continued treatment for the patient. Unfortunately it chose not to follow that lead in *O'Connor*, where a judgment that further treatment was not in the patient's interests could reasonably have been reached.

The New Jersey Supreme Court in *Conroy* partially accepted this approach when no explicit treatment directive or other clear evidence of a patient's past preferences was available. According to the court, if "the net burdens of the patient's life with the treatment . . . clearly and markedly outweigh the benefits that the patient derives from life" and "the recurring, unavoidable, and severe pain of the patient's life [are] such that the effect of administering life-sustaining treatment would be inhumane," life-sustaining treatment may be forgone.

In our view, however, *Conroy* articulates the benefit-burden analysis too narrowly to protect incompetent patients adequately, for it fails to include such factors as lack of awareness and relational capacity. Thus, it does not authorize non-treatment of permanently unconscious or barely conscious patients who obtain negligible benefits from life, but experience no pain and suffering. Moreover, *Conroy*, *Saikewicz*, and *Storar* limit the benefit-burden analysis to cases in which reliable evidence of the patients' competent treatment preferences is lacking, thus overlooking the possibility of conflict between such evidence and current interests. Nevertheless, the courts' partial recognition of the need to examine the incompetent patient's contemporaneous interests is encouraging, and may facilitate expanded acceptance of the current-interests standard.

DIFFICULTIES OF A CURRENT-INTERESTS APPROACH

The major difficulty in applying a current-interests approach lies in obtaining reliable information about a patient's subjective experiences and in evaluating their significance. The danger is that arbitrary assessments of patient interests will occur, to the detriment of patients and society's respect for life.

However, the difficulty in obtaining and evaluating data about the patient and thus determining her interests is surmountable in many cases. Even though these patients typically can furnish us with little or no verbal data on how they experience their lives, the observer can gain this information from assessing their behavior and physical condition. Evidence bearing on patients' perception of pain and other physical sensations, ability to interact with other persons and the environment, and ability to engage in cognitive activity are all relevant to the examination of what these patients' lives are like for them.

More daunting is the next step: to determine whether these experiences provide "a life worth living" to the patient and a corresponding obligation by family or society to preserve it, despite the burdens that doing so entails. Yet here too it is possible to make considerable progress before facing the toughest questions about quality of life and trade-offs with other interests.

For example, a wide consensus already exists that certain states of being are not in a patient's interest, and therefore need not be provided if the family requests non-treatment. One such situation exists when the patient can experience only unremitting pain, without any countervailing pleasure and enjoyment. With modern techniques of pain relief, however, few patients may be in this category.

Permanently unconscious patients comprise a larger agreed-upon category of individuals lacking significant interests in prolonged life. All available medical evidence indicates that these individuals have no mental awareness. Although they suffer no pain or distress, they cannot experience any benefit from continued life. For them, there is only the remote possibility of restoration in the event of a mistaken diagnosis or an as yet undiscovered cure that supplies a reason for maintenance. With the exception of the *Cruzan* case in Missouri, every state court that has faced the question has permitted non-treatment of these individuals under the orthodox approach. It is likely that these decisions were influenced by the view that continued life fails to confer a significant benefit on such patients, although the opinions fail explicitly to incorporate this analysis.

Assessment of current interests of other groups of patients may also reasonably occur. "Barely conscious" individuals who cannot initiate purposeful activity, whose experiences are limited to physical sensations, and whose medical prognosis holds no reasonable chance of improvement, have clear interests in avoiding pain and discomfort. Their interests in continued life seem small, however, because they lack the cognitive capacity to interact with others and to appreciate being alive. Although some will argue that any minimally conscious human being has a significant stake in being maintained, it is difficult to see how life without greater awareness of self and others can confer a genuine benefit on these patients. Families who take this position and request non-treatment would not therefore be violating the right to life of such patients.

In contrast, conscious incompetent patients who can experience enjoyment and pleasure, and whose conditions and necessary treatment interventions impose on them small or moderate burdens, have more significant interests in obtaining life-sustaining care. The "pleasantly senile" and other debilitated individuals who appear to receive benefits from their restricted lives fall into this category. Even though their activities may seem unduly limited to some observers, these individuals appear to retain sufficient mental capacity for continued life to hold material value for them. If society is committed to a patient-centered approach, it should be willing to provide the resources necessary to protect these patients' lives. It should also find that these patients' former competent preferences against treatment and family distress are inadequate to override the patients' interests in receiving continued care.

The hardest cases will fall between those who are barely conscious and the pleasantly senile. For those patients it may be difficult to ascertain or meaningfully discuss their interests in living from their own limited perspective. "Objective" quality of life assessments are inevitably crude and subject to dispute. Disagreement and controversy may be unavoidable. In some cases, it will be impossible to reach a clear decision on what outcome would best serve the patient's existing interests. Moreover, extensive debate may be required to determine what level of awareness and benefit is sufficient to give incompetent patients a significant interest in continued life, notwithstanding the patients' former competent preferences against treatment and the burdens imposed on family and society.

But these problems are no greater than the problems under the orthodox approach of determining what the patient would choose if competent when that approach is scrupulously applied. The comparative advantage of the current-interests standard is that quality of life assessments and the conflicts they pose with other interests are faced openly, rather than in the guise of family or proxy decision of what the patient would choose if competent. In our view this openness constitutes a great advantage.

THE INEVITABILITY OF QUALITY OF LIFE ASSESSMENTS

Applying the current-interests test necessarily involves assessing the value of a particular existence to the incompetent patient in question, and its value relative to the burdens that providing it poses for family and society. Ultimately, the current-interests test brings us to the controversial task of making quality of life judgments—of deciding whether the duty to sustain life in marginalized states is obligatory, notwithstanding the burdens on others of doing so.

Although balancing patient quality of life against other interests has long been a taboo subject, we believe that an honest, direct approach to these issues is both warranted and manageable. Since quality of life judgments must inevitably be made, it is preferable to make them openly so that arbitrary or unjustified assessments can be identified. The alternative is a conceptually flawed approach that allows those judgments to be made covertly, thus risking even greater likelihood of damage to incompetent patients, their families, and society.

How do these considerations apply to actual decision-making for incompetent patients? Families will still retain primary decision-making authority, deciding whether the patient has further interests in living. In the great majority of instances their choices will reflect general societal judgments about the value to patients of greatly diminished states of existence. In cases that are less clear, the family or proxy's choice should be reviewed in light of the current-interests standard. If an objective viewer finds that the patient has significant interests in continued existence, then treatment providing that existence should continue unless the community at large reevaluates its overriding commitment to a patient-centered approach to these questions.

CONCLUSION

As the non-treatment debate moves to hard questions concerning conscious incompetent patients, it is essential that the issues be clearly posed and carefully analyzed. The orthodox judicial approach, which substitutes the fiction of a competent decision-maker for the reality of an incompetent person, is inadequate to this task and should be abandoned.

That fiction confuses the issue, misleads families, doctors, and others struggling with treatment decisions, and harms the patients and families most directly affected.

An approach that focuses on the current interests of the incompetent patient—on her quality of life—is far preferable. Open assessment of quality of life will give incompetent patients their due, while at the same time acknowledging a proper role for family and cost concerns. While difficult questions will remain, the central normative questions will be directly faced. What quality of diminished life should be protected? At what cost? These are the questions that must be faced in decision-making at the margins of life.

THE LIMITS OF LEGAL OBJECTIVITY

Nancy K. Rhoden

PRIOR DIRECTIVES AND THE OBJECTIVE ENTERPRISE

The objective standard as articulated in *Conroy* was, of course, intended only for those situations in which the patient's prior beliefs were not determinative. If taken to its logical extension, however, the

From *North Carolina Review* 68, no. 5 (June 1990): 845–865. Copyright © 1990 North Carolina Law Review Association. Reprinted with permission.

Editors' note: Professor Rhoden's article has been substantially edited and most of the notes have been cut. Students who want to follow up on sources should consult the original article. Deleted sections noted the problems with the "subjective" tests articulated in the *Conroy* case (reprinted in this section) and challenged the adequacy of the "objective" tests on the grounds that they (1) set a standard that can almost never be met, and (2) focus narrowly on pain to the exclusion of other important subjective values. In the sections reprinted here, Rhoden argues that the objective approach advocated in the preceding article by Professors Dresser and Robertson also threatens the validity of prior directives.

quest for a person-neutral standard may come to clash with the widespread acceptance of clear-cut prior directives as controlling. This conflict arises because if we focus solely on the incompetent's present interests, we so radically distinguish her from the author of the prior directive that it's hard to see why the prior choice should govern.

To illustrate how a completely present-oriented test can undermine the justification for honoring living wills, imagine for a moment that after the court evaluated Ms. Conroy objectively, her nephew discovered a valid and clearly applicable living will rejecting all medical treatment if "barely conscious." Given its preference for a subjective test, the *Conroy* court almost certainly would want to reconsider and let the document control. But this hypothetical discovery creates a "past-present" conflict, in which Ms. Conroy's present interests support treatment, while her prior choice is to forgo it. Although the court could simply hold that an applicable living will trumps current interests, this decision procedure seems rather arbitrary in light of the just-completed assessment of current interests. Why, one might ask, should a prior directive control if it thwarts a patient's present interests?

One answer to this is that it should not. Dresser, as the most logical and consistent advocate of a present best interests test, essentially rejects living wills, except to the extent they provide useful reassurance in cases in which the objective choice would be to terminate treatment, so that the wills are largely redundant.[1] Hence my first task is to analyze her arguments and rebut them by setting forth a rights-based justification for honoring prior directives. . . .

The Impairment of the Incompetent's Interests

. . . [Dresser argues] that honoring a living will can compromise unacceptably the interests of an incompetent person. One cannot be sure that what the person chose then is what he would choose now, because views about what constitutes an acceptable level of functioning may change radically as function declines. Active, healthy persons often say they would never want to live if wheelchair-bound, on dialysis, or whatever, and then later embrace life despite their disabilities. Likewise, once capacity for complex intellectual pleasures is gone, simpler things take on greater importance. As Dresser and Robertson put it:

> If we truly could determine the choice that these patients would make if suddenly able to speak—if they could tell us what their interests in their compromised states are—such choices would be most likely to reflect their current and future interests as incompetent individuals, not their past preferences.[2]

Thus prior directives reflect competent persons' former interests, but the better, more caring way to make choices for incompetents is to focus on their current interests. The law should not allow someone to make a binding future choice for death, because to do so gives an unacceptable degree of primacy to the interests of competent persons over incompetent ones.

The strength of this argument is reinforced by a very troubling sort of example. Suppose a highly intellectual person makes a prior directive stating that if he

becomes even somewhat mentally impaired, he wants no medical treatment. He then suffers a mild stroke and is in a nursing home. While he cannot comprehend his prior directive, and hence can neither affirm nor rescind it, he appears to enjoy his simple existence, watching television and sharing meals with other patients. Then he gets pneumonia. His directive clearly rejects antibiotics. If it is controlling, the staff must simply watch him die. But, Dresser quite reasonably argues, he has substantial present interests in life, and they must prevail. This sort of case may well incline us toward a Parfit-type view*—that this happy incompetent person *is* someone different from the intellectual who made the document—or, at least, should make us question the wisdom of necessarily subordinating present interests to prior choices, no matter how explicit and strongly held.

All this makes a strong case against prior directives. It suggests that the reason living wills have been so widely accepted is not that we have an abiding faith in future-oriented choices, but that the substantive choice in most living wills is an objectively reasonable one (to avoid prolongation of the dying process, or treatment when persistently vegetative). Hence a prior directive may well help bolster a decision to stop treatment for a patient who lacks present interests in living, but it should not justify termination when the patient has such interests. I will later deal with the case in which the incompetent patient has clear-cut and substantial interests in living and will suggest that the right to make binding future choices should be less absolute than the right to make present ones. But first I must resurrect prior directives in general as reflecting a moral preference for individual choice rather than merely reinforcing objective decisions. To do so, I will show that rejecting future-oriented choices threatens present ones.

The Continuum with Contemporaneous Choices

Assume that George is a Christian Scientist who rejects all surgical interventions. He makes a prior directive refusing surgery at any time for any

---

*Editors' note: See Dresser/Robertson article, this section.

condition. He subsequently develops a brain tumor which impairs his cognitive processes so that he is incapable of either affirming or rejecting his prior directive. He is happily watching television, and the brain tumor could be removed, extending his life (though not restoring his competency). Dresser undoubtedly would say that decision makers should authorize surgery, on the grounds that the prior religious faith is no longer relevant and that his present interests in his happy, albeit limited, life should control.

George's case seems very similar to the intellectual's, except of course that his prior beliefs are religious rather than "merely" secular. A truly "hard-core" believer in prior directives may feel that in even these cases, the directive should prevail. Some proponents of precedent autonomy may feel otherwise, because the incompetent patients: (1) have such clear-cut interests in life; and (2) are so unlikely to retain beliefs in the primacy of the intellect or the tenets of the Christian Science faith. Hence some supporters of prior directives may wish to disavow them in one or both of these cases. To show, however, that this should not lead to a wholesale rejection of precedent autonomy, we merely need alter one of two variables. The first is the time frame; the second is the patient's mental status at the time of initial diagnosis and decision making.

First, the time frame. Assume our intellectual is also psychic—or at least aware that his blood pressure is 210 over 190. He anticipates his stroke and one day before it makes his prior directive. Although the stroke affects only his brain, one week later he contracts pneumonia. Despite his recent choice, made in anticipation of disability, a proponent of current interests undoubtedly still would protect the incompetent's present interests. After all, interests can change gradually over twenty years, or in one fell swoop when one's neocortex is damaged.

If this feels somewhat less comfortable to the proponent of patient autonomy, it is because the rapidity of the developments has blurred the distinction between present- and future-oriented choice. We can blur this distinction even further if, returning to George, the brain tumor is diagnosed while he is still competent. As a Christian Scientist, he refuses surgery. Because he knows incompe-

tency may soon ensue, he makes a prior directive. One week later, he is incompetent. Rethinking his choice now seems to me like a wrong to George—the George who competently chose, based on considered religious beliefs, to reject treatment. Yet from the present-oriented perspective, I cannot see why this is any different from the other cases. *Now* George is an incompetent whose life could be prolonged by medical intervention. And *now* he lacks the mental structure to hold his former beliefs. Under a present-oriented view, we would respect choice as long as the person was competent, but then, once his powers dimmed, we would rethink it if treatment was still potentially efficacious. In other words, a competent choice will lose its force once the person is incapable of realizing it has been made, because now—whether this occurs gradually or suddenly—the incompetent is the only player in town.

If we accept this present focus, then the competent patient's "right" to refuse treatment will be upheld only for the few months, weeks, days, or hours she remains competent. After that, the treatment decision will be made on the basis of the objectively assessed present interests of the incompetent. Taken to an extreme, this could mean that a Jehovah's Witness could refuse a blood transfusion until he "bled out" and became incompetent, after which he could be transfused.

However an objective test would decide cases of intermittent incompetency, such as the typical Jehovah's Witness scenario, it seems to commit us to a wholesale reassessment of contemporaneous treatment refusals upon subsequent incompetency. Not all refusals will impair the interests of the now-incompetent: if he is terminally ill, he may be better-off dying more quickly. But many treatment refusals will, especially those based upon minority views about religion or modern medicine. Minority beliefs are usually considered to be precisely those for which protection of autonomy is most crucial. Once we recognize that present autonomy and precedent autonomy are simply two ends of a continuum, along which are choices initially made when competent, reaffirmed repeatedly, but subject to reexamination after the person becomes incompetent, we see that rejecting precedent autonomy threatens a fairly broad spectrum of present, prior, and mixed present/prior choices.

Viewing the Incompetent

This returns us to the dilemma of how to view incompetent patients. They can, of course, be viewed just in the present, with only their current, highly truncated interests taken into account. As so viewed, the prior directive clearly impairs the incompetent's interests. Back when the directive was made, however, the person was acting as a moral agent, and it is harder to take a completely present-oriented view toward moral agents and their interests. As Christine Korsgaard, who criticizes Parfit for viewing persons in a peculiarly passive sense as essentially the experiencers of various sensations, puts it:

> Perhaps it is natural to think of the present self as necessarily concerned with present satisfaction. But it is mistaken. In order to make deliberative choices, your present self must identify with something from which you will derive your reasons, but not necessarily with something present. The sort of thing you identify yourself with may carry you automatically into the future; and I have been suggesting that this will very likely be the case. Indeed, the choice of any action, no matter how trivial, takes you some way into the future. And to the extent that you regulate your choices by identifying yourself as the one who is implementing something like a particular plan of life, you need to identify with your future in order to be *what you are even now*. When the person is viewed as an agent, no clear content can be given to the idea of a merely present self.[3]

Dresser criticizes prior directives as giving moral and legal primacy to competent persons over incompetent ones. While incompetent persons of course warrant respect, I think it is nonetheless perfectly appropriate to give primacy to competent persons—at least if the incompetent person inhabits the formerly competent person's body. The competent person's primacy derives from his status as moral agent. Moral agency is inherently future-directed, and the future may, unfortunately, encompass one's incompetency. Prior directives are the tools for projecting one's moral and spiritual values into the future. These values seem to me worthy of respect even when they conflict with the subsequent, purely physical, interests of an incompetent. (I must admit here, though, that there may be an irreconcilable clash of instincts about whether the incompetent should be viewed as the moral agent

he was or the more passive experiencer of physical sensations he is now.)

Another problem with the purely present perspective is that prior directives reflect concern for others. Many people make living wills because they do not want their family's resources to be consumed in sustaining a barely sentient existence. Consider another example of other-directed values. Suppose a pregnant woman is stricken with cancer. Her prognosis is better if she aborts, but she refuses, because having this baby is the most important thing to her. She makes out a document specifying this, and then lapses into incompetency. An abortion still could be performed. Someone who rejects prior directives would, it seems, have to reopen the issue of the abortion and endorse it if it promoted the now-incompetent woman's physical interests. Yet just as it is difficult to view moral agents only in the present, it is difficult to view them in total isolation. Surely it is misleading to view *this* woman in complete isolation. Her most cherished goal—to leave the legacy of a child—is attainable only via a prior directive that harms the incompetent. It reflects the values of the competent person she was, and these values warrant a degree of moral primacy.

All this suggests that while it may be true that the incompetent person, if suddenly able to speak, would choose based on her current interests, this should not be determinative, because her former values, though no longer consciously held, have not lost their moral force. Among other reasons, such values are still important because the formerly competent person made a choice—an exercise of her autonomy. Her living will should not be seen simply as evidence of what she (as an incompetent) might now want. Seen as mere evidence, a prior directive inevitably will fail, because even the most devastatingly impaired patient could now, at least hypothetically, want something else. Viewed as an actual choice, a living will can function fairly well. It of course has limitations, as do other prior choices such as testamentary wills. Much as one cannot know one's precise medical plight in advance, one cannot anticipate the changes in conduct, lifestyle, or fortune of one's heirs. A regular will clearly is not evidence of most recent desires, but is an actual choice, and a change in circumstances is simply the risk one runs in making future choices. The alternative is not to make such choices (or to designate a proxy rather than make a substantive choice). But if we believe in the right to make future choices, we should not complain about their inherent and inescapable limitations.

The analogy with testamentary wills, however, returns us to the troubling example of the intellectual's idiosyncratic directive, because a living will, unlike a testamentary will, can severely compromise a person's present interests. Are there no limits to the harmful future choices a person can make? It does not seem inconsistent with accepting precedent autonomy to place some limits on it. In a few cases, competent contemporaneous choices are overruled, because, for example, they place medical professionals in such an untenable position. This was the impetus for denying Elizabeth Bouvia the relief sought in her first lawsuit—the right to refuse food and water by mouth while receiving hygienic care in the psychiatric ward of a hospital. The court held, essentially, that individual autonomy could not transform medical professionals into attendants at a suicide parlor. Prior directives are made with far less knowledge of the medical situation and the patient's future interests than are current choices. Hence some restrictions could be placed on them (as the law currently does), so that the former intellectual could not demand that nursing home staff let a happy, otherwise healthy, but "pleasantly senile" person die. We can thus concede that such an unusual prior directive need not control— because other concerns can override our prima facie duty to honor it—without rejecting the basic principle of prior control. After all, challenging as this philosophical puzzle is, no one (at least at present) makes such directives. People make prior directives to avoid being tethered to medical technology when unconscious or in a state such as Claire Conroy's. When they start saying, "If I can't do higher mathematics, kill me," we will have to worry in earnest about the limits of precedent autonomy.

Finally, I do not deny that we can, when pressed, make quality-of-life assessments from a present-oriented perspective. Decision makers must do this for infants and for the never-competent. Something is wrong, however, when we treat formerly competent patients as if they were never competent. Someone who makes a prior directive sees herself as the unified subject of a human life. She sees her concern for her body, her goals, or her family as transcending her incapacity. It is at least one, if not an overriding, component of treating persons with respect, that we view them as they view themselves. If we are to do this, we must not ignore their prior choices and values.

Actual prior choices are an exercise of autonomy and hence deserve far more weight than informally expressed preferences. This is not only because of evidentiary concerns, but because a person who makes a living will has exercised her right to decide—a right that imposes upon others a prima facie duty to honor her choice. We have, however, no similar right that informally expressed preferences be honored. Yet many of the same reasons that make prior directives morally relevant also make prior preferences relevant. Primary among them is the sense that most persons, when competent, see their preferences, goals, and values as relevant to future choices about them, because they see themselves as unified subjects of their lives. Were we all Parfitians, this conclusion would change. But, I hazard to say, we are not. Hence, when making moral choices for formerly competent persons who left no explicit directives we should still consider their probable desires, although we should avoid succumbing to the illusion that such desires will necessarily be unambiguous or determinative.

THE ANALOGY TO WILLS AND THE PROBLEM OF THE SUBJECT

Someone might object that all this boils down to the claim that because many people feel that if they become incompetent they would want others to think of them as they were in their prime, the law should accept and reinforce this delusion. In other words, if there is no competent person there who will notice the dishonoring of his prior wishes, then thinking we must honor them is just as silly as thinking of the dead as they were when alive and imagining we have duties to them. The "problem of the subject"—the question of just who is harmed by posthumous betrayals—has received substantial philosophical consideration. I cannot treat it adequately here, but can offer some suggestions that relate back to the unconscious or barely conscious. One solution that is easy—perhaps too easy—is just to emphasize that competent people care about their future, and if word gets out that choices will be reassessed upon incompetency, everyone will be anxious and uneasy. This rule-utilitarian approach does yield a duty to honor prior directives, albeit one that does not run to anyone in particular. It clearly would be acceptable to someone whose general moral theory is a rule-utilitarian one. It is less satisfactory to a rights-based theorist, because it means that while failure to honor a present choice wrongs the chooser, failure to honor a prior choice is, in Joel Feinberg's words, merely a "diffuse public harm."

Because Feinberg believes that the dead can be wronged (and, indeed, harmed), he tackles this problem of who is harmed by a posthumous betrayal. Feinberg distinguishes two ways of conceptualizing the dead: as dead bodies ("postmortem persons") and as the persons they were when alive ("antemortem persons"). Postmortem persons cannot be harmed; they are mere corpses. But, Feinberg argues, antemortem persons can be harmed, because they can have "surviving interests" that can be invaded. Hence posthumous betrayals can count as harms to antemortem persons. Holding that the subject of the harm is the antemortem person is an attempt, and probably a successful one, to solve the problem of the subject.

Joan Callahan argues that although in postulating antemortem persons, Feinberg has devised a proper subject of harm, he faces another problem—that of "backward causation," or the implication that an event after a person's death can harm him prior to his death.[4] Feinberg seeks to avoid this implication by holding that the antemortem subject of posthumous harm was harmed all along, or at least at the point when he acquired the interest that would subsequently be defeated. It is just that until the harmful event actually occurs, no one could know of his harmed condition. As Feinberg puts it:

> [T]he financial collapse of the life-insurance company through which I have protected my loved dependents, occurring, let us imagine, five minutes after my death, several years in the future, makes it true that my present interest in my children's security is harmed, and therefore, that *I* am harmed too, though I know it not. When that time comes, my friends might feel sorry not only for my children but for me too, though I am dead.[5]

According to Feinberg, believing that the antemortem person is harmed before the event is no different from believing that a father whose son has just been killed is immediately harmed, even though he has not yet received the bad news.

Several closely related and, it seems, telling criticisms have been made of this notion that a person whose interests will be defeated after his death is in a harmed state from the time he acquires such interests. W. J. Waluchow notes that we do not think this way about future harms to existing persons; we do not consider ourselves already harmed by events that will happen in the future.[6] It seems he is correct that future harms should have the same logical structure whether the victim will be dead or alive when the harmful event occurs. As Callahan points out, Feinberg's theory implies that a person who will later perform a harmful action is, long before doing so, responsible for placing the victim in a harmed (though as-of-yet unrecognizably so) position. Sympathetic as I find Feinberg's overall approach, this particular aspect does seem to smack of predestination. If before a decedent's demise his future betrayer had not even formed his evil intent, it seems very strange to maintain that the decedent while alive was in a harmed state. Despite Feinberg's attempt to equate this with a father's lack of awareness of his son's recent death, there does seem to be a crucial asymmetry between being unaware of an event that has occurred, and being unaware of a future event that, unless we are fatalists, may not happen after all.

Even if Feinberg's attempted solution to the problem of backward causation fails, I believe that the basic moral intuition that we wrong the promisee when we breach a promise, even posthumously, remains firm, as Callahan's discussion itself illustrates. Callahan first tries to defend this duty by claiming that testamentary bequests generally merit respect in their own right; that we feel obligated to honor them because they usually coincide with other values we hold important, such as the good of individual heirs. To support this, she notes that we would feel less obligation to carry out an iniquitous or wasteful request (that all the paintings of a great artist be burned). But surely we don't feel that giving an estate to the decedent's spoiled, self-indulgent son (to whom it was bequeathed) is objectively preferable to giving it to his hard-working, saintly (but disinherited) daughter. If honoring his will is morally obligatory, this is because we believe the deceased had a right to distribute his estate as he saw fit, even if we abhor the end result. If truly heinous requests are not binding upon us, it is simply because other moral principles can sometimes override prima facie rights.

Callahan does admit that the independent moral value of bequests cannot fully account for what she recognizes as the genuine moral conviction that persons have a right to dispose of their property as they see fit. However, she claims that right yields a duty not to the decedent, but only to his heirs. That sounds initially plausible, but how would it apply to other promises made to a decedent? Suppose I leave my friend ten thousand dollars in my will in return for his promise to care for my cat. If, as soon as I die, he has my cat euthanized, it is hard not to think that he has breached a duty to me, rather than to my cat. It becomes even harder if the promise was to nurture my stamp collection. Moreover, when we turn to living wills, holding that the duty runs to the relatives is clearly unworkable, because surely the absence of family would not negate the duty to respect the prior directive. (And suggesting that duties run to persistently vegetative patients, viewed just in the present, is no more plausible than saying they run to corpses.) Thus Callahan is left recognizing the moral force of the duty to honor wills, but failing either to ground or direct such a duty.

The perplexities about harm predating the harmful event, and the opposite problem of being unable to justify the belief that there are duties to the dead, can each be avoided if we simply extrapolate from the observation that a right-holder need not have either the capacity or potential to discover a breach of duty. Clearly, if a person who has contracted for a statue to be erected in her honor moves to Australia, failure of the promisor to erect the statue is a breach of duty to the person in Australia, even if she never finds out. Why should the analysis change if the promisor procrastinates and breaches the contract after the emigrant has died? It is still a breach of duty, and of a duty that ran to the person who, while alive, held the right to performance. In other words, rights and duties, although correlative, need not be temporally coextensive.

This analysis relates back to the various ways persons can view themselves. Someone seeking a future-oriented promise sees herself as caring how her body, or property, or heirs, are treated. The promisor in turn incurs a duty of performance that entails an obligation to see the promisee as she envisioned herself. Thus the promisor cannot legitimately focus only upon the consequences of a breach (reasoning "she's a corpse now, she cannot care"), but instead must think of the promisee as she was in the past, and as she projected her goals and interests into the future. This duty in some sense runs backward: the object of its fulfillment or breach is most appropriately viewed as the person as she was when alive (Feinberg's "antemortem person"). But recognizing duties to antemortem persons does not mean we have to agree that dead persons can be harmed or that future victims of harms are harmed from the moment they acquire interests that will be defeated. All we need affirm is that living persons can have rights of future performance, and that breaches of duties to perform after death count as wrongs to the right-holder, thought of as she was when alive.

Although duties to persons who previously held the correlative right but who no longer exist are admittedly an unusual case, we might think of this as similar to other future-oriented promises made in anticipation of incapacity. Suppose Joe, a manic-depressive given to extravagant and disastrous business deals in his manic phase, makes a contract (during a lucid period) with a friend whereby the friend promises not to let him make any business deals while manic. Then Joe becomes manic. In adhering to the contract, the friend is upholding his duty to view Joe (and Joe's interests) as Joe saw things when lucid. This case differs from wills or living wills, because Joe himself will benefit in the future from having his present desires thwarted. But the cases are not so completely different, because each involves a duty to act upon wishes of a person that are no longer held and indeed to view the person, for moral purposes, as he viewed himself at a previous time, and as he projected the values held then into the future. The solution of saying a duty exists *now,* and breach of it is a breach of duty, and thus a wrong, to the person as he was *then,* is not unproblematic. If one accepts a rights-based justification for present and precedent autonomy, however, the backward-looking solution seems preferable to holding that upon death or incapacity, a formerly grounded duty suddenly runs in no direction at all.

CONCLUSION

Thus we must reject the premise of the present-oriented objective test—that if a subjective analysis does not yield a definitive answer, a fully objective approach must be used. Viewing the patient only in the present divides her from her history, her values, and her relationships—from all those things that made her a moral agent. It likewise undermines living wills. Living wills are not as unproblematic as often assumed: they are subject to the criticism that they subjugate the interests of incompetent persons to the values of competent ones. But as we have seen, many or most autonomous choices take the chooser some way into the future. Denying the right of future choice thus threatens the right of present choice. Hence the mirror image of the asserted problem with living wills is giving so much primacy to incompetents that one acts as if they never were competent. If a person has stated, "Treat me, when incompetent, as if my competent values still hold," respect for persons demands that we do so. This does give primacy to the competent person, but it is, after all, competent persons who have the considered moral values, life plans, and

treatment preferences that underlie our respect. Finally, this analysis can apply, albeit less strongly, to formerly competent patients who did not make prior directives, because they, too, most likely held relevant views. If we believe that a competent person is, more likely than not, to see her values as still being relevant during incapacity, then respect for persons suggests that we consider those values in making treatment decisions, even while recognizing that they may be more difficult to assess, and hence far less determinative, than actual prior choices.

NOTES

1. R. Dresser, "Life, Death, and Incompetent Patients: Conceptual Infirmities and Hidden Values in the Law," 373 *Ariz v. Rev.* at 379–82, 394–95; Dresser, "Relitigating Life and Death," 51 *Ohio St. L. J.* 425 (1990), at 433.

2. "Quality of Life and Non-Treatment Decisions for Incompetent Patients: A Critique of the Orthodox Approach," 17 *Law, Med. & Health Care* 234, 236–37 (1989) [*supra* this section].

3. C. Korsgaard, "Personal Identity and the Unity of Agency: A Kantian Response to Parfit," 18 *Phil. & Pub. Aff.* 101, 113–14 (1989) (footnotes omitted).

4. *See* J. Callahan, "On Harming the Dead," 97 *Ethics* 341, 345 (1987).

5. J. Feinberg, *Harm to Others*. 91 (1984).

6. W. Waluchow, "Feinberg's Theory of 'Preposthumous' Harm," 25 *Dialogue* 727, 732–33 (1986).

CHOOSING FOR NEVER-COMPETENT PATIENTS

TERMINATION OF LIFE-SUPPORT FOR A NEVER-COMPETENT PATIENT: THE CASE OF SHEILA POULIOT

Alicia R. Ouellette

Many disputes involving medical care for an incompetent patient pit a patient's family or surrogate against her health-care providers. Sometimes a family refuses treatment over the objection of a physician. Other times, the family demands treatment that the medical team deems futile or otherwise inappropriate. Sheila Pouliot's case was different. Pouliot's family, court-appointed surrogate, health-care providers, ethicists, and clergy all agreed on the appropriate treatment for Ms. Pouliot. The conflict arose because the laws in Ms. Pouliot's home state did not allow the family or the health-care providers to implement their agreed-upon plan.

Sheila Pouliot had lived with mental and physical disabilities for 42 years after she suffered serious complications from the mumps as an infant.

Her disabilities left her wholly dependent on others for all her basic life functions. She had profound mental retardation and severe cerebral palsy, which was manifested by incomplete quadriparesis and partial blindness. Unable to ingest food orally, Pouliot received nutrition through a feeding tube for most of her life. By the time she was in her early forties, Pouliot had become chronically ill. She had a seizure disorder, osteoporosis, several dislocated joints, and widespread flexion contractures in her elbows, knees, and hips. The tube feedings caused aspiration pneumonia, episodes of gastrointestinal bleeding, and chronic, severe constipation.

Pouliot's mother cared for her in the family home for 20 years. At home, Pouliot's older sister and brother doted upon her. When her mother became afflicted with Alzheimer's disease and was no longer able to care for her, Pouliot became a resident of a group home operated by the state of

Printed by permission of Alicia R. Ouellette.

New York, where she lived for the next 22 years. Pouliot's family visited with her every Sunday, birthdays, and holidays. Although she was not verbal, Ms. Pouliot appeared to enjoy the visits. She also enjoyed listening to music.

Ms. Pouliot was acutely ill when she was admitted to University Hospital in Syracuse at 42 years old. By the time she reached the hospital, she was near death. She was feverish, had low oxygen levels, hypotension, aspiration pneumonia, internal bleeding, severe abdominal pain, and a non-functioning intestine. Because of gastrointestinal bleeding, she could no longer tolerate tube feeding. She was in obvious pain, and communicated her discomfort by groaning. Pouliot's family met with the medical staff, SUNY Hospital's Ethics Committee, and clergy. All agreed that her condition was terminal, and that the appropriate treatment was the provision of palliative care involving the intravenous delivery of morphine only. The group also agreed that neither artificial nutrition and hydration nor antibiotics would be administered because such treatment would merely prolong Pouliot's suffering. One of Pouliot's treating physicians explained the group's decision in a progress note:

> After one hour discussion with team, family, social worker, nursing staff, chaplain and ethics consultant, we are in full agreement that this may be Ms. Pouliot's terminal illness. We agree that the most humane course is to provide comfort in the way of [morphine sulfate] as needed and to refrain from invasive resuscitative and recovery measures.[1]

With the family's agreement, the treatment team terminated artificial nutrition and hydration and provided comfort care. Ms. Pouliot rested comfortably for several days. A week after her admission to the hospital, however, the University Hospital's administration brought the case to the attention of the New York State Office of Mental Retardation and Developmental Disabilities. That agency instructed the hospital to obtain a court-appointed guardian for Ms. Pouliot, and asked the state Attorney General to intervene to enforce New York law on behalf of Ms. Pouliot.

New York law, like that of some other states,[2] did not allow a family member or surrogate to withhold artificial nutrition or hydration from a person like Sheila Pouliot who was never capable of understanding or making a reasoned decision about medical treatment. While the State recognized the fundamental right of *competent* patients to refuse medical treatment of all types, the state courts had steadfastly held that the right to refuse treatment is personal to the patient, and that "no person or court should substitute its judgment as to what would be an acceptable quality of life for another."[3] The only situation in which the courts would permit the termination of life-sustaining treatment for a patient who lacked competence was when the evidence clearly and convincingly showed that the patient intended to decline the treatment under the particular circumstances he or she was ultimately facing. Thus the law provided no mechanism to allow a decision to terminate treatment for people who never had competence, or for those formerly competent patients who had failed to express their wishes while competent.

In addition, New York law treated people like Pouliot, adults who have never had capacity to make medical choices, as though they were infants.[4] Specifically, the law allowed the parent or guardian of an infant to give effective consent for medical treatment in the best interest of the child, but did not allow a parent or guardian to deprive a child of life-saving treatment, however well-intended or ethically justified the decision to withhold might have been. New York's policy was—and continues to be—to err on the side of life: "Even when the parents' [or guardians'] decision is based on constitutional grounds, such as religious beliefs, it must yield to the State's interests, as *parens patriae*, in

---

1. Blouin v. Spitzer, 356 F.3d 348, 352 (2004).

2. Missouri and Michigan have similar laws to those in place in New York when Sheila Pouliot was dying. Wisconsin, Arizona, Hawaii, Mississippi, Ohio, and Utah also place limitations on surrogate decision makers that may not be warranted by the best interest of the patient. See Alicia Ouellette, "When Vitalism is Dead Wrong," 79 Ind. L. J. 1 (2004) for a discussion of the parameters of those laws.

3. In re Westchester County Med. Ctr. Ex rel O'Connor, 531 N.E.2d 607, 613 (N.Y. 1988).

4. *See* Matter of Storar, 52 N.Y.2d at 380.

protecting the health and welfare of the child."[5] The only way to protect a child's health and welfare, in the view of New York Courts, is to provide nutrition and hydration in all cases. Thus parents and guardians could not make "decisions that would result in [the incompetent patient] starving to death, if such could be medically avoided, regardless of how soon [the patient] may or may not succumb from other causes."[6]

Nine days after Pouliot was admitted to the hospital, a New York trial judge held a hearing at the hospital. The court appointed a guardian ad litem, who in turn petitioned the court to terminate all nutrition and hydration. The court heard testimony from Pouliot's doctors. All the providers agreed that providing any nutrition would be difficult because the bleeding in Pouliot's GI tract made tube feeding impossible. The doctors also agreed that providing any further treatment to Ms. Pouliot would prolong "her agony without any significant health or medical benefits."[7] Nonetheless, the court ordered the continuing provision of hydration and 900 calories of nutrition a day based on a straightforward application of New York law.

Doctors made efforts to provide Ms. Pouliot with the planned 900 calories a day, but the effort was ineffective. The blood vessels through which the doctors tried to infuse sustenance shut down, and the introduction of protein caused projectile vomiting and intractable hiccups. As a result, the only sustenance that Pouliot could sustain was IV hydration with sugar water. The IV provided 300 calories a day but no protein.

The provision of 300 calories a day without protein devastated Pouliot's body over the next two and a half months. The nutrition contained in the fluids was sufficient to maintain life (heart and lung function), but it could not prevent protein starvation, which caused Ms. Pouliot's body to catabolize, or break down and use energy from her own tissue, damaging her organs and causing her severe pain. Further, it caused her severe edema (swelling), which stretched her skin to the point where it fell off, leaving raw painful areas.

Pouliot's physicians used aggressive efforts to control her pain, but their efforts failed. Sheila Pouliot was in agony, dying inch by inch. She communicated her pain by moaning and crying, by furrowing her forehead, and by flexing her extremities. She got no relief despite the fact that she was on the equivalent of approximately 5000 mg of oral morphine a day. Her family could console her only by stroking her forehead or placing a musical angel next to her head on her pillow.

The physicians became increasingly convinced that the court-ordered treatment that kept Pouliot alive was actually making her condition worse. On February 29, 2000, more than two months after Ms. Pouliot entered the hospital, one of her treating physicians entered the following progress note in her chart: "[T]he intravenous fluids promote that the patient is kept alive for her own body to consume/eat itself. . . . [T]his current plan of IV hydration promotes an increase in patient suffering, does not promote life quality, and maintains her heart/lung capacity only. And, indeed, therefore this current tact is clearly outside of acceptable medical bounds, in effect worsening her condition, since she is consuming herself calorically. It is thus not medically indicated."[8]

Another of Ms. Pouliot's physicians stated in a consultation note, "Sheila is edematous, with total body bloating from hydration in the absence of protein. Hydration . . . . has resulted in severe . . . cardiac muscle breakdown. She will die a slow lingering death from protein malnutrition."[9] The treating physician also noted that the provision of artificial hydration ordered by the Court was "inhumane and is causing suffering. . . . From a medical standpoint, it is outside the bounds of . . . medically indicated care."[10]

Finally, the guardian decided to take action. He went back to court seeking an order that would allow the physicians to withdraw the IV fluids despite New York's laws. At the hearing, Ms. Pouliot's physicians testified that "the continuation of hydration for this patient is affirmatively causing

5. *Storar* at 380–381.

6. In re Matthews, 650 N.Y.S.2d 373, 377 (N.Y. App. Div. 1996).

7. Blouin v. Spitzer, 213 F. Supp. at 187.

8. Blouin v. Spitzer. 356 F.3d at 355.

9. Id.

10. Id., at 355.

significant physical harm to the patient in that it is bringing about unnatural and painful decomposition of her body tissues. . . ."[11] The hearing made clear that further treatment would only make the pain worse, but it would sustain her life. Terminating nutrition and hydration would lessen Pouliot's pain, but it would also cause her death. At this point Ms. Pouliot's life expectancy was approximately two to four months if hydration were continued. She would die within three to fourteen days if hydration was discontinued.

Trial Judge Tormey was therefore faced with a dilemma. Apply settled law and continue the treatment because it was technically "life sustaining," or buck the law. At this point, Judge Tormey did an unusual thing; he visited Sheila Pouliot in the hospital. There, he ordered the termination of all nutrition and hydration. He acknowledged that New York law did not allow his order, but he explained: "There's the law, and there's what's right." The State of New York appealed the decision, but the appeal was never heard. Sheila Pouliot died on March 6, 2000, just before the appellate court was to hear oral argument.

New York's laws for ending life support are some of the most restrictive in the country. New York's top court established the law in a series of cases that came before it during the 1980s. In the cases, the judges purposefully imposed the most rigorous burden of proof available in civil cases out of concern that each individual's "right to life" be protected by a standard that ensures that "if an error occurs it [will] be made on the side of life."[12] But the judges also struggled with their professional and personal roles in deciding the cases. The opinions themselves are replete with calls to the state legislature to set up a statutory framework to allow families and doctors [to] decide end-of-life cases without court involvement. And the judge who wrote the majority opinion in the seminal *O'Connor* case admitted that a family dispute over his own mother's medical care had convinced him that New York needed strict standards to prevent family members from making the wrong decisions for loved ones.[13]

The state legislature had every opportunity to change the law in the years between the court decisions and the Pouliot case, but it refused to do so. A bill that would allow surrogates to make treatment decisions based on the patient's wishes or, if the patient's wishes are not known, based on the patient's best interests has been proposed and rejected annually since 1993. The primary forces against the bill have been religious groups. The Catholic Conference, for example, opposed the bill throughout the 1990s on the ground that New York's rigorous clear and convincing evidence standard appropriately protects the sanctity of life and death. Its opposition was rooted in Catholic teaching that "the intrinsic value and personal dignity of every human being do not change, no matter what the concrete circumstances of his or her life." No matter how sick a person is, explained Pope John Paul II, he or she always has the right to the administration of water and food, even if by artificial means, because the administration of water and food "always represents a natural means of preserving life" and is, as such, "morally obligatory."[14] More recently, the New York Catholic Conference has opposed surrogate medical decision making bills that afford no special protection to the fetuses of pregnant patients.[15]

Representatives of Orthodox Jewish groups have also opposed changes to New York laws based on Jewish teachings. Under Jewish law, nutrition and hydration are not medical treatment, but are supportive care like washing, turning or grooming. These treatments must be provided, as must all medical intervention that might increase the longevity of a patient. Moreover, representatives of Orthodox Jewish groups have testified about potential conflicts-of-interest by family members, including those who would benefit financially from a patient's death.

---

11. Id.

12. O'Connor, 531 N.E.2d at 613.

13. Richard D. Simons, Oral History, 1 N.Y. Legal History 53, 86–87 (2005).

---

14. Address of Pope John Paul II to the participants in the International Congress on Life-Sustaining Treatments and Vegetative State: Scientific Advances and Ethical Dilemmas (March 20, 2004).

15. A 2006 version of the bill was acceptable to the Catholic Conference, but was opposed by pro-choice legislators because it made specific reference to the fetus of a dying pregnant woman.

The position of the Catholic Church and the Orthodox Jewish groups is consistent [with] that of many disability-rights groups, who advocate for laws like New York's that would make it impossible for families to terminate life-sustaining treatment for people who lack the legal capacity to make that decision for themselves. The disability rights groups argue that such laws are needed to protect disabled patients from unscrupulous doctors and family members who do not recognize the value of people who live with disabilities.

Sheila Pouliot's family was understandably angry after her death. They sued the State Attorney General and his assistants for constitutional and other wrongs allegedly inflected by them against their sister. The lawsuit was unsuccessful. The Attorney General is protected from lawsuits for enforcing the law. The federal appellate court agreed that the Attorney General's hands were tied by New York's laws. It also upheld as constitutional those laws. Thus, the only written precedent that followed from Sheila Pouliot's case upheld laws that limit treatment choices for people with profound disabilities, even when there is consensus on

the part of family and medical providers that those choices are medically appropriate and in the best interest of the patient.

Pouliot's doctors were equally appalled that New York's laws forced them to inflict what can fairly be characterized as an inhumane and torturous death on Sheila Pouliot. They engaged in a lobbying effort to change New York's law regarding medical decision-making for incompetent patients. That effort was mildly successful. In 2002, New York passed the Health Care Decisions Act for Persons with Mental Retardation, which allows the duly appointed surrogate of a person with mental retardation to terminate life-sustaining treatment under the very narrow circumstances that Sheila Pouliot faced.[16] The Act might have helped Sheila Pouliot, but it does nothing to change the New York laws for children, formerly competent adults, or the mentally ill, all of whom could still face medical torture in the name of sanctity of life.

---

16. *See* N.Y. Surr. Ct. Proc. Act § 1750-b (McKinney Supp. 2003).

EXTREME PREMATURITY AND PARENTAL RIGHTS AFTER *BABY DOE*

John A. Robertson

Contemporary ethical and legal norms hold that all human beings born alive should be treated equally, regardless of disability. Yet there is a strong sense

From *Hastings Center Report* 34, no. 4 (2004): 32–39. Reprinted by permission of The Hastings Center.

Editors' note: Some author's notes have been cut. Students who want to follow up on sources should consult the original article.

that some lives are so diminished in capacity for interaction or experience that little good is achieved by providing medical treatments necessary to keep them alive. In addition, many persons believe that the parents who have the chief responsibility to provide care should have a dominant say in whether their children are treated.

Before 1970, the question of whether to withhold treatment from such newborns was rarely contested. The ancient Spartan practice of exposing babies on hillsides and keeping those that survived had a contemporary counterpart in the common medical practice of simply not treating those born with major handicaps. As late as 1972, some doctors and parents thought it appropriate to withhold from children with Down Syndrome or spina bifida surgery necessary for their survival. Noted pediatricians published articles in major medical journals reporting the withholding of life-saving treatment from infants with many kinds of disabilities. Surveys of doctors showed that these practices were not exceptions.

In the mid-1970s, the emerging discipline of bioethics began to question the ethics and legality of these practices even as they were publicized. Courts became more willing to order treatment over parental wishes, though neither a uniform response nor clear guidelines emerged. It took the Baby Doe controversy of 1981 and the federal Child Abuse Amendments (CAA) of 1984 to produce a rough consensus about the norms and practices that would govern this area. Since passage of the CAA, ethical and legal controversy over parental authority to withhold treatment from handicapped or disabled newborns, although still featured in bioethics courses and texts, has largely ceased.

Yet one aspect of the controversy was never directly resolved. Because the Baby Doe controversy had focused on infants with genetic and chromosomal anomalies, the extent to which the CAA norms might require changes in practices with very premature and low birth weight infants remained open, even though it was occasionally mentioned in articles. As a result, physicians and hospitals that insisted on treating premature newborns over parental objections were vulnerable to tort actions by parents. In January 1998, a Houston jury awarded $43 million in damages to parents whose daughter, born at twenty-three weeks and weighing 614 grams, was resuscitated and initially treated without their consent, leading to a life with severe mental and physical impairments. Texas appellate courts eventually reversed that decision, but in the five-year interim, hospitals and physicians faced the prospect of huge damage awards if they sought to treat cases of extreme prematurity in accordance with CAA standards against the parents' wishes. This article reviews the controversy and assesses the extent to which parents should

have the right to decide not to treat severely premature newborns.

THE BABY DOE CONTROVERSY

The Baby Doe controversy, which played such a key role in clarifying norms and practices in this area, arose in 1981 in Bloomington, Indiana. Parents of a newborn child with Down Syndrome and a trachealesophageal fistula refused to consent to a standard operation that would enable the child to take food and water by mouth. The hospital and doctors sought approval from a family court to perform surgery against the parents' wishes. A probate court denied the request on the ground that the parents had the right to make the decision. The child's guardian *ad litem* appealed the case unsuccessfully to the Indiana and then to the United States Supreme Court. While the case was pending, it drew wide media coverage and the attention of right-to-life and disability rights groups. Before the United States Supreme Court could rule on the guardian's appeal, Baby Doe died.

Groups opposed to the outcome in the Baby Doe case sought relief from federal officials in the Reagan administration sympathetic to right to life concerns. Soon after, the Department of Health and Human Services issued regulations that required newborn nurseries and neonatal intensive care units receiving federal funds to post notice of a hotline number to report cases of discrimination in treatment based on handicap. When reports came in, "Baby Doe squads" of doctors, nurses, and social workers were dispatched to hospitals, demanding medical records to determine whether treatment was inappropriately denied.

Greatly disturbed by these interventions, the pediatric and hospital community sued to invalidate them on the ground that they were beyond federal regulatory authority. A federal district court enjoined enforcement because of the government's failure to follow legal requirements for new regulations. The administration then complied with those requirements and issued slightly less intrusive regulations. Further litigation ensued. The United States Supreme Court eventually ruled, in *Bowen v. American Hospital Association*, that Congress had not authorized federal agencies to regulate nontreatment decisions in hospitals and newborn nurseries.

The battleground shifted to Congress. The resulting tussle among the administration, right to life, disability, hospital and physician groups produced a compromise bill, the Child Abuse Amendments of 1984. Under this legislation, direct federal intervention in newborn nurseries and neonatal intensive care units would cease. Instead, states, as a condition of receiving federal child abuse prevention funds, would agree to set up systems, including infant care review committees, to make sure that all newborn children were protected against discrimination on the basis of disability. The only exceptions recognized to equal treatment of children with handicaps were for children who were permanently comatose, near death, or for whom treatment would be inhumane because futile or virtually futile.

A CONSENSUS OF SORTS

The Child Abuse Amendments of 1984 ended the political controversy over the federal role in decisions to withhold treatment from handicapped newborns. In terms of substantive norms, right to life and disability groups could claim victory. The substantive provisions of the CAA were strongly protective of the rights and interests of those with disabilities and left little room for nontreatment decisions to be based on expected low quality of life or the interests of parents. All children, whatever the extent of their disabilities, were to be provided medical treatment unless they met the narrowly defined exceptions.

Procedurally, however, physician and hospital groups could also claim victory. As a legal matter, the CAA substantive provisions were not directly imposed on any individual or institution, nor did they directly amend federal or state substantive law. They did not, for example, make it a federal crime or a civil wrong for a doctor, parent, or hospital not to treat a child who did not meet the narrow exceptions. Nor did the CAA require hospitals to comply with its standards in order to receive Medicare and Medicaid funds. Instead, it obligated the states to set up protective procedures in order to receive child abuse funds. Any regulatory action

would thus be the responsibility of individual states, which were less well equipped than the federal government for strong enforcement action. This was a far cry from federal hotlines and intrusive Baby Doe squads.

But while the CAA imposed no legal duties directly on doctors and hospitals, many doctors, hospital administrators, and even lawyers perceived its passage as creating a legal presumption in favor of treating children likely to have disabilities. Technically this was inaccurate, but it was not an unreasonable conclusion. At the very least, the CAA could be perceived as setting the standard of care to which hospitals and doctors would be held, both by accrediting bodies and by courts hearing challenges to nontreatment decisions. In addition, the ethical controversy over nontreatment decisions had convincingly shown the importance of respecting the life and interests of disabled children and recognizing limits on parental rights. The values incorporated in the CAA showed a deep ethical commitment to respecting human life regardless of disability.

Whatever its actual legal reach, passage of the CAA awakened pediatricians, neonatologists, and hospitals to the problem of discrimination against handicapped newborns. The norms of practice shifted: most physicians and hospitals were now more reluctant to defer automatically to parental wishes. Parents could no longer deny needed surgery to children with Down Syndrome or spina bifida, as had occurred in the much publicized Baby Jane Doe case at Stony Brook. If treatment were to be denied, a parent would have to show that the child was comatose, terminally ill, or that treatment would be futile or virtually futile. In borderline cases, some quality of life judgments might unavoidably occur, but overall a high degree of compliance followed passage of the CAA. Indeed, both the American Academy of Pediatrics and the American Medical Association, which had fought the Baby Doe rules, issued policies calling for equal treatment of newborns regardless of disability and low quality of life and recommended the use of institutional ethics committees to review contested cases.

With further experience, however, some physicians, ethicists, and parents caught up in such situations came to question whether the CAA and medical reactions to them had gone too far in favoring treatment regardless of quality of life. Yet there was little overt controversy or litigation until the issue arose in the context of extreme prematurity.

THE PROBLEM OF PREMATURITY AND VERY LOW BIRTH WEIGHT INFANTS

The area with the least consensus and the most uncertainty about the reach of the CAA was that of extreme prematurity. Due to a large investment of public resources, regionalization of perinatal intensive care units, and growing technical abilities, treatment of premature newborns had shown great success. The line for viability and successful survival has been continuously pushed back to earlier and earlier ages. Before 1980, few babies born in the 1000–1500 gram range before twenty-eight weeks would do well. Now they are routinely saved and restored to a relatively normal life. Great success is also occurring with smaller babies. It is now routine to save babies as young as twenty-five weeks and as little as 750 grams. Under twenty-five weeks, however, results are much more mixed. At the margins of viability, twenty-three to twenty-four weeks' gestation, mortality occurs in half or more of the cases, and survivors often have significant physical and mental handicaps, including blindness, hydrocephalus, cerebral palsy, limited use of language, and learning disabilities.

Newborns born under 750 grams and before twenty-five weeks pose a major problem under the CAA. On their face, the CAA standards leave no room for discretion. All conscious, viable premature newborns must be treated, even if they are likely to have severe physical and mental disabilities. Not to treat them would be to discriminate against them on the ground of expected disability.

In effect, the CAA supplied an ethical and legal justification for the intense efforts of neonatologists to push back the limits of viability. Most hospitals and neonatal programs treated premature newborns in conformity with the CAA, with neonatologists present at all premature deliveries and likely to resuscitate newborns born alive, regardless of parental wishes.

Not all neonatal programs complied equally strictly with the CAA standards in cases of very low birth weight, however. In more marginal cases, under twenty-five weeks or where Grade IV intraventricular hemorrhaging or other major problems had occurred, some programs would provide "compassionate care" or nontreatment only if parents requested it (usually without ethics committee or legal review of the decision). A 1991 *New York Times* survey found that two programs in the same New York county had completely different attitudes toward treatment in marginal cases, one treating aggressively, the other deferring to parental wishes. A 1994 *Chicago Tribune Sunday Magazine* survey showed similar disparities. In most cases the disparity in approach was due to the personal philosophy of the NICU director or perceptions of legal risk.

The aggressive approach to treatment of low birth weight infants in some programs has led to conflicts between parents and doctors and hospitals. Many parents reported being given little choice about treatment of their premature newborns, with the result that infants born at twenty-three to twenty-six weeks' gestation were resuscitated and vigorously treated, in some cases over parental wishes. While half or more of these children survived, many survivors were likely to have serious disabilities, including cerebral palsy, blindness, mental retardation, and learning disabilities. Increasingly, parents have requested that no resuscitation or treatment occur in these cases, thus pitting parental wishes against the neonatology ethic of trying to save all premature newborns and the no-discrimination requirements of the CAA.

MILLER V. HCA AS THE CATALYST FOR REEXAMINATION

In a litigation-oriented society, it is no surprise that this conflict is now played out in lawsuits brought by parents claiming violation of their rights to control the medical care provided to their children. Such suits shift the forum for defining treatment norms from Congress and the federal judiciary, which played a major role in the Baby Doe controversy, to state juries and trial and appellate judges. The jury award in the recent case of *Miller v. HCA* suggests that there is popular support for recognizing some parental right to have treatment withheld in low birth weight cases. Although the award was eventually overturned, the question remains whether parents should have a right to deny life-saving medical treatment to low birth weight newborns because of the high probability that they will have severe mental or physical disabilities.

The *Miller* case arose in Houston, Texas, when a twenty-eight-year-old woman twenty-three weeks into her first pregnancy in 1990 experienced contractions and possible rupture of membranes. The medical team attempted to stop her contractions with tocolytic therapy, but she developed chorionamnionitis, and prompt delivery appeared necessary. After discussing the child's prospects with the couple's obstetrician and a neonatology fellow, the father informed them that he and his wife did not want any "extraordinary, heroic" steps to be taken because of the child's extreme prematurity. Their physician consulted the head of obstetrics and they concluded that a neonatologist should be present at birth and that the child should be resuscitated if it were born alive. A meeting was held with the father to discuss a treatment plan. The need to have a neonatologist present and initial treatment provided was explained. All parties present except the father thought there was a consensus that the child, if born alive and vigorous, would be resuscitated, and that later management decisions would be based on the child's postbirth condition. The father denied that he had agreed to this plan.

Pitocin was started to induce labor, and the mother delivered a 614-gram girl, Sidney Miller, six hours later. The neonatologist present at delivery immediately treated the infant, first bagging and then intubating her. Her Apgar scores were three at one minute and six at five minutes. Some 90 minutes after birth, after central lines were inserted and surfactant administered, she was transferred to the NICU. The father, who was present at the birth, voiced no objections to the neonatologist's presence or treatment. He signed consents for injections of Vitamin E, surfactant, and a blood transfusion within the first two hours after birth. On the fourth day after birth the child suffered a Grade III/IV intraventricular hemorrhage. Later he or his wife consented to surgical cutdowns to insert other lines, and at five weeks consented to insertion of a cerebroventricular shunt to relieve her hydrocephalus.

After two months in the NICU, the child was transferred to Texas Children's Hospital, and six months after birth was released from the hospital. Her parents have cared for her since discharge at home. She has had numerous surgeries to repair or replace the shunt. She is now fourteen years old and has severe mental and physical disabilities: she has cerebral palsy, does not walk or talk, and is blind and incontinent. She smiles and appears to interact with parents to some minimal extent, although she seems to lack the capacity for symbolic interaction. With good care she could live to age seventy.

The parents sued the hospital and its corporate owners, but not the physicians, for treating the child at birth without their consent. After a two-week trial in January 1998, a jury awarded the family $30 million in compensatory and $13 million in punitive damages. The compensatory damages were based in part on the cost of providing care to Sidney until age seventy.

Even though it was reversed on appeal, *Miller* raised the question of whether parents have the right to have treatment withheld immediately at birth, prior to any resuscitation or evaluation of the child. The plaintiffs claimed that the hospital was aware of the parents' refusal of resuscitation and treatment at birth and knowingly chose to override their wishes, possibly to profit from the sale of expensive neonatal services. The hospital defendant argued first that the parents had in fact consented to the treatment—or at least gave a reasonable person the impression that they had consented. Second, the hospital argued that it was following its duty under Texas and federal law and the applicable standard of care to treat all newborns alike regardless of expected disability. In finding for the parents, the jury was necessarily finding that they had not consented to treatment, and that their consent was essential to the treatment, thus squarely posing the question of whether they had a right to deny treatment to a viable newborn who was likely to have substantial disabilities.

MODIFYING THE SUBSTANTIVE STANDARD

Some persons might argue that the jury verdict in *Miller* in favor of the parents was appropriate because of the great burdens that treatment against their wishes imposed on them. According to this view, the substantive norms for treatment reflected in the CAA and the law of many states (including Texas, as clarified on appeal) are too strict; they should be modified to privilege the parents' reluctance to take on those burdens. The parents' wishes should trump arguments that focus narrowly on the interests of a severely impaired child with little chance of a normal life. Because parents (and other children) will bear the burdens of caring for the child with severe impairments, they should have the right to refuse resuscitation or treatment in such cases.

Few would not have deep sympathy for a family faced with an extremely premature child and the great burdens that rearing the child could impose. In addition, many would find that the CAA standards are too demanding, given the realities that families face in these situations and the importance of respecting family autonomy. Yet modifying the equal treatment standards of the CAA and the law of most states to allow parental choices to trump the severely impaired child's interest in treatment would deviate from the principle that all persons who are conscious and not imminently dying should have equal access to needed medical services.

Given these competing concerns, the ethical and legal challenge is to uphold the general principle that all children born alive are to be treated equally regardless of disability while also recognizing the importance of parental decisional authority. The problem is that any modification of the equal treatment standards may be seen as opening the door to full-scale quality-of-life-based decisions, yet anything that clearly does not permit some quality-of-life decisions may still seem to improperly restrain the rightful sphere of parental choice.

One way to try to reconcile these competing concerns is to declare that treatment against the parents' wishes is required only if the child possesses some threshold level of cognitive ability. A second strategy would be to clarify the burden of proof so that parents are recognized as the primary decision-makers, with the burden of proof on caregivers or others to establish that the child has the required level of cognitive ability. Finally, a decision is needed as to whether parental choices made *before* birth should have the same presumptive weight as those made after birth (the issue in the *Miller* case).

How, then, to think about the threshold level of cognitive ability? One route would be to adopt a change that recognizes that some states of consciousness rest on such limited cognitive ability as to call into question whether the child's putative interest in continued life is substantial enough to warrant protection. In that case, denial of treatment could be justified under a patient-centered approach as not harming the child because the child simply lacks strong interests in continued life. Some threshold of cognitive ability beyond mere consciousness—such as the capacity for language or meaningful symbolic interaction—is needed to endow a person with interests in living and thus a duty to treat.

A standard based on relational ability is consistent with mainstream ethical writing on the subject. Father Richard McCormick, the highly regarded Catholic bioethicist, recognized in 1974 that treatment need not be provided if the child lacks the ability for interaction or human relationship.[1] Professor Nancy Rhoden argued in 1986 that there should be an additional category for withholding treatment under the CAA when the infant or child "lacks potential *for human interaction* as a result of profound retardation."[2] The President's Commission for the Study of Ethical Problems in Medicine and Biomedical [and Behavioral] Research and many bioethicists also supported such a standard.[3] Indeed, even authors who have strongly supported the right of handicapped newborns to be treated at birth have recognized that an exception in cases of extreme prematurity or lack of meaningful interests should also exist.[4]

None of these commentators, however, has specified more precisely what lack of "interaction or relationship" means. Under such a standard, treatment would still be required for premature infants who have suffered or might suffer intraventricular hemorrhaging and severe brain damage because such infants are still capable of some interaction with others. Despite their severe physical and mental disabilities, such children do respond to stimuli and appear to experience pleasure when touched or rubbed—arguably a form of "interaction or relationship" because it leads to further touching or rubbing. In the *Miller* case, for example, there was evidence that Sidney smiled and responded favorably to physical contact.

If interaction or relationship is taken to mean the human capacity for meaningful symbolic interaction or communication, then some greater mental capacity would be required than such severely damaged children have. If one lacks altogether the capacity for meaningful symbolic interaction, then one lacks the characteristics that make humans the object of moral duties beyond that of not imposing gratuitous suffering on them. We value humans in large part because of the capacity to have conscious interests and experiences, including meaningful symbolic interaction with others.

A modification in the CAA's substantive standards and in similar state laws to permit nontreatment in extreme cases would necessarily rest on quality of life assessments based on disability. But the mental disability in such cases is so extreme, so far from those cases in which children may be said to have valid interests in living, that they arguably do not threaten or harm the important values underlying the injunction against quality of life assessments in cases of disability. We could adopt such a standard without encouraging discrimination against disabled persons who have the capacity for symbolic thought and interaction. In contrast to nontreatment of a child with Down Syndrome or spina bifida, or indeed, children born at twenty-five weeks gestation and weighing over 750 grams, nontreatment in these cases does little damage to norms calling for respect for life and to equal treatment regardless of disability. If this modification of the CAA standards is too permissive, then no modification of those standards is likely to be acceptable.

PROCESS SOLUTIONS AND THE BURDEN OF PROOF

Substantive norms are not easily separated in practice from the procedures by which they are implemented. Another way to give greater deference to parental interests while upholding the norm of equal treatment would be to devise a procedural approach that better balances the interests of each. Both the American Academy of Pediatrics and the President's Commission for the Study of Bioethical Problems in Medicine recommended that institutional ethics committees review such decisions, particularly when there was disagreement or uncer-

tainty about whether the child's interests required treatment. Thomas Murray and Alan Fleischman have also supported this approach and even discussed the burden of proof to be followed in such cases.[5]

Although the Baby Doe rules included review by "infant care review committees," none was used in the *Miller* case. The hospital had not established such a committee, and even if it had, the rapidity with which events developed, and the fact that they all occurred on a Saturday, left little room for using it. Furthermore, since the administrator, social worker, the head of obstetrics, and other hospital personnel who had met with Mr. Miller on the afternoon before Sydney was born to explain the hospital policy of treating all newborns at birth all had the impression that he had accepted the policy, no emergency ethics committee or probate court review would have been called. If emergency permission to treat at birth had been sought, it is likely that an ethics committee or judge would have erred on the side of keeping the child alive while a more thorough assessment of the child's condition was made.

In future cases, the burden of proof that must be met to have a child treated over the parents' wishes should be clarified. Parents should have a presumptive right to have their decisions about the child's welfare respected unless a clear need to protect the child is shown. The burden would lie with physicians, hospitals, and other caregivers to challenge the parents' decision against treatment. If the "symbolic capacity" standard were employed, then the caregivers would have the burden of establishing, by at least a preponderance of the evidence, that the child is likely to have the minimum cognitive ability for symbolic interactions. In less certain cases, the parents' wishes would control.

An essential part of a burden-shifting approach is the effect it has on the rights and duties of the parties. Under the approach suggested here, neither the parents nor the physicians and hospitals would be liable if the parents made a good-faith judgment that treatment would not serve the child's interests and the physicians and hospital respected their choice. However, caregivers should also be free to challenge the parents' decision because of a good-faith belief that the child would possess the capacity for symbolic interactions. They should not be liable for questioning the parental decision or for seeking institutional ethics committee or judicial review of the decision. An initial decision to err on the side of life, as Fleischman and Murray recommended in 1983, would limit parental discretion in the short run, but facilitate and protect its exercise at a later stage.

DECIDING AFTER BIRTH

Any modification of the CAA's nontreatment standard and clarification of the burden of proof should also specify the point at which increased deference to the parents is appropriate. Parental autonomy is important, but it is not so robust that parents have the right to deny a disabled child the medical resources necessary for life regardless of the child's interests in living or ability to interact with others.

Determining whether those conditions are met will be difficult enough when they occur after birth but before physicians can determine how the child will fare, particularly if intraventricular bleeds have occurred or are expected. It is even more difficult to make those determinations before birth on the basis of gestational age estimates and expected birth weight. Whether the child lacks the capacity for symbolic interaction and whether the parents are making a reasonable judgment about them will require full information about the child's conditions and prospects. That can be obtained only after birth, because assessments about gestational age and its effects are too prone to error.

The question presented in *Miller* and other cases is whether parents should be free to decide against treatment in advance of birth by, for example, issuing a prenatal do-not-resuscitate order that has legal effect once the child has been born, so that if the child were alive at birth, no resuscitation or other efforts would be made on its behalf. Recall that in *Miller* the parents never objected to treatment once the child was born. They based their suit solely on the hospital's refusal to honor their pre-birth rejection of treatment—on the resuscitation by the neonatologist present at delivery.

To determine whether a particular infant lacks or is reasonably certain to lack the mental capacity for symbolic interaction or relationship one must first assess the child and its condition. But this can be

known only after birth, when a full assessment of the child's situation and likely capacity is possible. Doing so will require immediate treatment to stabilize the situation and a full work-up by neonatologists to determine the child's condition and prospects.

As a result, parents' directions not to resuscitate at birth should not be given effect until a medical assessment of the child's condition and prognosis justifying nontreatment has been made. Doctors and hospitals should be legally free to have neonatologists resuscitate and treat for a limited period after birth to assess the child's capacity regardless of parental consent or orders not to resuscitate. Under this standard, the initial medical response in the *Miller* case—resuscitation at birth if the child is alive—was reasonable. If medical evaluation after resuscitation shows that the child is likely to develop the capacity for meaningful symbolic interaction and the parents continue to refuse life-sustaining treatment, then ethics committee and judicial review should be sought to determine whether to treat the child over the parents' wishes.

A rule that permits initial treatment pending assessment admittedly carries burdens for parents. It means that closure on a difficult and trying event in their lives may be postponed for a few days. Also, it is easier to say no to treatment for an abstract child than for one that has a personal presence for them. The parents may find themselves bonding with the child during the assessment period, making it harder for them to refuse treatment later, even if doing so would be justified. Unless resuscitation and initial treatment occurs, however, there will be no firm basis for finding that the child lacks the relevant capacity that must be shown to justify denying treatment. Allowing parents to refuse resuscitation at birth based on prebirth estimates of age and size risks denying infants who are unexpectedly large or vigorous the chance for life.

Based on this analysis, the Texas Supreme Court decision affirming the reversal of the jury's finding for the parents rests on sound ethical and legal grounds.[6] While recognizing that parents ordinarily have the right to consent to or refuse medical care for their children, the Court also recognized that an exception to the parental consent requirement arises when an emergent condition exists and treatment must occur immediately to prevent the death of the child. The Court found that the doctor's initial resuscitation in *Miller* was justified because the situation was an emergency and there was not enough time necessary to get consent from the parents or from a court. As the Court noted, a nontreatment decision made prior to birth and postbirth evaluation would be based on "speculation" that would not promote the child's best interests.

A ruling in favor of the parents would have meant that parents always have the right in advance of birth to refuse treatment for premature newborns. Unless physicians and hospitals were first able to get a court to rule otherwise, the threat of *Miller* like damages would strongly incline them to follow the parents' wishes, depriving some newborns who could have meaningful lives of treatment they need to survive.

REFERENCES

1. R. McCormick, "To Save or Let Die—The Dilemma of Modern Medicine," *JAMA* 229 (1974): 172–75.
2. N. Rhoden, "Treatment Dilemmas for Imperiled Newborns: Why Quality of Life Counts," *Southern California Law Review* 1283, no. 58 (1985): 1322–23.
3. President's Commission for the Study of Ethical Problems in Medicine and Biomedical and Behavioral Research, *Deciding to Forego Life-Sustaining Treatment* (Washington, D.C.: U.S. Government Printing Office, 1983), 227–33; Hastings Center Special Project, "Imperiled Newborns," *Hastings Center Report* 17, no. 6 (1987): 14–16.
4. Compare J.A. Robertson, "Involuntary Euthanasia of Defective Newborns: A Legal Analysis," *Stanford Law Review* 29 (1975); with J.A. Robertson, "Dilemma in Danville," *Hastings Center Report* 11, no. 5 (1981): 5–8.
5. A.R. Fleischman and T.H. Murray, Ethics Committees for Infants Doe?, *Hastings Center Report* 13, no. 6 (1983): 5–9.
6. *Miller v. HCA, Inc.*, 47 Texas Supreme Court Journal 12 (2003).

RESUSCITATION OF THE PRETERM INFANT AGAINST PARENTAL WISHES

John J. Paris, Michael D. Schreiber, and Alun C. Elias-Jones

In a recent commentary in *The New England Journal of Medicine,* George Annas reviews a Texas Supreme court opinion, Miller v HCA, in which that court became the first to authorise a physician to resuscitate an extremely premature infant over parental objections.[1] The case raises anew an issue that the EPICure study describes as among the most diffi-

cult and trying clinical problems for obstetricians and paediatricians—the care of the fetus considered to be at the threshold of viability. More specifically, it examines one of the unresolved questions in that area: who decides for the extremely premature newborn, and on what basis, when there is a conflict between parents and physicians?

Although over the past 40 years, the norms on who is to make these treatment decisions and on what standard have been significantly altered and revised, there is now a strong consensus in the medical and bioethics community that for extremely premature infants—where the risk of mortality or morbidity is significant and the prospects of benefit is suffused in ambiguity and uncertainty—the decision on whether or not to institute medical treatment properly belongs to the parents. Reflecting

From John J. Paris, Michael D. Schreiber, and Alun C. Elias-Jones, "Resuscitation of the Preterm Infant against Parental Wishes," *Archives of Disease in Childhood, Fetal Neonatal Edition* 90, no. 3 (May 2005): F208–F210. Published with permission from the BMJ Publishing Group Ltd.

Editors' note: Some of the authors' notes have been cut. Students who want to follow up on sources should consult the original article.

on that consensus, Jerold F Lucey, the Editor in Chief of *Pediatrics,* recently wrote, "We should admit how little we know, explain the present bleak outlook, and ask [the parents] for their help. Some will choose active resuscitation, others will not.[2] The widespread agreement in both North America and the United Kingdom with that approach has come under challenge with the Texas Supreme Court's ruling in Miller v HCA.[3]

THE CASE

The case arose when Kara Miller presented at Woman's Hospital of Texas in premature labour. The ultrasound assessment was an estimated fetal weight of 629 g and a gestational age of 23 weeks. Tocolytics were administered to stop the labour, but were discontinued when it was learned that the mother had a life threatening infection. Labour inducing drugs were then begun. The attending obstetrician and a hospital neonatologist informed the parents that there was little chance of the infant being delivered alive. They also informed the parents that if the child were born alive, "it would most probably suffer severe impairments, including cerebral palsy, brain hemorrhaging, blindness, lung disease, pulmonary infections and mental retardation."

With that background, the obstetrician and neonatologist asked the parents whether they wanted their infant daughter treated aggressively if, as anticipated, they would have to induce delivery. The parents informed the doctors that they did not want any attempts at treatment. The parents' decision was recorded in the medical record, and the obstetrician informed the medical staff that no neonatologist would be needed at the delivery.

After the parents' decision had been agreed to, someone on the nursing staff informed other hospital personnel that no neonatologist would be present for the delivery. At a meeting called to discuss objections to that decision, the administrator of the neonatal intensive care unit stated that hospital policy required resuscitation of any baby weighing over 500 g. (A later investigation revealed that, although the statement had been made, no such law or policy existed). Once that claim had been made, it was agreed by the staff that a neonatologist would be present at the delivery to assess

the baby's age and weight. To prevent further compromise to the mother's condition, labour inducing drugs were administered. Some 11 hours later Kara Miller delivered a 23.1 week gestational age infant girl weighing 615 g. The neonate was limp, blue, had a "below normal" heart rate, but gasped for air and cried spontaneously. The infant was immediately "bagged," intubated, and placed on a ventilator. The Apgar scores were 3 at one minute and 6 at 10 minutes.

At some point during the first days of life, the infant suffered a significant brain haemorrhage which, in the Court's words, "caused [her] to suffer severe physical and mental impairments." The Court described her condition at the time of trial as: "[S]he was seven years old and could not walk, talk, feed herself, or sit up on her own. [She] was legally blind, suffered from mental retardation, cerebral palsy, seizures, and spastic quadriparesis in her limbs. She could not be toilet-trained and required a shunt in her brain to drain fluids that accumulate there and needed care twenty-four hours a day. The evidence further demonstrated that her circumstances will not change."

The Millers sued the hospital and its parent corporation Columbia/HCA Healthcare Corporation (HCA), the largest for-profit healthcare system in the United States. A jury found that the hospital, without the consent of the parents, had resuscitated their infant. It also found that negligent action was the cause of their daughter's injuries. The jury awarded the family $29 400 000 in actual damages for medical expenses, $17 503 066 in prejudgment interest, and $13 500 000 in punitive damages. The latter payment was designed as punishment for improper behaviour of the hospital and a deterrent to others from engaging in similar behaviour. The jury verdict was overturned by the Texas Supreme Court.

TEXAS SUPREME COURT OPINION

The Texas Supreme Court posed the question raised in Miller v HCA as follows: "This case requires us to determine the respective roles that parents and health care providers play in deciding whether to treat an infant who is born alive but in distress and is so premature that despite advancements in neonatal care, has a largely uncertain prognosis." In arriving at that question, the Court relied heavily on the testimony of the neonatal fellow who had attended the delivery as to why he had overridden the parents' refusal of treatment. When asked if he could predict where on the continuum from still-born to a normal child the Miller child would fall, the neonatal fellow replied, "No." He then continued, "This is a baby that is not necessarily going to have problems later on. There are babies that survive at this gestational age—with this birth-weight—that go on and do well."

Consent in cases involving infants has till now been the prerogative of the parents. The state, acting as parens patriae, can and does intervene to protect children from neglect and abuse or to prevent parental choices that would produce such results. But as long as parents choose from a professionally accepted option, the choice is rarely challenged or supervened. The Texas Supreme Court acknowledged that parental role, but in this instance the Court ruled that when a doctor is confronted in a case where there are "emergent circumstances"—that is, where death of a child is likely to result immediately unless treatment is administered—he/she can intervene even over parental objections.

The Texas Court, citing the testimony of the neonatal fellow, ruled that the infant "could only be properly evaluated when she was born." Consequently, in the Court's view, "Any decision by the Millers before [the infant's] birth would necessarily be based on speculation." Further, the Court opined, a pre-delivery decision would "not have been a fully informed one." As the Texas Supreme Court saw it, the doctor present at the delivery had to make "a split second decision on whether to provide life-sustaining treatment." In that situation, it held, "there simply was no time to obtain [the parents'] consent to treatment or to institute legal proceedings to challenge their withholding of consent without jeopardizing [the infant's] life."

DISCUSSION

This is a ruling of enormously sweeping scope, albeit in a narrowly circumscribed situation. It applies, as the Court would have it, only to children and "only when there is no time to consult

the parents, or seek court intervention if the parents withhold consent before death is likely to result." In reaching that conclusion, the Texas Supreme Court rejected the policies of the American Academy of Pediatrics and the "Good Medical Practice" guidelines of the Royal College of Paediatricians and Child Health (RCPCH) of counselling parents on the survival and outcome prospects of strikingly premature deliveries and involving them in decisions for their infants. And although Lord Donaldson in In Re R highlighted the doctor's duty to treat in an emergency without consent if in the doctor's judgment such a treatment would be in the best interests of the child, in the case of a baby with only a small chance of survival and even then with a high risk of handicap, it would not be unreasonable under the standards of the RCPCH's *Framework of practice* sections on "No purpose" or the "Unbearable situation" not to initiate resuscitation.

The "facts" adopted by the Texas Supreme Court from statements given at the trial by the neonatology fellow who attended the delivery of Baby Miller are strikingly at variance with the data found in the literature on mortality and morbidity of 23 week gestational age infants. Further, they do not reflect the general practice of neonatologists regarding delivery room decisions for infants at the threshold of viability. A recent survey of level 2/3 neonatologists by Harvard researchers reveals that "at or below 23 0/7 weeks gestation 93% of respondents considered treatment futile."[4] At 23 1/7–6/7 weeks gestation, almost 90% of respondents considered treatment to be of uncertain benefit—that is, neither clearly beneficial nor futile. In those circumstances, the overwhelming majority (76%) stated that they would follow the parents' decision to forego treatment and allow such infants to die. There was a similar response to a United Kingdom survey of paediatricians/neonatologists which found that, at less than 23 weeks gestation and under 500 g, 85% would be deterred from resuscitation.[5]

A helpful framework for decision making in these types of cases is found in an essay by Tyson and colleagues[6] on viability and morbidity of very low birthweight neonates. Rather than an either/or designation of parent or doctor as the decision maker, the authors propose that the treatment options should be governed by the prospects for the individual infant. To make that assessment, the authors divide treatment decisions for newborns into four categories: mandatory, optional, investigational, and unreasonable. They are explained as follows.

- Mandatory: if the parents ask the physician to withhold or withdraw ventilatory support that has a very high likelihood of benefiting a child, the treating physician's independent obligation to foster the best interests of the patient prohibits following the parent's request. An example would be parents who ask the physician to remove ventilation from a full term newborn unless the physician can guarantee that their child will be "normal."
- Optional: when the risks are very high and the benefits are at best uncertain or extremely low, the parents have the option of accepting or rejecting the proposed resuscitation. In this "grey zone" the parents' decision to either accept or reject ventilatory support should be followed.
- Investigational: for resuscitation for babies of very low birth weight, the outcome data are such that, in the words of Lantos *et al*, "The best we can tell parents is that this intervention is so new or its effects on this class of patients so unproven that it is an 'innovative' or 'experimental' procedure."[7] Such procedures, as the Nuremberg standards inform us, necessarily require patient or proxy consent.
- Unreasonable: if the parents are demanding attempts at resuscitation, when in the physician's best judgment there is no expectation of efficacy—for example, on a child born with Potter's syndrome or a 20 week, 298 g delivery, there is no obligation to attempt resuscitation. Indeed to attempt resuscitation or other medical treatment when there is no possibility of benefit to the patient would constitute an assault or battery.

A newborn's prospects vary from the complete uncertainty of a "normal" future for a full term baby experiencing a post-delivery respiratory episode, to the very high probability of mortality and significant morbidity awaiting a 23 week 614 g infant. The EPICure study, for example, reports a survival rate to discharge at 23 weeks—the age of the Miller child—of 11%. The most recent outcome data on extremely premature infants, the 2004 Vermont/Oxford Network study of 4172 infants born with very, very low birth weights, notes an increase in the percentage of survivors (17%), but in the words of the authors, the results are "not encouraging."[8] The vast majority (83%) died before discharge, and over half of those (52%) did so in the delivery room. Those who did survive almost always suffered from severe complications. As the effectiveness of neonatal intensive care technology for this class of newborns is "essentially unknown," the authors conclude that treatment of those infants is "a large, uncontrolled experiment."

Contrary to the ruling of the Texas Supreme Court, ventilation is not necessarily justified simply because it offers a modest chance of survival. As Francis Moore, the distinguished Harvard surgeon, reminds us, imposing a medical procedure on a patient requires a greater justification than mere survival. In his words, "There must be a rationale on which the desperately ill patient may be offered not merely pain, suffering and cost, but also true hope of prolonged survival [without devastating sequelae]."[9]

Although clearly premature infants will die without mechanical ventilation, the decision whether or not to initiate resuscitation ought not be based solely on a doctor's assessment of potential viability. Survivability is not the only issue at stake. Although death is unquestionably a bad outcome, imposing mechanical ventilation can make for a worse situation—demise after days or months of predictable morbidity so severe it might be judged an even greater tragedy than death.

To avoid that possibility, resuscitation decisions for extremely premature neonates should be based on the prospects for a particular child. To achieve that goal, as the EPICure study group put it, professionals must provide parents with "reliable outcome data based on gestational age that will allow the parents to plan care around the time of birth." Evaluating the significance of those data in an individual case and determining whether or not the risks and benefits warrant the use of aggressive technology is a value judgment, not a medical assessment. As such, it properly belongs to those who, along with the infant, will bear the burden of a decision to resuscitate: the parents.

CONCLUSION

The Miller case confirms the adage that "bad facts make bad law." The mis-statement of institutional policy by a hospital administrator led the medical staff to abandon the well thought through parent-physician decision to omit resuscitation of an infant at the very margins of viability, a decision that was well within the standard of care. The determination to resuscitate was based on the mistaken belief that the law required the resuscitation of any infant with a delivery weight >500 g. The record does not indicate why once the child was resuscitated and subsequently suffered significant neurological insult that the use of aggressive medical interventions was not re-evaluated and discontinued.

The only issue raised in the case and addressed by the Texas Supreme Court was whose decision is it to determine whether or not to omit resuscitation for an extremely premature infant. In the Court's view, that role belongs exclusively to the physician. The Court did not mandate that physicians resuscitate all potentially viable newborns. It did, however, authorise physicians to decide whether or not to resuscitate in these cases when the outcome is "essentially uncertain and when failure to resuscitate would result in the infant's death." In such instances, the physician may resuscitate the extremely preterm infant even over parental objections.

In the United Kingdom when there is disagreement between the medical staff and the parents and the opinion of a court has been sought, such as in the recent cases of Charlotte Wyatt and Luke Winston-Jones, judges have normally ruled in favour of the medical viewpoint, and have applied the RCPCH framework for practice as in the "no chance situation" applied with Baby C with spinal muscular atrophy type 1. Only rarely has the sincerely held view of caring parents won the ruling against unanimous medical opinion. However, in the Miller case it appears as though the disagreement was less with the parents than between members of the medical and nursing staff involved.

And although it might have been reasonable for the neonatal fellow in the obstetrical suite to have opted to resuscitate on the basis of a post-delivery assessment of potential viability, there appears to have been no attempt to reassess the clinical situation and the likely outcome after birth, particularly when a major intraventricular haemorrhage had been identified.

The danger with the Texas Supreme Court's ruling in Miller v HCA is that, under it, a physician who wants to resuscitate a neonate may do so no matter how premature, how unlikely to survive, how likely to incur severe disabilities, or how strongly the parents object. This substitution of the physician's values for those of the parents of infants delivered at the extreme margins of viability is a significant shift from present standards in neonatology. We believe such a change is neither good policy nor good medicine.

REFERENCES

1. Annas GJ. Extremely preterm birth and parental authority to refuse treatment: the case of Sidney Miller. *N Engl J Med* 2004;351:2118–23.
2. Lucey JF. Fetal infants: thoughts about what to do. *Pediatrics* 2004; 113:1819.
3. Miller v HCA, Inc. 118 S. W. 3rd 75, 2003.
4. Peerzada JM, Richardson DK, Burns JP. Delivery room decision-making at the threshold of viability. *J Pediatr* 2004;145:492–8.
5. Elias-Jones AC. Legal implications of the withdrawal of neonatal intensive care. University of Wales Library, 1996.
6. Tyson JE, Younes N., Verter J, et al. Viability, morbidity, and resource use among newborns of 501- to 800-g birth weight. *JAMA* 1996;276: 1645–51.
7. Lanlos J, Miles SH, Silverstein MD, et al. Survival after cardiopulmonary resuscitation in babies of very low birthweight. *N Engl J Med* 1988; 318:91–5.
8. Lucey JF, Rowan CA, Shiomo P, et al. Fetal infants: the fate of 4172 infants with birth weights of 401 to 500 grams—the Vermont Oxford Network experience (1996–2000). *Pediatrics* 2004;113:1559–6.
9. Moore F. The desperate case: CARE (costs, applicability, research, ethics). *JAMA* 1989; 261:1483–4.

PHYSICIAN-ASSISTED DEATH

DEATH AND DIGNITY: A CASE OF INDIVIDUALIZED DECISION MAKING

Timothy E. Quill

Diane was feeling tired and had a rash. A common scenario, though there was something subliminally worrisome that prompted me to check her blood count. Her hematocrit was 22, and the white-cell count was 4.3 with some metamyelocytes and unusual white cells. I wanted it to be viral, trying to deny what was staring me in the face. Perhaps in a repeated count it would disappear. I called Diane and told her it might be more serious than I had initially thought—that the test needed to be repeated and that if she felt worse, we might have to move quickly. When she pressed for the possibilities, I reluctantly opened the door to leukemia. Hearing

the word seemed to make it exist. "Oh, shit!" she said. "Don't tell me that." Oh, shit! I thought, I wish I didn't have to.

Diane was no ordinary person (although no one I have ever come to know has been really ordinary). She was raised in an alcoholic family and had felt alone for much of her life. She had vaginal cancer as a young woman. Through much of her adult life, she had struggled with depression and her own alcoholism. I had come to know, respect, and admire her over the previous eight years as she confronted these problems and gradually overcame them. She was an incredibly clear, at times brutally honest, thinker and communicator. As she took control of her life, she developed a strong sense of independence and confidence. In the previous three-and-one-half years, her hard work had paid off. She was completely abstinent from alcohol, she had established much deeper connections

From *New England Journal of Medicine* 324, no. 10 (March 7, 1991): 691–694.

with her husband, college-age son, and several friends, and her business and her artistic work were blossoming. She felt she was really living fully for the first time.

Not surprisingly, the repeated blood count was abnormal, and detailed examination of the peripheral blood smear showed myelocytes. I advised her to come into the hospital, explaining that we needed to do a bone marrow biopsy and make some decisions relatively rapidly. She came to the hospital knowing what we would find. She was terrified, angry, and sad. Although we knew the odds, we both clung to the thread of possibility that it might be something else.

The bone marrow confirmed the worst: acute myelomonocytic leukemia. In the face of this tragedy, we looked for signs of hope. This is an area of medicine in which technological intervention has been successful, with cures 25 percent of the time—long-term cures. As I probed the costs of these cures, I heard about induction chemotherapy (three weeks in the hospital, prolonged neutropenia, probable infectious complications, and hair loss; 75 percent of patients respond, 25 percent do not). For the survivors, this is followed by consolidation chemotherapy (with similar side effects; another 25 percent die, for a net survival of 50 percent). Those still alive, to have a reasonable chance of long-term survival, then need bone marrow transplantation (hospitalization for two months and whole-body irradiation, with complete killing of the bone marrow, infectious complications, and the possibility for graft-versus-host disease—with a survival of approximately 50 percent, or 25 percent of the original group). Though hematologists may argue over the exact percentages, they don't argue about the outcome of no treatment—certain death in days, weeks, or at most a few months.

Believing that delay was dangerous, our oncologist broke the news to Diane and began making plans to insert a Hickman catheter and begin induction chemotherapy that afternoon. When I saw her shortly thereafter, she was enraged at his presumption that she would want treatment, and devastated by the finality of the diagnosis. All she wanted to do was go home and be with her family. She had no further questions about treatment and in fact had decided that she wanted none. Together we lamented her tragedy and the unfairness of life.

Before she left, I felt the need to be sure that she and her husband understood that there was some risk in delay, that the problem was not going to go away, and that we needed to keep considering the options over the next several days. We agreed to meet in two days.

She returned in two days with her husband and son. They had talked extensively about the problem and the options. She remained very clear about her wish not to undergo chemotherapy and to live whatever time she had left outside the hospital. As we explored her thinking further, it became clear that she was convinced she would die during the period of treatment and would suffer unspeakably in the process (from hospitalization, from lack of control over her body, from the side effects of chemotherapy, and from pain and anguish). Although I could offer support and my best effort to minimize her suffering if she chose treatment, there was no way I could say any of this would not occur. In fact, the last four patients with acute leukemia at our hospital had died very painful deaths in the hospital during various stages of treatment (a fact I did not share with her). Her family wished she would choose treatment but sadly accepted her decision. She articulated very clearly that it was she who would be experiencing all the side effects of treatment and that odds of 25 percent were not good enough for her to undergo so toxic a course of therapy, given her expectations of chemotherapy and hospitalization and the absence of a closely matched bone marrow donor. I had her repeat her understanding of the treatment, the odds, and what to expect if there were no treatment. I clarified a few misunderstandings, but she had a remarkable grasp of the options and implications.

I have been a longtime advocate of active, informed patient choice of treatment or nontreatment, and of a patient's right to die with as much control and dignity as possible. Yet there was something about her giving up a 25 percent chance of long-term survival in favor of almost certain death that disturbed me. I had seen Diane fight and use her considerable inner resources to overcome alcoholism and depression, and I half expected her to change her mind over the next week. Since the window of time in which effective treatment can be initiated is rather narrow, we met several times that week. We obtained a second hematology consultation and talked at length about the meaning and implications of treatment and nontreatment. She talked to a psychologist she had seen in the past. I gradually understood the decision from her perspective and became convinced that it was the right decision for her. We arranged for home hospice care (although at that time Diane felt reasonably well, was active, and looked healthy), left the door open for her to change her mind, and tried to anticipate how to keep her comfortable in the time she had left.

Just as I was adjusting to her decision, she opened up another area that would stretch me profoundly. It was extraordinarily important to Diane to maintain control of herself and her own dignity during the time remaining to her. When this was no longer possible, she clearly wanted to die. As a former director of a hospice program, I know how to use pain medicines to keep patients comfortable and lessen suffering. I explained the philosophy of comfort care, which I strongly believe in. Although Diane understood and appreciated this, she had known of people lingering in what was called relative comfort, and she wanted no part of it. When the time came, she wanted to take her life in the least painful way possible. Knowing of her desire for independence and her decision to stay in control, I thought this request made perfect sense. I acknowledged and explored this wish but also thought that it was out of the realm of currently accepted medical practice and that it was more than I could offer or promise. In our discussion, it became clear that preoccupation with her fear of a lingering death would interfere with Diane's getting the most out of the time she had left until she found a safe way to ensure her death. I feared the effects of a violent death on her family, the consequences of an ineffective suicide that would leave her lingering in precisely the state she dreaded so much, and the possibility that a family member would be forced to assist her, with all the legal and personal repercussions that would follow. She discussed this at length with her family. They believed that they should respect her choice. With this in mind, I told Diane that information was available from the Hemlock Society that might be helpful to her.

A week later she phoned me with a request for barbiturates for sleep. Since I knew that this was an essential ingredient in a Hemlock Society suicide,

I asked her to come to the office to talk things over. She was more than willing to protect me by participating in a superficial conversation about her insomnia, but it was important to me to know how she planned to use the drugs and to be sure that she was not in despair or overwhelmed in a way that might color her judgment. In our discussion, it was apparent that she was having trouble sleeping, but it was also evident that the security of having enough barbiturates available to commit suicide when and if the time came would leave her secure enough to live fully and concentrate on the present. It was clear that she was not despondent and that in fact she was making deep, personal connections with her family and close friends. I made sure that she knew how to use the barbiturates for sleep, and also that she knew the amount needed to commit suicide. We agreed to meet regularly, and she promised to meet with me before taking her life, to ensure that all other avenues had been exhausted. I wrote the prescription with an uneasy feeling about the boundaries I was exploring—spiritual, legal, professional, and personal. Yet I also felt strongly that I was setting her free to get the most out of the time she had left, and to maintain dignity and control on her own terms until her death.

The next several months were very intense and important for Diane. Her son stayed home from college, and they were able to be with one another and say much that had not been said earlier. Her husband did his work at home so that he and Diane could spend more time together. She spent time with her closest friends. I had her come into the hospital for a conference with our residents, at which she illustrated in a most profound and personal way the importance of informed decision making, the right to refuse treatment, and the extraordinarily personal effects of illness and interaction with the medical system. There were emotional and physical hardships as well. She had periods of intense sadness and anger. Several times she became very weak, but she received transfusions as an outpatient and responded with marked improvement of symptoms. She had two serious infections that responded surprisingly well to empirical courses of oral antibiotics. After three tumultuous months, there were two weeks of relative calm and well-being, and fantasies of a miracle began to surface.

Unfortunately, we had no miracle. Bone pain, weakness, fatigue, and fevers began to dominate her life. Although the hospice workers, family members, and I tried our best to minimize the suffering and promote comfort, it was clear that the end was approaching. Diane's immediate future held what she feared the most—increasing discomfort, dependence, and hard choices between pain and sedation. She called up her closest friends and asked them to come over to say goodbye, telling them that she would be leaving soon. As we had agreed, she let me know as well. When we met, it was clear that she knew what she was doing, that she was sad and frightened to be leaving, but that she would be even more terrified to stay and suffer. In our tearful goodbye, she promised a reunion in the future at her favorite spot on the edge of Lake Geneva, with dragons swimming in the sunset.

Two days later her husband called to say that Diane had died. She had said her final goodbyes to her husband and son that morning, and asked them to leave her alone for an hour. After an hour, which must have seemed an eternity, they found her on the couch, lying very still and covered by her favorite shawl. There was no sign of struggle. She seemed to be at peace. They called me for advice about how to proceed. When I arrived at their house, Diane indeed seemed peaceful. Her husband and son were quiet. We talked about what a remarkable person she had been. They seemed to have no doubts about the course she had chosen or about their cooperation, although the unfairness of her illness and the finality of her death were overwhelming to us all.

I called the medical examiner to inform him that a hospice patient had died. When asked about the cause of death, I said, "acute leukemia." He said that was fine and that we should call a funeral director. Although acute leukemia was the truth, it was not the whole story. Yet any mention of suicide would have given rise to a police investigation and probably brought the arrival of an ambulance crew for resuscitation. Diane would have become a "coroner's case," and the decision to perform an autopsy would have been made at the discretion of the medical examiner. The family or I could have

been subject to criminal prosecution, and I to professional review, for our roles in support of Diane's choices. Although I truly believe that the family and I gave her the best care possible, allowing her to define her limits and directions as much as possible, I am not sure the law, society, or the medical profession would agree. So I said "acute leukemia" to protect all of us, to protect Diane from an invasion into her past and her body, and to continue to shield society from the knowledge of the degree of suffering that people often undergo in the process of dying. Suffering can be lessened to some extent, but in no way eliminated or made benign, by the careful intervention of a competent, caring physician, given current social constraints.

Diane taught me about the range of help I can provide if I know people well and if I allow them to say what they really want. She taught me about life, death, and honesty and about taking charge and facing tragedy squarely when it strikes. She taught me that I can take small risks for people that I really know and care about. Although I did not assist in her suicide directly, I helped indirectly to make it possible, successful, and relatively painless. Although I know we have measures to help control pain and lessen suffering, to think that people do not suffer in the process of dying is an illusion. Prolonged dying can occasionally be peaceful, but more often the role of the physician and family is limited to lessening but not eliminating severe suffering.

I wonder how many families and physicians secretly help patients over the edge into death in the face of such severe suffering. I wonder how many severely ill or dying patients secretly take their lives, dying alone in despair. I wonder whether the image of Diane's final aloneness will persist in the minds of her family, or if they will remember more the intense, meaningful months they had together before she died. I wonder whether Diane struggled in that last hour, and whether the Hemlock Society's way of death by suicide is the most benign. I wonder why Diane, who gave so much to so many of us, had to be alone for the last hour of her life. I wonder whether I will see Diane again, on the shore of Lake Geneva at sunset, with dragons swimming on the horizon.

PHYSICIAN-ASSISTED SUICIDE: A TRAGIC VIEW

John D. Arras

INTRODUCTION

For many decades now, the call for physician-assisted suicide (PAS) and euthanasia have been perennial lost causes in American society. Each generation has thrown up an assortment of earnest reformers and cranks who, after attracting their fifteen minutes of fame, inevitably have been defeated by the combined weight of traditional law and morality. Incredibly, two recent federal appellate court decisions suddenly changed the legal landscape in this area, making the various states within their respective jurisdictions the first governments in world history, excepting perhaps the Nazi regime in Germany, to officially sanction PAS. Within the space of a month, both an eight to three majority of the United States Court of Appeals for the Ninth Circuit[1] on the West Coast, and a three-judge panel in the United States Court of Appeals for the Second Circuit,[2] in the Northeast, struck down long-standing state laws forbidding physicians to aid or abet their patients in acts of suicide. Within a virtual blink of an eye, the unthinkable had come to pass: PAS and euthanasia had emerged from their exile beyond the pale of law to occupy center stage in a dramatic public debate that eventually culminated in the United States Supreme Court's unanimous reversal of both lower court decisions in June 1997. . . .[3]

As a firm believer in patient autonomy, I find myself to be deeply sympathetic to the central values motivating the case for PAS and euthanasia; I have concluded, however, that these practices pose too great a threat to the rights and welfare of too many people to be legalized in this country at the present time. Central to my argument in this paper will be the claim that the recently overturned decisions of the circuit courts employ a form of case-based reasoning that is ill-suited to the development of sound social policy in this area. I shall argue that in order to do justice to the very real threats posed by the widespread social practices of PAS and euthanasia, we need to adopt precisely the kind of policy perspective that the circuit courts rejected on principle. Thus, this essay presents the case for a forward-looking, legislative approach to PAS and euthanasia, as opposed to an essentially backward-looking, judicial or constitutional approach.[4] Although I suggest below that the soundest legislative policy at the present time would be to extend the legal prohibition of PAS into the near future, I remain open to the possibility that a given legislature, presented with sufficient evidence of the reliability of various safeguards, might come to a different conclusion.

ARGUMENTS AND MOTIVATIONS IN FAVOR OF PAS/EUTHANASIA

Let us begin, then, with the philosophical case for PAS and euthanasia, which consists of two distinct prongs, both of which speak simply, directly, and powerfully to our commonsensical intuitions. First, there is the claim of autonomy, that all of us possess a right to self-determination in matters profoundly touching on such religious themes as life, death, and the meaning of suffering. . . . Second, PAS and/or euthanasia are merciful acts that deliver terminally ill patients from painful and protracted death. . . . For patients suffering from the final ravages of end-stage AIDS or cancer, a doctor's lethal prescription or injection can be, and often is, welcomed as a blessed relief. Accordingly, we should treat human beings at least as well as we treat grievously ill or injured animals by putting them, at their own request, out of their misery.

From *Journal of Contemporary Health Law and Policy* 13 (1997): 361–389. Reprinted by permission.

Editors' note: This article has been heavily edited and many notes have been cut. Students who want to follow up on sources should consult the original article.

These philosophical reflections can be supplemented with a more clinical perspective addressed to the motivational factors lying behind many requests to die. Many people advocate legalization because they fear a loss of control at the end of life. They fear falling victim to the technological imperative; they fear dying in chronic and uncontrolled pain; they fear the psychological suffering attendant upon the relentless disintegration of the self; they fear, in short, a bad death. All of these fears, it so happens, are eminently justified. Physicians routinely ignore the documented wishes of patients and all-too-often allow patients to die with uncontrolled pain.[5] Studies of cancer patients have shown that over fifty percent suffer from unrelieved pain,[6] and many researchers have found that uncontrolled pain, particularly when accompanied by feelings of hopelessness and untreated depression, is a significant contributing factor for suicide and suicidal ideation.

Clinical depression is another major factor influencing patients' choice of suicide. Depression, accompanied by feelings of hopelessness, is the strongest predictor of suicide for both individuals who are terminally ill and those who are not. Yet most doctors are not trained to notice depression, especially in complex cases such as the elderly suffering from terminal illnesses. Even when doctors succeed in diagnosing depression, they often do not successfully treat it with readily available medications in sufficient amounts.

Significantly, the New York Task Force found that the vast majority of patients who request PAS or euthanasia can be treated successfully both for their depression and their pain, and that when they receive adequate psychiatric and palliative care, their requests to die usually are withdrawn.[7] In other words, patients given the requisite control over their lives and relief from depression and pain usually lose interest in PAS and euthanasia.

With all due respect for the power of modern methods of pain control, it must be acknowledged that a small percentage of patients suffer from conditions, both physical and psychological, that currently lie beyond the reach of the best medical and humane care. Some pain cannot be alleviated short of inducing a permanent state of unconsciousness in the patient, and some depression is unconquerable. For such unfortunate patients, the present law on PAS/euthanasia can represent an insuperable barrier to a dignified and decent death.[8]

OBJECTIONS TO PAS/EUTHANASIA

Opponents of PAS and euthanasia can be grouped into three main factions. One strongly condemns both practices as inherently immoral, as violations of the moral rule against killing the innocent. Most members of this group tend to harbor distinctly religious objections to suicide and euthanasia, viewing them as violations of God's dominion over human life. They argue that killing is simply wrong in itself, whether or not it is done out of respect for the patient's autonomy or out of concern for her suffering. Whether or not this position ultimately is justifiable from a theological point of view, its imposition on believers and non-believers alike is incompatible with the basic premises of a secular, pluralistic political order.

A second faction primarily objects to the fact that physicians are being called upon to do the killing. While conceding that killing the terminally ill or assisting in their suicides might not always be morally wrong for others to do, this group maintains that the participation of physicians in such practices undermines their role as healers and fatally compromises the physician-patient relationship.

Finally, a third faction readily grants that neither PAS nor active euthanasia, practiced by ordinary citizens or by physicians, are always morally wrong. On the contrary, this faction believes that in certain rare instances early release from a painful or intolerably degrading existence might constitute both a positive good and an important exercise of personal autonomy for the individual. Indeed, many members of this faction concede that should such a terrible fate befall them, they would hope to find a thoughtful, compassionate, and courageous physician to release them from their misery. But in spite of these important concessions, the members of this faction shrink from endorsing or regulating PAS and active euthanasia due to fears bearing on the social consequences of liberalization. This view is based on two distinct kinds of so-called "slippery slope" arguments: one bears on the inability to cabin PAS/euthanasia within the confines envisioned by its proponents; the other focuses on the likelihood of abuse, neglect, and mistake.

An Option Without Limits

The first version of the slippery slope argument contends that a socially sanctioned practice of PAS would in all likelihood prove difficult, if not impossible, to cabin within its originally anticipated boundaries. Proponents of legalization usually begin with a wholesomely modest policy agenda, limiting their suggested reforms to a narrow and highly specified range of potential candidates and practices. "Give us PAS," they ask, "not the more controversial practice of active euthanasia, for presently competent patients who are terminally ill and suffering unbearable pain." But the logic of the case for PAS, based as it is upon the twin pillars of patient autonomy and mercy, makes it highly unlikely that society could stop with this modest proposal once it had ventured out on the slope. As numerous other critics have pointed out, if autonomy is the prime consideration, then additional constraints based upon terminal illness or unbearable pain, or both, would appear hard to justify. Indeed, if autonomy is crucial, the requirement of unbearable suffering would appear to be entirely subjective. Who is to say, other than the patient herself, how much suffering is too much? Likewise, the requirement of terminal illness seems an arbitrary standard against which to judge patients' own subjective evaluation of their quality of life. If my life is no longer worth living, why should a terminally ill cancer patient be granted PAS but not me, merely because my suffering is due to my "non-terminal" amyotrophic lateral sclerosis (ALS) or intractable psychiatric disorder?

Alternatively, if pain and suffering are deemed crucial to the justification of legalization, it is hard to see how the proposed barrier of contemporaneous consent of competent patients could withstand serious erosion. If the logic of PAS is at all similar to that of forgoing life-sustaining treatments, and we have every reason to think it so, then it would seem almost inevitable that a case soon would be made to permit PAS for incompetent patients who had left advance directives. That would then be followed by a "substituted judgment" test for patients who "would have wanted" PAS, and finally an "objective" test would be developed for patients (including newborns) whose best interests would be served by PAS or active euthanasia even in the absence of any subjective intent (see Part 3, Section 5 above).

In the same way, the joint justifications of autonomy and mercy combine to undermine the plausibility of a line drawn between PAS and active euthanasia. As the authors of one highly publicized proposal have come to see, the logic of justification for active euthanasia is identical to that of PAS.[9] Legalizing PAS, while continuing to ban active euthanasia, would serve only to discriminate unfairly against patients who are suffering and wish to end their lives, but cannot do so because of some physical impairment. Surely these patients, it will be said, are "the worst-off group," and therefore they are the most in need of the assistance of others who will do for them what they can no longer accomplish on their own.

None of these initial slippery slope considerations amount to knock-down objections to further liberalization of our laws and practices. After all, it is not obvious that each of the highly predictable shifts (e.g., from terminal to "merely" incurable, from contemporaneous consent to best interests, and from PAS to active euthanasia), are patently immoral and unjustifiable. Still, in pointing out this likely slippage, the consequentialist opponents of PAS/euthanasia are calling on society to think about the likely consequences of taking the first tentative step onto the slope. If all of the extended practices predicted above pose substantially greater risks for vulnerable patients than the more highly circumscribed initial liberalization proposals, then we need to factor in these additional risks even as we ponder the more modest proposals.[10]

The Likelihood of Abuse

The second prong of the slippery slope argument argues that whatever criteria for justifiable PAS and active euthanasia ultimately are chosen, abuse of the system is highly likely to follow. In other words, patients who fall outside the ambit of our justifiable criteria will soon be candidates for death. This prong resembles what I have elsewhere called an "empirical slope" argument, as it is based not on the close logical resemblance of concepts or justifications, but rather on an empirical prediction of what is likely to happen when we insert a particular social practice into our existing social system.

In order to reassure skeptics, the proponents of PAS/euthanasia concur that any potentially justifiable social policy in this area must meet at least the following three requirements. The policy would have to insist first, that all requests for death be truly voluntary; second, that all reasonable alternatives to PAS and active euthanasia must be explored before acceding to a patient's wishes; and, third, that a reliable system of reporting all cases must be established in order to effectively monitor these practices and respond to abuses. As a social pessimist on these matters, I believe, given social reality as we know it, that all three assumptions are problematic.

With regard to the voluntariness requirement, we pessimists contend that many requests would not be sufficiently voluntary. In addition to the subtly coercive influences of physicians and family members, perhaps the most slippery aspect of this slope is the highly predictable failure of most physicians to diagnose reliably and treat reversible clinical depression, particularly in the elderly population. As one geriatric psychiatrist testified before the New York Task Force, we now live in the "golden age" of treating depression, but the "lead age" of diagnosing it. We have the tools, but physicians are not adequately trained and motivated to use them. Unless dramatic changes are effected in the practice of medicine, we can predict with confidence that many instances of PAS and active euthanasia will fail the test of voluntariness.

Second, there is the lingering fear that any legislative proposal or judicial mandate would have to be implemented within the present social system marked by deep and pervasive discrimination against the poor and members of minority groups. We have every reason to expect that a policy that worked tolerably well in an affluent community like Scarsdale or Beverly Hills, might not work so well in a community like Bedford-Stuyvesant or Watts, where your average citizen has little or no access to basic primary care, let alone sophisticated care for chronic pain at home or in the hospital.

There is also reason to worry about any policy of PAS initiated within our growing system of managed care, capitation, and physician incentives for delivering less care. Expert palliative care no doubt is an expensive and time-consuming proposition, requiring more, rather than less, time spent just talking with patients and providing them with humane comfort. It is highly doubtful that the context of physician-patient conversation within this new dispensation of "turnstile medicine" will be at all conducive to humane decisions untainted by subtle economic coercion.

In addition, given the abysmal and shameful track record of physicians in responding adequately to pain and suffering,[11] we also can confidently predict that in many cases all reasonable alternatives will not have been exhausted. Instead of vigorously addressing the pharmacological and psychosocial needs of such patients, physicians no doubt will continue to ignore, undertreat or treat many of their patients in an impersonal manner. The result is likely to be more depression, desperation, and requests for physician-assisted death from patients who could have been successfully treated. The root causes of this predictable failure are manifold, but high on the list is the inaccessibility of decent primary care to over thirty-seven million Americans. Other notable causes include an appalling lack of training in palliative care among primary care physicians and cancer specialists alike; discrimination in the delivery of pain control and other medical treatments on the basis of race and economic status; various myths shared by both physicians and patients about the supposed ill effects of pain medications; and restrictive state laws on access to opioids.

Finally, with regard to the third requirement, pessimists doubt that any reporting system would adequately monitor these practices. A great deal depends here on the extent to which patients and practitioners will regard these practices as essentially private matters to be discussed and acted upon within the privacy of the doctor-patient relationship. As the Dutch experience has conclusively demonstrated, physicians will be extremely loath to report instances of PAS and active euthanasia to public authorities, largely for fear of bringing the harsh glare of publicity upon the patients' families at a time when privacy is most needed. The likely result of this predictable lack of oversight will be society's inability to respond appropriately to disturbing incidents and long-term trends. In other words, the practice most likely will not be as amenable to regulation as the proponents contend.

The moral of this story is that deeply seated inadequacies in physicians' training, combined with structural flaws in our health care system, can be reliably predicted to secure the premature deaths of many people who would in theory be excluded by the criteria of most leading proposals to legalize PAS. If this characterization of the status quo is at all accurate, then the problem will not be solved by well meaning assurances that abuses will not be tolerated, or that patients will, of course, be offered the full range of palliative care options before any decision for PAS is ratified.[12] While such regulatory solutions are possible in theory, and may well justly prevail in the future, we should be wary of legally sanctioning any negative right to be let alone by the state when the just and humane exercise of that right will depend upon the provision of currently nonexistent services. The operative analogy here, I fear, is our failed and shameful policy of "deinstitutionalization," which left thousands of vulnerable and defenseless former residents of state psychiatric hospitals to fend for themselves on the streets, literally "rotting with their rights on." It is now generally agreed that the crucial flaw in this well-intended but catastrophic policy was our society's willingness to honor such patients' negative right to be free of institutional fetters without having first made available reliable local alternatives to institutionalization. The operative lesson for us here is that judges and courts are much better at enunciating negative rights than they are at providing the services required for their successful implementation. . . .

TOWARDS A POLICY OF PRUDENT (LEGAL) RESTRAINT AND AGGRESSIVE (MEDICAL) INTERVENTION

In contrast to the judicial approach, which totally vindicates the value of patient autonomy at the expense of protecting the vulnerable, my own preferred approach to a social policy of PAS and euthanasia conceives of this debate as posing an essentially "tragic choice."[13] It frankly acknowledges that whatever choice we make, whether we opt for a reaffirmation of the current legal restraints or for a policy of legitimization and regulation, there are bound to be "victims." The victims of the current policy are easy to identify: They are on the news, the talk shows, the documentaries, and often on Dr. Kevorkian's roster of so-called "patients." The victims of legalization, by contrast, will be largely hidden from view; they will include the clinically depressed eighty-year-old man who could have lived for another year of good quality if only he had been adequately treated, and the fifty-year-old woman who asks for death because doctors in her financially stretched HMO cannot, or will not, effectively treat her unrelenting, but mysterious, pelvic pain. Perhaps eventually, if we slide far enough down the slope, the uncommunicative stroke victim, whose distant children deem an earlier death to be a better death, will fall victim. There will be others besides these, many coming from the ranks of the uninsured and the poor. To the extent that minorities and the poor already suffer from the effects of discrimination in our health care system, it is reasonable to expect that any system of PAS and euthanasia will exhibit similar effects, such as failure to access adequate primary care, pain management, and psychiatric diagnosis and treatment. Unlike Dr. Kevorkian's "patients," these victims will not get their pictures in the papers, but they all will have faces and they will all be cheated of good months or perhaps even years.

This "tragic choice" approach to social policy on PAS/euthanasia takes the form of the following argument formulated at the legislative level. First, the number of "genuine cases" justifying PAS, active euthanasia, or both, will be relatively small. Patients who receive good personal care, good pain relief, treatment for depression, and adequate psychosocial supports tend not to persist in their desire to die.

Second, the social risks of legalization are serious and highly predictable. They include the expansion of these practices to nonvoluntary cases, the advent of active euthanasia, and the widespread failure to pursue readily available alternatives to suicide motivated by pain, depression, hopelessness, and lack of access to good primary medical care.

Third, rather than propose a momentous and dangerous policy shift for a relatively small number of "genuine cases"—a shift that would surely involve a great deal of persistent social division and strife analogous to that involved in the abortion controversy—we should instead attempt to redirect the public debate toward a goal on which we can and should all agree, namely the manifest and urgent need to reform the way we die in America. Instead of pursuing a highly divisive and dangerous campaign for PAS, we should attack the problem at its root with an ambitious program of reform in the areas of access to primary care and the education of physicians in palliative care. At least as far as the "slippery slope" opponents of PAS are concerned, we should thus first see to it that the vast majority of people in this country have access to adequate, affordable, and nondiscriminatory primary and palliative care. At the end of this long and arduous process, when we finally have an equitable, effective, and compassionate health care system in place, one that might be compared favorably with that in the Netherlands, then we might well want to reopen the discussion of PAS and active euthanasia.

Finally, there are those few unfortunate patients who truly are beyond the pale of good palliative, hospice, and psychiatric care. The opponents of legalization must face up to this suffering remnant and attempt to offer creative and humane solutions. One possibility is for such patients to be rendered permanently unconscious by drugs until such time, presumably not a long time, as death finally claims them. Although some will find such an option to be aesthetically unappealing, many would find it a welcome relief. Other patients beyond the reach of the best palliative and hospice care could take their own lives, either by well-known traditional means, or with the help of a physician who could sedate them while they refused further food and (life extending) fluids. Finally, those who find this latter option to be unacceptable might still be able to find a compassionate physician who, like Dr. Timothy Quill, will ultimately be willing, albeit in fear and trembling, to "take small risks for people they really know and care about." Such actions will continue to take place within the privacy of the patient-physician relationship, however, and thus will not threaten vulnerable patients and the social fabric to the same extent as would result from full legalization and regulation.

As the partisans of legalized PAS correctly point out, the covert practice of PAS will not be subject to regulatory oversight, and is thus capable of generating its own abuses and slippery slope. Still, I believe that the ever-present threat of possible criminal sanctions and revocation of licensure will continue to serve, for the vast majority of physicians, as powerful disincentives to abuse the system. Moreover, as suggested earlier, it is highly unlikely that the proposals for legalization would result in truly effective oversight.

CONCLUSION

Instead of conceiving this momentous debate as a choice between, on the one hand, legalization and regulation with all of their attendant risks, and on the other hand, the callous abandonment of patients to their pain and suffering, enlightened opponents must recommend a positive program of clinical and social reforms. On the clinical level, physicians must learn how to really listen to their patients, to unflinchingly engage them in sensitive discussions of their needs and the meaning of their requests for assisted death, to deliver appropriate palliative care, to distinguish fact from fiction in the ethics and law of pain relief; to diagnose and treat clinical depression, and finally, to ascertain and respect their patients' wishes for control regarding the forgoing of life-sustaining treatments. On the social level, opponents of PAS must aggressively promote major initiatives in medical and public education regarding pain control, in the sensitization of insurance companies and licensing agencies to issues of the quality of dying, and in the reform of state laws that currently hinder access to pain-relieving medications.

In the absence of an ambitious effort in the direction of aggressive medical and social reform, I fear that the medical and nursing professions will have lost whatever moral warrant and credibility they might still have in continuing to oppose physician-assisted suicide and active euthanasia. As soon as these reforms are in place, however, we might then wish to proceed slowly and cautiously with experiments in various states to test the overall benefits of a policy of legalization. Until that time, however, we are not well served as a society by court decisions allowing for legalization of PAS. The Supreme Court has thus reached a sound decision in ruling out a constitutional right to PAS. As the Justices acknowledged, however, this momentous decision will not end the moral debate over PAS and euthanasia. Indeed, it should and hopefully will intensify it.

NOTES

1. *Compassion in Dying* v. *Washington*, 79 F.3d 790, 838 (9th Cir. 1996).
2. *Quill* v. *Vacco*, 80 F.3d 716, 731 (2nd Cir. 1996).
3. *Vacco, Attorney General of New York. et al.* v. *Quill et al.* certiorari to the United States Court of Appeals for the Second Circuit, No. 95–1858. Argued January 8, 1997—Decided June 26, 1997. *Washington et al.* v. *Glucksberg et al.*, certiorari to the United States Court of Appeals for the Ninth Circuit, No. 96–110. Argued January 8, 1997—Decided June 26, 1997.
4. My stance on these issues has been profoundly influenced by my recent work with the New York State Task Force on Life and the Law (hereinafter "Task Force") to come to grips with this issue.
5. "A Controlled Trial to Improve Care for Seriously Ill Hospitalized Patients: The Study to Understand Prognoses and Preferences for Outcomes and Risks of Treatments" (SUPPORT), *Journal of the American Medical Association* 274 (Nov. 22, 1995): 1591–92.
6. Task Force, *When Death Is Sought*, x–xi.
7. Task Force, *When Death Is Sought*, xiv.
8. The preceding section thus signals two important points of agreement with the so-called "Philosophers' Brief" submitted to the Supreme Court in *Compassion in Dying* and *Vacco* by Ronald Dworkin, Thomas Nagel, Robert Nozick, John Rawls, Thomas Scanlon, and Judith Jarvis Thomson [in this volume, 488–96]. I agree that individuals in the throes of a painful or degrading terminal illness may well have a very strong moral and even legal interest in securing PAS. I also agree that the pain and suffering of a small percentage of dying patients cannot be adequately controlled by currently available medical interventions. As we shall see, however, I disagree with the philoso-

phers' conclusion that this interest is sufficiently strong in the face of current medical and social inadequacies as to justify a legal right that would void the reasonably cautious prohibitions of PAS and euthanasia in effect in every state.

9. Cassel et al., "Care of the Hopelessly Ill," 1380–84. See also Franklin G. Miller et al., "Regulating Physician-Assisted Death," *New England Journal of Medicine* 331(1994): 199–23 (conceding by the untenability of the previous distinction).
10. Professors Dworkin, et al. consistently fail to mention the possibility, let alone the high likelihood, of this first sort of slippage; I take this to be a serious omission both in their joint brief and in Dworkin's individually authored articles on this subject. These authors simply assume (with the plaintiffs and circuit court majority opinions) that this right will be restricted by means of procedural safeguards to presently competent, incurably ill individuals manifesting great pain and suffering due to physical illness. (For evidence of Dworkin's continuing failure to acknowledge this problem, see his assessment of the Supreme Court opinions in "Assisted Suicide: What the Court Really Said," *New York Review of Books* 44, no. 14 (Sept. 25, 1997): 40–44. Failure to notice this sort of dynamic might be due either to the philosophers' lack of familiarity with the recent history of bioethics or to their belief that the social risks of PAS are equivalent to the risks inherent in the widely accepted practice of forgoing life-sustaining treatments, and thus that such slippage would not present any additional risk. The latter assumption is, of course, vigorously contested by the opponents of PAS and euthanasia.
11. Task Force, *When Death Is Sought*, 43–47. "Despite dramatic advances in pain management, the delivery of pain relief is grossly inadequate in clinical practice . . . Studies have shown that only 2 to 60 percent of cancer pain is treated adequately." *Ibid.*, 43.
12. See, e.g., Ronald Dworkin, "Introduction to the Philosophers' Brief," *New York Review of Books*, 41–42 [in this volume, 484–87]; and Dworkin, "Assisted Suicide: What the Court Really Said," 44.
13. For an explication of the notion of a "tragic choice" in the sense that I employ here, see Guido Calabresi and Philip Bobbit, *Tragic Choices* (New York: W.W. Norton, 1978).

ASSISTED SUICIDE: THE PHILOSOPHERS' BRIEF

Ronald Dworkin

INTRODUCTION

The laws of all but one American state now forbid doctors to prescribe lethal pills for patients who want to kill themselves.* These cases[1] began when groups of dying patients and their doctors in Washington State and New York each sued asking that these prohibitions be declared unconstitutional so that the patients could be given, when and if they asked for it, medicine to hasten their death. The pleadings described the agony in which the patient plaintiffs were dying, and two federal Circuit Courts of Appeal—the Ninth Circuit in the Washington case and the Second Circuit in the New York case—agreed with the plaintiffs that the Constitution forbids the government from flatly prohibiting doctors to help end such desperate and pointless suffering.[2]

Washington State and New York appealed these decisions to the Supreme Court, and a total of sixty amicus briefs were filed, including briefs on behalf of the American Medical Association and the United States Catholic Conference urging the Court to reverse the circuit court decisions, and on behalf of the American Medical Students Association and the Gay Men's Health Crisis urging it to affirm them. The justices' comments during oral argument

persuaded many observers that the Court would reverse the decisions, probably by a lopsided majority. The justices repeatedly cited two versions—one theoretical, the other practical—of the "slippery slope" argument: that it would be impossible to limit a right to assisted suicide in an acceptable way, once that right was recognized.

The theoretical version of the argument denies that any principled line can be drawn between cases in which proponents say a right of assisted suicide is appropriate and those in which they concede that it is not. The circuit courts recognized only a right for competent patients already dying in great physical pain to have pills prescribed that they could take themselves. Several justices asked on what grounds the right once granted could be so severely limited. Why should it be denied to dying patients who are so feeble or paralyzed that they cannot take pills themselves and who beg a doctor to inject a lethal drug into them? Or to patients who are not dying but face years of intolerable physical or emotional pain, or crippling paralysis or dependence? But if the right were extended that far, on what ground could it be denied to anyone who had formed a desire to die—to a sixteen-year-old suffering from a severe case of unrequited love, for example?

The philosophers' brief answers these questions in two steps. First, it defines a very general moral and constitutional principle—that every competent person has the right to make momentous personal decisions which invoke fundamental religious or philosophical convictions about life's value for himself. Second, it recognizes that people may make such momentous decisions impulsively or out of emotional depression, when their act does not reflect their enduring convictions; and it therefore allows that in some circumstances a state has the constitutional power to override that right in order to protect citizens from mistaken but irrevocable acts of self-destruction. States may be allowed to prevent assisted suicide by people who—it is plausible to think—would later be grateful if they were prevented from dying.

Introduction to "Assisted Suicide: The Philosophers' Brief" by Ronald Dworkin, *The New York Review of Books* 44, no. 5 (March 27, 1997): 41–47. Reprinted with permission from The New York Review of Books. Copyright © 1997 NYREV, Inc.

Editors' note: In June 1997 the Supreme Court decided two cases (*State of Washington* v. *Glucksberg* and *Vacco* v. *Quill*) posing the question whether dying patients have a right to physician-assisted suicide. We present here the amicus curiae brief of six moral philosophers, with an introduction by Ronald Dworkin.

*In November 1997, Oregon voters rejected Measure 51, which would have reversed Measure 16 (approved by the voters in 1994), thereby legalizing physician-assisted suicide in that state.

That two-step argument would justify a state's protecting a disappointed adolescent from himself. It would equally plainly not justify forcing a competent dying patient to live in agony a few weeks longer. People will of course disagree about the cases in between these extremes, and if the Court adopted this argument, the federal courts would no doubt be faced with a succession of cases in years to come testing whether, for example, it is plausible to assume that a desperately crippled patient in constant pain but with years to live, who has formed a settled and repeatedly stated wish to die, would one day be glad he was forced to stay alive. But though two justices dwelled, during the oral argument, on the unappealing prospect of a series of such cases coming before the courts, it seems better that the courts do assume that burden, which they could perhaps mitigate through careful rulings, than that they be relieved of it at the cost of such terrible suffering. The practical version of the slippery slope argument is more complex. If assisted suicide were permitted in principle, every state would presumably adopt regulations to insure that a patient's decision for suicide is informed, competent, and free. But many people fear that such regulations could not be adequately enforced, and that particularly vulnerable patients—poor patients dying in overcrowded hospitals that had scarce resources, for example—might be pressured or hustled into a decision for death they would not otherwise make. The evidence suggests, however, that such patients might be better rather than less well protected if assisted suicide were legalized with appropriate safeguards.

More of them could then benefit from relief that is already available—illegally—to more fortunate people who have established relationships with doctors willing to run the risks of helping them to die. The current two-tier system—a chosen death and an end of pain outside the law for those with connections and stony refusals for most other people—is one of the greatest scandals of contemporary medical practice. The sense many middle-class people have that if necessary their own doctor "will know what to do" helps to explain why the political pressure is not stronger for a fairer and more open system in which the law acknowledges for everyone what influential people now expect for themselves.

For example, in a recent study in the State of Washington, which guaranteed respondents anonymity, 26 percent of doctors surveyed said they had received explicit requests for help in dying, and had provided, overall, lethal prescriptions to 24 percent of patients requesting them.[3] In other studies, 40 percent of Michigan oncologists surveyed reported that patients had initiated requests for death, 18 percent said they had participated in assisted suicide, and 4 percent in "active euthanasia"—injecting lethal drugs themselves. In San Francisco, 53 percent of the 1,995 responding physicians said they had granted an AIDS patient's request for suicide assistance at least once.[4] These statistics approach the rates at which doctors help patients die in Holland, where assisted suicide is in effect legal.

The most important benefit of legalized assisted suicide for poor patients however, might be better care while they live. For though the medical experts cited in various briefs disagreed sharply about the percentage of terminal cases in which pain can be made tolerable through advanced and expensive palliative techniques, they did not disagree that a great many patients do not receive the relief they could have. The Solicitor General who urged the Court to reverse the lower court judgments conceded in the oral argument that 25 percent of terminally ill patients actually do die in pain. That appalling figure is the result of several factors, including medical ignorance and fear of liability, inadequate hospital funding, and (as the Solicitor General suggested) the failure of insurers and health care programs to cover the cost of special hospice care. Better training in palliative medicine, and legislation requiring such coverage, would obviously improve the situation, but it seems perverse to argue that the patients who would be helped were better pain management available must die horribly because it is not; and, as Justice Breyer pointed out, the number of patients in that situation might well increase as medical costs continue to escalate.

According to several briefs, moreover, patients whose pain is either uncontrollable or uncontrolled are often "terminally sedated"—intravenous drugs (usually barbiturates or benzodiazepenes) are injected to induce a pharmacologic coma during which the patient is given neither water nor nutrition and dies sooner than he otherwise would.[5] Terminal sedation is widely accepted as legal, though it advances death.[6] But it is not subject to regulations nearly as stringent as those that a state forced to allow assisted suicide would enact, because such regulations would presumably include a requirement that hospitals, before accepting any request for assistance in suicide, must demonstrate that effective medical care including state-of-the art pain management had been offered. The guidelines recently published by a network of ethics committees in the Bay Area of California, for example, among other stringent safeguards, provide that a primary care physician who receives a request for suicide must make an initial referral to a hospice program or to a physician experienced in palliative care, and certify in a formal report filed in a state registry, signed by an independent second physician with expertise in such care, that the best available pain relief has been offered to the patient.[7]

Doctors and hospitals anxious to avoid expense would have very little incentive to begin a process that would focus attention on their palliative care practices. They would be more likely to continue the widespread practice of relatively inexpensive terminal care which is supplemented, perhaps, with terminal sedation. It is at least possible, however, that patients' knowledge of the possibility of assisted suicide would make it more difficult for such doctors to continue as before. That is the view of the Coalition of Hospice Professionals, who said, in their own amicus brief, "Indeed, removing legal bans on suicide assistance will enhance the opportunity for advanced hospice care for all patients because regulation of physician-assisted suicide would mandate that all palliative measures be exhausted as a condition precedent to assisted suicide."

So neither version of the slippery slope argument seems very strong. It is nevertheless understandable that Supreme Court justices are reluctant, particularly given how little experience we have so far with legalized assisted suicide, to declare that all but one of the states must change their laws to allow a practice many citizens think abominable and sacrilegious. But as the philosophers' brief that follows emphasizes, the Court is in an unusually difficult position. If it closes the door to a constitutional right to assisted suicide it will do substantial damage to constitutional practice and precedent, as well as to thousands of people in great suffering. It would face a dilemma in justifying any such decision, because it would be forced to choose between the two unappealing strategies that the brief describes.

The first strategy—declaring that terminally ill patients in great pain do not have a constitutional right to control their own deaths, even in principle—seems alien to our constitutional system, as the Solicitor General himself insisted in the oral argument. It would also undermine a variety of the Court's own past decisions, including the carefully constructed position on abortion set out in its 1993 decision in Casey. Indeed some amicus briefs took the occasion of the assisted suicide cases to criticize the abortion decisions—a brief filed on behalf of Senator Orrin Hatch of Utah and Representatives Henry Hyde of Illinois and Charles Canady of Florida, for example, declared that the abortion decisions were "of questionable legitimacy and even more questionable prudence." Protecting the abortion rulings was presumably one of the aims of the Clinton administration in arguing, through the Solicitor General, for the second strategy instead.

The first strategy would create an even more evident inconsistency within the practice of terminal medicine itself. Since the Cruzan decision discussed in the brief, lawyers have generally assumed that the Court would protect the right of any competent patient to have life sustaining equipment removed from his body even though he would then die. In the oral argument, several justices suggested a "common-sense" distinction between the moral significance of acts, on the one hand, and omissions, on the other. This distinction, they suggested, would justify a constitutional distinction between prescribing lethal pills and removing life support; for, in their view, removing support is only a matter of "letting nature take its course," while prescribing pills is an active intervention that brings death sooner than natural processes would.

The discussion of this issue in the philosophers' brief is therefore particularly significant. The brief insists that such suggestions wholly misunderstand the "common-sense" distinction, which is not between acts and omissions, but between acts or omissions that are designed to cause death and those that are not. One justice suggested that a patient who insists that life support be disconnected is not committing suicide. That is wrong: he is committing suicide if he aims at death, as most such patients do, just as someone whose wrist is cut in an accident is committing suicide if he refuses to try to stop the bleeding. The distinction between acts that aim at death and those that do not cannot justify a constitutional distinction between assisting in suicide and terminating life support. Some doctors, who stop life support only because the patient so demands, do not aim at death. But neither do doctors who prescribe lethal pills only for the same reason, and hope that the patient does not take them. And many doctors who terminate life support obviously do aim at death, including those who deny nutrition during terminal sedation, because denying nutrition is designed to hasten death, not to relieve pain.

There are equally serious objections, however, to the second strategy the philosophers' brief discusses. This strategy concedes a general right to assisted suicide but holds that states have the power to judge that the risks of allowing any exercise of that right are too great. It is obviously dangerous for the Court to allow a state to deny a constitutional right on the ground that the state lacks the will or resource to enforce safeguards if it is exercised, particularly when the case for the practical version of the "slippery slope" objection seems so weak and has been little examined.

NOTES

1. *State of Washington et al.* v. *Glucksberg et al.* and *Vacco et al.* v. *Quill et al.,* argued January 8, 1997.
2. I described the circuit court decisions in an earlier article, "Sex and Death in the Courts," *The New York Review,* August 8, 1996.
3. Anthony L. Back et al., "Physician-Assisted Suicide and Euthanasia in Washington State," *Journal of the American Medical Association,* Volume 275, No. 2, pp. 919, 920, 922 (1996).
4. See David I. Doukas et al., "Attitudes and Behaviors on Physician Assisted Death: A Study of Michigan Oncologists," *Clinical Oncology,* Volume 13, p. 1055 (1995); and L. Slome et al., "Attitudes Toward Assisted Suicide in AIDS: A Five Year Comparison Study," conference abstract now available on the World Wide Web (1996). The amicus brief of the Association of Law School Professors offers other statistics to the same effect taken from other states and from nurses.
5. According to one respondent's brief, "Despite some imprecision in the empirical evidence, it has been estimated that between 5 percent and 52 percent of dying patients entering home palliative care units have been terminally sedated." The brief cites Paul Rousseau, "Terminal Sedation in the Care of Dying Patients," *Archives of Internal Medicine,* Volume 156, p. 1785 (1996).
6. The amicus brief of the Coalition of Hospice Professionals raised a frightening question about terminal sedation. "Unfortunately, while a terminally sedated patient exhibits an outwardly peaceful appearance, medical science cannot verify that the individual ceases to experience pain and suffering. To the contrary, studies of individuals who have been anaesthetized (with the same kinds of drugs used in terminal sedation) for surgery (and who are in a deeper comatose state than terminally sedated patients since their breathing must be sustained by a respirator) have demonstrated that painful stimuli applied to the patient will cause a significant increase in brain activity, even though there is no external physical response." See, e.g., Orlando R. Hung et al., "Thiopental Pharmacodynamics: Quantitation of Clinical and Electroencephalographic Depth of Anesthesia," *Anesthesiology,* Volume 77, p. 237 (1992).
7. *BANEC-Generated Guidelines for Comprehensive Care of the Terminally Ill.* Bay Area Network of Ethics Committees, September 1996.

THE PHILOSOPHERS' BRIEF

Ronald Dworkin, Thomas Nagel, Robert Nozick, John Rawls, Thomas Scanlon, and Judith Jarvis Thomson

Amici are six moral and political philosophers who differ on many issues of public morality and policy. They are united, however, in their conviction that respect for fundamental principles of liberty and justice, as well as for the American constitutional tradition, requires that the decisions of the Courts of Appeals be affirmed.

INTRODUCTION AND SUMMARY OF ARGUMENT

These cases do not invite or require the Court to make moral, ethical, or religious judgments about how people should approach or confront their death or about when it is ethically appropriate to hasten one's own death or to ask others for help in doing so. On the contrary, they ask the Court to recognize that individuals have a constitutionally protected interest in making those grave judgments for themselves, free from the imposition of any religious or philosophical orthodoxy by court or legislature. States have a constitutionally legitimate interest in protecting individuals from irrational, ill-informed, pressured, or unstable decisions to hasten their own death. To that end, states may regulate and limit the assistance that doctors may give individuals who express a wish to die. But states may not deny people in the position of the patient-plaintiffs in these cases the opportunity to demonstrate, through whatever reasonable procedures the state might institute— even procedures that err on the side of caution—that their decision to die is indeed informed, stable, and fully free. Denying that opportunity to terminally ill patients who are in agonizing pain or otherwise doomed to an existence they regard as intolerable could only be justified on the basis of a religious or ethical conviction about the value or meaning of life itself. Our Constitution forbids government to impose such convictions on its citizens.

Petitioners [i.e., the state authorities of Washington and New York] and the amici who support them offer two contradictory arguments. Some deny that the patient-plaintiffs have any constitutionally protected liberty interest in hastening their own deaths. But that liberty interest flows directly from this Court's previous decisions. It flows from the right of people to make their own decisions about matters "involving the most intimate and personal choices a person may make in a lifetime, choices central to personal dignity and autonomy." *Planned Parenthood* v. *Casey,* 505 U.S. 833, 851 (1992).

The Solicitor General, urging reversal in support of Petitioners, recognizes that the patient-plaintiffs do have a constitutional liberty interest at stake in these cases. *See* Brief for the United States as Amicus Curiae Supporting Petitioners at 12, *Washington* v. *Vacco* (hereinafter Brief for the United States) ("The term 'liberty' in the Due Process Clause . . . is broad enough to encompass an interest on the part of terminally ill, mentally competent adults in obtaining relief from the kind of suffering experienced by the plaintiffs in this case, which includes not only severe physical pain, but also the despair and distress that comes from physical deterioration and the inability to control basic bodily functions."); *see also id.* at 13 ("*Cruzan* . . . supports the conclusion that a liberty interest is at stake in this case.").

The Solicitor General nevertheless argues that Washington and New York properly ignored this profound interest when they required the patient-plaintiffs to live on in circumstances they found intolerable. He argues that a state may simply declare that it is unable to devise a regulatory scheme that would adequately protect patients whose desire to die might be ill informed or unstable or foolish or not fully free, and that a state may therefore fall back on a blanket prohibition. This Court has never accepted that patently dangerous rationale for denying protection altogether to a conceded fundamental constitutional interest. It would be a serious mistake to do so now. If that rationale were accepted, an interest acknowledged to be constitutionally protected would be rendered empty.

ARGUMENT

I. THE LIBERTY INTEREST ASSERTED HERE IS PROTECTED BY THE DUE PROCESS CLAUSE

The Due Process Clause of the Fourteenth Amendment protects the liberty interest asserted by the patient-plaintiffs here.

Certain decisions are momentous in their impact on the character of a person's life decisions about religious faith, political and moral allegiance, marriage, procreation, and death, for example. Such deeply personal decisions pose controversial questions about how and why human life has value. In a free society, individuals must be allowed to make those decisions for themselves, out of their own faith, conscience, and convictions. This Court has insisted, in a variety of contexts and circumstances, that this great freedom is among those protected by the Due Process Clause as essential to a community of "ordered liberty." *Palko* v. *Connecticut*, 302 U.S. 319, 325 (1937). In its recent decision in *Planned Parenthood* v. *Casey*, 505 U.S. 833, 851 (1992), the Court offered a paradigmatic statement of that principle:

> matters [] involving the most intimate and personal choices a person may make in a lifetime, choices central to a person's dignity and autonomy, are central to the liberty protected by the Fourteenth Amendment.

That declaration reflects an idea underlying many of our basic constitutional protections. As the Court explained in *West Virginia State Board of Education* v. *Barnette*, 319 U.S. 624, 642 (1943):

> If there is any fixed star in our constitutional constellation, it is that no official . . . can prescribe what shall be orthodox in politics, nationalism, religion, or other matters of opinion or force citizens to confess by word or act their faith therein.

A person's interest in following his own convictions at the end of life is so central a part of the more general right to make "intimate and personal choices" for himself that a failure to protect that particular interest would undermine the general right altogether. Death is, for each of us, among the most significant events of life. As the Chief Justice said in *Cruzan* v. *Missouri*, 497 U.S. 261, 281 (1990), "[t]he choice between life and death is a deeply personal decision of obvious and overwhelming finality." Most of us see death—whatever we think will follow it—as the final act of life's drama, and we want that last act to reflect our own convictions, those we have tried to live by, not the convictions of others forced on us in our most vulnerable moment.

Different people, of different religious and ethical beliefs, embrace very different convictions about which way of dying confirms and which contradicts the value of their lives. Some fight against death with every weapon their doctors can devise. Others will do nothing to hasten death even if they pray it will come soon. Still others, including the patient-plaintiffs in these cases, want to end their lives when they think that living on, in the only way they can, would disfigure rather than enhance the lives they had created. Some people make the latter choice not just to escape pain. Even if it were possible to eliminate all pain for a dying patient—and frequently that is not possible—that would not end or even much alleviate the anguish some would feel at remaining alive, but intubated, helpless, and often sedated near oblivion.

None of these dramatically different attitudes about the meaning of death can be dismissed as irrational. None should be imposed, either by the pressure of doctors or relatives or by the fiat of government, on people who reject it. Just as it would be intolerable for government to dictate that doctors never be permitted to try to keep someone alive as long as possible, when that is what the patient wishes, so it is intolerable for government to dictate that doctors may never, under any circumstances, help someone to die who believes that further life means only degradation. The Constitution insists that people must be free to make these deeply personal decisions for themselves and must not be forced to end their lives in a way that appalls them, just because that is what some majority thinks proper.

II. THIS COURT'S DECISIONS IN *CASEY* AND *CRUZAN* COMPEL RECOGNITION OF A LIBERTY INTEREST HERE

A. Casey *Supports the Liberty Interest Asserted Here.* In *Casey*, this Court, in holding that a state cannot constitutionally proscribe abortion in all cases, reiterated that the Constitution protects a sphere of autonomy in which individuals must be permitted to make certain decisions for themselves. The Court began its analysis by pointing out that "[a]t the heart of liberty is the right to define one's own concept of existence, of meaning, of the universe, and of the mystery of human life." 505 U.S. at 851. Choices flowing out of these conceptions, on matters "involving the most intimate and personal choices a person may make in a lifetime, choices central to personal dignity and autonomy, are central to the liberty protected by the Fourteenth Amendment." *Id.* "Beliefs about these matters," the Court continued, "could not define the attributes of personhood were they formed under compulsion of the State." *Id.*

In language pertinent to the liberty interest asserted here, the Court explained why decisions about abortion fall within this category of "personal and intimate" decisions. A decision whether or not to have an abortion, "originat[ing] within the zone of conscience and belief," involves conduct in which "the liberty of the woman is at stake in a sense unique to the human condition and so unique to the law." *Id.* at 852. As such, the decision necessarily involves the very "destiny of the woman" and is inevitably "shaped to a large extent on her own conception of her spiritual imperatives and her place in society." *Id.* Precisely because of these characteristics of the decision, "the State is [not] entitled to proscribe [abortion] in all instances." *Id.* Rather, to allow a total prohibition on abortion would be to permit a state to impose one conception of the meaning and value of human existence on all individuals. This the Constitution forbids.

The Solicitor General nevertheless argues that the right to abortion could be supported on grounds other than this autonomy principle, grounds that would not apply here. He argues, for example, that the abortion right might flow from the great burden an unwanted child imposes on its mother's life. Brief for the United States at 14–15. But whether or not abortion rights could be defended on such grounds, they were not the grounds on which this Court in fact relied. To the contrary, the Court explained at length that the right flows from the constitutional protection accorded all individuals to "define one's own concept of existence, of meaning, of the universe, and of the mystery of human life." *Casey*, 505 U.S. at 851.

The analysis in *Casey* compels the conclusion that the patient-plaintiffs have a liberty interest in this case that a state cannot burden with a blanket prohibition. Like a woman's decision whether to have an abortion, a decision to die involves one's very "destiny" and inevitably will be "shaped to a large extent on [one's] own conception of [one's] spiritual imperatives and [one's] place in society." *Id.* at 852. Just as a blanket prohibition on abortion would involve the improper imposition of one conception of the meaning and value of human existence on all individuals, so too would a blanket prohibition on assisted suicide. The liberty interest asserted here cannot be rejected without undermining the rationale of *Casey*. Indeed, the lower court opinions in the Washington case expressly recognized the parallel between the liberty interest in *Casey* and the interest asserted here. *See Compassion in Dying* v. *Washington*, 79 F.3d 790, 801(9th Cir. 1996) (en banc) ("In deciding right-to-die cases, we are guided by the Court's approach to the abortion cases. *Casey* in particular provides a powerful precedent, for in that case the Court had the opportunity to evaluate its past decisions and to determine whether to adhere to its original judgment."), *aff'g.* 850 F. Supp. 1454, 1459 (W. D. Wash. 1994) ("[T]he reasoning in *Casey* [is] highly instructive and almost prescriptive . . ."). This Court should do the same.

B. Cruzan *Supports the Liberty Interest Asserted Here.* We agree with the Solicitor General that this Court's decision in "*Cruzan* . . . supports the conclusion that a liberty interest is at stake in this case." Brief for the United States at 8. Petitioners, however, insist that the present cases can be distinguished because the right at issue in *Cruzan* was limited to a right to reject an unwanted invasion of one's body.[1] But this Court repeatedly has held that in appropriate circumstances a state may require individuals to accept unwanted invasions of the body. *See, e.g., Schmerber* v. *California*, 384 U.S. 757 (1966) (extraction of blood sample from individual suspected of driving while intoxicated, notwithstanding defendant's objection, does not violate privilege against self-incrimination or other constitutional rights); *Jacobson* v. *Massachusetts*, 197 U.S. 11 (1905) (upholding compulsory vaccination for smallpox as reasonable regulation for protection of public health).

The liberty interest at stake in *Cruzan* was a more profound one. If a competent patient has a constitutional right to refuse life-sustaining treatment, then, the Court implied, the state could not override that right. The regulations upheld in *Cruzan* were designed only to ensure that the individual's wishes were ascertained correctly. Thus, if *Cruzan* implies a right of competent patients to refuse life-sustaining treatment, that implication must be understood as resting not simply on a right to refuse bodily invasions but on the more profound right to refuse medical intervention when what is at stake is a momentous personal decision, such as the timing and manner of one's death. In her concurrence, Justice O'Connor expressly recognized that the right at issue involved a "deeply personal decision" that is "inextricably intertwined" with our notion of "self-determination." 497 U.S. at 287–89.

Cruzan also supports the proposition that a state may not burden a terminally ill patient's liberty interest in determining the time and manner of his death by prohibiting doctors from terminating life support. Seeking to distinguish *Cruzan*, Petitioners insist that a state may nevertheless burden that right in a different way by forbidding doctors to assist in the suicide of patients who are not on life-support machinery. They argue that doctors who remove life support are only allowing a natural process to end in death whereas doctors who prescribe lethal drugs are intervening to cause death. So, according to this argument, a state has an independent justification for forbidding doctors to assist in suicide that it does not have for forbidding them to remove life support. In the former case though not the latter, it is said, the state forbids an act of killing that is morally much more problematic than merely letting a patient die.

This argument is based on a misunderstanding of the pertinent moral principles. It is certainly true that when a patient does not wish to die, different acts, each of which foreseeably results in his death, nevertheless have very different moral status. When several patients need organ transplants and organs are scarce, for example, it is morally permissible for a doctor to deny an organ to one patient, even though he will die without it, in order to give it to another. But it is certainly not permissible for a doctor to kill one patient in order to use his organs to save another. The morally significant difference between those two acts is not, however, that killing is a positive act and not providing an organ is a mere omission, or that killing someone is worse than merely allowing a "natural" process to result

in death. It would be equally impermissible for a doctor to let an injured patient bleed to death, or to refuse antibiotics to a patient with pneumonia—in each case the doctor would have allowed death to result from a "natural" process—in order to make his organs available for transplant to others. A doctor violates his patient's rights whether the doctor acts or refrains from acting, against the patient's wishes, in a way that is designed to cause death.

When a competent patient does want to die, the moral situation is obviously different, because then it makes no sense to appeal to the patient's right not to be killed as a reason why an act designed to cause his death is impermissible. From the patient's point of view, there is no morally pertinent difference between a doctor's terminating treatment that keeps him alive, if that is what he wishes, and a doctor's helping him to end his own life by providing lethal pills he may take himself, when ready, if that is what he wishes—except that the latter may be quicker and more humane. Nor is that a pertinent difference from the doctor's point of view. If and when it is permissible for him to act with death in view, it does not matter which of those two means he and his patient choose. If it is permissible for a doctor deliberately to withdraw medical treatment in order to allow death to result from a natural process, then it is equally permissible for him to help his patient hasten his own death more actively, if that is the patient's express wish.

It is true that some doctors asked to terminate life support are reluctant and do so only in deference to a patient's right to compel them to remove unwanted invasions of his body. But other doctors, who believe that their most fundamental professional duty is to act in the patient's interests and that, in certain circumstances, it is in their patient's best interests to die, participate willingly in such decisions: they terminate life support to cause death because they know that is what their patient wants. *Cruzan* implied that a state may not absolutely prohibit a doctor from deliberately causing death, at the patient's request, in that way and for that reason. If so, then a state may not prohibit doctors from deliberately using more direct and often more humane means to the same end when that is what a patient prefers. The fact that failing to provide life-sustaining treatment may be regarded as "only letting nature take its course" is no more morally significant in this context, when the patient wishes to die, than in the other, when he wishes to live. Whether a doctor turns off a respirator in accordance with the patient's request or prescribes pills that a patient may take when he is ready to kill himself, the doctor acts with the same intention: to help the patient die.

The two situations do differ in one important respect. Since patients have a right not to have life-support machinery attached to their bodies, they have, in principle, a right to compel its removal. But that is not true in the case of assisted suicide: patients in certain circumstances have a right that the state not forbid doctors to assist in their deaths, but they have no right to compel a doctor to assist them. The right in question, that is, is only a right to the help of a willing doctor.

III. STATE INTERESTS DO NOT JUSTIFY A CATEGORICAL PROHIBITION ON ALL ASSISTED SUICIDE

The Solicitor General concedes that "a competent, terminally ill adult has a constitutionally cognizable liberty interest in avoiding the kind of suffering experienced by the plaintiffs in this case." Brief for the United States at 8. He agrees that this interest extends not only to avoiding pain, but to avoiding an existence the patient believes to be one of intolerable indignity or incapacity as well. *Id.* at 12. The Solicitor General argues, however, that states nevertheless have the right to "override" this liberty interest altogether, because a state could reasonably conclude that allowing doctors to assist in suicide, even under the most stringent regulations and procedures that could be devised, would unreasonably endanger the lives of a number of patients who might ask for death in circumstances when it is plainly not in their interests to die or when their consent has been improperly obtained.

This argument is unpersuasive, however, for at least three reasons. *First*, in *Cruzan*, this Court noted that its various decisions supported the recognition of a general liberty interest in refusing medical treatment, even when such refusal could result in death. 497 U.S. at 278–79. The various risks described by the Solicitor General apply equally to those situations. For instance, a patient kept alive only by an elaborate and disabling life-support

system might well become depressed, and doctors might be equally uncertain whether the depression is curable: such a patient might decide for death only because he has been advised that he will die soon anyway or that he will never live free of the burdensome apparatus, and either diagnosis might conceivably be mistaken. Relatives or doctors might subtly or crudely influence that decision, and state provision for the decision may (to the same degree in this case as if it allowed assisted suicide) be thought to encourage it.

Yet there has been no suggestion that states are incapable of addressing such dangers through regulation. In fact, quite the opposite is true. In *McKay* v. *Bergstedt*, 106 Nev. 808, 801 P.2d 617 (1990), for example, the Nevada Supreme Court held that "competent adult patients desiring to refuse or discontinue medical treatment" must be examined by two nonattending physicians to determine whether the patient is mentally competent, understands his prognosis and treatment options, and appears free of coercion or pressure in making his decision. *Id.* at 827–28, 801 P.2d at 630. See also: *id.* (in the case of terminally ill patients with natural life expectancy of less than six months, [a] patient's right of self-determination shall be deemed to prevail over state interests, whereas [a] non-terminal patient's decision to terminate life-support systems must first be weighed against relevant state interests by trial judge); [and] *In re Farrell*, 108 N.J. 335, 354, 529 A.2d 404, 413 (1987) ([which held that a] terminally-ill patient requesting termination of life-support must be determined to be competent and properly informed about [his] prognosis, available treatment options and risks, and to have made decision voluntarily and without coercion). Those protocols served to guard against precisely the dangers that the Solicitor General raises. The case law contains no suggestion that such protocols are inevitably insufficient to prevent deaths that should have been prevented.

Indeed, the risks of mistake are overall greater in the case of terminating life support. *Cruzan* implied that a state must allow individuals to make such decisions through an advance directive stipulating either that life support be terminated (or not initiated) in described circumstances when the individual was no longer competent to make such a decision himself, or that a designated proxy be allowed to make that decision. All the risks just described are present when the decision is made through or pursuant to such an advance directive, and a grave further risk is added: that the directive, though still in force, no longer represents the wishes of the patient. The patient might have changed his mind before he became incompetent, though he did not change the directive, or his proxy may make a decision that the patient would not have made himself if still competent. In *Cruzan*, this Court held that a state may limit these risks through reasonable regulation. It did not hold—or even suggest—that a state may avoid them through a blanket prohibition that, in effect, denies the liberty interest altogether.

Second, nothing in the record supports the [Solicitor General's] conclusion that no system of rules and regulations could adequately reduce the risk of mistake. As discussed above, the experience of states in adjudicating requests to have life-sustaining treatment removed indicates the opposite. The Solicitor General has provided no persuasive reason why the same sort of procedures could not be applied effectively in the case of a competent individual's request for physician-assisted suicide.

Indeed, several very detailed schemes for regulating physician-assisted suicide have been submitted to the voters of some states and one has been enacted. In addition, concerned groups, including a group of distinguished professors of law and other professionals, have drafted and defended such schemes. *See, e.g.*, Charles H. Baron, *et al.*, *A Model State Act to Authorize and Regulate Physician-Assisted Suicide*, 33 Harv. J. Legis. 1 (1996). Such draft statutes propose a variety of protections and review procedures designed to insure against mistakes, and neither Washington nor New York attempted to show that such schemes would be porous or ineffective. Nor does the Solicitor General's brief: it relies instead mainly on flat and conclusory statements. It cites a New York Task Force report, written before the proposals just described were drafted, whose findings have been widely disputed and were implicitly rejected in the opinion of the Second Circuit below. *See generally Quill v. Vacco*, 80 F.3d 716 (2d Cir. 1996). The weakness of the Solicitor General's argument is signaled by his strong reliance on the experience in the Netherlands which, in effect, allows assisted suicide pursuant to published guidelines. Brief for the United States at 23–24. The Dutch guidelines are more permissive than the proposed and model American statutes, however. The Solicitor General deems the Dutch practice of ending the lives of people like neonates who cannot consent particularly noteworthy, for example, but that practice could easily and effectively be made illegal by any state regulatory scheme without violating the Constitution.

The Solicitor General's argument would perhaps have more force if the question before the Court were simply whether a state has any rational basis for an absolute prohibition; if that were the question, then it might be enough to call attention to risks a state might well deem not worth running. But as the Solicitor General concedes, the question here is a very different one: whether a state has interests sufficiently compelling to allow it to take the extraordinary step of altogether refusing the exercise of a liberty interest of constitutional dimension. In those circumstances, the burden is plainly on the state to demonstrate that the risk of mistakes is very high, and that no alternative to complete prohibition would adequately and effectively reduce those risks. Neither of the Petitioners has made such a showing.

Nor could they. The burden of proof on any state attempting to show this would be very high. Consider, for example, the burden a state would have to meet to show that it was entitled altogether to ban public speeches in favor of unpopular causes because it could not guarantee, either by regulations short of an outright ban or by increased police protection, that such speeches would not provoke a riot that would result in serious injury or death to an innocent party. Or that it was entitled to deny those accused of crime the procedural rights that the Constitution guarantees, such as the right to a jury trial, because the security risk those rights would impose on the community would be too great. One can posit extreme circumstances in which some such argument would succeed. *See, e.g., Korematsu v. United States*, 323 U.S., 214 (1944) (permitting United States to detain individuals of Japanese ancestry during wartime). But these circumstances would be extreme indeed, and the *Korematsu* ruling has been widely and severely criticized.

Third, it is doubtful whether the risks the Solicitor General cites are even of the right character to serve as justification for an absolute prohibition on the exercise of an important liberty interest. The risks fall into two groups. The first is the risk of medical mistake, including a misdiagnosis of competence or terminal illness. To be sure, no scheme of regulation, no matter how rigorous, can altogether guarantee that medical mistakes will not be made. But the Constitution does not allow a state to deny patients a great variety of important choices, for which informed consent is properly deemed necessary, just because the information on which the consent is given may, in spite of the most strenuous efforts to avoid mistake, be wrong. Again, these identical risks are present in decisions to terminate life support, yet they do not justify an absolute prohibition on the exercise of the right.

The second group consists of risks that a patient will be unduly influenced by considerations that the state might deem it not in his best interests to be swayed by, for example, the feelings and views of close family members. Brief for the United States at 20. But what a patient regards as proper grounds for such a decision normally reflects exactly the judgments of personal ethics—of why his life is important and what affects its value—that patients have a crucial liberty interest in deciding for themselves. Even people who are dying have a right to hear and, if they wish, act on what others might wish to tell or suggest or even hint to them, and it would be dangerous to suppose that a state may prevent this on the ground that it knows better than its citizens when they should be moved by or yield to particular advice or suggestion in the exercise of their right to make fateful personal decisions for themselves. It is not a good reply that some people may not decide as they really wish—as they would decide, for example, if free from the "pressure" of others. That possibility could hardly justify the most serious pressure of all—the criminal law which tells them that they may not decide for death if they need the help of a doctor in dying, no matter how firmly they wish it.

There is a fundamental infirmity in the Solicitor General's argument. He asserts that a state may reasonably judge that the risk of "mistake" to some persons justifies a prohibition that not only risks but insures and even aims at what would undoubtedly be a vastly greater number of "mistakes" of the opposite kind—preventing many thousands of competent people who think that it disfigures their lives to continue living, in the only way left to them, from escaping that—to them—terrible injury. A state grievously and irreversibly harms such people when it prohibits that escape. The Solicitor General's argument may seem plausible to those who do not agree that individuals are harmed by being forced to live on in pain and what they regard as indignity. But many other people plainly do think that such individuals are harmed, and a state may not take one side in that essentially ethical or religious controversy as its justification for denying a crucial liberty.

Of course, a state has important interests that justify regulating physician-assisted suicide. It may be legitimate for a state to deny an opportunity for assisted suicide when it acts in what it reasonably judges to be the best interests of the potential suicide, and when its judgment on that issue does not rest on contested judgments about "matters involving the most intimate and personal choices a person may make in a lifetime, choices central to personal dignity and autonomy." *Casey,* 505 U.S. at 851. A state might assert, for example, that people who are not terminally ill, but who have formed a desire to die, are, as a group, very likely later to be grateful if they are prevented from taking their own lives. It might then claim that it is legitimate, out of concern for such people, to deny any of them a doctor's assistance [in taking their own lives].

This Court need not decide now the extent to which such paternalistic interests might override an individual's liberty interest. No one can plausibly claim, however—and it is noteworthy that neither Petitioners nor the Solicitor General does claim—that any such prohibition could serve the interests of any significant number of terminally ill patients. On the contrary, any paternalistic justification for an absolute prohibition of assistance to such patients would of necessity appeal to a widely contested religious or ethical conviction many of them, including the patient-plaintiffs, reject. Allowing *that* justification to prevail would vitiate the liberty interest.

Even in the case of terminally ill patients, a state has a right to take all reasonable measures to insure that a patient requesting such assistance has made an informed, competent, stable and uncoerced decision. It is plainly legitimate for a state to establish procedures through which professional and administrative judgments can be made about these matters, and to forbid doctors to assist in suicide when its reasonable procedures have not been satisfied. States may be permitted considerable leeway in designing such procedures. They may be permitted, within reason, to err on what they take to be the side of caution. But they may not use the bare possibility of error as justification for refusing to establish any procedures at all and relying instead on a flat prohibition.

CONCLUSION

Each individual has a right to make the "most intimate and personal choices central to personal dignity and autonomy." That right encompasses the right to exercise some control over the time and manner of one's death.

The patient-plaintiffs in these cases were all mentally competent individuals in the final phase of terminal illness and died within months of filing their claims.

Jane Doe described how her advanced cancer made even the most basic bodily functions such as swallowing, coughing, and yawning extremely painful and that it was "not possible for [her] to reduce [her] pain to an acceptable level of comfort and to retain an alert state." Faced with such circumstances, she sought to be able to "discuss freely with [her] treating physician [her] intention of hastening [her] death through the consumption of drugs prescribed for that purpose." *Quill* v. *Vacco*, 80 F.2d 716, 720 (2d Cir. 1996) (quoting declaration of Jane Doe).

George A. Kingsley, in advanced stages of AIDS which included, among other hardships, the attachment of a tube to an artery in his chest which made even routine functions burdensome and the development of lesions on his brain, sought advice from his doctors regarding prescriptions which could hasten his impending death. *Id.*

Jane Roe, suffering from cancer since 1988, had been almost completely bedridden since 1993 and experienced constant pain which could not be alleviated by medication. After undergoing counseling for herself and her family, she desired to hasten her death by taking prescription drugs. *Compassion in Dying* v. *Washington*, 850 F. Supp. 1454, 1456 (1994).

John Doe, who had experienced numerous AIDS-related ailments since 1991, was "especially cognizant of the suffering imposed by a lingering terminal illness because he was the primary caregiver for his long-term companion who died of AIDS" and sought prescription drugs from his physician to hasten his own death after entering the terminal phase of AIDS. *Id.* at 1456–57.

James Poe suffered from emphysema which caused him "a constant sensation of suffocating" as well as a cardiac condition which caused severe leg pain. Connected to an oxygen tank at all times but unable to calm the panic reaction associated with his feeling of suffocation even with regular doses of morphine, Mr. Poe sought physician-assisted suicide. *Id.* at 1457.

A state may not deny the liberty claimed by the patient-plaintiffs in these cases without providing them an opportunity to demonstrate, in whatever way the state might reasonably think wise and necessary, that the conviction they expressed for an early death is competent, rational, informed, stable, and uncoerced.

Affirming the decisions by the Courts of Appeals would establish nothing more than that there is such a constitutionally protected right in principle. It would establish only that some individuals, whose decisions for suicide plainly cannot be dismissed as irrational or foolish or premature, must be accorded a reasonable opportunity to show that their decision for death is informed and free. It is not necessary to decide precisely which patients are entitled to that opportunity. If, on the other hand, this Court reverses the decisions below, its decision could only be justified by the momentous proposition—a proposition flatly in conflict with the spirit and letter of the Court's past decisions—that an American citizen does not, after all, have the right, even in principle, to live and die in the light of his own religious and ethical beliefs, his own convictions about why his life is valuable and where its value lies.

NOTE

1. In that case, the parents of Nancy Cruzan, a woman who was in a persistent vegetative state following an automobile accident, asked the Missouri courts to authorize doctors to end life support and therefore

her life. The Supreme Court held that Missouri was entitled to demand explicit evidence that Ms. Cruzan had made a decision that she would not wish to be kept alive in those circumstances, and to reject the evidence the family had offered as inadequate.

But a majority of justices assumed, for the sake of the argument, that a competent patient has a right to reject life-preserving treatment, and it is now widely assumed that the Court would so rule in an appropriate case.

EUTHANASIA: THE WAY WE DO IT, THE WAY THEY DO IT
End-of-Life Practices in the Developed World

Margaret P. Battin

Because we tend to be rather myopic in our discussions of death and dying, especially about the issues of active euthanasia and assisted suicide, it is valuable to place the question of how we go about dying in an international context. We do not always see that our own cultural norms may be quite different from those of other nations and that our background assumptions and actual practices differ dramatically—even when the countries in question are all developed industrial nations with similar cultural ancestries, religious traditions, and economic circumstances. I want to explore the three rather different approaches to end-of-life dilemmas prevalent in the United States, the Netherlands, and Germany—developments mirrored in Australia, Belgium, Switzerland, and elsewhere in the developed world—and consider how a society might think about which model of approach to dying is most appropriate for it.

THREE BASIC MODELS OF DYING

The Netherlands, Germany, and the United States are all advanced industrial democracies. They all

have sophisticated medical establishments and life expectancies over 75 years of age; their populations are all characterized by an increasing proportion of older persons. They are all in what has been called the fourth stage of the epidemiologic transition[1]—that stage of societal development in which it is no longer the case that the majority of the population dies of acute parasitic or infectious diseases, often with rapid, unpredictable onsets and sharp fatality curves (as was true in earlier and less developed societies); rather, in modern industrial societies, the majority of a population—as much as perhaps 70–80%—dies of degenerative diseases, especially delayed-degenerative diseases that are characterized by late, slow onset and extended decline. This is the case throughout the developed world. Accidents and suicide claim some, as do infectious diseases like AIDS, pneumonia, and influenza, but most people in highly industrialized countries die from heart disease (by no means always suddenly fatal); cancer; atherosclerosis; chronic obstructive pulmonary disease; diabetes; liver, kidney, or other organ disease; or degenerative neurological disorders. In the developed world, we die not so much from attack by outside diseases but from gradual disintegration. Thus, all three of these modern industrial countries—the United States, the Netherlands, and Germany—are alike in facing a common problem: how to deal with the characteristic new ways in which we die.

Reprinted from *Journal of Pain and Symptom Management* vol. 65, no. 5, Margaret Battin, "Euthanasia: The Way We Do It, the Way They Do It,"pp. 298–305, Copyright © 1991, with permission from the U.S. Cancer Pain Relief Committee.

Dealing with Dying in the United States

In the United States, we have come to recognize that the maximal extension of life-prolonging treatment in these late-life degenerative conditions is often inappropriate. Although we could keep the machines and tubes—the respirators, intravenous lines, feeding tubes—hooked up for extended periods, we recognize that this is inhumane, pointless, and financially impossible. Instead, as a society we have developed a number of mechanisms for dealing with these hopeless situations, all of which involve withholding or withdrawing various forms of treatment.

Some mechanisms for withholding or withdrawing treatments are exercised by the patient who is confronted by such a situation or who anticipates it. These include refusal of treatment, the patient-executed Do Not Resuscitate (DNR) order, the Living Will, and the Durable Power of Attorney. Others are mechanisms for decision by second parties about a patient who is no longer competent or never was competent, reflected in a long series of court cases from *Quinlan; Saikewicz; Spring; Eichner; Barber; Bartling; Conroy; Brophy;* the trio *Farrell, Peter,* and *Jobes,* to *Cruzan.* These cases delineate the precise circumstances under which it is appropriate to withhold or withdraw various forms of therapy, including respiratory support, chemotherapy, dialysis, antibiotics in intercurrent infections, and artificial nutrition and hydration. Thus, during the past quarter-century, roughly since *Quinlan* (1976), the U.S. has developed an impressive body of case law and state statutes that protects, permits, and facilitates the characteristic American strategy of dealing with end-of-life situations. These cases provide a framework for withholding or withdrawing treatment when physicians and family members believe there is no medical or moral point in going on. This has sometimes been termed *passive euthanasia;* more often, it is simply called *allowing to die.*

Indeed, "allowing to die" has become ubiquitous in the United States. For example, a 1988 study found that of the 85% of deaths in the United States that occurred in health care institutions, including hospitals, nursing homes, and other facilities, about 70% involved electively withholding some form of life-sustaining treatment.[2] A 1989 study found that 85–90% of critical care professionals said they were

withholding or withdrawing life-sustaining treatments from patients who were "deemed to have irreversible disease and are terminally ill."[3] A 1997 study of limits to life-sustaining care found that between 1987–88 and 1992–93, recommendations to withhold or withdraw life support prior to death increased from 51% to 90% in the intensive-care units studied.[4] Rates of withholding therapy such as ventilator support, surgery, and dialysis were found in yet another study to be substantial, and to increase with age.[5] A 1994/95 study of 167 intensive-care units—all the ICUs associated with U.S. training programs in critical care medicine or pulmonary and critical care medicine—found that in 75% of deaths, some form of care was withheld or withdrawn.[6] It has been estimated that 1.3 million American deaths a year follow decisions to withhold life support;[7] this is a majority of the just over 2 million American deaths per year.

In recent years, the legitimate use of withholding and withdrawing treatment has increasingly been understood to include practices likely or certain to result in death. The administration of escalating doses of morphine in a dying patient, which, it has been claimed, will depress respiration and so hasten death, is acceptable under the (Catholic) principle of double effect provided the medication is intended to relieve pain and merely foreseen but not intended to result in death; this practice is not considered killing or active hastening of death. The use of "terminal sedation," in which a patient dying in pain is sedated into unconsciousness while artificial nutrition and hydration are withheld, is also recognized as medically and legally acceptable; it too is understood as a form of "allowing to die," not active killing. With the single exception of Oregon, where physician-assisted suicide became legal in 1997,[8] withholding and withdrawing treatment and related forms of allowing to die are the only legally recognized ways we in the United States go about dealing with dying. A number of recent studies have shown that many physicians—in all states studied—do receive requests for assistance in suicide or active euthanasia and that a substantial number of these physicians have complied with one or more such requests; however, this more direct assistance in dying takes place entirely out of sight of the law. Except in Oregon, *allowing to die,* but not *causing to die,* has been the only legally protected alternative to maximal treatment legally recognized in the United States; it remains America's—and American medicine's—official posture in the face of death.

Dealing with Dying in the Netherlands

In the Netherlands, although the practice of withholding and withdrawing treatment is similar to that in the United States, voluntary active euthanasia and physician assistance in suicide are also available responses to end-of-life situations.[9] Active euthanasia is the more frequent form of assistance in dying and most discussion in the Netherlands has concerned it rather than assistance in suicide, though the conceptual difference is not regarded as great: many cases of what the Dutch term *voluntary active euthanasia* involve initial self-administration of the lethal dose by the patient but procurement of death by the physician, and many cases of what is termed *physician-assisted suicide* involve completion of the lethal process by the physician if a self-administered drug does not prove fully effective. Although until 2001 they were still technically illegal under statutory law, and even with legalization remain an "exception" to those provisions of the Dutch Penal Code which prohibit killing on request and intentional assistance in suicide, active euthanasia and assistance in suicide have long been widely regarded as legal, or rather *gedoogd*, legally "tolerated," and have in fact been deemed justified (not only nonpunishable) by the courts when performed by a physician if certain conditions were met. Voluntary active euthanasia (in the law, called "life-ending on request") and physician-assisted suicide are now fully legal by statute under these guidelines. Dutch law protects the physician who performs euthanasia or provides assistance in suicide from prosecution for homicide if these guidelines, known as the conditions of "due care," are met.

Over the years, the guidelines have been stated in various ways. They contain six central provisions:

1. that the patient's request be voluntary and well-considered;
2. that the patient be undergoing or about to undergo intolerable suffering, that is, suffering which is lasting and unbearable;
3. that all alternatives acceptable to the patient for relieving the suffering have been tried, and that the patient believes there is no other reasonable solution;
4. that the patient have full information about his situation and prospects;
5. that the physician consult with a second physician who has examined the patient and whose judgment can be expected to be independent;
6. that in performing euthanasia or assisting in suicide, the physician act with due care.

Of these criteria, it is the first that is held to be central: euthanasia may be performed only at the *voluntary* request of the patient. This criterion is also understood to require that the patient's request be a stable, enduring, reflective one—not the product of a transitory impulse. Every attempt is to be made to rule out depression, psychopathology, pressures from family members, unrealistic fears, and other factors compromising voluntariness, though depression is not in itself understood to preclude such choice. Euthanasia may be performed *only* by a physician, not by a nurse, family member, or other party.

In 1990, a comprehensive, nationwide study requested by the Dutch government, popularly known as the Remmelink Commission report, provided the first objective data about the incidence of euthanasia.[10] This study also provided information about other medical decisions at the end of life: withholding or withdrawal of treatment; the use of life-shortening doses of opioids for the control of pain; and direct termination, including not only voluntary active euthanasia and physician-assisted suicide but life-ending procedures not termed euthanasia. The Remmelink study was supplemented by a second empirical examination, focusing particularly carefully on the characteristics of patients and the nature of their euthanasia requests.[11] Five years later, the researchers from these two studies jointly conducted a major new nationwide study replicating much of the previous Remmelink inquiry, providing empirical data both about current practice in the Netherlands and change over a five-year period.[12] A third such study is to be published in fall 2003.

About 135,000 people die in the Netherlands every year, and of these deaths, about 30% are acute and unexpected, while about 70% are predictable and foreseen, usually the result of degenerative illness comparatively late in life. Of the total deaths in the Netherlands, about 20% involve decisions to withhold or withdraw treatment in situations where continuing treatment would probably have prolonged life; another 20% involve the "double effect" use of opioids to relieve pain but in dosages probably sufficient to shorten life.[13]

The 1990 study revealed that about 2,300 people, 1.8% of the total deaths in the Netherlands at that time, died by euthanasia—understood as the termination of the life of the patient at the patient's explicit and persistent request; close to another 400 people, 0.3% of the total, chose physician-assisted suicide. However, the study also revealed that another 0.8% of patients who died did so as the result of life-terminating procedures not technically called euthanasia, without explicit, current request. These cases, known as "the 1000 cases," unleashed highly exaggerated claims that patients were being killed against their wills. In fact, in about half of these cases, euthanasia had been previously discussed with the patient or the patient had expressed in a previous phase of the disease a wish for euthanasia if his or her suffering became unbearable ("Doctor, please don't let me suffer too long"); and in the other half, the patient was no longer competent and was near death, clearly suffering grievously although verbal contact had become impossible.[14] In 91% of these cases without explicit, current request, life was shortened by less than a week, and in 33% by less than a day.

By 1995, although the proportion of cases of assisted suicide had remained about the same, the proportion of cases of euthanasia had risen to about 2.4% (associated, the authors conjectured, with the aging of the population and an increase in the proportion of deaths due to cancer, that condition in which euthanasia is most frequent). However, the proportion of cases of life termination without current explicit request had declined slightly to 0.7%. In 1990, a total of 2.9% of all deaths had involved euthanasia and related practices; by 1995 this total was 3.3%. Not all cases are reported as required, though there has been a dramatic gain since the physician has no longer been required to report them directly to the police or the Ministry of Justice. However, there are no major differences between reported and unreported cases in terms of the

patient's characteristics, clinical conditions, or reasons for the action.[15] Euthanasia is performed in about 1:25 of deaths that occur at home, about 1:75 of hospital deaths, and about 1:800 of nursing home deaths.

Although euthanasia is thus not frequent, a small fraction of the total annual mortality, it is nevertheless a conspicuous option in terminal illness, well-known to both physicians and the general public. There has been very widespread public discussion of the issues that arise with respect to euthanasia during the last quarter-century, and surveys of public opinion show that public support for a liberal euthanasia policy has been growing: from 40% in 1966 to 81% in 1988,[16] then to about 90% by 2000. Doctors, too, support the practice, and although there has been a vocal opposition group, it has remained in the clear minority. Some 53% of Dutch physicians say that they have performed euthanasia or provided assistance in suicide, including 63% of general practitioners. An additional 35% of all physicians said that although they had not actually done so, they could conceive of situations in which they would be prepared to do so. Nine percent say they would never perform it, and just 3% say they not only would not do so themselves but would not refer a patient who requested it to a physician who would. Thus, although many physicians who had practiced euthanasia mentioned that they would be most reluctant to do so again and that "only in the face of unbearable suffering and with no alternatives would they be prepared to take such action,"[17] both the 1990 and 1995 studies showed that the majority of Dutch physicians accept the practice in some cases. Surveying the changes over the 5-year period between 1990–1995, the study authors also commented that the data do not support claims of a slippery slope.[18]

In general, pain alone is not the basis for deciding upon euthanasia, since pain can, in most cases, be effectively treated. Rather, the "intolerable suffering" mentioned in the second criterion is understood to mean suffering that is intolerable in the patient's (rather than the physician's) view and can include a fear of or unwillingness to endure *entluistering,* that gradual effacement and loss of personal identity that characterizes the end stages of many terminal illnesses. In very exceptional circumstances, the Supreme Court ruled in the

Chabot case of 1994, physician-assisted suicide may be justified for a patient with non-somatic, psychiatric illness like intractable depression, but such cases are extremely rare. Of patients who do receive euthanasia or physician-assisted suicide, about 80% have cancer, while just 3% have cardiovascular disease and 4% neurological disease.

In a year, almost 35,000 patients seek reassurance from their physicians that they will be granted euthanasia if their suffering becomes severe; there are about 9,700 explicit requests, and about two-thirds of these are turned down, usually on the grounds that there is some other way of treating the patient's suffering. In 14% of cases in 1990, the denial was based on the presence of depression or psychiatric illness.

In the Netherlands, many hospitals now have protocols for the performance of euthanasia; these serve to ensure that the legal guidelines have been met. However, euthanasia is often practiced in the patient's home, typically by the general practitioner who is the patient's long-term family physician. Euthanasia is usually performed after aggressive hospital treatment has failed to arrest the patient's terminal illness; the patient has come home to die, and the family physician is prepared to ease this passing. Whether practiced at home or in the hospital, it is believed that euthanasia usually takes place in the presence of the family members, perhaps the visiting nurse, and often the patient's pastor or priest. Many doctors say that performing euthanasia is never easy but that it is something they believe a doctor ought to do for his or her patient when the patient genuinely wants it and nothing else can help.

Thus, in the Netherlands a patient who is facing the end of life has an option not openly practiced in the United States: to ask the physician to bring his or her life to an end. Although not everyone does so—indeed, almost 97% of people who die in a given year do not do so—it is a choice legally recognized and widely understood.

Facing Death in Germany

In part because of its very painful history of Nazism, Germany medical culture has insisted that doctors should have no role in directly causing death. As in the other countries with advanced medical systems, withholding and withdrawing of care is widely used to avoid the unwanted or inappropriate prolongation of life when the patient is already dying, but there has been vigorous and nearly universal opposition in German public discourse to the notion of active euthanasia, at least in the horrific, politically-motivated sense associated with Nazism. In the last ten years, some Germans have begun to approve of euthanasia in the Dutch sense, based on the Greek root *eu-thanatos,* or "good death," a voluntary choice by the patient for an easier death, but many Germans still associate euthanasia with the politically-motivated exterminations by the Nazis, and view the Dutch as stepping out on a dangerously slippery slope.

However, although under German law killing on request (including voluntary euthanasia) is illegal, German law has not prohibited assistance in suicide since the time of Frederick the Great (1742), provided the person is *tatherrschaftsfähig,* capable of exercising control over his or her actions, and also acting out of *freiverantwortliche Wille,* freely responsible choice. Doctors are prohibited from assistance in suicide not by law but by the policies and code of ethics of the *Bundesärztekammer,* the German medical association. Furthermore, any person, physician or otherwise, has a duty to rescue a person who is unconscious. Thus, assistance in suicide is limited, but it is possible for a family member or friend to assist in a person's suicide, for instance by providing a lethal drug, as long as the person is competent and acting freely and the assister does not remain with the person after unconsciousness sets in.

Taking advantage of this situation, there has developed a private organization, the *Deutsche Gesellschaft für Humanes Sterben* (DGHS), or German Society for Dying with Dignity, which provides support to its very extensive membership in many end-of-life matters, including choosing suicide as an alternative to terminal illness. Of course, not all Germans are members of this organization and many are not sympathetic with its aims, yet the notion of self-directed ending of one's own life in terminal illness is widely understood as an option. Although the DGHS does not itself supply such information, it tells its members how to obtain a booklet published in Scotland with information about ending life, if they request it, provided they have not received medical or psychotherapeutic treatment for depression or other psychiatric illness during the last two years. The information includes a list of prescription drugs, together with the specific dosages necessary for producing a certain, painless death. The DGHS does not itself sell or supply lethal drugs;[19] rather, it recommends that the member approach a physician for a prescription for the drug desired, asking, for example, for a barbiturate to help with sleep. If necessary, the DGHS has been willing to arrange for someone to obtain drugs from neighboring countries, including France, Italy, Spain, Portugal, and Greece, where they may be available without prescription. It also makes available the so-called Exit Bag, a plastic bag used with specific techniques for death by asphyxiation. The DGHS provides and trains family members in what it calls *Sterbebegleitung* (accompaniment in dying), which may take the form of simple presence with a person who is dying, but may also involve direct assistance to a person who is committing suicide, up until unconsciousness sets in. The *Sterbebegleiter* is typically a layperson, not someone medically trained, and physicians play no role in assisting in these cases of suicide. Direct active *Sterbehilfe*—active euthanasia—is illegal under German law. But active indirect *Sterbehilfe,* understood as assistance in suicide, is not illegal, and the DGHS provides counseling in how a "death with dignity" may be achieved in this way.

To preclude suspicion by providing evidence of the person's intentions, the DGHS also provides a form—printed on a single sheet of distinctive purple paper—to be signed once when joining the organization, documenting that the person has reflected thoroughly on the possibility of "free death" *(Freitod)* or suicide in terminal illness as a way of releasing oneself from severe suffering, and expressing the intention to determine the time and character of one's own death. The person then signs this form again at the time of the suicide, leaving it beside the body as evidence that the act is not impetuous or coerced. The form also requests that, if the person is discovered before the suicide is complete, no rescue measures be undertaken. Because assisting suicide is not illegal in Germany (provided the person is competent and in control of his or her own will, and thus not already unconscious), there is no legal risk for family members, the

Sterbebegleiter, or others in reporting information about the methods and effectiveness of suicide attempts, and at least in the past the DGHS has encouraged its network of regional bureaus, located in major cities throughout the country, to facilitate feedback. On this basis, it has regularly updated and revised the drug information provided.

Open, legal assistance in suicide is supported by a feature of the German language that makes it possible to conceptualize it in a comparatively benign way. While English, French, Spanish, and many other languages have just a single primary word for suicide, German has four: *Selbstmord, Selbsttötung, Suizid,* and *Freitod,* of which the latter has comparatively positive, even somewhat heroic connotations.[20] Thus German-speakers can think about the deliberate termination of their lives in a linguistic way not easily available to speakers of other languages. The negatively-rooted term *Selbstmord* ("self-murder") can be avoided; the comparatively neutral terms *Selbsttötung* ("self-killing") and *Suizid* ("suicide") can be used, and the positively-rooted term *Freitod* ("free death") can be reinforced. The DGHS has frequently used *Freitod* rather than German's other, more negative terms to describe the practice with which it provides assistance. No reliable figures are available about the number of suicides with which this organization has assisted, and, as in the Netherlands, the actual frequency of directly assisted death is probably small. Yet it is fair to say, both because of the legal differences and the different conceptual horizons of German-speakers, that the option of self-produced death outside the medical system is more clearly open in Germany than it has been in the Netherlands or the United States.

In recent years, the DGHS has decreased its emphasis on suicide, now thinking of it as a "last resort" when pain control is inadequate—and turned much of its attention to the development of other measures for protecting the rights of the terminally ill, measures already available in many other countries. It distributes newly legalized advance directives, including living wills and durable powers of attorney, as well as organ-donation documents. It provides information about pain control, palliative care, and Hospice. It offers information about suicide prevention. Yet it remains steadfast in defense of the terminally ill patient's right to self-determination, including the right to suicide, and continues to be supportive of patients who make this choice.

To be sure, assisted suicide is not the only option open to terminally ill patients in Germany, and the choice may be infrequent. Reported suicide rates in Germany are only moderately higher than in the Netherlands or the United States,[21] though there is reason to think that terminal-illness suicides in all countries are often reported as deaths from the underlying disease. Although there is political pressure from right-to-die organizations to change the law to permit voluntary active euthanasia in the way understood in the Netherlands, Germany is also seeing increasing emphasis on help in dying, like that offered by Hospice, that does not involve direct termination. Whatever the pressures, the DGHS is a conspicuous, widely known organization, and many Germans appear to be aware that assisted suicide is available and not illegal even if they do not use its services.

OBJECTIONS TO THE THREE MODELS OF DYING

In response to the dilemmas raised by the new circumstances of death, in which the majority of people in the advanced industrial nations die after an extended period of terminal deterioration, different countries develop different practices. The United States, with the sole exception of Oregon, legally permits only withholding and withdrawal of treatment conceived of as "allowing to die," understood to include "double effect" uses of high doses of opiates and terminal sedation. The Netherlands permits these, but also permits voluntary active euthanasia and physician-assisted suicide. Germany rejects physician-performed euthanasia, but it permits assisted suicide not assisted by a physician. These three serve as the principal types or models of response to end-of-life dilemmas in the developed world. To be sure, all of these practices are currently undergoing evolution, and in some ways they are becoming more alike: Germany is paying new attention to the rights of patients to execute advance directives and thus to have treatment withheld or withdrawn, and public surveys reveal considerable support for euthanasia in the Dutch

sense, voluntary active aid-in-dying under careful controls. In the Netherlands, a 1995 policy statement of the Royal Dutch Medical Association expressed a careful preference for physician-assisted suicide in preference to euthanasia, urging that physicians encourage patients who request euthanasia to administer the lethal dose themselves as a further protective of voluntary choice. And, in the United States, the Supreme Court's 1997 ruling there is no constitutional right to physician-assisted suicide has been understood to countenance the emergence of a "laboratory of the states" in which individual states, following the example of Oregon, may in the future move to legalize physician-assisted suicide, though following an attempt in 2001 by the U.S. Attorney General to undercut Oregon's law by prohibiting the use of scheduled drugs for the purpose of causing death, it appears that the issue will return to the U.S. Supreme Court. Nevertheless, among these three countries that serve as the principal models of approaches to dying, there remain substantial differences, and while there are ethical and practical advantages to each approach, each approach also raises serious moral objections.

Objections to the German Practice

German law does not prohibit assisting suicide, but postwar German culture and the Germany physicians' code of ethics discourages physicians from taking an active role in causing death. This gives rise to distinctive moral problems. For one thing, if the physician is not permitted to assist in his or her patient's suicide, there may be little professional help or review provided for the patient's choice about suicide. If patients make such choices essentially outside the medical establishment, medical professionals may not be in a position to detect or treat impaired judgment on the part of the patient, especially judgment impaired by depression. Similarly, if the patient must commit suicide assisted only by persons outside the medical profession, there are risks that the patient's diagnosis and prognosis will be inadequately confirmed, that the means chosen for suicide will be unreliable or inappropriately used, that the means used for suicide will fall into the hands of other persons, and that the patient will fail to recognize or be able to resist intrafamilial pressures and manipulation. While it now makes efforts to counter most of these objections, even the DGHS itself has been accused in the past of promoting rather than simply supporting choices of suicide. Finally, as the DGHS now emphasizes, assistance in suicide can be a freely chosen option only in a legal context that also protects the many other choices a patient may make—declining treatment, executing advance directives, seeking Hospice care—about how his or her life shall end.

Objections to the Dutch Practice

The Dutch practice of physician-performed active voluntary euthanasia and physician-assisted suicide also raises a number of ethical issues, many of which have been discussed vigorously both in the Dutch press and in commentary on the Dutch practices from abroad. For one thing, it is sometimes said that the availability of physician-assisted dying creates a disincentive for providing good terminal care. There is no evidence that this is the case; on the contrary, Peter Admiraal, the anesthesiologist who has been perhaps the Netherlands' most vocal defender of voluntary active euthanasia, insists that pain should rarely or never be the occasion for euthanasia, as pain (in contrast to suffering) is comparatively easily treated.[22] In fact, pain is the primary reason for the request in only about 5% of cases. Instead, it is a refusal to endure the final stages of deterioration, both mental and physical, that primarily motivates the majority of requests.

It is also sometimes said that active euthanasia violates the Hippocratic Oath. The original Greek version of the Oath does prohibit the physician from giving a deadly drug, even when asked for it; but the original version also prohibits the physician from performing surgery and from taking fees for teaching medicine, neither of which prohibitions has survived into contemporary medical practice. At issue is whether deliberately causing the death of one's patient—killing one's patient, some claim—can ever be part of the physician's role. "Doctors must not kill," insist opponents,[23] but Dutch physicians often say that they see performing euthanasia—where it is genuinely requested by the patient and nothing else can be done to relieve the

patient's condition—as part of their duty to the patient, not as a violation of it. As the 1995 Remmelink report commented, "a large majority of Dutch physicians consider euthanasia an exceptional but accepted part of medical practice."[24] The Dutch do worry, however, that too many requests for euthanasia or assistance in suicide are refused—only about 1/3 of explicit requests are actually honored. One well-known Dutch commentator points to another, seemingly contrary concern: that some requests are made too early in a terminal course, even shortly after diagnosis, when with good palliative care the patient could live a substantial amount of time longer.[25] However, these are concerns about how euthanasia and physician-assisted suicide are practiced, not whether they should be legal at all.

The Dutch are also often said to be at risk of starting down the slippery slope, that is, that the practice of voluntary active euthanasia for patients who meet the criteria will erode into practicing less-than-voluntary euthanasia on patients whose problems are not irremediable and perhaps by gradual degrees will develop into terminating the lives of people who are elderly, chronically ill, handicapped, mentally retarded, or otherwise regarded as undesirable. This risk is often expressed in vivid claims of widespread fear and wholesale slaughter—claims based on misinterpretation of the 1,000 cases of life-ending treatment without explicit, current request, claims that are often repeated in the right-to-life press in both the Netherlands and the U.S. although they are simply not true. However, it is true that the Dutch have begun to agonize over the problems of the incompetent patient, the mentally ill patient, the newborn with serious deficits, and other patients who cannot make voluntary choices, though these are largely understood as issues about withholding or withdrawing treatment, not about direct termination.[26]

What is not often understood is that this new and acutely painful area of reflection for the Dutch—withholding and withdrawing treatment from incompetent patients—has already led in the United States to the emergence of a vast, highly developed body of law: namely, that long series of cases beginning with *Quinlan* and culminating in *Cruzan*. Americans have been discussing these issues for a long time and have developed a broad set of practices that are regarded as routine in with-holding and withdrawing treatment from persons who are no longer or never were competent. The Dutch see Americans as much further out on the slippery slope than they are because Americans have already become accustomed to second-party choices that result in death for other people. Issues involving second-party choices are painful to the Dutch in a way they are not to Americans precisely because *voluntariness* is so central in the Dutch understanding of choices about dying. Concomitantly, the Dutch see the Americans' squeamishness about first-party choices—voluntary euthanasia, assisted suicide—as evidence that we are not genuinely committed to recognizing voluntary choice after all. For this reason, many Dutch commentators believe that the Americans are at a much greater risk of sliding down the slippery slope into involuntary killing than they are.

Objections to the American Practice

The German, Dutch, and American practices all occur within similar conditions—in industrialized nations with highly developed medical systems where a majority of the population die of illnesses exhibiting characteristically extended downhill courses—but the issues raised by the American response to this situation—relying on withholding and withdrawal of treatment—may be even more disturbing than those of the Dutch or the Germans. We Americans often assume that our approach is "safer" because, except in Oregon, it involves only letting someone die, not killing them; but it, too, raises very troubling questions.

The first of these issues is a function of the fact that withdrawing and especially withholding treatment are typically less conspicuous, less pronounced, less evident kinds of actions than direct killing, even though they can equally well lead to death. Decisions about nontreatment have an invisibility that decisions about directly causing death do not have, even though they may have the same result, and hence there is a much wider range of occasions in which such decisions can be made. One can decline to treat a patient in many different ways, at many different times—by not providing oxygen, by not instituting dialysis, by not correcting

electrolyte imbalances, and so on—all of which will cause the patient's death. Open medical killing also brings about death, but is much more overt and conspicuous. Consequently, letting die invites many fewer protections. In contrast to the standard slippery-slope argument, which sees killing as riskier than letting die, the more realistic slippery-slope argument warns that because our culture relies primarily on decisions about nontreatment and practices like terminal sedation construed as "allowing to die," grave decisions about living or dying are not as open to scrutiny as they are under more direct life-terminating practices, and hence are more open to abuse. Indeed, in the view of one well-known commentator, the Supreme Court's 1997 decision in effect legalized active euthanasia, voluntary and nonvoluntary, in the form of terminal sedation, even as it rejected physician-assisted suicide.[27]

Second, reliance on withholding and withdrawal of treatment invites rationing in an extremely strong way, in part because of the comparative invisibility of these decisions. When a health care provider does not offer a specific sort of care, it is not always possible to discern the motivation; the line between believing that it would not provide benefit to the patient and that it would not provide benefit worth the investment of resources in the patient can be very thin. This is a particular problem where health care financing is decentralized, profit-oriented, and nonuniversal, as in the United States, and where rationing decisions without benefit of principle are not always available for easy review.

Third, relying on withholding and withdrawal of treatment can often be cruel. Even with hospice or with skilled palliative care, it requires that the patient who is dying from one of the diseases that exhibits a characteristic extended, downhill course (as the majority of patients in the developed world all do) must, in effect, wait to die until the absence of a certain treatment will cause death. For instance, the cancer patient who forgoes chemotherapy or surgery does not simply die from this choice; he or she continues to endure the downhill course of the cancer until the tumor finally destroys some crucial bodily function or organ. The patient with amyotrophic lateral sclerosis who decides in advance to decline respiratory support does not die at the time this choice is made but continues to endure increasing paralysis until breathing is impaired and suffocation occurs.

Of course, attempts are made to try to ameliorate these situations by administering pain medication or symptom control at the time treatment is withheld—for instance, by using opiates and paralytics as a respirator is withdrawn—but these are all ways of disguising the fact that we are letting the disease kill the patient rather than directly bringing about death. But the ways diseases kill people can be far more cruel than the ways physicians kill patients when performing euthanasia or assisting in suicide.

END-OF-LIFE PRACTICES
IN OTHER COUNTRIES

In most of the developed world dying looks much the same. As in the United States, the Netherlands, and Germany, the other industrialized nations also have sophisticated medical establishments, enjoy extended life expectancies, and find themselves in the fourth stage of the epidemiological transition, in which the majority of their populations die of diseases with extended downhill courses. Dying takes place in much the same way in all these countries, though the exact frequency of withholding and withdrawing treatment, of double-effect use of opiates, and euthanasia and physician-assisted suicide varies among them. Indeed, new data is rapidly coming to light.

In Australia, a replication of the Remmelink Commission study originally performed in the Netherlands found that of deaths in Australia that involved a medical end-of-life decision, 28.6% involved withholding or withdrawing treatment; 30.9% involved the use of opiates under the principle of double effect, and 1.8% involved voluntary active euthanasia (including 0.1% physician-assisted suicide), though neither are legal.[28] But the study also found—this is the figure that produced considerable surprise—that some 3.5% of deaths involved termination of the patient's life without the patient's concurrent explicit request. This figure is five times as high as that in the Netherlands. In slightly more than a third of these cases (38%), there was some discussion with the patient, though not an explicit request for death to be hastened, and in virtually all of the rest, the doctor did not consider the patient competent or capable of making such a decision. In 0.5% of all deaths involving medical end-of-life decisions, doctors did not discuss the choice of hastening of death with the patient because they thought it was "clearly the best one for the patient" or that "discussion would have done more harm than good."[29]

Replication of the same study in Flanders, Belgium, revealed a similar picture. Withholding and/or withdrawing treatment was involved in 16.4% of deaths; the double-effect use of opiates in 18.5%, euthanasia and physician-assisted suicide in 1.3%, and—a figure just slightly lower than that of Australia, but substantially higher than that of the Netherlands, termination of life without current, explicit consent from the patient in 3.2%.[30] While data is not yet available for actual end-of-life decision-making and practices for the full range of developed countries, a thorough study of end-of-life decisions in five European countries will be published in 2003.

End-of-life practices in other developed countries tend to follow one of the three models explored here. For example, Canada's practices are much like those of the United States, in that it relies on withholding and withdrawing treatment and other forms of allowing to die, but, in the 1993 case *Rodriquez* v. *British Columbia,* the Canadian Supreme Court narrowly rejected physician-assisted suicide. Australia's Northern Territory briefly legalized assisted dying in 1997, but the law was overturned after just four cases. The United Kingdom, the birthplace of the Hospice movement, stresses palliative care but also rejects physician-assisted suicide and active euthanasia. Late in 2001, Belgium's parliament voted to legalize voluntary active euthanasia and physician-assisted suicide; Belgium's law is patterned fairly closely after the Dutch law. Switzerland's law, like that of Germany, does not criminalize assisted suicide, but does not impose a duty to rescue that makes assistance in suicide difficult. The Swiss organization Exit, the analogue of Germany's DGHS, follows the same general model as the German organization in providing information, counseling, and other support to terminally ill patients who choose suicide, *Freitod,* but the Swiss group also provides such a patient an accompaniment team which consults with the patient to make sure that the choice of suicide is voluntary, secures a prescription from a sympathetic physician, and delivers the lethal medication to the person at a preappointed time. It encourages family members to be present when the patient takes the drug, if he or she still wants to use it, and operates at least one "safe house" for patients traveling from abroad for this purpose. In general, the Swiss organization provides extensive help to the patient who chooses this way of dying, though in keeping with Swiss law, it insists that the patient take the drug him- or herself: assisted suicide is legal, but euthanasia is not.

In contrast, practices in less developed countries look very, very different. In these countries, especially the least developed, background circumstances are different: lifespans are significantly shorter, health care systems are only primitively equipped and grossly underfunded, and many societies have not passed through to the fourth stage of the epidemiologic transition: in these countries, people die earlier, they are more likely to die of infectious and parasitic disease, and degenerative disease is more likely to be interrupted early by death from pneumonia, sepsis, malnutrition, and other factors in what would otherwise have been a long downhill course. Dying in the poorer countries remains different from dying in the richer countries, and the underlying ethical problem in the richer countries—what practices concerning the end of life to adopt when the majority of a population dies of late-life degenerative diseases with long downhill courses—is far less applicable in the less developed parts of the world.

THE PROBLEM:
A CHOICE OF CULTURES

In the developed world, we see three sorts of models in the three countries we've examined in detail. While much of medical practice in them is similar, they do offer three quite different basic options in approaching death. All three of these options generate moral problems; none of them, nor any others we might devise, is free of moral difficulty. The question, then, is this: for a given society, which practices about dying are, morally and practically speaking, best?

It is not possible to answer this question in a less-than-ideal world without attention to the specific characteristics and deficiencies of the society in question. In asking which of these practices is best, we must ask which is best *for us.* That we currently employ one set of these options rather than others does not prove that it is best for us; the question is, would practices developed in other cultures or those not yet widespread in any culture be better for our own culture than that which has so far developed here? Thus, it is necessary to consider the differences between our own society and these other societies in the developed world that have real bearing on which model of approach to dying we ought to adopt. This question can be asked by residents of any country or culture: which model of dying is best *for us?* I have been addressing this question from the point of view of an American, but the question could be asked by any member of any culture, anywhere.

First, notice that different cultures exhibit different degrees of closeness between physicians and patients—different patterns of contact and involvement. The German physician is sometimes said to be more distant and more authoritarian than the American physician; on the other hand, the Dutch physician is often said to be closer to his or her patients than either the American or the German is. In the Netherlands, basic primary care is provided by the *huisarts,* the general practitioner or family physician, who typically lives in the neighborhood, makes house calls frequently, and maintains an office in his or her own home. This physician usually also provides care for the other members of the patient's family and will remain the family's physician throughout his or her practice. Thus, the patient for whom euthanasia becomes an issue—say, the terminal cancer patient who has been hospitalized in the past but who has returned home to die—will be cared for by the trusted family physician on a regular basis. Indeed, for a patient in severe distress, the physician, supported by the visiting nurse, may make house calls as often as once a day, twice a day, or even more frequently (after all, the physician's office is right in the neighborhood) and is in continuous contact with the family. In contrast, the traditional American institution of the family doctor who makes house calls has largely become a thing of the past, and although some patients who die at home have access to hospice services and receive house calls from their long-term physician, many have no such long-term care and receive most of it from staff at a clinic or from house staff rotating through the services of a hospital. Most Americans die in institutions, including hospitals and nursing homes; in the Netherlands, in contrast, the majority of people die at home. The degree of continuing contact that the patient can have with a familiar, trusted physician and the degree of institutionalization clearly influence the nature of his or her dying and also play a role in whether physician-performed active euthanasia, assisted suicide, and/or withholding and withdrawing treatment is appropriate.

Second, the United States has a much more volatile legal climate than either the Netherlands or Germany; its medical system is highly litigious, much more so than that of any other country in the world. Fears of malpractice actions or criminal prosecution color much of what physicians do in managing the dying of their patients. Americans also tend to develop public policy through court decisions and to assume that the existence of a policy puts an end to any moral issue. A delicate legal and moral balance over the issue of euthanasia, as has been the case in the Netherlands throughout the time it was understood as *gedoogd,* tolerated but not fully legal, would hardly be possible here.

Third, we in the United States have a very different financial climate in which to do our dying. Both the Netherlands and Germany, as well as virtually every other industrialized nation, have systems of national health insurance or national health care. Thus the patient is not directly responsible for the costs of treatment, and consequently the patient's choices about terminal care and/or euthanasia need not take personal financial considerations into account. Even for the patient who does have health insurance in the United States, many kinds of services are not covered, whereas the national health care or health insurance programs of many other countries provide multiple relevant services, including at-home physician care, home-nursing care, home respite care, care in a nursing home or other long-term facility, dietitian care, rehabilitation care, physical therapy, psychological counseling, and so on. The patient in the United States needs to attend to the financial aspects of dying in a way that patients in many other countries do not, and in this country both the patient's choices and the recommendations of the physician are very often shaped by financial considerations.

There are many other differences between the United States, on the one hand, and the Netherlands and Germany, with their different options for dying, on the other hand, including differences in degrees of paternalism in the medical establishment, in racism, sexism, and ageism in the general culture, and in awareness of a problematic historical past, especially Nazism. All of these cultural, institutional, social, and legal differences influence the appropriateness or inappropriateness of practices such as active euthanasia and assisted suicide. For instance, the Netherlands' tradition of close physician-patient contact, its absence of malpractice-motivated medicine, and its provision of comprehensive health insurance, together with its comparative lack of racism and ageism and its experience in resistance to Nazism, suggest that this culture is able to permit the practice of voluntary active euthanasia, performed by physicians, as well as physician-assisted suicide, without risking abuse. On the other hand, it is sometimes said that Germany still does not trust its physicians, remembering the example of Nazi experimentation, and given a comparatively authoritarian medical climate in which the contact between physician and patient is quite distanced, the population could not be comfortable with the practice of physician-performed active euthanasia or physician-assisted suicide. There, only a wholly patient-controlled response to terminal situations, as in non-physician-assisted suicide, is a reasonable and prudent practice.

But what about the United States? This is a country where (1) sustained contact with a personal physician has been decreasing, (2) the risk of malpractice action is perceived as substantial, (3) much medical care is not insured, (4) many medical decisions are financial decisions as well, (5) racism has been on the rise, and (6) the public has not experienced direct contact with Nazism or similar totalitarian movements. Thus, the United States is in many respects an untrustworthy candidate for practicing active euthanasia. Given the pressures on individuals in an often atomized society, encouraging solo suicide, assisted if at all only by nonprofessionals, might well be open to considerable abuse too.

However, there are several additional differences between the United States and both the Netherlands and Germany that may seem peculiarly relevant here. First, American culture is more confrontational than many others, including Dutch culture. While the Netherlands prides itself rightly on a long tradition of rational discussion of public issues and on toleration of others' views and practices, the United States (and to some degree also Germany) tends to develop highly partisan, moralizing oppositional groups, especially over social issues like abortion. In general, this is a disadvantage, but in the case of euthanasia it may serve to alert the public to issues and possibilities it might not otherwise consider, especially the risks of abuse. Here the role of religious groups may be particularly strong, since in discouraging or prohibiting suicide and euthanasia (as many, though by no means all, religious groups do), they may invite their members to reinspect the reasons for such choices and encourage families, physicians, and health care institutions to provide adequate, humane alternatives.

Second, though this may at first seem to be not only a peculiar but a trivial difference, it is Americans who are particularly given to self-analysis. This tendency not only is evident in the United States' high rate of utilization of counseling services, including religious counseling, psychological counseling, and psychiatry, but also is more clearly evident in its popular culture: its diet of soap operas, situation comedies, and pop psychology books. It is here that the ordinary American absorbs models for analyzing his or her personal relationships and individual psychological characteristics. While, of course, things are changing rapidly and America's cultural tastes are widely exported, the fact remains that the ordinary American's cultural diet contains more in the way of professional and do-it-yourself amateur psychology and self-analysis than anyone else's. This long tradition of self-analysis may put Americans in a better position for certain kinds of end-of-life practices than many other cultures. Despite whatever other deficiencies U.S. society has, we live in a culture that encourages us to inspect our own motives, anticipate the impact of our actions on others, and scrutinize our own relationships with others, including our physicians. This disposition is of importance in euthanasia and assisted-suicide contexts because these are the kinds of fundamental choices about which one may have somewhat mixed motives, be subject to various interpersonal and situational pressures, and so on. If the voluntary character of choices about one's own dying is to be

protected, it may be a good thing to inhabit a culture in which self-inspection of one's own mental habits and motives, not to mention those of one's family, physician, and others who might affect one's choices, is culturally encouraged. Counseling specifically addressed to end-of-life choices is not yet easily or openly available, especially if physician-assisted suicide is at issue—though some groups like Seattle-based Compassion in Dying now provide it—but I believe it will become more frequent in the future as people facing terminal illnesses characterized by long downhill, deteriorative courses consider how they want to die.

Finally, the United States population, varied as it is, is characterized by a kind of do-it-yourself ethic, an ethic that devalues reliance on others and encourages individual initiative and responsibility. (To be sure, this ethic is little in evidence in the series of court cases from *Quinlan* to *Cruzan*, but these were all cases about patients who had become or always were incapable of decisionmaking.) This ethic seems to be coupled with a sort of resistance to authority that perhaps also is basic to the American temperament, even in all its diversity. If this is really the case, Americans might be especially well-served by end-of-life practices that emphasize self-reliance and resistance to authority.

These, of course, are mere conjectures about features of American culture relevant to the practice of euthanasia or assisted suicide. These are the features that one would want to reinforce should these practices become general, in part to minimize the effects of the negative influences. But, of course, these positive features will differ from one country and culture to another, just as the negative features do. In each country, a different architecture of antecedent assumptions and cultural features develops around end-of-life issues, and in each country the practices of euthanasia and assisted or physician-assisted suicide, if they are to be free from abuse, must be adapted to the culture in which they take place.

What, then, is appropriate for the United States' own cultural situation? Physician-performed euthanasia, even if not in itself morally wrong, is morally jeopardized where legal, time-related, and especially financial pressures on both patients and physicians are severe; thus, it is morally problematic in our culture in a way that it is not in the

Netherlands. Solo suicide outside the institution of medicine (as in Germany) may be problematic in a country (like the United States) that has an increasingly alienated population, offers deteriorating and uneven social services, is increasingly racist and classist, and in other ways imposes unusual pressures on individuals, despite opportunities for self-analysis. Reliance only on withholding and withdrawing treatment and allowing to die (as in the United States) can be cruel, and its comparative invisibility invites erosion under cost-containment and other pressures. These are the three principal alternatives we have considered, but none of them seems wholly suited to our actual situation for dealing with the new fact that most of us die of extended-decline, deteriorative diseases.

Perhaps, however, there is one that would best suit the United States, certainly better than its current reliance on allowing to die, and better than the Netherlands' more direct physician involvement or Germany's practices entirely outside medicine. The "arm's-length" model of physician-assisted suicide—permitting physicians to supply their terminally ill patients who request it with the means for ending their own lives (as has become legal in Oregon) still grants physicians some control over the circumstances in which this can happen—only, for example, when the prognosis is genuinely grim and the alternatives for symptom control are poor—but leaves the fundamental decision about whether to use these means to the patient alone. It is up to the patient then—the independent, confrontational, self-analyzing, do-it-yourself, authority-resisting patient—and his or her advisors, including family members, clergy, the physician, and other health care providers, to be clear about whether he or she really wants to use these means or not. Thus, the physician is involved but not directly, and it is the patient's decision, although the patient is not making it alone. Thus also it is the patient who performs the action of bringing his or her own life to a close, though where the patient is physically incapable of doing so or where the process goes awry the physician must be allowed to intercede. We live in an imperfect world, but of the alternatives for facing death—which we all eventually must—I think that the practice of permitting this somewhat distanced though still medically supported form of physician-assisted suicide is the one most nearly suited to the current state of our own flawed society. This is a model not yet central in any of the three countries examined here—the Netherlands, Germany, or (except in Oregon) the United States, or any of the other industrialized nations with related practices—but it is the one, I think, that suits us best.

NOTES

1. S. J. Olshansky and A. B. Ault, "The Fourth Stage of the Epidemiological Transition: The Age of Delayed Degenerative Diseases," *Milbank Memorial Fund Quarterly Health and Society* 64 (1986): 355–91.
2. S. Miles and C. Gomez, *Protocols for Elective Use of Life-Sustaining Treatment* (New York: Springer-Verlag, 1988).
3. C. L. Sprung, "Changing Attitudes and Practices in Forgoing Life-Sustaining Treatments," *JAMA* 262 (1990):2213.
4. T. J. Prendergast and J. M. Luce, "Increasing Incidence of Withholding and Withdrawal of Life Support from the Critically Ill," *American Journal of Respiratory and Critical Care Medicine* 155 (1):1–2 (January 1997).
5. M. B. Hamel et al. (SUPPORT Investigators), "Patient age and decisions to withhold life-sustaining treatments from seriously ill, hospitalized adults," *Annals of Internal Medicine* 130(2):116–125 (Jan. 19, 1999).
6. John M. Luce, "Withholding and Withdrawal of Life Support: Ethical, Legal, and Clinical Aspects," *New Horizons* 5(1):30–37 (Feb. 1997).
7. *New York Times*, 23 July 1990. A13.
8. Accounts of the use of Measure 16 in Oregon are to be found in A. E. Chin, K. Hedberg, G. K. Higginson, D. W. Fleming, "Legalized Physician-Assisted Suicide in Oregon—the first year's experience," *New England Journal of Medicine* 340:577–83 (1999); A. D. Sullivan, K. Hedberg, D. W. Fleming, "Legalized Physician-Assisted Suicide in Oregon—the second year," *New England Journal of Medicine* 342:598–604 (2000); and A. D. Sullivan, K. Hedberg, D. Hopkins, "Legalized Physician-Assisted Suicide in Oregon, 1998–2000," *New England Journal of Medicine* 344:605 (2001). The 70 cases of legal physician-assisted suicide that have taken place in the first three years since it became legal in Oregon—a three-year period during which a total of about 6 million deaths occurred in the U.S.—represent at most about 0.00116% of the total annual mortality. As of this writing new legal challenges have been directed against this law; the outcome remains in question.
9. For a fuller account, see my remarks "A Dozen Caveats Concerning the Discussion of Euthanasia in the Netherlands," in Margaret P. Battin, *The Least Worst Death: Essays in Bioethics on the End of Life* (New York and London: Oxford University Press, 1994): 130–44.

10. P. J. van der Maas, J. J. M. van Delden, L. Pijnenborg, "Euthanasia and Other Medical Decisions Concerning the End of Life," published in full in English as a special issue of *Health Policy*, 22, nos. 1–2 (1992) and, with C. W. N. Looman, in summary in *The Lancet* 338 (1991):669–674.

11. G. van der Wal et al., "Euthanasie en hulp bij zelfdoding door artsen in de thuissituatie," parts 1 and 2, *Nederlands Tijdschrift voor Geneesekunde* 135 (1991): 1593–98, 1600–03.

12. P. J. van der Maas, G. van der Wal, et al., "Euthanasia, Physician-Assisted Suicide, and Other Medical Practices Involving the End of Life in the Netherlands, 1990–1995," *New England Journal of Medicine* 335:22 (1996): 1699–1705.

13. The precise figures are 17.9% (1990) and 20.2% (1995) deaths involving decisions to forgo treatment; 18.8% (1990) and 19.1% (1995) deaths involving opioids in large doses; 1.7% (1990) and 2.4% (1995) euthanasia; 0.2% (1990) and 0.2 (1995) physician-assisted suicide; and 0.8% (1990) and 0.7% (1995), life-ending without patient's explicit request. Source: van der Maas et al., Table 1, p. 1701.

14. L. Pijnenborg, P. J. van der Maas, J. J. M. van Delden, C. W. N. Looman, "Life Terminating Acts without Explicit Request of Patient, *The Lancet* 341 (1993):1196–99.

15. G. van der Wal et al., "Evaluation of the Notification Procedure for Physician-Assisted Death in the Netherlands," *New England Journal of Medicine* 335:22 (1996):1706–1711.

16. E. Borst-Eilers, "Euthanasia in the Netherlands: Brief Historical Review and Present Situation," in Robert I. Misbin, ed., *Euthanasia: The Good of the Patient, the Good of Society* (Frederick, Md.: University Publishing Group, 1992): 59.

17. van der Maas et al., "Euthanasia and other Medical Decisions Concerning the End of Life," 673.

18. van der Maas et al., "Euthanasia, Physician-Assisted Suicide, and Other Medical Practices Involving the End of Life in the Netherlands, 1990–1995," p. 1705.

19. That is, it no longer sells or supplies such drugs. A scandal in 1992–93 engulfed the original founder and president of the DGHS, Hans Hennig Atrott, who had been secretly providing some members cyanide in exchange for substantial contributions; he was convicted of violating the drug laws and tax evasion, though not charged with or convicted of assisting suicides.

20. See my "Assisted Suicide: Can We Learn from Germany?" in Margaret P. Battin, *The Least Worst Death: Essays in Bioethics on the End of Life* (New York and London: Oxford University Press, 1994): 254–70.

21. The World Health Organization provides the following data concerning suicide rates, provided here for the years indicated for the various countries discussed in this paper:
Australia (1997) 14.3 (per 100,000 population)
Austria (1999) 19.2
Belgium (1995) 21.3
Canada (1997) 12.3
Germany (1998) 14.2
Netherlands (1997) 10.1
Switzerland (1996) 20.2
USA (1998) 11.3
Courtesy of John L. McIntosh, American Association of Suicidology.

22. P. Admiraal, "Euthanasia in a General Hospital," paper read at the Eighth World Congress of the International Federation of Right-to-Die Societies, Maastricht, the Netherlands, June 8, 1990.

23. See the editorial "Doctors Must Not Kill," *Journal of the American Medical Association* 259:2139–40 (1988), signed by Willard Gaylin, M.D., Leon R. Kass, M.D., Edmund D. Pellegrino, M.D., and Mark Siegler, M.D.

24. van der Maas et al., "Euthanasia, Physician-Assisted Suicide, and Other Medical Practices," 1705.

25. Govert den Hartogh, personal communication.

26. H. ten Have, "Coma: Controversy and Consensus," *Newsletter of the European Society for Philosophy of Medicine and Health Care* (May 1990): 19–20.

27. David Orentlicher, "The Supreme Court and Terminal Sedation: Rejecting Assisted Suicide, Embracing Euthanasia," *Hastings Constitutional Law Quarterly* 24(4):947–968 (1997); see also *The New England Journal of Medicine* 337(17): 1236–39 (1997).

28. Physician-assisted suicide was briefly legal in the Northern Territory of Australia in 1997 and four cases were performed before the law was overturned, but these cases did not occur during the study period.

29. Helga Kuhse, Peter Singer, Peter Baume, Malcolm Clark, and Maurice Rickard, "End-of-life Decisions in Australian Medical Practice," *The Medical Journal of Australia* 166:191–196 (1997).

30. Luc Deliens, Freddy Mortier, Johan Bilsen, Marc Cosyns, Robert Vander Stichele, Johan Vanoverloop, Koen Ingels, "End-of-life Decisions in Medical Practice in Flanders, Belgium: a nationwide survey," *The Lancet* 356:1806–11 (2000).

IS THERE A DUTY TO DIE?

John Hardwig

Many people were outraged when Richard Lamm claimed that old people had a duty to die. Modern medicine and an individualistic culture have seduced many to feel that they have a right to health care and a right to live, despite the burdens and costs to our families and society. But in fact there are circumstances when we have a duty to die. As modern medicine continues to save more of us from acute illness, it also delivers more of us over to chronic illnesses, allowing us to survive far longer than we can take care of ourselves. It may be that our technological sophistication coupled with a commitment to our loved ones generates a fairly widespread duty to die.

When Richard Lamm made the statement that old people have a duty to die, it was generally shouted down or ridiculed. The whole idea is just too preposterous to entertain. Or too threatening. In fact, a fairly common argument against legalizing physician-assisted suicide is that if it were legal, some people might somehow get the idea that they have a duty to die. These people could only be the victims of twisted moral reasoning or vicious social pressure. It goes without saying that there is no duty to die.

But for me the question is real and very important. I feel strongly that I may very well some day have a duty to die. I do not believe that I am idiosyncratic, mentally ill, or morally perverse in thinking this. I think many of us will eventually face precisely this duty. But I am first of all concerned with my own duty. I write partly to clarify my own convictions and to prepare myself. Ending my life might be a very difficult thing for me to do.

This notion of a duty to die raises all sorts of interesting theoretical and metaethical questions. I intend to try to avoid most of them because I hope my argument will be persuasive to those holding a wide variety of ethical views. Also, although the claim that there is a duty to die would ultimately require theoretical underpinning, the discussion needs to begin on the normative level. As is appropriate to my attempt to steer clear of theoretical commitments, I will use "duty" "obligation," and "responsibility" interchangeably, in a pretheoretical or preanalytic sense.[1]

CIRCUMSTANCES AND A DUTY TO DIE

Do many of us really believe that no one ever has a duty to die? I suspect not. I think most of us probably believe that there is such a duty, but it is very uncommon. Consider Captain Oates, a member of Admiral Scott's expedition to the South Pole. Oates became too ill to continue. If the rest of the team stayed with him, they would all perish. After this had become clear, Oates left his tent one night, walked out into a raging blizzard, and was never seen again.[2] That may have been a heroic thing to do, but we might be able to agree that it was also no more than his duty. It would have been wrong for him to urge—or even to allow—the rest to stay and care for him.

This is a very unusual circumstance—a "lifeboat case"—and lifeboat cases make for bad ethics. But I expect that most of us would also agree that there have been cultures in which what we would call a duty to die has been fairly common. These are relatively poor, technologically simple, and especially nomadic cultures. In such societies, everyone knows that if you manage to live long enough, you will eventually become old and debilitated. Then you will need to take steps to end your life. The old people in these societies regularly did precisely that. Their cultures prepared and supported them in doing so.

Those cultures could be dismissed as irrelevant to contemporary bioethics; their circumstances are so different from ours. But if that is our response, it is instructive. It suggests that we assume a duty to die is irrelevant to us because our wealth and technological sophistication have purchased exemption

From *Hastings Center Report* 27, no. 2 (1997): 34–42. Reprinted by permission of The Hastings Center.

for us . . . except under very unusual circumstances like Captain Oates's.

But have wealth and technology really exempted us? Or are they, on the contrary, about to make a duty to die common again? We like to think of modern medicine as all triumph with no dark side. Our medicine saves many lives and enables most of us to live longer. That is wonderful, indeed. We are all glad to have access to this medicine. But our medicine also delivers most of us over to chronic illnesses and it enables many of us to survive longer than we can take care of ourselves, longer than we know what to do with ourselves, longer than we even are ourselves.

The costs—and these are not merely monetary—of prolonging our lives when we are no longer able to care for ourselves are often staggering. If further medical advances wipe out many of today's "killer diseases"—cancers, heart attacks, strokes,—ALS, AIDS, and the rest—then one day most of us will survive long enough to become demented or debilitated. These developments could generate a fairly widespread duty to die. A fairly common duty to die might turn out to be only the dark side of our life-prolonging medicine and the uses we choose to make of it.

Let me be clear. I certainly believe that there is a duty to refuse life-prolonging medical treatment and also a duty to complete advance directives refusing life-prolonging treatment. But a duty to die can go well beyond that. There can be a duty to die before one's illnesses would cause death, even if treated only with palliative measures. In fact, there may be a fairly common responsibility to end one's life in the absence of any terminal illness at all. Finally, there can be a duty to die when one would prefer to live. Granted, many of the conditions that can generate a duty to die also seriously undermine the quality of life. Some prefer not to live under such conditions. But even those who want to live can face a duty to die. These will clearly be the most controversial and troubling cases; I will, accordingly, focus my reflections on them.

THE INDIVIDUALISTIC FANTASY

Because a duty to die seems such a real possibility to me, I wonder why contemporary bioethics has dismissed it without serious consideration. I believe that most bioethics still shares in one of our deeply embedded American dreams: the individualistic fantasy. This fantasy leads us to imagine that lives are separate and unconnected, or that they could be so if we chose. If lives were unconnected, things that happened in my life would not or need not affect others. And if others were not (much) affected by my life, I would have no duty to consider the impact of my decisions on others. I would then be free morally to live my life however I please, choosing whatever life and death I prefer for myself. The way I live would be nobody's business but my own. I certainly would have no duty to die if I preferred to live.

Within a health care context, the individualistic fantasy leads us to assume that the patient is the only one affected by decisions about her medical treatment. If only the patient were affected, the relevant questions when making treatment decisions would be precisely those we ask: What will benefit the patient? Who can best decide that? The pivotal issue would always be simply whether the patient wants to live like this and whether she would consider herself better off dead.[3] "Whose life is it, anyway?" we ask rhetorically.

But this is morally obtuse. We are not a race of hermits. Illness and death do not come only to those who are all alone. Nor is it much better to think in terms of the bald dichotomy between "the interests of the patient" and "the interests of society" (or a third-party payer), as if we were isolated individuals connected only to "society" in the abstract or to the other, faceless members of our health maintenance organization.

Most of us are affiliated with particular others and most deeply, with family and loved ones. Families and loved ones are bound together by ties of care and affection, by legal relations and obligations, by inhabiting shared spaces and living units, by interlocking finances and economic prospects, by common projects and also commitments to support the different life projects of other family members, by shared histories, by ties of loyalty. This life together of family and loved ones is what defines and sustains us; it is what gives meaning to most of our lives. We would not have it any other way. We would not want to be all alone, especially when we are seriously ill, as we age, and when we are dying.

But the fact of deeply interwoven lives debars us from making exclusively self-regarding decisions, as the decisions of one member of a family may dramatically affect the lives of all the rest. The impact of my decisions upon my family and loved ones is the source of many of my strongest obligations and also the most plausible and likeliest basis of a duty to die. "Society," after all, is only very marginally affected by how I live, or by whether I live or die.

A BURDEN TO MY LOVED ONES

Many older people report that their one remaining goal in life is not to be a burden to their loved ones. Young people feel this, too: when I ask my undergraduate students to think about whether their death could come too late, one of their very first responses always is, "Yes, when I become a burden to my family or loved ones." Tragically, there are situations in which my loved ones would be much better off—all things considered, the loss of a loved one notwithstanding—if I were dead.

The lives of our loved ones can be seriously compromised by caring for us. The burdens of providing care or even just supervision twenty-four hours a day, seven days a week are often overwhelming.[4] When this kind of caregiving goes on for years, it leaves the caregiver exhausted, with no time for herself or life of her own. Ultimately, even her health is often destroyed. But it can also be emotionally devastating simply to live with a spouse who is increasingly distant, uncommunicative, unresponsive, foreign, and unreachable. Other family members' needs often go unmet as the caring capacity of the family is exceeded. Social life and friendships evaporate, as there is no opportunity to go out to see friends and the home is no longer a place suitable for having friends in.

We must also acknowledge that the lives of our loved ones can be devastated just by having to pay for health care for us. One part of the recent SUPPORT study documented the financial aspects of caring for a dying member of a family. Only those who had illnesses severe enough to give them less than a 50 percent chance to live six more months were included in this study. When these patients survived their initial hospitalization and were discharged about one-third required considerable caregiving from their families; in 20 percent of cases a family member had to quit work or make some other major lifestyle change; almost one-third of these families lost all of their savings; and just under 30 percent lost a major source of income.[5]

If talking about money sounds venal or trivial, remember that much more than money is normally at stake here. When someone has to quit work, she may well lose her career. Savings decimated late in life cannot be recouped in the few remaining years of employability, so the loss compromises the quality of the rest of the caregiver's life. For a young person, the chance to go to college may be lost to the attempt to pay debts due to an illness in the family, and this decisively shapes an entire life.

A serious illness in a family is a misfortune. It is usually nobody's fault; no one is responsible for it. But we face choices about how we will respond to this misfortune. That's where the responsibility comes in and fault can arise. Those of us with families and loved ones always have a duty not to make selfish or self-centered decisions about our lives. We have a responsibility to try to protect the lives of loved ones from serious threats or greatly impoverished quality, certainly an obligation not to make choices that will jeopardize or seriously compromise their futures. Often, it would be wrong to do just what we want or just what is best for ourselves; we should choose in light of what is best for all concerned. That is our duty in sickness as well as in health. It is out of these responsibilities that a duty to die can develop.

I am not advocating a crass, quasi-economic conception of burdens and benefits, nor a shallow, hedonistic view of life. Given a suitably rich understanding of benefits, family members sometimes do benefit from suffering through the long illness of a loved one. Caring for the sick or aged can foster growth, even as it makes daily life immeasurably harder and the prospects for the future much bleaker. Chronic illness or a drawn-out death can also pull a family together, making the care for each other stronger and more evident. If my loved ones are truly benefiting from coping with my illness or debility, I have no duty to die based on burdens to them.

But it would be irresponsible to blithely assume that this always happens, that it will happen in my family, or that it will be the fault of my family if they cannot manage to turn my illness into a positive experience. Perhaps the opposite is more common: a hospital chaplain once told me that he could not think of a single case in which a family was strengthened or brought together by what happened at the hospital.

Our families and loved ones also have obligations, of course—they have the responsibility to stand by us and to support us through debilitating illness and death. They must be prepared to make significant sacrifices to respond to an illness in the family. I am far from denying that. Most of us are aware of this responsibility and most families meet it rather well. In fact, families deliver more than 80 percent of the long-term care in this country, almost always at great personal cost. Most of us who are a part of a family can expect to be sustained in our time of need by family members and those who love us.

But most discussions of an illness in the family sound as if responsibility were a one-way street. It is not, of course. When we become seriously ill or debilitated, we too may have to make sacrifices. To think that my loved ones must bear whatever burdens my illness, debility, or dying process might impose upon them is to reduce them to means to my well-being. And that would be immoral. Family solidarity, altruism, bearing the burden of a loved one's misfortune, and loyalty are all important virtues of families, as well. But they are all also two-way streets.

OBJECTIONS TO A DUTY TO DIE

To my mind, the most serious objections to the idea of a duty to die lie in the effects on my loved ones of ending my life. But to most others, the important objections have little or nothing to do with family and loved ones. Perhaps the most common objections are: (1) there is a higher duty that always takes precedence over a duty to die; (2) a duty to end one's own life would be incompatible with a recognition of human dignity or the intrinsic value of a person; and (3) seriously ill, debilitated, or dying people are already bearing the harshest burdens and so it would be wrong to ask them to bear the additional burden of ending their own lives.

These are all important objections; all deserve a thorough discussion. Here I will only be able to suggest some moral counterweights—ideas that might provide the basis for an argument that these objections do not always preclude a duty to die.

An example of the first line of argument would be the claim that a duty to God, the giver of life, forbids that anyone take her own life. It could be argued that this duty always supersedes whatever obligations we might have to our families. But what convinces us that we always have such a religious duty in the first place? And what guarantees that it always supersedes our obligations to try to protect our loved ones?

Certainly, the view that death is the ultimate evil cannot be squared with Christian theology. It does not reflect the actions of Jesus or those of his early followers. Nor is it clear that the belief that life is sacred requires that we never take it. There are other theological possibilities.[6] In any case, most of us—bioethicists, physicians, and patients alike—do not subscribe to the view that we have an obligation to preserve human life as long as possible. But if not, surely we ought to agree that I may legitimately end my life for other-regarding reasons, not just for self-regarding reasons.

Secondly, religious considerations aside, the claim could be made that an obligation to end one's own life would be incompatible with human dignity or would embody a failure to recognize the intrinsic value of a person. But I do not see that in thinking I had a duty to die I would necessarily be failing to respect myself or to appreciate my dignity or worth. Nor would I necessarily be failing to respect you in thinking that you had a similar duty. There is surely also a sense in which we fail to respect ourselves if in the face of illness or death, we stoop to choosing just what is best for ourselves. Indeed, Kant held that the very core of human dignity is the ability to act on a self-imposed moral law, regardless of whether it is in our interest to do so.[7] We shall return to the notion of human dignity.

A third objection appeals to the relative weight of burdens and thus, ultimately, to considerations of fairness or justice. The burdens that an illness creates for the family could not possibly be great enough to justify an obligation to end one's life—the sacrifice of life itself would be a far greater burden than any involved in caring for a chronically ill family member.

But is this true? Consider the following case:

An 87-year-old woman was dying of congestive heart failure. Her APACHE score predicted that she had less than a 50 percent chance to live for another six months.

She was lucid, assertive, and terrified of death. She very much wanted to live and kept opting for rehospitalization and the most aggressive life-prolonging treatment possible. That treatment successfully prolonged her life (though with increasing debility) for nearly two years. Her 55-year-old daughter was her only remaining family, her caregiver, and the main source of her financial support. The daughter duly cared for her mother. But before her mother died, her illness had cost the daughter all of her savings, her home, her job, and her career.

This is by no means an uncommon sort of case. Thousands of similar cases occur each year. Now, ask yourself which is the greater burden:

(a) To lose a 50 percent chance of six more months of life at age 87?

(b) To lose all your savings, your home, and your career at age 55?

Which burden would you prefer to bear? Do we really believe the former is the greater burden? Would even the dying mother say that (a) is the greater burden? Or has she been encouraged to believe that the burdens of (b) are somehow morally irrelevant to her choices?

I think most of us would quickly agree that (b) is a greater burden. That is the evil we would more hope to avoid in our lives. If we are tempted to say that the mother's disease and impending death are the greater evil, I believe it is because we are taking a "slice of time" perspective rather than a "lifetime perspective."[8] But surely the lifetime perspective is the appropriate perspective when weighing burdens. If (b) is the greater burden, then we must admit that we have been promulgating an ethics that advocates imposing greater burdens on some people in order to provide smaller benefits for others just because they are ill and thus gain our professional attention and advocacy.

A whole range of cases like this one could easily be generated. In some, the answer about which burden is greater will not be clear. But in many it is. Death—or ending your own life—is simply not the greatest evil or the greatest burden.

This point does not depend on a utilitarian calculus. Even if death were the greatest burden (thus disposing of any simple utilitarian argument), serious questions would remain about the moral justifiability of choosing to impose crushing burdens on

loved ones in order to avoid having to bear this burden oneself. The fact that I suffer greater burdens than others in my family does not license me simply to choose what I want for myself, nor does it necessarily release me from a responsibility to try to protect the quality of their lives.

I can readily imagine that, through cowardice, rationalization, or failure of resolve, I will fail in this obligation to protect my loved ones. If so, I think I would need to be excused or forgiven for what I did. But I cannot imagine it would be morally permissible for me to ruin the rest of my partner's life to sustain mine or to cut off my sons' careers, impoverish them, or compromise the quality of their children's lives simply because I wish to live a little longer. This is what leads me to believe in a duty to die.

WHO HAS A DUTY TO DIE?

Suppose, then, that there can be a duty to die. Who has a duty to die? And when? To my mind, these are the right questions, the questions we should be asking. Many of us may one day badly need answers to just these questions.

But I cannot supply answers here, for two reasons. In the first place, answers will have to be very particular and contextual. Our concrete duties are often situated, defined in part by the myriad details of our circumstances, histories, and relationships. Though there may be principles that apply to a wide range of cases and some cases that yield pretty straightforward answers, there will also be many situations in which it is very difficult to discern whether one has a duty to die. If nothing else, it will often be very difficult to predict how one's family will bear up under the weight of the burdens that a protracted illness would impose on them. Momentous decisions will often have to be made under conditions of great uncertainty.

Second and perhaps even more importantly, I believe that those of us with family and loved ones should not define our duties unilaterally, especially not a decision about a duty to die. It would be isolating and distancing for me to decide without consulting them what is too much of a burden for my loved ones to bear. That way of deciding about my moral duties is not only atomistic, it also treats my family and loved ones paternalistically.

They must be allowed to speak for themselves about the burdens my life imposes on them and how they feel about bearing those burdens.

Some may object that it would be wrong to put a loved one in a position of having to say, in effect, "You should end your life because caring for you is too hard on me and the rest of the family." Not only will it be almost impossible to say something like that to someone you love, it will carry with it a heavy load of guilt. On this view, you should decide by yourself whether you have a duty to die and approach your loved ones only after you have made up your mind to say good-bye to them. Your family could then try to change your mind, but the tremendous weight of moral decision would be lifted from their shoulders.

Perhaps so. But I believe in family decisions. Important decisions for those whose lives are interwoven should be made together, in a family discussion. Granted, a conversation about whether I have a duty to die would be a tremendously difficult conversation. The temptations to be dishonest could be enormous. Nevertheless, if I am contemplating a duty to die, my family and I should, if possible, have just such an agonizing discussion. It will act as a check on the information, perceptions, and reasoning of all of us. But even more importantly, it affirms our connectedness at a critical juncture in our lives and our life together. Honest talk about difficult matters almost always strengthens relationships.

However, many families seem unable to talk about death at all, much less a duty to die. Certainly most families could not have this discussion all at once, in one sitting. It might well take a number of discussions to be able to approach this topic. But even if talking about death is impossible, there are always behavioral clues—about your caregiver's tiredness, physical condition, health, prevailing mood, anxiety, financial concerns, outlook, overall well-being, and so on. And families unable to talk about death can often talk about how the caregiver is feeling, about finances, about tensions within the family resulting from the illness, about concerns for the future. Deciding whether you have a duty to die based on these behavioral clues and conversation about them honors your relationships better than deciding on your own about how burdensome you and your care must be.

I cannot say when someone has a duty to die. Still, I can suggest a few features of one's illness, history, and circumstances that make it more likely that one has a duty to die. I present them here without much elaboration or explanation.

(1) A duty to die is more likely when continuing to live will impose significant burdens—emotional burdens, extensive caregiving, destruction of life plans, and, yes, financial hardship—on your family and loved ones. This is the fundamental insight underlying a duty to die.

(2) A duty to die becomes greater as you grow older. As we age, we will be giving up less by giving up our lives, if only because we will sacrifice fewer remaining years of life and a smaller portion of our life plans. After all, it's not as if we would be immortal and live forever if we could just manage to avoid a duty to die. To have reached the age of, say, seventy-five or eighty years without being ready to die is itself a moral failing, the sign of a life out of touch with life's basic realities.[9]

(3) A duty to die is more likely when you have already lived a full and rich life. You have already had a full share of the good things life offers.

(4) There is greater duty to die if your loved ones' lives have already been difficult or impoverished, if they have had only a small share of the good things that life has to offer (especially if through no fault of their own).

(5) A duty to die is more likely when your loved ones have already made great contributions—perhaps even sacrifices—to make your life a good one. Especially if you have not made similar sacrifices for their well-being or for the well-being of other members of your family.

(6) To the extent that you can make a good adjustment to your illness or handicapping condition, there is less likely to be a duty to die. A good adjustment means that smaller sacrifices will be required of loved ones and there is more compensating interaction for them. Still, we must also recognize that some diseases—Alzheimer [*sic*] or Huntington [*sic*] chorea—will eventually take their toll on your loved ones no matter how courageously, resolutely, even cheerfully you manage to face that illness.

(7) There is less likely to be a duty to die if you can still make significant contributions to the lives of others, especially your family. The burdens to family members are not only or even primarily financial, neither are the contributions to them. However, the old and those who have terminal illnesses must also bear in mind that the loss their family members will feel when they die cannot be avoided, only postponed.

(8) A duty to die is more likely when the part of you that is loved will soon be gone or seriously compromised. Or when you soon will no longer be capable of giving love. Part of the horror of dementing disease is that it destroys the capacity to nurture and sustain relationships, taking away a person's agency and the emotions that bind her to others.

(9) There is a greater duty to die to the extent that you have lived a relatively lavish lifestyle instead of saving for illness or old age. Like most upper middle-class Americans, I could easily have saved more. It is a greater wrong to come to your family for assistance if your need is the result of having chosen leisure or a spendthrift lifestyle. I may eventually have to face the moral consequences of decisions I am now making.

These, then, are some of the considerations that give shape and definition to the duty to die. If we can agree that these considerations are all relevant, we can see that the correct course of action will often be difficult to discern. A decision about when I should end my life will sometimes prove to be every bit as difficult as the decision about whether I want treatment for myself.

CAN THE INCOMPETENT HAVE A DUTY TO DIE?

Severe mental deterioration springs readily to mind as one of the situations in which I believe I could have a duty to die. But can incompetent people have duties at all? We can have moral duties we do not recognize or acknowledge, including duties that we never recognized. But can we have duties we are unable to recognize? Duties when we are unable to understand the concept of morality at all? If so, do others have a moral obligation to help us carry out

this duty? These are extremely difficult theoretical questions. The reach of moral agency is severely strained by mental incompetence.

I am tempted to simply bypass the entire question by saying that I am talking only about competent persons. But the idea of a duty to die clearly raises the specter of one person claiming that another—who cannot speak for herself—has such a duty. So I need to say that I can make no sense of the claim that someone has a duty to die if the person has never been able to understand moral obligation at all. To my mind, only those who were formerly capable of making moral decisions could have such a duty.

But the case of formerly competent persons is almost as troubling. Perhaps we should simply stipulate that no incompetent person can have a duty to die, not even if she affirmed belief in such a duty in an advance directive. If we take the view that formerly competent people may have such a duty, we should surely exercise extreme caution when claiming a formerly competent person would have acknowledged a duty to die or that any formerly competent person has an unacknowledged duty to die. Moral dangers loom regardless of which way we decide to resolve such issues.

But for me personally, very urgent practical matters turn on their resolution. If a formerly competent person can no longer have a duty to die (or if other people are not likely to help her carry out this duty), I believe that my obligation may be to die while I am still competent, before I become unable to make and carry out that decision for myself. Surely it would be irresponsible to evade my moral duties by temporizing until I escape into incompetence. And so I must die sooner than I otherwise would have to. On the other hand, if I could count on others to end my life after I become incompetent, I might be able to fulfill my responsibilities while also living out all my competent or semicompetent days. Given our society's reluctance to permit physicians, let alone family members, to perform aid-in-dying, I believe I may well have a duty to end my life when I can see mental incapacity on the horizon.

There is also the very real problem of sudden incompetence—due to a serious stroke or automobile accident, for example. For me, that is the real nightmare. If I suddenly become incompetent, I will fall into the hands of a medical-legal system that will conscientiously disregard my moral beliefs and do what is best for me, regardless of the consequences for my loved ones. And that is not at all what I would have wanted!

SOCIAL POLICIES AND A DUTY TO DIE

The claim that there is a duty to die will seem to some a misplaced response to social negligence. If our society were providing for the debilitated, the chronically ill, and the elderly as it should be, there would be only very rare cases of a duty to die. On this view, I am asking the sick and debilitated to step in and accept responsibility because society is derelict in its responsibility to provide for the incapacitated.

This much is surely true: there are a number of social policies we could pursue that would dramatically reduce the incidence of such a duty. Most obviously, we could decide to pay for facilities that provided excellent long-term care (not just health care!) for all chronically ill, debilitated, mentally ill, or demented people in this country. We probably could still afford to do this. If we did, sick, debilitated, and dying people might still be morally required to make sacrifices for their families. I might, for example, have a duty to forgo personal care by a family member who knows me and really does care for me. But these sacrifices would only rarely include the sacrifice of life itself. The duty to die would then be virtually eliminated.

I cannot claim to know whether in some abstract sense a society like ours should provide care for all who are chronically ill or debilitated. But the fact is that we Americans seem to be unwilling to pay for this kind of long-term care, except for ourselves and our own. In fact, we are moving in precisely the opposite direction—we are trying to shift the burdens of caring for the seriously and chronically ill onto families in order to save costs for our health care system. As we shift the burdens of care onto families, we also dramatically increase the number of Americans who will have a duty to die.

I must not, then, live my life and make my plans on the assumption that social institutions will protect my family from my infirmity and debility.

To do so would be irresponsible. More likely, it will be up to me to protect my loved ones.

A DUTY TO DIE AND THE MEANING OF LIFE

A duty to die seems very harsh, and often it would be. It is one of the tragedies of our lives that someone who wants very much to live can nevertheless have a duty to die. It is both tragic and ironic that it is precisely the very real good of family and loved ones that gives rise to this duty. Indeed, the genuine love, closeness, and supportiveness of family members is a major source of this duty: we could not be such a burden if they did not care for us. Finally, there is deep irony in the fact that the very successes of our life-prolonging medicine help to create a widespread duty to die. We do not live in such a happy world that we can avoid such tragedies and ironies. We ought not to close our eyes to this reality or pretend that it just doesn't exist. We ought not to minimize the tragedy in any way.

And yet, a duty to die will not always be as harsh as we might assume. If I love my family, I will want to protect them and their lives. I will want not to make choices that compromise their futures. Indeed, I can easily imagine that I might want to avoid compromising their lives more than I would want anything else. I must also admit that I am not necessarily giving up so much in giving up my life: the conditions that give rise to a duty to die would usually already have compromised the quality of the life I am required to end. In any case, I personally must confess that at age fifty-six, I have already lived a very good life, albeit not yet nearly as long a life as I would like to have.

We fear death too much. Our fear of death has led to a massive assault on it. We still crave after virtually any life-prolonging technology that we might conceivably be able to produce. We still too often feel morally impelled to prolong life—virtually any form of life—as long as possible. As if the best death is the one that can be put off longest.

We do not even ask about meaning in death, so busy are we with trying to postpone it. But we will not conquer death by one day developing a technology so magnificent that no one will have to die.

Nor can we conquer death by postponing it ever longer. We can conquer death only by finding meaning in it.

Although the existence of a duty to die does not hinge on this, recognizing such a duty would go some way toward recovering meaning in death. Paradoxically, it would restore dignity to those who are seriously ill or dying. It would also reaffirm the connections required to give life (and death) meaning. I close now with a few words about both of these points.

First, recognizing a duty to die affirms my agency and also my moral agency. I can still do things that make an important difference in the lives of my loved ones. Moreover, the fact that I still have responsibilities keeps me within the community of moral agents. My illness or debility has not reduced me to a mere moral patient (to use the language of the philosophers). Though it may not be the whole story, surely Kant was onto something important when he claimed that human dignity rests on the capacity for moral agency within a community of those who respect the demands of morality.

By contrast, surely there is something deeply insulting in a medicine and an ethic that would ask only what I want (or would have wanted) when I become ill. To treat me as if I had no moral responsibilities when I am ill or debilitated implies that my condition has rendered me morally incompetent. Only small children, the demented or insane, and those totally lacking in the capacity to act are free from moral duties. There is dignity, then, and a kind of meaning in moral agency, even as it forces extremely difficult decisions upon us.

Second, recovering meaning in death requires an affirmation of connections. If I end my life to spare the futures of my loved ones, I testify in my death that I am connected to them. It is because I love and care for precisely these people (and I know they care for me) that I wish not to be such a burden to them. By contrast, a life in which I am free to choose whatever I want for myself is a life unconnected to others. A bioethics that would treat me as if I had no serious moral responsibilities does what it can to marginalize, weaken, or even destroy my connections with others.

But life without connection is meaningless. The individualistic fantasy, though occasionally liberating, is deeply destructive. When life is good and vitality seems unending, life itself and life lived for yourself may seem quite sufficient. But if not life,

certainly death without connection is meaningless. If you are only for yourself, all you have to care about as your life draws to a close is yourself and your life. Everything you care about will then perish in your death. And that—the end of everything you care about—is precisely the total collapse of meaning. We can, then, find meaning in death only through a sense of connection with something that will survive our death.

This need not be connections with other people. Some people are deeply tied to land (for example, the family farm), to nature, or to a transcendent reality. But for most of us, the connections that sustain us are to other people. In the full bloom of life, we are connected to others in many ways—through work, profession, neighborhood, country, shared faith and worship, common leisure pursuits, friendship. Even the guru meditating in isolation on his mountain top is connected to a long tradition of people united by the same religious quest.

But as we age or when we become chronically ill, connections with other people usually become much more restricted. Often, only ties with family and close friends remain and remain important to us. Moreover, for many of us, other connections just don't go deep enough. As Paul Tsongas has reminded us, "When it comes time to die, no one says, 'I wish I had spent more time at the office.'"

If I am correct, death is so difficult for us partly because our sense of community is so weak. Death seems to wipe out everything when we can't fit it into the lives of those who live on. A death motivated by the desire to spare the futures of my loved ones might well be a better death for me than the one I would get as a result of opting to continue my life as long as there is any pleasure in it for me. Pleasure is nice, but it is meaning that matters.

· · ·

I don't know about others, but these reflections have helped me. I am now more at peace about facing a duty to die. Ending my life if my duty required might still be difficult. But for me, a far greater horror would be dying all alone or stealing the futures of my loved ones in order to buy a little more time for myself. I hope that if the time comes when I have a duty to die, I will recognize it, encourage my loved ones to recognize it too, and carry it out bravely.

ACKNOWLEDGMENTS

I wish to thank Mary English, Hilde Nelson, Jim Bennett, Tom Townsend, the members of the Philosophy Department at East Tennessee State University, and anonymous reviewers of the *Report* for many helpful comments on earlier versions of this paper. In this paper, I draw on material in John Hardwig, "Dying at the Right Time; Reflections on (Un)Assisted Suicide" in *Practical Ethics*, ed. H. LaFollette (London: Blackwell, 1996), with permission.

NOTES

1. Given the importance of relationships in my thinking, "responsibility"—rooted as it is in "respond"—would perhaps be the most appropriate word. Nevertheless, I often use "duty" despite its legalistic overtones, because Lamm's famous statement has given the expression "duty to die" a certain familiarity. But I intend no implication that there is a law that grounds this duty, nor that someone has a right corresponding to it.

2. For a discussion of the Oates case, see Tom L. Beauchamp, "What Is Suicide?" in *Ethical Issues in Death and Dying*, ed. Tom L. Beauchamp and Seymour Perlin (Englewood Cliffs, N.J.: Prentice-Hall, 1978).

3. Most bioethicists advocate a "patient-centered ethics"—an ethics which claims only the patient's interests should be considered in making medical treatment decisions. Most health care professionals have been trained to accept this ethic and to see themselves as patient advocates. For arguments that a patient-centered ethics should be replaced by a family-centered ethics see John Hardwig, "What About the Family?" *Hastings Center Report* 20, no. 2 (1990): 5–10; Hilde L. Nelson and James L. Nelson, *The Patient in the Family* (New York: Routledge, 1995).

4. A good account of the burdens of caregiving can be found in Elaine Brody, *Women in the Middle: Their Parent-Care Years* (New York: Springer Publishing Co., 1990). Perhaps the best article-length account of these burdens is Daniel Callahan, "Families as Caregivers; the Limits of Morality" in *Aging and Ethics: Philosophical Problems in Gerontology*, ed. Nancy Jecker (Totowa N.J.: Humana Press, 1991).

5. Kenneth E. Covinsky et al., "The Impact of Serious Illness on Patients' Families," *JAMA* 272 (1994): 1839–44.

6. Larry Churchill, for example, believes that Christian ethics takes us far beyond my present position: "Christian doctrines of stewardship prohibit the extension of one's own life at a great cost to the neighbor . . . And such a gesture should not appear to us a sacrifice, but as the ordinary virtue entailed by a just, social conscience." Larry Churchill, *Rationing Health Care in America* (South Bend, Ind.: Notre Dame University Press, 1988), p. 112.

7. Kant, as is well known, was opposed to suicide. But he was arguing against taking your life out of self-interested motives. It is not clear that Kant would or we should consider taking your life out of a sense of duty to be wrong. See Hilde L. Nelson, "Death with Kantian Dignity," *Journal of Clinical Ethics* 7 (1996): 215–21.

8. Obviously, I owe this distinction to Norman Daniels. Norman Daniels, *Am I My Parents' Keeper? An Essay on Justice Between the Young and the Old* (New York: Oxford University Press, 1988). Just as obviously, Daniels is not committed to my use of it here.

9. Daniel Callahan, *The Troubled Dream of Life* (New York: Simon & Schuster, 1993).

"FOR NOW HAVE I MY DEATH"[1]: THE "DUTY TO DIE" VERSUS THE DUTY TO HELP THE ILL STAY ALIVE

Felicia Nimue Ackerman

For the last three days he screamed incessantly. It was unendurable. I cannot understand how I bore it; you could hear him three rooms off. Oh, what I have suffered![2]

I

Suppose you are a sixty-year-old who has worked hard and made sacrifices for your family. Now you are ill and the care necessary to keep you alive is taking up a lot of time and money, including almost all your spouse's free time and much of the money you previously set aside for your child's college education. You and your family still love one another, but you all have strong self-interested desires as well. You want to stay alive as long as possible. Your spouse, a dedicated amateur athlete who used to spend much time playing tennis, is tired of being your caregiver. Your child wants to go to college. Who has a duty to do what? Here are four possible answers.

1. You have a duty to die (possibly including a duty to commit suicide) in order to avoid burdening your family.
2. Your spouse has a duty to accept the loss of leisure time and take care of you (that is why "in sickness and in health" is in the marriage vows) and your child has a duty to accept the loss of your financial contribution to his education, in order to avoid burdening you with the premature loss of your life.
3. Either course of action can be justified; it is not a matter of duty.
4. It depends.

From Felicia Nimue Ackerman, "For Now Have I My Death": The "Duty to Die" Versus the Duty to Help the Ill Stay Alive, *Midwest Studies in Philosophy* 24 (2000), Blackwell Publishers.

Editors' note: Some author's notes have been cut. Students who want to follow up on sources should consult the original article.

John Hardwig has recently argued in favor of (1), at least in some circumstances. This paper will criticize his views and argue for alternatives.

One way Hardwig seeks to support his view is by pointing out that

> [m]any older people report that their one remaining goal in life is not to be a burden to their loved ones. Young people feel this, too: when I ask my undergraduate students to think about whether their death could come too late, one of their very first responses always is, "Yes, when I become a burden to my family or loved ones."[3]

Hardwig thinks this reflects "moral wisdom." He does not consider the possibility that it reflects our society's bias against and systematic devaluation of the old and ill, a devaluation some old people accept uncritically, just as many women used to accept the idea that women should be subordinate to men. After all, it would hardly be surprising to discover that fifty years ago, most married women reported that they did not want careers that would burden their families. But people (or at least liberals) nowadays would have second thoughts about calling this moral wisdom, let alone using it to support an argument that married women had a duty to avoid careers that would burden their families. We now recognize two factors. First, fifty years ago there was so much social pressure on married women, if they worked outside the home at all, not to let their work inconvenience their families that any woman who dissented from this outlook risked being instantly condemned as selfish (which is not to deny that some women genuinely felt this way). Second, there was bias involved in seeing women's careers, but not men's, as a burden to their families. Many people recognize these things nowadays. But how many recognize that the same factors apply to Hardwig's uncritical report of present-day expressions of attitudes toward old age and illness? To illustrate the first factor, imagine the social reaction to a sick old person who said, "I'm sorry if it burdens my family, but my life comes first." The fact that sick old people do make "burdensome" choices often enough to give the question of a duty to die practical as well as theoretical interest suggests that many of the old and ill are less self-sacrificing than the sentiments they pay lip service to may suggest. To illustrate the second factor, consider the (deliberate) oddness of my formulation of (2), above. Sick old people are routinely called burdens to their families, but college-bound teenagers are not. It is surprising that someone who believes "life without connection is meaningless" would think it shows moral wisdom for people to talk as though they did not realize that accepting the burdens of taking care of one another is part of what a family is all about. If Hardwig really holds, as much of his writing claims, the more moderate position that there are *limits* to the burdens families can be expected to assume (although I will argue that his limits are unacceptably stringent), then why does he think it shows moral wisdom to speak as though any burden, no matter how small, would be unacceptable?

Similar concerns apply to Hardwig's use of such loaded words as 'individualistic' and 'selfish.' I doubt that anyone actually believes what he condemns as "the individualistic fantasy . . . that the patient is the only one affected by decisions about her medical treatment." And few would find fault, except on grounds of triteness, with his claim that "[t]hose of us with families and loved ones always have a duty not to make selfish . . . decisions about our lives." We normally use the pejorative term 'selfish' only for things we want to condemn. But in order to see what sorts of decisions Hardwig condemns as selfish or unduly individualistic, we must look at the family burdens he thinks can give rise to a duty to die. He says:

> The lives of our loved ones can be seriously compromised by caring for us. The burdens of providing care or even just supervision twenty-four hours a day, seven days a week are often overwhelming. When this kind of caregiving goes on for years, it leaves the caregiver exhausted, with no time for herself or life of her own. Ultimately, even her health is often destroyed. But it can also be emotionally devastating simply to live with a spouse who is increasingly distant, uncommunicative, unresponsive, foreign, and unreachable. Other family members' needs often go unmet as the

caring capacity of the family is exceeded. Social life and friendships evaporate, as there is no opportunity to go out to see friends and the home is no longer a place suitable for having friends in.

> We must also acknowledge that the lives of our loved ones can be devastated just by having to pay for health care for us. One part of [a] recent . . . study documented the financial aspects of caring for a dying member of a family. Only those who had illnesses severe enough to give them less than a 50 percent chance to live six more months were included in this study. When these patients survived their initial hospitalization and were discharged about one-third required considerable caregiving from their families; in 20 percent of cases a family member had to quit work or make some other major lifestyle change; almost one-third of these families lost all of their savings; and just under 30 percent lost a major source of income.

> If talking about money sounds venal or trivial, remember that much more than money is normally at stake here. When someone has to quit work, she may well lose her career. Savings decimated late in life cannot be recouped in the few remaining years of employability, so the loss compromises the quality of the rest of the caregiver's life. For a young person, the chance to go to college may be lost to the attempt to pay debts due to an illness in the family, and this decisively shapes an entire life.

These remarks cry out for critical examination. For one thing, Hardwig's conception of what can constitute an unacceptable family burden seems astonishingly weak. Several questions immediately arise. Should being "distant, uncommunicative, unresponsive, foreign, and unreachable" really be a capital offense anywhere, let alone in a "loving" family? Does a loving family really welcome a beloved member's suicide in order to keep a young person from having to work and/or borrow his way through college? Does the view that you have a duty to spend your hard-earned money to put your able-bodied child through college rather than to prolong your own life reflect a devaluation of the old and the ill that will someday be as offensive to liberals as 1950s attitudes toward women are today?

Hardwig's bias is also reflected in his failure to extend his criticism of selfishness and individualism to a teenager's decision to accept the college tuition money that could be used to extend his father's life or to a husband's self-interested encouragement of the suicide of his ailing wife. Such failure illustrates how terms like 'selfish' and 'individualistic' can serve in a worldview promoting not altruism, but the favoring of the interests of some *individuals* over those of others. Hardwig says, "We fear death too much." But to the extent that his views are widespread, I think that what we fear too much is having our lives and plans disrupted by the medical needs of our loved ones. This fear may cause us to magnify such disruptions out of proportion, to the point where having to work and borrow one's way through college or live with a distant and uncommunicative spouse seems so terrible that the sick person's death seems preferable and perhaps even obligatory.

There are other elements of bias in the quoted passage. The burden of providing "care or even just supervision twenty-four hours a day, seven days a week," far from being unbearable or unique to caretakers of the ill, is routine for many stay-at-home single mothers of babies and toddlers (and for stay-at-home married mothers whose husbands do no child care). . . . It is likewise common for "a family member [to have] to quit work or make some other major lifestyle change" or for a family to lose "a major source of income" when a baby is born. (Of course, people are aware of such needs when they choose to have children, but people who choose to marry are likewise aware of the strong possibility that their spouse will someday be ill and need care. I will discuss this matter more in the next section.) And Hardwig's claim that "[s]ocial life and friendships evaporate, as there is no opportunity to go out to see friends and the home is no longer a place suitable for having friends in" raises three questions. First, hasn't Hardwig ever heard of the telephone or e-mail? Why is he so ready to see the hardships of taking care of a sick person as reasons why that sick person has a duty to die, rather than as practical problems open to practical remedies? Second, precisely why is a home with a seriously ill person "no longer a place suitable for having friends in"? Suppose that person is unpredictable and incontinent. Is a home with a rambunctious toddler who is not yet toilet trained no longer a suitable place for having friends in? Third, does a loving spouse really welcome the suicide of a beloved partner in order to preserve the spouse's social life? What sort of values and what sort of love would this priority indicate?

The foregoing may make Hardwig look like a bigot with respect to age and health. So it is important to consider other aspects of his arguments, including the following case:

> An 87-year-old woman was dying of congestive heart failure. [The prognosis was] that she had less than a 50 percent chance to live for another six months. She was lucid, assertive, and terrified of death. She very much wanted to live and kept opting for rehospitalization and the most aggressive life-prolonging treatment possible. That treatment successfully prolonged her life (though with increasing debility) for nearly two years. Her 55-year-old daughter was her only remaining family, her caregiver, and the main source of her financial support. The daughter duly cared for her mother. But before her mother died, her illness had cost the daughter all of her savings, her home, her job, and her career.

I will return to this case after looking at some general features of Hardwig's views.

II

Hardwig's approach has one great strength: he acknowledges the existence of genuine conflicts of interest between patients and their families. This contrasts favorably with the sentimentality of the hospice approach, on which "[p]atients, their families and loved ones are the unit of care."[4] In contrast, Hardwig points out that "[t]he conflicts of interests, beliefs, and values among family members are often too real and too deep to treat all members as 'the patient.'"[5] He also refuses to hide behind the claim that many of the conditions he thinks can generate a duty to die can also impair patients' lives to the point where they have self-interested reasons for wanting to die. He recognizes that the most problematic cases are those where the burdensome patient wants to live. I follow him in focusing on such cases. In fact, unless otherwise specified, I assume as a background condition that the patient *greatly* wants to stay alive, and that the family's competing wants are equally strong.

Elsewhere, however, Hardwig is not so clear-headed. He uses the phrase 'duty to die' indiscriminately to apply to a duty to eschew aggressive life-prolonging medical care and a duty to commit suicide. He holds that "[t]here can be a duty to die before one's illness would cause death, even if treated only with palliative measures," and that "there may be a fairly common responsibility to end one's life in the absence of any terminal illness at all," and he offers a detailed discussion of whether a person with a duty to die should carry out his own suicide or solicit suicide assistance from his loving family or from doctors.

Hardwig's use of the phrase 'duty to die' to cover both a duty to commit suicide and a duty to eschew aggressive life-prolonging medical treatment leads him to exaggerate the originality and daringness of his position. The view that sick people can have a duty to commit suicide may indeed strike people as "just too preposterous to entertain. Or too threatening." But this is hardly true of the view that the old and/or terminally ill have a duty not to burden their families and society by insisting on the most aggressive life-prolonging treatment possible, regardless of financial and other costs. This latter view is popular nowadays to the point of cliché. It occurs with varying degrees of explicitness in numerous newspaper and magazine pieces, as well as in highly praised, widely read, and widely influential books by Daniel Callahan[6] and Sherwin B. Nuland,[7] the latter a *New York Times* bestseller and National Book Award winner. The *denial* of this latter view is what strikes people as "just too preposterous to entertain. Or too threatening." (When did you last hear anyone, bioethicist or otherwise, say that terminally ill old people are entitled to extend their lives as long as possible and by the most aggressive care possible, regardless of the cost to their families and society?) Hardwig is conventional, not original, when he says that "we must now face the fact: deaths that come too late are only the other side of our miraculous, life-prolonging modern medicine."[8] What is amazing is his claim (in 1996!) that "[w]e have so far avoided looking at this dark side of our medical triumphs."[9]

Unsurprisingly, Daniel Callahan, who is hostile to aggressive life-extending care for the old and ill but to whom suicide is anathema, has criticized Hardwig's moral equation of suicide and the refusal of aggressive life-prolonging medical care. Since I accept neither Callahan's views about suicide nor his views about aggressive life-prolonging medical care, I will not defend this sort of criticism. Instead, I find Callahan and Hardwig similar in the low value they place on the lives of the old and the ill. Callahan's objection to Hardwig that

> it trivializes the relationship of family members to each other to act as if their mutual obligations to each other are to be judged by some benefit-burden calculus. Hardwig seems to be saying in effect: "for better or worse, in sickness and in health—well, sort of, it all depends"[10]

should be read in light of things he says elsewhere. For example:

> It is not improper for people to worry about being a burden on their families. . . . A family member should reject [a technologically extended death] for the sake of the family's welfare after he or she is gone.[11]

Callahan even says that "the *primary* aspiration of the old [should be] to serve the young."[12] He also says, "We do not need a . . . set of moral values that will impose upon families the drain of extended illness and death."[13] (Note the bias in Callahan's use of "we" here. Who are the "we" who do not need such a set of moral values? Families eager to free themselves of burdensome sick "loved ones" do not need such a set of moral values, but the sick people themselves may, if they want to stay alive. What "we" (i.e., such actual and potential sick people) do not need is a set of moral values that impose on us the drain of being pressured to forgo high-tech life-extending care and die sooner than necessary, in order to avoid burdening our families—a description of the situation that is no more biased than Callahan's own. "We" old people also do not need a set of moral values that tell us our primary aspiration should be to serve the young.) Callahan's real objection thus seems to be to suicide, rather than to a benefit-burden calculation. In contrast, I have only a practical reason for finding Hardwig's views about the duty to commit suicide more objectionable than Callahan's views about the duty to refuse aggressive life-prolonging medical care: the former duty casts a much wider net. This paper will not distinguish further between these two possible duties, but will follow Hardwig's practice of using 'duty to die' to apply indiscriminately to both.

Hardwig's second conflation is also interesting. He makes no distinction between the duty to die in order to avoid burdening your children and the duty to die in order to avoid burdening your spouse.

(Interestingly, none of his examples mentions young adults with a duty to die in order to avoid burdening their caregiving parents.) But there are obvious differences between parental and "adult child" cases, on the one hand, and spousal cases on the other. Parents have often made great sacrifices for their children, including an approximation of the hyperbolically described "twenty-four hours a day, seven days a week" care that Hardwig considers so onerous in the case of the old and the ill. There is a large literature on what, if anything, grown children owe their parents, but, to my mind, nothing that refutes Joel Feinberg's "My benefactor once freely offered me his services when I needed them. . . . But now circumstances have arisen in which he needs help, and I am in a position to help him. Surely I *owe* my services now, and he would be entitled to resent my failure to come through."[14] He would also be entitled to resent my hypocrisy if I claimed to love him. (What if I have significant obligations elsewhere? This issue will be touched upon later.)

Marriages differ from parent-child relationships in two ways that are relevant here. First, they do not normally begin with a long period of one-sided caregiving, let alone one-sided caregiving by the party most likely to need care later on. Second, marriages are freely entered into by both parties. This gives couples the opportunity for prenuptial discussions and agreements that will generate their own agreed-upon caregiving duties. Of course, such an approach has its own problems. The first, which also applies to living wills, is that it may be virtually impossible for many healthy young people to enter imaginatively into hypothetical situations in which they would be seriously ill and debilitated. As Ellen Goodman puts it, "No one . . . wants to live to be senile. But once senile, he may well want to live."[15] The second problem, which also applies to prenuptial financial agreements, is that such an arrangement may seem cold-blooded and destructive to the loving spirit of the marriage. Hardwig also advocates discussions in families. He even advocates having them once a person is ill, which avoids the first problem and enables people to consider the "particular and contextual" details of their actual situation. But it enormously intensifies the second problem. Hardwig's sentimental claim that "[h]onest talk about difficult matters almost always strengthens

relationships" raises the question of just how it would strengthen a relationship to say to your father, even in response to his query, "Well, Dad, you're not pleasant to have around anymore, and if you don't die soon, your care will use up all the money you saved for my college education, so I'd really appreciate it if you killed yourself now or at least stopped getting treatment." This may be a crude formulation, but what could be a better one of such a crude thought? The plain fact is that letting your father know you value his life less than your college tuition is unlikely to strengthen your relationship. It is surprising that someone hardheaded enough to see that the slogan "the patient is the family" glosses over genuine conflicts of interest (see the material leading up to note [5]) would slip into the sentimentality of supposing that honest discussion of such conflicts will almost always strengthen relationships. Prenuptial agreements may seem cold-blooded, but at least they do not involve the cruelty of telling a sick and vulnerable person that you would welcome his death. Prenuptial discussions also give a couple the option of calling off the wedding if they find that their values are too far apart.

III

Hardwig realizes that a duty to die may seem harsh. "And yet," he says, "a duty to die will not always be as harsh as we might assume. If I love my family, I will want to protect them and their lives. I will not want to make choices that compromise their futures." But if he loves his ill wife, will he want to protect her and her life? Will he want to avoid compromising her future by encouraging her to commit suicide so he will be free of the burden of caregiving? Hardwig says that "there is something deeply insulting in . . . an ethic that . . . [treats] me as if I had no moral responsibilities when I am ill or debilitated." Will he also be insulted if his ill wife commits suicide because she thinks he is the sort of person who would rather have her dead than take care of her? I would be enormously insulted if a loved one had such a view of me. Hardwig tells us that his "own grandfather committed suicide after his heart attack as a final gift to his wife—he had plenty of life insurance but not nearly enough health insurance, and he feared that she would be left homeless and destitute if he lingered on in an incapacitated state."[16] Hardwig does not tell us whether his grandmother appreciated this "gift." What sort of person would she be if she did? If she welcomed this sacrifice, how could she be worth it? What sort of love could she have felt for her husband? What sort of love could he have thought she felt for him? And was there no one else in this loving family who could help his grandmother so she would not have to be left "homeless and destitute" if her husband lingered on?

This brings me to a discussion of what I have elsewhere called "the paradox of the selfless invalid." In its most extreme form, the paradox goes as follows. Either the patient's loved ones want him to die quickly in order to save money or otherwise make their lives easier, or they do not. If they do not, the patient does not respect them by dying for their sake. If they do, then why is the patient sacrificing what would otherwise be left of his life for people who love him so little that they value his life less than money and/or freedom from encumbrance? Wouldn't a truly loving family find such a sacrifice appalling? Of course, families can have mixed feelings, which include both the desire to have the patient stay alive and the self-interested desire to get it all over with and to keep expenses down. But the basic point remains. Decent and loving families, as part of their decency and lovingness, will recognize the latter desire as ignoble and, on balance, will not want patients to pander to it.

This extreme view is itself open to objections. Just as it is inhumane to suppose a sick person has a duty to forgo an extra year of life in order to conserve money for a child's college tuition, it is unreasonable to suppose there are no limits to what a loving family can be expected to do for a sick member, even to the point of selling literally everything they own in order to give him a minute of extra life. The devil is in the details, or, as Hardwig puts it, "the really serious moral questions are . . . how far family and friends can be asked to support and sustain the patient."[17] I have argued that some of Hardwig's answers are ludicrous. Where should we draw the line? I hardly have an exact answer, nor does Hardwig. But here are his general guidelines.

(1) A duty to die is more likely when continuing to live will impose significant burdens—emotional burdens, extensive caregiving, destruction of life plans, and yes, financial hardship—on your family and loved ones. This is the fundamental insight underlying a duty to die.

(2) A duty to die becomes greater as you grow older. As we age, we will be giving up less by giving up our lives, if only because we will sacrifice fewer remaining years of life and a smaller portion of our life plans. After all, it's not as if we would be immortal and live forever if we could just manage to avoid a duty to die. To have reached the age of, say, seventy-five or eighty years without being ready to die is itself a moral failing, the sign of a life out of touch with life's basic realities.

(3) A duty to die is more likely when you have already lived a full and rich life. You have already had a full share of the good things life offers.

(4) There is a greater duty to die if your loved ones' lives have already been difficult or impoverished, if they have had only a small share of the good things that life has to offer (especially if through no fault of their own).

(5) A duty to die is more likely when your loved ones have already made great contributions—perhaps even sacrifices—to make your life a good one. Especially if you have not made similar sacrifices for their well-being or for the well-being of other members of your family.

(6) To the extent that you can make a good adjustment to your illness or handicapping condition, there is less likely to be a duty to die. A good adjustment means that smaller sacrifices will be required of loved ones and there is more compensating interaction for them. Still, we must also recognize that some diseases—Alzheimer [*sic*] or Huntington [*sic*] chorea—will eventually take their toll on your loved ones no matter how courageously, resolutely, even cheerfully you manage to face that illness.

(7) There is less likely to be a duty to die if you can still make significant contributions to the lives of others, especially your family.

The burdens to family members are not only or even primarily financial, neither are the contributions to them. However, the old and those who have terminal illnesses must also bear in mind that the loss their family members will feel when they die cannot be avoided, only postponed.

(8) A duty to die is more likely when the part of you that is loved will soon be gone or seriously compromised. Or when you soon will no longer be capable of giving love. Part of the horror of dementing disease is that it destroys the capacity to nurture and sustain relationships, taking away a person's agency and the emotions that bind her to others.

(9) There is a greater duty to die to the extent that you have lived a relatively lavish lifestyle instead of saving for illness or old age. . . . It is a greater wrong to come to your family for assistance if your need is the result of having chosen leisure or a spendthrift lifestyle.

I suggest we reconceptualize the problem by asking how these and related conditions might affect the duty to make sacrifices in order to extend the life of a burdensomely ill loved one. I will call this "a duty to aid." Here are nine conditions parallel to Hardwig's.

1. A duty to aid is more likely when failing to do so will impose significant burdens, when the ill loved one wants very much to go on living and needs your help. This is the fundamental insight underlying a duty to aid.

2. Perhaps a duty to aid becomes greater as you grow older, because you will be sacrificing a smaller portion of your life plans. Alternatively, a duty to aid may be greater when you are young, because you have more stamina as well as more life ahead of you, with more opportunity to recoup your losses. At any rate, to have reached adulthood without being ready to undertake major financial burdens and changes in "lifestyle" in order to aid a seriously ill loved one is itself a moral failing, a sign of a life out of touch with life's basic realities.

3. A duty to aid is more likely when you are living a full and rich life that will provide you with substantial goods and pleasures to counterbalance the burden of aiding.

4. There is a greater duty to aid if your ill loved one's life has already been difficult or impoverished, if he has had only a small share of the good things that life has to offer (especially if through no fault of his own).

5. A duty to aid is more likely when your loved one has already made great contributions—perhaps even sacrifices—to make your life a good one. Especially if you have not made similar sacrifices for his well-being. This imbalance frequently exists between grown children and the parents who raised them.

6. To the extent that there are others able to share the burden of aiding, there is less you have a duty to do. To the extent that you cannot make a good adjustment to the duty of aiding, there is less of a duty to aid. Still, we must also recognize that unwillingness to make a good adjustment does not constitute inability to do so, nor does making a good adjustment mean you must enjoy aiding.

7. There is less of a duty to aid if you have significant obligations elsewhere. However, you must also bear in mind that your obligations to your children do not automatically outweigh your obligations to your parents. The popular slogan "The best thing you can do for your parents is to take good care of their grandchildren" is obviously false if your father needs and wants a heart transplant, which he cannot afford without your help, and your son "needs" and wants four years at Yale.

8. A duty to aid is more likely when your loved one is painfully aware that the part of him that was loved will soon be gone or seriously compromised and is terrified that his loved ones will abandon him. And if you genuinely love your "loved one," then to the extent that the part that is loved is *not* compromised, you will have a strong self-interested reason for wanting to help him stay alive; you would hate never seeing him again.

9. There is a greater duty to provide physical care to the extent that you have lived a relatively lavish "lifestyle" that has prevented you from saving enough to provide financial help.

These guidelines are not formally incompatible with Hardwig's. He grants that families "must be prepared to make significant sacrifices to respond to an illness in the family, although his examples I quoted earlier of what can constitute an intolerable family burden raise the question of just what sort of "significant sacrifices" he has in mind. His statement "I cannot imagine that it would be morally permissible for me to . . . compromise the quality of [my grandchildren's] lives simply because I wish to live a little longer" illustrates the importance of this question. What deprivation could *not* be said to compromise the quality of one's grandchildren's lives? Going without private schooling? Going without summer camp? Going without tennis lessons? At any rate, my guidelines and Hardwig's reflect (although they do not entail) different orientations. Hardwig believes we can find meaning in death by recognizing our duty to die, thus engaging in an "affirmation of connections." I am less inclined to find meaning in death at all. I find Malory's "Let me lie down and wail with you"[18] a much more humane response to adversity than today's relentless tendency to insist we turn adversity into an opportunity for "growth," a tendency Hardwig at any rate follows very selectively. His selectivity reflects his characteristic bias. After all, if we are going to urge people to regard death and dying as opportunities for growth and "affirmation of connections," why not urge families to seize the opportunity to grow and "affirm connections" by making loving sacrifices to prolong the life of a seriously ill loved one? Hardwig says, "Caring for the sick or aged can foster growth. . . . But it would be irresponsible to blithely assume that this always happens, that it will happen in my family, or that it will be the fault of my family if they cannot manage to turn my illness into a positive experience." He does not criticize such unsuccessful families for having a "sense of community [that] is so weak." He reserves this harsh judgment for old and/or ill people who are unwilling to unburden their families by dying (although he does grant that "[a] man who can leave his wife the day after she learns she has cancer, on the grounds that he has his own life to live, is to be deplored").[19]

Hardwig's guidelines, as well as his whole approach, raise another question. Why does he fail to consider cases where the sacrificial suicide of someone who is healthy and far from old could benefit his (not overly) loving family? Suppose you are a forty-year-old mid-level executive who has been

downsized. The only job you can get pays the minimum wage, not enough to support your family, even with the added income of your wife, who now has to work fifty hours a week as a home health aide, doing the caregiving Hardwig finds so onerous when done for a family member. Your family is about to lose their home; you will all have to move to a rat-infested apartment in an unsafe inner-city, neighborhood. "For [your children], the chance to go to college [will] be lost" (if we assume, as Hardwig inexplicably does in cases involving illness, that young people's working and/or borrowing their way through college is not an option). There is, however, a solution. Like Hardwig's grandfather, you have excellent life insurance. (If your life insurance has the common two-year "suicide clause" denying payment if the insured person commits suicide within two years of purchasing the policy, that clause has long since expired.) In accord with Hardwig's guidelines, we can build in that your life so far has been rich and full, your wife has had a difficult, impoverished childhood, and your family has made sacrifices for your career (your wife sacrificed her own career and also spent much time in the tedious pseudosocializing necessary to further your ambitions, and your children endured the dislocation of frequent moves). We can even say that you lost your job not through downsizing but through your own fault and that you have little in the way of savings because you lived a "relatively lavish lifestyle instead of saving." Would Hardwig then say you could have a duty to commit suicide instead of burdening your family by depriving them of your life insurance money? If not, why not?

Like Hardwig, I cannot lay down a series of precise rules saying who owes whom what when a sick family member needs care. In Hardwig's case of the eighty-seven-year-old woman, for example, I think much hinges on her prior relationship with her daughter. How much did that mother sacrifice for her daughter? Did the mother pay, and make sacrifices to pay, for the education that enabled the daughter to have the career Hardwig is so distressed about her losing? What was their relationship like once the daughter grew up? Did the mother, like many parents nowadays, give her daughter some of the money that enabled the daughter to buy the home Hardwig is so distressed about her losing? What happened after the mother died? Did the daughter ever find another job? Hardwig does not tell us any of these things. But I think it is clear that in my own example with which I opened this paper, alternative (2) is the right answer. A teenager should work and borrow his way through college in order to free up money to prolong the life of a beloved parent who raised him and sacrificed for him. A spouse should forgo tennis (even if it is not a trivial recreation but an important part of his life) in order to take care of the beloved partner "that he promised his faith unto."[20] "Sometimes, it's simply the only loving thing to do."[21]

NOTES

1. Sir Thomas Malory, *Le Morte D'Arthur* (London: Penguin, 1969), v.2, 515.
2. Leo Tolstoy, *The Death of Ivan Ilych* (New York: New American Library of World Literature, 1960), 10. Tolstoy, of course, intended this remark (by a cancer patient's widow) to show monumental selfishness and callousness.
3. John Hardwig, "Is There a Duty to Die?" *Hastings Center Report* 27, no. 2 (1997), 36.
4. See B. Manard and C. Perrone, *Hospice Care: An Introduction and Review of the Evidence* (Arlington, VA: National Hospice Organization, 1994), 4.
5. John Hardwig, "What about the Family?" *Hastings Center Report* (March/April 1990), 5.
6. See Daniel Callahan, *Setting Limits* (Washington, DC: Georgetown University Press, 1987), *What Kind of Life?* (Washington, DC: Georgetown University Press, 1990), and *The Troubled Dream of Life* (New York: Simon and Schuster, 1993).
7. Sherwin B. Nuland, *How We Die* (New York: Knopf, 1994).
8. Hardwig, "Dying at the Right Time," 63.
9. Ibid.
10. Callahan, letter to the editor, *Hastings Center Report* (November/December 1997), 4.
11. Callahan, *The Troubled Dream of Life,* 218–19.
12. Callahan, *Setting Limits,* 43 (italics in original).
13. Callahan, *The Troubled Dream of Life,* 218–9.
14. Joel Feinberg, "Duties, Rights, and Claims," *American Philosophical Quarterly* 3, no. 2 (1966), 139 (italics in original).
15. Ellen Goodman, "Who Lives? Who Dies? Who Decides?" in E. Goodman, *At Large* (New York: Simon and Schuster, 1981), 161. (The first part of Goodman's statement is false. I want to live to be senile. I would rather be mentally intact than senile, of course, but I would rather be senile than dead.)
16. Hardwig, "What about the Family?" 6.
17. Hardwig, "What about the Family?" 6.
18. Malory, *Le Morte D'Arthur,* v.2, 172.
19. Hardwig, "What about the Family?" 7.
20. Malory, *Le Morte D'Arthur,* v. 2, 426.
21. This is a claim Hardwig makes about killing yourself in order to avoid burdening your loved ones: "Dying at the Right Time," 57.

RECOMMENDED SUPPLEMENTARY READING

GENERAL WORKS

Annas, George J. *Standard of Care: The Law of American Bioethics.* Oxford: Oxford University Press, 1993.

Beauchamp, Tom L., and Robert M. Veatch, eds. *Ethical Issues in Death and Dying.* 2nd ed. Upper Saddle River, NJ: Prentice Hall, 1996.

Brock, Dan. *Life and Death: Philosophical Essays in Biomedical Ethics.* New York: Cambridge University Press, 1993.

Brody, Baruch. *Life and Death Decision Making.* New York: Oxford University Press, 1988.

Buchanan, Allen, and Dan Brock. *Deciding for Others: The Ethics of Surrogate Decision Making.* Cambridge: Cambridge University Press, 1989.

Byock, Ira. *Dying Well: The Prospect for Growth at the End of Life.* New York: Riverhead Books, 1997.

Cantor, Norman L. *Legal Frontiers of Death and Dying.* Bloomington: Indiana University Press, 1987.

———. "Twenty-Five Years after *Quinlan:* A Review of the Jurisprudence of Death and Dying." *Journal of Law, Medicine & Ethics* 29 (2001): 182–196.

Englehardt, H. Tristram, Jr. *The Foundations of Bioethics.* New York: Oxford University Press, 1986.

Gorovitz, Samuel. *Drawing the Line: Life, Death, and Ethical Choice in an American Hospital.* Oxford: Oxford University Press, 1991.

Kamm, F. M. *Morality, Mortality.* 2 vols. New York: Oxford University Press, 1993–1996.

Lynn, Joanne. "Serving Patients Who May Die Soon and Their Families: The Role of Hospice and Other Services." *Journal of the American Medical Association* 285 (February 21, 2001): 925–932.

McMahan, Jeff. *The Ethics of Killing: Killing at the Margins of Life.* New York: Oxford University Press, 2001.

Meisel, Alan. *The Right to Die.* New York: Wiley, 1989.

Moller, David Wendell. *Confronting Death.* New York: Oxford University Press, 1996.

President's Commission for the Study of Ethical Problems in Medicine and Biomedical and Behavioral Research. *Deciding to Forego Life-Sustaining Treatment.* Washington, DC: U.S. Government Printing Office, 1983.

Ramsey, Paul. *Ethics at the Edges of Life, Part Two.* New Haven, CT: Yale University Press, 1978.

Thomasma, David C., and Thomasine Kushner, eds. *Birth to Death: Science and Bioethics.* New York: Cambridge University Press, 1996.

Veatch, Robert. *Death, Dying, and the Biological Revolution.* 2nd ed. New Haven, CT: Yale University Press, 1989.

Weir, Robert F. *Abating Treatment with Critically Ill Patients.* New York: Oxford University Press, 1989.

———, ed. *Ethical Issues in Death and Dying.* 2nd ed. New York: Columbia University Press, 1986.

THE DEFINITION OF DEATH

Agich, George, and Royce P. Jones. "Personal Identity and Brain Death: A Critical Response." *Philosophy & Public Affairs* 15 (Summer 1986): 267–274.

Baron, L., S. D. Shemie, J. Teitelbaum, and C. J. Doig. "Brief Review: History, Concept and Controversies in the Neurological Determination of Death." *Canadian Journal of Anethesia* 53, no. 6 (June 2006): 602–608.

Bernat, James L. "Refinements in the Definition and Criterion of Death." In *The Definition of Death: Contemporary Controversies,* edited by Stuart J. Youngner, Robert M. Arnold, and Renie Schapiro. Baltimore: Johns Hopkins University Press, 1999.

Brody, Baruch. "Special Ethical Issues in the Management of PVS Patients." *Law, Medicine & Health Care* 20 (1992): 104–115.

Capron, Alexander M. "Anencephalic Donors: Separate the Dead from the Dying." *Hastings Center Report* 17, no. 1 (1987): 5–9.

———. "Brain Death—Well Settled Yet Still Unresolved." *New England Journal of Medicine* 344 (2001): 1244–1246.

Cole, David. "Statutory Definitions of Death and the Management of Terminally Ill Patients Who May Become Organ Donors after Death." *Kennedy Institute of Ethics Journal* 3, no. 2 (1993): 145–155.

Cranford, Ronald E. "The Persistent Vegetative State: The Medical Reality (Getting the Facts Straight)." *Hastings Center Report* 18, no. 1 (1988): 27–32.

Eberl, J. T. "Review of John P. Lizza: Persons, Humanity, and the Definition of Death." *American Journal of Bioethics* 7, no. 3 (March 2007): 55–57.

Emanuel, Linda L. "Reexamining Death: The Asymptomatic Model and a Bounded Zone Definition." *Hastings Center Report* (July–August 1995): 27–35.

Gervais, Karen Grandstrand. "Advancing the Definition of Death: A Philosophical Essay," *Medical Humanities Review* 3, no. 2 (1989): 7–19.

———. *Redefining Death.* New Haven, CT: Yale University Press, 1986.

Green, Michael, and Daniel Wikler. "Brain Death and Personal Identity." *Philosophy & Public Affairs* 9, no. 2 (Winter 1980): 105–133.

Greenberg, Gary. "As Good as Dead." *The New Yorker* August 13, 2001: 36–41.

Hammer, M. D., and D. Crippen. "Brain Death and Withdrawal of Support." *Surgical Clinics of North America* 86, no. 6 (December 2006): 1541–1551.

Harvard Medical School Committee to Examine the Definition of Brain Death. "A Definition of Irreversible Coma." *Journal of the American Medical Association* 205, no. 6 (August 5, 1968): 337–340.

McMahan, Jeff. "The Metaphysics of Brain Death." *Bioethics* 9, no. 2 (April 1995): 91–126.

Pernick, Martin S. "Brain Death in a Cultural Context: The Reconstruction of Death, 1967–1981." In *The Definition of Death: Contemporary Controversies,* edited by Stuart J. Youngner, Robert M. Arnold, and Renie Schapiro. Baltimore: Johns Hopkins University Press, 1999.

Potts, Michael, Paul A. Byrne, and Richard G., Nilges, eds. *Beyond Brain Death: The Case against Brain Based Criteria for Human Death.* Dordrecht, The Netherlands: Kluwer Academic, 2000.

Shewmon, D. A., A. M. Capron, W. J. Peacock, and B. L. Shulman. "The Use of Anencephalic Infants as Organ Sources: A Critique. *Journal of the American Medical Association* 261, no. 12 (March 24–31, 1989): 1773–1781.

Shinnar, Shlomo, and John Arras. "Ethical Issues in the Use of Anencephalic Infants as Organ Donors." *Neurologic Clinics* 7, no. 4 (November 1989): 729–743.

Steinbock, Bonnie. "Recovery from Persistent Vegetative State? The Case of Carrie Coons." *Hastings Center Report* 19, no. 4 (1989): 14–15.

Tomlinson, Tom. "The Irreversibility of Death: Reply to Cole." *Kennedy Institute of Ethics Journal* 3, no. 2 (1993): 157–165.

Truog, Robert D. "Is It Time to Abandon Brain Death?" *Hastings Center Report* 27 (1997): 29–37.

Veatch, Robert M. "The Impending Collapse of the Whole-Brain Definition of Death." *Hastings Center Report* 23, no. 4 (July 1, 1993): 18–25.

Whetstine, L. M. "Bench-to-Bedside Review: When Is Dead Really Dead—On the Legitimacy of Using Neurologic Criteria to Determine Death." *Critical Care* 11, no. 2 (March 13, 2007): 208.

———. "Not Dead, Not Dying? Ethical Categories and Persistent Vegetative State." *Hastings Center Report* 18, no. 1 (1988): 41–47.

Wijdicks, Eelco F. M. "The Diagnosis of Brain Death." *New England Journal of Medicine* 344 (2001): 1215–1221.

Wikler, Daniel. "Brain Death: A Durable Consensus?" *Bioethics* 7, nos. 2–3 (1993): 239–246.

Youngner, Stuart et al. "'Brain Death' and Organ Retrieval: A Cross-Sectional Survey of Knowledge and Concepts among Health Professionals." *Journal of the American Medical Association* 261 (1989): 2205–2210.

Youngner, Stuart J., Robert M. Arnold, and Renie Schapiro, eds. *The Definition of Death: Contemporary Controversies.* Baltimore: Johns Hopkins University Press, 1999.

Zaner, Richard M., ed. *Death: Beyond Whole-Brain Criteria.* Dordrecht, The Netherlands: Kluwer Academic, 1988.

DECISIONAL CAPACITY AND THE RIGHT TO REFUSE TREATMENT

Brink, Susan. "Taking Charge." *U.S. News & World Report,* July 28, 1997: 17–21 (an update on the Dax Cowart Story).

Brock, Dan W. "Decision-Making Competence and Risk." *Bioethics* 5, no. 2 (1991): 105–112.

Callahan, Daniel. "Terminating Life-Sustaining Treatment of the Demented." *Hastings Center Report* (November–December 1995): 25–31.

Connors, Russell B., Jr., and Martin L. Smith. "Religious Insistence on Medical Treatment: Christian Theology and Imagination." *Hastings Center Report* (July–August 1996): 23–30.

Freedman, Benjamin. "Competence, Marginal and Otherwise: Concepts and Ethics." *International Journal of Law and Psychiatry* 4 (1981): 53–72.

Kliever, Lonnie D., ed. *Dax's Case: Essays in Medical Ethics and Human Meaning.* Dallas, TX: Southern Methodist University Press, 1989.

Kopehnan, Loretta M. "On the Evaluative Nature of Competency and Capacity Judgments." *International Journal of Law and Psychiatry* (1990): 309–329.

Macklin, Ruth. "Consent, Coercion and Conflicts of Rights." *Perspectives in Biology and Medicine* 20, no. 3 (1977): 360–371.

May, Larry. "Challenging Medical Authority: The Refusal of Treatment by Christian Scientists." *Hastings Center Report* (January–February 1995): 15–21.

Meisel, Alan. "Legal Myths about Terminating Life Support." *Archives of Internal Medicine* 109 (1991):1497–1502.

Powell, Tia, and Bruce Lowenstein. "Refusing Life-Sustaining Treatment after Catastrophic Injury: Ethical Implications." *Journal of Law, Medicine & Ethics* 24, no. 1 (Spring 1996): 54–61.

Roth, Loren H., Alan Meisel, and Charles Lidz. "Tests of Competency to Consent to Treatment." *American Journal of Psychiatry* 134, no. 3 (March 1977): 279–284.

Sheldon, Mark. "Ethical Issues in the Forced Transfusion of Jehovah's Witness Children." *The Journal of Emergency Medicine* 14, no. 2 (1996): 251–257.

Skene, Loane. "Risk-Related Standard Inevitable in Assessing Competence." *Bioethics* 5, no. 2 (1991): 113–122.

Wicclair, Mark R. "Patient Decision-Making Capacity and Risk." *Bioethics* 5, no. 2 (1991): 91–104.

ADVANCE DIRECTIVES

"Advance Directives: Expectations, Experience, and Future Practice." *Journal of Clinical Ethics* 4, no. 1 (1993): 1–104.

Brett, Allan S. "Limitations of Listing Specific Medical Interventions in Advance Directives," *Journal of the American Medical Association* 266, no. 6 (August 14, 1991): 825–828.

———. "Advance Directives and the Personal Identity Problem." *Philosophy & Public Affairs* 17 (Fall 1988): 277–302.

Cantor, Norman. *Advance Directives and the Pursuit of Death with Dignity.* Bloomington: Indiana University Press, 1993.

———. "Making Advance Directives Meaningful." *Psychology, Public Policy, and Law* 4 (1998): 629–652.

Dresser, Rebecca. "Confronting the Near Irrelevance of Advance Directives." *Journal of Clinical Ethics* 5 (1994): 55–56.

Hackler, C. R., R. Moseley, and D. E. Vawter, eds. *Advance Directives in Medicine.* New York: Praeger, 1989.

Kirschner, K. L. "When Written Advance Directives Are Not Enough." *Clinical Geriatric Medicine* 21, no. 1 (February 2005): 193–209.

Matesanz, Mateu B. "Advance Statements: Legal and Ethical Implications." *Nursing Standard* 21, no. 2 (September 2006): 41–45.

"Patient Self-Determination Act." *Cambridge Quarterly of Healthcare Ethics* 2, no. 2 (special section, 1992): 97–126.

Robertson, John. "Second Thoughts on Living Wills." *Hastings Center Report* 21, no. 6 (1991): 6–9.

Teno, Joan et al. "Do Formal Advance Directives Affect Resuscitation Decisions and the Use of Resources for Seriously Ill Patients?" *Journal of Clinical Ethics* 5, no. 1 (Spring 1994): 23–30.

CHOOSING FOR ONCE-COMPETENT AND NEVER-COMPETENT PATIENTS

Allen, W. "Erring Too Far on the Side of Life: Deja Vu All Over Again in the Schiavo Saga." *Stetson Law Review* 35, no. 1 (Fall 2005): 123–145.

Arras, John. "Beyond Cruzan: Individual Rights, Family Autonomy and the Persistent Vegetative State." *Journal of the American Geriatrics Society* 39 (1991): 1018–1024.

Blustein, Jeffrey. "The Family in Medical Decisionmaking." *Hastings Center Report* 23, no. 3 (May–June 1993): 6–13.

Cantor, Norman. "Discarding Substituted Judgment and Best Interests: Toward a Constructive Preference Standard for Dying, Previously Competent Patients without Advance Instructions." *Rutgers Law Review* 48 (1996): 1193–1272.

Capron, Alexander M., ed. "Medical Decision-Making and the 'Right to Die' after Cruzan." *Law, Medicine & Health Care* 19, nos. 1–2 (Spring/Summer 1991): 5–104.

"Children and Bioethics: Uses and Abuses of the Best Interests Standard." *Journal of Medicine and Philosophy* 22, no. 3 (Symposium, June 1997).

Dresser, Rebecca. "Missing Persons: Legal Perceptions of Incompetent Patients." *Rutgers Law Review* 46, no. 2 (Winter 1994): 609–719.

———. "Dworkin on Dementia: Elegant Theory, Questionable Policy." *Hastings Center Report* (November–December 1995): 32–38.

Emanuel, Ezekiel J. *The Ends of Human Life: Medical Ethics in a Liberal Polity.* Cambridge, MA: Harvard University Press, 1991.

Emanuel, Ezekiel J., and Linda L. "Decisions at the End of Life: Guided by Communities of Patients." *Hastings Center Report* 23, no. 5 (1993): 6–14.

Fins, J. J. "Affirming the Right to Care, Preserving the Right to Die: Disorders of Consciousness and Neuroethics after Schiavo." *Palliative Support Care* 4, no. 2 (June 2006): 169–178.

Freedman, Benjamin. "Respectful Service and Reverent Obedience: A Jewish View on Making Decisions for Incompetent Parents." *Hastings Center Report* (July–August 1996): 31–37.

Kadish, Sanford H. "Letting Patients Die: Legal and Moral Reflections." *California Law Review* 80, no. 4 (1992): 857–888.

Kopelman, L. M. "The Best Interests Standard for Incompetent on Incapacitated Persons of All Ages." *Journal of Law and Medical Ethics* 35, no. 1 (Spring 2007): 187–196.

Li, L. L., K. Y. Cheong, L. K. Yaw, and E. H. Liu. "The Accuracy of Surrogate Decisions in Intensive Care Scenarios." *Anesthesia Intensive Care* 35, no. 1 (Fall 2007): 46–51.

Lynn, Joanne, ed. *By No Extraordinary Means: The Choice to Forego Life-Sustaining Food and Water.* Bloomington: Indiana University Press, 1986.

May, William E. et al. "Feeding and Hydrating the Permanently Unconscious and Other Vulnerable Persons." *Issues in Law and Medicine* 3, no. 3 (1987): 203–211.

Meisel, Alan. "The Legal Consensus about Forgoing Life-Sustaining Treatment: Its Status and Prospects." *Kennedy Institute of Ethics Journal* 2, no. 4 (December 1992): 309–342.

Nelson, James Lindermann. "Taking Families Seriously." *Hastings Center Report* 22, no. 4 (1992): 6–12.

———. "Critical Interests and Sources of Familial Decision-Making Authority for Incapacitated Patients." *Journal of Law, Medicine & Ethics* 23, no. 2 (Summer 1995): 143–148.

New York State Task Force on Life and the Law. *Life-Sustaining Treatment: Making Decisions and Appointing a Health Care Agent.* 1987.

———. *When Others Must Choose: Deciding for Patients without Capacity.* 1992.

"Pediatric Decision Making." *Journal of Law, Medicine & Ethics* 23, no. 1 (symposium; Spring 1995).

Rhoden, Nancy K. "Litigating Life and Death." *Harvard Law Review* 102, no. 2 (December 1988): 375–446.

Solomon, Mildred Z. et al. "Decisions Near the End of Life: Professional Views on Life-Sustaining Treatments." *American Journal of Public Health* 83, no. 1 (January 1993): 14–23.

Veatch, Robert M. "Forgoing Life-Sustaining Treatment: Limits to the Consensus." *Kennedy Institute of Ethics Journal* 3, no. 1 (March 1993): 1–19.

Weyrauch, S. "Decision Making for Incompetent Patients: Who Decides and By What Standards?" *Tulsa Law Journal* 35, no. 3–4 (Spring–Summer 2000): 765–789.

White, Patricia D., ed. "Essays in the Aftermath of Cruzan." *Journal of Medicine and Philosophy* 17, no. 6 (December 1992): 563ff.

Wolfson, J. "Defined by Her Dying, Not Her Death: The Guardian Ad Litem's View of Schiavo." *Death Studies* 30, no. 2 (March 2006): 113–120.

PHYSICIAN-ASSISTED DEATH

"Aid in Dying: The Supreme Court and the Public Response." *Hastings Center Report* (September–October, 1997).

Arras, John D. "The Right to Die on the Slippery Slope." *Social Theory and Practice* 8, no. 3 (Fall 1982): 285–328.

Battin, Margaret P. *The Least-Worst Death: Essays in Bioethics on the End of Life.* New York: Oxford University Press, 1994.

———. *The Death Debate: Ethical Issues in Suicide.* Englewood Cliffs, NJ: Prentice Hall, 1996.

———. "A Dozen Caveats Concerning the Discussion of Euthanasia in the Netherlands." In *Arguing Euthanasia:*

The Controversy over Mercy Killing, Assisted Suicide and the Right to Die, edited by Jonathan Moreno. New York: Simon and Schuster, 1995.

Battin, Margaret P., Rosamond Rhodes, and Anita Silvers. *Physician-Assisted Suicide: Expanding the Debate.* New York and London: Routledge, 1998.

Beauchamp, Tom L., ed. *Intending Death: The Ethics of Assisted Suicide and Euthanasia.* Upper Saddle River, NJ: Prentice Hall, 1996.

Brock, Dan W. "Voluntary Active Euthanasia." *Hastings Center Report* (March–April 1992).

Brody, Baruch. *Suicide and Euthanasia.* Dordrecht, The Netherlands: Kluwer Academic, 1989.

Brody, Howard. "Assisted Death: A Compassionate Response to Medical Failure." *New England Journal of Medicine* 327, no. 19 (November 5, 1992): 1384–1388.

Callahan, Daniel. *The Troubled Dream of Life: Living with Mortality.* New York: Simon and Schuster, 1993.

Cohen, Cynthia B. "Christian Perspectives on Assisted Suicide and Euthanasia: The Anglican Tradition." *Journal of Law, Medicine & Ethics* 24, no. 4 (Winter 1996): 369–379.

Downing, A. B., and Barbara Smoker. *Voluntary Euthanasia: Experts Debate the Right to Die.* London: Peter Owen, 1986.

Dworkin, Gerald, R. G. Frey, and Sissela Bok. *Euthanasia and Physician-Assisted Suicide: For and Against.* Cambridge: Cambridge University Press, 1998.

Dworkin, Ronald. *Life's Dominion: An Argument about Abortion, Euthanasia, and Individual Freedom.* New York: Knopf, 1993.

"Dying Well? A Colloquy on Euthanasia and Assisted Suicide." *Hastings Center Report* 22, no. 2 (special issue, 1992): 6–55.

"Euthanasia and Physician-Assisted Suicide: Murder or Mercy." *Cambridge Quarterly of Healthcare Ethics* 2, no. 1 (special section, 1993): 9–88.

Feinberg, Joel. "Voluntary Euthanasia and the Inalienable Right to Life." *Philosophy & Public Affairs* 7, no. 2 (Winter 1978): 93–123.

Foot, Philippa. "Euthanasia." *Philosophy & Public Affairs* 6, no. 2 (Winter 1977): 85–112.

Gaylin, Willard et al. "Doctors Must Not Kill." *Journal of American Medical Association* 259, no. 14 (April 8, 1988): 2139–2140.

Glover, Jonathan. *Causing Death and Saving Lives.* New York: Penguin Books, 1977.

Jennings, Bruce. "Active Euthanasia and Forgoing Life-Sustaining Treatment: Can We Hold the Line?" *Journal of Pain and Symptom Management* 6, no. 5 (July 1991): 312–316.

Kamisar, Yale. "Some Non-Religious Views against Proposed 'Mercy-Killing' Legislation." *Minnesota Law Review* 42 (1958): 969–1042.

———. "Are Laws against Assisted Suicide Unconstitutional?" *Hastings Center Report* 23, no. 3 (1993): 32–41.

Kass, Leon. "Is There a Right to Die?" *Hastings Center Report* 23, no. 1 (1993): 34–43.

Kevorkian, Jack. *Prescription Medicine: The Goodness of Planned Death.* Buffalo, NY: Prometheus Books, 1991.

Kuhse, Helga. "Voluntary Euthanasia and Other Medical End-of-Life Decisions: Doctors Should Be Permitted to Give Death a Helping Hand." In *Birth to Death: Science and Bioethics,* edited by David C. Thomasma and Thomasine Kushner. Cambridge: Cambridge University Press, 1996.

Mappes, Thomas A., and Jane S. Zembaty, "Patient Choices, Family Interests, and Physician Obligations." *Kennedy Institute of Ethics Journal* 4 (1994): 27–46.

Momeyer, Richard. "Does Physician-Assisted Suicide Violate the Integrity of Medicine?" *Journal of Medicine and Philosophy* 20, no. 1 (February 1995): 13–24.

Moreno, Jonathan D. *Arguing Euthanasia: The Controversy over Mercy Killing, Assisted Suicide, and the "Right to Die."* New York: Simon and Schuster, 1995.

New York State Task Force on Life and the Law. *When Death Is Sought: Assisted Suicide and Euthanasia in the Medical Context.* 1994.

———. *When Death Is Sought: Assisted Suicide and Euthanasia in the Medical Context, Supplement to Report.* April 1997.

Orentlicher, David. "The Legalization of Physician-Assisted Suicide: A Very Modest Revolution." *Boston College Law Review* 38, no. 3 (1997): 443–475.

"Physician-Assisted Suicide in Context: Constitutional, Regulatory, and Professional Challenges." *Journal of Law, Medicine & Ethics* 24, no. 3 (symposium, Fall 1996): 181–242.

Pratt, David A. "Too Many Physicians: Physician-Assisted Suicide after Glucksberg/Quill." *Albany Journal of Law, Science & Technology* 9 (1999): 161–234.

Pratt, David A., and Bonnie Steinbock. "Death with Dignity or Unlawful Killing: The Ethical and Legal Debate Over Physician-Assisted Death." *Criminal Law Bulletin* (May–June 1997): 226–261.

Quill, Timothy E. *Death and Dignity: Making Choices and Taking Charge.* New York: Oxford University Press, 1986.

———. "The Ambiguity of Clinical Intentions." *New England Journal of Medicine* 329 (1992): 1039–1040.

———. *A Midwife through the Dying Process: Stories of Healing and Hard Choices at the End of Life.* Baltimore: Johns Hopkins University Press, 1996.

Quill, Timothy E., Christine K. Cassel, and Diane E. Meier, "Care of the Hopelessly Ill: Proposed Clinical Criteria for Physician-Assisted Suicide." *New England Journal of Medicine* 327, no. 19 (November 5, 1992): 1380–1384.

Rachels, James. *The End of Life: Euthanasia and Morality.* New York: Oxford University Press, 1986.

Steinbock, Bonnie, and Alastair Norcross, eds. *Killing and Letting Die*. 2nd ed. New York: Fordham University Press, 1994.

Symposium on Assisted Suicide. *Hastings Center Report* (May–June 1995).

Thomasma, David C., Thomasine Kimbrough-Kushner, Gerrit K. Kimsma, and Chris Cisesielski-Carlucci. *Asking to Die: Inside the Dutch Debate about Euthanasia*. Dordrecht, The Netherlands: Kluwer Academic, 1998.

Velleman, J. David. "Against the Right to Die." *Journal of Medicine and Philosophy* 17, no. 6 (December 1992): 664–681.

Weir, R. F. "The Morality of Physician-Assisted Suicide." *Law, Medicine & Health Care* 20 (1992): 116–126.

PART FOUR

REPRODUCTION

THE MORALITY OF ABORTION

Law and Policy

More than thirty years have passed since the Supreme Court struck down restrictive abortion statutes in the landmark decision of *Roe* v. *Wade* (1973), yet the moral battle over abortion continues to rage. On the one side are those who defend the unborn child's right to life; on the other, those who insist that women must be able to make their own decisions about whether to bear a child.

In recent years, the battle over abortion has focused on late-term abortions, which many Americans, even the majority who generally support abortion rights, find morally troubling. In a procedure described by its opponents as "partial-birth abortion" (known medically as intact dilation and extraction), the fetus is partly delivered and its brain suctioned out in order to collapse the skull so that it can pass through the cervix. Congress twice attempted to ban partial-birth abortions, and twice the legislation was vetoed by President Clinton. A number of states passed laws banning partial-birth abortions, laws which were challenged in court. On June 29, 2000, the Supreme Court, in a 5 to 4 decision (*Stenberg* v. *Carhart*), invalidated a Nebraska law banning partial-birth abortions, a decision that rendered similar laws in thirty other states unconstitutional as well. The Court ruled that because the procedure may be the most medically appropriate way of terminating some pregnancies, it cannot constitutionally be banned.

At present, then, the law on abortion is clear. As the Supreme Court has consistently ruled, the constitutional right of privacy protects a woman's decision to terminate her pregnancy up until viability, and even thereafter when necessary to protect her life or health. The morality of abortion, however, remains hotly debated.

Moral Perspectives

The five selections in Section 1 offer philosophical discussions that illuminate the basic moral structure behind the issue of abortion. The abortion controversy poses two fundamental and extraordinarily difficult ethical questions. The first question relates to the moral status of the fetus, and is usually framed as asking whether the fetus is a "human being" or a "person" with a right to life. The second question relates to the moral obligation of a pregnant woman to continue gestating the fetus. It has often been assumed that the answer to the first question determines the answer to the second. That is, it is assumed that if the fetus is a person with a right to life, then abortion is morally wrong. As we will see, things are not that simple. Nevertheless, if the fetus is a full-fledged person, with a right to life, the usual reasons for supporting abortion—that the world is already overpopulated, that children are better off if they are wanted, that bearing and raising unwanted children imposes serious burdens on women—would appear to be inadequate. We do not think it is right to kill people to prevent overpopulation, nor that parents can kill their unwanted newborns. As for the burdens imposed on women by unwanted pregnancies, it may be objected that the situation is not unique. For example, women are the primary caretakers of elderly parents, but no one thinks that old and senile people may be killed to relieve the burden on their daughters. If abortion is different, it must be because of a difference in moral status between born human beings and fetuses. At the core of the abortion debate is the question of the moral status of the fetus.

This issue is addressed in the first three selections of Section 1. The traditional conservative position is represented in the first selection, which comes from the *Evangelium Vitae* by Pope John Paul II. Abortion, according to the pope, is an "unspeakable crime" because it is "the deliberate and direct killing of a human being." The pope acknowledges that the decision to have an abortion is often made not for selfish reasons or out of convenience, but to protect important values such as the woman's own health, or to procure a decent standard of living for her family. Nevertheless, he maintains that such reasons "can never justify the deliberate killing of an innocent human being." As for the claim that a fertilized egg is not yet a human being, the pope responds, "It would never be made human if it were not human already." Nor does this claim rest on religious views such as the occurrence of ensoulment. Rather, "modern genetic science" demonstrates that at fertilization there is a new, individual human being. This human being is to be respected and treated as a person, with a right to life, from the moment of conception.

The classic article by Mary Anne Warren, "On the Moral and Legal Status of Abortion," has set the stage for contemporary debates on abortion, and requires a summary here. Warren argues that the conservative position on abortion fails to notice that the term "human being" has two different meanings. The genetic or biological meaning ascribes species membership to an entity. Human embryos and fetuses clearly are human beings in this sense; they are not members of any other species. However,

there is another sense of "human being," the moral sense. To ascribe moral humanity to a being is to say that it has full membership in the moral community and is the possessor of certain rights (human rights). Warren thinks that the conservative position confuses these two meanings, and that this confusion is responsible for the view that all genetic humans, even human embryos, are moral humans.

In the second selection, "Why Abortion Is Immoral," Don Marquis agrees that it is hard to see why it is reasonable to base moral status on something as arbitrary as the number of chromosomes in one's cells. At the same time, the "person view," which holds that moral status is based on such abilities as self-consciousness, rationality, and language use, has its own difficulties. Proponents of the person view have to explain why their principle, which justifies abortion, does not justify the killing of newborn infants, or elderly senile or severely mentally impaired individuals.

Whatever else might be said for the person view, it certainly does not seem to square with or explain our repugnance to infanticide. For this reason, a number of theorists (Steinbock 1992; Sumner 1981) have suggested a weaker criterion of moral status, namely, sentience—the ability to experience pain and pleasure. Sentience theorists maintain that sentience is a necessary condition for having interests and a welfare, and that only beings that have interests and a welfare have moral status. In the third selection, "Why Most Abortions Are Not Wrong," Steinbock outlines this conception of moral status, calling it "the interest view." The implications of the interest view for abortion depend on the factual question: when do fetuses become sentient? Undoubtedly the onset of sentience is gradual, but it probably occurs during the second trimester. Prior to the onset of sentience, abortion is not seriously wrong. Any reason why a woman does not want to become a mother suffices to justify abortion: After the fetus becomes sentient, its interests must be balanced against those of the pregnant woman. This accords with a moderate view on abortion in which the reasons for having an abortion must be proportionately more compelling as the fetus develops and acquires more of the characteristics of born human beings.

One difficulty for sentience theorists is the status of nonhuman animals. Just as the challenge for person theorists is to explain why it would be wrong to kill human infants, the challenge for sentience theorists is to explain why it is not seriously wrong to kill (most) animals. Some theorists in both camps are willing to "bite the bullet" and accept the counterintuitive implications of their views. Michael Tooley, a person theorist, thinks infanticide is not generally wrong (Tooley 1983), and Peter Singer, a sentience theorist, thinks the killing of animals is usually wrong (Singer 1975). Sentience theorists who want to ascribe a greater moral status to sentient human beings than to animals must explain why this is rational. One possibility is to differentiate among sentient beings, giving greater moral status to sentient beings who are also persons or potentially persons because of the centrality of personhood to moral agency and responsibility (Steinbock 1992).

Marquis maintains that the sentience view is no improvement over the person view, and both are as flawed as the genetic humanity criterion for moral status. The solution, Marquis suggests, is to stop looking for what gives an entity human moral status. Instead, we should develop a general account of the wrongness of killing people, and then see if abortion is included in this account. What makes killing wrong is the loss of the victim's future—in particular, a future like ours (or FLO, as it has come to be called). This principle differs from the traditional pro-life position in two ways. First, it is not based on the special value of human life; it is not "speciesist." If there are nonhuman aliens or animals with a future like ours, however that is interpreted, they too have a right to life. Second, Marquis notes that his principle does not rule out practices opposed by most pro-lifers. For example, on Marquis's view, it might not be wrong to kill someone in a persistent vegetative state (PVS), who will never regain consciousness, because such a person no longer has a valuable future. A fetus, however, usually does have a valuable future and therefore abortion is almost always immoral. It is immoral for the same reason that it would be wrong to kill you or me: to do so would deprive us of our valuable futures.

Marquis thinks that the FLO account is superior to the interest view because the FLO account can explain what is wrong with killing people who are temporarily unconscious, while the interest view, he says, cannot. Steinbock responds to this objection by saying that someone who is temporarily unconscious has had desires and preferences in the past, which

form the basis for saying he would not want to be killed now. However, even if the FLO account is the correct account of the wrongness of killing, it is not clear it has the implications for abortion that Marquis claims. Steinbock argues that this depends on the theory of personal identity one accepts. On a psychological theory of identity, it is not clear that the adult is "the same person" as the preconscious fetus, as it lacks any thoughts, memories, or experiences that could connect them. There is continuous physical development between the fetus and the adult, and this could justify the claim that they are "the same individual," given a physical continuity view of identity. However, there is also physical continuity between the fetus and the embryo, and between the embryo and the gametes that combined to produce it. Why, then, is it only fetuses that have FLO; why not gametes? But if gametes have FLO, then Marquis, it seems, is committed to regarding contraception as being as morally wrong as abortion—a consequence that Marquis strenuously wishes to avoid.

So far, we have been looking only at arguments that focus on the status of the fetus. This leaves out entirely the pregnant woman whose body sustains the fetus. Judith Jarvis Thomson's novel contribution to the abortion debate is to point out that settling the moral status of the fetus does not necessarily determine the morality of abortion. In "A Defense of Abortion," Thomson argues that the antiabortion argument based on the fetus's right-to-life argument is logically flawed. The conclusion—that abortion is wrong—does not follow from the premise that the fetus is a person, with a right to life. For the argument does not show that killing the fetus *violates* its right to life. This may sound paradoxical: If the fetus has a right to life, and abortion kills it, surely its right to life is violated? But this is precisely what Thomson wishes to deny. The core of her argument is that a right to life does not carry with it the right to whatever one may need to stay alive. Much of Thomson's article discusses whether the woman's (partial) responsibility for the fetus's existence in her body does give the fetus-person a right to use her body. If her responsibility for the fetus does give it a right to use her body, then her refusal to let it remain in her body could be seen as depriving the fetus of what it has a right to, and this would make abortion unjust killing. Somewhat ironically, although Thomson's article is intended as a defense of abortion, her argument has great appeal for people who think that abortion is generally wrong, but wish to make an exception in the case of rape. If the woman was clearly not responsible for her pregnancy, as in the case of rape, then she cannot be said to have given the fetus a right to use her body. Thus, abortion in the case of rape is not unjust killing, and does not violate the fetus's right to life.

Thomson tries to show that nonresponsibility extends beyond the rape scenario; that, for example, a woman who has a contraceptive failure also has not given the fetus a right to use her body. She then goes on to consider whether a woman *ought*—out of common decency—to allow the fetus-person to use her body, even if it has no right to do so. Thomson rejects this suggestion, however, saying that the sacrifice on the part of the pregnant woman is too great. No one is morally required to make large sacrifices in order to keep another person alive. This part of Thomson's article inspired an "equal protection" argument against restrictive abortion laws, on the grounds that requiring women, but not men, to be "Good Samaritans" violates equal protection (Regan 1979). Despite its title, Thomson's article is best read not as a general defense of abortion, but rather as a focused critique of the conservative argument against abortion, in particular, the claim that abortion is immoral because the fetus has a right to life. However, even if Thomson is correct about the limitations of rights in general, and the right to life in particular, it could still be possible to argue that abortion is wrong. If the fetus is a person, then it is a special person, namely, the pregnant woman's child. Parents have special obligations, that strangers do not, to nurture and protect their children.

Margaret Olivia Little takes up this issue in "The Morality of Abortion," the last selection. She maintains that even if abortion is not a "wrongful interference," as Thomson has argued, it might still be morally wrong. "If fetuses are persons, the question we really need to decide is what positive responsibilities, if any, do pregnant women have to continue gestational assistance? This is a question that takes us into far richer, and far more interesting, territory than that occupied by discussions of murder." In part, this is a question of what we owe others as a matter of general beneficence. It is much more than that, however, due to the unique nature of gestation. This has been virtually ignored in mainstream philosophical discussions of abortion, and this "has ended up deeply underselling the moral complexity of abortion." Just as pro-lifers oversimplify the situation by assuming that the wrongness of abortion follows from the personhood of the fetus, so too pro-choicers oversimplify matters by assuming that it follows from the nonpersonhood of the fetus that abortion is morally neutral. Even if fetuses are not persons, and not owed the respect due to persons, they still might be, as Little put it, *"respect-worthy."*

OBLIGATIONS TO THE NOT-YET-BORN

The central question posed by abortion is whether a pregnant woman has the right to terminate her pregnancy, ending the life of (that is, killing) the fetus she is carrying. But what if the woman does not want to terminate her pregnancy, but instead to carry to term? What obligations does she have to protect the health and well-being of her future, not-yet-born child? As Howard Minkoff and Lynn M. Paltrow emphasize in "The Rights of 'Unborn Children' and the Value of Pregnant Women," pregnant women are typically "the most powerful advocates for the wellbeing of unborn children." At the same time, women can make choices during pregnancy that pose risks to the health of future children. A woman who smokes during pregnancy is more likely to have a child who is premature or of low birth weight and at increased risk of morbidity and mortality; if she binge drinks, she puts the child at risk of fetal alcohol syndrome, characterized by a range of mental problems from learning disabilities to severe and irreversible mental retardation. The use of other drugs during pregnancy also increases health risks and neurological deficits. It might be thought that if a woman has the moral and legal right to terminate a pregnancy, killing the fetus, then it is inconsistent to be concerned about her infliction of harms less serious than death, such as disability. However, this does not follow. The argument for abortion is based, in part, on the claim that fetuses are not persons and do not have full moral status. By contrast, born children are people with the same moral and legal rights that everyone else has not to be harmed. Thus, if a woman intends to carry a pregnancy to term, and knows (or should know) that an avoidable act is likely to cause serious harm to the child she will bring into the world, then she has a prima facie obligation to that future child not to harm it prenatally. The *timing* of the behavior (i.e., that it occurs before the full-fledged person exists) is not relevant. As regards the obligation not to inflict harm, remoteness in time, in itself, has no more significance than remoteness in space (Parfit 1984).

It follows that there can be obligations to prevent harm to future actual children that do not exist in the case of merely possible children (embryos and fetuses). At the same time, the existence of prima facie obligations to not-yet-born children does not imply that pregnant women must do whatever they can to avoid any risk to the fetus at whatever the cost to themselves. Nor are medical practitioners, legislators, judges, or prosecutors entitled to diminish the rights of women in the name of protecting fetuses.

In the next selection in Section 2 Allen Buchanan, Dan W. Brock, Norman Daniels, and Daniel Wikler raise the question of whether parents might have a moral obligation to use genetic testing to avoid the birth of a child with a severe genetic impairment. When, if ever, is it wrong to have a child who might have a serious disability? This question raises both practical and conceptual questions. The practical question is, what are prospective parents morally required to do to avoid the birth of a severely disabled child? As we have already argued, prospective parents should take reasonable steps to prevent the not-yet-born child from developing a disability (Steinbock 1992). But should prospective parents use genetic testing to learn if they are at risk of having a child with a genetic disease, and if so, either avoid conception or terminate a pregnancy to avoid that outcome? Buchanan et al. argue that there is a moral obligation to prevent the births of people with serious genetic diseases. The deeply philosophical issue is the explanation of that obligation.

In the Introduction of *From Chance to Choice*, the book from which the last selection is taken, the authors say, "we argue that the most straightforward and compelling case for developing and using genetic interventions is to fulfill one of the most basic moral obligations human beings have: the obligation to prevent harm" (Buchanan et al. 2000, 18). However, in many cases, the only way to prevent the genetic harm is to prevent the child's birth. That is, the choice facing a couple at risk of transmitting a genetic disease to their offspring is *not* between having this child in an impaired condition and having this child "healthy and whole." The choice is rather between having this child in an impaired condition and not having this child. This raises the troubling questions: Can one protect a child by preventing it from being born? Can birth in an impaired condition be unfair to the child?

This problem has been much discussed in the philosophical literature, notably by Derek Parfit, so that it is often referred to as "the Parfit problem." It is also the basis of a novel tort, the tort of "wrongful life." The tort is very controversial, for reasons that are legal, philosophical, and political, and it is recognized as a cause of action in only three states (New Jersey, California, and Washington). From a philosophical perspective, the wrong to the child is based on the idea that when life is filled with suffering and bereft of compensating pleasures, life is not a benefit but a harm (Feinberg 1986; Steinbock 1986). The child has been wronged by being given a life that is not a good to the child, from his or her own perspective. Some would argue that life is *always* worth living, no matter how great the suffering, no matter how limited the child's existence. But this seems to be more a matter of faith (or perhaps a failure of imagination) than a defensible position. Nevertheless, as Asch points out in Part 5 of this text, and Buchanan et al. agree, most people with disabilities, even severe disabilities, find their lives worth living. Buchanan et al. term such cases "wrongful disabilities" to distinguish them from "wrongful life" cases. The challenge is to say what the "wrong" is in "wrongful disability" cases. Why is it wrong to have children who will have lives that are, on balance, worth living?

John Robertson has forcefully argued that, as long as the child can be expected to have a life worth living, procreation is not a wrong to the child (Robertson 1994). He concludes that protecting offspring is never, or hardly ever, a rationale for restricting procreative choice. This may sound startling. Surely, it may be asked, we should think about the welfare of children when assessing new reproductive technologies? (This is an explicit requirement of the Human Fertilization and Embryology Authority, which licenses fertility clinics in the United Kingdom.) For example, if a reproductive technique was found to be associated with a higher incidence of disability in offspring, that would presumably be a reason to ban it.

Suppose we discovered that intracytoplasmic sperm injection (ICSI), in which a single sperm is injected directly into the egg, increased the risk of having a child with cystic fibrosis. One theory is that some men are infertile because they have a mild case of CF. They do not have any of the lung or digestive problems associated with CF, but only infertility. Enabling them to reproduce via ICSI, when ordinarily they would not be able to reproduce, means that some of them will transmit the mutated allele to their child, and (if the mother is also a carrier) might result in the birth of a child with CF. Robertson does not think that this would justify banning ICSI. The decision to use ICSI, or any other reproductive technology, should be up to the infertile couple. They may, of course, wish to avoid having a child with CF, and they should be told of the risk so that they can make an informed decision. However, it does not make sense to ban the technique in order to protect *the child,* for banning the technique would also prevent the child, who has no other way of getting born, from existing. As Robertson puts it, "But for the technique in question, the child never would have been born. Whatever psychological or social problems arise, they hardly rise to the level of severe handicap or disability that would make the child's very existence a net burden, and hence a wrongful life" (Robertson 1994, 122).

In other words, Robertson is willing to acknowledge that birth can be seen as a harm and a wrong to the child if, but only if, the child's life is likely to be so awful that it constitutes "wrongful life" (a life that, from the child's own perspective, is not worth living). Buchanan et al. agree. Such cases are likely to be rare, but in these few cases, they conclude that "it would be clearly and seriously morally wrong for individuals to risk conceiving and having . . . a child." They hasten to add that they do not support forced abortion, which would be "so deeply invasive of [the woman's] reproductive freedom, bodily integrity, and right to decide about her own health care as to be virtually never morally justified."

What about wrongful disability cases? Again, Buchanan et al. agree with Robertson: The child in a wrongful disability case has not been harmed in the ordinary sense of harm. However, they disagree that no serious moral wrong has been done. The wrong is allowing the birth of a child in a harmful condition, when this could have been prevented. This is brought out in their example, P1, in which a woman can avoid having a child with moderate mental retardation by taking medication and delaying pregnancy for one month. However, delaying pregnancy means that a different child will be born, one conceived from a different egg (and sperm). Thus, delaying pregnancy changes the identity of the child, making this a "nonidentity" problem. If the woman decides not to wait, she cannot be said to have harmed the child who gets born, for that child could not have been born any other way, and moderate mental retardation is not a plausible candidate for wrongful life. Nevertheless, the harm is "avoidable by substitution" (Peters 1989). That is, the woman could have a mentally normal child simply by taking the medication and delaying pregnancy for one month. Since this imposes virtually no hardship on her, and prevents the birth of a moderately retarded child, waiting is the right thing to do. This suggests that we need to revise or extend our conception of harm to fit wrongful disability cases by including in our moral theory some non-person-affecting principles.

In "Cheap Listening—Reflections on the Concept of Wrongful Disability," Richard J. Hull argues against the wrongful disability approach and the principle of substitution. Hull thinks that the problem with the substitution principle is that it attempts to show what is wrong with having a child who will suffer unavoidably by comparing that child's life with the life of a different possible child who will suffer less. The focus should instead be on notions such as parental responsibility and agency. Parents aspire to providing the best possible conditions in which to raise a child, not just what is above an acceptable minimum. This aspiration is relevant to the morality of procreation. Thus, even while a life of some suffering is better than no life at all in many cases, "we can make good sense of the claim that one may not want to take responsibility for creating avoidable suffering, even at the cost of creating no life at all." This approach is intended to explain why prospective parents are justified in terminating a pregnancy, but it does not explain the moral obligation to terminate—precisely what the substitution principle is intended to explain—since Hull apparently does not think there is such a moral obligation. Thus, the fundamental difference between the two approaches turns on whether it is merely morally permissible for prospective parents to avoid having children with serious disabling conditions or whether they have a moral obligation to avoid this outcome.

ASSISTED REPRODUCTION

Approximately 10 percent of American couples are infertile, usually defined as the inability to conceive a child after a year of unprotected intercourse. For many, infertility is a source of great pain and disappointment, leading them to seek medical help to enable them to have a child and build a family. The help they need may be as low tech as advice about optimal times to have intercourse or the prescribing of fertility drugs, or it may involve more high-tech procedures, such as in vitro fertilization (IVF) and the freezing of embryos, and more recently eggs. All of these procedures are relatively expensive and often are not covered by insurance. A single attempt at IVF costs anywhere from $5,000 to $12,000, and most couples attempt more than one cycle in the pursuit of parenthood. There have been notable improvements in the efficacy of assisted reproduction (AR). When we prepared the last edition, even the best clinics treating the least-impaired couples reported success rates only in the mid-30 percent range. Today, a woman who uses donor eggs and fresh (nonfrozen) embryos has a 50 percent chance of having a live birth (CDC, 2004). But even as efficacy and safety have improved, there are still health concerns. One such concern is the dramatic rise in the rate of multiple births—twins, triplets, and even quadruplets and quintuplets. Multiples are more likely to have health problems, and to pose greater risks for the mother.

In addition to concerns about efficacy and safety, there are also philosophical questions about the commercialization of reproduction; the commodification of gametes, embryos, and possibly children; the exploitation of women (and the opposite danger of paternalism); and the protection of children and families. These questions are difficult enough when AR is used by traditional couples: infertile men and women. Today, however, AR is sought by single men and women who are not infertile but do not have a partner, as well as gay men and lesbian women who cannot reproduce with their partners. Indeed, someday it may be possible to have a child by cloning one's own (or someone else's) genetic material.

To understand the complex issues surrounding assisted reproduction, we begin Section 3 with a selection titled "The Presumptive Primacy of Procreative Liberty" from *Children of Choice* by John A. Robertson (1994). Robertson is perhaps the most prominent defender of the rights of infertile couples to have biologically related offspring. He supports allowing individuals to make their own reproductive decisions, including decisions about fertility treatments and collaborative reproduction. He believes that attempts to ban or restrict reproductive rights violate the constitutional rights of infertile people, in the absence of demonstrable proof that such techniques would cause tangible harm to existing people. By contrast, the Catholic Church opposes virtually every assisted reproductive technique, including artificial insemination by husband (AIH), at least where AIH is a substitute for, as opposed to a facilitator of, the conjugal act, or sexual intercourse within marriage. The usual objections to AR, such as commercialization of reproduction and the introduction of a "third party" into the marital relationship, are not present in AIH. Nevertheless, the church objects to AIH for the same reason it objects to contraception: Both are seen as severing the connection between procreation and the conjugal act. The one AR technique the Vatican appears willing to accept is a variation on the IVF protocol that begins with the infertile couple undergoing intercourse while the husband wears a special condom in which small holes have been cut, so as not to violate the Church's edict against contraception. After intercourse, sperm are retrieved from the condom and placed in a laboratory dish next to eggs that have been retrieved from the wife's ovary. Then the whole mixture is quickly inserted back into the wife's fallopian tube so that fertilization can take place inside her body. "This protocol has been given the acronym GIFT, not only to distinguish it from the morally suspect IVF technology, but also to provide the image of a 'gift of life' that comes directly from God" (Silver, 1997, 76).

A different criticism of Robertson's approach comes from Thomas H. Murray, who maintains that the procreative liberty paradigm is the wrong way to think about the ethics of assisted reproduction. In his selection titled "What Are Families For? Getting to an Ethics of Reproductive Technology" he writes, "The most egregious defect of procreative liberty is its nearly complete disregard of the interests of children created through reproductive technologies." The standard for justifying restrictions on procreative liberty based on the interests of the child is a "wrongful life" standard: that is, the reproductive technology unavoidably creates a child in so wretched a condition that the child would have been better off never having been born. Since this standard is rarely, if ever, met, restrictions on reproductive technology are hardly ever justified. The procreative liberty approach, Murray argues, "prohibits or condemns almost nothing." A saner approach, he maintains, is a framework that acknowledges "the moral significance and interests of the children created through reproductive technologies, and [does] so in a full and robust manner, not as a side-constraint that proves meaningless in practice."

Robertson would undoubtedly respond that his approach *does* take into consideration the interests of children born of reproductive technology. For even if certain technologies expose children to risks, these risks are not always avoidable. The choice for the child is birth with the harmful condition or not getting born at all. The question then becomes whether the child's own interests are best served by allowing it to be born with impairments or by preventing its birth. Robertson notes that most people with disabilities find their lives worth living. They do not agree that they would be better off if they had never been born. Because of this, Robertson maintains that the wrongful life standard is not only *unopposed* to the interests of children created by AR, but rather it is the standard we must use if we are to take the interests of future children seriously. This does not mean that there are no reasons to restrict AR, in Robertson's view, but rather that the reasons for such restrictions are unlikely to be derived from the interests of children born using AR technologies.

Another concern raised by AR is the potential for "collaborative reproduction" or using the reproductive parts and abilities of several people in the production of one child. Such arrangements as surrogate motherhood and gamete donation make it possible for a child to have as many as five potential parents: a rearing mother and father, a biological father, a genetic mother, who donates the egg, and a gestational mother, who provides the womb. Indeed, with a technique known as "ooplasmic transfer," two women can provide one egg, one providing the nucleus containing most of the DNA and one providing the cytoplasm. Nor is the multiplication of parents merely a theoretical possibility. It actually happened in a 1998 California case, *In re Buzzanca,* in which the couple, both of whom had fertility problems, used sperm donation, egg donation, and a surrogate. Before the child, Jaycee, was born, the couple divorced and the husband, John Buzzanca, refused to pay child support, arguing that the resulting child was not a child of the marriage. The trial court agreed. Indeed, it held that Jaycee Buzzanca, *had* no legal parents. Since Luanne Buzzanca, who had cared for the child from birth, had neither contributed an egg nor gestated Jaycee, she was not Jaycee's mother and would have to adopt her to become her legal mother. The appeals court disagreed. It overturned the decision, holding that the intent to parent made John and Luanne the lawful parents of Jaycee. Luanne Buzzanca was given legal custody of Jaycee, while the matter of child support was remanded. The court issued a plea to the legislature "to sort out the parent rights and responsibilities of those involved in artificial reproduction," saying:

> No matter what one thinks of artificial insemination, traditional and gestational surrogacy (in all its permutations), and—as now appears in the not-too-distant future, cloning and even gene splicing—courts are still going to be faced with the problem of determining legal parentage. A child cannot be ignored. Even if all means of artificial reproduction were outlawed with draconian criminal penalties visited on the doctors and parties involved, courts will still be called upon to decide who the lawful parents really are and who—other than the taxpayers—is obligated to provide maintenance and support for the child. These cases will not go away. (In re Marriage of John A. and Luanne H. Buzzanca, 61 Cal App. 4th 1410)

One of the biggest concerns arising from collaborative reproduction stems from its commercial aspect.

In the fourth selection in Section 3, "Grade A: The Market for a Yale Woman's Eggs," Jessica Cohen discusses her own experience with egg donation, which has become a significant part of the $2-billion-a-year infertility industry. Not only can couples select a child that resembles them (as adoptive couples have done for years), but they can also request information about the donor's ethnicity, educational attainments, and SAT scores. "Should couples be able to pay a premium on an open market for their idea of the perfect egg?" Cohen asks. What if their perfect and expensive egg results in an average child? Cohen worries about the creation of a child "encumbered with too many expectations." In the fifth selection, "Payment for Egg Donation," Bonnie Steinbock looks at the pros and cons of commercial egg donation. She rejects the view that there should not be any payments to women who provide eggs. Why should everyone else involved—the doctors, the nurses, the lawyers, the receptionists—get paid, but not the woman who undergoes the considerable burden of egg retrieval? However, while fairness indicates compensation of some sort, too high a price poses a different risk: that dangling large sums of money in front of college students or young professionals might lead them to discount the risks, making their decision to donate (or sell) less than fully voluntary. While Steinbock acknowledges that this is a legitimate concern, she is more worried about the exploitation that occurs when clinics do not reveal all of the risks and potential costs (if something goes wrong) to potential donors, for fear they will not donate.

REPRODUCTIVE CLONING

In July 1997, Dr. Ian Wilmut announced that he had successfully cloned a lamb, Dolly, using SCNT cloning. Wilmut's team took the DNA from a somatic cell (in this case, a mammary cell) of an adult ewe and placed it in an egg cell from another ewe, from which the nucleus had been removed. The resulting embryo was carried to term by yet a third sheep, creating Dolly who was a (nearly) identical genetic copy, or "delayed" genetic twin, of the sheep whose mammary cell was used. (She was not totally identical to the sheep from whom she was cloned because a small amount of mitchondrial DNA remained in the enucleated egg cell.)

President Clinton immediately imposed a temporary ban on federal funding of human cloning research. He directed the National Bioethics Advisory Commission (NBAC) to undertake a thorough review of the legal and ethical issues and to report back to him within ninety days with recommendations on possible federal actions to prevent the abuse of this new technology. To no one's surprise, the NBAC

report recommended that the president's moratorium be continued. It held, almost exclusively on the basis of safety considerations, that it was morally unacceptable at this time for anyone, privately or publicly funded, to engage in SCNT cloning research aimed at creating a child. The report stressed the medical and scientific potential of cloning technology for such uses as the creation of tissue for burn victims or bone marrow for transplantation, and it emphasized the need to make a distinction between "human cloning" (now usually called "therapeutic cloning") and "cloning a human being" ("reproductive cloning") so as not to hinder important areas of scientific research. As for the use of SCNT cloning to create human beings, the report recommended further dialogue on the nonsafety objections (ethical, religious, and policy) and suggested that the issue be revisited in three to five years.

Under President George W. Bush, NBAC was replaced by the President's Council on Bioethics, which issued a report, *Human Cloning and Human Dignity,* in 2002 covering the science and ethics of therapeutic cloning (or as they call it, cloning-for-biomedical-research) and reproductive cloning (cloning-to-produce-children). The first selection in Section 4, "The Case against Cloning-to-Produce-Children," comes from *Human Cloning and Human Dignity* written by the Presidents Council. Much of the case stems from concerns about safety, in particular, the risks imposed on the children who would be born. This concern involves several empirical questions: What would be the likely rate of miscarriage and stillbirth? Would liveborn children created by cloning be more susceptible than children created by coitus or IVF to birth defects, and how severe are the defects likely to be? So far, we have only animal data to go by (primarily cattle), which is not necessarily predictive of what would happen with humans. Indeed, as no primates have yet been cloned, it is not clear that human reproductive cloning is even possible. In addition to the empirical questions, there is the ethical question, how safe is safe enough? (Peters 2004). Some maintain that reproductive cloning would be ethically acceptable when researchers are reasonably sure that clones would have no more likelihood of birth defects than do children produced by sexual reproduction (about 2 percent). Others maintain that a more reasonable comparison would be with IVF, which has a

5 percent risk of serious defect. The President's Council, however, takes the view that not only would it be unethical to attempt to clone a child at present, based on safety concerns, but that any attempts to make cloning safer would constitute unethical experimentation on the child-to-be. Therefore, on safety grounds alone, cloning-to-produce-children is now and will always be unethical. Moreover, even if cloning were entirely safe, the council rejects it as a means to produce a child on other grounds, including individuality, commodification of children, eugenics, and the likelihood of damage to families and to society at large.

In the next selection, Bonnie Steinbock looks at both safety and nonsafety objections to reproductive cloning. In "Reproductive Cloning: Another Look," Steinbock notes that a relatively high rate of miscarriage, stillbirth, and neonatal mortality has plagued animal cloning, making this currently an ethically unacceptable reproductive technique in human beings. Another question is whether clones that made it to birth would be more likely to have birth defects, and how severe these might be. There is some evidence that the birth defects in cloned nonhuman animals may be due to the particular cloning technique used, and not cloning per se. If this proves to be the case, then reproductive cloning might be made much safer, even as safe as other AR techniques. Steinbock rejects the council's wholesale conclusion that cloning could never be safe enough to warrant clinical trials in humans. She turns next to the nonsafety objections, including those marshaled by the President's Council, and concludes that none of these is terribly persuasive, certainly not persuasive enough to justify an absolute and permanent ban on human cloning. When not based on safety concerns, the ethics of reproductive cloning seems to depend on the motivation for wanting to clone a child. The last selection in Section 3, "Even If It Worked, Cloning Wouldn't Bring Her Back," is a moving article by

Thomas H. Murray that rejects one possible motivation for reproductive cloning, namely, to replace a dead or dying child.

REFERENCES

Buchanan, Allen, Dan W. Brock, Norman Daniels, and Daniel Wikler. 2000. *From chance to choice: Genetics & justice.* Cambridge: Cambridge University Press.

CDC (Centers for Disease Control and Prevention). 2004. Assisted Reproductive Technology (ART) Report, http://www.cdc.gov.ART2004/index.htm.

Feinberg, Joel. 1986. Abortion. In *Matters of life and death,* ed. Tom Regan, 2nd ed. New York: Random House.

Parfit, Derek. 1984. *Reasons and persons.* Oxford: Clarendon Press.

Peters, Philip G. 1989. Protecting the unconceived: Nonexistence, avoidability, and reproductive technology. *Arizona Law Review* 31 (3):487–548.

Peters, Philip G. Jr. 2004. *How safe is safe enough? Obligations to the children of reproductive technology.* New York: Oxford University Press.

Regan, Donald. 1979. Rewriting *Roe* v. *Wade. Michigan Law Review* 77.

Robertson, John A. 1994. *Children of choice: Freedom and the new reproductive technologies.* Princeton, NJ: Princeton University Press.

Silver, Lee M. 1997. *Remaking Eden: How genetic engineering and cloning will transform the American family.* New York: Avon Books.

Singer, Peter. 1975. *Animal liberation.* New York: Avon Books.

Steinbock, Bonnie. 1986, April. The logical case for "wrongful life." *Hastings Center Report* 16 (2): 15–20.

Steinbock, Bonnie. 1992. *Life before birth: The moral and legal status of embryos and fetuses.* New York: Oxford University Press.

Sumner, L. W. 1981. *Abortion and moral theory.* Princeton, NJ: Princeton University Press.

Tooley, Michael. 1983. *Abortion and infanticide.* New York: Oxford University Press.

Warren, M. A. 1973. On the moral and legal status of abortion. *Monist* 57:43–61.

THE MORALITY
OF ABORTION

THE UNSPEAKABLE CRIME OF ABORTION

Pope John Paul II

Among all the crimes which can be committed against life, procured abortion has characteristics making it particularly serious and deplorable. The Second Vatican Council defines abortion, together with infanticide, as an "unspeakable crime."[1]

But today, in many people's consciences, the perception of its gravity has become progressively obscured. The acceptance of abortion in the popular mind, in behaviour and even in law itself, is a telling sign of an extremely dangerous crisis of the moral sense, which is becoming more and more incapable of distinguishing between good and evil, even when the fundamental right to life is at stake. Given such a grave situation, we need now more than ever to have the courage to look the truth in the eye and *to call things by their proper name*, without yielding to convenient compromises or to the temptation of self-deception. In this regard the reproach of the Prophet is extremely straightforward: "Woe to those who call evil good and good evil, who put darkness for light and light for darkness" (*Is* 5:20). Especially in the case of abortion there is a widespread use of ambiguous terminology, such as "interruption of pregnancy," which tends to hide abortion's true nature and to attenuate its seriousness in public opinion. Perhaps this linguistic phenomenon is itself a symptom of an uneasiness of conscience. But no word has the power to change the reality of things: procured abortion is *the deliberate and direct killing, by whatever means it is carried out, of a human being in the initial phase of his or her existence, extending from conception to birth*.

The moral gravity of procured abortion is apparent in all its truth if we recognize that we are dealing with murder and, in particular, when we consider the specific elements involved. The one eliminated is a human being at the very beginning of life. No one more absolutely *innocent* could be imagined. In no way could this human being ever be considered an aggressor, much less an unjust

From John Paul II. *Evangelium Vitae*, Encyclical Letter, August 16, 1993. Copyright © 1993 Liberia Editrice Vaticana. *Editors' note:* Some text has been cut. Students who want to read the article in its entirety should consult the original.

aggressor! He or she is *weak*, defenseless, even to the point of lacking that minimal form of defence consisting in the poignant power of a newborn baby's cries and tears. The unborn child is *totally entrusted* to the protection and care of the woman carrying him or her in the womb. And yet sometimes it is precisely the mother herself who makes the decision and asks for the child to be eliminated, and who then goes about having it done.

It is true that the decision to have an abortion is often tragic and painful for the mother, insofar as the decision to rid herself of the fruit of conception is not made for purely selfish reasons or out of convenience, but out of a desire to protect certain important values such as her own health or a decent standard of living for the other members of the family. Sometimes it is feared that the child to be born would live in such conditions that it would be better if the birth did not take place. Nevertheless, these reasons and others like them, however serious and tragic, can never justify the deliberate killing of an innocent human being.

As well as the mother, there are often other people too who decide upon the death of the child in the womb. In the first place, the father of the child may be to blame, not only when he directly pressures the woman to have an abortion, but also when he indirectly encourages such a decision on her part by leaving her alone to face the problems of pregnancy:[2] in this way the family is thus mortally wounded and profaned in its nature as a community of love and in its vocation to be the "sanctuary of life." Nor can one overlook the pressures which sometimes come from the wider family circle and from friends. Sometimes the woman is subjected to such strong pressure that she feels psychologically forced to have an abortion: certainly in this case moral responsibility lies particularly with those who have directly or indirectly obliged her to have an abortion. Doctors and nurses are also responsible, when they place at the service of death skills which were acquired for promoting life.

But responsibility likewise falls on the legislators who have promoted and approved abortion laws, and, to the extent that they have a say in the matter, on the administrators of the health-care centres where abortions are performed. A general and no less serious responsibility lies with those who have encouraged the spread of an attitude of sexual permissiveness and a lack of esteem for motherhood,

and with those who should have ensured—but did not—effective family and social policies in support of families, especially larger families and those with particular financial and educational needs. Finally, one cannot overlook the network of complicity which reaches out to include international institutions, foundations and associations which systematically campaign for the legalization and spread of abortion in the world. In this sense abortion goes beyond the responsibility of individuals and beyond the harm done to them, and takes on a distinctly social dimension. It is a most serious *wound* inflicted on society and its culture by the very people who ought to be society's promoters and defenders. As I wrote in my *Letter to Families,* "we are facing an immense threat to life: not only to the life of individuals but also to that of civilization itself."[3] We are facing what can be called a *"structure of sin" which opposes human life not yet born.*

Some people try to justify abortion by claiming that the result of conception, at least up to a certain number of days, cannot yet be considered a personal human life. But in fact, "from the time that the ovum is fertilized, a life is begun which is neither that of the father nor the mother; it is rather the life of a new human being with his own growth. It would never be made human if it were not human already. This has always been clear, and . . . modern genetic science offers clear confirmation. It has demonstrated that from the first instant there is established the programme of what this living being will be: a person, this individual person with his characteristic aspects already well determined. Right from fertilization the adventure of a human life begins, and each of its capacities requires time—a rather lengthy time—to find its place and to be in a position to act."[4] Even if the presence of a spiritual soul cannot be ascertained by empirical data, the results themselves of scientific research on the human embryo provide "a valuable indication for discerning by the use of reason a personal presence at the moment of the first appearance of a human life: how could a human individual not be a human person?"[5]

Furthermore, what is at stake is so important that, from the standpoint of moral obligation, the mere probability that a human person is involved would suffice to justify an absolutely clear prohibition of any intervention aimed at killing a human embryo. Precisely for this reason, over and above all scientific debates and those philosophical affirmations to which the Magisterium has not expressly committed itself, the Church has always taught and continues to teach that the result of human procreation, from the first moment of its existence, must be guaranteed that unconditional respect which is morally due to the human being in his or her totality and unity as body and spirit: *"The human being is to be respected and treated as a person from the moment of conception;* and therefore from that same moment his rights as a person must be recognized, among which in the first place is the inviolable right of every innocent human being to life."[6] . . .

NOTES

1. Pastoral Constitution on the Church in the Modern World *Gaudium et Spes.* 51: "Abortius necnon infanticidium nefanda sunt crimina."
2. Cf. John Paul II. Apostolic Letter *Muliens Dignitatem* (15 August 1988), 14:*AAS* 80 (1988), 1686.
3. No. 21:*AAS* 86 (1994), 920.
4. Congregation for the Doctrine of the Faith, *Declaration on Procured Abortion* (18 November 1974), Nos. 12–13: *AAS* 66 (1974), 738.
5. Congregation for the Doctrine of the Faith, Instruction on Respect for Human Life in Its Origin and on the Dignity of Procreation *Donum vitae* (22 February 1987), I, No. 1:*AAS* 80 (1988), 78–79.
6. *Ibid., loc. cit:.,* 79.

WHY ABORTION IS IMMORAL

Don Marquis

I

. . . Consider the way a typical anti-abortionist argues. She will argue or assert that life is present from the moment of conception or that fetuses look like babies or that fetuses possess a characteristic such as a genetic code that is both necessary and sufficient for being human. Anti-abortionists seem to believe that (1) the truth of all of these claims is quite obvious, and (2) establishing any of these claims is sufficient to show that abortion is morally akin to murder.

A standard pro-choice strategy exhibits similarities. The pro-choicer will argue or assert that fetuses are not persons or that fetuses are not rational agents or that fetuses are not social beings. Pro-choicers seem to believe that (1) the truth of any of these claims is

From Don Marquis, *Journal of Philosophy* 86, no. 4 (April 1989): 183–202. Reprinted by permission.

Editors' note: Some text and all author's notes have been cut. Students who want to read the article in its entirety should consult the original.

quite obvious, and (2) establishing any of these claims is sufficient to show that an abortion is not a wrongful killing.

In fact, both the pro-choice and the anti-abortion claims do seem to be true, although the "it looks like a baby" claim is more difficult to establish the earlier the pregnancy. We seem to have a standoff. How can it be resolved? . . .

Note what each partisan will say. The anti-abortionist will claim that her position is supported by such generally accepted moral principles as "It is always prima facie seriously wrong to take a human life" or "It is always prima facie seriously wrong to end the life of a baby." Since these are generally accepted moral principles, her position is certainly not obviously wrong. The pro-choicer will claim that her position is supported by such plausible moral principles as, "Being a person is what gives an individual intrinsic moral worth," or, "It is only seriously prima facie wrong to take the life of a member of the human community." Since these are generally accepted moral principles, the pro-choice position is certainly not obviously wrong. Unfortunately, we have again arrived at a standoff.

Now, how might one deal with this standoff? The standard approach is to try to show how the moral principles of one's opponent lose their plausibility under analysis. It is easy to see how this is possible. On the one hand, the anti-abortionist will defend a moral principle concerning the wrongness of killing which tends to be broad in scope in order that even fetuses at an early stage of pregnancy will fall under it. The problem with broad principles is that they often embrace too much. In this particular instance, the principle, "It is always prima facie wrong to take a human life," seems to entail that it is wrong to end the existence of a living human cancer-cell culture, on the grounds that the culture is both living and human. Therefore, it seems that the anti-abortionist's favored principle is too broad.

On the other hand, the pro-choicer wants to find a moral principle concerning the wrongness of killing which tends to be narrow in scope in order that fetuses will *not* fall under it. The problem with narrow principles is that they often do not embrace enough. Hence, the needed principles such as, "It is prima facie seriously wrong to kill only persons," or, "It is prima facie wrong to kill only rational agents," do not explain why it is wrong to kill infants or young children or the severely retarded or even perhaps the severely mentally ill. Therefore, we seem again to have a standoff. The anti-abortionist charges, not unreasonably, that pro-choice principles concerning killing are too narrow to be acceptable; the pro-choicer charges, not unreasonably, that anti-abortionist principles concerning killing are too broad to be acceptable.

Attempts by both sides to patch up the difficulties in their positions run into further difficulties. The anti-abortionist will try to remove the problem in her position by reformulating her principle concerning killing in terms of human beings. Now we end up with: "It is always prima facie seriously wrong to end the life of a human being." This principle has the advantage of avoiding the problem of the human cancer-cell culture counterexample. But this advantage is purchased at a high price. For although it is clear that a fetus is both human and alive, it is not at all clear that a fetus is a human *being*. There is at least something to be said for the view that something becomes a human being only after a process of development, and that, therefore, first trimester fetuses, and perhaps all fetuses, are not yet human beings.

Hence, the anti-abortionist, by this move, has merely exchanged one problem for another.

The pro-choicer fares no better. She may attempt to find reasons why killing infants, young children, and the severely retarded is wrong which are independent of her major principle that is supposed to explain the wrongness of taking human life, but which will not also make abortion immoral. This is no easy task. Appeals to social utility will seem satisfactory only to those who resolve not to think of the enormous difficulties with a utilitarian account of the wrongness of killing and the significant social costs of preserving the lives of the unproductive. A pro-choice strategy that extends the definition of 'person' to infants or even to young children seems just as arbitrary as an anti-abortion strategy that extends the definition of 'human being' to fetuses. Again, we find symmetries in the two positions and we arrive at a standoff.

There are even further problems that reflect symmetries in the two positions. In addition to counterexample problems, or the arbitrary application problems that can be exchanged for them, the standard anti-abortionist principle, "It is prima facie seriously wrong to kill a human being," or one of its variants, can be objected to on the grounds of ambiguity. If 'human being' is taken to be a *biological* category, then the anti-abortionist is left with the problem of explaining why a merely biological category should make a moral difference. Why, it is asked, is it any more reasonable to base a moral conclusion on the number of chromosomes in one's cells than on the color of one's skin? If 'human being', on the other hand, is taken to be a *moral* category, then the claim that a fetus is a human being cannot be taken to be a premise in the anti-abortion argument, for it is precisely what needs to be established. Hence, either the anti-abortionist's main category is a morally irrelevant, merely biological category, or it is of no use to the anti-abortionist in establishing (noncircularly, of course) that abortion is wrong.

Although this problem with the anti-abortionist position is often noticed, it is less often noticed that the pro-choice position suffers from an analogous problem. The principle, "Only persons have the right to life" also suffers from an ambiguity. The term 'person' is typically defined in terms of psychological characteristics, although there will certainly be disagreement concerning which characteristics are most important. Supposing that this matter can be settled, the pro-choicer is left with the problem of explaining why *psychological* characteristics should make a *moral* difference. If the pro-choicer should attempt to deal with this problem by claiming that an explanation is not necessary, that in fact we do treat such a cluster of psychological properties as having moral significance, the sharp-witted anti-abortionist should have a ready response. We do treat being both living and human as having moral significance. If it is legitimate for the pro-choicer to demand that the anti-abortionist provide an explanation of the connection between the biological character of being a human being and the wrongness of being killed (even though people accept this connection), then it is legitimate for the anti-abortionist to demand that the pro-choicer provide an explanation of the connection between psychological criteria for being a person and the wrongness of being killed (even though that connection is accepted).

[Joel] Feinberg has attempted to meet this objection (he calls psychological personhood "commonsense personhood"):

> The characteristics that confer commonsense personhood are not arbitrary bases for rights and duties, such as race, sex or species membership; rather they are traits that make sense out of rights and duties and without which those moral attributes would have no point or function. It is because people are conscious; have a sense of their personal identities; have plans, goals, and projects; experience emotions; are liable to pains, anxieties, and frustrations; can reason and bargain, and so on—it is because of these attributes that people have values and interests, desires and expectations of their own, including a stake in their own futures, and a personal well-being of a sort we cannot ascribe to unconscious or nonrational beings. Because of their developed capacities they can assume duties and responsibilities and can have and make claims on one another. Only because of their sense of self, their life plans, their value hierarchies, and their stakes in their own futures can they be ascribed fundamental rights. There is nothing arbitrary about these linkages.

The plausible aspects of this attempt should not be taken to obscure its implausible features. There is a great deal to be said for the view that being a psychological person under some description is a necessary condition for having duties. One cannot have a duty unless one is capable of behaving morally, and a being's capability of behaving morally will require having a certain psychology. It is far from obvious, however, that having rights entails consciousness or rationality, as Feinberg suggests. We speak of the rights of the severely retarded or the severely mentally ill, yet some of these persons are not rational. We speak of the rights of the temporarily unconscious. The New Jersey Supreme Court based their decision in the Quinlan case on Karen Ann Quinlan's right to privacy, and she was known to be permanently unconscious at that time. Hence, Feinberg's claim that having rights entails being conscious is, on its face, obviously false. . . .

There is a way out of this apparent dialectical quandary. . . .

II

. . . We can start from the following unproblematic assumption concerning our own case: it is wrong to kill us. Why is it wrong? Some answers can be easily eliminated. It might be said that what makes killing us wrong is that a killing brutalizes the one who kills. But the brutalization consists of being inured to the performance of an act that is hideously immoral; hence, the brutalization does not explain the immorality. It might be said that what makes killing us wrong is the great loss others would experience due to our absence. Although such hubris is understandable, such an explanation does not account for the wrongness of killing hermits, or those whose lives are relatively independent and whose friends find it easy to make new friends.

A more obvious answer is better. What primarily makes killing wrong is neither its effect on the murderer nor its effect on the victim's friends and relatives, but its effect on the victim. The loss of one's life is one of the greatest losses one can suffer. The loss of one's life deprives one of all the experiences, activities, projects, and enjoyments that would otherwise have constituted one's future. Therefore, killing someone is wrong, primarily because the killing inflicts (one of) the greatest possible losses on the victim. . . . When I am killed, I am deprived both of what I now value which would have been part of my future personal life, but also what I would come to value. Therefore, when I die, I am deprived of all of the value of my future. Inflicting this loss on me is ultimately what makes killing me wrong. This being the case, it would seem that what makes killing *any* adult human being prima facie seriously wrong is the loss of his or her future. . . .

The claim that what makes killing wrong is the loss of the victim's future is directly supported by two considerations. In the first place, this theory explains why we regard killing as one of the worst of crimes. Killing is especially wrong, because it deprives the victim of more than perhaps any other crime. In the second place, people with AIDS or cancer who know they are dying believe, of course, that dying is a very bad thing for them. They believe that the loss of a future to them that they would otherwise have experienced is what makes their premature death a very bad thing for them. A better theory of the wrongness of killing would require a different natural property associated with killing which better fits with the attitudes of the dying. What could it be?

The view that what makes killing wrong is the loss to the victim of the value of the victim's future gains additional support when some of its implications are examined. In the first place, it is incompatible with the view that it is wrong to kill only beings who are biologically human. It is possible that there exists a different species from another planet whose members have a future like ours. Since having a future like that is what makes killing someone wrong, this theory entails that it would be wrong to kill members of such a species. Hence, this theory is opposed to the claim that only life that is biologically human has great moral worth, a claim which many anti-abortionists have seemed to adopt. This opposition, which this theory has in common with personhood theories, seems to be a merit of the theory.

In the second place, the claim that the loss of one's future is the wrong-making feature of one's being killed entails the possibility that the futures of some actual nonhuman mammals on our own planet are sufficiently like ours that it is seriously wrong to kill them also. Whether some animals do have the same right to life as human beings depends on adding to the account of the wrongness of killing some additional account of just what it is about my future or the futures of other adult human beings which makes it wrong to kill us. No such additional account will be offered in this essay. Undoubtedly, the provision of such an account would be a very difficult matter. Undoubtedly, any such account would be

quite controversial. Hence, it surely should not reflect badly on this sketch of an elementary theory of the wrongness of killing that it is indeterminate with respect to some very difficult issues regarding animal rights.

In the third place, the claim that the loss of one's future is the wrong-making feature of one's being killed does not entail, as sanctity-of-human-life theories do, that active euthanasia is wrong. Persons who are severely and incurably ill, who face a future of pain and despair, and who wish to die will not have suffered a loss if they are killed. It is, strictly speaking, the value of a human's future which makes killing wrong in this theory. This being so, killing does not necessarily wrong some persons who are sick and dying. Of course, there may be other reasons for a prohibition of active euthanasia, but that is another matter. Sanctity-of-human-life theories seem to hold that active euthanasia is seriously wrong even in an individual case where there seems to be good reason for it independently of public policy considerations. This consequence is most implausible, and it is a plus for the claim that the loss of a future of value is what makes killing wrong that it does not share this consequence.

In the fourth place, the account of the wrongness of killing defended in this essay does straightforwardly entail that it is prima facie seriously wrong to kill children and infants, for we do presume that they have futures of value. Since we do believe that it is wrong to kill defenseless little babies, it is important that a theory of the wrongness of killing easily account for this. Personhood theories of the wrongness of killing, on the other hand, cannot straightforwardly account for the wrongness of killing infants and young children. Hence, such theories must add special ad hoc accounts of the wrongness of killing the young. The plausibility of such ad hoc theories seems to be a function of how desperately one wants such theories to work. The claim that the primary wrong-making feature of a killing is the loss to the victim of the value of its future accounts for the wrongness of killing young children and infants directly; it makes the wrongness of such acts as obvious as we actually think it is. This is a further merit of this theory. Accordingly, it seems that this value of a future-like-ours theory of the wrongness of killing shares strengths of both sanctity-of-life and personhood accounts while avoiding weaknesses of both.

In addition, it meshes with a central intuition concerning what makes killing wrong.

The claim that the primary wrong-making feature of a killing is the loss to the victim of the value of its future has obvious consequences for the ethics of abortion. The future of a standard fetus includes a set of experiences, projects, activities, and such which are identical with the futures of adult human beings and are identical with the futures of young children. Since the reason that is sufficient to explain why it is wrong to kill human beings after the time of birth is a reason that also applies to fetuses, it follows that abortion is prima facie seriously morally wrong.

This argument does not rely on the invalid inference that, since it is wrong to kill persons, it is wrong to kill potential persons also. The category that is morally central to this analysis is the category of having a valuable future like ours; it is not the category of personhood. The argument that abortion is prima facie seriously morally wrong proceeded independently of the notion of person or potential person or any equivalent. Someone may wish to start with this analysis in terms of the value of a human future, conclude that abortion is, except perhaps in rare circumstances, seriously morally wrong, infer that fetuses have the right to life, and then call fetuses "persons" as a result of their having the right to life. Clearly, in this case, the category of person is being used to state the *conclusion* of the analysis rather than to generate the *argument* of the analysis. . . .

III

How complete an account of the wrongness of killing does the value of a future-like-ours account have to be in order that the wrongness of abortion is a consequence? This account does not have to be an account of the necessary conditions for the wrongness of killing. Some persons in nursing homes may lack valuable human futures, yet it may be wrong to kill them for other reasons. Furthermore, this account does not obviously have to be the sole reason killing is wrong where the victim did have a valuable future. This analysis claims only that, for any killing where the victim did have a valuable future like ours, having that future by itself is sufficient to create the strong presumption that the killing is seriously wrong.

One way to overturn the value of a future-like-ours argument would be to find some account of the wrongness of killing which is at least as intelligible and which has different implications for the ethics of abortion. Two rival accounts possess at least some degree of plausibility. One account is based on the obvious fact that people value the experience of living and wish for that valuable experience to continue. Therefore, it might be said, what makes killing wrong is the discontinuation of that experience for the victim. Let us call this the *discontinuation account*. Another rival account is based upon the obvious fact that people strongly desire to continue to live. This suggests that what makes killing us so wrong is that it interferes with the fulfillment of a strong and fundamental desire, the fulfillment of which is necessary for the fulfillment of any other desires we might have. Let us call this the *desire account*. . . .

One problem with the desire account is that we do regard it as seriously wrong to kill persons who have little desire to live or who have no desire to live or, indeed, have a desire not to live. We believe it is seriously wrong to kill the unconscious, the sleeping, those who are tired of life, and those who are suicidal. The value-of-a-human-future account renders standard morality intelligible in these cases; these cases appear to be incompatible with the desire account.

The desire account is subject to a deeper difficulty. We desire life, because we value the goods of this life. The goodness of life is not secondary to our desire for it. If this were not so, the pain of one's own premature death could be done away with merely by an appropriate alteration in the configuration of one's desires. This is absurd. Hence, it would seem that it is the loss of the goods of one's future, not the interference with the fulfillment of a strong desire to live, which accounts ultimately for the wrongness of killing.

It is worth noting that, if the desire account is modified so that it does not provide a necessary, but only a sufficient, condition for the wrongness of killing, the desire account is compatible with the value of a future-like-ours account. The combined accounts will yield an anti-abortion ethic. This suggests that one can retain what is intuitively plausible about the desire account without a challenge to the basic argument of this paper.

It is also worth noting that, if future desires have moral force in a modified desire account of the wrongness of killing, one can find support for an anti-abortion ethic even in the absence of a value of a future-like-ours account. If one decides that a morally relevant property, the possession of which is sufficient to make it wrong to kill some individual, is the desire at some future time to live—one might decide to justify one's refusal to kill suicidal teenagers on these grounds, for example—then, since typical fetuses will have the desire in the future to live, it is wrong to kill typical fetuses. Accordingly, it does not seem that a desire account of the wrongness of killing can provide a justification of a pro-choice ethic of abortion which is nearly as adequate as the value of a human-future justification on an anti-abortion ethic.

The discontinuation account looks more promising as an account of the wrongness of killing. It seems just as intelligible as the value of a future-like-ours account, but it does not justify an anti-abortion position. Obviously, if it is the continuation of one's activities, experiences, and projects, the loss of which makes killing wrong, then it is not wrong to kill fetuses for that reason, for fetuses do not have experiences, activities, and projects to be continued or discontinued. Accordingly, the discontinuation account does not have the anti-abortion consequences that the value of a future-like-ours account has. Yet, it seems as intelligible as the value of a future-like-ours account, for when we think of what would be wrong with our being killed, it does seem as if it is the discontinuation of what makes our lives worthwhile which makes killing us wrong.

Is the discontinuation account just as good an account as the value of a future-like-ours account? The discontinuation account will not be adequate at all, if it does not refer to the *value* of the experience that may be discontinued. One does not want the discontinuation account to make it wrong to kill a patient who begs for death and who is in severe pain that cannot be relieved short of killing. (I leave open the question of whether it is wrong for other reasons.) Accordingly, the discontinuation account must be more than a bare discontinuation account. It must make some reference to the positive value of the patient's experiences. But, by the same token, the value of a future-like-ours account cannot be a bare future account either. Just having a future surely does not itself rule out killing the above patient. This account must make some reference to the value of

the patient's future experiences and projects also. Hence, both accounts involve the value of experiences, projects, and activities. So far we still have symmetry between accounts.

The symmetry fades, however, when we focus on the time period of the value of the experiences, etc., which has moral consequences. Although both accounts leave open the possibility that the patient in our example may be killed, this possibility is left open only in virtue of the utterly bleak future for the patient. It makes no difference whether the patient's immediate past contains intolerable pain, or consists in being in a coma (which we can imagine is a situation of indifference), or consists in a life of value. If the patient's future is a future of value, we want our account to make it wrong to kill the patient. If the patient's future is intolerable, whatever his or her immediate past, we want our account to allow killing the patient. Obviously, then, it is the value of that patient's future which is doing the work in rendering the morality of killing the patient intelligible.

This being the case, it seems clear that whether one has immediate past experiences or not does no work in the explanation of what makes killing wrong. The addition the discontinuation account makes to the value of a human future account is otiose. Its addition to the value-of-a-future account plays no role at all in rendering intelligible the wrongness of killing. Therefore, it can be discarded with the discontinuation account of which it is a part.

IV

The analysis of the previous section suggests that alternative general accounts of the wrongness of killing are either inadequate or unsuccessful in getting around the anti-abortion consequences of the value of a future-like-ours argument. A different strategy for avoiding these anti-abortion consequences involves limiting the scope of the value of a future argument. More precisely, the strategy involves arguing that fetuses lack a property that is essential for the value-of-a-future argument (or for any anti-abortion argument) to apply to them.

One move of this sort is based upon the claim that a necessary condition of one's future being valuable is that one values it. Value implies a valuer.

Given this one might argue that, since fetuses cannot value their futures, their futures are not valuable to them. Hence, it does not seriously wrong them deliberately to end their lives.

This move fails, however, because of some ambiguities. Let us assume that something cannot be of value unless it is valued by someone. This does not entail that my life is of no value unless it is valued by me. I may think, in a period of despair, that my future is of no worth whatsoever, but I may be wrong because others rightly see value—even great value—in it. Furthermore, my future can be valuable to me even if I do not value it. This is the case when a young person attempts suicide, but is rescued and goes on to significant human achievements. Such young people's futures are ultimately valuable to them, even though such futures do not seem to be valuable to them at the moment of attempted suicide. A fetus's future can be valuable to it in the same way. Accordingly, this attempt to limit the anti-abortion argument fails.

Another similar attempt to reject the anti-abortion position is based on [Michael] Tooley's claim that an entity cannot possess the right to life unless it has the capacity to desire its continued existence. It follows that, since fetuses lack the conceptual capacity to desire to continue to live, they lack the right to life. Accordingly, Tooley concludes that abortion cannot be seriously prima facie wrong. . . .

What could be the evidence for Tooley's basic claim? Tooley once argued that individuals have a prima facie right to what they desire and that the lack of the capacity to desire something undercuts the basis of one's right to it. . . . This argument plainly will not succeed in the context of the analysis of this essay, however, since the point here is to establish the fetus's right to life on other grounds. Tooley's argument assumes that the right to life cannot be established in general on some basis other than the desire for life. This position was considered and rejected in the preceding section of this paper.

One might attempt to defend Tooley's basic claim on the grounds that, because a fetus cannot apprehend continued life as a benefit, its continued life cannot be a benefit, or cannot be something it has a right to, or cannot be something that is in its interest. This might be defended in terms of the general proposition that, if an individual is literally incapable of caring about or taking an interest in some X, then one does not have a right to X, or X is not a benefit, or X is not something that is in one's interest.

Each member of this family of claims seems to be open to objections. As John C. Stevens has pointed out, one may have a right to be treated with a certain medical procedure (because of a health insurance policy one has purchased), even though one cannot conceive of the nature of the procedure. And, as Tooley himself has pointed out, persons who have been indoctrinated, or drugged, or rendered temporarily unconscious may be literally incapable of caring about or taking an interest in something that is in their interest, or is something to which they have a right, or is something that benefits them. Hence, the Tooley claim that would restrict the scope of the value of a future-like-ours argument is undermined by counterexamples.

Finally, Paul Bassen has argued that, even though the prospects of an embryo might seem to be a basis for the wrongness of abortion, an embryo cannot be a victim and therefore cannot be wronged. An embryo cannot be a victim, he says, because it lacks sentience. His central argument for this seems to be that, even though plants and the permanently unconscious are alive, they clearly cannot be victims. What is the explanation of this? Bassen claims that the explanation is that their lives consist of mere metabolism and mere metabolism is not enough to ground victimizability. Mentation is required.

The problem with this attempt to establish the absence of victimizability is that both plants and the permanently unconscious clearly lack what Bassen calls "prospects" or what I have called "a future life like ours." Hence, it is surely open to one to argue that the real reason we believe plants and the permanently unconscious cannot be victims is that killing them cannot deprive them of a future life like ours; the real reason is not their absence of present mentation.

Bassen recognizes that his view is subject to this difficulty, and he recognizes that the case of children seems to support this difficulty, for "much of what we do for children is based on prospects." He argues, however, that, in the case of children and in other such cases, "potentiality comes into play only where victimizability has been secured on other grounds." . . .

Bassen's defense of his view is patently question-begging, since what is adequate to secure victimizability is exactly what is at issue. His examples do not support his own view against the thesis of this essay. Of course, embryos can be victims: when their lives are deliberately terminated, they are deprived of their futures of value, their prospects. This makes them victims, for it directly wrongs them.

The seeming plausibility of Bassen's view stems from the fact that paradigmatic cases of imagining someone as a victim involve empathy, and empathy requires mentation of the victim. The victims of flood, famine, rape, or child abuse are all persons with whom we can empathize. That empathy seems to be part of seeing them as victims.

In spite of the strength of these examples, the attractive intuition that a situation in which there is victimization requires the possibility of empathy is subject to counterexamples. Consider a case that Bassen himself offers: "Posthumous obliteration of an author's work constitutes a misfortune for him only if he had wished his work to endure." . . . The conditions Bassen wishes to impose upon the possibility of being victimized here seem far too strong. Perhaps this author, due to his unrealistic standards of excellence and his low self-esteem, regarded his work as unworthy of survival, even though it possessed genuine literary merit. Destruction of such work would surely victimize its author. In such a case, empathy with the victim concerning the loss is clearly impossible.

Of course, Bassen does not make the possibility of empathy a necessary condition of victimizability; he requires only mentation. Hence, on Bassen's actual view, this author, as I have described him, can be a victim. The problem is that the basic intuition that renders Bassen's view plausible is missing in the author's case. In order to attempt to avoid counterexamples, Bassen has made his thesis too weak to be supported by the intuitions that suggested it.

Even so, the mentation requirement on victimizability is still subject to counterexamples. Suppose a severe accident renders me totally unconscious for a month, after which I recover. Surely killing me while I am unconscious victimizes me, even though I am incapable of mentation during that time. It thus follows that Bassen's thesis fails. Apparently, attempts to restrict the value of a future-like-ours argument so that fetuses do not fall within its scope do not succeed.

V

In this essay, it has been argued that the correct ethic of the wrongness of killing can be extended to fetal life and used to show that there is a strong presumption that any abortion is morally impermissible. If the ethic of killing adopted here entails, however, that contraception is also seriously immoral, then there would appear to be a difficulty with the analysis of this essay.

But this analysis does not entail that contraception is wrong. Of course, contraception prevents the actualization of a possible future of value. Hence, it follows from the claim that futures of value should be maximized that contraception is prima facie immoral. This obligation to maximize does not exist, however; furthermore, nothing in the ethics of killing in this paper entails that it does. The ethics of killing in this essay would entail that contraception is wrong only if something were denied a human future of value by contraception. Nothing at all is denied such a future by contraception, however.

Candidates for a subject of harm by contraception fall into four categories: (1) some sperm or other, (2) some ovum or other, (3) a sperm and an ovum separately, and (4) a sperm and an ovum together. Assigning the harm to some sperm is utterly arbitrary, for no reason can be given for making a sperm the subject of harm rather than an ovum. Assigning the harm to some ovum is utterly arbitrary, for no reason can be given for making an ovum the subject of harm rather than a sperm. One might attempt to avoid these problems by insisting that contraception deprives both the sperm and the ovum separately of a valuable future like ours. On this alternative, too many futures are lost. Contraception was supposed to be wrong, because it deprived us of one future of value, not two. One might attempt to avoid this problem by holding that contraception deprives the combination of sperm and ovum of a valuable future like ours. But here the definite article misleads. At the time of contraception, there are hundreds of millions of sperm, one (released) ovum and millions of possible combinations of all of these. There is no actual combination at all. Is the subject of the loss to be a merely possible combination? Which one? This alternative does not yield an actual subject of harm either. Accordingly, the immorality of contraception is not entailed by the loss of a future-like-ours argument simply because there is no nonarbitrarily identifiable subject of the loss in the case of contraception.

VI

The purpose of this essay has been to set out an argument for the serious presumptive wrongness of abortion subject to the assumption that the moral permissibility of abortion stands or falls on the moral status of the fetus. Since a fetus possesses a property, the possession of which in adult human beings is sufficient to make killing an adult human being wrong, abortion is wrong. This way of dealing with the problem of abortion seems superior to other approaches to the ethics of abortion, because it rests on an ethics of killing which is close to self-evident, because the crucial morally relevant property clearly applies to fetuses, and because the argument avoids the usual

equivocations on 'human life', 'human being', or 'person'. The argument rests neither on religious claims nor on papal dogma. It is not subject to the objection of "speciesism." Its soundness is compatible with the moral permissibility of euthanasia and contraception. It deals with our intuitions concerning young children.

Finally, this analysis can be viewed as resolving a standard problem—indeed, *the* standard problem—concerning the ethics of abortion. Clearly, it is wrong to kill adult human beings. Clearly, it is not wrong to end the life of some arbitrarily chosen single human cell. Fetuses seem to be like arbitrarily chosen human cells in some respects and like adult humans in other respects. The problem of the ethics of abortion is the problem of determining the fetal property that settles this moral controversy. The thesis of this essay is that the problem of the ethics of abortion, so understood, is solvable.

WHY MOST ABORTIONS ARE NOT WRONG

Bonnie Steinbock

I.   INTRODUCTION

The focus of this chapter is the morality of abortion, not whether it should be legal. Some people who believe that many or even most abortions are morally wrong take a prochoice stance as regards the law. They think that the decision to abort properly belongs to the woman herself because the state ought not to be involved in so personal and intimate a decision as whether to bear a child. Such people maintain that women should think long and hard about whether their circumstances justify abortion,

From *Advances in Bioethics* 5: 245–267. Copyright © 1999 by JAI Press Inc. All rights of reproduction in any form reserved. ISBN: 0-7623-0559-2.

Editors' note: Most author's notes have been cut. Students who want to follow up on sources should consult the original article.

but they want the choice to remain the woman's, as it is she who will bear the burden of an unwanted pregnancy. Other arguments for keeping abortion safe and legal are based on the horrendous health consequences of illegal abortion or the inequalities that result when women, especially poor and minority women, are unable to control their fertility (Graber, 1996). Someone can cite these reasons for keeping abortion legal without believing, as I do, that abortion is almost always a morally permissible option. My belief that abortion is not wrong is based on two considerations: the moral status of the embryo and fetus and the burdens imposed by pregnancy and childbirth on women. I begin by presenting briefly the view of moral status that I take to be correct, that is, the interest view. The interest view limits moral status to beings who have interests and restricts the possession of interests to conscious, sentient beings. The implication for abortion is that it is not seriously wrong to kill a nonconscious, nonsentient fetus where there is an adequate reason for doing so, such as not wanting to be pregnant. Next I discuss Don Marquis' challenge to the interest view (Marquis, 1989). According to Marquis, killing is prima facie wrong when it deprives a being of a valuable future like ours. If a being has a valuable future, the fact that it is now nonconscious and nonsentient is irrelevant. Marquis' account of the wrongness of killing implies that abortion is almost always wrong. I try to show that his view has serious problems, in particular, that it applies to gametes as well as fetuses, and it makes contraception as well as abortion seriously wrong.

I then discuss whether abortion can be a serious moral issue at all, given the interest view, and conclude by addressing some problematic abortions that many people, prochoice as well as prolife, have considered to be morally wrong.

II. THE MORAL STATUS OF THE FETUS

I use the term "fetus" to refer to the unborn at all stages of pregnancy, even though this is not, strictly speaking, correct. Between conception and 8 weeks, the correct term is "embryo"; the term "fetus" is correctly used between 8 weeks gestation age and birth. I will use the term "fetus" throughout, both in order to avoid the inconvenience of the phrase "embryo or fetus" and because using the term "embryo" which refers to the earliest weeks of pregnancy, might convey an unfair advantage to my argument. Everything I have to say about abortion in this essay applies as much to a 12-week-old fetus as it does to a newly fertilized egg.

I will not discuss the morality of abortion beyond the first trimester of pregnancy (approximately 12 weeks long) since the vast majority of abortions (approximately 90 percent) take place by then. I am quite willing to accept that late abortions, especially those that occur after 24 weeks, are morally problematic; but since these are quite rare (about one percent of all abortions) and almost always done for very serious moral reasons such as to preserve the life or health of the mother or to prevent the birth of an infant with a serious disability, I will not discuss these abortions. Instead, I will focus on so-called elective abortions, those chosen to avoid the burdens of pregnancy, childbearing, and childrearing.

Most opponents of abortion say that abortion is wrong because it is the killing of an innocent human being. They see no morally relevant difference between an early gestation fetus and a newborn baby. If it would be wrong to kill a newborn because it is unwanted (something on which there is virtually unanimous agreement), then, according to this thinking, it is equally wrong to perform an abortion, which deliberately kills the fetus.

The question, then, is whether an early gestation fetus (or simply "fetus" as I will say from now on) is morally equivalent to a newborn baby. This seems to me completely implausible. A newborn can feel, react, and perceive. It cries when it is hungry or stuck with needles. Very soon after birth it cries from boredom or loneliness as well and can be soothed by being rocked and held. By contrast, the first-trimester fetus cannot think, feel, or perceive anything. It is certainly alive and human, but it feels and is aware of nothing; it is more like a gamete (a sperm or an ovum), which is also alive and human, than a baby. While early abortion is not the psychological equivalent of contraception, it is morally closer to contraception than to homicide.

My thesis is that killing fetuses is morally different from killing babies because fetuses are not, and babies are, sentient. By sentience, I mean the ability to experience pain and pleasure. But what is the moral significance of sentience? I have argued (Steinbock, 1992) that sentience is important because nonsentient beings, whether mere things (e.g., cars and rocks and works of art) or living things without nervous systems (e.g., plants), lack interests of their own. Therefore, nonsentient beings are not among those beings whose interests we are required to consider. To put it another way, nonsentient beings lack moral status. I refer to this view of moral status as "the interest view."

Critics of the interest view ask why a being has to feel or experience anything to have interests. Leaving a bicycle out in the rain will cause it to rust, affecting adversely both its appearance and its performance. Why can we not say that this is contrary to its interests? Stripping the bark off a tree will cause it to die. Why can't we say that this is against the tree's interest? Limiting interests to sentient beings (namely, animals—human and otherwise) seems to limit unduly the arena of our concern. What about rivers and forests and mountains? What about the environment?

However, this objection misconceives the interest view. The claim is not that we should be concerned to protect and preserve only sentient beings, but rather that only sentient beings can have an interest or a stake in their own existence. It is only sentient beings to whom anything matters, which is quite different from saying that only sentient beings matter. The interest view can acknowledge the value of many nonsentient beings, from works of art to wilderness areas. It recognizes that we have all kinds of reasons—economic, aesthetic, symbolic, even moral reasons—to protect or preserve nonsentient beings. The difference between sentient and nonsentient beings is not that sentient beings have value and nonsentient ones lack value. Rather, it is that since nonsentient beings cannot be hurt or made to suffer, it does not matter *to them* what is done to them. In deciding what we should do, we cannot consider *their* interests since they do not have any. It might be wrong to deface a work of art or to burn a flag, but it is not a wrong *to* the painting or the flag. Put another way "golden rule"–type reasons do not apply to nonsentient beings. That is, no one would explain opposition to burning the flag of the United States of America by saying, "How would you like it if you were a flag and someone burned you?" Instead, such opposition would have to be based on the symbolic importance of the flag and the message that is conveyed when it is burned in a political demonstration. (I am not saying that flag-burning *is* wrong, only contrasting an intelligible reason for opposing flag-burning, based on the symbolic value of the flag, with an absurd reason.)

The interest view is a general theory about moral status, but it has implications for the morality of abortion. During early gestation, fetuses are nonsentient beings and, as such, they do not have interests. Scientists do not agree on precisely when fetuses become sentient, but most agree that first-trimester fetuses are not sentient. The reason is that, in the first trimester, the fetal nervous system is not sufficiently developed to transmit pain messages to the brain. Since the brain cannot receive pain messages, the first-trimester fetus is not sentient; it cannot feel anything. The synaptic connections necessary for pain perception are established in the fetal brain between

20 and 24 weeks of gestation (Anand and Hickey, 1987). This means not only that premature infants *are* capable of experiencing pain—something that doctors rejected until very recently—but also that, throughout the first and most of the second trimester, fetuses do not experience pain or any other sensation. Despite the claims of propaganda films like *The Silent Scream,* first-trimester fetuses do not suffer when they are aborted.

Prolifers may think that I have missed the point of their opposition to abortion. They need not claim that abortion *hurts* the fetus, or causes it to experience pain, but rather that abortion deprives the fetus of its *life.* I quite agree that this is the important issue, but I maintain that a nonsentient being is not deprived of anything by being killed. In an important sense, it does not have a life to lose.

Now this claim may strike some people as odd. If the fetus is alive, then surely it has a life to lose? But this is just what I am denying. It seems to me that unless there is conscious awareness of some kind, a being does not have a life to lose. Consider all the living cells in our bodies which die or are killed. Surely it would be absurd to speak of all of them as losing their lives or being deprived of their lives. Or consider those in a state of permanent unconsciousness, with no hope of regaining consciousness. I would say that such persons have already lost their lives in any sense that matters, even though they are still biologically alive. It is not biological life that matters, but rather conscious existence. Killing the fetus before it becomes conscious and aware deprives it of nothing. To put it another way, the first-trimester fetus has a biological life, but its biographical life has not yet begun (Rachels, 1986). The interest view suggests that it is *prima facie* wrong to deprive beings of their biographical lives, but not wrong to end merely biological lives, at least where there are good reasons for doing so, such as not wanting to bear a child.

III.   THE ARGUMENT FROM POTENTIAL

Of course, there is one difference between a human fetus and any other living, nonsentient being, namely, that if the fetus is not killed, but allowed to develop and grow, it will become a person, just like you or me. Some opponents of abortion cite the potential of the fetus to become a sentient being, with interests and a welfare of its own, as the reason for ascribing to it the moral status belonging to sentient beings. Equally, on this view, the potential of the fetus to become a person gives it the same rights as other persons, including the right to life.

The potentiality principle has been criticized on several grounds. Firstly, it does not follow from the fact that something is a potential *x* that it should be treated as an actual *x*. This is often called "the logical problem with potentiality." As John Harris (1985) puts it, we're all potentially dead, but that's no reason to treat living people as if they were corpses. Secondly, it is not clear why potential personhood attaches only to the fertilized egg. Why aren't unfertilized eggs and sperm also potential people? If certain things happen to them (like meeting a gamete) and certain other things do not (like meeting a contraceptive), they too will develop into people. Admittedly, the chance of any particular sperm becoming a person is absurdly low, but why should that negate its potential? Isn't every player a potential winner in a state lottery, even though the chances of winning are infinitesmal? We should not confuse potentialities with probabilities. So if abortion is wrong because it kills a potential person, then using a spermicide as a contraceptive is equally wrong because it also kills a potential person. Few opponents of abortion are willing to accept this conclusion, which means either giving up the argument from potential or finding a way to differentiate morally between gametes and embryos.

IV. MARQUIS' ARGUMENT

Don Marquis (1989) argues that traditional arguments on abortion, both those of opponents of abortion and those of proponents of a woman's right to choose, are seriously flawed. His argument against abortion derives from a general principle about the wrongness of killing. Killing adult human beings is *prima facie* wrong because it deprives them of their worthwhile future. Marquis writes:

> The loss of one's life is one of the greatest losses one can suffer. The loss of one's life deprives one of all the experiences, activities, projects, and enjoyments that would otherwise have constituted one's future. Therefore, killing someone is wrong, primarily because the

killing inflicts (one of) the greatest possible losses on the victim. . . . When I am killed, I am deprived both of what I now value which would have been part of my future personal life, but also what I would come to value. Therefore, when I die, I am deprived of all of the value of my future. Inflicting this loss on me is ultimately what makes killing me wrong. This being the case, it would seem that what makes killing *any* adult human being *prima facie* seriously wrong is the loss of his or her future (Marquis, 1989, p. 592; in this volume, pp. 549–550).

This argument for the wrongness of killing applies only to those who in fact have a future with experiences, activities, projects, and enjoyments. In Marquis' view, it might not be wrong to kill someone in a persistent vegetative state (PVS), for example, who will never regain consciousness, because such a person no longer has a valuable future. (There might be other reasons against killing PVS patients, but these would not refer to the loss inflicted on the patient.) Similarly, persons who are severely and incurably ill and who face a future of pain and despair and who wish to die may not be wronged if they are killed, because the future of which they are deprived is not considered by them to be a valuable one. However, most fetuses (leaving aside those with serious anomalies) do have valuable futures. If they are not aborted, they will come to have lives they will value and enjoy, just as you and I value and enjoy our lives. Therefore, abortion is seriously wrong for the same reason that killing an innocent adult human being is seriously wrong: it deprives the victim of his or her valuable future.

Marquis' argument against abortion is similar to arguments based on the principle of potentiality in that the wrongness of killing is derived from the loss of the valuable future the fetus will have, if allowed to grow and develop, rather than being based on any characteristic, such as genetic humanity, the fetus now has. However, Marquis' view differs from traditional potentiality arguments in two ways. Firstly, most arguments from potential maintain that it is wrong not only to kill persons, but also to kill potential persons. Though a human fetus is not now a person, it will develop into one if allowed to grow and develop. By contrast, Marquis' argument says nothing about the wrongness of killing persons and therefore nothing about the wrongness of killing potential persons. Marquis is explicit about his argument not necessarily being limited to persons but applying to any beings who have valuable futures like ours. Some nonpersons (e.g., some animals) also might have such futures, and so it might be wrong to kill them in Marquis' account. Admittedly, the concept of a person is not coextensive with the capacity to have a valuable future, and there are heated debates about what it is to be a person. However, if we use the term "person" simply to mean an individual with a valuable future like ours and hence one it would be seriously wrong to kill, we can reword Marquis' account in terms of the wrongness of killing persons.

Another way in which Marquis differs from potentiality theorists is that his argument is not based on the potential of the fetus to become something different from what it is now. Rather, it is wrong to kill a fetus because killing it deprives it of its valuable future—the very same reason why it is wrong to kill you or me. Thus, although Marquis focuses on a certain kind of potential, namely, the fetus's potential to have experiences in the future, this potential is no different from the potential that any born human being has to have future experiences. Thus, he cannot be accused of basing the wrongness of killing born human beings on a feature that we actually possess, while basing the wrongness of abortion on a (merely) potential feature of the fetus.

Marquis thinks that his view is superior to other accounts of moral status in that it is able to explain what is wrong with killing people who are temporarily unconscious, something the interest view seems incapable of doing. If it is morally permissible to kill nonsentient beings, why is it wrong to kill someone in a reversible coma? Such a person is not now conscious or sentient. And if we appeal to his future conscious states, the same argument seems to apply to the fetus, who will become conscious and sentient if we just leave it alone.

Two responses can be made to this objection to the interest view. The first is to note an important difference between a temporarily unconscious person and a fetus. The difference is that the person who is now unconscious has had experiences, plans, beliefs, desires, etc. in the past. These past experiences are relevant because they form the basis for saying that the comatose person wants not to be killed while unconscious. "He valued his life," we might say. "Of course he would not want to be killed." This desire or preference is the basis for saying that the temporarily

unconscious person has an interest in not being killed. But the same cannot be said of a nonsentient fetus. A nonsentient fetus cannot be said to want anything, and so cannot be said to want not to be killed. By contrast, if I am killed while sleeping or temporarily comatose, I am deprived of something I want very much, namely, to go on living. This is not an *occurrent* desire; that is, it is rarely if ever a desire of which I am consciously aware, but it is certainly one of my desires. We have all sorts of desires of which we are not at any particular moment consciously aware, and it would be absurd to limit our desires to what we are actually thinking about. Nor do our desires, plans, and goals, or the interests composing them, vanish when we fall into dreamless sleep.

However, our interests are not limited to what we take an interest in, as Tom Regan (1976) has correctly noted. Our interests also include what is *in* our interest, whether or not we are interested in it. For example, getting enough sleep, eating moderately, and forgoing tobacco might be in the interest of a person who has no interest in following such a regime. Now even if the nonconscious fetus is not interested in continuing to live, could we not say that continued existence is *in* its interest? If the fetus will go on to have a valuable future, is not that future in its interest?

The issue raised here is whether the future the fetus will go on to have is in an important sense *its* future. Marquis considers the existence of past experiences to be entirely irrelevant to the question of whether an entity can be deprived of its future. But this is not at all clear. Killing embryos or early gestation fetuses differs from killing adult human beings because adult human beings have a life that they (ordinarily) value and which they would prefer not to lose: a biographical as opposed to merely biological life. How might the idea of having a biographical life be connected with the possibility of having a personal future, a future of one's own? In an unpublished manuscript, "The Future-Like-Ours Argument Against Abortion and The Problem of Personal Identity," David Boonin[1996] uses a plausible theory of personal identity—the psychological continuity account—to argue that nonsentient fetuses do not have a personal future.[1] According to the psychological continuity account of personal identity, having a certain set of past experiences is what makes me the person I am, and the experiences that I have, *my* experiences. What makes experiences at two different times experiences of the same person is that they are appropriately related by a chain of memories, desires, intentions, and the like. So an individual's past experiences are not, as Marquis claims, otiose to an account of the value of his future; indeed, they are precisely what makes his future *his*.

On this account of personal identity, then, there is an important difference between someone who is temporarily unconscious and a fetus. The difference is this: when the unconscious person regains consciousness, "there will be a relationship of continuity involving memories, intentions, character traits, and so on between his subsequent experiences and those which he had before he lapsed into the coma" (Boonin, 1996, p. 11).

This is what makes his future experiences (those he will have if he is not killed) *his*. The situation of the preconscious fetus is quite different.

> When he gains (rather than regains) consciousness, there will be no relationship of continuity involving memories, intentions, character traits, and so on between his subsequent experiences and those which he had before he gained consciousness precisely because he *had* no experiences before he gained consciousness. This is what permits us to say of the preconscious fetus that it is not he who will have these later experiences if he is not killed. And this, in turn, is what permits us to deny that *he* will be harmed if we prevent those experiences from occurring (Boonin, 1996, p. 12).

If we accept the psychological continuity account of personal identity, then past experiences do matter because without past experiences there is no one with a personal future. This is not to say that this provides us with a reason to kill the presentient fetus but rather that we lack the strong reason for not killing it that we have in the case of people like you and me. The justificatory reason for killing the fetus stems from the woman's rights to bodily autonomy and self-determination, to which I will return in the next section.

However, perhaps the psychological continuity account is wrong. Perhaps personal identity is better based on physical continuity. In that case, even if the born human being has no memories connecting her to the fetal stage, we can still say that she is the same individual because there is physical continuity between the born human and the fetal human.

There are certain advantages to a physical continuity account of personal identity. It allows us to say of someone who develops total amnesia that he has a history of which he has absolutely no memory, and this seems to be a plain statement of fact. Similarly, most people have very few memories about anything that occurred before the ages of four or five; yet most of us are convinced that we are the same individuals we were when very young. Of course, there could be psychological connections of which we have no memory. For example, providing an infant with secure, loving experiences as opposed to terrifying or traumatic ones is likely to affect the psychological development of the eventual adult, whether or not she remembers what happened. So it may be that a more sophisticated psychological account, one that is not entirely dependent on memory, is the better account of identity, but I will not pursue that issue.

Boonin argues that the trouble with basing identity on physical continuity is that this implies that contraception is as wrong as abortion, something most people, including Marquis, want to reject. Thus, the claim that contraception prevents a gamete from enjoying a future like ours takes the form of a *reductio ad absurdum*: the argument (allegedly) commits one to an absurd (or at least unacceptable) conclusion. A physical continuity account of personal identity is vulnerable to the objection that it makes contraception as wrong as abortion because there seems to be no reason why embryos have and gametes do not have valuable futures. For the embryo does not appear *ex nihilo*. Its physical history goes back to the conjoining of the sperm and ovum. Thus, if you prevent the sperm and ovum from conjoining, you deprive each of them of the future they would have had if fertilization had taken place.

Marquis says that his view does not apply to contraception because, prior to fertilization, there is no entity that has a future. It is only after fertilization, when there is a being with a specific genetic code, that there is an individual with a future who can be deprived of that future by being killed. But why should this be so? Admittedly, neither gamete can have a future all by itself, but that is also true of the embryo, which cannot develop all by itself. It needs a uterus and adequate nutrients to develop into a fetus and a baby. Admittedly, the future the sperm will have is not its future alone; it shares its future with the ovum it fertilizes. This makes the situation of gametes unusual, perhaps unique, but does not seem to provide a reason why gametes cannot have futures if the criterion of identity is physical continuity.

Sometimes it is said that a sperm is not a unique individual in the way that a fetus is. For who the sperm turns out to be depends on which ovum it unites with. Why, however, should this lack of uniqueness deprive the sperm of being a potential person, or to use Marquis' language, why should its lack of uniqueness prevent it from having "a future like ours"? Although we cannot specify which future existence the sperm will have, if it is allowed to fertilize an egg, it will become *somebody* and that somebody will have a valuable future.

I think the reason we do not usually think of sperm as having futures is that, in the ordinary reproductive context, literally millions of sperm are released, and only one can fertilize the egg. The rest are doomed. So it seems implausible to say that by killing sperm, we are depriving them of a future. Still, *one* of them might fertilize the egg, even though we cannot say which one it will be, and that one sperm will not get to develop into an embryo and eventual person if it is killed before conception occurs.

Moreover, assisted reproductive technology (ART) facilitates the tracing of an embryo back to its constituent gametes in a way never before possible. In the context of *in vitro* fertilization (IVF), where an egg and sperm are placed in a petri dish for fertilization to occur, we *can* identify the particular gametes who might unite. If dumping out the contents of the petri dish after fertilization has occurred would be immoral because doing that deprives the fertilized egg of "a future like ours," why is it not equally wrong to dump out the contents of the petri dish seconds before fertilization occurs? The ability to identify which gametes make up the embryo is even greater in the micromanipulation technique known as intracytoplasmic sperm injection (ICSI). The ICSI technique enables patients with male factor infertility, where not enough motile sperm can be recovered for ordinary *in vitro* fertilization (IVF), to be considered for assisted reproductive intervention. In ICSI, a single sperm is injected directly into the egg. The isolation of a single sperm makes it possible for us to identify with certainty which sperm conjoined with the egg in the resultant embryo. Thus, the individual who comes to be after fertilization is physically

continuous with the sperm in the pipette and the egg in the petri dish. Killing the gametes before fertilization deprives both of them of the future they would have had.

Marquis might respond to the ART examples by maintaining, in his account, that embryos *in vitro* do not have valuable futures like ours. It is only after implantation, when twinning is no longer possible, that we have an individual who can be said to have a personal future. Thus, Marquis need not be backed into claiming a moral difference between dumping out a petri dish just before or just after conception. Equally, his view is compatible with allowing contraceptives and abortifacients that kill the embryo before implantation occurs. These are seen as importantly morally different from terminating a clinical pregnancy, that is, after implantation occurs. Certainly most of us do regard abortion, even in the first trimester, as morally different from contraception or even a morning-after pill. It seems to me, however, that the reason is not that the status of the embryo radically changes with implantation. Rather, it is that most people have very different feelings toward the termination of a pregnancy than they have toward the prevention of pregnancy. I will return to this point later.

In any event, I do not think Marquis has adequately explained why embryos have valuable futures and gametes do not. For this reason, I consider his account of why abortion is immoral to be vulnerable to the usual objection to potentiality arguments, namely, that they make contraception seriously wrong. The interest view avoids this difficulty. As for its alleged difficulty with explaining why it is wrong to kill sleeping and temporarily comatose people, I maintain that this can be explained in terms of the interests of the nonconscious person, interests that a fetus does not yet have. For these reasons, the interest view seems to me a better account of moral status than the future-like-ours account.

V.   THE ARGUMENT FROM BODILY SELF-DETERMINATION

Suppose I am right about the first trimester fetus's lack of moral status. This does not mean, as I said earlier, that this gives us a reason for killing the fetus. Wantonly killing living things, even if they lack moral status, may well be wrong. To show that most abortions are not wrong, I have to do more than show that fetuses lack moral status. I have to explain why there are good reasons for killing them. These reasons stem from the fact that sustaining the life of a fetus requires the pregnant woman to serve as its life-support system. Thus, the morality of abortion depends not only on whether the fetus is the kind of being it is seriously wrong to kill, but also on whether women have serious moral obligations to sustain the lives of presentient fetuses by not terminating their pregnancies.

The first person to make this point about abortion was Judith Thomson (1971). Thomson argues that even if the fetus is a person with a right to life, it does not follow that abortion is wrong. For the right to life does not give its possessor an unlimited right to whatever it needs to stay alive. In particular, the right to life does not give anyone a right to use another person's body without permission. In at least some cases of pregnancy (e.g., rape and possibly also unintended pregnancy due to contraceptive failure), the fetus was not given even tacit permission to use the woman's body, and therefore it has no right to use it. Having an abortion does not violate the fetus's right to life, even though it kills it.

Thomson's main concern is with the anti-abortion argument based on the fetus's right to life. Therefore, she is primarily interested in whether abortion violates the fetus's right to life. However, she acknowledges that even if no right of the fetus is violated, abortion might still be wrong if the woman has a moral obligation to let the fetus stay in her body until it can survive in the world. After all, we can and do have obligations to help others that do not stem from their rights. Whether the pregnant woman is morally obligated to allow the fetus to stay inside her body depends, according to Thomson, on the degree of burden and sacrifice this imposes on her. For no one is morally obligated, Thomson says, to make large sacrifices to keep another person alive; and pregnancy—unwanted pregnancy—does impose very great sacrifices.

Firstly, there are the physical complaints of pregnancy: weight gain, soreness in the breasts, tiredness, nausea, heartburn, leg cramps, the need to urinate frequently, the difficulty of sleeping in the last trimester, and so forth. Then there is labor and delivery, which can be protracted and painful.

These are not insignificant burdens even in a normal pregnancy where there is no serious risk of harm to the pregnant woman. In "problem pregnancies," the woman may experience much more serious difficulties, including death. Don Regan (1979) argues that outside the abortion context there is no situation in which anyone is required to undergo significant risks and burdens to preserve another person's life. Restrictive abortion laws thus impose burdens on pregnant women that are not imposed on others in comparable situations and so violate the principle of "equal protection."

Although this argument may be successful in showing that abortion should remain legal, its moral force is less clear. Consider the moral obligations of parents to their children, and the sacrifices we think parents should be willing to make for their sakes. In the context of parenthood, it seems false to maintain that no one is morally obligated to make large sacrifices to keep another person alive. Would we think that a parent was under no obligation to take a dying child to the doctor if this were very inconvenient? Suppose the child needed a bone marrow or even a kidney transplant and the parent was a match. Would it be morally permissible for the parent to refuse because of the pain, inconvenience, or bodily invasion? We might not want a society in which judges could force parents to be donors, but surely there *is* a moral obligation to undergo even large sacrifices involving bodily invasion for the sake of one's children. If the fetus is a person, then it presumably has the same status as any other child, and the same claim on its parents that any born children have, including the obligation to make significant sacrifices on its behalf. Of course the burden falls primarily on the woman, since only women can be pregnant (so far), but that biological fact is not intrinsically unfair.

However, if the fetus is importantly different from a born child, as I argued in the last section, then it is hard to see why a woman is morally required to undertake significant risks and burdens to keep the fetus alive. These burdens are not all physical. If abortion is morally wrong, then either the woman will have to raise a child when she does not want to do so, or she will have to endure the pregnancy, labor, and delivery and give the baby up for adoption. Some prolifers talk as if this should be easy enough; after all, she was ready to kill her baby. Why should giving it away upset her? But this cruel attitude ignores the realities. Terminating a pregnancy—especially in the first trimester—is nothing like giving a child up for adoption, in terms of the grief the mother is likely to feel. I can imagine few sacrifices more difficult. One might be morally obligated to make a sacrifice of this magnitude for one's *child*, but no one has a moral obligation to make this huge sacrifice for a merely potential person.

VI.   IS ABORTION A SERIOUS MORAL ISSUE?

Some people think not merely that a woman has the right to decide whether to have an abortion, but that no decision she makes can be criticized on moral grounds. For example, Mary Anne Warren (1973) once claimed that abortion is a "morally neutral" issue, comparable to the decision to have one's hair cut. Most people, regardless of their position on abortion, find this extremely implausible, even outrageous. Are we forced to view abortion this way, if we deny that the fetus has moral status? Surely not. In the first place, terminating a pregnancy is typically connected with powerful emotions in a way that deciding to get one's hair cut is not. The pregnant woman may feel ashamed, embarrassed, or guilty about her pregnancy; and all of these feelings may influence how she feels about an abortion. Her feelings about her partner and their relationship, her attitudes toward sexuality and motherhood are all likely to play a part in her decision; and these topics are fraught with emotional significance in a way that a decision to cut one's hair generally is not. She may be ambivalent about the pregnancy, wishing she could keep the baby, although recognizing that she would make a better mother if she waits until she is older or married or more established in a career. Even a woman who is certain she does not want a child (now) may experience some sadness (as well as relief) at ending a pregnancy—sadness at not being able to welcome and enjoy what is ideally a joyous occasion and something to be celebrated. All of these factors help to explain why so many people do not have the same emotional attitudes toward abortion that they have toward contraception. For most people, even most American Catholics, contraception is likely to be regarded as morally neutral,

a sensible preventive health habit, like flossing your teeth. It has none of the sadness or sense of loss that may accompany abortions.

These are all reasons why abortion feels different from contraception; but does this emotional difference support a moral difference if fetuses lack moral status? The answer depends on one's conception of morality. In one conception of morality, actions are wrong only if they harm others. On a different conception of morality, virtue ethics, the morality of actions is not limited to the harm they are likely to cause, but includes our assessment of the character traits or attitudes of the agent. It is possible that some people have abortions too casually or for unimportant reasons, and this may affect our moral appraisal of what they do. For example, I once heard a 15-year-old girl announce that she was about to have her third abortion. Surprised that so young a girl had had so many unwanted pregnancies when birth control was readily available, I asked her why she kept getting pregnant. "Oh," she said, "I can never remember to put in a diaphragm, and the pill makes me fat." Such an offhand attitude toward sex and pregnancy seems immature, callow, and superficial. Young people should not become sexually active until they are prepared to take precautions to prevent pregnancy. In addition, this girl's insouciant attitude toward having abortions, which would not be necessary if she were more responsible about contraception, indicates a cavalier, indeed, wanton attitude toward potential human life.

Nevertheless, though I deplore the attitudes revealed by the girl's easy acceptance of abortion, I do not think that her decision to have an abortion was wrong. In fact, the very opposite is true. We hear today that quite a lot of young teenagers of 15 or 16 decide to keep their babies because they want the status and prestige that comes with being a mother, or they want the unconditional love they think a baby will provide, or they hope that this will induce a straying boyfriend to stick around. All of these are, in my opinion, terrible reasons for having a child. Before committing oneself to the responsibilities of parenthood, one should have reasonable grounds for thinking that one will be able to be a good—or good enough—parent. Although some 15-year-olds may be capable of being good mothers, most lack the maturity this requires: the patience, experience, knowledge, and ability to put the interests of someone else first. In my view, a 15-year-old who knows that she cannot be a "good enough" parent and has an abortion partly for this reason acts more responsibly, more morally, than the girl who has a baby without thinking about her responsibilities to her future child.

VII.   WHICH ABORTIONS ARE IMMORAL?

As the title of my essay suggests, I believe that most abortions are not wrong. Most abortions occur because the woman does not want to have a child, and I think that this is a very good reason to terminate a pregnancy. However, some abortions may be immoral for a variety of reasons.

A.   Trivial Reasons

Consider the following story. A man learns that his girlfriend is pregnant. He is ecstatic and would like to marry her and raise the child together. However, she tells him that she does not want to continue the pregnancy because she does not want to be pregnant in the summer when she would be unable to wear a bikini. This is certainly a very trivial reason for having an abortion. Would the triviality of the reason make the abortion morally wrong? Certainly her willingness to abort for so slight a reason reflects very badly on her character, but perhaps we should be glad that someone so ditzy is not planning on motherhood, just as we are glad when the immature girl in the previous section decides to abort. There is one difference between this case and the one discussed above, namely, that in this case the girl's partner is willing to take on the childrearing responsibilities by himself if necessary. Assuming that he will be a good parent, bringing the child into the world would not be unfair to the child. If it were really the case that she has no other reason for wanting to avoid pregnancy (such as the usual risks and burdens) and is only worried about not being able to wear a bikini, we might reasonably judge her abortion to be immoral. So trivial a reason does not seem to justify killing a fetus or depriving a man of his desperately wanted child. However, it is scarcely plausible that this could ever be a woman's sole reason for wishing to avoid pregnancy.

B.   Sex Selection

A more realistic example is abortion for sex selection. In some cultures, the desire for a male child is so strong that women will request prenatal diagnosis for the sole purpose of learning the sex of the fetus in order to abort if it is a girl. Most people in our culture consider the destruction of a healthy fetus just because of its sex to be immoral, either because of the sexist attitude it expresses or because such abortions reflect insufficient respect for potential human life, or both. However, it is not clear that abortion for sex selection is always or necessarily wrong. Imagine a woman in her late 40s who has already borne five sons and finds to her amazement that she is again pregnant. If she were to decide to abort, few people would regard her decision as unjustified or her reason—that she has completed her family and is through with childbearing and rearing—as trivial. Now suppose that the woman has always wanted a girl. She could face a sixth child, she thinks, if it were the longed-for daughter. If it is morally permissible for her to terminate the pregnancy, I do not see why it would be wrong for her to terminate if the fetus would be another son. Wanting a daughter after five boys is not an unreasonable or sexist preference. It seems to me that it is up to the woman to decide if another pregnancy would be too burdensome, and that the decision that it would not be if the child were a girl does not demonstrate insufficient respect for prenatal life.

In some countries, the desire for a son is so strong that women undergo numerous pregnancies in order to have a male child. We may regard such a preference as sexist and unenlightened, but it exists and has large implications for the lives of women living in these cultures. Repeated pregnancies take a serious toll on their health and force them to bear more children than they can adequately feed and clothe. The lives of the girls who are born in the attempt to get a son are often substandard as they typically receive less food and medical attention than their brothers. Preventing the births of girls by abortion seems a morally preferable option to requiring that they be born, then neglected, or allowed to starve to death. So while we may regard abortion for sex selection to be generally wrong, at least in our country, the automatic and absolute rejection of sex selection fails to take into consideration the social realities in which it may occur.

C.   Fetal Reduction

Most fetal reductions are done when there are more fetuses than can be safely expected to be carried to term. Typically, this is due to the woman's having taken fertility drugs, which greatly increases the chance of having multiple fetuses. Fertility drugs were responsible for the first surviving set of septuplets born in Iowa in November 1997 to Bobbi and Kenny McCaughey. Doctors usually advise women pregnant with more than three fetuses to undergo selective reduction. The reasoning behind fetal reduction is that if some of the fetuses are not killed, the chances that any of them will survive, especially without disability, are greatly reduced. If a reduction is not performed, the couple may lose the entire pregnancy. The mother's health is also put at risk in a multiple pregnancy.

Fetal reduction of a much-wanted pregnancy is likely to be a heartrending choice, even though this improves the chances of survival of the remaining fetuses. For some, like the McCaugheys, selective reduction may be completely unacceptable. Some people criticized the McCaugheys for their decision not to reduce, arguing that while Bobbi McCaughey was entitled to risk her own life and health by carrying seven fetuses, she had no right to subject her future children to the substantial risks of mental retardation, cerebral palsy, and blindness. These critics say that the fact that "the gamble paid off," and all the babies appear to be healthy so far (although it may be some time before any damage is evident), does not make the risk-taking more justifiable. Indeed, some doctors who have had very bad outcomes with multiple births are no longer willing to prescribe fertility drugs for women who would not consider selective reduction. Others think that the choice must remain that of the individual patient.

The choice to reduce a multiple pregnancy to twins is invariably regarded as permissible by those who think that abortion can ever be justified, since the aim is to preserve the life and health of the mother and remaining fetuses. What if the pregnant woman wants a fetal reduction from twins to a singleton, not because of the objective risk of a multiple birth, but because she would prefer to have just one baby? In August 1996, Dr. Phillip Bennett of Queen Charlotte's Hospital in London told *The Sunday Express* that he had recommended abortion of one fetus as a solution when the woman told him she could not continue her 16-week-old pregnancy if it meant having twins. He felt that it would be better to do the reduction and leave one alive than to lose two babies.

The first reports of the story maintained that the woman was a 28-year-old single mother with one child, who was too poor to raise twins. The public reacted with shock, anger, and dismay. Life, a British national charity, said it was deluged with calls and was able immediately to offer the woman upward of $16,000 to give birth to both twins and give one up for adoption. Many commentators were appalled by the doctor's willingness to perform a selective reduction in this situation. One called it selective murder, saying, "I mean, we know they have aborted healthy babies before, but to leave one and kill the other is abhorrent" (Ibrahim, 1996).

As it later turned out, the woman was a middle-class professional who was not motivated by lack of funds. Apparently, she simply did not want to cope with twins. This does not seem unduly callous or selfish. Even carrying twins puts considerable extra burdens on the pregnant woman, and caring for twins is a great deal more work than caring for one child. The justification for abortion in this case is very similar to the standard case: it is based on the amount of sacrifice and burden the pregnancy will impose. In this case, as in all the rest, only the woman herself can judge if the burdens are too great for her to bear. If aborting both twins is both legally and morally permissible (and indeed would have passed unnoticed), it is hard to see why aborting one of the twins would be morally wrong. If the woman had felt she had no choice but to abort one fetus because of poverty, that would indeed have been tragic—though no more tragic than the decision to abort a single fetus due to poverty. Yet such cases, which surely occur, do not get written up in the newspapers; and no one offers these poor women money so they will be able to keep their babies.

D.   Vengeful Abortion

Abortion could also be immoral if done for morally bad, as opposed to trivial, reasons. For example, imagine a woman who has an abortion to take revenge on her husband when she learns that he was unfaithful to her earlier in the marriage. She does not want to end the marriage, or even not to have his child, but only to make him suffer as she has suffered. Once she feels that he has adequately made amends, she intends to get pregnant again. Let us further imagine that she already has two children to whom she has been an excellent mother. This variation of the *Medea* story, with its jealousy, vengefulness, spite, and cruelty, is a pretty clear example of an immoral abortion. My qualification is due to the fact that the woman seems psychotic and thus possibly not morally responsible.

VIII.   CONCLUSION

Of course, most women do not have abortions for the bizarre reasons given above. A very common reason for abortion, perhaps the most common, is birth control failure. Women get pregnant using diaphragms, IUDs, even on the pill. The possibility of birth control failure makes abortion a necessity if women are to have genuine choice about when and whether they reproduce. Even if the pregnancy is someone's "fault," that is, due to a failure to use birth control, that bears no relation to the morality of abortion. Given that fetuses are not the sorts of entities whom it is seriously wrong to kill, women have the moral right to decide for themselves if they are willing to endure the burdens of pregnancy and childbirth. In most cases, their reasons for wishing to terminate their pregnancies are sensible ones. In fact, in light of the number of abused and neglected children in the world, it might make more sense to ask that people justify their decisions to have children, instead of their decisions to terminate pregnancies.

NOTES

1. For a more recent statement of Boonin's critique of Marquis's argument, see his book, *A Defense of Abortion* (Cambridge University Press, 2003, section 2.8).

REFERENCES

Anand, K.J.S. & Hickey, P.R. (1987). Pain and its effects in the human neonate and fetus. N. Engl. J. Med. 317, 1322.

Boonin, D. (1996). The future-like-ours argument against abortion and the problem of personal identity. (Unpublished.)

Graber, M.A. (1996). Rethinking Abortion: Equal Choice, the Constitution, and Reproductive Politics. Princeton University Press, Princeton, NJ.

Harris, J. (1985). The Value of Life: An Introduction to Medical Ethics. Routledge & Kegan Paul, London.

Ibrahim, Y.M. (1996). Planned abortion of one twin stirs furor in Britain. The New York Times, August 6, p. A3.

Marquis, D. (1989). Why abortion is immoral. J. of Phil. 76, 183–202.

McCormick, J. and Kantrowitz, B. (1997). The magnificent seven. Newsweek, December 1, pp. 58–62.

Rachels, J. (1986). The End of Life: Euthanasia and Morality. Oxford University Press, New York.

Regan, D. (1979). Rewriting *Roe* v. *Wade*. Mich. L. Rev. 77.

Regan, T. (1976). Feinberg on what sorts of beings can have rights. Southern J. of Phil. 14, 485–498.

Robertson, J.A. (1994). Children of Choice: Freedom and the New Reproductive Technologies. Princeton University Press, Princeton, NJ.

Steinbock, B. (1992). Life Before Birth: The Moral and Legal Status of Embryos and Fetuses. Oxford University Press, New York.

Thomson, J. (1971). A defense of abortion. Phil. & Pub. Affairs 1, 47–66.

Warren, M.A. (1973). On the moral and legal status of abortion. Monist 57, 43–61.

A DEFENSE OF ABORTION[1]

Judith Jarvis Thomson

Most opposition to abortion relies on the premise that the fetus is a human being, a person, from the moment of conception. The premise is argued for, but, as I think, not well. Take, for example, the most common argument. We are asked to notice that the development of a human being from conception through birth into childhood is continuous; then it is said that to draw a line, to choose a point in this development and say "before this point the thing is not a person, after this point it is a person" is to make an arbitrary choice, a choice for which in the nature of things no good reason can be given. It is concluded that the fetus is, or anyway that we had better say it is, a person from the moment of conception. But this conclusion does not follow. Similar things might be said about the development of an acorn into an oak tree, and it does not follow that acorns are oak trees, or that we had better say they are. Arguments of this form are sometimes called "slippery slope arguments"—the phrase is perhaps self-explanatory—and it is dismaying that opponents of abortion rely on them so heavily and uncritically.

I am inclined to agree, however, that the prospects for "drawing a line" in the development of the fetus look dim. I am inclined to think also that we shall probably have to agree that the fetus has already become a human person well before birth. Indeed, it comes as a surprise when one first learns how early in its life it begins to acquire human characteristics. By the tenth week, for example, it already has a face, arms and legs, fingers and toes; it has internal organs, and brain activity is detectable.[2] On the other hand, I think that the premise is false, that the fetus is not a person from the moment of conception. A newly fertilized ovum, a newly implanted clump of cells, is no more a person than an acorn is an oak tree. But I shall not discuss any of this. For it seems to me to be of great interest to ask what happens if, for

the sake of argument, we allow the premise. How, precisely, are we supposed to get from there to the conclusion that abortion is morally impermissible? Opponents of abortion commonly spend most of their time establishing that the fetus is a person, and hardly any time explaining the step from there to the impermissibility of abortion. Perhaps they think the step too simple and obvious to require much comment. Or perhaps instead they are simply being economical in argument. Many of those who defend abortion rely on the premise that the fetus is not a person, but only a bit of tissue that will become a person at birth; and why pay out more arguments than you have to? Whatever the explanation, I suggest that the step they take is neither easy nor obvious, that it calls for closer examination than it is commonly given, and that when we do give it this closer examination we shall feel inclined to reject it.

I propose, then, that we grant that the fetus is a person from the moment of conception. How does the argument go from here? Something like this, I take it. Every person has a right to life. So the fetus has a right to life. No doubt the mother has a right to decide what shall happen in and to her body; everyone would grant that. But surely a person's right to life is stronger and more stringent than the mother's right to decide what happens in and to her body, and so outweighs it. So the fetus may not be killed; an abortion may not be performed.

It sounds plausible. But now let me ask you to imagine this. You wake up in the morning and find yourself back to back in bed with an unconscious violinist. A famous unconscious violinist. He has been found to have a fatal kidney ailment, and the Society of Music Lovers has canvassed all the available medical records and found that you alone have the right blood type to help. They have therefore kidnapped you, and last night the violinist's circulatory system was plugged into yours, so that your kidneys can be used to extract poisons from his blood as well as your own. The director of the hospital now tells you, "Look, we're sorry the Society of Music Lovers did this to you—we would never

From Judith Jarvis Thomson, "A Defense of Abortion," *Philosophy & Public Affairs* 1, no. 1 (1971): 47–66, Blackwell Publishers.

have permitted it if we had known. But still, they did it, and the violinist now is plugged into you. To unplug you would be to kill him. But never mind, it's only for nine months. By then he will have recovered from his ailment, and can safely be unplugged from you." Is it morally incumbent on you to accede to this situation? No doubt it would be very nice of you if you did, a great kindness. But do you *have* to accede to it? What if it were not nine months, but nine years? Or longer still? What if the director of the hospital says, "Tough luck, I agree, but you've now got to stay in bed, with the violinist plugged into you, for the rest of your life. Because remember this. All persons have a right to life, and violinists are persons. Granted you have a right to decide what happens in and to your body, but a person's right to life outweighs your right to decide what happens in and to your body. So you cannot ever be unplugged from him." I imagine you would regard this as outrageous, which suggests that something really is wrong with that plausible-sounding argument I mentioned a moment ago.

In this case, of course, you were kidnapped; you didn't volunteer for the operation that plugged the violinist into your kidneys. Can those who oppose abortion on the ground I mentioned make any exception for a pregnancy due to rape? Certainly. They can say that persons have a right to life only if they didn't come into existence because of rape; or they can say that all persons have a right to life, but that some have less of a right to life than others, in particular, that those who came into existence because of rape have less. But these statements have a rather unpleasant sound. Surely the question of whether you have a right to life at all, or how much of it you have, shouldn't turn on the question of whether or not you are the product of a rape. And in fact the people who oppose abortion on the ground I mentioned do not make this distinction, and hence do not make an exception in case of rape.

Nor do they make an exception for a case in which the mother has to spend the nine months of her pregnancy in bed. They would agree that would be a great pity, and hard on the mother; but all the same, all persons have a right to life, the fetus is a person, and so on. I suspect, in fact, that they would not make an exception for a case in which, miraculously enough, the pregnancy went on for nine years, or even the rest of the mother's life.

Some won't even make an exception for a case in which continuation of the pregnancy is likely to shorten the mother's life; they regard abortion as impermissible even to save the mother's life. Such cases are nowadays very rare, and many opponents of abortion do not accept this extreme view. All the same, it is a good place to begin: a number of points of interest come out in respect to it.

1. Let us call the view that abortion is impermissible even to save the mother's life "the extreme view." I want to suggest first that it does not issue from the argument I mentioned earlier without the addition of some fairly powerful premises. Suppose a woman has become pregnant, and now learns that she has a cardiac condition such that she will die if she carries the baby to term. What may be done for her? The fetus, being a person, has a right to life, but as the mother is a person too, so has she a right to life. Presumably they have an equal right to life. How is it supposed to come out that an abortion may not be performed? If mother and child have an equal right to life, shouldn't we perhaps flip a coin? Or should we add to the mother's right to life her right to decide what happens in and to her body, which everybody seems to be ready to grant—the sum of her rights now outweighing the fetus's right to life?

The most familiar argument here is the following. We are told that performing the abortion would be directly killing[3] the child, whereas doing nothing would not be killing the mother, but only letting her die. Moreover, in killing the child, one would be killing an innocent person, for the child has committed no crime, and is not aiming at his mother's death. And then there are a variety of ways in which this might be continued. (1) But as directly killing an innocent person is always and absolutely impermissible, an abortion may not be performed. Or, (2) as directly killing an innocent person is murder, and murder is always and absolutely impermissible, an abortion may not be performed.[4] Or, (3) as one's duty to refrain from directly killing an innocent person is more stringent than one's duty to keep a person from dying, an abortion may not be performed. Or, (4) if one's only options are directly killing an innocent person or letting a person die, one must prefer letting the person die, and thus an abortion may not be performed.[5]

Some people seem to have thought that these are not further premises which must be added if the conclusion is to be reached, but that they follow from the very fact that an innocent person has a right to life.[6] But this seems to me to be a mistake, and perhaps the simplest way to show this is to bring out that while we must certainly grant that innocent persons have a right to life, the theses in (1) through (4) are all false. Take (2), for example. If directly killing an innocent person is murder, and thus is impermissible, then the mother's directly killing the innocent person inside her is murder, and thus is impermissible. But it cannot seriously be thought to be murder if the mother performs an abortion on herself to save her life. It cannot seriously be said that she *must* refrain, that she *must* sit passively by and wait for her death. Let us look again at the case of you and the violinist. There you are, in bed with the violinist, and the director of the hospital says to you "It's all most distressing, and I deeply sympathize, but you see this is putting an additional strain on your kidneys, and you'll be dead within the month. But you *have* to stay where you are all the same. Because unplugging you would be directly killing an innocent violinist, and that's murder, and that's impermissible." If anything in the world is true, it is that you do not commit murder, you do not do what is impermissible, if you reach around to your back and unplug yourself from that violinist to save your life. . . .

2. The extreme view could of course be weakened to say that while abortion is permissible to save the mother's life, it may not be performed by a third party, but only by the mother herself. But this cannot be right either. For what we have to keep in mind is that the mother and the unborn child are not like two tenants in a small house which has, by an unfortunate mistake, been rented to both: the mother *owns* the house. The fact that she does adds to the offensiveness of deducing that the mother can do nothing from the supposition that third parties can do nothing. But it does more than this: it casts a bright light on the supposition that third parties can do nothing. Certainly it lets us see that a third party who says "I cannot choose between you" is fooling himself if he thinks this is impartiality. If Jones has found and fastened on a certain coat, which he needs to keep him from freezing, but which Smith also needs to keep him from freezing, then it is not impartiality that says "I cannot choose between you" when Smith owns the coat. Women have said again and again "This body is *my* body!"

and they have reason to feel angry, reason to feel that it has been like shouting into the wind. Smith, after all, is hardly likely to bless us if we say to him, "Of course it's your coat, anybody would grant that it is. But no one may choose between you and Jones who is to have it."

We should really ask what it is that says "no one may choose" in the face of the fact that the body that houses the child is the mother's body. It may be simply a failure to appreciate this fact. But it may be something more interesting, namely the sense that one has a right to refuse to lay hands on Jones, a right to refuse to do physical violence to people, even where it would be just and fair to do so, even where justice seems to require that somebody do so. Thus justice might call for somebody to get Smith's coat back from Jones, and yet you have a right to refuse to be the one to lay hands on Jones, a right to refuse to do physical violence to him. This, I think, must be granted. But then what should be said is not "no one may choose" but only "I cannot choose," and indeed not even this, but "*I will not act*," leaving it open that somebody else can or should, and in particular that anyone in a position of authority, with the job of securing people's rights, both can and should. So this is no difficulty. I have not been arguing that any given third party *must* accede to the mother's request that he perform an abortion to save her life, but only that he *may*.

I suppose that in some views of human life the mother's body is only on loan to her, the loan not being one which gives her any prior claim to it. One who held this view might well think it impartiality to say "I cannot choose." But I shall simply ignore this possibility. My own view is that if a human being has any just, prior claim to anything at all, he has a just, prior claim to his own body. And perhaps this needn't be argued for here anyway, since, as I mentioned, the arguments against abortion we are looking at do grant that the woman has a right to decide what happens in and to her body.

But although they do grant it, I have tried to show that they do not take seriously what is done in granting it. I suggest the same thing will reappear even more clearly when we turn away from cases in which the mother's life is at stake, and attend, as I propose we now do, to the vastly more common cases in which a woman wants an abortion for some less weighty reason than preserving her own life.

3. Where the mother's life is not at stake, the argument I mentioned at the outset seems to have a much stronger pull. "Everyone has a right to life, so the unborn person has a right to life." And isn't the child's right to life weightier than anything other than the mother's own right to life, which she might put forward as ground for an abortion?

This argument treats the right to life as if it were unproblematic. It is not, and this seems to me to be precisely the source of the mistake.

For we should now, at long last, ask what it comes to, to have a right to life. In some views having a right to life includes having a right to be given at least the bare minimum one needs for continued life. But suppose that what in fact *is* the bare minimum a man needs for continued life is something he has no right at all to be given? If I am sick unto death, and the only thing that will save my life is the touch of Henry Fonda's cool hand on my fevered brow, then all the same, I have no right to be given the touch of Henry Fonda's cool hand on my fevered brow. It would be frightfully nice of him to fly in from the West Coast to provide it. It would be less nice, though no doubt well meant, if my friends flew out to the West Coast and carried Henry Fonda back with them. But I have no right at all against anybody that he should do this for me. Or again, to return to the story I told earlier, the fact that for continued life that violinist needs the continued use of your kidneys does not establish that he has a right to be given the continued use of your kidneys. He certainly has no right against you that *you* should give him continued use of your kidneys. For nobody has any right to use your kidneys unless you give him such a right; and nobody has the right against you that you shall give him this right—if you do allow him to go on using your kidneys, this is a kindness on your part, and not something he can claim from you as his due. Nor has he any right against anybody else that *they* should give him continued use of your kidneys. Certainly he had no right against the Society of Music Lovers that they should plug him into you in the first place. And if you now start to unplug yourself, having learned that you will otherwise have to spend nine years in bed with him, there is nobody in the world who must try to prevent you, in order to see to it that he is given something he has a right to be given.

Some people are rather stricter about the right to life. In their view, it does not include the right to be given anything, but amounts to, and only to, the right not to be killed by anybody. But here a related difficulty arises. If everybody is to refrain from killing that violinist, then everybody must refrain from doing a great many different sorts of things. Everybody must refrain from slitting his throat, everybody must refrain from shooting him—and everybody must refrain from unplugging you from him. But does he have a right against everybody that they shall refrain from unplugging you from him? To refrain from doing this is to allow him to continue to use your kidneys. It could be argued that he has a right against us that *we* should allow him to continue to use your kidneys. That is, while he has no right against us that we should give him the use of your kidneys, it might be argued that he anyway has a right against us that we shall not now intervene and deprive him of the use of your kidneys. I shall come back to third-party interventions later. But certainly the violinist has no right against you that *you* shall allow him to continue to use your kidneys. As I said, if you do allow him to use them, it is a kindness on your part, and not something you owe him.

The difficulty I point to here is not peculiar to the right to life. It reappears in connection with all the other natural rights; and it is something which an adequate account of rights must deal with. For present purposes it is enough just to draw attention to it. But I would stress that I am not arguing that people do not have a right to life—quite to the contrary, it seems to me that the primary control we must place on the acceptability of an account of rights is that it should turn out in that account to be a truth that all persons have a right to life. I am arguing only that having a right to life does not guarantee having either a right to be given the use of or a right to be allowed continued use of another person's body—even if one needs it for life itself. So the right to life will not serve the opponents of abortion in the very simple and clear way in which they seem to have thought it would.

4. There is another way to bring out the difficulty. In the most ordinary sort of case, to deprive someone of what he has a right to is to treat him unjustly. Suppose a boy and his small brother are jointly given a box of chocolates for Christmas. If the older boy takes the box and refuses to give his brother any of the chocolates, he is unjust to him, for the brother has been given a right to half of them. But suppose that, having learned that otherwise it means nine years in bed with that violinist, you unplug yourself from him. You surely are not being unjust to him, for you gave him no right to use your kidneys, and no one else can have given him any such right. But we have to notice that in unplugging yourself, you are killing him; and violinists, like everybody else, have a right to life, and thus in the view we were considering just now, the right not to be killed. So here you do what he supposedly has a right you shall not do, but you do not act unjustly to him in doing it.

The emendation which may be made at this point is this: the right to life consists not in the right not to be killed, but rather in the right not to be killed unjustly. This runs a risk of circularity, but never mind: it would enable us to square the fact that the violinist has a right to life with the fact that you do not act unjustly toward him in unplugging yourself, thereby killing him. For if you do not kill him unjustly, you do not violate his right to life, and so it is no wonder you do him no injustice.

But if this emendation is accepted, the gap in the argument against abortion stares us plainly in the face: it is by no means enough to show that the fetus is a person, and to remind us that all persons have a right to life—we need to be shown also that killing the fetus violates its right to life, i.e., that abortion is unjust killing. And is it?

I suppose we may take it as a datum that in a case of pregnancy due to rape the mother has not given the unborn person a right to the use of her body for food and shelter. Indeed, in what pregnancy could it be supposed that the mother has given the unborn person such a right? It is not as if there were unborn persons drifting about the world, to whom a woman who wants a child says "I invite you in."

But it might be argued that there are other ways one can have acquired a right to the use of another person's body than by having been invited to use it by that person. Suppose a woman voluntarily indulges in intercourse, knowing of the chance it will issue in pregnancy, and then she does become pregnant; is she not in part responsible for the presence, in fact the very existence, of the unborn person inside her? No doubt she did not invite it in. But doesn't her partial responsibility for its being there

itself give it a right to the use of her body?[7] If so, then her aborting it would be more like the boy's taking away the chocolates, and less like your unplugging yourself from the violinist—doing so would be depriving it of what it does have a right to, and thus would be doing it an injustice.

And then, too, it might be asked whether or not she can kill it even to save her own life: If she voluntarily called it into existence, how can she now kill it, even in self-defense?

The first thing to be said about this is that it is something new. Opponents of abortion have been so concerned to make out the independence of the fetus, in order to establish that it has a right to life, just as its mother does, that they have tended to overlook the possible support they might gain from making out that the fetus is *dependent* on the mother, in order to establish that she has a special kind of responsibility for it, a responsibility that gives it rights against her which are not possessed by any independent person—such as an ailing violinist who is a stranger to her.

On the other hand, this argument would give the unborn person a right to its mother's body only if her pregnancy resulted from a voluntary act, undertaken in full knowledge of the chance a pregnancy might result from it. It would leave out entirely the unborn person whose existence is due to rape. Pending the availability of some further argument, then, we would be left with the conclusion that unborn persons whose existence is due to rape have no right to the use of their mothers' bodies, and thus that aborting them is not depriving them of anything they have a right to and hence is not unjust killing.

And we should also notice that it is not at all plain that this argument really does go even as far as it purports to. For there are cases and cases, and the details make a difference. If the room is stuffy, and I therefore open a window to air it, and a burglar climbs in, it would be absurd to say, "Ah, now he can stay, she's given him a right to the use of her house—for she is partially responsible for his presence there, having voluntarily done what enabled him to get in, in full knowledge that there are such things as burglars, and that burglars burgle." It would be still more absurd to say this if I had had bars installed outside my windows, precisely to prevent burglars from getting in, and a burglar got in only because of a defect in the bars. It remains equally absurd if we imagine it is not a burglar who climbs in, but an innocent person who blunders or falls in. Again, suppose it were like this: people-seeds drift about in the air like pollen, and if you open your windows, one may drift in and take root in your carpets or upholstery. You don't want children, so you fix up your windows with fine mesh screens, the very best you can buy. As can happen, however, and on very, very rare occasions does happen, one of the screens is defective; and a seed drifts in and takes root. Does the person-plant who now develops have a right to the use of your house? Surely not—despite the fact that you voluntarily opened your windows, you knowingly kept carpets and upholstered furniture, and you knew that screens were sometimes defective. Someone may argue that you are responsible for its rooting, that it does have a right to your house, because after all you *could* have lived out your life with bare floors and furniture, or with sealed windows and doors. But this won't do—for by the same token anyone can avoid a pregnancy due to rape by having a hysterectomy, or anyway by never leaving home without a (reliable!) army.

It seems to me that the argument we are looking at can establish at most that there are *some* cases in which the unborn person has a right to the use of its mother's body, and therefore *some* cases in which abortion is unjust killing. There is room for much discussion and argument as to precisely which, if any. But I think we should sidestep this issue and leave it open, for at any rate the argument certainly does not establish that all abortion is unjust killing.

5. There is room for yet another argument here, however. We surely must all grant that there may be cases in which it would be morally indecent to detach a person from your body at the cost of his life. Suppose you learn that what the violinist needs is not nine years of your life, but only one hour: all you need do to save his life is to spend one hour in that bed with him. Suppose also that letting him use your kidneys for that one hour would not affect your health in the slightest. Admittedly you were kidnapped. Admittedly you did not give anyone permission to plug him into you. Nevertheless it seems to me plain you *ought* to allow him to use your kidneys for that hour—it would be indecent to refuse.

Again, suppose pregnancy lasted only an hour, and constituted no threat to life or health. And suppose that a woman becomes pregnant as a result of rape. Admittedly she did not voluntarily do anything to bring about the existence of a child. Admittedly she did nothing at all which would give the unborn person a right to the use of her body. All the same it might well be said, as in the newly emended violinist story, that she *ought* to allow it to remain for that hour—that it would be indecent of her to refuse.

Now some people are inclined to use the term "right" in such a way that it follows from the fact that you ought to allow a person to use your body for the hour he needs, that he has a right to use your body for the hour he needs, even though he has not been given that right by any person or act. They may say that it follows also that if you refuse, you act unjustly toward him. This use of the term is perhaps so common that it cannot be called wrong; nevertheless it seems to me to be an unfortunate loosening of what we would do better to keep a tight rein on. Suppose that box of chocolates I mentioned earlier had not been given to both boys jointly, but was given only to the older boy. There he sits, stolidly eating his way through the box, his small brother watching enviously. Here we are likely to say "You ought not to be so mean. You ought to give your brother some of those chocolates." My own view is that it just does not follow from the truth of this that the brother has any right to any of the chocolates. If the boy refuses to give his brother any, he is greedy, stingy, callous—but not unjust. I suppose that the people I have in mind will say it does follow that the brother has a right to some of the chocolates, and thus that the boy does act unjustly if he refuses to give his brother any. But the effect of saying this is to obscure what we should keep distinct, namely the difference between the boy's refusal in this case and the boy's refusal in the earlier case, in which the box was given to both boys jointly, and in which the small brother thus had what was from any point of view clear title to half.

A further objection to so using the term "right" that from the fact that A ought to do a thing for B, it follows that B has a right against A that A do it for him, is that it is going to make the question of whether or not a man has a right to a thing turn on how easy it is to provide him with it; and this seems not merely unfortunate, but morally unacceptable.

Take the case of Henry Fonda again. I said earlier that I had no right to the touch of his cool hand on my fevered brow even though I needed it to save my life. I said it would be frightfully nice of him to fly in from the West Coast to provide me with it, but that I had no right against him that he should do so. But suppose he isn't on the West Coast. Suppose he has only to walk across the room, place a hand briefly on my brow—and lo, my life is saved. Then surely he ought to do it; it would be indecent to refuse. Is it to be said, "Ah, well, it follows that in this case she has a right to the touch of his hand on her brow, and so it would be an injustice for him to refuse"? So that I have a right to it when it is easy for him to provide it, though no right when it's hard? It's rather a shocking idea that anyone's rights should fade away and disappear as it gets harder and harder to accord them to him.

So my own view is that even though you ought to let the violinist use your kidneys for the one hour he needs, we should not conclude that he has a right to do so—we should say that if you refuse, you are, like the boy who owns all the chocolates and will give none away, self-centered and callous, indecent in fact, but not unjust. And similarly, that even supposing a case in which a woman pregnant due to rape ought to allow the unborn person to use her body for the hour he needs, we should not conclude that he has a right to do so; we should conclude that she is self-centered, callous, indecent, but not unjust, if she refuses. The complaints are no less grave; they are just different. However, there is no need to insist on this point. If anyone does wish to deduce "he has a right" from "you ought," then all the same he must surely grant that there are cases in which it is not morally required of you that you allow that violinist to use your kidneys, and in which he does not have a right to use them, and in which you do not do him an injustice if you refuse. And so also for mother and unborn child. Except in such cases as the unborn person has a right to demand it—and we were leaving open the possibility that there may be such cases— nobody is morally *required* to make large sacrifices, of health, of all other interests and concerns, of all other duties and commitments, for nine years, or even for nine months, in order to keep another person alive.

6. We have in fact to distinguish between two kinds of Samaritan: the Good Samaritan and what we might call the Minimally Decent Samaritan.

The story of the Good Samaritan, you will remember, goes like this:

> A certain man went down from Jerusalem to Jericho, and fell among thieves, which stripped him of his raiment, and wounded him, and departed, leaving him half dead.
>
> And by chance there came down a certain priest that way; and when he saw him, he passed by on the other side.
>
> And likewise a Levite, when he was at the place, came and looked on him, and passed by on the other side.
>
> But a certain Samaritan, as he journeyed, came where he was; and when he saw him he had compassion on him.
>
> And went to him, and bound up his wounds, pouring in oil and wine, and set him on his own beast, and brought him to an inn, and took care of him.
>
> And on the morrow, when he departed, he took out two pence, and gave them to the host, and said unto him, "Take care of him; and whatsoever thou spendest more, when I come again, I will repay thee."
>
> (Luke 10:30–35)

The Good Samaritan went out of his way, at some cost to himself, to help one in need of it. We are not told what the options were, that is, whether or not the priest and the Levite could have helped by doing less than the Good Samaritan did, but assuming they could have, then the fact they did nothing at all shows they were not even Minimally Decent Samaritans, not because they were not Samaritans, but because they were not even minimally decent.

These things are a matter of degree, of course, but there is a difference, and it comes out perhaps most clearly in the story of Kitty Genovese, who, as you will remember, was murdered while thirty-eight people watched or listened, and did nothing at all to help her. A Good Samaritan would have rushed out to give direct assistance against the murderer. Or perhaps we had better allow that it would have been a Splendid Samaritan who did this, on the ground that it would have involved a risk of death for himself. But the thirty-eight not only did not do this, they did not even trouble to pick up a phone to call the police. Minimally

Decent Samaritanism would call for doing at least that, and their not having done it was monstrous.

After telling the story of the Good Samaritan, Jesus said, "Go, and do thou likewise." Perhaps he meant that we are morally required to act as the Good Samaritan did. Perhaps he was urging people to do more than is morally required of them. At all events it seems plain that it was not morally required of any of the thirty-eight that he rush out to give direct assistance at the risk of his own life, and that it is not morally required of anyone that he give long stretches of his life—nine years or nine months—to sustaining the life of a person who has no special right (we were leaving open the possibility of this) to demand it.

Indeed, with one rather striking class of exceptions, no one in any country in the world is *legally* required to do anywhere near as much as this for anyone else. The class of exceptions is obvious. My main concern here is not the state of the law in respect to abortion, but it is worth drawing attention to the fact that in no state in this country is any man compelled by law to be even a Minimally Decent Samaritan to any person; there is no law under which charges could be brought against the thirty-eight who stood by while Kitty Genovese died. By contrast, in most states in this country women are compelled by law to be not merely Minimally Decent Samaritans, but Good Samaritans to unborn persons inside them. This doesn't by itself settle anything one way or the other, because it may well be argued that there should be laws in this country—as there are in many European countries—compelling at least Minimally Decent Samaritanism.[8] But it does show that there is a gross injustice in the existing state of the law. And it shows also that the groups currently working against liberalization of abortion laws, in fact working toward having it declared unconstitutional for a state to permit abortion, had better start working for the adoption of Good Samaritan laws generally, or earn the charge that they are acting in bad faith.

I should think, myself, that Minimally Decent Samaritan laws would be one thing, Good Samaritan laws quite another, and in fact highly improper. But we are not here concerned with the law. What we should ask is not whether anybody should be compelled by law to be a Good Samaritan, but whether we must accede to a situation in which somebody is being compelled—by nature, perhaps—to be a Good Samaritan. We have, in other words, to look now at third-party interventions. I have been arguing that no person is morally required to make large sacrifices to sustain the life of another who has no right to demand them, and this even where the sacrifices do not include life itself; we are not morally required to be Good Samaritans or anyway Very Good Samaritans to one another. But what if a man cannot extricate himself from such a situation? What if he appeals to us to extricate him? It seems to me plain that there are cases in which we can, cases in which a Good Samaritan would extricate him. There you are, you were kidnapped, and nine years in bed with that violinist lie ahead of you. You have your own life to lead. You are sorry, but you simply cannot see giving up so much of your life to the sustaining of his. You cannot extricate yourself, and ask us to do so. I should have thought that—in light of his having no right to the use of your body—it was obvious that we do not have to accede to your being forced to give up so much. We can do what you ask. There is no injustice to the violinist in our doing so.

7. Following the lead of the opponents of abortion, I have throughout been speaking of the fetus merely as a person, and what I have been asking is whether or not the argument we began with, which proceeds only from the fetus's being a person, really does establish its conclusion. I have argued that it does not.

But of course there are arguments and arguments, and it may be said that I have simply fastened on the wrong one. It may be said that what is important is not merely the fact that the fetus is a person, but that it is a person for whom the woman has a special kind of responsibility issuing from the fact that she is its mother. And it might be argued that all my analogies are therefore irrelevant—for you do not have that special kind of responsibility for that violinist, Henry Fonda does not have that special kind of responsibility for me. And our attention might be drawn to the fact that men and women both *are* compelled by law to provide support for their children.

I have in effect dealt (briefly) with this argument in section 4 above; but a (still briefer) recapitulation now may be in order. Surely we do not have any such "special responsibility" for a person unless we have assumed it, explicitly or implicitly. If a set of parents do not try to prevent pregnancy, do not obtain an abortion, and then at the time of birth of the child do not put it out for adoption, but rather take it home with them, then they have assumed responsibility for it, they have given it rights, and they cannot *now* withdraw support from it at the cost of its life because they now find it difficult to go on providing for it. But if they have taken all reasonable precautions against having a child, they do not simply by virtue of their biological relationship to the child who comes into existence have a special responsibility for it. They may wish to assume responsibility for it, or they may not wish to. And I am suggesting that if assuming responsibility for it would require large sacrifices, then these parents may refuse. A Good Samaritan would not refuse— or anyway, a Splendid Samaritan, if the sacrifices that had to be made were enormous. But then so would a Good Samaritan assume responsibility for that violinist; so would Henry Fonda, if he is a Good Samaritan, fly in from the West Coast and assume responsibility for me.

8. My argument will be found unsatisfactory on two counts by many of those who want to regard abortion as morally permissible. First, while I do argue that abortion is not impermissible, I do not argue that it is always permissible. There may well be cases in which carrying the child to term requires only Minimally Decent Samaritanism of the mother, and this is a standard we must not fall below. I am inclined to think it a merit of my account precisely that it does *not* give a general yes or a general no. It allows for and supports our sense that, for example, a sick and desperately frightened fourteen-year-old schoolgirl, pregnant due to rape, may *of course* choose abortion, and that any law which rules this out is an insane law. And it also allows for and supports our sense that in other cases resort to abortion is even positively indecent. It would be indecent in the woman to request an abortion, and indecent in a doctor to perform it, if she is in her seventh month, and wants the abortion just to avoid the nuisance of postponing a trip abroad. The very fact that the arguments I have been drawing attention to treat all cases of abortion, or even all cases of abortion in which the mother's life is not at stake, as morally on a par ought to have made them suspect at the outset.

Secondly, while I am arguing for the permissibility of abortion in some cases, I am not arguing for the right to secure the death of the unborn child.

It is easy to confuse these two things in that up to a certain point in the life of the fetus it is not able to survive outside the mother's body; hence removing it from her body guarantees its death. But they are importantly different. I have argued that you are not morally required to spend nine months in bed, sustaining the life of that violinist; but to say this is by no means to say that if, when you unplug yourself, there is a miracle and he survives, you then have a right to turn round and slit his throat. You may detach yourself even if this costs him his life; you have no right to be guaranteed his death, by some other means, if unplugging yourself does not kill him. There are some people who will feel dissatisfied by this feature of my argument. A woman may be utterly devastated by the thought of a child, a bit of herself, put out for adoption and never seen or heard of again. She may therefore want not merely that the child be detached from her, but more, that it die. Some opponents of abortion are inclined to regard this as beneath contempt— thereby showing insensitivity to what is surely a powerful source of despair. All the same, I agree that the desire for the child's death is not one which anybody may gratify, should it turn out to be possible to detach the child alive.

At this place, however, it should be remembered that we have only been pretending throughout that the fetus is a human being from the moment of conception. A very early abortion is surely not the killing of a person, and so is not dealt with by anything I have said here.

NOTES

1. I am very much indebted to James Thomson for discussion, criticism, and many helpful suggestions.
2. Daniel Callahan, *Abortion: Law, Choice and Morality* (New York, 1970), p. 373. This book gives a fascinating survey of the available information on abortion. The Jewish tradition is surveyed in David M. Feldman, *Birth Control in Jewish Law* (New York, 1968), Part 5, the Catholic tradition in John T. Noonan, Jr., "An Almost Absolute Value in History," in *The Morality of Abortion,* ed. John T. Noonan, Jr. (Cambridge, Mass., 1970).
3. The term "direct" in the arguments I refer to is a technical one. Roughly, what is meant by "direct killing" is either killing as an end in itself, or killing as a means to some end; for example, the end of saving someone else's life. See note 5 below, for an example of its use.

4. Cf. *Encyclical Letter of Pope Pius XI on Christian Marriage,* St. Paul Editions (Boston, n.d.), p. 32: "however much we may pity the mother whose health and even life is gravely imperiled in the performance of the duty allotted to her by nature, nevertheless what could ever be a sufficient reason for excusing in any way the direct murder of the innocent? This is precisely what we are dealing with here." Noonan (*The Morality of Abortion,* p. 43) reads this as follows: "What cause can ever avail to excuse in any way the direct killing of the innocent? For it is a question of that."

5. The thesis in (4) is in an interesting way weaker than those in (1), (2), and (3): they rule out abortion even in cases in which both mother *and* child will die if the abortion is not performed. By contrast, one who held the view expressed in (4) could consistently say that one needn't prefer letting two persons die to killing one.

6. Cf. the following passage from Pius XII, *Address to the Italian Catholic Society of Midwives:* "The baby in the maternal breast has the right to life immediately from God.—Hence there is no man, no human authority, no science, no medical, eugenic, social, economic or moral 'indication' which can establish or grant a valid juridical ground for a direct deliberate disposition of an innocent human life, that is a disposition which looks to its destruction either as an end or as a means to another end perhaps in itself not illicit.—The baby, still not born, is a man in the same degree and for the same reason as the mother" (quoted in Noonan, *The Morality of Abortion,* p. 45).

7. The need for a discussion of this argument was brought home to me by members of the Society for Ethical and Legal Philosophy, to whom this paper was originally presented.

8. For a discussion of the difficulties involved, and a survey of the European experience with such laws, see *The Good Samaritan and the Law,* ed. James M. Ratcliffe (New York, 1966).

THE MORALITY OF ABORTION

Margaret Olivia Little

INTRODUCTION

It is often noted that the public discussion of abortion's moral status is disappointingly crude. The positions staked out and the reasoning proffered seem to reflect little of the subtlety and nuance—not to mention ambivalence—that mark more private reflections on the subject. Despite attempts by various parties to find middle ground, the debate remains largely polarized—at its most dramatic, with extreme conservatives claiming abortion the moral equivalent of murder even as extreme liberals think it devoid of moral import.

To some extent, this polarization is due to the legal battle that continues to shadow moral discussions: admission of ethical nuance, it is feared, will

From Margaret Olivia Little, "The Morality of Abortion," in *A Companion to Applied Ethics,* edited by Christopher Wellman and Ray Frey, 2003, Blackwell Publishers.

play as concession on the deeply contested question of whether abortion should be a legally protected option for women. But to some extent, blame for the continued crudeness can be laid at the doorstep of moral theory itself.

For one thing, the ethical literature on abortion has focused its attention almost exclusively on the thinnest moral assessment—on whether and when abortion is "morally permissible." That question is, of course, a crucial one, its answer often desperately sought. But many of our deepest struggles with the morality of abortion concern much more textured questions about its placement on the scales of *decency, respectfulness,* and *responsibility.* It is one thing to decide that an abortion was permissible, quite another to decide that it was *honorable;* one thing to decide that an abortion was impermissible, quite another to decide that it was *monstrous.* It is these latter categories that determine what we might call the thick moral interpretation of the act—and, with it, the meaning the woman must live with, and the reactive attitudes such as disgust, forbearance, or admiration that she and others think the act deserves. A moral theory that moves too quickly or focuses too exclusively on moral permissibility won't address these crucial issues.

Moreover, the tools that mainstream moral theory has used for analyzing abortion fit only awkwardly to this subject-matter. Many treatments analyze abortion in the same terms used for assessing when war is justified, or the extent of our obligations to needy strangers, or the protection owed Da Vinci paintings. While there is some overlap of issues, such treatments end up leaving to the side many of the most important themes relevant to the ethics of gestation: what it means to play a role in *creating* a person, how to assess responsibilities that involve *sharing*, not just risking, one's body and life, what follows from the fact that the entity in question is or would be *one's child*. Nor are such lacunae incidental glitches. As theorists such as Catharine MacKinnon (1991) and Robin West (1993) have pointed out, our moral and political theories have been forged, by and large, to deal with interactions between independently situated and relatively equal strangers. However well this might work for soldierly heroism and barroom brawls (a question worth pressing in its own right), such a theory might not be expected to do well with moral questions dealing with the sort of intertwinement at issue in pregnancy.

If this is right, it means it is especially important not to focus all our energies, as many treatments are wont to do, arbitrating the question of fetal personhood. The question certainly matters: the moral contours of abortion, as we shall see, are importantly different depending on the answer we give it. The question is, moreover, a genuinely complex one, pressing, in essence, on the extent to which moral status is a function of the sort of being something already is, as judged by its occurrent properties, and the sort of creature it would become if it developed. (My own view, which I won't defend here, is that full moral status is in part anticipatory and in part something achieved; the fetus's status becomes progressively more weighty as pregnancy continues.) Complex as the issue of personhood is, though, the temptation to think our work done if only we could settle it—as though the moral status of abortion follows lockstep from the moral status of the fetus—has led theorists to ignore the rich ethical issues that

are raised by the, shall we say, rather distinctive situation in which the fetus is located.

To make progress on abortion's moral status, it thus turns out, requires us not just to arbitrate already familiar controversies in metaphysics and ethics, but to attend to the distinctive aspects of pregnancy that often stand at their margins. In the following, I want to argue that if we acknowledge gestation as an *intimacy,* motherhood as a *relationship,* and creation as a *process,* we will be in a far better position to appreciate the moral textures of abortion. I explore these textures, in the first half on stipulation that the fetus is a person, in the second half under supposition that early human life has an important value worthy of respect.

FETAL PERSONHOOD: FROM WRONGFUL INTERFERENCE TO POSITIVE RESPONSIBILITIES

If fetuses are persons, then abortion is surely an enormously serious matter: What is at stake is nothing less than the life of a creature with full moral standing. To say that the stakes are high, though, is not to say that moral analysis is obvious (which is why elsewhere in moral theory, conversation usually starts, not stops, once we realize people's lives are at issue). I think the most widely held objection to abortion is badly misguided; more importantly, it obscures the deeper ethical question at issue.

On the usual view, it is perfectly obvious what to say about abortion on supposition of fetal personhood: if fetuses are persons, then abortion is murder. Persons, after all, have a fundamental right to life, and abortion, it would seem, counts as its gross violation. On this view, we can assess the status of abortion quite cleanly. In particular, we needn't delve too deeply into the burdens that continued gestation might present for women—not because their lives don't matter or because we don't sympathize with their plight, but because we don't take hardship as justification for murder.

In fact, though, abortion's assimilation to murder will seem clear-cut only if we have already ignored key features of gestation. While certain metaphors depict gestation as passive carriage—as though the fetus were simply occupying a room until it is born—the truth is of course far different.

One who is gestating is providing the fetus with sustenance—donating nourishment, creating blood, delivering oxygen, providing hormonal triggers for development—without which it could not live. For a fetus, to live *is* to be receiving aid. And whether the assistance is delivered by way of intentional activity (as when the woman eats or takes her prenatal vitamins) or by way of biological mechanism, assistance it plainly is. But this has crucial implications for abortion's alleged status as murder. To put it simply, the right to life, as Judith Thomson famously put it, does not include the right to have all assistance needed to maintain that life (Thomson, 1971). Ending gestation will, at early stages at least, certainly lead to the fetus's demise, but that does not mean that doing so would constitute murder.

Now Thomson herself illustrated the point with an (in)famous thought experiment in which one person is kidnapped and used as life support for another: staying connected to the Famous Violinist, she points out, may be the kind thing to do, but disconnecting oneself does not violate the Violinist's rights. The details of this rather esoteric example have led to widespread charges that Thomson's point ignores the distinction between killing and letting die, and would apply at any rate only to cases in which the woman was not responsible for procreation occurring. In fact, though, I think the central insight here is broader than the example, or Thomson's own analysis, indicates.

As Frances Kamm's work points out (Kamm, 1992), in the usual case of a killing—if you stab a person on the street, for instance—you interfere with the trajectory the person had independently of you. She faced a happy enough future, we'll say; your action changed that, taking away from her something she would have had but for your action. In ending gestation, though, what you are taking away from this person is something she wouldn't have had to begin with without your aid. She comes to you with a downward trajectory, as it were: but for you she would already be dead. In removing that assistance, you are not violating the person's right to life, judged in the traditional terms of a right against interference. While all killings are tragedies, then, not all are alike: some killings, as Kamm puts it, share the crucial "formal" feature of letting die, which is that they leave the person no worse off than before she encountered you.

The argument is not some crude utilitarian one, according to which you get to kill the person because you saved her life (as though, having given you a nice lamp for your birthday, I may therefore later steal it with impunity). The point, rather, is that where I am still in the process of saving—or sustaining or enabling—your life, and that life cannot be thusly saved or sustained by anyone else, ending that assistance, even by active means, does not violate your right to life.

Now some, of course, will argue that matters change when the woman is causally responsible for procreation. In such cases, it will be said, she is responsible for introducing the person's need. She isn't like someone happening by an accident on the highway who knows CPR; she's like the person who *caused* the accident. Her actions introduced a set of vulnerabilities or needs, and we have a special duty to lessen vulnerabilities and repair harms we have inflicted on others.

But there is a deep disanalogy between causing the accident and procreating. The fact of causing a crash itself introduces a harm to surrounding drivers: they are in a worse position for having encountered that driver. But the simple act of procreating does not worsen the fetus's position: without procreation, the fetus wouldn't exist at all; and the mere fact of being brought into existence is not a bad thing. To be sure, creating a human is creating someone who comes with needs. But this, crucially, is not the same as inflicting a need *onto* someone (see Silverstein, 1987). It isn't as though the fetus already existed with one level of needs and the woman added a new one (as does happen, for instance, if a woman takes a drug after conception that increases the fetus's vulnerability to, say, certain cancers). The woman is (partially) responsible for creating a life, and it's a life that necessarily includes needs, but that is not the same as being responsible for the person being needy rather than not. The pregnant woman has not made the fetus more vulnerable than it would otherwise have been: absent her procreative actions, it wouldn't have existed at all.

Even if the fetus is a person, then, abortion would not be murder. More broadly put, abortion, whatever its rights and wrongs, isn't a species of *wrongful interference*.

None of this, though, is to say that abortion under such supposition is therefore unproblematic.

It is to argue, instead, that the crucial moral issue needs to be re-located. Wrongful interference is a central concern in morality, but it isn't the only one. We are also concerned with notions of *neglect, abandonment* and *disregard*. These are issues that involve abrogations of positive responsibilities to help others, not injunctions against interfering with them. If fetuses are persons, the question we really need to decide is what positive responsibilities, if any, do pregnant women have to continue gestational assistance? This is a question that takes us into far richer, and far more interesting, territory than that occupied by discussions of murder.

One issue it raises is: what do pregnant women owe to the fetuses they carry as a matter of *general beneficence*? Philosophers, of course, familiarly divide over the ambitions of beneficence, generically construed; but abortion raises distinct difficulties of its own. On the one hand, the beneficence called for here is of a particularly urgent kind: the stakes are life and death, and the pregnant woman is the *only* one who can render the assistance needed. It's a rare (and, many of us will think, dreadful) moral theory that will think she faces no responsibilities to assist here: passing a drowning person for mere convenience when no one else is within shouting distance is a very good example of moral indecency. On the other hand, gestation is not just any activity. It involves sharing one's very body. It brings with it an emotional intertwinement that can reshape one's entire life. It brings another person into one's family. Being asked to gestate another person, that is, isn't like being asked to write a check to support an impoverished child; it's like being asked to adopt the child. Doing so is a caring, compassionate act; it is also an enormous undertaking that has reverberations for an entire lifetime. Deciding whether, and if so when, such action is obligatory rather than admirable is no light matter.

I don't think moral theory has begun to address the rich questions at issue here. When are intimate actions owed to generic others? How do we weigh the sacrifice morality requires of us when it is measured, not in terms of risk, but of intertwinement? What should we think of such obligations if the required acts would be performed under conditions of profound self-alienation? The *type* of issue paradigmatically represented by gestation—an assistance that combines life and death stakes with deep

intimacy— is virtually nowhere discussed in ethical theory. (We aren't called upon in the usual course of events to save people's lives by, say, having sexual intercourse with them.) By ignoring these issues, mainstream moral theory has ended up deeply underselling the moral complexity of abortion.

Difficult as these questions are, though, it is actually a second issue, I suspect, that is responsible for much of the passion that surrounds abortion on supposition of fetal personhood. On reflection, many will say, the issues confronting the pregnant woman aren't about generic beneficence at all. The considerations she faces are not just those that would face someone uniquely well placed to serve as Good Samaritan to some stranger—as when one passes the drowning person: for the pregnant woman and fetus, crucially, aren't strangers. If the fetus is a person, many will say, it is *her child;* and for this reason she has special responsibilities to meet its needs. In the end, I believe, much of the animating concern with abortion is not about what we owe to generic others; it's about what parents owe their children.

But if it's parenthood that is carrying normative weight, then we need an ethics of parenthood—a theory of what makes someone a parent in this thickly normative sense and what the contours of its responsibilities really are. This should raise something of a warning flag. Philosophers, it must be said, have by and large done a rather poor job when it comes to parenthood—variously avoiding it, romanticizing it, or assimilating it to categories, like contractual relations, to which it stands in paradigmatic contrast. This general shortcoming is evident in discussions of abortion, where two remarkably unhelpful models dominate.

One position, advocated by Judith Thomson and some of the most recent treatments of abortion, is a classically liberal one. It agrees that special responsibilities attach to parenthood but argues that parenthood is thereby a status that is entered into only by consent. That consent is usually tacit, to be sure— taking the baby home from the hospital qualifies; nonetheless, special responsibilities to a child accrue only when one voluntarily assumes them.

Such a model is surely an odd one. The model yields the plausible view that the rape victim does not face the very same set of duties as many other pregnant women, but it does so by implying that a man who fathers a child during a one-night stand has no special responsibilities toward that child unless he decides he does. Perhaps most strikingly, such a view has no resources for acknowledging that there may be moral reasons why one *should* consent to the status. Those who sustain a biological connection may have a tendency to enter the role of parent, but on this scheme it's a mere psychological proclivity that rides atop nothing normative.

Another position is classically conservative. According to this view, the special responsibilities of parenthood are grounded in biological progenitorship. It is blood ties, to use the old-fashioned vernacular—"passing on one's genes," in more current translation—that makes one a parent and grounds heightened responsibilities. This view has its own blind spot. It has the resources for agreeing that a man who fathers a child from a one-night stand faces special responsibilities for the child whether he likes it or not, but none for distinguishing between the responsibilities of someone who has served as the special steward for a child—who has engaged for years in the *activity* of parenting—and the responsibilities of someone who bears literally no connection beyond a genetic or causal contribution to existence. On this view, a sperm donor faces all the responsibilities of a social father.

What both positions have in common is the supposition that parenthood is an all or nothing affair. Applied to pregnancy, the gestating woman either owes everything we imagine we owe to the children we love and rear or she owes nothing beyond general beneficence unless she decides she does. But parenthood—like all familial relations—is surely a more complicated moral notion than this. Parenthood, and its attendant responsibilities, admit of *layers*. It has a crucial existence as a social *role*—something with institutionally defined entrances, exits, and expectations that can attach to us quite independently of what our self-conceptions might say. It also has a crucial existence as a *relationship*—an emotional connection, a shared history, an intertwinement of lives. It is because of that intertwinement that parents' motivation to sacrifice is so often immediate. But it is also because of that relationship that even especially ambitious sacrifices are legitimately expected, and why failure to undertake them would be so problematic: absent unusual circumstances,

it becomes a betrayal of the relationship itself. In short, parenthood is not monolithic: some of the responsibilities we paradigmatically associate as parental attach, not to the role, but to the relationship that so often accompanies it.

These layers matter especially when we get to gestation, for the pregnant woman stands precisely at their intersection. If a fetus is a person, then there is surely an important sense in which she is its mother: to regard her as just a passing stranger uniquely able to help it would grossly distort the situation. But she is not yet a mother most thickly described—a mother in standing relationship with a child, with the responsibilities born of shared history and the enterprise of caretaking.

These demarcations are integral, I think, to understanding the distinctive sorts of conflicts that pregnancy can represent—including, most notably, the conflicts it can bring *within* the mantle of motherhood. Women sometimes decide to abort even though they regard the fetus they carry as their child, because they realize, grimly, that bringing this child into the world will leave too little room to care adequately for the children they are already raising. This is a conflict we cannot even name, much less arbitrate, on standard views—if the fetus is her child, how could she possibly choose to sacrifice its life unless the stakes are literally equivalent for the others? But this is to ignore the layers of parenthood. She occupies the *role* of mother to the fetus, but with the other children, she is, by dint of time, interaction, and intertwinement, in a *relationship* of motherhood. The fetus is her baby, then,—not just some passing stranger she alone can help—which is why this conflict brings the kind of agony it does. But if it is her child in the role sense only, she does not yet owe all that she owes to her other children. Depending on the circumstances, other family members with whom she is already in relationship may, tragically, come first.

None of this is to make light of the responsibilities pregnant women face on supposition of fetal personhood. If fetuses are persons, such responsibilities are surely profound. It is, rather, to insist that they admit of layer and degree, and that these distinctions, while delicate, are crucial to capturing the *types* of tragedy—and the types of moral compromise—abortion can here represent.

THE SANCTITY OF LIFE: RESPECT REVISITED

Just as we cannot assume that abortion is monstrous if fetuses are persons, so too we cannot assume that abortion is empty of moral import if they are not. Given all the ink that has been spilt on arbitrating the question of fetal personhood, one might be forgiven for having thought so: on some accounts, decisions about whether to continue or end a pregnancy really are, from a moral point of view, just like decisions about whether to cut one's hair.

But as Ronald Dworkin has urged (Dworkin, 1993), to think abortion morally weighty does not require supposition that the fetus is a person, or even a creature with interests in continued life. Destruction of a Da Vinci painting, he points out, is not bad *for the painting*—the painting has no interests. Instead, it is regrettable because of the deep value it has. So, too, one of the reasons we might regard abortion as morally weighty does not have to do with its being bad for *the fetus*—a setback to its interests, for it may not satisfy the criteria of having interests. Abortion may be weighty, instead, because there is something precious and significant about germinating human life that deserves our deep respect. This, as Dworkin puts it, locates issues of abortion in a different neighborhood of our moral commitments: namely, the accommodation we owe to things of value. That an organism is a potential person may not make it a claims-bearer, but it does mean it has a kind of stature that is worthy of respect.

This intuition, dismissed by some as mere sentimentality, is, I think, both important and broadly held. Very few people regard abortion as the moral equivalent of contraception. Most think a society better morally—not just by public health measures—if it regards abortion as a backup to failed contraception rather than as routine birth control. Reasons adequate for contracepting do not translate transparently as reasons adequate for aborting. Indeed, there is a telling shift in presumption: for most people, it takes no reason at all to justify contracepting; it takes *some* reason to justify ending a pregnancy. That a human life has now begun matters morally.

Burgeoning human life, we might put it, is *respect-worthy*. This is why we care not just whether, but how, abortion is done—while crass jokes are made or with solemnity, and why we care how the fetal remains are treated. It is why the thought of someone aborting for genuinely trivial reasons—to fit into a favorite party dress, say—makes us morally queasy. Perhaps most basically, it is why the thought of someone aborting with casual indifference fills us with misgiving. Abortion involves loss. Not just loss of the hope that various parties might have invested, but loss of something valuable in its own right. To respect something is to appreciate fully the value it has and the claims it presents to us; someone who aborts but never gives it a second thought hasn't exhibited genuine appreciation of the value and moral status of that which is now gone.

But if many share the intuition that early human life has a value deserving of respect, there is considerable disagreement about what that respect looks like. There is considerable conflict, that is, over what accommodation we owe to burgeoning human life. In part, of course, this is due to disagreement over the *degree* of value such life should be accorded: those for whom it is thoroughly modest will have very different views on issues, from abortion to stem cell research, than those for whom it is transcendent. But this is only part of the story. Obscured by analogies to Da Vinci paintings, some of the most important sources of conflict, especially for the vast middle rank of moderates, ride atop rough agreement on fetal value. If we listen to women's own struggles about when it is morally decent to end pregnancy, what we hear are themes about *motherhood* and *respect for creation*. These themes are enormously complex, I want to argue; for they enter stories on both sides of the ledger—for some women, as reasons to continue, and for some, as reasons to end, pregnancy. Let me start with motherhood.

For many women who contemplate abortion, the desire to end pregnancy is not, or not centrally, a desire to avoid the nine months of pregnancy; it is to avoid what lies on the far side of those months—namely, motherhood. If gestation were simply a matter of rendering, say, somewhat risky assistance to help a burgeoning human life they've come across—if they could somehow render that assistance without thereby adding a member to their family—the decision faced would be a far different one. But gestation doesn't just allow cells to become a person; it turns one into a mother.

One of the most common reasons women give for wanting to abort is that they do not want to become a mother—now, ever, again, with this partner, or no reliable partner, with these few resources, or these many that are now, after so many years of mothering, slated finally to another cause. Nor does adoption represent a universal solution. To give up a child would be for some a life-long trauma; others occupy fortunate circumstances that would, by their own lights, make it unjustified to give over a child for others to rear. Or again—and most frequently—she doesn't want to raise a child just now but knows that if she *does* carry the pregnancy to term, she won't *want* to give up the child for adoption. Gestation, she knows, is likely to reshape her heart and soul, transforming her into a mother emotionally, not just officially; and it is precisely that transformation she does not want to undergo. It is because continuing pregnancy brings with it this new identity and, likely, relationship, then, that many feel it legitimate to decline.

But pregnancy's connection to motherhood also enters the phenomenology of abortion in just the opposite direction. For some women, that it would be her child is precisely why she feels she must continue the pregnancy—even if motherhood is not what she desired. To be pregnant is to have one's potential child knocking at one's door; to abort is to turn one's back on it, a decision, many women say, that would haunt them forever. On this view, the desire to avoid motherhood, so compelling as a reason to contracept, is uneasy grounds to abort: for once an embryo is on the scene, it isn't about rejecting motherhood, it's about rejecting one's *child*. Not literally, of course, since there is no child yet extant to stand as the object of rejection. But the stance one should take to pregnancy, sought or not, is one of *acceptance:* when a potential family member is knocking at the door, one should move over, make room, and welcome her in.

These two intuitive stances represent just profoundly different ways of gestalting the situation of ending pregnancy. On the first view, abortion is closer to contraception—hardly equivalent, because it means the demise of something of value. But the desire to avoid the enterprise and identity of motherhood is an understandable and honorable basis for deciding to end a pregnancy. Given that there is no child yet on the scene, one does not owe special

openness to the relationship that stands at the end of pregnancy's trajectory. On the second view, abortion is closer to exiting a parental relationship—hardly equivalent, for one of the key relata is not yet fully present. But one's decision about whether to continue the pregnancy already feels specially constrained: that one would be related to the resulting person exerts now some moral force. It would take especially grave reasons to refuse assistance here, for the norms of parenthood already have a toehold. Assessing the moral status of abortion, it turns out, then, is not just about assessing the contours of generic respect owed to burgeoning human life, it's about assessing the salience of *impending relationship*. And this is an issue that functions in different ways for different women—and, sometimes, in one and the same woman.

In my own view, until the fetus is a person, we should recognize a moral prerogative to decline parenthood and end the pregnancy. Not because motherhood is necessarily a burden (though it can be); but because it so thoroughly changes what we might call one's fundamental practical identity. The enterprise of mothering restructures the self—changing the shape of one's heart, the primary commitments by which one lives one's life, the terms by which one judges one's life a success or a failure. If the enterprise is eschewed and one decides to give the child over to another, the identity of mother still changes the normative facts that are true of one, as there is now someone by whom one does well or poorly. And either way—whether one rears the child or lets it go—to continue a pregnancy means that a piece of one's heart, as the saying goes, will forever walk outside one's body. As profound as the respect we should have for burgeoning human life, we should acknowledge moral prerogatives over identity-constituting commitments and enterprises as profound as motherhood.

But I also don't think this is the whole of the moral story. If women find themselves with different ways of gestalting the prospective relationship involved in pregnancy, it is in part because they have different identities, commitments, and ideals that such a prospect intersects with—commitments which, while permissibly idiosyncratic, are morally authoritative for *them*. If a woman feels already duty-bound by the norms of parenthood to nurture this creature, it may be for the very good reason that, in an important personal sense, she already *is* its mother. She finds herself—perhaps to her surprise, happy or otherwise—with a maternal commitment to this creature. As philosophers forget but women and men have long known, something can be your child even if it is not yet a person. But taking on the identity of mother towards something just *is* to take on certain imperatives about its well-being as categorical. Her job is thus clear—it's to help this creature reach its fullest potential. For other women, the identity is still something that can be assessed—tried on, perhaps accepted, but perhaps declined: in which case respect is owed, but is saved, or confirmed, for others—other relationships, other projects, other passions.

And again, if a woman feels she owes a stance of welcome to burgeoning human life that comes her way, it may be, not because she thinks such a stance authoritative for all, but because of the virtues around which her practical identity is now oriented: receptivity to life's agenda, for instance, or responsiveness to that which is most vulnerable. For another woman, the executive virtues to be exercised tug in just the other direction: loyalty to treasured life plans, a commitment that it be she, not the chances of biology, that should determine her life's course, bolstering self-direction after a life too long ruled by serendipity and fate.

Deciding when it is morally decent to end a pregnancy, it turns out, is an admixture of settling impersonally or universally authoritative moral requirements, and of discovering and arbitrating—sometimes after agonizing deliberation, sometimes in a decision no less deep for its immediacy—one's own commitments, identity, and defining virtues.

A similarly complex story appears when we turn to the second theme. Another thread that appears in many women's stories in the face of unsought pregnancy is respect for the weighty responsibility involved in creating human life. Once again, it is a theme that pulls and tugs in different directions.

In its most familiar direction, it shows up in many stories of why an unsought pregnancy is continued. Many people believe that one's responsibility to nurture new life is importantly amplified if one is responsible for bringing about its existence in the first place. Just what it takes to count as responsible here is a point on which individuals diverge (whether voluntary but contracepted intercourse is

different from intercourse without use of birth control, and again from intentionally deciding to become pregnant at the IVF clinic). But triggering the relevant standard of responsibility for creation, it is felt, brings with it a heightened responsibility to nurture: it is disrespectful to create human life only to allow it to wither. Put more rigorously, one who is responsible for bringing about a creature that has intrinsic value in virtue of its potential to become a person has a special responsibility to enable it to reach that end state.

But the idea of respect for creation is also, if less frequently acknowledged, sometimes the reason why women are moved to *end* pregnancies. As Barbara Katz Rothman (1989) puts it, decisions to abort often represent, not a decision to destroy, but a refusal to create. Many people have deeply felt convictions about the circumstances under which they feel it right for them to bring a child into the world—can it be brought into a decent world, an intact family, a society that can minimally respect its agency? These considerations may persist even after conception has taken place; for while the *embryo* has already been created, a person has not. Some women decide to abort, that is, not because they do not *want* the resulting child—indeed, they may yearn for nothing more, and desperately wish that their circumstances were otherwise—but because they do not think bringing a child into the world the right thing for them to do.

These are abortions marked by moral language. A woman wants to abort because she knows she couldn't give up a child for adoption but feels she couldn't give the child the sort of life, or be the sort of parent, she thinks a child *deserves*; a woman who would have to give up the child thinks it would be *unfair* to bring a child into existence already burdened by rejection, however well grounded its reasons; a woman living in a country marked by poverty and gender apartheid wants to abort because she decides it would be *wrong* for her to bear a daughter whose life, like hers, would be filled with so much injustice and hardship.

Some have thought that such decisions betray a simple fallacy: unless the child's life were literally going to be worse than non-existence, how can one abort out of concern for the future child? But the worry here isn't that one would be imposing a *harm* on the child by bringing it into existence (as though children who are in the situations mentioned have lives that aren't worth living). The claim is that bringing about a person's life in these circumstances would do violence to her ideals of creating and parenthood. She does not want to bring into existence a daughter she cannot love and care for, she does not want to bring into existence a person whose life will be marked by disrespect or rejection.

Nor does the claim imply judgment on women who *do* continue pregnancies in similar circumstances—as though there were here an obligation to abort. For the norms in question, once again, need not be impersonally authoritative moral chums. Like ideals of good parenting, they mark out considerations all should be sensitive to, perhaps, but equally reasonable people may adhere to different variations and weightings. Still, they are normative for those who do have them; far from expressing mere matters of taste, the ideals one does accept carry an important kind of categoricity, issuing imperatives whose authority is not reducible to mere desire. These are, at root, issues about *integrity,* and the importance of maintaining integrity over one's participation in this enterprise precisely because it is so normatively weighty.

What is usually emphasized in the morality of abortion is the ethics of destruction; but there is a balancing ethics of creation. And for many people, conflict about abortion is a conflict *within* that ethics. On the one hand, we now have on hand an entity that has a measure of sanctity: that it has begun is reason to help it continue—perhaps especially if one had a role in its procreation—which is why even early abortion is not normatively equivalent to contraception. On the other hand, not to end a pregnancy *is* to do something else, namely, to continue creating a person, and for some women, pregnancy strikes in circumstances in which they cannot countenance that enterprise. For some, the sanctity of developing human life will be strong enough to tip the balance towards continuing the pregnancy; for others, their norms of respectful creation will hold sway. For those who believe that the norms governing creation of a person are mild relative to the normative telos of embryonic life, being a responsible creator means continuing to gestate, and doing the best one can to bring about the conditions under which that creation will be more respectful. For others, though, the normativity of fetal telos is mild and their standards of respectful creation high, and the lesson goes in just the other direction: it is a sign of respect not to continue creating when certain background conditions, such as a loving family or adequate resources, are not in place.

However one thinks these issues settle out, they will not be resolved by austere contemplation of the value of human life. They require wrestling with the rich meanings of creation, responsibility, and kinship. And these issues, I have suggested, are just as much issues about one's integrity as they are about what is impersonally obligatory. On many treatments of abortion, considerations about whether or not to continue a pregnancy are exhausted by preferences, on the one hand, and universally authoritative moral demands, on the other; but some of the most important terrain lies in between.

REFERENCES

Dworkin, R. (1993). *Life's dominion: an argument about abortion, euthanasia, and individual freedom.* New York: Alfred A. Knopf.

Kamm, F. M. (1992). *Creation and abortion: a study in moral and legal philosophy.* New York: Oxford University Press.

MacKinnon, C. A. Reflections on sex equality under law. *The Yale Law Journal,* 100:5 (March 1991), 1281–1328, p. 1314.

Rothman, B. K. (1989). *Recreating motherhood: ideology and technology in a patriarchal society.* New York: Norton.

Silverstein, H. S. (1987). On a woman's 'responsibility' for the fetus. *Social Theory and Practice,* 13, 103–19.

Thomson, J. J. (1971) A defense of abortion. *Philosophy and Public Affairs,* 1, 47–66.

West, R. (1993). Jurisprudence and gender. In D. Kelly Weisberg (Ed.). *Feminist legal theory: foundations* (pp. 75–98). Philadelphia: Temple University Press.

OBLIGATIONS TO THE NOT-YET-BORN

THE RIGHTS OF "UNBORN CHILDREN" AND THE VALUE OF PREGNANT WOMEN

Howard Minkoff and Lynn M. Paltrow

A quarter century after the "International Year of the Child," we now seem to be in the era of the "Unborn Child." Partly this is because of medical advances: highly refined imaging techniques have made the fetus more visually accessible to parents. In good measure, however, the new era is a product of political shifts. In 2004, President Bush signed into law the Unborn Victims of Violence Act, which makes it a separate federal offense to bring about the death or bodily injury of a "child in utero" while committing certain crimes, and recognizes everything from a zygote to a fetus as an independent "victim" with legal rights distinct from the woman who has been harmed. In 2002, the Department of Health and Human Services adopted new regulations expanding the definition of "child" in the State Children's Health Insurance Program "so that a State may elect to make individuals in the period between conception and birth eligible for coverage." Finally, Senator Brownback and thirty-one cosponsors have proposed the Unborn Child Pain Awareness Act, a scientifically dubious piece of legislation that would require physicians performing the exceedingly rare abortions after twenty weeks to inform pregnant women of "the option of choosing to have anesthesia or other pain-reducing drug or drugs administered directly to the pain-capable unborn child."

The legislative focus on the unborn is aimed at women who choose abortion, but it may also have adverse consequences for women who choose not to have an abortion, and it challenges a central tenet of human rights—namely, that no person can be required to submit to state enforced surgery for the benefit of another.

The historical context of fetal rights legislation should make the most fervent proponents of fetal rights—pregnant women—wary. Often, in the past, expansions of fetal rights have been purchased through the diminution of pregnant women's rights. The fetal "right" to protection from environmental

From *Hastings Center Report* 36, no. 2 (2006): 26–28. Reprinted by permission of The Hastings Center.

toxins cost pregnant women the right to good jobs: for nearly ten years before the U.S. Supreme Court ruled against such polices in 1991, companies used "fetal protection" policies as a basis for prohibiting fertile women from taking high-paying blue collar jobs that might expose them to lead. The fetal "right" to health and life has cost women their bodily integrity (women have been forced to undergo cesarean sections or blood transfusion), their liberty (women have been imprisoned for risking harm to a fetus through alcohol or drug use), and in some cases their lives (a court-ordered cesarean section probably accelerated the death in 1987 of Angela Carder, who had a recurrance of bone cancer that had metastasized to her lung). The fetal "right" not to be exposed to pharmaceutical agents has cost pregnant women their right to participate in drug trials that held out their only hope of cure from lethal illnesses. The vehicle for these infringements on pregnant women's rights has been third parties' assertions that they, rather than the mother, have the authority to speak for the fetus in securing these newly defined rights. For example, employers have argued for the right to speak for the fetus in determining when a work environment is inappropriate for the fetus. In mandating cesarean section, the courts have apparently concluded that the judiciary is better positioned to speak for the fetus and that a competent but dying mother's wishes to refuse surgery are no longer worthy of consideration. Most recently, a state's attorney has taken up the cudgel for the fetus by charging a woman with murder for her refusal to consent to a cesarean section.

It is within the context of these attempts to wrest the right to speak for the fetus from mothers that legislation that will expand the rights of the fetus—such as the Unborn Victims of Violence Act—must be considered. The act makes the injury or death of a fetus during commission of a crime a federal offense, the punishment for which "is the same as the punishment . . . for that conduct had that injury or death occurred to the unborn child's mother."[1] As written, the law appears unambiguously to immunize pregnant women against legal jeopardy should any act of theirs result in fetal harm: "Nothing in this section shall be construed to permit the prosecution . . . of any woman with respect to her unborn child." But similar statutory guarantees proffered in the past have not been decisive. In 1970 the California

Legislature created the crime of "fetal murder" and specifically excluded the conduct of the pregnant woman herself, but women who suffered stillbirths were nevertheless prosecuted under the statute. The prosecutor explained that "The fetal murder law was never intended to protect pregnant women from assault by third parties which results in death of the fetus. The purpose was to protect the unborn child from murder."[2]

In Missouri cases, a woman who admitted to smoking marijuana once while pregnant and a pregnant woman who tested positive for cocaine were charged with criminal child endangerment on the basis of a statute that declares the rights of the unborn—yet also includes an explicit exception for the pregnant woman herself in language strikingly similar to that used in the Unborn Victims Act ("nothing in this section shall be interpreted as creating a cause of action against a woman for indirectly harming her unborn child by failing to properly care for herself"[3]). The state argued that this language did not preclude prosecution of the pregnant women because "the pregnant woman is not in a different position than a third-party who injures the unborn child" and because her drug use "'directly' endangered the unborn child."[4]

Even if the historical record did not contain these examples of a legislative bait and switch, the principles codified by the new federal statute would be worrisome. When laws create parity between harming pregnant women and harming members "of the species Homo sapiens" of any gestational age (as the Unborn Victims of Violence Act specifies), they establish symmetry between the rights of pregnant women and those of fetuses. In so doing, they suggest a need to balance rights when those rights appear to conflict with each other, and potentially to subordinate the rights of the women to those of the fetus. But to take this stance is not merely to elevate the rights of the unborn to parity with those of born individuals. It is in fact to grant them rights previously denied to born individuals: courts have allowed forced surgery to benefit the unborn, but have precluded forced surgery to benefit born persons. In 1978 Robert McFall sought a court order to force his cousin David Shimp, the only known compatible donor, to submit to a transplant. The court declined, explaining: "For our law to compel the Defendant to submit to an intrusion of his body would change every concept and principle upon which our society is founded. To do so would defeat the sanctity of the individual and would impose a rule which would know no limits."[5]

The Unborn Child Pain Awareness Act is yet another example of a law focused on the fetus that devalues pregnant women and children and sets the stage for further erosion of their human rights. It mandates that prior to elective terminations, physicians deliver a precisely worded, though scientifically questionable, monologue that details the purported pain felt by the fetus and allows for fetal pain management. In so doing, it introduces two damaging concepts. First, it makes women and abortion providers a unique class, excluded from the standard medical model in which counseling is provided by a physician who uses professional judgment to determine what a reasonable individual would need in order to make an informed choice about a procedure. Instead, legislators' judgment is substituted for a physician's determination of the appropriate content of counseling.

Second, it elevates the rights of the midtrimester fetus beyond those of term fetuses, as well as those of its born siblings. Congress has never mandated that mothers be told that there may be fetal pain associated with fetal scalp electrodes or forceps deliveries. Nor have doctors been compelled to speak to the pain that accompanies circumcision or, for that matter, numerous medical conditions for which people are prevented from receiving adequate palliative care. Indeed, there is no federal law scripting counseling about the pain that could accompany any procedure to any child, or indeed any person, after birth. Society has generally relied on professionals to exercise medical judgment in crafting the content of counseling, and on medical societies to assure that counseling evolves as science progresses.

While support for fetal rights laws is now *de rigueur* among politicians, there is apparently no similar mandate to address the social issues that truly threaten pregnant women and victimize their fetuses. Although states increasingly are seeking ways to arrest and punish women who won't undergo recommended surgery or who are unable to find drug rehabilitation programs that properly treat pregnant women and families, no means have been found to guarantee paid maternity leave or to proffer more than quite limited employment protections

from discrimination for women when they are pregnant. Many of our nation's tax and social security policies, rather than bolstering women's social standing, help to ensure mothers' economic vulnerability. Hence, the opposition to the Unborn Victims of Violence Act from some activists must be recognized as the logical consequence of years of having mothers beatified in words and vilified in deeds.

These arguments should not be misconstrued as evidence of a "maternal-fetal" conflict. Unless stripped of their rights, pregnant women will continue to be the most powerful advocates for the wellbeing of unborn children. Clashes between the rights of mothers and their fetuses are used as Trojan horses by those who would undermine the protections written into law by *Roe*. Proponents of the right-to-life agenda recognize that when fetal rights expand, the right to abortion will inevitably contract. Furthermore, the responsibilities of physicians in this environment are clear and are grounded in the principles of professionalism—primacy of patient welfare, patient autonomy, and social justice.[6] Those principles require that patients' needs be placed before any "societal pressures" and that "patients' decisions about their care must be paramount."[7] These words are bright line guideposts for clinicians who may at times feel caught in a balancing act. Whether the counterclaim to a pregnant woman's right to autonomy is a societal demand for drug test results obtained in labor, an administrator's request to get a court order to supersede an informed woman's choice, or a colleague's plea to consider fetal interests more forcefully, these principles remind us that no other concern should dilute physicians' commitment to the pregnant woman.[8]

The argument that women should not lose their civil and human rights upon becoming pregnant is predicated neither on the denial of the concept that an obstetrician has two patients, nor on the acceptance of any set position in the insoluble debate as to when life begins. The courts have provided direction for those dealing with the competing interests of two patients, even if one were to concede that the fetus in this regard is vested with rights equal to that of a born person. A physician who had both Robert McFall (potential marrow recipient) and David Shimp (potential donor) as patients may well have shared the judge's belief that Shimp's refusal to donate his marrow, and thereby to condemn McFall to death, was "morally reprehensible." But the clinician would ultimately have to be guided by the judge's decision to vouchsafe David Shimp's sanctity as an individual. Pregnancy does not diminish that sanctity or elevate the rights of the fetus beyond that of Robert McFall or any other born person. Thus, while the obstetrician's commitment to his "other" patient (the fetus) should be unstinting, it should be so only to a limit set by those, to quote Justice Blackman, "who conceive, bear, support, and raise them."[9] To do otherwise would be to recruit the medical community into complicity with those who would erode the rights of women in the misguided belief that one can champion the health of children by devaluing the rights of their mothers.

NOTES

1. 18 U.S.C. s. 1841(a)(2)(A).
2. *Jaurigue v. California,* Reporter's Transcript, Hearing August 21, 1992, Case No. 18988, Justice Court Cr. No. 23611, Sup. Court of California for the County of San Benito, Honorable Donald Chapman, Judge, p. 2823.
3. *Missouri v. Smith,* Jackson County Circuit Court, No. CR2000–00964 (June 23, 2000).
4. *Missouri v. Smith,* Jackson County Circuit Court, Case No. CR2000–00964, State's Response to Motion to Dismiss the Indictment (Aug 10, 2002) at 2.
5. *McFall v. Shimp,* 10 Pa. D.&C. 3d 90 (Allegheny Cty. 1978).
6. ABIM Foundation, American Board of Internal Medicine, ACP-ASIM Foundation, American College of Physicians-American Society of Internal Medicine, European Federation of Internal Medicine, "Medical Professionalism in the New Millennium: A Physician Charter," *Annals of Internal Medicine* 136, no. 3 (2002): 243–46.
7. Ibid.
8. ACOG Committee on Ethics, "Maternal Decision Making, Ethics, and the Law," *Obstetrics & Gynecology* 106 (2005): 1127–37.
9. *Int'l Union v. Johnson Controls, Inc.,* 499 U.S. 197–206 (1991).

REPRODUCTIVE FREEDOM AND PREVENTION OF GENETICALLY TRANSMITTED HARMFUL CONDITIONS

Allen Buchanan, Dan W. Brock, Norman Daniels, and Daniel Wikler

Public Policy and Wrongful Life Issues   It is perhaps fortunate that despite the great expansion of genetic information that will be available in the future both from pre-conception testing for genetic risks to potential offspring and from prenatal diagnosis of the genetic condition of a fetus, public policy may be able largely to avoid the most contentious and intractable wrongful life issues for at least two reasons. First, only a very small proportion of genetic abnormalities and diseases are both compatible with life and also so severe as to result in the affected child having a life not worth living. Second, courts and legislatures are likely to continue to be reluctant to permit wrongful life legal suits, both because damages covering the child's medical and extra care expenses can usually be obtained by a suit brought in the name of the parents instead of a wrongful life suit in the name of the child, and because uncertainty exists about how to assess damages for wrongful life. But regardless of what occurs in the courts, moral choice about whether conceiving a child or carrying a pregnancy to term would constitute an action of wrongful life will be increasingly faced in the future by parents or would-be parents.

Reprinted with permission of the authors and publisher from their book, *From Chance to Choice,* Cambridge: Cambridge University Press, 2000.

Editors' note: Some text has been cut. Students who want to read the article in its entirety should consult the original.

A complicating factor is that the woman or couple making the choice will often face only a risk, not a certainty, that the child will not have a life worth living and that risk can vary from very low to approaching certainty. Whether it is morally wrong to conceive in the face of such risks' will depend in part on the woman's willingness and intention to do appropriate prenatal genetic testing and to abort her fetus if it is found to have a disease or condition incompatible with a worthwhile life.

As noted before, pursuing the moral complexities of abortion would take us too far afield here. Nevertheless, suppose, as the authors of this book believe, that the fetus at least through the first two trimesters is not a person and so aborting it then is morally permissible. Aborting a fetus found during the first two trimesters to have a disease that would make life a burden to the child prevents the creation of a person with a life not worth living; no wrongful life then occurs, so there is no question of moral wrongdoing. Even conceiving when there is a relatively high risk of genetic transmission of a disease incompatible with a life worth living could be morally acceptable so long as the woman firmly intends to test the fetus for the disease and to abort it if the disease is present.

On the other hand, a woman may intend not to test her fetus and abort it if such a disease is present, either because she considers abortion morally wrong or for other reasons. In that case, the higher the risk that the child will have a genetic disease or condition incompatible with a life worth living, the stronger the moral case that she does a serious moral wrong to that child in conceiving it and carrying it to term.

If a mother or anyone else knowingly and responsibly caused harm to an already born child so serious as to make its life no longer worth living, that would constitute extremely serious child abuse and be an extremely serious moral and legal wrong. In that case, however, the child would have had a worthwhile life that was taken away by whomever was guilty of the child abuse; the wrong to the child then is depriving it of a worthwhile life that it otherwise would have had. That is a different and arguably more serious wrong than wrongful life, where the alternative to the life not worth living is never having a life at all, and so not having a worthwhile life taken away. The wrong in nearly all cases of wrongful life

is bringing into existence a child who will have a short life dominated by severe and unremitting suffering—that is, being caused to undergo that suffering without compensating benefits.

How high must the risk be of a child having a genetic disease incompatible with a worthwhile life be for it to be morally wrong for the parents to conceive it and allow it to be born? There is, of course, no precise probability at which the risk of the harm makes it morally wrong to conceive or not to abort; different cases fall along a spectrum in the degree to which undertaking the risk is morally justified. How seriously wrong, if a wrong at all, it is to risk the conception and birth of a child with such a life will depend on several factors. How bad is the child's life, and in particular how severe and unremitting is its suffering? How high is the probability of the child having a genetic disease incompatible with a worthwhile life? How weighty are its parents' interests in having the child? For example, is this likely its parents' only opportunity to become parents, or are they already parents seeking to have additional children? How significant is the possibility of the parents having an unaffected child if this pregnancy is terminated and another conception pursued? How willing and able are the parents to support and care for the child while it lives?

These factors, and no doubt others unique to specific cases, will determine how strong the moral case is against individuals risking having a child who will not have a life worth living. It is worth underlining that any case for the wrongness of parents conceiving and bringing to term such a child depends on their having reasonable access to genetic testing, contraception, and abortion services, and this can require public provision and funding of these services for those who otherwise cannot afford them.

We hope that our analysis so far makes it clear why we believe that there are some cases, albeit very few, in which it would be clearly and seriously morally wrong for individuals to risk conceiving and having such a child. However, use of government power to force an abortion on an unwilling woman would be so deeply invasive of her reproductive freedom, bodily integrity, and right to decide about her own health care as to be virtually never morally justified. Allowing the child to be born and then withholding life support even over its parents' objections would probably be morally preferable. The government's doing this forcibly and over the parents' objections would be extraordinarily controversial, both morally and legally, but in true cases of wrongful life, the wrong done is sufficiently serious as to possibly justify doing so in an individual case. However, at the present time as a practical matter, the common and strong bias in favor of life, even in the face of serious suffering, makes it nearly inconceivable that public policy might authorize the government forcibly to take an infant from its parents, not for the purpose of securing beneficial treatment for it, but instead to allow it to die because it could not have a worthwhile life. Moreover, the risk of abuse of such a governmental power to intervene forcibly in reproductive choices to prevent a wrongful life is too great to warrant granting that power.

There is a stronger moral case for the use of government coercive power to prevent conception in some wrongful life cases. Similar power is now exercised by government over severely mentally disabled people who are sterilized to prevent them from conceiving. In such cases, the individual sterilized is typically deemed incompetent to make a responsible decision about conception, as well as unable to raise a child. Forced sterilization of a competent individual is more serious morally, but the harm to be prevented of wrongful life is more serious than the harm prevented in typical involuntary sterilization cases where the child would have a worthwhile life if raised by others. Nevertheless, the historical abuses of "eugenic sterilizations" . . . are enough to warrant not giving government the coercive power to prevent wrongful life conceptions unless their occurrence was very common and widespread. Wrongful life conceptions are sufficiently uncommon, and practical and moral difficulties in using the coercive power of government to prevent them sufficiently great, to rule out policies that prevent people from conceiving wrongful lives. Coercive government intrusion into reproductive freedom to prevent wrongful life would be wrong.

PRE-CONCEPTION INTERVENTIONS TO PREVENT CONDITIONS COMPATIBLE WITH A WORTHWHILE LIFE

The Human Genome Project and related research will produce information permitting genetic screening for an increasing number of genetically transmitted diseases, or susceptibilities to diseases and other harmful conditions. In the foreseeable future, our capacities for conception and prenatal screening for these diseases and conditions will almost certainly far outstrip our capacities for genetic or other therapy to correct for the harmful genes and their effects. The vast majority of decisions faced by prospective parents, consequently, will not be whether to pursue genetic or other therapy for their fetus or child, but instead whether to test for particular genetic risks and/or conditions and, when they are found to be present, whether to avoid conception or to terminate a pregnancy. Moreover, the vast majority of genetic risks that will be subject to testing will not be for conditions incompatible with a life worth living—the wrongful life cases—but rather for less severe conditions compatible with having a life well worth living.

These genetically transmitted conditions and diseases will take different forms. Sometimes their disabling features will be manifest during much of the individual's life, but still will permit a worthwhile life, as with most cases of Down syndrome, which is caused by a chromosomal abnormality. Sometimes the disease or condition will result in significant disability and a significantly shorter than normal life span, but not so disabling or short as to make the life not worth living, as with cystic fibrosis. Sometimes the disease or condition; although devastating in its effects on the afflicted individual's quality of life, will only manifest symptoms after a substantial period of normal life and unction, as with Huntington's chorea and Alzheimer's dementia.

When the genetically transmitted conditions could and should have been prevented, they will constitute what we have called cases of wrongful disability. But in which cases will the failure to prevent a genetically transmitted disability be morally wrong? Again, different cases fall along a spectrum in the degree of moral justification for undertaking or not undertaking to prevent the disability.

Whether failure to prevent a disability is wrong in specific cases will typically depend on many features of that case. For example, what is the relative seriousness of the disability for the child's well-being and opportunities? What measures are available to the child's parents to prevent the condition—such as abortion, artificial insemination by donor, or oocyte donation—how acceptable are these means to the prospective parents? Is it possible, and if so how likely, that they can conceive another child without the disabling condition, or will any child they conceive have or be highly likely to have the condition? If the disability can only be prevented by not conceiving at all, do the couple have alternative means, such as adoption, of becoming parents? When the condition can be prevented or its adverse impact compensated for, what means are necessary to do so?

These and other considerations can all bear on the threshold question: Is the severity of a genetically transmitted disability great enough that particular parents are morally obligated to prevent it, given the means necessary for them to do so; or is it sufficiently limited and minor that it need not be prevented, but is instead a condition that the child can reasonably be expected to live with?

Different prospective parents will answer this threshold question differently because they differ about such matters as the burdensomeness and undesirability of particular alternative methods of reproduction that may be necessary to prevent the disability, the seriousness of the impact of the particular disability on a person's well-being and opportunity, aspects of reproductive freedom such as the importance of having children and of having biologically related as opposed to adopted or only partially biologically related children, the extent of society's obligation and efforts to make special accommodations to eliminate or ameliorate the disability, and their willingness to assume the burdens of raising a child with the disability in question.

Because there are these multiple sources of reasonable disagreement bearing on the threshold question, and because the aspects of reproductive freedom at stake will usually be of substantial importance, public policy should usually permit prospective parents to make and act on their own judgments about whether they morally ought to prevent particular genetically transmitted disabilities for the sake of their child. But there is a systematic objection to all preconception wrongful disability cases that must be met in order to clear the way for individual judgments about specific cases.

To fix attention on the general problem in question, which is restricted to cases of genetically transmitted disease, let us imagine, a case, call it P1, in which a woman is told by her physician that she should not attempt to become pregnant now because she has a condition that is highly likely to result in

moderate mental retardation in her child. Her condition is easily and fully treatable by taking a safe medication for one month. If she takes the medication and delays becoming pregnant for a month, the risk to her child will be eliminated and there is every reason to expect that she will have a normal child. Because the delay would interfere with her vacation travel plans, however, she does not take the medication, gets pregnant now, and gives birth to a child who is moderately retarded.

According to commonsense moral views, this woman acts wrongly, and in particular, wrongs her child by not preventing its disability for such a morally trivial reason, even if for pragmatic reasons people would oppose government intrusion into her decision. According to commonsense morality, her action is no different morally if she failed to take the medicine in a case, P2, in which the condition is discovered, and so the medicine must be taken, after conception when she is already pregnant. Nor is it different morally than if she failed to provide a similar medication to her born child, in a case, P3, if doing so is again necessary to prevent moderate mental retardation in her child. It is worth noting that in most states in this country, her action in P3 would probably constitute medical neglect, and governmental child protection agencies could use coercive measures, if necessary, to ensure the child's treatment.

This suggests that it might only be because her reproductive freedom and her right to decide about her own health care are also involved in P1 that we are reluctant to coerce her decision, if necessary, there as well. On what Derek Parfit has called the "no difference" view, the view of commonsense morality, her failure to use the medication to prevent her child's mental retardation would be equally seriously wrong, and for the same reason, in each of the three cases (Parfit 1984). But her action in P1, which is analogous in relevant respects to preconception genetic screening to prevent disabilities, has a special feature that makes it not so easily shown to be wrong as commonsense morality might suppose.

What is the philosophical problem at the heart of wrongful disability cases like P1? As with wrongful life cases, in which the necessary comparison of life with nonexistence is thought to create both philosophical and policy problems, so also in wrongful disability cases do the philosophical and policy problems arise from having to compare a disabled existence with not having existed at all. But the nature of the philosophical problems in wrongful life and wrongful disability cases are in fact quite different. The philosophical objections we considered wrongful life cases centered on whether it is coherent to compare an individual's quality of life with never having existed at all—that is, with nonexistence—and whether merely possible persons can have moral rights or be owed moral obligations. In wrongful disability cases, a person's disability uncontroversially leaves him or her with a worthwhile life. The philosophical problem, as noted earlier, is how this is compatible with the commonsense view that it would be wrong to prevent the disability.

The special difficulty in wrongful disability cases, which Derek Parfit has called the "nonidentity problem," is that it would not be better for the person with the disability to have had it prevented, since that could only be done by preventing him or her from ever having existed at all. Preventing the disability would deny the disabled individual a worthwhile, although disabled life. That is because the disability could only have been prevented either by conceiving at a different time and/or under different circumstances (in which case a different child would have been conceived) or by terminating the pregnancy (in which case this child also never would have been born, although a different child may or may not have been conceived instead). None of these possible means of preventing the disability would be better for the child with the disability—all would deny him or her a worthwhile life.

But if the mother's failure to prevent the disability did not make her child worse off than he or she would have been without the intervention, then her failure to prevent it seems not to harm her child. And if she did not harm her child by not preventing its disability, then why does she wrong her child morally by failing to do so? How could making her child better off, or at least not worse off, by giving it a life worth living, albeit a life with a significant disability, wrong it? A wrong action must be bad for someone, but her choice to create her child with its disability is bad for no one, so she does no wrong. Of course, there is a sense in which it is bad for her child to have the disability, in comparison with being without it, but there is nothing the mother could have done to enable that child to be born without the disability, and so nothing she does or omits doing is bad for her child.

So actions whose harmful effects would constitute seriously wrongful child abuse if done to an existing child are no harm, and so not wrong, if their harmful effects on a child are inextricable from the act of bringing that child into existence with a worthwhile life! This argument threatens to undermine common and firmly held moral judgments, as well as public policy measures, concerning prevention of such disabilities for children.

Actual versus Possible Persons   David Heyd has accepted the implications of this argument and concludes that in all of what he calls "genesis" choices—that is, choices that inextricably involve whether a particular individual will be brought into existence—only the interest of actual persons, not those of possible persons such as the disabled child in case P1, are relevant to the choice (Heyd 1992). So in case P1, the effects on the parents and the broader society, such as the greater childrearing costs and burdens of having the moderately retarded child instead of taking the medication and having a normal child a month later are relevant to the decision. But the effects on and interests of the child who would be moderately retarded are not relevant. In cases P2 and P3, on the other hand, Heyd presumably would share the commonsense moral view that the fundamental reason the woman's action would be wrong is the easily preventable harm that she allows her child to suffer. In these situations, the preventable harm to her child is the basis of the moral wrong she does her child.

In Parfit's "no difference" view, the woman's action in P1 is equally wrong, and for the same reason, as her action in P2 and P3. We share with Parfit, in opposition to Heyd, the position that the woman's action in P1 is wrong because of the easily preventable effect on her child. But we do not accept the "no difference" thesis. We will suggest a reason why her action in P1 may not be as seriously wrong as in P2 or P3, and also suggest that the reason her action is wrong in P1 is similar to but nevertheless importantly different from the reason it is wrong in P2 and P3.

As Parfit notes, the difficulty is identifying and formulating a moral principle that implies that the woman's action in P1 is seriously wrong, but does not have unacceptable implications for other cases. Before proceeding further, we must emphasize that we cannot explore this difficulty fully here. The issues are extraordinarily complex and involve testing the implications of such a principle in a wide variety of cases outside of the genetic context that is our concern here (e.g., in population policy contexts and, in particular, avoiding what Parfit calls the "Repugnant Conclusion" and explaining what he calls the "Asymmetry"). Its relationship to other principles and features of a moral theory must also be explained, including that to the principle applicable to P2 and P3 (Parfit 1984).

The apparent failure to account for common and firmly held moral views in the genetics cases of wrongful disabilities like P1 constitutes one of the most important practical limitations (problems of population policy are another) of traditional ethical theories and of their principles of beneficence—doing good—and nonmaleficence—not causing or preventing harm. Where the commonsense moral judgment about cases like P1 is that the woman is morally wrong to go ahead and have the disabled child instead of waiting and having a normal child, the principles of traditional ethical theories apparently fail to support that judgment. New or revised moral principles appear to be needed. What alternatives and resources, either within or beyond traditional moral principles or theories, could account for and explain the wrong done in wrongful disability cases?

Person-Affecting Moral Principles Perhaps the most natural way to account for the moral wrongful disability cases like P1 is to abandon the specific feature of typical moral principles about obligations to prevent or not cause harm which generates difficulty when we move from standard cases of prevention of harm to existing persons, as in P3, to harm prevention in genesis cases like P1. That feature is what philosophers have called the "person-affecting" property of principles of beneficence and nonmaleficence. Recall that earlier we appealed to principle M: Those individuals responsible for a child's, or other dependent person's, welfare are morally required not to let her suffer a serious harm or disability or a serious loss of happiness or good that they could have prevented without imposing substantial burdens or costs or loss of benefits on themselves or others.

The person-affecting feature of M is that the persons who will suffer the harm if it is not prevented

and not suffer it if it is prevented must be one and the same distinct individual. If M is violated, a distinct child or dependent person is harmed without good reason, and so the moral wrong is done to that person. Since harms to persons must always be harms to some person, it may seem that there is no alternative to principles that are person-affecting, but that is not so. The alternative is clearest if we follow Derek Parfit by distinguishing "same person" from "same number" choices.

In same person choices, the same persons exist in each of the different alternative courses of action from which an agent chooses. Cases P2 and P3 above were same person choices (assuming in P2 that the fetus is or will become a person, though that is not essential to the point)—the harm of moderate retardation prevented is to the woman's fetus or born child. In same number choices, the same number of persons exist in each of the alternative courses of action from which an agent chooses, but the identities of some of the persons—that is, who exists in those alternatives—is affected by the choice. P1 is a same number but not a same person choice—the woman's choice affects which child will exist. If the woman does not take the medication and wait to conceive, she gives birth to a moderately retarded child, whereas if she takes the medication and waits to conceive, she gives birth to a different child who is not moderately retarded.

The concept of "harm," arguably, is necessarily comparative, so the concept of "harm prevention" may seem necessarily person-affecting; this is why harm prevention principles seem not to apply to same number, different person choices like P1. But it would be a mistake to think that non–person-affecting principles, even harm prevention principles, are not coherent. Suppose for simplicity that the harm in question in P1 from the moderate retardation is suffering and limited opportunity. Then in P1, if the woman chooses to have the moderately retarded child, she causes suffering and limited opportunity to exist that would be prevented and not exist if she chooses to take the medication and wait to conceive a different normal child. An example of a non–person-affecting principle that applies to P1 is:

N: Individuals are morally required not to let any child or other dependent person for whose welfare they are responsible experience serious suffering or limited opportunity or serious loss of happiness or good, if they can act so that, without affecting the number of persons who will exist and without imposing substantial burdens or costs or loss of benefits on themselves or others, no child or other dependent person for whose welfare they are responsible will experience serious suffering or limited opportunity or serious loss of happiness or good.

Any suffering and limited opportunity must, of course, be experienced by some person—they cannot exist in disembodied form—and so in that sense N remains person-affecting. But N does not require that the same individuals who experience suffering and limited opportunity in one alternative exist without the suffering and limited opportunity in the other alternative; it is a same number, not a same person, principle. N allows the child who does not experience the suffering and limited opportunity to be a different person from the child who does; that is why the woman's action in P1 is morally wrong according to N, but not according to M. If the woman in P1 does take the medication and wait to conceive a normal child, she acts so as to make the suffering and limited opportunity "avoidable by substitution," as Philip G. Peters, Jr. has put it (Peters 1989).

A different way of making the same point is to say that this principle for the prevention of suffering applies not to distinct individuals, so that the prevention of suffering must make a distinct individual better off than if he or she would have been, as M requires, but to the classes of individuals who will exist if the suffering is or is not prevented, as N does (Peters 1989; Bayles 1976). Assessing the prevention of suffering by the effect on classes of persons, as opposed to distinct individuals, also allows for avoidability by substitution—an individual who does not suffer if one choice is made is substituted for a different person who does suffer if the other choice is made. A principle applied to the classes of all persons who will exist in each of two or more alternative courses of action will be a non–person-affecting principle.

The preceding discussion referred only to the prevention of harm or loss of opportunity because that is the focus of this chapter. However, it should be noted that N allows, for the same reasons as does M, the weighing of securing happiness or good against preventing suffering and loss of opportunity. If it did not, but required only preventing serious suffering, then N would require not creating a child who would experience serious suffering, but also great happiness and good, in favor of creating a child who would suffer less, but experience no compensating happiness or good, even though the latter child on balance would have a substantially worse life. We note as well that we have not defined "serious" as it functions in either M or N; it is difficult to do so in a sufficiently general yet precise way to make the application of the principle simple and straightforward for a wide range of cases. Judgment must be used in applying N. The seriousness of suffering and loss of opportunity, or loss of happiness and good, that could be prevented must be assessed principally in light of their potential impact on the child's life, the probability of that impact, and the possibility and probability of compensatory measures to mitigate that impact. Applying N requires judgment as well regarding what are "substantial burdens or costs, or loss of benefits, on themselves or others." For example, how serious are possible moral objections by the parents to the use of abortion, and how great are the financial costs or medical risks of having an alternative child using assisted reproduction technologies, and so forth?

We do not claim that all moral principles concerning obligations to prevent harm, or of beneficence and nonmaleficence more generally, are non–person-affecting, and so we do not reject principle M. In typical cases of harm where a distinct individual is made worse off, the moral principles most straightforwardly applicable to them are person-affecting. Our claim is only that an adequate moral theory should include as well non–person-affecting principles like N. How these principles are related, as well as what principles apply to different number cases in a comprehensive moral theory, involves deep difficulties in moral theory that we cannot pursue here. In this respect, we do not propose a full solution to the nonidentity problem. . . .

REFERENCES

Bayles, M. 1976. "Harm to the Unconceived." *Philosophy and Public Affairs* 5(3): 292–304.

Heyd, D. 1992. *Genetics: Moral Issues in the Creation of People*. Berkeley, CA: University of California Press.

Parfit, D. 1984. *Reasons and Persons*. Oxford: Clarendon Press.

Peters, P.G. 1989. "Protecting the Unconceived: Nonexistence, Avoidability, and Reproductive Technology." *Arizona Law Review* 31(3): 487–548.

CHEAP LISTENING? REFLECTIONS ON THE CONCEPT OF WRONGFUL DISABILITY

Richard J. Hull

The intuition underlying principle N[1] is that 'it is good to prevent suffering and promote happiness (even if doing so reduces no person's suffering and increases no person's happiness).'[2] The desire to refrain from bringing about avoidable suffering is morally acceptable, if not admirable; and I think that consideration of termination on that basis requires no further justification. Indeed, it strikes me as odd to claim that refraining from bringing about avoidable suffering is only justified by then bringing about a life of less or no suffering. It is rather like saying that my desire to refrain from driving a car that pollutes the air obliges me to buy a helium-powered one.

However, if we claim that bringing about a life of less or no suffering is *not* what justifies refraining from bringing about avoidable suffering, then we seem to fall straight back into the non-identity problem. We seem to be committed once again to endorsing the problematic claim that non-existence is preferable to an existence of some suffering that is otherwise worthwhile. Now while we *could* claim that, on the basis of a very low threshold for what we considered to be wrongful life, I do not think that

it is inevitable that we must. Instead, we can commit ourselves to the claim that non-existence is preferable to our *becoming responsible for* bringing about a certain degree of avoidable suffering, not that non-existence is preferable to that suffering itself. Thus, I am suggesting that questions of wrongful disability do not simply involve a direct evaluation of existence(s) versus non-existence. They also involve an evaluation of parental responsibility: agency weighs in with utility.

In a straight comparison of existence versus non-existence, virtually all existence wins. That is what creates the problem that the idea of substitution attempts to solve in same number cases. It also leads to Parfit's repugnant conclusion in different number cases, where

> for any possible population of at least 10 billion people, all with a very high quality of life, there must be some much larger imaginable population whose existence, if other things are equal, would be better, even though its members have lives that are barely worth living.[3]

The fact that repugnant conclusions can follow in different number cases points, I think, to a problem with the substitution idea. It certainly fails to consider, or sufficiently consider, the moral agency of those responsible for bringing such conclusions about. In turn, the fact that our moral agency tends to aim high rather than low can explain why we find such conclusions to be repugnant. As prospective parents, for example, we tend to take a top down rather than a bottom up approach. We think of providing the best possible conditions (social, economic medical and emotional) in which to raise a child rather than being satisfied to ensure that such conditions are just somewhat above an acceptable minimum. As such, our aspirations with regard to what we are prepared to take responsibility for bringing about go way beyond the better-than-nothing

From Richard J. Hull, "Cheap Listening? Reflections on the Concept of Wrongful Disability," *Biothics* 20 (April 2006): 55–63, Blackwell Publishers.

Editors' note: Some text and author's notes have been cut. Students who want to read the article in its entirety should consult the original.

1. N: Individuals are morally required not to let any child or other dependent person for whose welfare they are responsible experience serious suffering or limited opportunity or serious loss of happiness or good, if they can act so that, *without affecting the number of persons who will exist* and without imposing substantial burdens or costs or loss of benefits on themselves or others, no child or other dependent person for whose welfare they are responsible will experience serious suffering or limited opportunity or serious loss of happiness or good. From A. Buchanan et al., *From Chance to Choice: Genetics and Justice* (Cambridge: Cambridge University Press, 2000), 254.

2. Ibid.

3. Ibid.

criterion set by the non-identity problem. Indeed, their point of comparison is more likely to be closer to the polar opposite: 'everything' rather than 'nothing'.[4] Assuming that we can legitimately add those aspirations to the equation, then while a life of some suffering is, strictly, better than no life at all in many cases, we can make good sense of the claim that one may not want to take responsibility for creating avoidable suffering, even at the cost of creating no life at all.

Thus, while questions about future children tend to focus, quite rightly, on the quality of life that those children are likely to have, this need not be at the expense of considering the aspirations of potential parents. Indeed, when focussing on quality of life, it would be incomplete not to also consider how the quality of life of those having to make reproductive choices and decisions might be affected in given cases. How a given decision might reflect and/or affect our moral integrity should therefore be factored into our moral appraisal.

That said, if we can plausibly give weight to, say, the desire not to be responsible for creating challenges for others that lie outside what is perceived to be an acceptable range, then we have found a justification for termination of pregnancy that neither commits us to a wrongful life claim, nor requires that we substitute a non-disabled child 'instead'. The former is true if we need not claim that a life is not worth living in order to justifiably refrain from bringing that life about. I have argued that we need not. We need merely be claiming that a particular life would be worse than that which we could be reasonably expected to take responsibility for bringing about. Indeed, given that we seem to be sympathetic to that sort of claim in more run-of-the-mill cases of termination where sub-optimal reasons abound, I fail to see why we should not be sympathetic to it in cases of projected disability.

Moreover, if the desire not to be responsible for creating challenges for others that lie outside what is

perceived to be an acceptable range acts as a justification for termination then, rather obviously, the morality of termination does not hinge on whether or not substitution takes place. By implication, the potentially 'repugnant' ramifications of the substitution idea in different number cases are avoided,[5] as are the theoretical difficulties with it in same number cases. That is, the reason to terminate is not as vulnerable to defeat by creative alternatives that score a marginal success on the scale of utility, as is the idea of substitution. The force of the reason is quite independent of available alternatives. Indeed, one of the attractions of this kind of justification of termination is that it is justified in different number cases where fewer people result: where, for example, a decision to refrain from bringing about a life of some suffering impacts on the desire to conceive another child. I think that the more our moral framework can account for and be sympathetic to that kind of case, the better it will be. Moreover, in the light of that, ideas of substitution can seem rather insensitive.

Given the arguments so far, 'avoidability by substitution' does not comprise the only justification of termination on the grounds of projected disability. Likewise, termination *without* substitution need not imply, nor be justified by, a wrongful life claim. What is not so clear is where that leaves the concept of wrongful disability.

Hitherto, I have tried to develop a justification of termination on the grounds of projected disability that avoids the counter-intuitive implications of Buchanan et al.'s principle N. Yet while it is a justification, it by no means denotes wrongful disability. Indeed, the more one takes account of things like the social aspect of what we perceive to be an 'acceptable range', the personal nature and potential impact of reproductive decisions, parental responsibilities and aspirations, and the Parfitian point about non-existence, the less one can describe having disabled children as 'wrongful'.

As I argued earlier, clear cases of wrongful disability potentially occur where choices exist that, if made, would result in the *same* child coming into the

---

4. This seems to be what Woodward is getting at, albeit from a different angle, when he writes 'people can think that their lives contain, on balance, a fairly large positive amount of welfare and yet also think that, good as this is, it is not good enough—it falls too far short of what they conceive of as an ideal life'. J. Woodward. The Non-Identity Problem. *Ethics* 1986; 96(4): p. 823.

5. For example, substituting disabled twins or triplets in the place of one non-disabled child could be favoured in a straight utility comparison, yet the very idea seems far removed from our moral sensibilities.

world in better circumstances. So, to reiterate, where a pre or postnatal intervention (without substantial risk) was available to alleviate an impairment but was not opted for, that deliberate failure to assist would be wrong. Other than to that kind of case, however, the term cannot be legitimately applied.

One of the implications of taking the Parfitian point about non-existence seriously is that it seems ever so difficult to maintain that bringing about a worthwhile although disabled life is wrong, when the only other option is not to bring it about at all. This carries through to pre-conception choices as well as to post-conception ones. Post-conception, where the only alternative to having a disabled child is termination, I have argued that we should be sympathetic to decisions to terminate pregnancy on the grounds of a desire not to be responsible for creating challenges for others that lie outside what is perceived to be an acceptable range. (Availability of substitution may or may not come into it.) However, that does not mean that choosing to continue with that pregnancy is wrongful. Indeed, such a claim is both insensitive and inaccurate. It is insensitive given the profoundly personal nature of reproductive decisions alluded to earlier: given, for example, the controversial nature of the issue of abortion and the deeply held beliefs that tend to attach to it. It is inaccurate if Parfit is right, that a worthwhile although disabled life is better than no life at all.

Likewise, pre-conception choices that result in the creation of a disabled child cannot be described as wrongful, for the very same reasons. An example would be where a prospective mother has a treatable condition that would be likely to result in her child suffering from some kind of impairment. If she delays conception for, say, a month, the condition will have cleared up and she will be able to conceive a non-disabled child. Now while we may not understand her choice not to delay conception, if she makes it, I do not think that we can say that it is wrong since a child with a worthwhile life will result who would otherwise not. Indeed, one of the implications of Parfit's non-identity problem more generally is that we can no longer claim that things are wrong that we have claimed are wrong up to now and perhaps would still quite like to. However, what we *can* legitimately claim here is that the decision of the mother not to delay conception is *irresponsible*, given the ease with which she can

bring about a state of affairs that entails less suffering (in a different person, same number sense).

In addition, we might want to claim that the decision, post-conception, to go ahead and have a disabled child rather than to terminate, while not wrongful, is irresponsible to the extent that, again, avoidable suffering is created. However, we have to be more careful with such a claim given the beliefs that some parents will have with regard to termination. For example, some parents will believe that having a disabled child is, in their circumstances, the *most responsible* thing they could do. With that in mind, we would do well to be more gentle with our moral judgements and our use of terminology. However, the more that the severity of a projected disability errs toward what could be considered to be wrongful life, the more I think that we can legitimately claim that it is irresponsible to bring that disability about.

If the morality of termination does not hinge on whether or not substitution takes place, as I have argued it does not, then neither should a concept of wrongful disability. Indeed, while the idea of substitution in same number cases may point to a preferable state of affairs, other considerations do rather suggest that it is unable to determine that one state of affairs is wrong and the other is right. Those other considerations include our responsibilities and aspirations as moral agents, the personal nature and potential impact of reproductive decisions and questions raised by the non-identity problem.

The non-identity problem, perhaps unwittingly, reminds us of the value or worth contained within a vast range of human life. Of increasing importance as genetic technologies develop is the question of what we consider to be an acceptable range of human capability. Continuing to think seriously about that question will help to determine where we might be sympathetic with respect to decisions not to bring certain types of life about and where we might be less so, or not at all. It might also equip us to more coherently and emphatically resist some of the potential excesses afforded by technological development. Moreover, in considering the critical question of what we perceive to be an acceptable range, I have argued throughout that we should be acutely aware of the social context that may help to define it, a context that need by no means be inevitable, or just.

ASSISTED REPRODUCTION

THE PRESUMPTIVE PRIMACY OF PROCREATIVE LIBERTY

John Robertson

Procreative liberty has wide appeal but its scope has never been fully elaborated and often is contested. The concept has several meanings that must be clarified if it is to serve as a reliable guide for moral debate and public policy regarding new reproductive technologies.

WHAT IS PROCREATIVE LIBERTY?

At the most general level, procreative liberty is the freedom either to have children or to avoid having them. Although often expressed or realized in the context of a couple, it is first and foremost an individual interest. It is to be distinguished from freedom in the ancillary aspects of reproduction, such as

liberty in the conduct of pregnancy or choice of place or mode of childbirth.

The concept of reproduction, however, has a certain ambiguity contained within it. In a strict sense, reproduction is always genetic. It occurs by provision of one's gametes to a new person, and thus includes having or producing offspring. While female reproduction has traditionally included gestation, in vitro fertilization (IVF) now allows female genetic and gestational reproduction to be separated. Thus a woman who has provided the egg that is carried by another has reproduced, even if she has not gestated and does not rear resulting offspring. Because of the close link between gestation and female reproduction, a woman who gestates the embryo of another may also reasonably be viewed as having a reproductive experience, even though she does not reproduce genetically.[1]

In any case, reproduction in the genetic or gestational sense is to be distinguished from child rearing. Although reproduction is highly valued in part because it usually leads to child rearing, one can produce offspring without rearing them and rear

Editors' note: Many of the author's notes have been cut. Students who want to follow up on sources should consult the original article.

children without reproduction. One who rears an adopted child has not reproduced, while one who has genetic progeny but does not rear them has.

In this book the terms "procreative liberty" and "reproductive freedom" will mean the freedom to reproduce or not to reproduce in the genetic sense, which may also include rearing or not, as intended by the parties. Those terms will also include female gestation whether or not there is a genetic connection to the resulting child.

Often the reproduction at issue will be important because it is intended to lead to child rearing. In cases where rearing is not intended, the value to be assigned to reproduction *tout court* will have to be determined. Similarly, when there is rearing without genetic or gestational involvement, the value of nonreproductive child rearing will also have to be assessed. In both cases the value assigned may depend on the proximity to reproduction where rearing is intended.

Two further qualifications on the meaning of procreative liberty should be noted. One is that "liberty" as used in procreative liberty is a negative right. It means that a person violates no moral duty in making a procreative choice, and that other persons have a duty not to interfere with that choice. However, the negative right to procreate or not does not imply the duty of others to provide the resources or services necessary to exercise one's procreative liberty despite plausible moral arguments for governmental assistance.

As a matter of constitutional law, procreative liberty is a negative right against state interference with choices to procreate or to avoid procreation. It is not a right against private interference, though other laws might provide that protection. Nor is it a positive right to have the state or particular persons providing the means or resources necessary to have or avoid having children. The exercise of procreative liberty may be severely constrained by social and economic circumstances. Access to medical care, child care, employment, housing, and other services may significantly affect whether one is able to exercise procreative liberty. However, the state presently has no constitutional obligation to provide those services. Whether the state should alleviate those conditions is a separate issue of social justice.

The second qualification is that not everything that occurs in and around procreation falls within

liberty interests that are distinctively procreative. Thus whether the father may be present during childbirth, whether midwives may assist birth, or whether childbirth may occur at home rather than in a hospital may be important for the parties involved, but they do not implicate the freedom to reproduce (unless one could show that the place or mode of birth would determine whether birth occurs at all). Similarly, questions about a pregnant woman's drug use or other conduct during pregnancy . . . implicates liberty in the course of reproduction but not procreative liberty in the basic sense. Questions about whether the use of a technology is distinctively procreative recur throughout this book.

THE IMPORTANCE OF PROCREATIVE LIBERTY

Procreative liberty should enjoy presumptive primacy when conflicts about its exercise arise because control over whether one reproduces or not is central to personal identity, to dignity, and to the meaning of one's life. For example, deprivation of the ability to avoid reproduction determines one's self-definition in the most basic sense. It affects women's bodies in a direct and substantial way. It also centrally affects one's psychological and social identity and one's social and moral responsibilities. The resulting burdens are especially onerous for women, but they affect men in significant ways as well.

On the other hand, being deprived of the ability to reproduce prevents one from an experience that is central to individual identity and meaning in life. Although the desire to reproduce is in part socially constructed, at the most basic level transmission of one's genes through reproduction is an animal or species urge closely linked to the sex drive. In connecting us with nature and future generations, reproduction gives solace in the face of death. As Shakespeare noted, "nothing 'gainst Time's scythe can make defense/save breed."[2] For many people "breed"—reproduction and the parenting that usually accompanies it—is a central part of their life plan, and the most satisfying and meaningful experience they have. It also has primary importance as an expression of a couple's love or unity. For many persons, reproduction also has religious significance and is experienced as a "gift from God." Its denial—through infertility or governmental restriction—is experienced as a great loss, even if one has already had children or will have little or no rearing role with them.

Decisions to have or to avoid having children are thus personal decisions of great import that determine the shape and meaning of one's life. The person directly involved is best situated to determine whether that meaning should or should not occur. An ethic of personal autonomy as well as ethics of community or family should then recognize a presumption in favor of most personal reproductive choices. Such a presumption does not mean that reproductive choices are without consequence to others, nor that they should never be limited. Rather, it means that those who would limit procreative choice have the burden of showing that the reproductive actions at issue would create such substantial harm that they could justifiably be limited. Of course, what counts as the "substantial harm" that justifies interference with procreative choice may often be contested, as the discussion of reproductive technologies in this book will show.

A closely related reason for protecting reproductive choice is to avoid the highly intrusive measures that governmental control of reproduction usually entails. State interference with reproductive choice may extend beyond exhortation and penalties to gestapo and police state tactics. Margaret Atwood's powerful futuristic novel *The Handmaid's Tale* expresses this danger by creating a world where fertile women are forcibly impregnated by the ruling powers and their pregnancies monitored to replenish a decimated population.[3]

Equally frightening scenarios have occurred in recent years when repressive governments have interfered with reproductive choice. In Romania and China, men and women have had their most private activities scrutinized in the service of state reproductive goals. In Ceaușescu's Romania, where contraception and abortion were strictly forbidden, women's menstrual cycles were routinely monitored to see if they were pregnant. Women who did not become pregnant or who had abortions were severely punished. Many women nevertheless sought illegal abortions and died, leaving their children orphaned and subject to sale to Westerners seeking children for adoption.

In China, forcible abortion and sterilization have occurred in the service of a one-child-per-family population policy. Village cadres have seized pregnant women in their homes and forced them to have abortions. A campaign of forcible sterilization in India in 1977 was seen as an "attack on women and children" and brought Indira Gandhi's government down. In the United States, state-imposed sterilization of "mental defectives," sanctioned in 1927 by the United States Supreme Court in *Buck* v. *Bell,* resulted in 60,000 sterilizations over a forty-year period. Many mentally normal people were sterilized by mistake, and mentally retarded persons who posed little risk of harm to others were subjected to surgery. It is no surprise that current proposals for compulsory use of contraceptives such as Norplant are viewed with great suspicion.

TWO TYPES OF PROCREATIVE LIBERTY

To see how values of procreative liberty affect the ethical and public policy evaluation of new reproductive technologies, we must determine whether the interests that underlie the high value accorded procreative liberty are implicated in their use. This is not a simple task because procreative liberty is not unitary, but consists of strands of varying interests in the conception and gestation of offspring. The different strands implicate different interests, have different legal and constitutional status, and are differently affected by technology.

An essential distinction is between the freedom to avoid reproduction and the freedom to reproduce. When people talk of reproductive rights, they usually have one or the other aspect in mind. Because different interests and justifications underlie each and countervailing interests for limiting each aspect vary, recognition of one aspect does not necessarily mean that the other will also be respected; nor does limitation of one mean that the other can also be denied.

However, there is a mirroring or reciprocal relationship here. Denial of one type of reproductive liberty necessarily implicates the other. If a woman is not able to avoid reproduction through contraception or abortion, she may end up reproducing, with all the burdens that unwanted reproduction entails. Similarly, if one is denied the liberty to reproduce through forcible sterilization, one is forced to avoid reproduction, thus experiencing the loss that absence of progeny brings. By extending reproductive options, new reproductive technologies present challenges to both aspects of procreative choice.

AVOIDING REPRODUCTION: THE LIBERTY NOT TO REPRODUCE

One sense in which people commonly understand procreative liberty is as the freedom to avoid reproduction—to avoid begetting or bearing offspring and the rearing demands they make. Procreative liberty in this sense could involve several different choices, because decisions to avoid procreation arise at several different stages. A decision not to procreate could occur prior to conception through sexual abstinence, contraceptive use, or refusal to seek treatment for infertility. At this stage, the main issues concern freedom to refrain from sexual intercourse, the freedom to use contraceptives, and the freedom to withhold gametes for use in noncoital conception. Countervailing interests concern societal interests in increasing population, a partner's interest in sexual intimacy and progeny, and moral views about the unity of sex and reproduction.

Once pregnancy has occurred, reproduction can be avoided only by termination of pregnancy. Procreative freedom here would involve the freedom to abort the pregnancy. Competing interests are protection of embryos and fetuses and respect for human life generally, the most heated issue of reproductive rights. They may also include moral or social beliefs about the connectedness of sex and reproduction, or views about a woman's reproductive and work roles.

Once a child is born, procreation has occurred, and the procreators ordinarily have parenting obligations. Freeing oneself from rearing obligations is not strictly speaking a matter of procreative liberty, though it is an important personal interest. Even if parents relinquish the child for adoption, the psychological reality that one has reproduced remains. Opposing interests at this stage involve the need to provide parenting, nurturing, and financial support to offspring. The right to be free of those obligations, as well as the right to assume them after birth occurs, is not directly addressed in this book except to the extent that those rights affect reproductive decisions.

Technology and the Avoidance of Reproduction

Many reproductive technologies raise questions about the scope of the liberty interest in avoiding reproduction. New contraceptive, contragestive, and abortion technologies raise avoidance issues directly, though the issues raised are not always novel. For example, an important issue in voluntary use of long-lasting contraceptives concerns access by minors and the poor, an issue of justice in the distribution of medical resources that currently exists with other contraceptives. The more publicized issue of whether the state may require child abusers or women on welfare to use Norplant implicates the target group's right to procreate, not their liberty interest in avoiding reproduction.

Contragestive agents such as RU486, which prevent reproduction after conception has occurred, raise many of the current issues of the abortion debate. Because RU486 operates so early in pregnancy, however, it focuses attention on the moral status of very early abortions and the moral differences, if any, between postcoital contraceptives and abortifacients. Ethical assessment and legal rights to use contragestives will depend on the ethical and legal status of early prenatal stages of human life.

More novel avoidance issues will arise with IVF and embryo cryopreservation technology. IVF often produces more embryos than can be safely implanted in the uterus. If couples must donate rather than discard unwanted embryos, they will become biologic parents against their will. This prospect raises the question of whether the liberty interest in avoiding reproduction includes avoiding genetic offspring when no rearing obligations will attach—reproduction *tout court*. Is one's fundamental interest in avoiding reproduction seriously implicated if one will never know or have contact with one's offspring? The resulting moral and policy issue is how to balance the interest in avoiding genetic offspring *tout court* with respect for preimplantation stages of human life.

Technologies of quality control and selection through genetic screening and manipulation will also raise novel questions about the right to avoid reproduction. Prenatal screening enables couples to avoid reproduction because of the genetic characteristics of expected offspring. Are the interests that support protecting the freedom to avoid reproduction present when that freedom is exercised selectively? Because some reasons for rejecting fetuses are more appealing than others, would devising criteria for such choices violate the right not to procreate? For example, should law or morality permit abortion of a fetus with Tay-Sachs disease or Down's syndrome but not female fetuses or fetuses with a disease of varying expressivity such as cystic fibrosis?

Legal Status of Avoiding Reproduction

Legally, the negative freedom to avoid reproduction is widely recognized, though great controversy over abortion persists, and there is no positive constitutional right to contraception and abortion. The freedom to avoid reproduction is clearest for men and women prior to conception. In the United States and most developed countries, marriage and sexual intercourse are a matter of choice. However, rape laws do not always effectively protect women, and some jurisdictions do not criminalize marital rape. Legal access to contraception and sterilization is firmly established, though controversy exists over providing contraception to adolescents because of fears that it would encourage nonmarital sexual intercourse.

Constitutional recognition of the right to use contraceptives—to have sex and not reproduce—occurred in the 1965 landmark case of *Griswold* v. *Connecticut*. The executive director of Planned Parenthood and its medical director, a licensed physician, challenged a Connecticut law that made it a crime to use or distribute contraceptives. The United States Supreme Court found that the law violated a fundamental liberty right of married couples, which it later extended to unmarried persons, to use contraceptives as a matter of personal liberty or privacy. Although the Court alluded to the unsavory prospect of police searching the marital bedroom for evidence of the crime as a reason for invalidating the law, it is clear that the Court was protecting the right of persons who engage in sexual intimacy to avoid unwanted reproduction. The right to avoid reproduction through contraception is thus firmly protected, even where fornication laws remain in effect.

Legal protection also exists for other activities tied to avoiding reproduction prior to pregnancy. Thus both men and women are deemed owners of gametes within or outside their bodies, so that they may prevent them from being used for reproduction without their permission. Men and women also have rights to prevent extracorporeal embryos formed from their gametes from being placed in women and brought to term without their consent.

Once conception has occurred, the right to avoid reproduction differs for the woman and man involved. In the United States and most of Western Europe, abortion in early stages of the pregnancy is widely permitted. Under *Roe* v. *Wade,* whose central holding was reaffirmed in 1992 in *Planned Parenthood* v. *Casey,* women, whether single or married, adult or minor, have a right to terminate pregnancy up to viability. However, the state may inform them of its views concerning the worth of the fetus and require them to wait 24 hours before obtaining an abortion. Parental consent or notification requirements can be imposed on minors, as long as a judicial bypass is provided in cases in which the minor does not wish to inform her parents. Also, because the right to abortion is a negative right, the state has no obligation to fund abortions for indigent women.

Although pregnancy termination usually kills the fetus, the right to end pregnancy does not protect the right to cause the death of a fetus that has emerged alive from the abortion process, or even to choose a method of abortion that is most likely to cause fetal demise. Nor does it give a woman the right to engage in prenatal conduct that poses unreasonable risks to the health of future offspring when she is choosing to go to term. After birth occurs, the mother and father have obligations to the child until custody is formally relinquished or transferred to others.

The father, once conception through sexual intercourse has occurred, has no right to require or prevent abortion, and cannot avoid rearing duties of financial support once birth occurs. This is true even if the woman has lied to him about her fertility or her use of contraceptives. However, he is free to relinquish custody and give up for adoption. He is also free to determine whether IVF embryos formed from his sperm should be implanted in the uterus.

The law's recognition of a right to avoid reproduction both prior to and after conception provides the legal framework for resolving conflicts presented by new reproductive technologies that affect interests in avoiding reproduction. While many technologies raise the same issues confronted in *Griswold* and *Roe,* new twists will arise that directly challenge the scope of that right. To resolve those conflicts, the separate elements that comprise the interest in avoiding reproduction must be analyzed and evaluated against the competing interests affected by those technologies.

THE FREEDOM TO PROCREATE

In addition to freedom to avoid procreation, procreative liberty also includes the freedom to procreate— the freedom to beget and bear children if one chooses. As with avoiding reproduction, the right to reproduce is a negative right against public or private interference, not a positive right to the services or the resources needed to reproduce. It is an important freedom that is widely accepted as a basic, human right. But its various components and dimensions have never been fully analyzed, as technologies of conception and selection now force us to do.

As with avoiding reproduction, the freedom to procreate involves the freedom to engage in a series of actions that eventuate in reproduction and usually in child rearing. One must be free to marry or find a willing partner, engage in sexual intercourse, achieve conception and pregnancy, carry a pregnancy to term, and rear offspring. Social and natural barriers to reproduction would involve the unavailability of willing or suitable partners, impotence or infertility, and lack of medical and child-care resources. State barriers to marriage, to sexual intercourse, to conception, to infertility treatment, to carrying pregnancies to term, and to certain child-rearing arrangements would also limit the freedom to procreate. The most commonly asserted reasons for limiting coital reproduction are overpopulation, unfitness of parents, harm to offspring, and costs to the state or others. Technologies that treat infertility raise additional concerns that are discussed below.

The moral right to reproduce is respected because of the centrality of reproduction to personal identity, meaning, and dignity. This importance makes the liberty to procreate an important moral right, both for an ethic of individual autonomy and for ethics of community or family that view the purpose of marriage and sexual union as the reproduction and rearing of offspring. Because of this importance, the right to reproduce is widely recognized as a prima facie moral right that cannot be limited except for very good reason.

Recognition of the primacy of procreation does not mean that all reproduction is morally blameless, much less that reproduction is always responsible and praiseworthy and can never be limited. However, the presumptive primacy of procreative liberty sets a very high standard for limiting those rights, tilting the balance in favor of reproducing but not totally determining its acceptability. A two-step process of analysis is envisaged here. The first question is whether a distinctively procreative interest is involved. If so, the question then is whether the harm threatened by reproduction satisfies the strict standard for overriding this liberty interest.

The personal importance of procreation helps answer questions about who holds procreative rights and about the circumstances under which the right to reproduce may be limited. A person's capacity to find significance in reproduction should determine whether one holds the presumptive right, though this question is often discussed in terms of whether persons with such a capacity are fit parents. To have a liberty interest in procreating, one should at a minimum have the mental capacity to understand or appreciate the meanings associated with reproduction. This minimum would exclude severely retarded persons from having reproductive interests, though it would not remove their right to bodily integrity. However, being unmarried, homosexual, physically disabled, infected with HIV, or imprisoned would not disqualify one from having reproductive interests, though they might affect one's ability to rear offspring. Whether those characteristics justify limitations on reproduction is discussed later. Nor would already having reproduced negate a person's interest in reproducing again, though at a certain point the marginal value to a person of additional offspring diminishes.

What kinds of interests or harms make reproduction unduly selfish or irresponsible and thus could justifiably limit the presumptive right to procreate? To answer this question, we must distinguish coital and noncoital reproduction. Surprisingly, there is a widespread reluctance to speak of coital reproduction as irresponsible, much less to urge public action to prevent irresponsible coital reproduction from occurring. If such a conversation did occur, reasons for limiting coital reproduction would involve the heavy costs that it imposed on others—costs that outweighed whatever personal meaning or satisfaction the person(s) reproducing experienced. With coital reproduction, such costs might arise if there were severe overpopulation, if the persons reproducing were unfit parents, if reproduction would harm offspring, or if significant medical or social costs were imposed on others.

Because the United States does not face the severe overpopulation of some countries, the main grounds for claiming that reproduction is irresponsible is where the person(s) reproducing lack the financial means to raise offspring or will otherwise harm their children. As later discussions will show, both grounds are seriously inadequate as justifications for interfering with procreative choice. Imposing rearing costs on others may not rise to the level of harm that justifies depriving a person of a fundamental moral right. Moreover, protection of offspring from unfit parenting requires that unfit parents not rear, not that they not reproduce. Offspring could be protected by having others rear them without interfering with parental reproduction.

A further problem, if coital reproduction were found to be unjustified, concerns what action should then be taken. Exhortation or moral condemnation might be acceptable, but more stringent or coercive measures would act on the body of the person deemed irresponsible. Past experience with forced sterilization of retarded persons and the inevitable focus on the poor and minorities as targets of coercive policies make such proposals highly unappealing. Because of these doubts, there have been surprisingly few attempts to restrict coital reproduction in the United States since the era of eugenic sterilization, even though some instances of reproduction—for example, teenage pregnancy, inability to care for offspring—appear to be socially irresponsible.

An entirely different set of concerns arises with noncoital reproductive techniques. Charges that noncoital reproduction is unethical or irresponsible arise because of its expense, its highly technological character, its decomposition of parenthood into genetic, gestational, and social components, and its potential effects on women and offspring. To assess whether these effects justify moral condemnation or public limitation, we must first determine whether noncoital reproduction implicates important aspects of procreative liberty.

The Right to Reproduce and Noncoital Technology

If the moral right to reproduce presumptively protects coital reproduction, then it should protect noncoital reproduction as well. The moral right of the coitally infertile to reproduce is based on the same desire for offspring that the coitally fertile have. They too wish to replicate themselves, transmit genes, gestate, and rear children biologically related to them. Their infertility should no more disqualify them from reproductive experiences than physical disability should disqualify persons from walking with mechanical assistance. The unique risks posed by noncoital reproduction may provide independent justifications for limiting its use, but neither the noncoital nature of the means used nor the infertility of their beneficiaries means that the presumptively protected moral interest in reproduction is not present.

A major question about this position, however, is whether the noncoital or collaborative nature of the means used truly implicates reproductive interests. For example, what if only one aspect of reproduction—genetic transfer, gestation, or rearing—occurs, as happens with gamete donors or surrogates who play no rearing role? Is a person's procreative liberty substantially implicated in such partial reproductive roles? The answer will depend on the value attributed to the particular collaborative contribution and on whether the collaborative enterprise is viewed from the donor's or recipient's perspective.

Gamete donors and surrogates are clearly reproducing even though they have no intention to rear. Because reproduction *tout court* may seem less important than reproduction with intent to rear, the donor's reproductive interest may appear less important. However, more experience with these practices is needed to determine the inherent value of "partial" reproductive experiences to donors and surrogates. Experience may show that it is independently meaningful, regardless of their contact with offspring. If not, then countervailing interests would more easily override their right to enter these roles.

Viewed from the recipient's perspective, however, the donor or surrogate's reproduction *tout court* does not lessen the reproductive importance of her contribution. A woman who receives an egg or embryo donation has no genetic connection with offspring but has a gestational relation of great personal significance. In addition, gamete donors and surrogates enable one or both rearing partners to have a biological relation with offspring. If one of them has no biological connection at all, they will still have a strong interest in rearing their partner's biologic offspring. Whether viewed singly through the eyes of the partner who is reproducing, or jointly as an endeavor of a couple seeking to rear children who are biologically related to at least one of the two, a significant reproductive interest is at stake. If so, noncoital, collaborative treatments for infertility should be respected to the same extent as coital reproduction is.

Questions about the core meaning of reproduction will also arise in the temporal dislocations that cryopreservation of sperm and embryos make possible. For example, embryo freezing allows siblings to be conceived at the same time, but born years apart and to different gestational mothers. Twins could be created by splitting one embryo into two. If one half is frozen for later use, identical twins could be born at widely different times. Sperm, egg, and embryo freezing also make posthumous reproduction possible.

Such temporally dislocative practices clearly implicate core reproductive interests when the ultimate recipient has no alternative means of reproduction. However, if the procreative interests of the recipient couple are not directly implicated, we must ask whether those whose gametes are used have an independent procreative interest, as might occur if they directed that gametes or embryos be thawed after their death for purposes of posthumous reproduction. In that case the question is whether the expectancy of posthumous reproduction is so central to an individual's procreative identity or life-plan that it should receive the same respect that one's reproduction when alive receives. The answer to such a question will be important in devising policy for storing and posthumously disposing of gametes and embryos. The answer will also affect inheritance questions and have implications for management of pregnant women who are irreversibly comatose or brain dead.

The problem of determining whether technology implicates a major reproductive interest also arises with technologies that select offspring characteristics. Some degree of quality control would seem logically to fall within the realm of procreative liberty. For many couples the decision whether to procreate depends on the ability to have healthy children. Without some guarantee or protection against the risk of handicapped children, they might not reproduce at all.

Thus viewed, quality control devices become part of the liberty interest in procreating or in avoiding procreation, and arguably should receive the same degree of protection. If so, genetic screening and selective abortion, as well as the right to select a mate or a source for donated eggs, sperm, or embryos should be protected as part of procreative liberty. The same arguments would apply to positive interventions to cure disease at the fetal or embryo stage. However, futuristic practices such as non-therapeutic enhancement, cloning, or intentional diminishment of offspring characteristics may so deviate from the core interests that make reproduction meaningful as to fall outside the protective canopy of procreative liberty.

Finally, technology will present questions of whether one may use one's reproductive capacity to produce gametes, embryos, and fetuses for non-reproductive uses in research or therapy. Here the purpose is not to have children to rear, but to get material for research or transplant. Are such uses of reproductive capacity tied closely enough to the values and interests that underlie procreative freedom to warrant similar respect? Even if procreative choice is not directly involved, other liberties may protect the activity.

Are Noncoital Technologies Unethical?

If this analysis is accepted, then procreative liberty would include the right to use noncoital and other technologies to form a family and shape the characteristics of offspring. Neither infertility nor the fact that one will only partially reproduce eliminates the existence of a prima facie reproductive experience for someone. However, judgments about the proximity of these partial reproductive experiences to the core meanings of reproduction will be required in balancing those claims against competing moral concerns.

Judgment about the reproductive importance of noncoital technologies is crucial because many people have serious ethical reservations about them, and are more than willing to restrict their use. The concerns here are not the fears of overpopulation, parental unfitness, and societal costs that arise with allegedly irresponsible coital reproduction. Instead, they include reduction of demand for hard-to-adopt children, the coercive or exploitive bargains that will be offered to poor women, the commodification of both children and reproductive collaborators, the objectification of women as reproductive vessels, and the undermining of the nuclear family.

However, often the harms feared are deontological in character. In some cases they stem from a religious or moral conception of the unity of sex and reproduction or the definition of family. Such a view characterizes the Vatican's strong opposition to IVF, donor sperm, and other noncoital and collaborative techniques. Other deontological concerns derive from a particular conception of the proper reproductive role of women. Many persons, for example, oppose paid surrogate motherhood because of a judgment about the wrongness of a woman's willingness to sever the mother-child bond for the sake of money. They also insist that the gestational mother is always morally entitled to rear, despite her preconception promise to the contrary. Closely related are dignitary objections to allowing any reproductive factors to be purchased, or to having offspring selected on the basis of their genes.

Finally, there is a broader concern that noncoital reproduction will undermine the deeper community interest in having a clear social framework to define boundaries of families, sexuality, and reproduction. The traditional family provides a container for the narcissism and irrationality that often drives human reproduction. This container assures commitments to the identifications and taboos that protect children from various types of abuse. The technical ability to disaggregate and recombine genetic, gestational, and rearing connections and to control the genes of offspring may thus undermine essential protections for offspring, couples, families, and society.

These criticisms are powerful ones that explain much of the ambivalence that surrounds the use of certain reproductive technologies. They call into question the wisdom of individual decisions to use them, and the willingness of society to promote or facilitate their use. Unless one is operating out of a specific religious or deontological ethic, however, they do not show that all individual uses of these techniques are immoral, much less that public policy should restrict or discourage their use.

These criticisms seldom meet the high standard necessary to limit procreative choice. Many of them are mere hypothetical or speculative possibilities. Others reflect moralisms concerning a "right" view of reproduction, which individuals in a pluralistic society hold or reject to varying degrees. In any event, without a clear showing of substantial harm to the tangible interests of others, speculation or mere moral objections alone should not override the moral right of infertile couples to use those techniques to form families. Given the primacy of procreative liberty, the use of these techniques should be accorded the same high protection granted to coital reproduction.

RESOLVING DISPUTES OVER PROCREATIVE LIBERTY

As this brief survey shows, new reproductive technologies will generate ethical and legal disputes about the meaning and scope of procreative liberty. Because procreative liberty has never been fully elaborated, the importance of procreative choice in many novel settings will be a question of first impression. The ultimate decision reached will reflect the value assigned to the procreative interest at stake in light of the effects causing concern. In an important sense, the meaning of procreative liberty will be created or constituted for society in the process of resolving such disputes.

If procreative liberty is taken seriously, a strong presumption in favor of using technologies that centrally implicate reproductive interests should be recognized. Although procreative rights are not absolute, those who would limit procreative choice should have the burden of establishing substantial harm. This is the standard used in ethical and legal analyses of restrictions on traditional reproductive decisions. Because the same procreative goals are involved, the same standard of scrutiny should be used for assessing moral or governmental restrictions on novel reproductive techniques.

In arbitrating these disputes, one has to come to terms with the importance of procreative interests relative to other concerns. The precise procreative interest at stake must be identified and weighed against the core values of reproduction. As noted, this will raise novel and unique questions when the technology deviates from the model of two-person coital reproduction, or otherwise disaggregates or alters ordinary reproductive practices. However, if an important reproductive interest exists, then use of the technology should be presumptively permitted. Only substantial harm to tangible interests of others should then justify restriction.

In determining whether such harm exists, it will be necessary to distinguish between harms to individuals and harms to personal conceptions of morality, right order, or offense, discounted by their probability of occurrence. As previously noted, many objections to reproductive technology rest on differing views of what "proper" or "right" reproduction is aside from tangible effects on others. For example, concerns about the decomposition of parenthood through the use of donors and surrogates, about the temporal alteration of conception, gestation and birth, about the alienation or commercialization of gestational capacity, and about selection and control of offspring characteristics do not directly affect persons so much as they affect notions of right behavior. Disputes over early abortion and discard or manipulation of IVF-created embryos also exemplify this distinction, if we grant that the embryo/previable fetus is not a person or entity with rights in itself.

At issue in these cases is the symbolic or constitutive meaning of actions regarding prenatal life, family, maternal gestation, and respect for persons over which people in a secular, pluralistic society often differ. A majoritarian view of "right" reproduction or "right" valuation of prenatal life, family, or the role of women should not suffice to restrict actions based on differing individual views of such preeminently personal issues. At a certain point, however, a practice such as cloning, enhancement, or intentional diminishment of offspring may be so far removed from even pluralistic notions of reproductive meaning that they leave the realm of protected reproductive choice. People may differ over where that point is, but it will not easily exclude most reproductive technologies of current interest.

To take procreative liberty seriously, then, is to allow it to have presumptive priority in an individual's life. This will give persons directly involved the final say about use of a particular technology, unless tangible harm to the interests of others can be shown. Of course, people may differ over whether an important procreative interest is at stake or over how serious the harm posed from use of the reproductive technology is. Such a focused debate, however, is legitimate and ultimately essential in developing ethical standards and public policy for use of new reproductive technologies.

THE LIMITS OF PROCREATIVE LIBERTY

The emphasis on procreative liberty that informs this book provides a useful but by no means complete or final perspective on the technologies in question. Theological, social, psychological, economic, and feminist perspectives would emphasize different aspects of reproductive technology, and might be much less sanguine about potential benefits and risks. Such perspectives might also offer better guidance in how to use these technologies to protect offspring, respect women, and maintain other important values.

A strong rights perspective has other limitations as well. Recognition of procreative liberty, whether in traditional or in new technological settings, does not guarantee that people will achieve their reproductive goals, much less that they will be happy with what they do achieve. Nature may be recalcitrant to the latest technology. Individuals may lack the will, the perseverance, or the resources to use effective technologies. Even if they do succeed, the results may be less satisfying than envisaged. In addition, many individual instances of procreative choice may cumulate into larger social changes that from our current vantage point seem highly undesirable. But these are the hazards and limitations of any scheme of individual rights.

Recognition of procreative liberty will protect the right of persons to use technology in pursuing their reproductive goals, but it will not eliminate the ambivalence that such technologies engender. Societal ambivalence about reproductive technology is recapitulated at the individual level, as individuals and couples struggle with whether to use the technologies in question. Thus recognition of procreative liberty will not eliminate the dilemmas of personal choice and responsibility that reproductive choice entails. The freedom to act does not mean that we will act wisely, yet denying that freedom may be even more unwise, for it denies individuals' respect in the most fundamental choices of their lives.

NOTES

1. Whether labeled reproductive or not, gestation is a central experience for women and should enjoy the special respect or protected status accorded reproductive activities. On this view, a woman who receives an embryo donation or who serves as a gestational surrogate is having a reproductive experience, whether or not she also rears.

2. Sonnet 12 ("When I do count the clock that tells the time/And see the brave day sunk in hideous night"). Sonnet 2 ("When forty winters shall besiege thy brow/And dig deep trenches in thy beauty's field") also sings the praises of reproduction as an answer to death and old age.

3. Margaret Atwood, *The Handmaid's Tale* (Boston: Houghton Mifflin, 1986).

INSTRUCTION ON RESPECT FOR HUMAN LIFE IN ITS ORIGIN AND ON THE DIGNITY OF PROCREATION

Vatican, Congregation for the Doctrine of the Faith

BIOMEDICAL RESEARCH AND THE TEACHING OF THE CHURCH

The gift of life which God the Creator and Father has entrusted to man calls him to appreciate the inestimable value of what he has been given and to take responsibility for it: This fundamental principle must be placed at the center of one's reflection in order to clarify and solve the moral problems raised by artificial interventions on life as it originates and on the processes of procreation.

Thanks to the progress of the biological and medical sciences, man has at his disposal ever more effective therapeutic resources; but he can also acquire new powers, with unforeseeable consequences, over human life at its very beginning and in its first stages. Various procedures now make it possible to intervene not only in order to assist, but also to dominate the processes of procreation. These techniques can enable man to "take in hand his own destiny," but they also expose him "to the temptation to go beyond the limits of a reasonable dominion over nature." They might constitute progress in the service of man, but they also involve serious risks. Many people are therefore expressing an urgent appeal that in interventions on procreation the values and rights of the human person be safeguarded. Requests for clarification and guidance are coming not only from the faithful, but also from those who recognize the church as "an expert in humanity" with a mission to serve the "civilization of love" and of life.

The church's magisterium [asserts] . . . the criteria of moral judgment as regards the applications of scientific research and technology, especially in relation to human life and its beginnings . . . to be the respect, defense and promotion of man, his "primary and fundamental right" to life, his dignity as a person who is endowed with a spiritual soul and with moral responsibility and who is called to beatific communion with God. . . .

From *Origins* 16, no. 40 (March 19, 1987). Abridged.

Editors' note: Some text and all notes have been cut. Students who want to read the article in its entirety should consult the original.

ANTHROPOLOGY AND PROCEDURES
IN THE BIOMEDICAL FIELD

Which moral criteria must be applied in order to clarify the problems posed today in the field of biomedicine? The answer to this question presupposes a proper idea of the nature of the human person in his bodily dimension.

For it is only in keeping with his true nature that the human person can achieve self-realization as a "unified totality"; and this nature is at the same time corporal and spiritual. By virtue of its substantial union with a spiritual soul, the human body cannot be considered as a mere complex of tissues, organs and functions, nor can it be evaluated in the same way as the body of animals; rather, it is a constitutive part of the person who manifests and expresses himself through it.

The natural moral law expresses and lays down the purposes, rights and duties which are based upon the bodily and spiritual nature of the human person. Therefore this law cannot be thought of as simply a set of norms on the biological level; rather, it must be defined as the rational order whereby man is called by the Creator to direct and regulate his life and actions and in particular to make use of his own body.

A first consequence can be deduced from these principles: An intervention on the human body affects not only the tissues, the organs and their functions, but also involves the person himself on different levels. It involves, therefore, perhaps in an implicit but nonetheless real way, a moral significance and responsibility. . . .

Applied biology and medicine work together for the integral good of human life when they come to the aid of a person stricken by illness and infirmity and when they respect his or her dignity as a creature of God. No biologist or doctor can reasonably claim, by virtue of his scientific competence, to be able to decide on people's origin and destiny. This norm must be applied in a particular way in the field of sexuality and procreation, in which man and woman actualize the fundamental values of love and life.

God, who is love and life, has inscribed in man and woman the vocation to share in a special way in his mystery of personal communion and in his work as Creator and Father. For this reason marriage possesses specific goods and values in its union and in procreation which cannot be likened to those existing in lower forms of life. Such values and meanings are of the personal order and determine from the moral point of view the meaning and limits of artificial interventions on procreation and on the origin of human life. These interventions are not to be rejected on the grounds that they are artificial. As such, they bear witness to the possibilities of the art of medicine. But they must be given a moral evaluation in reference to the dignity of the human person, who is called to realize his vocation from God to the gift of love and the gift of life.

FUNDAMENTAL CRITERIA
FOR A MORAL JUDGMENT

The fundamental values connected with the techniques of artificial human procreation are two: the life of the human being called into existence and the special nature of the transmission of human life in marriage. The moral judgment on such methods of artificial procreation must therefore be formulated in reference to these values.

Physical life, with which the course of human life in the world begins, certainly does not itself contain the whole of a person's value, nor does it represent the supreme good of man, who is called to eternal life. However it does constitute in a certain way the "fundamental" value of life precisely because upon this physical life all the other values of the person are based and developed. The inviolability of the innocent human being's right to life "from the moment of conception until death" is a sign and requirement of the very inviolability of the person to whom the Creator has given the gift of life.

By comparison with the transmission of other forms of life in the universe, the transmission of human life has a special character of its own, which derives from the special nature of the human person. "The transmission of human life is entrusted by nature to a personal and conscious act and as such is subject to the all-holy laws of God: immutable and inviolable laws which must be recognized and observed. For this reason one cannot use means and follow methods which could be licit in the transmission of the life of plants and animals."

Advances in technology have now made it possible to procreate apart from sexual relations through the meeting *in vitro* of the germ cells previously taken from the man and the woman. But what is technically possible is not for that very reason morally admissible. Rational reflection on the fundamental values of life and of human procreation is therefore indispensable for formulating a moral evaluation of such technological interventions on a human being from the first stages of his development. . . .

I. RESPECT FOR HUMAN EMBRYOS

What respect is due to the human embryo, taking into account his nature and identity?

The human being must be respected—as a person—from the very first instant of his existence. . . .

This congregation is aware of the current debates concerning the beginning of human life, concerning the individuality of the human being and concerning the identity of the human person. The congregation recalls the teachings found in the Declaration on Procured Abortion:

"From the time that the ovum is fertilized, a new life is begun which is neither that of the father nor of the mother; it is rather the life of a new human being with his own growth. It would never be made human if it were not human already. To this perpetual evidence . . . modern genetic science brings valuable confirmation. It has demonstrated that, from the first instant, the program is fixed as to what this living being will be: a man, this individual man with his characteristic aspects already well determined. Right from fertilization is begun the adventure of a human life, and each of its great capacities requires time . . . to find its place and to be in a position to act."

This teaching remains valid and is further confirmed, if confirmation were needed, by recent findings of human biological science which recognize that in the zygote (the cell produced when the nuclei of the two gametes have fused) resulting from fertilization the biological identity of a new human individual is already constituted.

Certainly no experimental datum can be in itself sufficient to bring us to the recognition of a spiritual soul; nevertheless, the conclusions of science regarding the human embryo provide a valuable indication for discerning by the use of reason a personal presence at the moment of this first appearance of a human life: How could a human individual not be a human person? The magisterium has not expressly committed itself to an affirmation of a philosophical nature, but it constantly reaffirms the moral condemnation of any kind of procured abortion. This teaching has not been changed and is unchangeable.

Thus the fruit of human generation from the first moment of its existence, that is to say, from the moment the zygote has formed, demands the unconditional respect that is morally due to the human being in his bodily and spiritual totality. The human being is to be respected and treated as a person from the moment of conception and therefore from that same moment his rights as a person must be recognized, among which in the first place is the inviolable right of every innocent human being to life. This doctrinal reminder provides the fundamental criterion for the solution of the various problems posed by the development of the biomedical sciences in this field: Since the embryo must be treated as a person, it must also be defended in its integrity, tended and cared for, to the extent possible, in the same way as any other human being as far as medical assistance is concerned. . . .

How is one to evaluate morally research and experimentation on human embryos and fetuses?

Medical research must refrain from operations on live embryos, unless there is a moral certainty of not causing harm to the life or integrity of the unborn child and the mother, and on condition that the parents have given their free and informed consent to the procedure. It follows that all research, even when limited to the simple observation of the embryo, would become illicit were it to involve risk to the embryo's physical integrity or life by reason of the methods used or the effects induced.

As regards experimentation, and presupposing the general distinction between experimentation for purposes which are not directly therapeutic and experimentation which is clearly therapeutic for the subject himself, in the case in point one must also distinguish between experimentation carried out on embryos which are still alive and experimentation carried out on embryos which are dead. *If the embryos are living, whether viable or not, they must be respected just like any other human person; experimentation on embryos which is not directly therapeutic is illicit.*

No objective, even though noble in itself such as a foreseeable advantage to science, to other human beings or to society, can in any way justify experimentation on living human embryos or fetuses, whether viable or not, either inside or outside the mother's womb. The informed consent ordinarily required for clinical experimentation on adults cannot be granted by the parents, who may not freely dispose of the physical integrity or life of the unborn child. Moreover, experimentation on embryos and fetuses always involves risk, and indeed in most cases it involves the certain expectation of harm to their physical integrity or even their death.

To use human embryos or fetuses as the object or instrument of experimentation constitutes a crime against their dignity as human beings having a right to the same respect that is due to the child already born and to every human person. . . .

In the case of experimentation that is clearly therapeutic, namely, when it is a matter of experimental forms of therapy used for the benefit of the embryo itself in a final attempt to save its life and in the absence of other reliable forms of therapy, recourse to drugs or procedures not yet fully tested can be licit.

The corpses of human embryos and fetuses, whether they have been deliberately aborted or not, must be respected just as the remains of other human beings. In particular, they cannot be subjected to mutilation or to autopsies if their death has not yet been verified and without the consent of the parents or of the mother. Furthermore, the moral requirements must be safeguarded that there be no complicity in deliberate abortion and that the risk of scandal be avoided. Also, in the case of dead fetuses, as for the corpses of adult persons, all commercial trafficking must be considered illicit and should be prohibited.

How is one to evaluate morally the use for research purposes of embryos obtained by fertilization "in vitro"?

Human embryos obtained *in vitro* are human beings and subjects with rights: Their dignity and right to life must be respected from the first moment of their existence. *It is immoral to produce human embryos destined to be exploited as disposable "biological material."*

In the usual practice of *in vitro* fertilization, not all of the embryos are transferred to the woman's body; some are destroyed. Just as the church condemns induced abortion, so she also forbids acts against the life of these human beings. *It is a duty to condemn the particular gravity of the voluntary destruction of human embryos obtained "in vitro" for the sole purpose of research, either by means of artificial insemination or by means of "twin fission." By acting in this way the researcher usurps the place of God; and, even though he may be unaware of this, he sets himself up as the master of the destiny of others inasmuch as he arbitrarily chooses whom he will allow to live and whom he will send to death and kills defenseless human beings.*

Methods of observation or experimentation which damage or impose grave and disproportionate risks upon embryos obtained *in vitro* are morally illicit for the same reasons. Every human being is to be respected for himself and cannot be reduced in worth to a pure and simple instrument for the advantage of others. *It is therefore not in conformity with the moral law deliberately to expose to death human embryos obtained "in vitro."* In consequence of the fact that they have been produced *in vitro*, those embryos which are not transferred into the body of the mother and are called "spare" are exposed to an absurd fate, with no possibility of their being offered safe means of survival which can be licitly pursued.

What judgment should be made on other procedures of manipulating embryos connected with the "techniques of human reproduction"?

Techniques of fertilization *in vitro* can open the way to other forms of biological and genetic manipulation of human embryos, such as attempts or plans for fertilization between human and animal gametes and the gestation of human embryos in the uterus of animals, or the hypothesis or project of constructing artificial uteruses for the human embryo. *These procedures are contrary to the human dignity proper to the embryo, and at the same time they are contrary to the right of every person to be conceived and to be born within marriage and from marriage. Also, attempts or hypotheses for obtaining a human being without any connection with sexuality through "twin fission," cloning or parthenogenesis are to be considered contrary to the moral law, since they are in opposition to the dignity both of human procreation and of the conjugal union.*

The freezing of embryos, even when carried out in order to preserve the life of an embryo—cryopreservation—*constitutes an offense against the respect due to human beings* by exposing them to grave risks of death or harm to their physical integrity and depriving them, at least temporarily, of maternal shelter and gestation, thus placing them in a situation in which further offenses and manipulation are possible.

Certain attempts to influence chromosomic or genetic inheritance are not therapeutic, but are aimed at producing human beings selected according to sex or other predetermined qualities. These manipulations are contrary to the personal dignity of the human being and his or her integrity and identity. . . .

II.   INTERVENTIONS UPON HUMAN PROCREATION

. . . A preliminary point for the moral evaluation of [*in vitro* fertilization and artificial insemination] is constituted by the consideration of the circumstances and consequences which those procedures involve in relation to the respect due the human embryo. Development of the practice of *in vitro* fertilization has required innumerable fertilizations and destructions of human embryos. Even today, the usual practice presupposes a hyperovulation on the part of the woman: A number of ova are withdrawn, fertilized and then cultivated *in vitro* for some days. Usually not all are transferred into the genital tracts of the woman; some embryos, generally called "spare," are destroyed or frozen. On occasion, some of the implanted embryos are sacrificed for various eugenic, economic or psychological reasons. Such deliberate destruction of human beings or their utilization for different purposes to the detriment of their integrity and life is contrary to the doctrine on procured abortion already recalled.

The connection between *in vitro* fertilization and the voluntary destruction of human embryos occurs too often. This is significant: Through these procedures, with apparently contrary purposes, life and death are subjected to the decision of man, who thus sets himself up as the giver of life and death by decree. This dynamic of violence and domination may remain unnoticed by those very individuals who, in wishing to utilize this procedure, become subject to it themselves. The facts recorded and the cold logic which links them must be taken into consideration for a moral judgment

on *in vitro* fertilization and embryo transfer: The abortion mentality which has made this procedure possible thus leads, whether one wants it or not, to man's domination over the life and death of his fellow human beings and can lead to a system of radical eugenics. . . .

A.   Heterologous* Artificial Fertilization

Why must human procreation take place in marriage?

Every human being is always to be accepted as a gift and blessing of God. However, from the moral point of view a truly responsible procreation vis-a-vis the unborn child must be the fruit of marriage.

For human procreation has specific characteristics by virtue of the personal dignity of the parents and of the children: The procreation of a new person, whereby the man and the woman collaborate with the power of the Creator, must be the fruit and the sign of the mutual self-giving of the spouses, of their love and of their fidelity. *The fidelity of the spouses in the unity of marriage involves reciprocal respect of their right to become a father and a mother only through each other.*

The child has the right to be conceived, carried in the womb, brought into the world and brought up within marriage: It is through the secure and recognized relationship to his own parents that the child can discover his own identity and achieve his own proper human development.

The parents find in their child a confirmation and completion of their reciprocal self-giving: The child is the living image of their love, the permanent sign of their conjugal union, the living and indissoluble concrete expression of their paternity and maternity.

By reason of the vocation and social responsibilities of the person, the good of the children and of the parents contributes to the good of civil society; the vitality and stability of society require that children come into the world within a family and that the family be firmly based on marriage.

---

* [Heterologous: involving sperm and egg from a man and woman who are not married to each other.]

The tradition of the church and anthropological reflection recognize in marriage and in its indissoluble unity the only setting worthy of truly responsible procreation.

Does heterologous artificial fertilization conform to the dignity of the couple and to the truth of marriage?

Through *in vitro* fertilization and embryo transfer and heterologous artificial insemination, human conception is achieved through the fusion of gametes of at least one donor other than the spouses who are united in marriage. *Heterologous artificial fertilization is contrary to the unity of marriage, to the dignity of the spouses, to the vocation proper to parents, and to the child's right to be conceived and brought into the world in marriage and from marriage.*

Respect for the unity of marriage and for conjugal fidelity demands that the child be conceived in marriage; the bond existing between husband and wife accords the spouses, in an objective and inalienable manner, the exclusive right to become father and mother solely through each other. Recourse to the gametes of a third person in order to have sperm or ovum available constitutes a violation of the reciprocal commitment of the spouses and a grave lack in regard to that essential property of marriage which is its unity.

Heterologous artificial fertilization violates the rights of the child; it deprives him of his filial relationship with his parental origins and can hinder the maturing of his personal identity. Furthermore, it offends the common vocation of the spouses who are called to fatherhood and motherhood: It objectively deprives conjugal fruitfulness of its unity and integrity; it brings about and manifests a rupture between genetic parenthood, gestational parenthood and responsibility for upbringing. Such damage to the personal relationships within the family has repercussions on civil society: What threatens the unity and stability of the family is a source of dissension, disorder and injustice in the whole of social life.

These reasons lead to a negative moral judgment concerning heterologous artificial fertilization: Consequently, fertilization of a married woman with the sperm of a donor different from her husband and fertilization with the husband's sperm of an ovum not coming from his wife are morally illicit. Furthermore, the artificial fertilization of a woman who is unmarried or a widow, whoever the donor may be, cannot be morally justified.

The desire to have a child and the love between spouses who long to obviate a sterility which cannot be overcome in any other way constitute understandable motivations; but subjectively good intentions do not render heterologous artificial fertilization conformable to the objective and inalienable properties of marriage or respectful of the rights of the child and of the spouses.

Is "surrogate" motherhood morally licit?

No, for the same reasons which lead one to reject heterologous artificial fertilization: For it is contrary to the unity of marriage and to the dignity of the procreation of the human person. . . .

B. Homologous* Artificial Fertilization

Since heterologous artificial fertilization has been declared unacceptable, the question arises of how to evaluate morally the process of homologous artificial fertilization: *in vitro* fertilization and embryo transfer and artificial insemination between husband and wife. First a question of principle must be clarified.

What connection is required from the moral point of view between procreation and the conjugal act?

(a) The church's teaching on marriage and human procreation affirms the "inseparable connection, willed by God and unable to be broken by man on his own initiative, between the two meanings of the conjugal act: the unitive meaning and the procreative meaning. Indeed, by its intimate structure the conjugal act, while most closely uniting husband and wife, capacitates them for the generation of new lives according to laws inscribed in the very being of man and of woman." . . . "By safeguarding both these essential aspects, the unitive and the procreative, the conjugal act preserves in its fullness the sense of

---

*[Homologous: involving sperm and egg from a man and woman who are married to each other.]

true mutual love and its ordination toward man's exalted vocation to parenthood."

The same doctrine concerning the link between the meanings of the conjugal act and between the goods of marriage throws light on the moral problem of homologous artificial fertilization, since "it is never permitted to separate these different aspects to such a degree as positively to exclude either the procreative intention or the conjugal relation."

Contraception deliberately deprives the conjugal act of its openness to procreation and in this way brings about a voluntary dissociation of the ends of marriage. Homologous artificial fertilization, in seeking a procreation which is not the fruit of a specific act of conjugal union, objectively effects an analogous separation between the goods and the meanings of marriage.

Thus . . . *from the moral point of view procreation is deprived of its proper perfection when it is not desired as the fruit of the conjugal act, that is to say, of the specific act of the spouses' union.*

(b) The moral value of the intimate link between the goods of marriage and between the meanings of the conjugal act is based upon the unity of the human being, a unity involving body and spiritual soul. Spouses mutually express their personal love in the "language of the body," which clearly involves both "spousal meanings" and parental ones. The conjugal act by which the couple mutually express their self-gift at the same time expresses openness to the gift of life. It is an act that is inseparably corporal and spiritual. It is in their bodies and through their bodies that the spouses consummate their marriage and are able to become father and mother. In order to respect the language of their bodies and their natural generosity, the conjugal union must take place with respect for its openness to procreation; and the procreation of a person must be the fruit and the result of married love. The origin of the human being thus follows from a procreation that is "linked to the union, not only biological but also spiritual, of the parents, made one by the bond of marriage." Fertilization achieved outside the bodies of the couple remains by this very fact deprived of the meanings and the values which are expressed in the language of the body and in the union of human persons.

(c) Only respect for the link between the meanings of the conjugal act and respect for the unity of the human being make possible procreation in conformity with the dignity of the person. In his unique and irrepeatable origin, the child must be respected and recognized as equal in personal dignity to those who give him life. The human person must be accepted in his parents' act of union and love; the generation of a child must therefore be the fruit of that mutual giving which is realized in the conjugal act wherein the spouses cooperate as servants and not as masters in the work of the Creator, who is love.

In reality, the origin of a human person is the result of an act of giving. The one conceived must be the fruit of his parents' love. He cannot be desired or conceived as the product of an intervention of medical or biological techniques; that would be equivalent to reducing him to an object of scientific technology. No one may subject the coming of a child into the world to conditions of technical efficiency which are to be evaluated according to standards of control and dominion.

The moral relevance of the link between the meanings of the conjugal act and between the goods of marriage, as well as the unity of the human being and the dignity of his origin, demand that the procreation of a human person be brought about as the fruit of the conjugal act specific to the love between spouses. . . .

Is homologous "in vitro" fertilization morally licit?

The answer to this question is strictly dependent on the principles just mentioned. Certainly one cannot ignore the legitimate aspirations of sterile couples. For some, recourse to homologous *in vitro* fertilization and embryo transfer appears to be the only way of fulfilling their sincere desire for a child. The question is asked whether the totality of conjugal life in such situations is not sufficient to ensure the dignity proper to human procreation. It is acknowledged that *in vitro* fertilization and embryo transfer certainly cannot supply for the absence of sexual relations and cannot be preferred to the specific acts of conjugal union, given the risks involved for the child and the difficulties of the procedure. But it is asked whether, when there is no other way of overcoming the sterility which is a source of suffering, homologous *in vitro* fertilization may not constitute an aid, if not a form of therapy, whereby its moral licitness could be admitted.

The desire for a child—or at the very least an openness to the transmission of life—is a necessary prerequisite from the moral point of view for responsible human procreation. But this good intention is not sufficient for making a positive moral evaluation of *in vitro* fertilization between spouses. The process of *in vitro* fertilization and embryo transfer must be judged in itself and cannot borrow its definitive moral quality from the totality of conjugal life of which it becomes part nor from the conjugal acts which may precede or follow it. . . .

[E]ven in a situation in which every precaution were taken to avoid the death of human embryos, homologous *in vitro* fertilization and embryo transfer dissociates from the conjugal act the actions which are directed to human fertilization. For this reason the very nature of homologous *in vitro* fertilization and embryo transfer also must be taken into account, even abstracting from the link with procured abortion.

Homologous *in vitro* fertilization and embryo transfer is brought about outside the bodies of the couple through actions of third parties whose competence and technical activity determine the success of the procedure. Such fertilization entrusts the life and identity of the embryo into the power of doctors and biologists and establishes the domination of technology over the origin and destiny of the human person. Such a relationship of domination is in itself contrary to the dignity and equality that must be common to parents and children.

Conception *in vitro* is the result of the technical action which presides over fertilization. *Such fertilization is neither in fact achieved nor positively willed as the expression and fruit of a specific act of the conjugal union. In homologous "in vitro" fertilization and embryo transfer, therefore, even if it is considered in the context of de facto existing sexual relations, the generation of the human person is objectively deprived of its proper perfection: namely, that of being the result and fruit of a conjugal act in which the spouses can become "cooperators with God for giving life to a new person."* . . .

Although the manner in which human conception is achieved with *in vitro* fertilization and embryo transfer cannot be approved, every child which comes into the world must in any case be accepted as a living gift of the divine Goodness and must be brought up with love.

How is homologous artificial insemination to be evaluated from the moral point of view?

Homologous artificial insemination within marriage cannot be admitted except for those cases in which the technical means is not a substitute for the conjugal act but serves to facilitate and to help so that the act attains its natural purpose. . . .

"In its natural structure, the conjugal act is a personal action, a simultaneous and immediate cooperation on the part of the husband and wife, which by the very nature of the agents and the proper nature of the act is the expression of the mutual gift which, according to the words of Scripture, brings about union 'in one flesh.'" Thus moral conscience "does not necessarily proscribe the use of certain artificial means destined solely either to the facilitating of the natural act or to ensuring that the natural act normally performed achieves its proper end." If the technical means facilitates the conjugal act or helps it to reach its natural objectives, it can be morally acceptable. If, on the other hand, the procedure were to replace the conjugal act, it is morally illicit.

Artificial insemination as a substitute for the conjugal act is prohibited by reason of the voluntarily achieved dissociation of the two meanings of the conjugal act. Masturbation, through which the sperm is normally obtained, is another sign of this dissociation: Even when it is done for the purpose of procreation the act remains deprived of its unitive meaning: "It lacks the sexual relationship called for by the moral order, namely the relationship which realizes 'the full sense of mutual self-giving and human procreation in the context of true love.'" . . .

What moral criterion can be proposed with regard to medical intervention in human procreation?

The medical act must be evaluated not only with reference to its technical dimension, but also and above all in relation to its goal, which is the good of persons and their bodily and psychological health. The moral criteria for medical intervention in procreation are deduced from the dignity of human persons, of their sexuality and of their origin.

Medicine which seeks to be ordered to the integral good of the person must respect the specifically human values of sexuality. The doctor is at the service of persons and of human procreation. He does not have the authority to dispose of them or to decide their fate. A medical intervention respects the dignity of persons when it seeks to assist the conjugal act either in order to facilitate its performance or in order to enable it to achieve its objective once it has been normally performed.

On the other hand, it sometimes happens that a medical procedure technologically replaces the conjugal act in order to obtain a procreation which is neither its result nor its fruit. In this case the medical act is not, as it should be, at the service of conjugal union, but rather appropriates to itself the procreative function and thus contradicts the dignity and the inalienable rights of the spouses and of the child to be born.

The humanization of medicine, which is insisted upon today by everyone, requires respect for the integral dignity of the human person first of all in the act and at the moment in which the spouses transmit life to a new person. It is only logical therefore to address an urgent appeal to Catholic doctors and scientists that they bear exemplary witness to the respect due to the human embryo and to the dignity of procreation. The medical and nursing staff of Catholic hospitals and clinics are in a special way urged to do justice to the moral obligations which they have assumed, frequently also, as part of their contract. Those who are in charge of Catholic hospitals and clinics and who are often religious will take special care to safeguard and promote a diligent observance of the moral norms recalled in the present instruction.

The suffering caused by infertility in marriage.

The suffering of spouses who cannot have children or who are afraid of bringing a handicapped child into the world is a suffering that everyone must understand and properly evaluate.

On the part of the spouses, the desire for a child is natural: It expresses the vocation to fatherhood and motherhood inscribed in conjugal love. This desire can be even stronger if the couple is affected by sterility which appears incurable. Nevertheless, marriage does not confer upon the spouses the right to have a child, but only the right to perform those natural acts which are per se ordered to procreation.

A true and proper right to a child would be contrary to the child's dignity and nature. The child is not an object to which one has a right nor can he be considered

as an object of ownership: Rather, a child is a gift, "the supreme gift" and the most gratuitous gift of marriage, and is a living testimony of the mutual giving of his parents. For this reason, the child has the right as already mentioned, to be the fruit of the specific act of the conjugal love of his parents; and he also has the right to be respected as a person from the moment of his conception.

Nevertheless, whatever its cause or prognosis, sterility is certainly a difficult trial. The community of believers is called to shed light upon and support the suffering of those who are unable to fulfill their legitimate aspiration to motherhood and fatherhood. Spouses who find themselves in this sad situation are called to find in it an opportunity for sharing in a particular way in the Lord's cross, the source of spiritual fruitfulness. Sterile couples must not forget that "even when procreation is not possible, conjugal life does not for this reason lose its value. Physical sterility in fact can be for spouses the occasion for other important services to the life of the human person, for example, adoption, various forms of educational work and assistance to other families and to poor or handicapped children." . . .

III. MORAL AND CIVIL LAW

The Values and Moral Obligations That Civil Legislation Must Respect and Sanction in This Matter

The inviolable right to life of every innocent human individual and the rights of the family and of the institution of marriage constitute fundamental moral values because they concern the natural condition and integral vocation of the human person; at the same time they are constitutive elements of civil society and its order.

For this reason the new technological possibilities which have opened up in the field of biomedicine require the intervention of the political authorities and of the legislator, since an uncontrolled application of such techniques could lead to unforeseeable and damaging consequences for civil society. Recourse to the conscience of each individual and to the self-regulation of researchers cannot be sufficient for ensuring respect for personal rights and public order. . . .

The intervention of the public authority must be inspired by the rational principles which regulate the relationships between civil law and moral law. The task of the civil law is to ensure the common good of people through the recognition of and the defense of fundamental rights and through the promotion of peace and of public morality. . . .

As a consequence of the respect and protection which must be ensured for the unborn child from the moment of his conception, the law must provide appropriate penal sanctions for every deliberate violation of the child's rights. The law cannot tolerate—indeed it must expressly forbid—that human beings, even at the embryonic stage, should be treated as objects of experimentation, be mutilated or destroyed with the excuse that they are superfluous or incapable of developing normally.

The political authority is bound to guarantee to the institution of the family, upon which society is based, the juridical protection to which it has a right. From the very fact that it is at the service of people, the political authority must also be at the service of the family. Civil law cannot grant approval to techniques of artificial procreation which, for the benefit of third parties (doctors, biologists, economic or governmental powers), take away what is a right inherent in the relationship between spouses; and therefore civil law cannot legalize the donation of gametes between persons who are not legitimately united in marriage.

Legislation must also prohibit, by virtue of the support which is due to the family, embryo banks, post-mortem insemination and "surrogate motherhood." . . .

WHAT ARE FAMILIES FOR? GETTING TO AN ETHICS OF REPRODUCTIVE TECHNOLOGY

Thomas H. Murray

Procreative liberty, as the regnant contemporary framework for thinking about the ethics of reproductive technologies, has its defects. It begins with a pair of confusions and disregards a central, vital interest; it ignores the values at the heart of family life and relies on a thin and unsatisfying conception of human flourishing.

Intellectual frameworks matter: They direct our attention toward certain moral considerations over others, and they implicitly tell us what, like the cents column on income tax returns, can be ignored. Once the shortcomings of procreative liberty as the dominant framework in ethical discourse on assisted reproduction become obvious, so does the need for a more fulsome and nuanced framework, one that begins with the moral significance of the

relationship between parents and children, the values at the heart of that relationship, and the ways in which people flourish, or shrivel—physically, emotionally, and morally.

I want to describe briefly the defects in procreative liberty as a framework for thinking about parents and children. I also want to propose a different starting point—a more challenging and complex one to be sure, that begins with what we value most highly and insists on keeping the broader picture in view, however difficult that may sometimes be. Finally, I want to explore what difference it would make to begin with one rather than the other framework.

AN IMPOVERISHED WORLDVIEW

The confusions in the standard account of procreative liberty are twofold. First, procreative liberty seems confused as to its purpose. Does it mean to

From *Hastings Center Report* 32, no. 3 (2002): 41–45. Reprinted by permission of The Hastings Center.

be an insightful ethical analysis that illuminates what is morally important about families, parents, and children? Or is it only a quasi-moral, quasi-legal algorithm for considering questions about law and policy in reproductive technologies? Its proponents often write as if procreative liberty was indeed a comprehensive moral account of the ethics of initiating parenthood and implicitly of parenthood in general.[1]

The second confusion abides in the claim that decisions about what sort of child to have and what means to employ to create a child are merely the flip side of decisions *whether* to have a child—that is, decisions about abortion and contraception. Advocates of procreative liberty fix on the free choices of presumably autonomous adults. But abortion and contraception are means *to not have* a child, at least not at this time, or not under these circumstances. The not-so-flip side is the decision *to have* a child, to create a new person who will have interests, hopes, and concerns of her or his own. It is also a decision to initiate a vital, life-long relationship.

The most egregious defect of procreative liberty is its nearly complete disregard of the interests of children created through reproductive technologies. Advocates of procreative liberty accept one side-constraint: it does not justify creating a child who is worse off than if he or she had never been born at all. I have described this as akin to trying to divide by zero—an arithmetic operation that cannot yield a meaningful answer. All we need agree here is that, as a practical matter, this supposed constraint in practice constrains far too little, if it constrains anything at all.

Imagine a couple who ask that the developing spinal column of their fetus be disrupted, making the child paraplegic. Why would they want to do such a thing? Perhaps they desire the experience of raising a child with a disability, perhaps they believe the demands of caring for such a child will help keep their failing marriage together, perhaps they already have a child with paraplegia, desire another, but do not want their older child to feel less capable than its younger sibling or the child-to-be to feel different from its older sibling. We may be curious about the reasons or motivations behind such a request, but procreative liberty disallows interest in reasons and motivation. It is none of your business, procreative liberty declares.

I want to be clear: I do not believe that proponents of procreative liberty embrace the prospect of prenatal mutilation. My point is rather that the conceptual framework they employ provides no firm support for morally condemning such an action. It permits adults to use virtually any reproductive means for virtually any end; it prohibits or condemns almost nothing. The test of an analytic moral framework cannot be limited to those cases for which it gives the answers one wants; if it provides morally dubious or outrageous answers in other cases, or feeble answers where moral judgments should be clear and ringing, then we have reason to doubt its insightfulness and completeness.

The third defect, procreative liberty's failure to acknowledge values at the heart of family life, is the most sweeping difficulty and at the same time the most difficult to remedy. Control and choice—the values at the heart of procreative liberty—are not entirely out of place in the relationship between parents and children. But they are hardly the entire story, or even the most important themes, and excesses of control and choice can distort and destroy what is most precious in families.

FAMILIES, VALUES, AND HUMAN FLOURISHING

The standard account of procreative liberty is truncated and impoverished. It limits its moral universe to a few values, primarily autonomous adult choice and control. Left out are the values served by parenthood and families, and the role that enduring relationships play in our flourishing as human beings.

Advocates of procreative liberty might argue that the decision about which particular values to pursue is left to the adults making the choice. They can point to the analogy with a woman's right to choose whether to become pregnant or to carry that pregnancy to term.

Here, I think, is where procreative liberty makes a fundamental mistake. Whatever one believes about women's moral rights concerning birth control or abortion, it is undeniable that becoming pregnant and giving birth to a child have an enormous impact on women's lives and on their possibilities for flourishing. Having, raising, and loving a child is a profoundly life-altering experience for both women and men. We must not lose sight of this. At the same time, unpredictable and uncontrolled fertility can restrict women's opportunities for education and work; it consigns some women to deep, enduring poverty.

Procreative liberty's problems began when it appropriated the abstract principle—the right to choose—and ripped it out of the rich context that provided its moral heft: women's prospects for flourishing are diminished when they have no control over their fertility. Procreative liberty then applied that abstracted idea to a very different context—parents, children, and families—with little or no reflection on how these affect our flourishing.

We need a richer ethical framework. We need a framework that acknowledges what should be obvious: decisions about *having* a child are not merely the other side of the moral/legal coin of decisions *not to have* a child. Many people—indeed, probably a robust majority of Americans—support women's access to abortion yet have qualms about the commercialization of reproduction, the growing powers of control over the traits of our children, and reproductive cloning. Our framework must acknowledge the moral significance and interests of the children created through reproductive technologies and do so in a full and robust manner, not as a side-constraint that proves meaningless in practice. And this framework must attend carefully to the values central to the relationship between parents and children, and not be satisfied with the valorization of choice and control in the hands of autonomous adults.

Having and raising children is not the only way to find the enduring, intimate relationships that typify families. But it is the path chosen by many, including those who use reproductive technologies. There are central human values that are either found only in the context of enduring, committed human relationships such as families, or that rely upon such relationships for their realization. Values such as love, loyalty, intimacy, steadfastness, acceptance, and forgiveness are crucial to well-functioning families, which are also the most robust settings in which to raise children to become confident, competent, loving, and emotionally resilient adults.

I do not mean to romanticize families: families can be riven by selfishness, betrayal, and mistrust, or shattered by injustice and oppression. Humans are fallible and all families are imperfect. Yet families are also astonishingly powerful communities of shared memory and experience. Those memories can be scorching and bitter—consider children who were victims of sexual abuse within their family. But they can also be sweet or, perhaps as powerful an emotional glue, a bittersweet mingling of disappointment and loss with love and enduring mutual constancy.

HOW WE GOT HERE

The roots of our current way of framing the ethics of reproduction are old and deep, manifested in the nascent bioethics movement in the latter half of the twentieth century. As bioethics began to gather steam as a field of scholarly inquiry with an accompanying commentary on practical ethical issues, there arose parallel social and political currents concerning women's reproductive capabilities, the emergence of effective and reasonably safe means for controlling those capabilities, and with those new means of control, new possibilities for women's lives. Women could now think about what a good life for them would entail, a good life that had no need to deny a central role to having, raising, and loving children, yet one that also envisioned creative work and other activities outside the household, activities that uncontrolled fertility made difficult or impossible.

The availability of reliable and reasonably safe and convenient contraception has been credited with leading to a sharp change in sexual mores. But that may be looking through the wrong end of the telescope. Contraception, and then in 1973 the legalization of abortion, gave women the means to avoid having a child when for whatever reason they did not want to. What also happened, particularly in the wake of the U.S. Supreme Court decision in *Roe V. Wade*, was that different views of women's nature and flourishing had now been laid out for all to see and had become pivotal in the fierce debates and policy battles over abortion.

Less attention has been paid to differences in the conceptions of men's flourishing, but those differences are every bit as important. As Kristen Luker has written, people's views about abortion were woven deeply into a complex fabric of beliefs, not least about what constituted flourishing for women and for men, and how disparate those two conceptions were from each other.[2] For several years when my children were very young, I cared for them as a single parent, and when Cynthia and I met and married, we cared together for them, including a daughter born from our marriage. The caring I experienced from my own parents—father as well as mother—prepared me well to care for—and enjoy profoundly—my children. A sharp division of capacities between men and women has never struck me as convincing. Women can be more or less competitive; so can men. Men can be better or worse nurturers; the same for women.

Reflections such as these have convinced me that we must take seriously conceptions of human flourishing if we are to have any chance for meaningful moral dialogue or robust and sensible public policy on a variety of issues concerning conceiving, bearing, and raising children. Any wise inquiry into ideas about human flourishing must acknowledge diversity. It must also, I believe, pay great attention to the similarities and the disparities between the conceptions held about flourishing for women and for men.

It would be unforgivably foolish to presume that all people everywhere shared the same notions of human flourishing. The Taliban, for one, made very sharp distinctions in their perceptions of good lives for women and for men, differences that are likely to reflect and be reflected by assumptions about the nature of women and men. As this example suggests, diversity must be given its due—but not more than its due. If you ask your neighbors where they find meaning in their lives, they will tell you in overwhelming numbers that it is in their families. If you talk with someone who has recently had their first child, as my daughter Kate and her husband Matt did with Grace Emilia, our first grandchild, they are likely to tell you—through the haze of exhaustion—that the experience is life-transforming and wondrous.

None of this is peculiar to post-industrial America. In his stunning scholarly tour de force, *The Kindness of Strangers: The Abandonment of Children in Western Europe from Late Antiquity to the Renaissance,* the late historian John Boswell wrote:

> Everywhere in Western culture, from religious literature to secular poetry, parental love is invoked as the ultimate standard of selfless and untiring devotion, central metaphors of theology and ethics presuppose this love as a universal point of reference, and language must devise special terms to characterize persons wanting in this "natural" affection.[3]

And I can agree with Thomas Jefferson who wrote to his daughter of his hope that his granddaughter "will make us all, and long, happy as the center of our common love."[4]

The awful price that must be paid for this profound attachment, when a child dies, is the enormous, life-long grief that comes in its wake. People say that the death of your child is the worst thing that can happen to a person. Our experience affirms the truth of that.

Of course, there are families in which deep affection never takes hold, or loses out to selfishness or indifference. And there are times and places when grinding poverty and uncontrolled fertility led to the abandonment of many children who could not be cared for. But the fact that all parents are imperfect and some downright awful, and that some families are blighted by poverty or illness or oppression or any of a multitude of factors that can stunt the growth of love and mutual concern, should not blind us to what is morally and emotionally important about families, to the central role families play in many people's flourishing.

We will find better insight about what it means to be human, I believe, by reflecting on the central relationships in our lives and the significance of those relationships for our flourishing, than by focusing exclusively on the liberty of autonomous adults. We must take care to acknowledge and understand differences among conceptions of flourishing, but we should not reflexively set aside the best and most broadly shared understandings of human flourishing simply because no single one commands universal accord.[5]

Those different conceptions lie barely beneath the surface of some of our most bitter public disputes, yet we regularly fail to acknowledge or probe for possible areas of agreement. The obvious example is the debate over abortion, where the disputants prefer to battle over intractable metaphysical questions about the moral status of fetuses and embryos or the limits of state control over women's bodies. These are important questions, to be sure, but they are not the only wedges into the broader disagreements. They are merely the ones that allow partisans on both sides to feel righteous.

It is neither likely nor desirable that only one rich, full-fledged conception of human flourishing prevail in our public policy debate. But I do believe that failing to engage each other about competing conceptions of human flourishing and the values central to family life results in a moral debate in which many of the most important elements remain hidden or scarcely noticed. It likewise results in public policies that are fiercely resisted—as in abortion—or virtually non-existent—regrettably true of reproductive technologies in the United States (a lack that makes us an object of curiosity in other countries). The divide between right-to-life and pro-choice factions in the United States has resulted in an enormous hole in American public policy. Any political leader who takes on the world of infertility treatment, IVF, and the like does so at risk of his or her political life.

WHERE TO START THINKING

In practice, procreative liberty and what we could call a flourishing-centered approach diverge especially in what moral considerations they include. Take, for example, the case of the Nash family. Their daughter, Molly, would die without a life-saving infusion of healthy, immunologically compatible blood stem cells. One possible source: the stem cell-rich umbilical cord blood from a new brother or sister. The Nashes used preimplantation genetic diagnosis for two simultaneous purposes—to avoid having another child with Fanconi anemia, a life-threatening illness, and to choose an embryo that might become, upon birth, a compatible cord blood donor for its older sister. Procreative liberty dictates a two-step analysis: Was this choice an authentic, informed expression of the prospective parents' autonomy? Would the child have been better off never being born at all? If the answers are, respectively, yes and no, then procreative liberty gives its blessing.

An approach centered on human flourishing requires much more. It begins with reflections on parents and children, on the values served by and intrinsic to this relationship, and on the significance of the proposed act, practice, or policy for the flourishing of children and parents. This is not a simple or easy task. It's more like a complex life-long inquiry.

The process is not mysterious, however. We must reflect on the values that are most important and most widely shared for parents, children, and families; on what makes for good lives for children, women, and men. There will not be one and only one morally defensible account of human flourishing. But not all accounts will be equally convincing. Some seek fulfillment and pleasure through tyranny and oppression or by inflicting physical or emotional cruelty, by employing manipulation and deceit, resulting in emotional emptiness. If someone wishes to defend that as a morally desirable form of human flourishing, let them try.

An insightful analysis will also acknowledge that institutions and practices shape the possibilities for flourishing—or its negation. The shaping factors include law and public policy of course, but also culture, economic circumstances, and professional norms. We must consider the implications of whatever choice confronts us for each of these factors, just as we ask how those factors themselves give shape to that choice—and how they might be refashioned to support human flourishing more vigorously.

Thinking about the Nash case by attending to values, flourishing, and context compels us to ask difficult questions. Does preimplantation testing and selection in this instance support or undermine the values central to parents and children? Will it strengthen that family's prospects for flourishing, or erode them? What effect will this case have on practices and policies in preimplantation genetic testing?

Each of these questions deserves extended reflection, more than I can provide here. My sense is that, in the end, we would conclude that the Nash family's choice was an ethically defensible action, born in compassion for the suffering of one child, and not an effort to exert excessive control over the traits of another. We could come to a very different conclusion about parents wanting to impose their preferences for less compelling ends. By contrast, procreative liberty has difficulty summoning the ethical will to curb the indulgence of almost any parental whim. That is a vitally important difference.

What are families for? This is the question we must ask when we think about the ethics of reproductive technologies. Choice and control are to be valued, but not limitlessly, and not as decisive moral panaceas. Choice is not the universal moral solvent, dissolving all moral dilemmas. We should turn first to that which shapes our lives and gives them meaning, and especially to those enduring relationships of mutual caring that grow between parents and children. Those relationships occupy crucial places in the grand tapestries of images and narratives that depict our richest and fullest images of human flourishing, as well as human failure, cruelty, and misery. When we avert our gaze from those tapestries, we blind ourselves to what ought to be our starting point for thinking insightfully about ethical issues in creating children.

REFERENCES

1. J.A. Robertson, *Children of Choice: Freedom and the New Reproductive Technologies* (Princeton, N.J.: Princeton University Press, 1994).

2. Kristen Luker describes these views, and the impact of recognizing that other people held quite different ones, on activists in both the pro-choice and right-to-life movements in *Abortion and the Politics of Motherhood* (Berkeley, Calif., University of California Press, 1984).

3. J. Boswell, *The Kindness of Strangers: The Abandonments of Children in Western Europe from Late Antiquity to the Renaissance* (New York, Pantheon Press, 1988), at 37–38.

4. Quoted in S.N. Randolph, *The Domestic Life of Thomas Jefferson* (New York: Frederick Ungar, 1958).

5. T.H. Murray, *The Worth of a Child* (Berkeley, Calif.: University of California Press, 1996).

GRADE A: THE MARKET FOR A YALE WOMAN'S EGGS

Jessica Cohen

Early in the spring of last year a classified ad ran for two weeks in the *Yale Daily News:* "Egg Donor Needed." The couple that placed the ad was picky, and for that reason was offering $25,000 for an egg from the right donor.

As a child I had a book called *Where Did I Come From?* It offered a full biological explanation, in cartoons, to answer those awkward questions that curious tots ask. But the book is now out of date. Replacing it is, for example, *Mommy, Did I Grow in Your Tummy?: Where Some Babies Come From,* which explains the myriad ways that children of the twenty-first century may have entered their families, including egg donation, surrogacy, *in vitro* fertilization, and adoption. When conception doesn't occur in the natural way, it becomes very complicated. Once all possible parties have been accounted for—egg donor, sperm donor, surrogate mother, paying couple—as many as five people can be involved in conceiving and carrying a child. No wonder a new book is necessary.

The would-be parents' decision to advertise in the *News*—and to offer a five-figure compensation—immediately suggested that they were in the market for an egg of a certain rarefied type. Beyond their desire for an Ivy League donor, they wanted a young woman over five feet five, of Jewish heritage, athletic, with a minimum combined SAT score of 1500, and attractive. I was curious—and I fit all the criteria except the SAT score. So I e-mailed Michelle and David (not their real names) and asked for more information about the process and how much the SAT minimum really meant to them. Then I waited for a reply.

Donating an egg is neither simple nor painless. Following an intensive screening and selection process the donor endures a few weeks of invasive medical procedures. First the donor and the woman who will carry the child must coordinate their menstrual cycles. Typically the donor and the recipient take birth-control pills, followed by shots of a synthetic hormone such as Lupron; the combination suppresses ovulation and puts their cycles in sync. After altering her cycle the donor must enhance her egg supply with fertility drugs in the same way an infertile woman does when trying to conceive. Shots of a fertility hormone are administered for seven to eleven days, to stimulate the production of an abnormally large number of egg-containing follicles. During this time the donor must have her blood tested every other day so that doctors can monitor her hormone levels, and she must come in for periodic ultrasounds. Thirty-six hours before retrieval day a shot of hCG, human chorionic gonadotropin, is administered to prepare the eggs for release, so that they will be ready for harvest.

The actual retrieval is done while the donor is under anesthesia. The tool is a needle, and the product, on average, is ten to twenty eggs. Doctors take that many because "not all eggs will be good," according to Surrogate Mothers Online, an informational Web site designed and maintained by experienced egg donors and surrogate mothers. "Some will be immature and some overripe."

Lisa, one of the hosts on Surrogate Mothers Online and an experienced egg donor, described the process as a "rewarding" experience. When she explained that once in a while something can go wrong, I braced myself for the fine print. On very rare occasions, she wrote, hyperstimulation of the ovaries can occur, and the donor must be hospitalized until the ovaries return to normal. In even rarer cases the ovaries rupture, resulting in permanent infertility or possibly even death. "I must stress that this is very rare," Lisa assured prospective donors. "I had two very wonderful experiences . . . The second [time] I stayed awake to help the doctor count how many eggs he retrieved."

David responded to my e-mail a few hours after I'd sent it. He told me nothing about himself, and only briefly alluded to the many questions I had asked about the egg-donation process. He spent the bulk of the e-mail describing a cartoon, and then requested photos of me. The cartoon was a scene with a "couple that is just getting married, he a nerd and she a beauty," he wrote. "They are kvelling about how wonderful their offspring will be with his brains and her looks." He went on to describe the punch line: the next panel showed a nerdy-looking baby thinking empty thoughts. The following paragraph was more direct. David let me know that he and his wife were flexible on most criteria but that Michelle was "a real Nazi" about "donor looks and donor health history."

This seemed to be a commentary of some sort on the couple's situation and how plans might go awry, but the message was impossible to pin down. I thanked him for the e-mail, asked where to send my pictures, and repeated my original questions about egg donation and their criteria.

In a subsequent e-mail David promised to return my photos, so I sent him dorm-room pictures, the kind that every college student has lying around. Now they assumed a new level of importance. I would soon learn what this anonymous couple, somewhere in the United States, thought about my genetic material as displayed in these photographs.

Infertility is not a modern problem, but it has created a modern industry. Ten percent of American couples are infertile, and many seek treatment from the $2-billion-a-year infertility industry. The approximately 370 fertility clinics across the United States help prospective parents to sift through their options. I sympathize with women who cannot use their own eggs to have children. The discovery must be a sober awakening for those who have always dreamed of raising a family. When would-be parents face this problem, however, their options depend greatly on their income. All over the world most women who can't have children must simply accept the fact and adopt, or find other roles in society. But especially here in the United States wealth can enable such couples to have a child of their own and to determine how closely that child will resemble the one they might have had—or the one they dream of having.

The Web site of Egg Donation, Inc, a program based in California, contains a database listing approximately 300 potential donors. In order to access the list interested parties must call the company and request the user ID and the password for the month. Once I'd given the receptionist my name and address, she told me the password "colorful," I hung up and entered the database. Potential parents can search for a variety of features, narrowing the pool as much as they like according to ethnic origin, religion of birth, state of residence, hair color, eye color, height, and weight. I typed in the physical and religious characteristics that Michelle and David were looking for and found four potential donors. None of them had a college degree.

The standard compensation for donating an egg to Egg Donation is $3,500 to $5,000, and additional funds are offered to donors who have advanced degrees or are of Asian, African-American, or Jewish descent. Couples searching for an egg at Egg Donation can be picky, but not as picky as couples advertising in the *Yale Daily News*. Should couples be able to pay a premium on an open market for their idea of the perfect egg? Maybe a modern-day Social Darwinist would say yes. Modern success is measured largely in financial terms, so why shouldn't the most successful couples, eager to pay more, have access to the most expensive eggs? Of course, as David illustrated in his first e-mail, input does not always translate perfectly into output—the donor's desirable characteristics may never actually be manifested in the child.

If couples choose not to find their eggs through an agency, they must do so independently. An Internet search turned up a few sites like Surrogate Mothers Online, where would-be donors and parents can post classified ads. More than 500 classifieds were posted on the site: a whole marketplace, an eBay for genetic material.

"Hi! My name is Kimberly," one of the ads read. "I am 24 years old, 5' 6" with blonde hair and green eyes. I previously donated eggs and the couple was blessed with BIG twin boys! The doctor told me I have perky ovaries!. . . . The doctor told me I had the most perfect eggs he had ever seen." The Web site provided links to photographs of Kimberly and an e-mail address. Would-be parents on the site offered "competitive" rates, generally from $5,000 to $10,000 for donors who fit their specifications.

About a week after I sent my pictures to David and Michelle, I received a third e-mail: "Got the pictures. You look perfect. I can't say this with any authority. That is my wife's department." I thought back to the first e-mail, where he'd written, "She's been known to disregard a young woman based on cheekbones, hair, nose, you name it." He then shifted the focus. "My department is the SAT scores. Can you tell me more about your academic performance? What are you taking at Yale? What high school did you attend?"

The whole thing seemed like a joke. I dutifully answered his questions, explaining that I was from a no-name high school in the Midwest, I couldn't do math or science, and my academic performance was, well, average; I couldn't help feeling a bit disconcerted by his particular interest in my SAT score.

Michelle and David now had my educational data as well as my photos. They were examining my credentials and trying to imagine their child. If I was accepted, a harvest of my eggs would be fertilized by the semen of the author of the disturbing e-mails I had received. A few embryos would be implanted; the remaining, if there were any, would be frozen; and then I would be out of the picture forever.

The modern embryo has been frozen, stolen, aborted, researched, and delivered weeks early, along with five or six instant siblings. The summer of 2001 was full of embryo news, and the first big story was President Bush's deliberation on stem-cell research. The embryos available for genetic research include those frozen by fertility clinics for later use by couples attempting *in vitro* fertilization.

Embryos took the spotlight again when Helen Beasley, a surrogate mother from Shrewsbury, England, decided to sue a San Francisco couple for parental rights to the twin fetuses she was carrying. The couple and Beasley had agreed that they would pay her $20,000 to carry one child created from a donated egg and the father's sperm. The agreement also called for selective reduction—the abortion of any additional embryos. Beasley claimed that there had been a verbal agreement that such reduction would occur by the twelfth week. The problem arose when Beasley, who had discovered she was carrying twins, was told to abort one, but the arrangements for the reduction weren't made until the thirteenth week. Fearing for her own health and objecting to the abortion of such a highly developed fetus, she refused. At that time she was suing for the right to put the babies up for adoption. She was also seeking the remainder of the financial compensation specified in the contract. The couple did not want the children, and yet had the rights to the genetic material; Beasley was simply a vessel. The case is only one of a multitude invited by modern fertility processes. On August 15, 2001, *The New York Times* reported that the New Jersey Supreme Court had upheld a woman's rights to the embryos that she and her ex-husband had created and frozen six years before. A strange case for child-custody lawyers.

Nearly ten years ago, at the University of California at Irvine's Center for Reproductive Health, doctors took the leftover frozen embryos from previous clients and gave them without consent to other couples and to research centers. Discovery of the scam resulted in more than thirty prosecutions; a group of children had biological parents who hadn't consented to their existence and active parents who had been given stolen goods. Who can say whether throwing the embryos away would have been any better?

Even if Michelle and David liked my data, I knew I'd have a long way to go before becoming an actual donor. The application on Egg Donation's Web site is twelve pages long—longer than Yale's entrance application. The first two pages cover the basics: appearance, name, address, age, and other mundane details. After that I was asked if I'd ever filed for bankruptcy or ever had counseling, if I drank, what my goals in life were, what two of my favorite books were, what my paternal grandfather's height and weight were, what hobbies I had, what kind of relationship I would want to have with the parents and child, and so forth. A few fill-in-the-blanks were thrown in at the end: "I feel strongly about ___. I am sorry I did not___. In ten years I want to be ___." Not even my closest friends knew all these things about me. If Egg Donation, offering about a fifth what Michelle and David were offering, wanted all this information, what might Michelle and David want?

Michelle and David were certainly trying hard. On one classified-ad site I came across a request that was strangely familiar: "Loving family seeks exceptional egg donor with 1500 SAT, great looks, good family health history, Jewish heritage and athletic. Height 5 4–5 9, Age 18–29. We will pay EXTREMELY well and will take care of all expenses. Hope to hear

from you." The e-mail address was David and Michelle's familiar AOL account. Theirs was the most demanding classified on the site, but also the only one that offered to pay "EXTREMELY well."

I kept dreaming about all the things I could do with $25,000. I had gone into the correspondence on a whim. But soon, despite David's casual tone and the optimistic attitude of all the classifieds and information I read, I realized that this process was something I didn't want to be a part of. I understand the desire for a child who will resemble and fit in with the family. But once a couple starts choosing a few characteristics, shooting for perfection is too easy—especially if they can afford it. The money might have changed my life for a while, but it would have led to the creation of a child encumbered with too many expectations.

After I'd brooded about these matters, I received the shortest e-mail of the correspondence. The verdict on my pictures was in: "I showed the pictures to [my wife] this AM. Personally, I think you look great. She said ho-hum."

David said he might reconsider, and that he was going to keep one of my pictures. That was it. No good-bye, no thanks for my willingness to be, in effect, the biological mother of their child. I guess I didn't fit their design; my genes weren't the right material for their *chef d'oeuvre*. So I was rejected as a donor. I keep imagining the day when David and Michelle's child asks where he or she came from. David will describe how hard they both worked on the whole thing, how many pictures they looked at, and how much money they spent. The child will turn to them and say, "Ho-hum."

PAYMENT FOR EGG DONATION

Bonnie Steinbock

Both payment for egg donation and payment for surrogacy raise ethical issues. I will address only egg donation, for two reasons. First, more has been written about surrogacy than about egg donation. Second, and more important, the two practices raise very different ethical issues. Surrogacy, or contract pregnancy as some prefer to call it, involves giving birth to a child and then waiving one's rights to custody of that child. In a few well-publicized cases, surrogates have changed their minds and attempted to keep the children. This has never, to my knowledge, occurred with egg donation. This is because there is a huge psychological and emotional difference between giving someone else your egg to gestate and deliver a baby, and gestating and delivering a baby yourself and then giving that baby to someone else. Indeed, in most cases, the egg donor does not even know if a child resulted from her donation. While a donor certainly should think about how she will feel about the possibility that there will be a child, or children, genetically linked to her out there in the world, she does not have to contemplate surrendering a child to whom she has given birth. Additionally, a child born from a surrogate arrangement may feel abandoned by the biological mother, just as an adopted child often does. The feelings of rejection by such children are likely to be compounded by the recognition that the birth mothers conceived them and relinquished them for money. It is implausible that a child conceived through egg donation would feel the same way. Finally, whatever may be wrong with commercial egg donation, it cannot plausibly be characterized as "baby selling."

Reprinted by permission from *The Mount Sinai Journal of Medicine* 71, no. 4 (2004): 255–265.

Editors' note: All author's notes have been cut. Students who want to follow up on sources should consult the original article.

A TERMINOLOGICAL POINT: "DONORS" VS. "VENDORS"

Some view the term "commercial egg donation" as an oxymoron. Thomas Murray writes, "Despite the repeated reference to 'donors' of both ovum and sperm, paying individuals for their biological products makes them vendors, not donors." He recommends that the term "AID" (artificial insemination by donor) should really be "AIV" (artificial insemination by vendor). In response, some maintain that paying gamete providers does not make them vendors, because they are not being paid for a product, but are being compensated for their time, inconvenience, and risk. I will have more to say about this later. In the meantime, I continue to use the term "donation" even when referring to the commercial enterprise, not because I want to prejudge the question of whether payment is for the product or compensation, still less to prejudge the question of moral acceptability, but simply because it is accepted usage.

LAW AND MORALITY

One important distinction is between the legality and the morality of egg donation. While legality and morality are not entirely separate, and arguments for making something illegal are often moral arguments, the two often raise different issues. In Germany, Norway, Sweden, and Japan, the use of donor eggs is illegal. It is unlikely that egg donation could be banned in the United States, because such a ban would probably violate the constitutional right to privacy. What about banning payments to egg donors? In Canada, there is proposed legislation to ban the "buying and selling of eggs, sperm and embryos, including their exchange for goods, services or other benefits. . . ." The Minister of Health adds, "This prohibition will come into force over a period of time to ease the transition from the current commercial system to an altruistic system." Legislation in the United States banning payment to egg donors might not withstand constitutional scrutiny. It would depend on whether or not banning payment is viewed as an undue restriction on procreative liberty. The point I am making is that even if there are serious moral objections to commercial egg donation, there could be constitutional barriers to making it illegal.

When the topic is the morality of a controversial practice, an important question is whether it is morally permissible. However, this is not the only question we can ask. Margaret Little characterizes moral permissibility as "the thinnest moral assessment." Writing about abortion, Little says, ". . . many of our deepest struggles with the morality of abortion concern much more textured questions about its placement on the scales of *decency, respectfulness,* and *responsibility.* It is one thing to decide that an abortion was permissible, quite another to decide that it was *honorable;* one thing to decide that an abortion was impermissible, quite another to decide that it was *monstrous.*" So even if paying egg donors is morally permissible, it does not follow that it is desirable, praiseworthy, or decent.

The practice of commercial egg donation has come under severe criticism, but before examining the ethics of paying donors, we need to see if there is something intrinsically wrong about donating one's gametes to others for the purposes of reproduction, even in the absence of any payment.

NONCOMMERCIAL GAMETE DONATION

The Roman Catholic Church opposes gamete (ovum or sperm) donation because of its views on the unity of sexual intercourse and procreation. Sexual intercourse without openness to procreation is wrong, the Church claims (hence its opposition to birth control), but equally so is procreation without sexual intercourse (hence its opposition to most forms of assisted reproduction). Even the "simple case" of *in vitro* fertilization (IVF), where the husband and wife provide the gametes and the resulting embryos are implanted in the wife's uterus, is impermissible, according to Catholic teaching. The wrong is compounded in gamete donation, as the introduction of "a third party" violates the unity of marriage. In addition, according to the Rev. Albert Moraczewski,

egg donation is demeaning to women. "A donor woman is not really being treated as a person," he said. "Whether she is paid or acts out of kindness, her egg is being used, so she is not fully treated as a person whose reproductive capacity should be expressed as a result of the love of her husband."

But why is egg donation demeaning? Presumably blood donation is not demeaning, and does not fail to treat the donor as a person. What is the difference? The answer, according to the Vatican, is that egg donation involves a wrongful use of reproductive capacity. But then to characterize egg donation as demeaning is not to give a reason why it is wrong; rather, egg donation is demeaning because it is wrong. To see egg donation as demeaning, one must accept the principle that reproductive capacity should be exercised only through a sexual act in the context of a loving marriage. And that principle is justified by the supposedly indissolvable unity of sex, love and procreation. There is nothing inconsistent or incoherent in this view, but it is unlikely to be persuasive to non-Catholics who accept contraception or assisted reproduction.

A different objection to gamete, specifically sperm, donation comes from Daniel Callahan. AID is "fundamentally wrong," according to Callahan, because a sperm donor is a father, who has all the duties of any other biological father, including rearing responsibilities. Sperm donation, according to Callahan, is as irresponsible as abandoning a woman when she becomes pregnant. He writes:

> The only difference between the male who impregnates a woman in the course of sexual liaison and then disappears, and the man who is asked to disappear voluntarily after providing sperm, is that the latter kind of irresponsibility is, so to speak, licensed and legitimated. Indeed, it is treated as a kindly, beneficent action. The effect on the child is of course absolutely identical—an unknown, absent father.

Certainly, it is true that the child born from sperm donation does not know his or her genetic father. But it is not true that these children are fatherless, as is true of most children whose fathers abandon their mothers. They do have fathers—the men who are raising them. Why, one may ask, is it irresponsible to enable an infertile man, who wants very much to parent a child, to become a father? Sperm donors, it may be said, do not evade or abandon their obligations, as do men who abandon women they have impregnated, but rather transfer their rearing rights and duties to others. These others may be men or they may be single women or lesbian couples, who are increasingly using sperm donation. Is it wrong to donate sperm if the resulting child will grow up in a fatherless home? Is this an abandonment of one's responsibility as a father? In my view, this depends on whether the child can be expected to have a reasonably good life. There is evidence that children in single-parent households are at a disadvantage (since it is usually more stressful to raise a child on one's own), but growing up in a lesbian family does not appear to have a negative impact on quality of parenting or children's psychological development. Many lesbian mothers attempt to mitigate the disadvantages of not having a father by making sure that there are other men in their child's life.

David Benatar acknowledges that "gamete donation is not a unilateral abandonment of responsibility," but rather a transference of responsibility. Nevertheless, Benatar thinks that the responsibility of child rearing is one that should not be transferred, that doing so shows a lack of moral seriousness. Certainly, transferring child-rearing responsibilities without much thought is reprehensible; one thinks of Rousseau, who took five illegitimate children he had with his mistress to an orphanage. But is that what gamete donors do? Sperm and ova are not, after all, children. In my opinion, gamete donors do not give others their children to raise. Rather, they enable people who very much want to have children of their own to do so by providing them with genetic material. A woman who does not have eggs can still experience gestation, birth, and lactation, giving her a biological, if not genetic, connection to her child. In addition, if her husband's sperm is used, he will also have a biological connection to the child.

THE NEED FOR EGG DONATION

Egg donation began in the early 1980s; the first pregnancy using this technique was reported in Australia in 1983. Ovum donation is offered to women with three types of reproductive problems. Women in the first group lack functioning ovaries. Those in the second group have no detectable ovarian failure, but they do not achieve pregnancy through IVF.

These include women for whom ovarian retrieval is unsuccessful and those who cannot undergo egg retrieval, usually because scarring or endometriosis prevents access to the ovaries. A third group of women use donated eggs for genetic reasons.

When egg donation was first introduced, the eggs came from either close friends or relatives, in a practice known as "known donation," or they came from women who were undergoing IVF themselves. Because the number of eggs retrieved exceeded the number of embryos that could be safely implanted, women undergoing IVF often had extra eggs, which they were often willing to make available for donation. This source greatly diminished when it became possible to freeze embryos (egg freezing is still experimental). Another source of eggs was from patients undergoing tubal ligation. However, the demand for donors soon outstripped these sources and programs began to recruit women from the public at large through advertising. Thus, commercial egg donation came into being.

The main reason for the increasing demand for egg donors is that, for some women, using an egg donor significantly improves their chances of becoming pregnant. "An infertile woman using her own eggs for *in vitro* fertilization has about a 15 to 20 percent chance of becoming pregnant, less if her ovaries are scarred by infection or endometriosis or are simply too old to function effectively. With an egg donor, her chances of bearing a child shoot up to 30 or even 40 percent." The older the woman, the greater are her chances of becoming pregnant if she uses donor eggs. According to one article, "a 44-year-old woman attempting IVF with her own eggs at Pacific Fertility has a 3.5 percent chance of becoming pregnant. If that same woman uses a donor egg from a younger woman, her chances of giving birth are 50 percent." For some women, therefore, egg donation provides the only realistic option for having a child.

WHAT IS INVOLVED
IN EGG DONATION?

The process is very time-consuming. First, the prospective donor must be accepted into a program; this may involve several visits. She will undergo physical and gynecological examinations, blood and urine tests, and a psychological examination, and participate in discussions of the responsibilities involved in becoming a donor. Because eggs cannot be frozen (or "banked"), the actual donation cycle will not occur unless the prospective donor is accepted, is matched with a recipient, and has given her consent.

The following is typical of the medical process undergone by donors. First, the donor may take a prescribed medication for one or more weeks to temporarily stop her ovaries' normal functioning. This makes it easier to control her response to fertility drugs which will be used later in the cycle. She will be given an injection by the physician or instructed in how to inject the medication daily at home. The medications may cause hot flashes, vaginal dryness, fatigue, sleep problems, body aches, mood swings, breast tenderness, headache and visual disturbances.

Next, medications must be injected over a period of about 10 days to stimulate her ovaries to mature a number of eggs (typically 25–30) for retrieval. Frequent early morning transvaginal ultrasound examinations and blood tests (about every 2–3 days) are needed to monitor the donor's response to the drugs, and adjust the dose as needed. While using injectable fertility drugs, the donor may experience mood swings, breast tenderness, enlarged ovaries and bloating. Occasionally, these medications result in ovarian hyperstimulation syndrome, in which the ovaries swell and fluid builds up in the abdominal cavity. If the hyperstimulation is mild, it will recede after the donor's next menstrual period. If the hyperstimulation is moderate, careful monitoring, bed rest, and pain medication may be necessary. Severe hyperstimulation is infrequent, but may cause serious medical complications, such as blood clots, kidney failure, fluid accumulation in the lungs, and shock. This condition can be life-threatening. Severe hyperstimulation occurs in about 1–10% of IVF cycles. It may result in one or both of the donor's ovaries having to be removed.

The mature eggs are removed from the ovaries in a minor surgical procedure called "transvaginal ovarian aspiration." It is usually done in the physician's office. First, the donor will be given painkillers or put under intravenous sedation. Then, the physician inserts a needle through the vagina to aspirate the eggs out of the follicles. According to one description, "The procedure takes 15 to 60 minutes

and, except for grogginess and some mild pelvic discomfort, there should be no after-effects." Some may experience more than mild pelvic discomfort: one egg donor described it (on a website for donors) as "feeling like somebody punched you in the stomach." Many donors find the actual retrieval less unpleasant than the side effects from the drugs.

WHY DO WOMEN WANT TO DONATE?

Given the rigors of egg donation, why would a woman who was not undergoing IVF or tubal ligation be willing to undergo egg donation for strangers? Some donors are curious about their own bodies and fertility. They want to know if their eggs are "good." Some have a personal reason for helping, such as having friends or relatives who have struggled with infertility or have undergone miscarriages. Others are attracted by the idea of giving "the gift of life," as the advertisements for egg donors put it. One donor explained it as follows, on a donor website: "I can't even describe how it felt to know that in some small way I helped this couple achieve a huge dream in their life." But while most egg donors are motivated in part by altruistic considerations, most women would not be egg donors for strangers without financial compensation. Many say that egg donation would be impossible if they were not compensated for lost work time, transportation, daycare costs, and the like. However, most donors think that reimbursement for pecuniary expenses alone is not enough. They think that it is only fair that they should receive reasonable compensation for what they go through in order to provide eggs: the inconvenience, burden, and medical risk they have endured.

HOW MUCH PAYMENT?

Compensation has been increasing rapidly over the years. In the mid-1980s, egg donors were paid only about $250 per cycle. Today, the payment is usually between $1,500 and $3,000—depending on the location of the clinic. In an effort to attract donors, some clinics offer substantially more. In 1998, Brooklyn IVF raised its donor compensation from $2,500 to $5,000 per cycle to keep pace with St. Barnabas

Medical Center is nearby Livingston, New Jersey. "It's obvious why we had to do it," says Susan Lobel, Brooklyn IVF's assistant director. "Most New York area IVF programs have followed suit."

Donors with particular attributes, such as enrollment in an Ivy League college, high SAT scores, physical attractiveness, or athletic or musical ability have allegedly been offered far larger sums. "The International Fertility Center in Indianapolis, Indiana, for instance, places ads in the *Daily Princetonian* offering Princeton women as much as $35,000 per cycle. The National Fertility Registry, which, like many egg brokerages, features an online catalogue for couples to browse in, advertises $35,000 to $50,000 for Ivy League eggs." In March 2000, an ad appeared in *The Daily Californian* (the campus newspaper for the University of California, Berkeley), which read, "Special Egg Donor Needed," and listed the following criteria for a "preferred donor"; "height approximately 5′ 6″, Caucasian, S.A.T. score around 1250 or high A.C.T., college student or graduate under 30, no genetic medical issues." The compensation was listed as $80,000 "paid to you and/or the charity of your choice." In addition, all related expenses would be paid. Extra compensation was available for someone especially gifted in athletics, science/mathematics or music.

Perhaps the most well-known instance of commercial egg donation is Ron Harris's web site, www.ronsangels.com, which offered models as egg donors, "auctioning their ova via the Internet to would-be parents willing to pay up to $150,000 in hopes of having a beautiful child." A subsequent story suggested that the "egg auction" might just be a publicity stunt to attract people to an erotic web site, a claim that a spokesman for Mr. Harris denied. Some infertility experts maintain that the ads offering large sums of money for special donors are not genuine offers, but rather a "bait and switch" tactic to recruit donors. Donors who respond are told that the ad has been filled, but that there are other recipients (offering substantially less money) seeking donors. *The Daily Californian* ad mentioned above specifically stated, "This ad is being placed for a particular client and is not soliciting eggs for a donor bank." I recently e-mailed the International Infertility Center in Indianapolis, asking them if the fee of $35,000 mentioned in the news report was actually paid to anyone. They responded that the "high-profile client" on whose behalf they had advertised did

not find an ovum donor meeting the requirements, and so no ovum donor was compensated $35,000 for a cycle. I have not been able to discover if any "special donors" have received the sums in the ads.

Most people would distinguish between reasonable compensation and offering $30,000 or more to special donors. What explains the negative reaction most people experience when learning of these huge offers? Perhaps we think that people who are so intent on getting superior eggs (or "designer genes") will be incompetent parents. Instead of anticipating having a child to love, it seems that the couple is focusing on the traits their child will have. They are not satisfied with having a healthy child, which is the reason for genetic screening of donors. Nor is their aim simply to have children who resemble them, something that adoptive parents also usually want. These are reasonable requests, whereas seeking donors from Ivy League schools, with high SATs and athletic ability, indicates something else. The placers of these ads want, and are willing to pay huge sums to get, a "superior" child, and this seems inconsistent with an ideal of unconditional parental love and acceptance.

Moreover, anyone who thinks that it is possible to guarantee that a child will be brilliant, athletic, musically talented, or even blond haired and blue eyed, is likely to be disappointed. According to several prominent geneticists writing in *The New Republic* "despite what your high school biology teacher told you, Mendelian rules do not apply even to eye color or hair color." Even genetic diseases widely considered to follow Mendelian rules, like sickle-cell anemia, may be more or less severe, due to the interaction with other genes in the genome. Predicting or determining non-disease-related traits like intelligence, athletic ability, or musical talent is even less likely, as there are probably thousands of genes that play a role. Finally, the interaction of genes and the environment makes it very difficult to know in advance what phenotypic traits an individual will have. This is not to deny that traits like intelligence or athletic ability have a genetic component, but only to say that they cannot be guaranteed by the choice of an egg donor (who, after all, only provides half the genes). We may well worry about the welfare of a child who fails to live up to parental expectations, after the parents have spent all that money.

The welfare of offspring is a legitimate concern, despite philosophical worries over how to conceptualize it. If commercial egg donation led to poor parenting or had adverse effects on the parent-child relationship, that would be an important moral objection. Yet such an objection might not justify the conclusion that the buying and selling of eggs is morally impermissible, still less that it should be legally banned. For we do not think that procreation is morally permissible only for ideal parents. Nevertheless, concern about effects on parenting and the parent-child relationship fall under the heading of "thick" moral assessments, and may be legitimate.

On the other hand, it is possible that couples who place the ads understand that they cannot determine their children's traits and that they do not have false expectations. Nevertheless, they might say, they want to give their child an advantage, a better chance at traits likely to help the child in life. It is not that they can only love a tall, brilliant, athletic child, they might say, but rather than they are well aware how advantageous such traits can be. Why, they might ask, if they have the money to spend, should they not use it to give their child the best chance in life? Indeed, some have argued that prospective parents are morally required to have the best child they can.

The Human Fertilization and Embryology Authority (HFEA) in the U.K. cited "the physical and psychological well-being of children born from egg donation" as a reason to ban all payments, not just large ones, to egg donors. According to one member of HFEA, "Children produced by egg donation could be adversely affected psychologically if they knew that payment had been made as part of their creation." This seems not only speculative, but implausible. Children may be psychologically harmed if they sense that their parents' love is contingent on their having certain traits, but why would a child be psychologically harmed by learning that the woman who provided the egg from which he or she was conceived received payment? It seems to me that this concern stems from an inappropriate analogy with commercial surrogacy. Children might well be upset to learn that their biological mothers gave them away for money, but it seems implausible that any child would have similar feelings about an egg donor. This being the case, it is hard to see why children would be affected by whether donors were paid or not.

Another moral objection to these ads is that they are elitist and violate a principle of equality. There is something offensive in the idea that the eggs of Princeton women are worth $50,000, while the eggs of women at Brooklyn College are worth only $5,000. (John Arras has jokingly suggested that perhaps *US News & World Report* should include how much their coeds can get for their eggs in their rankings of colleges [personal communication].) Yet it is not clear why we should be offended at the difference in the price put on eggs if we are not offended by differences in employment opportunities or salary.

Some people are disturbed not only by the payment of large sums to egg donors, but by any payment at all. Commercial egg donation is criticized on the grounds that this "commodifies" the human body or "commodifies" reproduction.

COMMODIFICATION

To commodify something is to give it a market price. That in itself is not a bad thing. We could not buy our groceries or clothes or the morning paper if they did not have a market price. If some things should not be commodified, we need a rationale for this. This is not always forthcoming. As the guest editors of a recent special issue on commodification in the *Kennedy Institute of Ethics Journal* say, "Unfortunately, a great deal of the talk about 'commodification' has been clumsy and sloppy. The term has been used as a magic bullet, as if saying, 'But that's commodification!' is the same as having made an argument."

The challenge is to distinguish legitimate activities in which the human body or its abilities are used, from those thought to be illegitimate. As Ruth Macklin has put it, "Every service in our economy is sold: academics sell their minds; athletes sell their bodies. . . . If a pretty actress can sell her appearance and skill for television, why should a fecund woman be denied the ability to sell her eggs? Why is one more demeaning than the other?"

Those who tend to oppose commodification typically portray those who are skeptical about its moral wrongness as being enamored of the market, of thinking that freedom of choice is the only or the most important moral value. They say, ". . . there are some categories of human activities that should not be for sale." But this, even if true, is unhelpful. We want to know *what* things and activities should not be for sale and *why*? Michael Walzer gives voting as an example of a market exchange that should be blocked. Citizens may not sell their votes or vote a certain way for a price. This is so even if the exchange is fully voluntary and even if it makes both parties better off. The reason why votes may not be sold is that this conflicts with the rationale for having the institution of voting in the first place. Voting is intended to express the will of the people in a democracy. Democracy is subverted if votes can be bought.

What we want, then, is a similarly persuasive rationale for the wrongness of selling human body parts. Suzanne Holland attempts to give one. She writes:

> For many of us, our sense of the dignity of humanity is fundamentally disturbed by the suggestion that that which bears the marks of personhood can somehow be equated with property. We do not wish to have certain aspects of that which we associate with our personhood sold off on the market for whatever the market will bear.

Eggs should not be seen as property, according to Holland, because the human body is "inalienable." But what does this mean? To call rights "inalienable" is to say that they cannot be taken away from us, though Joel Feinberg has argued that we can waive them. If calling the human body "inalienable" means that others cannot use my body or body parts without my permission, that is undeniable. But why does this imply that I may not sell my gametes? If "inalienable" just means "may not be treated like property," then Holland has not given a reason why eggs are not property, but rather a tautology.

The fact that something is a human body part does not make it obviously wrong to sell it. In the novel *Little Women*, Jo sells her hair to raise money for her father, who is serving as a chaplain in the Union Army. Surely that was not morally wrong of Jo, nor demeaning to her. Indeed, her willingness to part with "her one beauty" is an unselfish and noble gesture. If selling one's hair is morally permissible, but selling one's gametes is not, what is the moral difference?

It might be thought that I am missing an obvious point. Selling one's hair is not wrong because hair is unrelated to sex and reproduction. Selling one's eggs is akin to selling one's body in prostitution, and "we all know" that prostitution is wrong. Actually, prostitutes do not literally sell their bodies, since they do not relinquish control. It is more accurate to say that they rent them out, or rather that they perform sexual acts in exchange for money. Most of us believe that this is wrong, but this belief may be due in part to sexual puritanism. Perhaps the distaste we feel for prostitution stems (at least in part) from the way prostitutes have typically been regarded in patriarchal societies—as women of no value, undeserving of respect. Imagine a world in which those who provided sexual services were treated with as much respect as psychotherapists, trainers, and masseurs are in our society. It might be that, under such conditions, prostitution would not be as degrading. But even if this argument is invalid, there is a vast personal difference between these two types of "selling," and there is no obvious reason why paying egg donors is incompatible with treating them with respect.

There are two more reasons why selling eggs might be wrong. Providing eggs is both painful and risky. Perhaps offering money to women will lead them to take undue risks, opening up the potential for coercion or exploitation. In addition, some argue that payment for eggs inserts the values of the market into the family. I will consider these objections in turn.

THE POTENTIAL FOR COERCION OR EXPLOITATION

In its report on *Assisted Reproductive Technologies*, the New York State Task Force made the following recommendation:

> Gametes and embryos should not be bought and sold, but gamete and embryo donors should be offered compensation for the time and inconvenience associated with donation. Payments to egg donors should not be so high as to become coercive or so low that they provide inadequate reimbursement for time and inconvenience.

Can offering large sums of money for eggs be seen as coercive? That depends on the theory of coercion that one adopts. In one theory, to coerce is to make a threat: do this or I will make you worse off. The classic example is the highwayman who says, "Your money or your life." Clearly, potential egg donors are not coerced in this sense, no matter how much money is offered to them. They can turn down the offer and be no worse off than they were.

Perhaps this is too narrow a view of coercion. Perhaps there can be "coercive offers" as well as threats. Consider the following example:

The Lecherous Millionaire: Betty's child will die without expensive surgery, which is not covered by her insurance. Alan, a millionaire, offers to pay for the surgery if Betty will have sex with him.

Alan is not threatening Betty. He will not harm her if she refuses. Yet there is a very real sense in which she has "no choice," and for this reason we might see the offer as coercive. But even if this is true, and there can be "coercive offers," does this apply to egg donation? It might, if the money were offered to terribly poor women whose lives, or the lives of their children, depended on their donating eggs. A woman whose only choice was to give away her eggs or see her child die of starvation might well be seen as the victim of coercion. However, poor women are not usually sought out as egg donors. Typical egg donors are middle-class, often professional, young women. It is simply not true to say that they have no choice but to sell their eggs.

Very large offers of money could be quite tempting to any woman, not just those in desperate need of money. But, as Wertheimer points out, offers are not coercive just because they are tempting. And they are not coercive because they are so good that it would be irrational to refuse. It is not coercive to offer someone a great job at double the salary she is currently earning.

However, if offers of large sums of money are not coercive, they may still be criticized as being "undue inducements." Offering "too much" money may be an attempt to manipulate women into becoming donors. The lure of financial gain may lead them to discount the risks to themselves and to make decisions they will later regret. To take advantage of this is a form of exploitation.

It might be argued that we should not attempt to protect adults from irrational assessments or choices they will later regret, because this is paternalistic. However, paternalism involves preventing people from doing what they want on the grounds that this is in their best interest. It is not paternalistic to refrain from taking advantage of someone's susceptibility to temptation.

Some people have tried to meet the charge of commodification by distinguishing between compensating egg donors for their time, risk, and inconvenience, and payment for their eggs. This distinction has been challenged by several commentators, including Ruth Macklin, who writes. "If there is something suspect about commodifying human reproductive products, it is similarly suspect to commodify human reproductive services." However, I think there are two reasons to distinguish between payment for time, risk, and inconvenience, and payment for eggs. First, if payment is viewed as compensation for the burdens of egg retrieval, then large payments based on the donor's college, height, or SAT scores would be unjustified. It is as burdensome for a SUNY-Albany student as it is for a Princeton student to go through the egg retrieval process. Additionally, if payment is compensation for the donor's time, risk, and burden, then donors would be compensated regardless of the number or quality of eggs retrieved, whereas this makes no sense if payment is for the product (eggs). Despite Macklin's rejection of the product/service distinction, she makes precisely this recommendation.

If excessive payments exploit donors, so do payments that are too low. Justice would seem to require that the women who go through the rigors of egg retrieval be fairly compensated. Why are only egg donors expected to act altruistically, when everyone else involved in egg donation receives payment? In light of the sacrifices of time, risk, and burden that egg donors make, it seems only fair that they receive enough money to make the sacrifice worthwhile.

OTHER WORRIES ABOUT EXPLOITATION

Concerns about the exploitation of egg donors are not limited to payment issues. When the New York State Task Force on Life and the Law completed its report on assisted reproductive technologies, one of its findings was that there were serious omissions in the process of gaining informed consent of egg donors. Donors did not always know how strenuous donation would be, or how much time it would take. They often had only the vaguest idea about who would pay their expenses, should there be medical complications stemming from donation.

In one study, researchers were told by a number of women that all of their follow-up care was provided free of charge, but two women were billed for medical expenses for follow-up care and medical complications even though both were promised that the clinic would cover these costs:

> One woman was promised follow-up care prior to donating, but after the donation, that care was denied. She sought out her own personal physician for a sonogram and had to pay hundreds of dollars out of pocket because she was uninsured at the time.

Another woman fainted at work while taking hormonal injections. She had muscle spasms and started to convulse, and had to stay overnight in the hospital. "The clinic denied that her condition was related to the donation and refused to pay for her hospitalization. She is currently fighting with her own health insurance and worker's compensation over the $3500 bill."

One of the most significant sources of conflict in egg donation is the pressure on health care providers to hyperstimulate the donor to produce the maximum number of oocytes. The more eggs, the better the recipient's chances at implantation, but the greater the danger to the donor of suffering from hyperstimulation syndrome. One donor who testified before the advisory committee to the New York State Task Force on Life and the Law revealed that one of her cycles had been stopped, but she had no idea that this was due to excessive stimulation, which had posed health risks to her. She thought that the reason so many eggs had been retrieved was that she was "super-fertile." One of the fertility doctors on the committee said that it was not uncommon for clinics to "flatter" donors in this way, to get them to be repeat donors. Such deceptive treatment of donors is, in my view, a greater source of exploitation, and an area of greater moral concern, than offering payment.

Altruistic egg donation would not necessarily be immune from exploitation. In fact, the true risks and burdens of egg donation might be less likely to be revealed in a voluntary system than in a carefully regulated commercial market, if only because the counseling and screening of donors costs money. Yet altruism can be an appropriate factor. When egg donation imposes little or no extra burden, as in the case of women who are undergoing IVF themselves or women having tubal ligations, there is less reason to compensate women for donating. Altruism in such cases is morally appropriate, as is the case with blood donation, which also involves minimal time and risk. The greater the burdens and risks, the less appropriate is the expectation of altruistic donation.

For some critics, it is not concerns about vulnerable donors that lie at the heart of their objections to commercial egg donation, but rather the effects on the families that are created and ultimately on society at large.

THREATS TO FAMILIES

Tom Murray writes:

> New reproductive technologies are a challenge to our notions of family because they expose what has been at the core of the family to the vicissitudes of the market. At the heart of our often vague concerns about the impact of new reproductive technologies, such as those about the purchase of human eggs, is our sense that they threaten somehow what is valuable about families.

While Murray acknowledges that even noncommercial gamete donation raises "morally relevant difficulties" (presumably those raised by Callahan and Benatar, as well as the issue of the introduction of "a third party" into the marital relationship), he thinks it likely that these difficulties are outweighed by the good of creating new parent-child relationships. It is payment that Murray finds morally objectionable. He writes:

> If you believe that markets, the values markets exemplify, and the relationships that typify market interactions, celebrate human freedom, and that such freedom is the preeminent good, then none of this should bother you. If, however, you regard families as a sphere distinct from the marketplace, a sphere whose place in human flourishing requires that it be kept free of destructive incursions by the values of the market, paying gamete providers should trouble you.

I think we would all agree that families should be protected from destructive incursions by the values of the market—but which incursions are destructive? Presumably it is okay to pay the people who care for our children: day care workers, nannies, and babysitters. These transactions, supposedly, do not commercialize families. Also, presumably, there is nothing wrong with paying those who provide fertility treatment: doctors, nurses, receptionists, lawyers, and genetics counselors. So what is it about paying gamete providers that is threatening to families? Murray does not say. One can agree with his view that "thinking of children as property, and of family life as essentially a series of commercial transactions, is a grievous distortion," but it is unclear what this has to do with paying gamete donors. Eggs are not children, and buying eggs (or even embryos) is not buying children. Still less is it clear why reasonable compensation to egg providers should turn family life into a series of commercial transactions.

INCOMPLETE COMMODIFICATION: A REASONABLE COMPROMISE

Is there room for compromise between those who prefer an altruistic system of egg donation and those who think that egg donors should be paid? Suzanne Holland suggests we take an approach she calls "incomplete commodification":

> With respect to gamete donors, an incompletely commodified approach could recognize that donors are contributing to something that can be seen as a social and personal good (remedying infertility), even as they deserve a degree of compensation that constitutes neither a financial burden ([if they are paid] too little) nor a [temptation to undergo] health risk ([if paid] too much). I see no reason not to follow the suggestion of [the] ASRM [American Society for Reproductive Medicine] and cap egg donor compensation at $5000. . . . Allowing some compensation, but capping it at $5000, would reduce the competition for eggs and perhaps curb the lure of advertising that is targeted to college students in need of "easy money."

Not everyone agrees that $5,000 is appropriate compensation. Mark V. Sauer, a reproductive endocrinologist at Columbia-Presbyterian Medical Center, was "shocked" by the decision of St. Barnabas to double compensation from the community standard of $2,500 to $5,000 per cycle: "Even if one considers the time spent in traveling to the local office and waiting for an ultrasound exam to be 'work,' donors now will be earning in excess of $300 per hour. I find it hard to believe that anyone thinks this 'reasonable compensation' according to the recommendations of the Ethics Committee of the American Society for Reproductive Medicine." However, Sauer's figure apparently takes into consideration only the number of hours spent traveling to and waiting at the clinic, together with the time required for the procedure. It does not consider compensation for risk or discomfort, or the time that some donors will have to take off from work or classes due to side effects from the drugs they must take. When these factors are considered, reimbursement of $5,000 may not be an "indecent proposal." Perhaps if, like Sauer, doctors are worried that "most importantly, and most unfortunately, these expenses will have to be passed on directly to our patients, who are already spending considerable sums of money to seek this procedure," they might consider reducing their fees.

If compensation were completely banned, few women would agree to be egg donors. Very little egg donation would occur, and this would be unfortunate for those women who cannot have babies any other way. This is part of the justification for paying egg donors; the other part has to do with treating donors fairly. At the same time, legitimate concerns about the psychological welfare of the offspring created, and the potential for exploitation of donors, speaks to the need to limit payments to amounts that are reasonable and fair.

REPRODUCTIVE CLONING

THE CASE AGAINST CLONING-TO-PRODUCE-CHILDREN

The President's Council on Bioethics

A. THE ETHICS OF HUMAN EXPERIMENTATION

We begin with concerns regarding the safety of the cloning procedure and the health of the participants. We do so for several reasons. First, these concerns are widely, indeed nearly unanimously, shared. Second, they lend themselves readily to familiar modes of ethical analysis—including concerns about harming the innocent, protecting human rights, and ensuring the consent of all research subjects. Finally, if carefully considered, these concerns begin to reveal the important ethical principles that must guide our broader assessment of cloning-to-produce-children. They suggest that human beings, unlike inanimate matter or even animals, are in some way *inviolable*, and therefore challenge us to reflect on what it is

about human beings that makes them inviolable, and whether cloning-to-produce-children threatens these distinctly human goods.

In initiating this analysis, there is perhaps no better place to start than the long-standing international practice of regulating experiments on human subjects. After all, the cloning of a human being, as well as all the research and trials required before such a procedure could be expected to succeed, would constitute experiments on the individuals involved—the egg donor, the birthing mother, and especially the child-to-be. It therefore makes sense to consider the safety and health concerns that arise from cloning-to-produce-children in light of the widely shared ethical principles that govern experimentation on human subjects.

Since the Second World War, various codes for the ethical conduct of human experimentation have been adopted around the world. These codes and regulations were formulated in direct response to serious ethical lapses and violations committed by research scientists against the rights and dignity of individual human beings. Among the most important and widely accepted documents to emerge

---

This material is an excerpt. Full report can be accessed at http://www.bioethics.gov/reports/cloningreport/index.html.

Editors' note: Most notes have been cut. Students who want to follow up on sources should consult the original article.

were the Nuremberg Code of 1947 and the Helsinki Declaration of 1964. Influential in the United States is also the Belmont Report, published in 1978 by the National Commission for the Protection of Human Subjects of Biomedical and Behavioral Research.

The Nuremberg Code laid out ten principles for the ethical conduct of experiments, focusing especially on voluntary consent of research subjects, the principle that experiments should be conducted only with the aim of providing a concrete good for society that is unprocurable by other methods, and with the avoidance of physical or mental harm. The Helsinki Declaration stated, among other things, that research should be undertaken only when the prospective benefit clearly outweighs the expected risk, when the research subject has been fully informed of all risks, and when the research-subject population is itself likely to benefit from the results of the experiment.

Finally, the Belmont Report proposed three basic ethical principles that were to guide the treatment of human subjects involved in scientific research. The first of these is *respect for persons,* which requires researchers to acknowledge the autonomy and individual rights of research subjects and to offer special protection to those with diminished autonomy and capacity. The second principle is *beneficence.* Scientific research must not only refrain from harming those involved but must also be aimed at helping them, or others, in concrete and important ways. The third principle is *justice,* which involves just distribution of potential benefits and harms and fair selection of research subjects. When applied, these general principles lead to both a requirement for informed consent of human research subjects and a requirement for a careful assessment of risks and benefits before proceeding with research. Safety, consent, and the rights of research subjects are thus given the highest priority.

It would be a mistake to view these codes in narrow or procedural terms, when in fact they embody society's profound sense that human beings are not to be treated as experimental guinea pigs for scientific research. Each of the codes was created to address a specific disaster involving research science—whether the experiments conducted by Nazi doctors on concentration camp prisoners, or the Willowbrook scandal in which mentally retarded children were infected with hepatitis, or the Tuskegee scandal in which under-

privileged African-American men suffering from syphilis were observed but not treated by medical researchers—and each of the codes was an attempt to defend the inviolability and dignity of all human beings in the face of such threats and abuses. More simply stated, and codes attempt to defend the weak against the strong and to uphold the equal dignity of all human beings. In taking up the application of these codes to the case of cloning-to-produce-children, we would suggest that the proper approach is not simply to discover specific places where human cloning violates this or that stipulation of this or that code, but to grapple with how such cloning offends the spirit of these codes and what they seek to defend.

The ethics of research on human subjects suggest three sorts of problems that would arise in cloning-to-produce-children: (1) problems of safety; (2) a special problem of consent; and (3) problems of exploitation of women and the just distribution of risk. We shall consider each in turn.

1. Problems of Safety. First, cloning-to-produce-children is not now safe. Concerns about the safety of the individuals involved in a cloning procedure are shared by nearly everyone on all sides of the cloning debate. Even most proponents of cloning-to-produce-children generally qualify their support with a caveat about the safety of the procedure. Cloning experiments in other mammals strongly suggest that cloning-to-produce-children is, at least for now, far too risky to attempt. Safety concerns revolve around potential dangers to the cloned child, as well as to the egg donor and the woman who would carry the cloned child to birth.

(a) Risks to the child. Risks to the cloned child-to-be must be taken especially seriously, both because they are most numerous and most serious and because—unlike the risks to the egg donor and birth mother—they cannot be accepted knowingly and freely by the person who will bear them. In animal experiments to date, only a small percentage of implanted clones have resulted in live births, and a substantial portion of those live-born clones have suffered complications that proved fatal fairly quickly. Some serious though nonfatal abnormalities in cloned animals have also been observed, including substantially increased birth-size, liver and brain defects, and lung, kidney, and cardiovascular problems.

Longer-term consequences are of course not known, as the oldest successfully cloned mammal is only six years of age. Medium-term consequences, including premature aging, immune system failure, and sudden unexplained death, have already become apparent in some cloned mammals. Some researchers have also expressed concerns that a donor nucleus from an individual who has lived for some years may have accumulated genetic mutations that—if the nucleus were used in the cloning of a new human life—may predispose the new individual to certain sorts of cancer and other diseases.

(b) Risks to the egg donor and the birth mother. Accompanying the threats to the cloned child's health and well-being are risks to the health of the egg donors. These include risks to her future reproductive health caused by the hormonal treatments required for egg retrieval and general health risks resulting from the necessary superovulation.

Animal studies also suggest the likelihood of health risks to the woman who carries the cloned fetus to term. The animal data suggest that late-term fetal losses and spontaneous abortions occur substantially more often with cloned fetuses than in natural pregnancies. In humans, such late-term fetal losses may lead to substantially increased maternal morbidity and mortality. In addition, animal studies have shown that many pregnancies involving cloned fetuses result in serious complications, including toxemia and excessive fluid accumulation in the uterus, both of which pose risks to the pregnant animal's health. In one prominent cattle cloning study, just under one-third of the pregnant cows died from complications late in pregnancy.

Reflecting on the dangers to birth mothers in animal cloning studies, the National Academy report concluded:

> Results of animal studies suggest that reproductive cloning of humans would similarly pose a high risk to the health of both fetus or infant and mother and lead to associated psychological risks for the mother as a consequence of late spontaneous abortions or the birth of a stillborn child or a child with severe health problems.[1]

(c) An abiding moral concern. Because of these risks, there is widespread agreement that, at least for now, attempts at cloning-to-produce-children would constitute unethical experimentation on human subjects and are therefore impermissible. These safety considerations were alone enough to lead the National Bioethics Advisory Commission in June 1997 to call for a temporary prohibition of human cloning-to-produce-children. Similar concerns, based on almost five more years of animal experimentation, convinced the panel of the National Academy of Sciences in January 2002 that the United States should ban such cloning for at least five years.

Past discussions of this subject have often given the impression that the safety concern is a purely temporary one that can be allayed in the near future, as scientific advances and improvements in technique reduce the risks to an ethically acceptable level. But this impression is mistaken, for considerable safety risks are likely to be enduring, perhaps permanent. If so, there will be abiding ethical difficulties *even with efforts aimed at making human cloning safe.*

The reason is clear: experiments to develop new reproductive technologies are necessarily intergenerational, undertaken to serve the reproductive desires of prospective parents but practiced also and always upon prospective children. Any such experiment unavoidably involves risks to the child-to-be, a being who is both the *product* and also the most vulnerable human *subject* of the research. Exposed to risk during the extremely sensitive life-shaping processes of his or her embryological development, any child-to-be is a singularly vulnerable creature, one maximally deserving of protection against risk of experimental (and other) harm. If experiments to learn how to clone a child are ever to be ethical, the degree of risk to that child-to-be would have to be extremely low, arguably no greater than for children-to-be who are conceived from union of egg and sperm. It is extremely unlikely that this moral burden can be met, not for decades if at all.

In multiple experiments involving six of the mammalian species cloned to date, more than 89 percent of the cloned embryos transferred to recipient females did not come to birth, and many of the live-born cloned animals are or become abnormal. If success means achieving normal and healthy development not just at birth but throughout the life span, there is even less reason for confidence. The oldest cloned mammal (Dolly) is only six years old and has exhibited unusually early arthritis. The reasons for failure in animal cloning are not well understood. Also, no nonhuman primates have been cloned. It will be decades (at least) before we could obtain positive evidence that cloned primates might live a normal healthy (primate) life.

Even a high success rate in animals would not suffice by itself to make human trials morally acceptable. In addition to the usual uncertainties in jumping the gap from animal to human research, cloning is likely to present particularly difficult problems of interspecies difference. Animal experiments have already shown substantial differences in the reproductive success of identical cloning techniques used in different species. If these results represent species-specific differences in, for example, the ease of epigenetic reprogramming and imprinting of the donor DNA, the magnitude of the risks to the child-to-be of the first human cloning experiments would be unknown and potentially large, no matter how much success had been achieved in animals. There can in principle be no direct experimental evidence sufficient for assessing the degree of such risk.*

Can a highly reduced risk of deformity, disease, and premature death in animal cloning, coupled with the inherently unpredictable risk of moving from animals to humans, ever be low enough to meet the ethically acceptable standard set by reproduction begun with egg and sperm? The answer, as a matter of necessity, can never be better than "Just possibly." Given the severity of the possible harms involved in human cloning, and given that those harms fall on the very vulnerable child-to-be, such an answer would seem to be enduringly inadequate.

Similar arguments, it is worth noting, were made before the first attempts at human in vitro fertilization. People suggested that it would be unethical experimentation even to try to determine whether IVF could be safely done. And then, of course, IVF was accomplished. Eventually, it became a common procedure, and today the moral argument about its safety seems to many people beside the point. Yet the fact of success in that case does not establish precedent in this one, nor does it mean that the first attempts at IVF were not in fact unethical experiments upon the unborn, despite the fortunate results.†

Be this as it may, the case of cloning is genuinely different. With IVF, assisted fertilization of egg by sperm immediately releases a developmental process, linked to the sexual union of the two gametes, that nature has selected over millions of years for the entire mammalian line. But in cloning experiments to produce children, researchers would be transforming a sexual system into an asexual one, a change that requires major and "unnatural" reprogramming of donor DNA if there is to be any chance of success. They are neither enabling nor restoring a natural process, and the alterations involved are such that success in one species cannot be presumed to predict success in another. Moreover, any new somatic mutations in the donor cell's chromosomal DNA would be passed along to the cloned child-to-be and its offspring. Here we can see even more the truly intergenerational character of cloning experimentation, and this should justify placing the highest moral burden of persuasion on those who would like to proceed with efforts to make cloning safe for producing children. (By reminding us of the need to protect the lives and well-being of our children and our children's children, this broader analysis of the safety question points toward larger moral objections to producing cloned children, objections that we shall consider shortly.)

It therefore appears to us that, given the dangers involved and the relatively limited goods to be gained from cloning-to-produce-children, conducting

---

*It is of course true that there is always uncertainty about moving from animal to human experimentation or therapy. But in the usual case, what justifies the assumption of this added unknown risk is that the experimental subject is a likely beneficiary of the research, either directly or indirectly. And where this is not the case, risk may be assumed if there is informed and voluntary consent. Neither of these conditions applies for the child-to-be in human cloning experiments.

†Surprisingly, there has been very little systematic study of the offspring of in vitro fertilization. One recently published study has suggested that IVF (and especially intracytoplasmic sperm injection [ICSI]) may not be as benign as we had thought (Hansen, M., et al., "The Risk of Major Birth Defects after Intracytoplasmic Sperm Injection and In Vitro Fertilization," *New Eng. J. Med.* 346: 725–730, 2002).

experiments in an effort to make cloning-to-produce-children safer would itself be an unacceptable violation of the norms of the ethics of research. *There seems to be no ethical way to try to discover whether cloning-to-produce-children can become safe, now or in the future.*

2. A Special Problem of Consent. A further concern relating to the ethics of human research revolves around the question of consent. Consent from the cloned child-to-be is of course impossible to obtain, and because no one consents to his or her own birth, it may be argued that concerns about consent are misplaced when applied to the unborn. But the issue is not so simple. For reasons having to do both with the safety concerns raised above and with the social, psychological, and moral concerns to be addressed below, an attempt to clone a human being would potentially expose a cloned individual-to-be to great risks of harm, quite distinct from those accompanying other sorts of reproduction. Given the risks, and the fact that consent cannot be obtained, the ethically correct choice may be to avoid the experiment. The fact that those engaged in cloning cannot ask an unconceived child for permission places a burden on the cloners, not on the child. Given that anyone considering creating a cloned child must know that he or she is putting a newly created human life at exceptional risk, the burden on the would-be cloners seems clear: they must make a compelling case why the procedure should not be avoided altogether.*

Reflections on the purpose and meaning of seeking consent support this point. Why, after all, does society insist upon consent as an essential principle of the ethics of scientific research? Along with honoring the free will of the subject, we insist on consent to protect the weak and the vulnerable, and in particular to protect them from the powerful. It would therefore be morally questionable, at the very least, to choose to impose potentially grave harm on an individual, especially in the very act of

giving that individual life. Giving existence to a human being does not grant one the right to maim or harm that human being in research.

3. Problems of Exploitation of Women and Just Distribution of Risk. Cloning-to-produce-children may also lead to the exploitation of women who would be called upon to donate oocytes. Widespread use of the techniques of cloning-to-produce-children would require large numbers of eggs. Animal models suggest that several hundred eggs may be required before one attempt at cloning can be successful. The required oocytes would have to be donated, and the process of making them available would involve hormonal treatments to induce superovulation. If financial incentives are offered, they might lead poor women especially to place themselves at risk in this way (and might also compromise the voluntariness of their "choice" to make donations). Thus, research on cloning-to-produce-children could impose disproportionate burdens on women, particularly low-income women.

4. Conclusion. These questions of the ethics of research—particularly the issue of physical safety—point clearly to the conclusion that cloning-to-produce-children is unacceptable. In reaching this conclusion, we join the National Bioethics Advisory Commission and the National Academy of Sciences. But we go beyond the findings of those distinguished bodies in also pointing to the dangers that will *always* be inherent in the very process of trying to make cloning-to-produce-children safer. On this ground, we conclude that the problem of safety is not a temporary ethical concern. It is rather an enduring moral concern that might not be surmountable and should thus preclude work toward the development of cloning techniques to produce children. In light of the risks and other ethical concerns raised by this form of human experimentation, *we therefore conclude that cloning-to-produce-children should not be attempted.*

For some people, the discussion of ethical objections to cloning-to-produce-children could end here. Our society's established codes and practices in regard to human experimentation by themselves offer compelling reasons to oppose indefinitely attempts to produce a human child by cloning. But there *is* more to be said.

---

*The argument made in this paragraph is not unique to cloning. There may be other circumstances in which prospective parents, about to impose great risk of harm on a prospective child-to-be, might bear a comparable burden.

First, many people who are repelled by or opposed to the prospect of cloning human beings are concerned not simply or primarily because the procedure is unsafe. To the contrary, their objection is to the use of a *perfected* cloning technology and to a society that would embrace or permit the production of cloned children. The ethical objection based on lack of safety is *not* really an objection to cloning *as such*. Indeed, it may in time become a vanishing objection should people be allowed to proceed— despite insuperable ethical objections such as the ones we have just offered—with experiments to perfect the technique.* Should this occur, the ethical assessment of cloning-to-produce-children would need to address itself to the merits (and demerits) of cloning itself, beyond the safety questions tied to the techniques used to produce cloned children. Thus, anticipating the possibility of a perfected and usable technology, it is important to delineate the case against the practice itself.

Moreover, because the Council is considering cloning within a broad context of present and projected techniques that can affect human procreation or alter the genetic makeup of our children, it is important that we consider the full range and depth of ethical issues raised by such efforts.

How should these issues be raised, and within what moral framework? Some, but by no means all, of the deepest moral concerns connected to human cloning could be handled by developing a richer consideration of the ethics of human experimentation. Usually—and regrettably—we apply the ethical principles governing research on human subjects in a utilitarian spirit, weighing benefits versus harms, and moreover using only a very narrow notion of "harm." The calculus that weighs benefits versus harms too often takes stock only of bodily harm or violations of patient autonomy, though some serious efforts have been made in recent years to consider broader issues. In addition, we often hold a rather narrow view of what constitutes "an experiment." Yet cloning-to-produce-children would be a "human

experiment" in many senses, and risks of bodily harm and inadequate consent do not exhaust the ways in which cloning might do damage. As we have described, cloning-to-produce-children would be a *biological experiment*—with necessary uncertainties about the safety of the technique and the possibility of physical harm. But it would also be an *experiment in human procreation*—substituting asexual for sexual reproduction and treating children not as gifts but as our self-designed products. It would be an *experiment in human identity*—creating the first human beings to inherit a genetic identity lived in advance by another. It would be an *experiment in genetic choice and design*—producing the first children whose entire genetic makeup was selected in advance. It would be an *experiment in family and social life*—altering the relationships within the family and between the generations, for example, by turning "mothers" into "twin sisters" and "grandparents" into "parents," and by having children asymmetrically linked biologically to only one parent. And it would represent a *social experiment* for the entire society, insofar as the society accepted, even if only as a minority practice, this unprecedented and novel mode of producing our offspring.

By considering these other ways in which cloning would constitute an experiment, we could enlarge our analysis of the ethics of research with human subjects to assess possible *non-bodily* harms of cloning-to-produce-children. But valuable as this effort might be, we have not chosen to proceed in this way. Not all the important issues can be squeezed into the categories of harms and benefits. People can be mistreated or done an injustice whether they know it or not and quite apart from any experienced harm. Important human goods can be traduced, violated, or sacrificed without being registered in anyone's catalogue of harms. The form of bioethical inquiry we are attempting here will make every effort not to truncate the moral meaning of our actions and practices by placing them on the Procrustean bed of utilitarianism. To be sure, the ethical principles governing human research are highly useful in efforts to protect vulnerable individuals against the misconduct or indifference of the powerful. But a different frame of reference is needed to evaluate the human meaning of innovations that may affect the lives and humanity of everyone, vulnerable or not.

---

*Such improvements in technique could result in part from the practice of cloning-for-biomedical-research, were it to be allowed to go forward. This possibility is one of the issues we shall consider in evaluating the ethics of cloning-for-biomedical-research in Chapter Six.

Of the arguments developed below, some are supported by most Council Members, while other arguments are shared by only some Members. Even among the arguments they share, different Members find different concerns to be weightier. Yet we all believe that the arguments presented in the sections that follow are worthy of consideration in the course of trying to assess *fully* the ethical issues involved. We have chosen to err on the side of inclusion rather than exclusion of arguments because we acknowledge that concerns now expressed by only a few may turn out in the future to be more important than those now shared by all. Our fuller assessment begins with an attempt to fathom the deepest meaning of human procreation and thus necessarily the meaning of raising children. Our analysis will then move on to questions dealing with the effects of cloning on individuals, family life, and society more generally.

B.   THE HUMAN CONTEXT: PROCREATION AND CHILD-REARING

Were it to take place, cloning-to-produce-children would represent a challenge to the nature of human procreation and child-rearing. Cloning is, of course, not only a means of procreation. It is also a technology, a human experiment, and an exercise of freedom, among other things. But cloning would be most unusual, consequential, and most morally important as a new way of bringing children into the world and a new way of viewing their moral significance.

In Chapter One we outlined some morally significant features of human procreation and raised questions about how these would be altered by human cloning. We will now attempt to deepen that analysis, and begin with the salient fact that a child *is not made, but begotten*. Procreation is not making but the outgrowth of doing. A man and woman give themselves in love to each other, setting their projects aside in order to do just that. Yet a child results, arriving on its own, mysterious, independent, yet the fruit of the embrace.* Even were the

child wished for, and consciously so, he or she is the issue of their love, not the product of their wills; the man and woman in no way produce or choose a *particular* child, as they might buy a particular car. Procreation can, of course, be assisted by human ingenuity (as with IVF). In such cases, it may become harder to see the child solely as a gift bestowed upon the parents' mutual self-giving and not to some degree as a product of their parental wills. Nonetheless, because it is still sexual reproduction, the children born with the help of IVF begin—as do all other children—with a certain genetic independence of their parents. They replicate neither their fathers nor their mothers, and this is a salutary reminder to parents of the independence they must one day grant their children and for which it is their duty to prepare them.

Gifts and blessings we learn to accept as gratefully as we can. Products of our wills we try to shape in accord with our desires. Procreation as traditionally understood invites acceptance, rather than reshaping, engineering, or designing the next generation. It invites us to accept limits to our control over the next generation. It invites us even—to put the point most strongly—to think of the child as one who is not simply our own, our possession. Certainly, it invites us to remember that the child does not exist simply for the happiness or fulfillment of the parents.

To be sure, parents do and must try to form and mold their children in various ways as they inure them to the demands of family life, prepare them for adulthood, and initiate them into the human community. But, even then, it is only our sense that these children are not our possessions that makes such parental nurture—which always threatens not to nourish but to stifle the child—safe.

This concern can be expressed not only in language about the relation between the generations but also in the language of equality. The things we make are not just like ourselves; they are the products of our wills, and their point and purpose are ours to determine. But a begotten child comes into the world just as its parents once did, and is therefore their equal in dignity and humanity.

The character of sexual procreation shapes the lives of children as well as parents. By giving rise to genetically new individuals, sexual reproduction imbues all human beings with a sense of individual

---

*We are, of course, well aware that many children are conceived in casual, loveless, or even brutal acts of sexual intercourse, including rape and incest.

identity and of occupying a place in this world that has never belonged to another. Our novel genetic identity symbolizes and foreshadows the unique, never-to-be-repeated character of each human life. At the same time, our emergence from the union of two individuals, themselves conceived and generated as we were, locates us immediately in a network of relation and natural affection.

Social identity, like genetic identity, is in significant measure tied to these biological facts. Societies around the world have structured social and economic responsibilities around the relationship between the generations established through sexual procreation, and have developed modes of child-rearing, family responsibility, and kinship behavior that revolve around the natural facts of begetting.

There is much more to be said about these matters, and they are vastly more complicated than we have indicated. There are, in addition, cultural differences in the way societies around the world regard the human significance of procreation or the way children are to be regarded and cared for. Yet we have said enough to indicate that the character and nature of human procreation matter deeply. They affect human life in endless subtle ways, and they shape families and communities. A proper regard for the profundity of human procreation (including child-rearing and parent-child relations) is, in our view, indispensable for a full assessment of the ethical implications of cloning-to-produce-children.

C.   IDENTITY, MANUFACTURE, EUGENICS, FAMILY, AND SOCIETY

Beyond the matter of procreation itself, we think it important to examine the possible psychological and emotional state of individuals produced by cloning, the well-being of their families, and the likely effects on society of permitting human cloning. These concerns would apply even if cloning-to-produce-children were conducted on a small scale; and they would apply in even the more innocent-seeming cloning scenarios, such as efforts to overcome infertility or to avoid the risk of genetic disease. Admittedly, these matters are necessarily speculative, for empirical evidence is lacking.

Nevertheless, the importance of the various goods at stake justifies trying to think matters through in advance.

Keeping in mind our general observations about procreation, we proceed to examine a series of specific ethical issues and objections to cloning human children: (1) problems of identity and individuality; (2) concerns regarding manufacture; (3) the prospect of a new eugenics; (4) troubled family relations; and (5) effects on society.

1. Problems of Identity and Individuality. Cloning-to-produce-children could create serious problems of identity and individuality. This would be especially true if it were used to produce multiple "copies" of any single individual, as in one or another of the seemingly far-fetched futuristic scenarios in which cloning is often presented to the popular imagination. Yet questions of identity and individuality could arise even in small-scale cloning, even in the (supposedly) most innocent of cases, such as the production of a single cloned child within an intact family. Personal identity is, we would emphasize, a complex and subtle psychological phenomenon, shaped ultimately by the interaction of many diverse factors. But it does seem reasonably clear that cloning would at the very least present a unique and possibly disabling challenge to the formation of individual identity.

Cloned children may experience concerns about their distinctive identity not only because each will be genetically essentially identical to another human being, but also because they may resemble in appearance younger versions of the person who is their "father" or "mother." Of course, our genetic makeup does not by itself determine our identities. But our genetic uniqueness is an important source of our sense of who we are and how we regard ourselves. It is an emblem of independence and individuality. It endows us with a sense of life as a never-before-enacted possibility. Knowing and feeling that nobody has previously possessed our particular gift of natural characteristics, we go forward as genetically unique individuals into relatively indeterminate futures.

These new and unique genetic identities are rooted in the natural procreative process. A cloned child, by contrast, is at risk of living out a life overshadowed in important ways by the life of the "original"—general appearance being only the most obvious. Indeed, one of the reasons some people are interested in cloning is that the technique promises to produce in each case a particular individual whose traits and characteristics are already known. And however much or little one's genotype *actually* shapes one's natural capacities, it could mean a great deal to an individual's *experience* of life and the expectations that those who cloned him or her might have. The cloned child may be constantly compared to "the original," and may consciously or unconsciously hold himself or herself up to the genetic twin that came before. If the two individuals turned out to lead similar lives, the cloned person's achievements may be seen as derivative. If, as is perhaps more likely, the cloned person departed from the life of his or her progenitor, this very fact could be a source of constant scrutiny, especially in circumstances in which parents produced their cloned child to become something in particular. Living up to parental hopes and expectations is frequently a burden for children; it could be a far greater burden for a cloned individual. The shadow of the cloned child's "original" might be hard for the child to escape, as would parental attitudes that sought in the child's very existence to replicate, imitate, or replace the "original."

It may reasonably be argued that genetic individuality is not an indispensable human good, since identical twins share a common genotype and seem not to be harmed by it. But this argument misses the context and environment into which even a single human clone would be born. Identical twins have as progenitors two biological parents and are born together, before either one has developed and shown what his or her potential—natural or otherwise—may be. Each is largely free of the burden of measuring up to or even knowing in advance the genetic traits of the other, because both begin life together and neither is yet known to the world. But a clone is a genetic near-copy of a person who is already living or has already lived. This might constrain the clone's sense of self in ways that differ in kind from the experience of identical twins. Everything about the predecessor—from physical height and facial appearance, balding patterns and inherited diseases, to temperament and native talents, to shape of life and length of days, and even cause of death—will appear before the expectant eyes of the cloned person, always with at least the nagging concern that there, notwithstanding the grace of God, go I. The crucial matter, again, is not simply the truth regarding the extent to which genetic identity actually shapes us—though it surely does shape us to some extent. What matters is the cloned individual's *perception* of the significance of the "precedent life" and the way that perception cramps and limits a sense of self and independence.

2. Concerns regarding Manufacture. The likely impact of cloning on identity suggests an additional moral and social concern: the transformation of human procreation into human manufacture, of begetting into making. By using the terms "making" and "manufacture" we are not claiming that cloned children would be artifacts made altogether "by hand" or produced in factories. Rather, we are suggesting that they would, like other human "products," be brought into being in accordance with some preselected genetic pattern or design, and therefore in some sense "made to order" by their producers or progenitors.

Unlike natural procreation—or even most forms of assisted reproduction—cloning-to-produce-children would set out to create a child with a very particular genotype: namely, that of the somatic cell donor. Cloned children would thus be the first human beings whose entire genetic makeup is selected in advance. True, selection from among existing genotypes is not yet design of new ones. But the principle that would be established by human cloning is both far-reaching and completely novel: parents, with the help of science and technology, may determine in advance the genetic endowment of their children. To this point, parents have the right and the power to decide *whether* to have a child. With cloning, parents acquire the power, and presumably the right, to decide *what kind* of a child to have. Cloning would thus extend the power of one generation over the next—and the power of parents over their offspring—in ways that open the door, unintentionally or not, to a future project of genetic manipulation and genetic control.

Of course, there is no denying that we have already taken steps in the direction of such control. Preimplantation genetic diagnosis of embryos and prenatal diagnosis of fetuses—both now used to prevent the birth of individuals carrying genes for genetic diseases—reflect an only conditional acceptance of the next generation. With regard to *positive* selection for desired traits, some people already engage in the practice of sex selection, another example of conditional acceptance of offspring. But these precedents pale in comparison to the degree of control provided by cloning and, in any case, do not thereby provide a license to proceed with cloning. It is far from clear that it would be wise to proceed still farther in our attempts at control.

The problem with cloning-to-produce-children is not that artificial technique is used to assist reproduction. Neither is it that genes are being manipulated. We raise no objection to the use of the coming genetic technologies to treat individuals with genetic diseases, even in utero—though there would be issues regarding the protection of human subjects in research and the need to find boundaries between therapy and so-called enhancement (of this, more below). The problem has to do with the control of the entire genotype and the production of children to selected specifications.

Why does this matter? It matters because human dignity is at stake. In natural procreation, two individuals give life to a new human being whose endowments are not shaped deliberately by human will, whose being remains mysterious, and the open-endedness of whose future is ratified and embraced. Parents beget a child who enters the world exactly as they did—as an unmade gift, not as a product. Children born of this process stand equally beside their progenitors as fellow human beings, not beneath them as made objects. In this way, the uncontrolled beginnings of human procreation endow each new generation and each new individual with the dignity and freedom enjoyed by all who came before.

Most present forms of assisted reproduction imitate this natural process. While they do begin to introduce characteristics of manufacture and industrial technique, placing nascent human life for the first time in human hands, they do not control the final outcome. The end served by IVF is still the same as natural reproduction—the birth of a child from the union of gametes from two progenitors. Reproduction with the aid of such techniques still implicitly expresses a willingness to accept as a gift the product of a process we do not control. In IVF children emerge out of the same mysterious process from which their parents came, and are therefore not mere creatures of their parents.

By contrast, cloning-to-produce-children—and the forms of human manufacture it might make more possible in the future—seems quite different. Here, the process begins with a very specific final product in mind and would be tailored to produce that product. Even were cloning to be used solely to remedy infertility, the decision to clone the (sterile) father would be a decision, willy-nilly, that the child-to-be should be the near-twin of his "father." Anyone who would clone merely to ensure a "biologically related child" would be dictating a very specific form of biological relation: genetic virtual identity. In every case of cloning-to-produce-children, scientists or parents would set out to produce specific individuals for particular reasons. The procreative process could come to be seen increasingly as a means of meeting specific ends, and the resulting children would be products of a designed manufacturing process, products over whom we might think it proper to exercise "quality control." Even if, in any given case, we were to continue to think of the cloned child as a gift, *the act itself teaches a different lesson,* as the child becomes the continuation of a parental project. We would learn to receive the next generation less with gratitude and surprise than with control and mastery.

One possible result would be the industrialization and commercialization of human reproduction. Manufactured objects become commodities in the marketplace, and their manufacture comes to be guided by market principles and financial concerns. When the "products" are human beings, the "market" could become a profoundly dehumanizing force. Already there is commerce in egg donation for IVF, with ads offering large sums of money for egg donors with high SAT scores and particular physical features.

The concerns expressed here do not depend on cloning becoming a widespread practice. The introduction of the terms and ideas of production into the realm of human procreation would be troubling regardless of the scale involved; and the adoption of a market mentality in these matters could blind us to the deep moral character of bringing forth new life. Even were cloning children to be rare, the moral harms to a society that accepted it could be serious.

3. Prospect of a New Eugenics. For some of us, cloning-to-produce-children also raises concerns about the prospect of eugenics or, more modestly, about genetic "enhancement." We recognize that the term "eugenics" generally refers to attempts to improve the genetic constitution of a particular political community or of the human race through general policies such as population control, forced sterilization, directed mating, or the like. It does not ordinarily refer to actions of particular individuals attempting to improve the genetic endowment of their own descendants. Yet, although cloning does not in itself point to public policies by which the state would become involved in directing the development of the human gene pool, this might happen in illiberal regimes, like China, where the government already regulates procreation.* And, in liberal societies, cloning-to-produce-children could come to be used privately for individualized eugenic or "enhancement" purposes: in attempts to alter (with the aim of improving) the genetic constitution of one's own descendants—and, indirectly, of future generations.

Some people, in fact, see enhancement as the major purpose of cloning-to-produce-children. Those who favor eugenics and genetic enhancement were once far more open regarding their intentions to enable future generations to enjoy more advantageous genotypes. Toward these ends, they promoted the benefits of cloning: escape from the uncertain lottery of sex, controlled and humanly directed reproduction. In the present debate about cloning-to-produce-children, the case for eugenics and enhancement is not made openly, but it nonetheless remains an important motivation for some advocates. Should cloning-to-produce-children be introduced successfully, and should it turn out that the cloned humans do in fact inherit many of the natural talents of the "originals," some people may become interested in the prospects of using it to produce "enhanced children"—especially if other people's children were receiving comparable advantages.

Cloning can serve the ends of individualized enhancement either by avoiding the genetic defects that may arise when human reproduction is left to chance or by preserving and perpetuating outstanding genetic traits. In the future, if techniques of genetic enhancement through more precise genetic engineering became available, cloning could be useful for perpetuating the enhanced traits and for keeping any "superior" manmade genotype free of the flaws that sexual reproduction might otherwise introduce.

"Private eugenics" does not carry with it the dark implications of state despotism or political control of the gene pool that characterized earlier eugenic proposals and the racist eugenic practices of the twentieth century. Nonetheless, it could prove dangerous to our humanity. Besides the dehumanizing prospects of the turn toward manufacture that such programs of enhancement would require, there is the further difficulty of the lack of standards to guide the choices for "improvement." To this point, biomedical technology has been applied to treating diseases in patients and has been governed, on the whole, by a commonsense view of health and disease. To be sure, there are differing views about how to define "health." And certain cosmetic, performance-enhancing, or hedonistic uses of biomedical techniques have already crossed any plausible boundary between therapy and enhancement, between healing the sick and "improving" our powers.† Yet, for the most part, it is by some commonsense views of health that we judge who is in need of medical treatment and what sort of treatment might be most appropriate. Even today's practice of a kind of "negative" eugenics— through prenatal genetic diagnosis and abortion of fetuses with certain genetic abnormalities—is informed by the desire to promote health.

The "positive" eugenics that could receive a great boost from human cloning, especially were it to be coupled with techniques of precise genetic modification, would not seek to restore sick human

---

*According to official Chinese census figures for 2000, more than 116 male births were recorded for every 100 female births. It is generally believed that this is the result of the widespread use of prenatal sex selection and China's one-child policy, though it should be noted that even in a country such as South Korea, which has no such policy, the use of prenatal sex selection has skewed the sex ratio in favor of males.

---

†One thinks of certain forms of plastic surgery or recreational uses of euphoriant drugs, and the uses in athletics and schools of performance-enhancing drugs, such as anabolic steroids, erythropoietin, and Ritalin.

beings to natural health. Instead, it would seek to alter humanity, based upon subjective or arbitrary ideas of excellence. The effort may be guided by apparently good intentions: to improve the next generation and to enhance the quality of life of our descendants. But in the process of altering human nature, we would be abandoning the standard by which to judge the goodness or the wisdom of the particular aims. We would stand to lose the sense of what is and is not human.

The fear of a new eugenics is not, as is sometimes alleged, a concern born of some irrational fear of the future or the unknown. Neither is it born of hostility to technology or nostalgia for some premodern pseudo–golden age of superior naturalness. It is rather born of the rational recognition that once we move beyond therapy into efforts at enhancement, we are in uncharted waters without a map, without a compass, and without a clear destination that can tell us whether we are making improvements or the reverse. The time-honored and time-tested goods of human life, which we know to be good, would be put in jeopardy for the alleged and unknowable goods of a post-human future.

4. *Troubled Family Relations.* Cloning-to-produce-children could also prove damaging to family relations, despite the best of intentions. We do not assume that cloned children, once produced, would not be accepted, loved, or nurtured by their parents and relatives. On the contrary, we freely admit that, like any child, they might be welcomed into the cloning family. Nevertheless, the cloned child's place in the scheme of family relations might well be uncertain and confused. The usually clear designations of father and brother, mother and sister would be confounded. A mother could give birth to her own genetic twin, and a father could be genetically virtually identical to his son. The cloned child's relation to his or her grandparents would span one and two generations at once. Every other family relation would be similarly confused. There is, of course, the valid counter-argument that holds that the "mother" could easily be defined as the person who gives birth to the child, regardless of the child's genetic origins, and for social purposes that may serve to eliminate some problems. But because of the special nature of cloning-to-produce-children, difficulties may be expected.

The crucial point is not the *absence* of the natural biological connections between parents and children. The crucial point is, on the contrary, the *presence* of a unique, one-sided, and replicative biological connection to only *one* progenitor. As a result, family relations involving cloning would differ from all existing family arrangements, including those formed through adoption or with the aid of IVF. A great many children, after all, are adopted, and live happy lives in loving families, in the absence of any biological connections with their parents. Children conceived by artificial insemination using donor sperm and by various IVF techniques may have unusual relationships with their genetic parents, or no genetic relationships at all. But all of these existing arrangements attempt in important ways to emulate the model of the natural family (at least in its arrangement of the generations), while cloning runs contrary to that model.

What the exact effects of cloning-to-produce-children might be for families is highly speculative, to be sure, but it is still worth flagging certain troubling possibilities and risks. The fact that the cloned child bears a special tie to only one parent may complicate family dynamics. As the child developed, it could not help but be regarded as specially akin to only one of his or her parents. The sins or failings of the father (or mother), if reappearing in the cloned child, might be blamed on the progenitor, adding to the chances of domestic turmoil. The problems of being and rearing an adolescent could become complicated should the teenage clone of the mother "reappear" as the double of the woman the father once fell in love with. Risks of competition, rivalry, jealousy, and parental tension could become heightened.*

Even if the child were cloned from someone who is not a member of the family in which the child is raised, the fact would remain that he or she has been

---

*And there might be special complications in the event of divorce. Does the child rightfully or more naturally belong to the "genetic parent"? How would a single parent deal with a child who shares none of her genes but carries 100 percent of the genes of the person she chose to divorce? Whether such foreseeable complications would in fact emerge is, of course, an empirical question that cannot be answered in advance. But knowledge of the complexities of family life lead us not to want to dismiss them.

produced in the nearly precise genetic image of another and for some particular reason, with some particular design in mind. Should this become known to the child, as most likely it would, a desire to seek out connection to the "original" could complicate his or her relation to the rearing family, as would living consciously "under the *reason*" for this extra-familial choice of progenitor. Though many people make light of the importance of biological kinship (compared to the bonds formed through rearing and experienced family life), many adopted children and children conceived by artificial insemination or IVF using donor sperm show by their actions that they do not agree. They make great efforts to locate their "biological parents," even where paternity consists in nothing more than the donation of sperm. Where the progenitor is a genetic near-twin, surely the urge of the cloned child to connect with the unknown "parent" would be still greater.

For all these reasons, the cloning family differs from the "natural family" or the "adoptive family." By breaking through the natural boundaries between generations, cloning could strain the social ties between them.

5. Effects on Society. The hazards and costs of cloning-to-produce-children may not be confined to the direct participants. The rest of society may also be at risk. The impact of human cloning on society at large may be the least appreciated, but among the most important, factors to consider in contemplating the morality of this activity.

Cloning is a human activity affecting not only those who are cloned or those who are clones, but also the entire society that allows or supports such activity. For insofar as the society *accepts* cloning-to-produce-children, to that extent the society may be said to *engage* in it. A society that allows dehumanizing practices—especially when given an opportunity to try to prevent them—risks becoming an accomplice in those practices. (The same could be said of a society that allowed even a few of its members to practice incest or polygamy.) Thus the question before us is whether cloning-to-produce-children is an activity that we, *as a society*, should engage in. In addressing this question, we must reach well beyond the rights of individuals and the difficulties or benefits that cloned children or their families might encounter. We must consider what kind of a society we wish to be, and, in particular, what forms of bringing children into the world we want to encourage and what sorts of relations between the generations we want to preserve.

Cloning-to-produce-children could distort the way we raise and view children, by carrying to full expression many regrettable tendencies already present in our culture. We are already liable to regard children largely as vehicles for our own fulfillment and ambitions. The impulse to create "designer children" is present today—as temptation and social practice. The notion of life as a gift, mysterious and limited, is under siege. Cloning-to-produce-children would carry these tendencies and temptations to an extreme expression. It advances the notion that the child is but an object of our sovereign mastery.

A society that clones human beings thinks about human beings (and especially children) differently than does a society that refuses to do so. It could easily be argued that we have already in myriad ways begun to show signs of regarding our children as projects on which we may work our wills. Further, it could be argued that we have been so desensitized by our earlier steps in this direction that we do not recognize this tendency as a corruption. While some people contend that cloning-to-produce-children would not take us much further down a path we have already been traveling, we would emphasize that the precedent of treating children as projects cuts two ways in the moral argument. Instead of using this precedent to justify taking the next step of cloning, the next step might rather serve as a warning and a mirror in which we may discover reasons to reconsider what we are already doing. Precisely because the stakes are so high, precisely because the new biotechnologies touch not only our bodies and minds but also the very idea of our humanity, we should ask ourselves how we as a society want to approach questions of human dignity and flourishing.

D. CONCLUSION

Cloning-to-produce-children may represent a forerunner of what will be a growing number of capacities to intervene in and alter the human genetic endowment. No doubt, earlier human actions have produced changes in the human gene pool: to take only one example, the use of insulin to treat diabetics who otherwise would have died before reproducing has increased the genes for diabetes in the population. But different responsibilities accrue when one sets out to make such changes prospectively, directly, and deliberately. To do so without regard for the likelihood of serious unintended and unanticipated consequences would be the height of hubris. Systems of great complexity do not respond well to blunt human intervention, and one can hardly think of a more complex system—both natural and social—than that which surrounds human reproduction and the human genome. Given the enormous importance of what is at stake, we believe that the so-called "precautionary principle" should be our guide in this arena. This principle would suggest that scientists, technologists, and, indeed, all of us should be modest in claiming to understand the many possible consequences of any profound alteration of human procreation, especially where there are not compelling reasons to proceed. Lacking such understanding, no one should take action so drastic as the cloning of a human child. In the absence of the necessary human wisdom, prudence calls upon us to set limits on efforts to control and remake the character of human procreation and human life.

It is not only a matter of prudence. Cloning-to-produce-children would also be an *injustice* to the cloned child—from the imposition of the chromosomes of someone else, to the intentional deprivation of biological parents, to all of the possible bodily and psychological harms that we have enumerated in this chapter. It is ultimately the claim that the cloned child would be seriously wronged—and not only harmed in body—that would justify government intervention. It is to this question—the public policy question of what the government should and can do to prevent such injustice—that we will turn in Chapter Seven. But, regarding the ethical assessment, Members of the Council are in unanimous agreement that cloning-to-produce-children is not only unsafe but also morally unacceptable and ought not to be attempted.*

NOTE

1. National Academy of Sciences (NAS), *Scientific and Medical Aspects of Human Reproductive Cloning*, Washington, DC: National Academy Press, 2002.

---

*Not surprisingly, some of us feel more strongly than others about this conclusion. One or two of us might someday be willing to see cloning-to-produce-children occur in the rare defensible case, but then only if means were available to confine its use to such cases.

REPRODUCTIVE CLONING: ANOTHER LOOK

Bonnie Steinbock

Somatic cell nuclear transfer ("SCNT") in mammals involves removing the nucleus, which contains the DNA, from a somatic cell (any cell in the body other than a gamete, that is, sperm or oocyte [egg]), and putting it into an enucleated oocyte (that is, an oocyte from which the nucleus has been removed). Fusion of the donor somatic cell's nucleus and the recipient enucleated oocyte can be performed chemically or, more often, by a jolt of electricity (a process called electroporation). If the process is successful, the newly created cell will start to divide and become an embryo. SCNT for reproductive purposes is also known as human reproductive cloning.

In 1997, the Report of the National Bioethics Advisory Commission ("Report") entitled *Cloning Human Beings*[1] recommended "[a] continuation of the current moratorium on the use of federal funding in support of" research into SCNT cloning for reproductive purposes.[2] The National Bioethics Advisory Commission's ("NBAC") objection to human reproductive cloning was based primarily on safety grounds, such as the high probability of failure and consequent high risk of miscarriage, and the risk of developmental abnormalities in offspring. Critics of the Report alleged that in focusing primarily on safety issues, NBAC "duck[ed] the moral questions."[3] They had hoped that NBAC would give an unqualified rejection of human reproductive cloning based on moral concerns such as human individuality and dignity, the commodifi-cation of children, and the opportunity for genetic enhancement.

However, NBAC did not *duck* the moral issues; it simply was unable to reach a consensus on them. Given the diverse ethical and political views of the members of NBAC, it is not surprising that safety was the only factor on which all members could agree, especially within the ninety day time constraint President Clinton imposed. The Report recommended that the moral debate continue, so that when the five year moratorium ended, the moral issues would be better defined.

Eight years later, are we any clearer on the morality of human reproductive cloning (or as the President's Council on Bioethics ("President's Council") prefers to call it, "cloning-to-produce-children")? There is widespread, indeed nearly universal, agreement that human reproductive cloning should not proceed. In part, the vehement rejection of reproductive cloning can be seen as a political calculation on the part of supporters of therapeutic cloning that unless they completely dissociate themselves from reproductive cloning, they will be unable to garner support for what they regard as much more important: therapeutic cloning.

Therapeutic cloning refers to the use of SCNT cloning to create embryos from which embryonic stem cells are removed and stem cell lines created. The hope is that these embryonic stem cell lines could one day be used to cure a range of diseases and injuries, including diabetes, cancer, heart disease, Parkinson's, and spinal cord injuries. In both therapeutic and reproductive cloning, the same technique is used to create an embryo, but in reproductive cloning the embryo is gestated to become a fetus, and then a baby. In therapeutic cloning, the embryo is created as a source of embryonic stem cells. However, since removing the stem cells destroys the embryo, this research is unacceptable to those who regard human embryos as having the same moral status as born human beings.

From *University of Chicago Legal Forum* (2006): 87–111.

Editors' note: Some author's notes have been cut. Students who want to follow up on sources should consult the original article.

1. National Bioethics Advisory Commission ("NBAC"), *Cloning Human Beings* (1997).

2. Id at 109.

3. Gina Kolata, *Commission on Cloning: Ready-Made Controversy,* NY Times A12 (June 9, 1997) (attributing the criticism to George Annas, a law professor at Boston University).

Some believe the term "therapeutic cloning" is misleading. The President's Council noted that,

> [t]he act of cloning embryos may be undertaken with healing motives. But it is not *itself* an act of healing or therapy. The beneficiaries of any such acts of cloning are, at the moment, hypothetical and in the future. And if medical treatments do eventually result, the embryonic clone from which the treatment was derived will not itself be the beneficiary of any therapy. On the contrary, this sort of cloning actually takes apart (or destroys) the embryonic being that results from the act of cloning.[4]

To avoid any misleading implications, the President's Council recommended the term "research cloning" or "cloning-for-biomedical-research.

Many supporters of therapeutic cloning think that politically it would be wise to dissociate themselves from reproductive cloning. As Rudolph Jaenisch and Ian Wilmut put it, "[p]ublic reaction to human cloning failures could hinder research in embryonic stem cells for the repair of organs and tissues. . . . The potential benefit of this therapeutic cell cloning will be enormous, and this research should not be associated with the human cloning activists.[5] This could be a smart move. Should the promise of therapeutic cloning be realized, an extremely large number of people would benefit—many more than the number of people interested in reproductive cloning. But politics aside, are there well-founded moral arguments against human reproductive cloning?

I.   SAFETY ARGUMENTS

Arguments about the safety of certain research techniques or new technologies are clearly relevant to the morality of engaging in that research or using the new technology. Every code of ethics concerning research on human subjects emphasizes the importance of protecting subjects from undue risks of harm. While it may be controversial whether the information likely to be obtained from a particular research protocol justifies the risk of harm to human

subjects, there is no doubt that the imposition of risk always requires justification—the potential for harm is always an ethical reason against performing an experiment or using a certain technology.

Another advantage of focusing on the safety of a technique like cloning is that safety arguments are, or are usually thought to be, less subjective than other kinds of moral arguments because they are based on empirical evidence, as opposed to moral principles and values. Yet precisely because they are based on the current state of the science, safety arguments can only express contingent opposition to cloning: if cloning techniques become safe and effective, the safety argument evaporates. Because many opponents of reproductive cloning favor a flat ban on reproductive cloning, not a temporary or limited one, they are not satisfied with arguments from safety. Moreover, although safety claims are supposed to be scientific and empirical, critics have charged that they are often motivated by a moral aversion to cloning rather than by an objective assessment of the science involved.

A.   Is Human Reproductive Cloning Even Possible?

Since as yet no one has ever cloned and brought to full term a human being, we have no direct evidence about whether it can be done safely. In fact, there is some doubt about whether it is even possible to clone a human being. In 2004, a South Korean team, headed by Dr. Hwang Woo Suk, claimed to have cloned a human blastocyst.[6] In June 2005, his team claimed to have cloned human blastocysts using DNA from eleven patients, through an efficient new technique that required very few human eggs. However, it was later determined that Dr. Hwang had fabricated the evidence supporting his claims. While the Hwang debacle was undoubtedly something of a setback for therapeutic cloning, British scientists have since managed to clone

---

4. President's Council on Bioethics ("President's Council"), *Human Cloning and Human Dignity: An Ethical Inquiry* 44 (2002).

5. Rudolph Jaenisch and Ian Wilmut, *Don't Clone Humans!* 291 Science 2552, 2552 (Mar 30, 2001) at 2552.

6. Nicholas Wade and Choe Sang-Hun, *Human Cloning Was All Faked, Koreans Report*, NY Times A1 (Jan 10, 2006). See also NAS Panel, *Human Reproductive Cloning* at 260 (cited in note 1) (defining a blastocyst as "[a] preimplantation embryo in placental mammals . . . of about 30–150 cells").

human blastocysts for research purposes, demonstrating that it is indeed possible. However, neither British laboratory intends to transfer the cloned embryos to a uterus for gestation.

Reproductive cloning has also been attempted with nonhuman primates. In 2004, Dr. Gerald Schatten and his team from the University of Pittsburgh reported that they had cloned 135 monkey embryos using Dr. Hwang's technique, and transferred them into 25 mothers. However, none of them resulted in a pregnancy that lasted more than a month. Nor has anyone else succeeded in bringing a cloned primate to term. So far, there has been only one report of a birth of a cloned rhesus monkey, and that report has not been replicated. Dr. Schatten says that his research cannot be used as evidence that a cloned human baby could survive long in development.

B. Would Human Reproductive Cloning Be Safe?

At this point, it seems we must remain agnostic about whether human reproductive cloning is possible. The next question is whether it would be safe. To answer that question, we must look to the experience with cloning other animals, including mice, sheep, goats, pigs, cattle, cats, and, most recently, a dog. Such evidence is not perfect, since every species is different, but it is the best we have.

In *Remaking Eden*,[7] Lee Silver suggested that cloning might be *safer* than ordinary sexual reproduction, since many genetic diseases are the result of autosomal recessive genes which are transmitted to offspring only when both parents carry the recessive trait. For example, if two carriers of a gene for cystic fibrosis ("CF") mate, there is a 25 percent chance that the resulting child will have CF, a 25 percent chance the child will be disease-free, and a 50 percent chance the child will be a carrier. But if a carrier for CF, or any autosomal recessive trait, were cloned, he or she would not transmit the disease. For this reason, Silver argued that the rate of genetic defects in cloned animals

would be inherently lower than in animals created through sexual reproduction.[8]

However, when *Remaking Eden* was written, only one animal, a sheep called Dolly, had ever been cloned, and Silver did not anticipate the health problems that subsequently came to light. Dolly, Silver says, "was perfectly normal no matter what rumors you've heard."[9] Since Dolly, many healthy clones have been born and have survived to fertile adulthood.

Cloned cattle often suffer from "large offspring syndrome" ("LOS"), as well as "more drastic defects," such as placental malfunction, respiratory distress, and circulatory problems, the most common causes of neonatal death. "Even apparently healthy survivors may suffer from immune dysfunction, or kidney or brain malformation, which can contribute to death later. So, if human cloning is attempted, those embryos that do not die early may live to become abnormal children and adults; both are troubling outcomes.[10] Often cited as safety reasons not to pursue

---

7. Lee Silver, *Remaking Eden: How Genetic Engineering and Cloning Will Transform the American Family* (Avon 1997).

8. See Silver, *Remaking Eden* at 121 (cited in note 7) ("[B]irth defects in cloned children could occur less frequently than birth defects in naturally conceived children.").

9. E-mail from Lee Silver to Bonnie Steinbock (Oct 7, 2005) (on file with author). Actually, Dolly did suffer from arthritis, but Wilmut thinks that it is unlikely that it was a result of her having been cloned. Instead, he thinks it may have been caused by her standing on her back legs to greet visitors. Rick Weiss, *Middle-Aged Dolly Develops Arthritis: Questions on Clones' Aging Raised*, Wash Post A03 (Jan 5, 2002). She also developed a contagious lung disease that was spreading among the sheep at the Roslin Institute, which led to her being euthanized in 2003 at the age of 6 years. Again, the cause was probably not having been cloned, since sheep that live indoors—as was necessary in the case of Dolly for security reasons—are prone to developing lung infections of this kind. Kerry Lynn Macintosh, *Illegal Beings: Human Clones and the Law* 63 (Cambridge: Cambridge University Press 2005).

10. Jaenisch and Wilmut, 291 Science at 2552 (cited in note 5). See also Nadia Halim, *Scientists Show Cloning Leads to Severe Dysregulation of Many Genes*. Whitehead Institute for Biomedical Research (Sept 11, 2002), available at <http://www.wi.mit.edu/news/archives/2002/rj_0911.html> (last visited Apr 19, 2006) ("[E]ven seemingly 'normal-looking' clones may have serious underlying epigenetic abnormalities."); John Travis, *Dolly Was Lucky*, Science News Online, available at <http://www.geneimprint.com/articles/?y=Press&q=cloning/sciencenews/index.html> (last visited Apr 19, 2006) (describing a cloned sheep that had to be euthanized due to a severe respiratory problem, quoting Ian Wilmut. "Who would want to be responsible for a child born with an abnormality like that?").

human reproductive cloning are its inefficiency and the consequent risk of miscarriage and stillbirth, premature aging, and LOS. I will consider each of these in turn.

1. Inefficiency. Only a few percent of nuclear transfer embryos survive to birth, and of those, many die within the perinatal period. According to Jaenisch and Wilmut, "[t]here is no reason to believe that the outcomes of attempted human cloning will be any different.[11] In her recent book, *Illegal Beings,* law professor Kerry Lynn Macintosh argues that the inefficiency argument is a half truth. In particular, she objects to the way the media presented Dolly's story. It took Wilmut and his associates 277 attempts to get Dolly, but the story was often presented as if there were 277 miscarriages. For example, a congressional report recommending a complete ban on human reproductive cloning claimed that "[c]loning experiments produced 277 stillborn, miscarried or dead sheep before Dolly was successfully cloned. That failure rate, which has remained steady since 1997, is not acceptable for human beings." However, 277 actually refers to the number of enucleated eggs Wilmut used. "In fact, there were no miscarriages, no deformed lambs, and no deaths resulting from the transfer of the *adult* cell nuclei in the Dolly experiment."[12] Macintosh acknowledges that some of Wilmut's other experiments did end in miscarriages, but in those experiments he tried to clone sheep from embryonic and fetal cells. Macintosh maintains that it is not surprising that these attempts had a high failure rate. The majority of embryos and fetuses produced by sexual reproduction never make it to birth, so why should we expect a different result with cloning? By contrast, when a somatic cell from an adult animal is used, you are using DNA that has proven its ability to generate a healthy term birth.

Nevertheless, even if Dolly's case was misreported, a relatively high rate of miscarriage, stillbirth, and neonatal mortality has plagued animal cloning. As the National Academy of Sciences Panel put it, "across multiple species there are far more failures in the development of cloned fetuses than there are live normal births."[13] In animals, the low efficiency rate of cloning makes it an economically unfeasible reproductive technique. In human beings, a reproductive technique that resulted in a high rate of miscarriage would be ethically unacceptable, especially since the losses do not occur only in very early pregnancy, as is common in natural pregnancies. "Whereas most fetal losses in conventional zygotic pregnancies occur in the first trimester, with reproductive cloning, fetuses are lost throughout pregnancy and in the early neonatal period.[14] This is of great concern, not only because a late miscarriage is more likely to be emotionally more distressing to the mother than an early one, but also because of the increased risk of maternal morbidity and mortality. Cloning studies in animals show that there are often abnormalities in the placenta or the fetus, which probably cause the miscarriage. These pregnancy complications, along with pregnancy toxemia, also pose a risk to maternal health. What about the health of cloned animals that do manage to survive? According to some reports, the majority are "physiologically and reproductively normal." However, some health problems have been flagged.

2. Premature aging. It has been charged that nuclear transfer results in an animal with shortened telomeres. Telomeres are the caps on the ends of chromosomes, and they shorten as somatic cells age. Thus, there is a potential for cloned embryos, whose chromosomes come from somatic cells, to have shortened telomeres, producing an animal that is older than her chronological age. While this claim was made about Dolly, it is not clear that Dolly really had shortened telomeres, or that she suffered from premature aging. One reason to doubt that her telomeres were too short is that telomeres are very small, making it difficult to measure them accurately. The alleged difference between Dolly and other sheep of her age "could be within the range of natural

---

11. Id.

12. Macintosh, *Illegal Beings* at 48 (cited in note 9).

13. National Academy of Sciences ("NAS"), *Scientific and Medical Aspects of Human Reproductive Cloning* 40 (Natl Academy 2002).

14. Id.

variation in the telomere lengths of sheep."[15] In addition, such shortening has not been found in clones of other species, such as cattle. The report of the National Academies of Sciences Panel noted that the possibility of prematurely old clones "does not seem to be a major concern. Any shortening of telomeres in cloned sheep appears to be minor and can be minimized by judicious choice of the cell type used as a nucleus donor."[16] Moreover, human blastocysts have high levels of telomerase activity, which suggests that they might be able to rebuild telomeres after reproductive cloning.

3. Large offspring syndrome. Of greater concern than premature aging is the tendency of cloned cattle fetuses and newborns to grow to abnormally large sizes, jeopardizing their own health and that of the mothers who gestate and give birth to them. This defect is referred to as "large offspring syndrome" ("LOS"). In addition to LOS, abnormal placentas, maternal and fetal distress, and cardiovascular abnormalities have been observed. However, it is not clear that LOS would occur in cloned humans. Cows and sheep conceived through in vitro fertilization ("IVF") also have a tendency toward LOS, and this has not been observed in human babies. In fact, human babies conceived through IVF tend to be smaller than normal. Moreover, a team of scientists, led by Randy Jirtle, at Duke University claim to have discovered that a key gene restraining embryo growth, called insulin-like growth factor 2 receptor ("IGF2R"), cannot be switched off during human cloning. This, they allege, would make LOS in humans far less likely, and thus make human cloning safer than animal cloning. But other cloning experts call Jirtle's claim "ludicrous," noting that disruption of other imprinted genes might be just as important as the disruption of IGF2R.

At this point, no one really knows what causes LOS or why it occurs in some species and not others.

"All that can be said is that it probably results from abnormal gene expression in the early embryo, including the misexpression of imprinted genes."[17] Thus, to understand LOS and other abnormalities in cloned animals, we need to understand a little bit about embryonic development in sexual reproduction and cloning.

4. Genetic imprinting and reprogramming. In ordinary sexual reproduction, offspring receive two copies of each gene, one from the mother, the other from the father. In some cases, for normal development to occur, one of those copies must be silenced or switched off, so that only one copy of the gene is expressed. This silencing or switching off is known as genetic imprinting. Many people believe that the low efficiency of cloning, as well as the abnormalities observed in cloned animals, are due to imprinting failures that occur during the cloning process. These anomalies are epigenetic, that is, they concern the expression of genes.

After fertilization occurs, the fertilized egg, or zygote, begins to divide into many cells. Each of these cells is undifferentiated in that it can give rise to any of the cells in the body. Eventually, the cells become differentiated: distinct cell types. By contrast, the nucleus of a cloned embryo comes from a differentiated cell, a somatic cell of a specific type. If it retains its particular pattern of gene expression, it cannot develop into all the different cells of the body. The trick in SCNT cloning is to undo the cell-specific pattern of the donor somatic cell in a process known variously as genetic, nuclear, or genomic reprogramming.

Jaenisch and Wilmut argue that, in general, the defects in fetal clones and live-born cloned offspring are due to failures in genomic reprogramming. It is possible that successful genomic reprogramming requires that the cytoplasm receive two distinct sets of DNA—one from a sperm and one from an egg—as in ordinary sexual reproduction. Thus epigenetic errors in cloning may result from the fact that the egg cytoplasm, which does the reprogramming, is presented with two sets of DNA from a single somatic cell.

---

15. Macintosh, *Illegal Beings* at 61 (cited in note 9) ("The scientists admitted that this difference could be within the range of natural variation in the telomere lengths of sheep.")

16. NAS Panel, *Human Reproductive Cloning* at 48 (cited in note 13).

---

17. NAS Panel, *Human Reproductive Cloning* at 41 (cited in note 13).

Alternatively, the epigenetic errors may have to do with the timing of reprogramming. Epigenetic reprogramming normally is accomplished during spermatogenesis and oogenesis, "processes that in humans take months and years, respectively.[18] By contrast, in nuclear transfer, the reprogramming of the cloned embryos must occur "within minutes or, at most, hours." This time difference could cause reprogramming errors, which "could lead in turn to dysregulation of gene expression.

However, some have argued that the problem is not that the reprogramming occurs too quickly in nuclear transfer, but that it occurs too slowly. According to one author, nuclear reprogramming does not occur within the hours immediately following SCNT, but is a slow, ongoing process in the cloned embryo, and one that is likely not completed until the cells become committed to the inner cell mass lineage.

> This creates a paradoxical situation in which cloned embryo nuclei must sustain and direct their own reprogramming toward totipotentiality during cleavage and beyond. One significant consequence of this is that the phenotype of cloned embryos will be distinct from that of normal embryos, and will likely vary with donor cell type. Thus, cloned embryos likely exist in a poor state of health in standard embryo culture media, and this situation may persist or even worsen upon transfer to the reproductive tract.[19]

It is not known whether the temporally protracted nature of reprogramming is an unavoidable part of cloning, or whether it could be overcome by improvements in the technology. Improving the culture system might accelerate the pace of reprogramming, avoiding many of the epigenetic problems that are seen.

Some scientists think that cloning problems such as low efficiency and abnormalities are not due to reprogramming at all. One study compared the gene expression profiles of cow embryos obtained by artificial insemination ("AI"), IVF, and SCNT, and found that the SCNT embryos had undergone significant reprogramming by the blastocyst stage. Moreover, the cloned embryos resembled AI embryos much more closely than IVF embryos. This

suggests that the problems in cloning animals may not result from nuclear reprogramming, and that "problems may occur during redifferentiation for tissue genesis and organogenesis, and small reprogramming errors may be magnified downstream in development."[20] Another theory is that poor efficiency and defects in cloned offspring might be the result not of imprinting errors, but of mitochondrial heteroplasmy, in which the embryo inherits mitochondria from two different individuals, instead of just the mother.

Still another theory is that phenotypic anomalies could be due to the type of donor cell used. A study of cloned mice done by a group of Japanese scientists found that over 90 percent of newborn mice pups were normal, and that the paternal and maternal imprints on genes that direct embryonic development were faithfully maintained. The expression of imprinted genes was found to be normal in cloned fetuses, although some placentas were larger than normal and did exhibit some epigenetic alternations. The study suggested that previously reported abnormalities in cloned mice may have occurred because they were cloned from embryonic stem cells, instead of adult somatic cells. When the mice were cloned from adult somatic cells, they were indistinguishable from controls. "Epigenetic mutations accumulated during culture of [embryonic stem] cells, not the biological effects inherent to [SCNT], are therefore likely to have been the primary cause of anomalies in [embryonic stem] cell [nuclear transfer] clones . . . [embryonic stem] cells are perhaps a poor model with which to study [SCNT].[21] One commentator noted that

> the amazing thing . . . is that this paper that said that cloning was safer than previously thought was published in a top scientific journal, *Science,* and it didn't even make it into the newspapers. . . . Dolly sneezes

---

18. Jaenisch and Wilmut, 291 Science at 2552 (cited in note 5).

19. Keith E. Latham, *Cloning: Questions Answered and Unsolved,* 72 Differentiation 11, 13 (Feb 2004).

20. Sadie Smith, et al, *Global Gene Expression Profiles Reveal Significant Nuclear Reprogramming by the Blastocyst Stage After Cloning,* 102 Proceedings Natl Acad Sciences 17582, 17582 (Dec 6, 2005). For a general discussion, see NAS Panel, *Human Reproductive Cloning* at 47-48 (cited in note 13) (discussing the potential problems related to mitochondrial heteroplasmy).

21. Kimiko Inoue, et al, *Faithful Expression of Imprinted Genes in Cloned Mice,* 295 Science 297, 297 (Jan 11, 2002).

and its [sic] on the front page of the *New York Times,* but this paper saying clones are okay doesn't go anywhere. People don't want to hear this.[22]

In sum, we do not yet know what causes the problems observed in cloned animals, whether they would occur in human beings, or how they might be prevented. Clearly, it would be irresponsible at this point to attempt to clone human beings, but with more research into cloning nonhuman mammals, the problems may be circumvented. This, then, leads to the next question:

C. How Safe Is Safe Enough? Some of the literature suggests that human reproductive cloning would be ethically unacceptable if there were any chance of producing a child with a serious birth defect. For example, Cibelli, et al, argue that "until nuclear transfer is better characterized and understood—and the danger of generating a handicapped child *eliminated*—the unpredictability of the procedure strongly counsels against its application in human reproduction."[23] However, the danger of having a child with a disability will never be eliminated. Reproduction—natural or assisted—is not risk-free. Even ordinary sexual reproduction can result in miscarriage, stillbirth, birth defects, or maternal morbidity or mortality. So the issue should not be whether cloning is perfectly safe, but rather, how safe must cloning be in order to be ethically acceptable? According to Professor Macintosh, the animal data reveal that "an astonishing 77 percent of live born animals were healthy."[24] This may be "astonishing" to those convinced that all cloned animals must have serious defects. At the same time, a 77 percent rate of healthy offspring is not wonderful; a technique with a 23 percent rate of birth defects would not be medically or ethically acceptable for specialists in reproductive medicine.

If eliminating all risk is impossible, and a 23 percent risk of a serious defect is too high, what risk is acceptable? Some think the point of reference should be the rate of defects in ordinary nonmedically assisted reproduction. Approximately 2-3 percent of babies are born with a medically significant birth defect. However, this also seems too stringent a standard, for "in vitro fertilization carries roughly twice the risk of major birth defects and low weight in term singleton babies, and no one seriously suggests that using in vitro fertilization is unethical."[25] A more reasonable comparison, it seems, is with current assisted reproduction technology ("ART"). The figure usually given is that over 95 percent of children born through ART are normal, leaving a 5 percent risk of serious defect.

Suppose researchers managed to clone chimpanzees, our nearest relatives, with the risk of a serious defect below 5 percent. Would this be "safe enough" to begin clinical trials in humans? The President's Council thinks not. In fact, the President's Council categorically opposes doing any research on reproductive cloning with human beings, because this would entail doing unjustifiable experiments on human beings. There seems to be no ethical way to try to discover whether cloning-to-produce-children can become safe, now or in the future."[26]

This is a startling conclusion. If all cloning research involving humans is unjustifiable experimentation, why is not all research on assisted reproductive techniques equally unethical? The President's Council responds that the analogy does not hold because "the case of cloning is genuinely different." They argue that, unlike cloning, IVF is still sexual reproduction, the joining of two gametes "that nature has selected over millions of years for the entire mammalian line."[27] By contrast, cloning is asexual reproduction, which involves reprogramming. That is true, but it is a description of cloning, not a reason why it can never ethically be shown to be safe. There does not seem to be a reason why of all new techniques, cloning should be the only one incapable of being shown to be safe enough to warrant trials with informed and willing human subjects.

---

22. Lee Silver, *Public Policy Crafted in Response to Public Ignorance is Bad Public Policy,* (transcribed remarks), 53 Hastings L J 1037, 1042–43 (2002).

23. José B. Cibelli, et al, "The Health Profile of Cloned Animals," 20 *Nature Biotechnology* 13, 14 (Jan 2002) (emphasis added).

24. Macintosh, *Illegal Beings* at 58–59 (cited in note 9).

25. Philip G. Peters, Jr., *How Safe Is Safe Enough? Obligations to the Children of Reproductive Technology* 47 (Oxford 2004).

26. President's Council, *Human Cloning* at 94 (cited in note 4).

27. President's Council, *Human Cloning* at 93–94 (cited in note 4).

Another issue that has received a great deal of attention is whether any harm is done to a child by using a reproductive technique that causes the child to be born with a serious defect, if the child could not have been born otherwise. Many have argued that so long as the child has a life worth living, he or she has not been harmed or wronged by birth. Moreover, if the child has not been harmed or wronged, it is hard to see what wrong has been committed by those responsible for the child's birth. This complex issue is beyond the scope of this paper, but there can be very good reasons not to use techniques that will result in the birth of children with serious defects, even if those reasons do not refer to the child's having been wronged or harmed.

While the safety objections are clearly important, they cannot justify a categorical, permanent ban on human reproductive cloning. Should modifications in techniques turn out to make cloning in other mammals, especially primates, relatively safe (in other words, as safe as other reproductive technologies), there could not be safety objections to attempting to clone human beings. I turn now therefore to:

II.   NON-SAFETY OBJECTIONS

A.   Easily Dismissed Objections

Some of the objections to human reproductive cloning can be easily dismissed, such as the idea that human reproductive cloning is "playing God." All medical intervention is "playing God," in the sense that human intervention is changing the course of nature. By vaccinating children, by treating people with antibiotics, and by transplanting organs, we prevent the deaths of millions of people each year. It does not seem that there is any principled way to determine which of these practices counts as "playing God" and which do not—or as I prefer to put it, which instances of "playing God" are morally acceptable and which unacceptable. It seems that each new medical intervention is regarded with suspicion, as a human transgression on divine prerogative. This is true of organ transplantation, which is now an accepted part of modern medicine. To the extent that the "playing God" objection simply reflects the unfamiliarity of a medical intervention, it is

not a serious moral objection. On the other hand, if the objection is that we should be very careful about unforeseen and unwanted side effects of cloning, or any new technology, it deserves to be taken seriously. But if this is the correct interpretation of the "playing God" objection, it is only the safety objection restated.

Another easily dismissible objection to human reproductive cloning is that it would threaten the individuality of the cloned individual. This objection stems from a misunderstanding of what cloning is. It is not the creation of an exact copy of an individual, but rather that person's delayed genetic twin, no more a copy than identical twins are copies. They have the same genome, but they are not exactly alike, emotionally, mentally, or even physically; friends and relatives can usually tell them apart. To think that a clone would be a copy of the person who donates the somatic cell is to commit the fallacy of genetic determinism: that is, the fallacy of thinking that it is an individual's genome that is the sole determinant of what that person is or will be.

There is a related objection, however, that is not so easily dismissible, and this has to do with the numbers of individuals cloned. It is one thing to have one identical twin; it is another to have a hundred. It would be unsettling, to say the least, to encounter dozens of individuals who had your genome. This might be a reason to limit the number of human clones created from any particular donor. This in turn suggests that the morality of cloning human beings may well turn on the reasons for doing it, as we will see in the next section.

B.   Cloning and the Selection of Genetic Makeup

One concern expressed by the President's Council was that "[c]loned children would . . . be the first human beings whose entire genetic makeup is selected in advance."[28] The fear is that this would open the door to a future project of genetic manipulation and genetic control.

Cloning would enable people to know in advance their child's genome, which could be the reason why

---

28. President's Council, *Human Cloning* at 104 (cited in note 4).

some people would choose to clone: to get a child with a particular genome. This might be done for egotistical ends, for example, by someone who thought that he or she was a particularly fine specimen of humanity that ought to be replicated. Or cloning might be used by people who want to raise a child with someone else's genome—for example, Michael Jordan's—because they want to be the parents of the next basketball superstar. Or cloning might be used to "replace" a dead or dying child.

If those who use cloning expect to get an identical copy of the person cloned, they are likely to be greatly disappointed because, as noted above, a person's genome does not determine what that individual will be like emotionally, intellectually, or even physically. Michael Jordan's clone would undoubtedly be athletic, but there is no guarantee he would be good at or interested in basketball. He might be more interested in football or tennis or even (gasp!) ballet. To the extent that cloning is chosen because individuals believe that it can deliver a replica of the person cloned, it illustrates the fallacy of genetic determinism.

If reproductive cloning were to become safe and effective, it would be important not to mislead people into thinking that cloning would enable them to create a child "to spec." As Lee Silver put it, "all that anyone will ever get from the use of cloning, or any other reproductive technology, is an unpredictable son or daughter, who won't listen to his parents any more than my children will listen to me."[29]

Guarding against the fallacy of genetic determinism or the idea that cloning can create a replica would be especially important where the prospective parents were attempting to replace a dead or dying child. Grieving parents might believe or hope that cloning would enable them to have their child back again, and this is, of course, impossible. For clinics or physicians to suggest otherwise would be the height of irresponsibility. However, it is possible that some people might want to clone a deceased child, even with a clear understanding of its limits, and full recognition of the environmental and in utero factors that influence personality, behavior, and even physical characteristics. Autumn Fiester has considered this with respect to the cloning of pets. Responding to the objection that pet cloning is

a deceptive practice that exploits the grief of pet owners, she writes, "[t]he bereft pet owner might know full well that the clone will be nothing more than a genetic twin, and the decision to clone might be merely an attempt to preserve something important from the original animal, rather than *resurrect* it."[30] She suggests that the desire to clone a beloved pet is no more irrational than the desire to breed the pet. It may be argued that this demonstrates precisely what would be wrong with cloning a human being; that in cloning a human being, we would be treating the individual as it is permissible to treat pets, as something less than full human beings possessing human dignity.

C. The Human Dignity Objection

The President's Council also offers a human dignity objection. Contrasting cloning with sexual procreation, the Council states:

> Parents beget a child who enters the world exactly as they did—as an unmade gift, not as a product. Children born of this process stand equally beside their progenitors as fellow human beings, not beneath them as made objects. In this way, the uncontrolled beginnings of human procreation endow each new generation and each new individual with the dignity and freedom enjoyed by all who came before.[31]

The idea here seems to be that whereas begetting creates a *child*, cloning creates a *product*, a thing, a made object. This turns children into things, violating Kant's dictum that we are never to treat others merely as means to our ends, that is, merely as things or tools or props to be manipulated. But is this a fair objection? Would cloning create things instead of children? Would it be treating children as mere means to our ends?

It is important to emphasize that if cloning technology were developed to the point of being safe and effective in human beings, the clone would be a fellow human being, as much like you or I as Dolly

---

29. Silver, 53 Hastings L J at 1041 (cited in note 22).

30. Autumn Fiester, "Creating Fido's Twin: Can Pet Cloning Be Ethically Justified?" 35 *Hastings Center Report* 34, 37 (July/Aug 2005).

31. President's Council, *Human Cloning* at 105–06 (cited in note 4).

was like other sheep. The cloned baby would not be a product or a thing or a made object, but a human being with the same human dignity accorded any other human being.

However, the objection to cloning may not be that the cloned child would not be a fellow human being, but rather that the decision to clone suggests that the parents want a child with a specific genome, and that this in turn suggests an attempt to design the child. The attempt to design the child is what turns the child into a product. Parents are not supposed to want to design their children, nor is their love supposed to be contingent on the child's having certain traits or characteristics. Parents ought to accept their children for who they are. The attempt to select or control their genomes, and thus to some extent, their traits, is a form of parental tyranny. "When parents attempt to shape their children's characteristics to match their preferences and expectations, such an exercise of free choice on the parents' part may constrain their child's prospects for flourishing."[32]

While this objection has nothing to do with human dignity, it is not a trivial concern. It is important not to encourage parents to think that they can or should design their children, partly because this might constrain the child's development, and partly because the parents are likely to be disappointed, which may have further adverse effects on their ability to be good parents. However, it should be noted that many infertile couples already choose sperm and egg donors on the basis of traits they hope will be inherited by their offspring. Most often, they hope to get a child that "fits into" their family. Like adoptive couples, they seek to have a child similar to the child they would have had, but for their infertility. This selection of gametes has not led to parental tyranny, so it is unclear why cloning would.

Moreover, prospective parents might choose reproductive cloning not in [an] attempt to get a child with a specific genome, but simply to have a child with whom they have a genetic connection. Consider a couple who have not been able to have a child. Their infertility work-up reveals that the husband

has severe male factor infertility. In other words, he has no viable sperm at all. Their physician recommends sperm donation. However, the couple is reluctant to bring a "third party" into their marriage. They want their child to be biologically "theirs." That is why they are not (yet) willing to consider adoption—just like most couples who undergo assisted reproduction. Imagine now that cloning has been shown to be safe and effective—as safe and effective as IVF. The man could provide a somatic cell, from which his DNA would be extracted and inserted into an enucleated egg cell from his wife. The resulting embryo would be implanted in her uterus for gestation. She would give birth to a son who would be genetically related to his father (albeit with a small amount of mitochondrial DNA from his mother) and biologically (gestationally) related to his mother. It is difficult to see anything in this scenario that makes it morally distinct from other forms of assisted reproduction. Moreover, when we consider this use of reproductive cloning, there is no danger of dozens of copies, since human parents typically only want a few children.

The idea that a reproductive technology can threaten or violate human dignity is puzzling, and requires us to think about what human dignity consists of. We may think of "dignity" as having to do with a certain demeanor: acting with formal, grave, or noble bearing. This sense of dignity has little to do with any aspect of reproduction, sexual or asexual. Another sense of dignity is related to the Kantian requirement of respect for persons. Human dignity is clearly violated when people are tortured, demeaned, or humiliated, since such treatment reduces them to mere means to someone else's ends. Less extreme forms of dignity-violation, such as deception, coercion, and exploitation, also treat people in a way to which they could not in principle consent, and thus violates Kant's second formulation of the categorical imperative. But none of this has anything to do with methods by which children might be brought into the world. There is no reason why clones (or "monoparental children," as Silver prefers to call them[33]) would be treated any worse

---

32. Thomas H. Murray, *Enhancement*, in Bonnie Steinbock, ed, *The Oxford Handbook of Bioethics* (Oxford, 2007).

33. Silver, 53 Hastings L J at 1040 (cited in note 29).

than children created by assisted reproductive therapy—and they might even be cherished more than children who are the accidental result of a one-night stand.

CONCLUSION

None of the non-safety moral arguments against cloning is terribly persuasive. Either they are premised on the fallacy of genetic determinism—which should be rejected—or they are directed not against cloning itself, but against certain morally objectionable reasons for wanting to clone children, in other words, to get a child with certain specific traits. If the goal is simply to have a genetically related child, and due to gametic failure cloning is the only way to achieve this goal, it is difficult to see why cloning would be morally more suspect than other reproductive techniques. Other motives (for example, wanting a super-star athlete, attempting to replace a dead child) might be morally suspect, but such motives are not uniquely connected to cloning. Parents who force a child to become an athlete, or who treat a child as no more than a replacement for a dead child, are as blameworthy as individuals who use cloning to accomplish their purposes.

It seems then that the real problems with human reproductive cloning are safety-based. Clearly, at this point, the technology is not ready for prime time, and it would be irresponsible for any researcher to attempt to clone a human baby. However, as that may change, there is no justification for an absolute and permanent ban on human reproductive cloning, and ethics commissions ought to leave off suggesting that there is.

EVEN IF IT WORKED, CLONING WOULDN'T BRING HER BACK

Thomas H. Murray

Eleven days ago, as I awaited my turn to testify at a congressional hearing on human reproductive cloning, one of five scientists on the witness list took the microphone. Brigitte Boisselier, a chemist working with couples who want to use cloning techniques to create babies, read aloud a letter from "a father, (Dada)." The writer, who had unexpectedly become a parent in his late thirties, describes his despair over his 11-month-old son's death after heart surgery and 17 days of "misery and struggle." The room was quiet as Boisselier read the

man's words: "I decided then and there that I would never give up on my child. I would never stop until I could give his DNA—his genetic make-up—a chance.

I listened to the letter writer's refusal to accept the finality of death, to his wish to allow his son another opportunity at life through cloning, and I was struck by the futility and danger of such thinking. I had been asked to testify as someone who has been writing and teaching about ethical issues in medicine and science for more than 20 years; but I am also a grieving parent. My 20-year-old daughter's murder, just five months ago, has agonizingly reinforced what I have for years argued as an ethicist: Cloning can neither change the fact of death nor deflect the pain of grief.

Reprinted with permission from *The Washington Post*, April 8, 2001.

Only four years have passed since the birth of the first cloned mammal—Dolly the sheep—was announced and the possibility of human cloning became real. Once a staple of science fiction, cloning was now the stuff of scientific research. A presidential commission, of which I am a member, began to deliberate the ethics of human cloning; scientists disavowed any interest in trying to clone people; and Congress held hearings but passed no laws. A moratorium took hold, stable except for the occasional eruption of self-proclaimed would-be cloners such as Chicago-based physicist Richard Seed and a group led by a man named Rael who claims that we are all clones of alien ancestors.

Recently, Boisselier, Rael's chief scientist, and Panos Zavos, an infertility specialist in Kentucky, won overnight attention when they proclaimed that they would indeed create a human clone in the near future. The prospect that renegade scientists might try to clone humans reignited the concern of lawmakers, which led to the recent hearings before the House Energy and Commerce subcommittee on oversight and investigations.

Cloning advocates have had a difficult time coming up with persuasive ethical arguments. Indulging narcissism—so that someone can create many Mini-Me's—fails to generate much support for their cause. Others make the case that adults should have the right to use any means possible to have the child they want. Their liberty trumps everything else; the child's welfare barely registers, except to avoid a life that would be worse than never being born, a standard akin to dividing by zero—no meaningful answer is possible. The strategy that has been the most effective has been to play the sympathy card—and who evokes more sympathy than someone who has lost a child?

Sadly, I'm in a position to correct some of these misunderstandings. I'm not suggesting that my situation is the same as that of the letter's author. Not better. Not worse. Simply different. His son was with him for less than a year, our daughter for 20; his son died of disease in a hospital; Emily, daughter to Cynthia and me, sister to Kate and Matt, Nicky and Pete, was reported missing from her college campus in early November. Her body was found more than five weeks later. She had been abducted and shot.

As I write those words, I still want to believe they are about someone else, a story on the 11 o'clock news. Cynthia and I often ask each other, how can this be our life? But it is our life and Emily, as a physical, exuberant, loving presence, is not in the same way a part of it anymore. Death changes things and, I suspect, the death of a child causes more wrenching grief than any other death. So I am told; so my experience confirms.

I want to speak, then, to the author of that letter, father to father, grieving parent to grieving parent; and to anyone clinging to unfounded hope that cloning can somehow repair the arbitrariness of disease, unhappiness and death. I have nothing to sell you, I don't want your money, and I certainly don't want to be cruel. But there are hard truths here that some people, whether through ignorance or self-interest, are obscuring.

The first truth is that cloning does not result in healthy, normal offspring. The two scientific experts on animal cloning who shared the panel with Boisselier reported the results of the cattle, mice and other mammals cloned thus far: They have suffered staggering rates of abnormalities and death; some of the females bearing them have been injured and some have died. Rudolf Jaenisch, an expert on mouse cloning at MIT's Whitehead Institute for Biomedical Research, told the subcommittee that he did not believe there was a single healthy cloned mammal in existence—not even Dolly, the sheep that started it all, who is abnormally obese.

Scientists do not know why cloning fails so miserably. One plausible explanation begins with what we already know—that as the cells of an embryo divide and begin to transform into the many varieties of tissue that make up our bodies, most of the genes in each cell are shut down, leaving active only those that the cell needs to perform its specific role. A pancreatic islet cell, for example, needs working versions of the genes that recognize when a person needs the hormone insulin, then cobble it together and shunt it into the bloodstream. All of that individual's other genetic information is in that islet cell, but most of it is chemically locked, like an illegally parked car immobilized by a tire boot.

To make a healthy clone, scientists need to unlock every last one of those tire boots in the cell that is to be cloned. It is not enough to have the genes for islet cells; every gene will be needed sometime, somewhere. Unless and until scientists puzzle out how to restore all the genes to their original state, we will continue to see dead, dying and deformed clones.

You do not need to be a professional bioethicist, then, to see that trying to make a child by cloning, at this stage in the technology, would be a gross violation of international standards protecting people from overreaching scientists, a blatant example of immoral human experimentation.

Some scientists claim they can avoid these problems. Zavos, who spoke at the hearing, has promised to screen embryos and implant only healthy ones. But Zavos failed to give a single plausible reason to believe that he can distinguish healthy from unhealthy cloned embryos.

Now for the second truth: Even if cloning produced a healthy embryo, the result would not be the same person as the one whose genetic material was used. Each of us is a complex amalgam of luck, experience and heredity. Where in the womb an embryo burrows, what its mother eats or drinks, what stresses she endures, her age—all these factors shape the developing fetus. The genes themselves conduct an intricately choreographed dance, turning on and off, instructing other genes to do the same in response to their interior rhythms and to the pulses of the world outside. How we become who we are remains a mystery.

About the only thing we can be certain of is that we are much more than the sum of our genes. As I said in my testimony, perhaps the best way to extinguish the enthusiasm for human cloning would be to clone Michael Jordan. Michael II might well have no interest in playing basketball but instead long to become an accountant. What makes Michael I great is not merely his physical gifts, but his competitive fire, his determination, his fierce will to win.

Yet another hard truth: Creating a child to stand in for another—dead—child is unfair. No child should have to bear the oppressive expectation that he or she will live out the life denied to his or her idealized genetic avatar. Parents may joke about their specific plans for their children; I suspect their

children find such plans less amusing. Of course, we should have expectations for our children: that they be considerate, honest, diligent, fair and more. But we cannot dictate their temperament, talents or interest. Cloning a child to be a reincarnation of someone else is a grotesque, fun-house mirror distortion of parental expectations.

Which brings me to the final hard truth: There is no real escape from grief.

Cynthia and I have fantasized about time running backward so that we could undo Emily's murder. We would give our limbs, our organs, our lives to bring her back, to give her the opportunity to live out her dream of becoming an Episcopal priest, of retiring as a mesmerizing old woman sitting on her porch on Cape Cod, surrounded by her grandchildren and poodles.

But trying to recreate Emily from her DNA would be chasing an illusion. Massive waves of sorrow knock us down, breathless; we must learn to live with them. When our strength returns we stagger to our feet, summon whatever will we can, and do what needs to be done. Most of all we try to hold each other up. We can no more wish our grief away than King Canute could stem the ocean's tide.

So I find myself wanting to say to the letter writer, and to the scientists who offer him and other sorrowing families false hope: There are no technological fixes for grief; cloning your dear dead son will not repair the jagged hole ripped out of the tapestry of your life. Your letter fills me with sadness for you and you wife, not just for the loss of your child but also for the fruitless quest to quench your grief in a genetic replica of the son you lost.

It would be fruitless even—especially—if you succeeded in creating a healthy biological duplicate. But there is little chance of that.

Emily lived until a few months shy of her 21st birthday. In those years our lives became interwoven in ways so intricate that I struggle for words to describe how Cynthia and I now feel. We were fortunate to have her with us long enough to see her become her own person, to love her wholeheartedly and to know beyond question that she loved us. Her loss changes us forever. Life flows in one direction; science cannot reverse the stream or reincarnate the dead.

The Emily we knew and loved would want us to continue to do what matters in our lives, to love each other, to do good work, to find meaning. Not to forget her, ever: We are incapable of that. Why would we want to? She was a luminous presence in our family, an extraordinary friend, a promising young philosopher. And we honor her by keeping her memory vibrant, not by trying to manufacture a genetic facsimile. And that thought makes me address the letter's author once more: I have to think that your son, were he able to tell you, would wish for you the same.

RECOMMENDED SUPPLEMENTARY READING

GENERAL WORKS

Alpern, Kenneth D., ed. *The Ethics of Reproductive Technology.* New York: Oxford University Press, 1992.

Andrews, Lori B. *The Clone Age: Adventures in the New World of Reproductive Technology.* New York: Henry Holt, 1999.

Andrews, Lori B., Jane E. Fullarton, Neil A. Holtzman, and Arno G. Motulsky, eds. *Assessing Genetic Risks: Implications for Health and Social Policy.* Washington, DC: National Academy Press, 1994.

Bartels, Dianne M. et al., eds. *Beyond Baby M. Ethical Issues in the New Reproductive Technologies.* Clifton, NJ: Humana Press, 1990.

Buchanan, Allen, Dan W. Brock, Norman Daniels, and Daniel Wikler. *From Chance to Choice: Genetics and Justice.* Cambridge: Cambridge University Press, 2000.

Callahan, Joan C., ed. *Reproduction, Ethics, and the Law.* Bloomington: Indiana University Press, 1995.

Caulfield, Timothy A., and Bryn Williams-Jones, eds. *The Commercialization of Genetic Research: Legal, Ethical, and Policy Issues.* Dordrecht, The Netherlands: Kluwer Academic, 1999.

Cohen, Sherrill, and Nadine Taub. *Reproductive Laws for the 1990s.* Clifton, NJ: Humana Press, 1989.

Cranor, Carl F. *Are Genes Us? The Social Consequences of the New Genetics.* New Brunswick, NJ: Rutgers University Press, 1994.

Davis, Dena S. *Genetic Dilemmas: Reproductive Technology, Parental Choices, and Children's Futures.* New York and London: Routledge, 2001.

Dyson, Anthony, and John Harris, eds. *Ethics and Biotechnology.* London: Routledge, 1994

Elias, Sherman, and George J. Annas. *Reproductive Genetics and the Law.* Chicago: Year Book Medical Publishers, 1987.

Fotion, Nick, and Jan Heller, eds. *Contingent Future Persons: On the Ethics of Deciding* Who *Will Live, or Not, in the Future.* Dordrecht, The Netherlands: Kluwer Academic, 1997.

Glover, Jonathan. *What Sort of People Should There Be?* New York: Random House, 1977.

Harris, John. *Clones, Genes, and Immortality: Ethics and the Genetic Revolution.* New York: Oxford University Press, 1998.

————. *Enhancing Evolution: The Ethical Case for Making Better People.* Princeton: Princeton University Press, 2007.

————. *Wonderwoman and Superman: The Ethics of Human Biotechnology.* Oxford: Oxford University Press, 1992.

Harris, John, and Soren Holm, eds. *The Future of Human Reproduction.* Oxford: Clarendon Press, 1998.

Heyd, David. *Genethics: Moral Issues in the Creation of People.* Berkeley: University of California Press, 1992.

Kelves, Daniel J. *In the Name of Eugenics: Genetics and the Uses of Human Heredity.* New York: Knopf, 1985.

Kitcher, Philip. *The Lives to Come: The Genetic Revolution and Human Possibilities.* New York: Simon and Schuster, 1996.

McCullough, Laurence B., and Frank A. Chervenak. *Ethics in Obstetrics and Gynecology.* New York: Oxford University Press, 1994.

Mehlman, Maxwell J. and Jeffrey R. Botkin. *Access to the Genome: The Challenge to Equality.* Washington, DC: Georgetown University Press, 1998.

Murray, Thomas H. *The Worth of a Child.* Berkeley: University of California Press, 1996.

Murray, Thomas H., and Maxwell J. Mehlman, eds. *Encyclopedia of Ethical, Legal, and Policy Issues in Biotechnology.* Vols. 1 and 2. New York: John Wiley & Sons, Inc., 2000.

Parfit, Derek. *Reasons and Persons.* Oxford: Clarendon Press, 1984.

Purdy, Laura. *Reproducing Persons: Issues in Feminist Bioethics.* Ithaca, New York: Cornell University Press, 1996.

Roberts, Melinda. *Child versus Childmaker: Future Persons and Present Duties in Ethics and the Law.* Lanham, MD: Rowman & Littlefield, 1998.

Robertson, John A. *Children of Choice: Freedom and the New Reproductive Technologies.* Princeton, NJ: Princeton University Press. 1994.

Rothman, Barbara Katz. *Recreating Motherhood: Ideology and Technology in a Patriarchal Society.* New York: Norton, 1989.

————. *The Tentative Pregnancy. How Amniocentesis Changes the Experience of Motherhood.* New York: Norton, 1993.

Silver, Lee M. *Remaking Eden: How Genetic Engineering and Cloning Will Transform the American Family.* New York: Avon Books, 1997.

Singer, Peter. *Animal Liberation.* New York: Avon Books, 1975.

Singer, Peter, and Deane Wells. *Making Babies: The New Science and Ethics of Conception.* New York: Scribner's, 1985.

Steinbock, Bonnie. *Life Before Birth: The Moral and Legal Status of Embryos and Fetuses.* New York: Oxford University Press, 1992.

————, ed. *Legal and Ethical Issues in Human Reproduction.* Hampshire, UK: Ashgate Publishing Ltd., 2002.

Strong, Carson. *Ethics in Reproductive and Perinatal Medicine: A New Framework.* New Haven, CT: Yale University Press, 1997.

Warren, Mary Anne. *Moral Status: Obligations to Persons and Other Living Things.* New York: Oxford University Press, 1997.

Wolf, Susan M., ed. *Feminism and Bioethics.* New York: Oxford University Press, 1996.

THE MORALITY OF ABORTION

Bassen, Paul. "Present Stakes and Future Prospects: The Status of Early Abortion." *Philosophy & Public Affairs* 11, no. 4 (1982): 314–337.

Bayertz, Kurt, ed. *Sanctity of Life and Human Dignity.* Dordrecht, The Netherlands: Kluwer Academic, 1996.

Boonin, David. *A Defense of Abortion.* Cambridge: Cambridge University Press, 2003.

Callahan, Sidney, and Daniel Callahan, eds. *Abortion: Understanding Differences.* New York: Plenum Press, 1984.

Davis, Nancy Ann. "Abortion and Self-Defense." *Philosophy & Public Affairs* 13, no. 3 (Summer 1984): 516–539.

————. "The Abortion Debate: The Search for Common Ground." 2 parts. *Ethics* 103 (April/July 1993): 731–778.

Dworkin, Ronald. *Life's Dominion: An Argument about Abortion, Euthanasia, and Individual Freedom.* New York: Knopf, 1993.

Dwyer, Susan, and Joel Feinberg, eds. *The Problem of Abortion.* 3rd ed. Belmont, CA: Wadsworth, 1997.

Feinberg, Joel. "Abortion." In *Matters of Life and Death,* edited by Tom Regan, 2nd ed. New York: Random House, 1986.

Garrow, David J. *Liberty and Sexuality: The Right to Privacy and the Making of* Roe v. Wade. New York: Macmillan, 1994.

Gorney, Cynthia. *Articles of Faith: A Frontline History of the Abortion Wars.* New York: Simon and Schuster, 1998.

Graber, Mark A. *Rethinking Abortion: Equal Choice, the Constitution, and Reproductive Politics.* Princeton, NJ: Princeton University Press, 1996.

Hursthouse, Rosalind. *Beginning Lives.* Oxford: Basil Blackwell, 1987.

————. "Virtue Theory and Abortion." *Philosophy & Public Affairs* 20, no. 3 (Summer 1991): 223–246.

Kamm, Frances Myrna. *Creation and Abortion: A Study in Moral and Legal Philosophy.* New York: Oxford University Press, 1992.

Little, Margaret. "Abortion, Intimacy, and the Duty to Gestate." *Ethical Theory and Moral Practice* 2 (1999): 295–312.

Luker, Kristin. *Abortion and the Politics of Motherhood.* Berkeley: University of California Press, 1984.

Marquis, Don. "Why Most Abortions Are Wrong." In *Advance in Bioethics,* edited by Rem B. Edwards and E. Edward Bittar, vol. 5. Stamford, CT: JAI Press, 1999: 215–244.

McDonaugh, Eileen. *Breaking the Abortion Deadlock.* New York: Oxford University Press, 1996.

Norcross, Alastair. "Killing, Abortion, and Conttraception: A Reply to Marquis." *Journal of Philosophy* (1990): 268–278.

Petchesky, Rosalind P. *Abortion and Woman's Choice: The State, Sexuality and Reproductive Freedom.* Rev. ed. Boston: Northeastern Press, 1990.

Regan, Donald. "Rewriting *Roe v. Wade.*" *Michigan Law Review* 77 (1979).

Robertson, John A. "*Casey* and the Resuscitation of *Roe v. Wade.*" *Hastings Center Report* 22, no. 5 (1992): 24–29.

Summer, L. W. *Abortion and Moral Theory.* Princeton, NJ: Princeton University Press, 1981.

Tooley, Michael. *Abortion and Infanticide.* New York: Oxford University Press, 1983.

Tribe, Laurence. *Abortion: The Clash of Absolutes.* New York: Norton, 1990.

OBLIGATIONS TO THE NOT-YET-BORN

Botkin, Jeffrey R. "Fetal Privacy and Confidentiality." *Hastings Center Report* (September–October 1995): 32–39.

Copelon, R., C. Zampas, E. Brusie, and J. Devore. "Human Rights Begin at Birth: International Law and the Claim of Fetal Rights." *Reproductive Health Matters* 13, no. 26 (November 2005): 120–129.

————. "Prenatal Screening: Professional Standards and the Limits of Parental Choice." *Obstetrics and Gynecology* 75, no. 5 (1990): 328–329.

Green, Ronald M. "Paternal Autonomy and the Obligation Not to Harm One's Child Genetically." *Journal of Law, Medicine and Ethics* 25 (1997): 5–15.

Harris, J. "The Concept of the Person and the Value of Life." *Kennedy Institute of Ethics Journal* (December 1999): 293–308.

Lugosi, Charles I. "Respecting Human Life in 21st Century America: A Moral Perspective to Extend Civil Rights to the Unborn from Creation to Natural Death." *Issues in Law & Medicine* 20, no. 3 (March 22, 2005): 211–259.

Peters, Philip G. "Harming Future Persons: Obligations to the Children of Reproductive Technology," *Southern California Interdisciplinary Law Journal* 8 (1999): 375–400.

———. "Protecting the Unconceived: Nonexistence, Avoidability, and Reproductive Technology." *Arizona Law Review* 31, no. 3. (1989): 487–548.

———. "Rethinking Wrongful Life: Bridging the Boundary Between Tort and Family Law." *Tulane Law Review* 67, no. 2 (1992): 397–454.

Sakaihara, M. "Claims Made by Children in Japan for Injuries Caused Before Birth." *Medicine, Science, and the Law* 47, no. 1 (January 2007): 61–63.

Schroedel, Jean Reith. *Is the Fetus a Person?: A Comparison of Policies Across the Fifty States.* Ithaca NY: Cornell University Press, 2000.

Steinbock, Bonnie. "The Logical Case for 'Wrongful Life.'" *Hastings Center Report* 16, no. 2 (April 1986): 15–20.

Steinbock, Bonnie, and Ron McClamrock. "When Is Birth Unfair to the Child?" *Hastings Center Report* 24, no. 6 (November 1994): 15–21.

ASSISTED REPRODUCTION

Anderson, Elizabeth. "Is Women's Labor a Commodity?" *Philosophy & Public Affairs* 19, no. 1 (Winter 1990).

Annas, George J. "Baby M: Babies (and Justice) for Sale." *Hastings Center Report* 17, no. 3 (1987).

Arneson, Richard J. "Commodification and Commercial Surrogacy." *Philosophy & Public Affairs* 21, no. 2 (Spring 1992).

Charo, R. Alta. "And Baby Makes Three—Or Four, Or Five, Or Six: Redefining the Family After the Reprotech Revolution." *Wisconsin Women's Law Journal* 7 (1992–1993): 1–23.

Callahan, Daniel. "Bioethics and Fatherhood," *Utah Law Review* (1992): 735–746.

Check, E. "Ethicists and Biologists Ponder the Price of Eggs." *Nature* 442, no. 7103 (August 10, 2006): 606–607.

Cohen, Cynthia B. "'Give Me Children or I Shall Die!' New Reproductive Technologies and Harm to Children." *Hastings Center Report* (March– April 1996): 19–29.

———, ed. *New Ways of Making Babies.* Bloomington: Indiana University Press, 1996.

———. "Unmanaged Care: The Need to Regulate New Reproductive Technologies in the United States." *Bioethics* 11, nos. 3 & 4 (1997): 348–365.

Congregation for the Doctrine of the Faith. "Instruction on Respect for Human Life in Its Origin and on the Dignity of Procreation: Replies to Certain Questions of the Day." Rome, Italy: The Vatican, March 10, 1987.

Corea, Gena. *The Mother Machine: Reproductive Technologies from Artificial Insemination to Artificial Wombs.* New York: Harper, 1985.

Field, Martha A. *Surrogate Motherhood: The Legal and Human Issues.* Cambridge, MA: Harvard University Press, 1988.

Glover, Jonathan. *Ethics of New Reproductive Technologies: The Glover Report to the European Commission.* DeKalb: Northern Illinois University Press, 1989.

Gorovitz, Samuel. "Progeny, Progress, and Primrose Paths." In *Doctors' Dilemmas: Moral Conflict and Medical Care.* New York: Oxford University Press, 1982.

Gostin, Laurence O., ed. *Surrogate Motherhood: Politics and Privacy.* Bloomington: Indiana University Press, 1990.

Holland, Suzanne. "Contested Commodities at Both Ends of Life: Buying and Selling Gametes, Embryos, and Body Tissues." *Kennedy Institute of Ethics Journal* 11, no. 3 (2001).

Holland, Suzanne, and Dena S. Davis, Guest Editors. "Who's Afraid of Commodification?" Special issue, *Kennedy Institute of Ethics Journal* 11, no. 3 (September 2001).

Johnston, J. "Paying Egg Donors: Exploring the Arguments." *Hastings Center Report* 36, no. 1 (January–February 2006): 28–31.

Kalfoglou, Andrea, and Gail Geller. "Navigating Conflict of Interest in Oocyte Donation: An Analysis of Donors' Experiences." *Women's Health Issues* 10, no. 5 (2000): 226–239.

Keefe, D. L., and J. P. Parry. "New Approaches to Assisted Reproductive Technologies." *Seminars in Reproductive Medicine* 23, no. 4 (November 2005): 301–308.

Lauritzen, Paul. *Pursuing Parenthood: Ethical Issues in Assisted Reproduction.* Bloomington: Indiana University Press, 1993.

Macklin, Ruth. "Artificial Means of Reproduction and Our Understanding of the Family." *Hastings Center Report* 21, no. 1 (1991): 5–11.

Mahoney, Julia D. "The Market for Human Tissue." *Virginia Law Review* 86, no. 2 (March 2000): 163–223.

New York State Task Force on Life and the Law. *Assisted Reproductive Technologies: Analysis and Recommendations for Public Policy,* 1998.

———. *Surrogate Parenting,* 1988.

Radin, Margaret Jane. "Market-Inalienability." *Harvard Law Review* 100 (1987): 1839–1947.

Robertson, J. A. "Compensation and Egg Donation for Research." *Fertility and Sterility* 86, no. 6 (December 2006): 1573–1575.

Robertson, John A. "Posthumous Reproduction." *Indiana Law Journal* 69, no. 4 (1994): 1027–1065.

———. "Legal Issues in Human Egg Donation and Gestational Surrogacy." *Seminars in Reproductive Endocrinology* 13, no. 3 (1995): 210–218.

Satz, Debra. "Markets in Women's Reproductive Labor." *Philosophy & Public Affairs* 21 (1992): 107–131.

Seibel, Michelle M., and Susan Crockin, eds. *Family Building Through Egg and Sperm Donation: Medical, Legal and Ethical Issues.* Sudbury, MA: Jones and Bartlett, 1996.

Steinbock, Bonnie. "Surrogate Motherhood as Prenatal Adoption." *Law, Medicine and Health Care* 16 (1988): 44–50.

Wertheimer, Alan. "Two Questions about Surrogacy and Exploitation." *Philosophy Public Affairs* 21, no. 3 (Summer 1992): 211–239.

REPRODUCTIVE CLONING

Allmers, H., and S. Kenwright. "Ethics of Cloning." *Lancet* 349, no. 9062 (May 10, 1997): 1401.

Andrews, Lori B. "Mom, Dad, Clone: Implications for Reproductive Privacy." *Cambridge Quarterly of Healthcare Ethics* 7, no. 2 (1998): 176–186.

Annas, George J. "Regulatory Models for Human Embryo Cloning: The Free Market, Professional Guidelines, and Government Restrictions." *Kennedy Institute of Ethics Journal* 4 (1994): 235–249.

Brannigan, Michael C., ed. *Ethical Issues in Human Cloning.* New York and London: Seven Bridges Press, 2001.

Callahan, Daniel. "The Puzzle of Profound Respect." *Hastings Center Report* 25 (1995): 39–40.

Capron, Alexander Morgan. "Inside the Beltway Again: A Sheep of a Different Feather." *Kennedy Institute of Ethics Journal* 7 (1997): 171–179.

Charo, R. Alta. "The Hunting of the Snark: The Moral Status of Embryos, Right-to-lifers, and Third World Women." *Stanford Law & Policy Review* 6 (1995): 11–37.

"Cloning Human Beings: Responding to the National Bioethics Advisory Commission's Report." *Hastings Center Report* (September–October 1997).

Cloning Symposium, *Jurimetrics* 38, no. 1 (1997).

Elsner, D. "Just Another Reproductive Technology? The Ethics of Human Cloning as an Experimental Medical Procedure." *Journal of Medical Ethics* 32, no. 10 (October 2006): 596–600.

Humber, James M., and Robert Almeder. *Human Cloning.* Totowa, NJ: Humana Press, 1998.

Kass, Leon. "The Wisdom of Repugnance: Why We Should Ban the Cloning of Humans." *The New Republic* (June 2, 1997): 17–26.

Klotzko, Arlene Judith. *The Cloning Sourcebook.* New York: Oxford University Press, 2001.

Kolata, Gina. *Clone: The Road to Dolly and the Path Ahead.* New York: William Morrow, 1998.

Lauritzen, Paul, ed. *Cloning and the Future of Human Embryo Research.* New York: Oxford University Press, 2001.

Lester, Lane P., and James C. Hefley. *Human Cloning.* Ada, MI: Baker, 1998.

Lewontin, Richard. "The Confusion over Cloning." *New York Review of Books* 44 (October 23, 1997).

Lewontin, Richard, with Harold T. Shapiro, James F. Childress, and Thomas H. Murray. "'The Confusion over Cloning': An Exchange." *New York Review of Books* 45, no. 4 (March 5, 1998): 46–47.

Mackinnon, Barbara, ed. *Human Cloning: Science, Ethics, and Public Policy.* Urbana: University of Illinois Press, 2000.

Macklin, Ruth. "Splitting Embryos on the Slippery Slope: Ethics and Public Policy." *Kennedy Institute of Ethics Journal* 4, no. 3 (September 1994): 209–225.

McCormick, R. A. "Should We Clone Humans?" *The Christian Century*, November 17–24, 1993: 1148–1149.

McGee, Glenn. *The Human Cloning Debate.* Berkeley, CA: Berkeley Hills Books, 1998.

Meilaender, Gilbert. "The Point of a Ban." *Hastings Center Report* 31, no. 1 (2001): 9–16.

National Bioethics Advisory Commission. *Cloning Human Beings: Report and Recommendations.* Rockville, MD: National Bioethics Advisory Commission, 1997.

Nussbaum, Martha C., and Cass R. Sunstein, eds. *Clones and Clones: Facts and Fantasies about Human Cloning.* New York: Norton, 1998.

Pence, Gregory. *Flesh of My Flesh: The Ethics of Cloning—A Reader.* Lanham, MD: Rowman & Littlefield, 1998.

———. *Who's Afraid of Human Cloning?* Lanham, MD: Rowman & Littlefield, 1998.

Rantala, M. L., and Arthur J. Milgram, eds. *Cloning: For and Against.* Chicago: Open Court, 1999.

Rhodes, Rosamond. "Clones, Harms, and Rights." *Cambridge Quarterly of Healthcare Ethics* 4 (1995): 285–290.

Roberts, Melinda. "Human Cloning: A Case of No Harm Done?" *Journal of Medicine and Philosophy* 21 (1996): 537–554.

Robertson, John A. "Liberty, Identity, and Human Cloning." *Texas Law Review* 76, no. 6 (1998).

———. "The Question of Human Cloning." *Hastings Center Report* 24, no. 2 (March–April 1994): 6–14.

———. "Two Models of Human Cloning." *Hofstra Law Review* 27 (1999): 609–638.

Verhey, A. "Playing God and Invoking a Perspective." *Journal of Medicine and Philosophy* 20 (1995): 347–364.

———. "Cloning: Revisiting an Old Debate." *Kennedy Institute of Ethics Journal* 4, no. 3 (September 1994): 227–234.

Winter, Paul A. *Cloning.* San Diego, CA: Greenhaven, 1998.

PART FIVE

GENETICS

Approximately 3 percent of all children are born with a severe disorder that is presumed to be genetic in origin, and several thousand definite or suspected "single-gene" diseases have been described. Among the better known are cystic fibrosis (CF), Tay-Sachs disease, and Huntington's disease (HD). Most genetic diseases manifest early in life, though some inherited diseases—and many others that have a genetic component—have their onset later in life: for example, HD and hemochromatosis. There are many disorders in which both genetic and environmental factors play major roles, including coronary heart disease, breast cancer, obesity, schizophrenia, depression, and hypertension. The more we learn about genetics, the more we learn about the genetic causes of disease. At the same time, we have learned that only a few disorders and traits are linked to a single gene. Most are the result of several genes acting together as well as gene–environment interactions (Conrad 2005, 7).

Since 1990, much of our understanding of "the new genetics" has been propelled by the Human Genome[1] Project (HGP), a thirteen-year effort coor-dinated by the U.S. Department of Energy and the National Institutes of Health. The project originally was planned to last fifteen years, but rapid techno-logical advances accelerated the completion date to 2003, and a draft of the human genome was completed in 2000. The goals of the project included identifying all the approximately 20,000–25,000 genes in human DNA, determining the sequences of the 3 billion chemical base pairs that make up human DNA, storing this information in data-bases, improving tools for data analysis, transfer-ring related technologies to the private sector, and addressing the ethical, legal, and social issues (ELSI) that may arise from the project. It is hoped that the HGP will help scientists find the source of nearly 4,000 known genetic disorders, as well as diseases that are produced in part by genetic mal-functions, and various normal human traits. At the same time, genetic medicine remains largely promissory. Although we have known about the specific genes for cystic fibrosis and Huntington's disease for a decade, these have yet to translate into specific improvements in treatment (Conrad 2005, 7). Nevertheless, most experts agree that genomics will become an increasingly important part of med-icine in the future. Although advances in genetics pose important questions in their own right, they are also inextricably bound up with some of the most controversial and socially divisive issues in medical ethics, such as genetic interventions for the sake of enhancement, as opposed to prevention or treatment of disease (treated in this part). Another

---

1. "A **genome** is all the DNA in an organism, including its genes. Genes carry information for making all the proteins required by all organisms. These proteins determine, among other things, how the organism looks, how well its body metabolizes food or fights infection, and sometimes even how it behaves." Human Genome Project Information, http://www.ornl.gov/sci/techresources/Human_Genome/project/about.shtml.

controversial issue is the use of genetic tests to predict (and wean out) undesirable behaviors. Both enhancement and behavioral genetics are covered in Part 7.

In the United States, it is standard practice that pregnant women over the age of thirty-five be offered prenatal testing for Down syndrome, because the risk of having a child with Down syndrome increases dramatically as the mother ages. In 2007, the American College of Obstetricians and Gynecologists (ACOG) recommended that *all* pregnant women, regardless of age, be offered prenatal testing for Down syndrome. This is because most babies (80 percent) with Down syndrome are born to women *under* the age of thirty-five, for the simple reason that younger women are the ones having the most babies.

Geneticists distinguish between genetic screening and genetic testing. Genetic screening is usually understood to refer to a public health program performed on a whole population, or some subset, such as an ethnic group at high risk for a particular disease. An example of screening a whole population would be performing colonoscopies on everyone over fifty. Colon cancer always starts out as a polyp, which can be detected by a colonoscopy. The disease is very treatable if caught in the early stages, and nearly always fatal in the later stages. So population screening will prevent many cases of colon cancer and save a lot of lives. An example of screening an ethnic group would be carrier screening of Ashkenazi Jews for Tay-Sachs disease, a neuromuscular disease that manifests itself in infancy and nearly always causes death between the ages of three and five. Those who are carriers for the disease will not get it themselves, but if two carriers reproduce, there is a 25 percent chance in every pregnancy that the infant will be afflicted. Tay-Sachs used to have a much higher prevalency among Ashkenazi Jews (that is, Jews of Eastern European descent) than in the general population. Screening the Ashkenazi Jewish population to see which people are carriers has enabled carriers to avoid marrying other carriers, and thus passing on the disease. In fact, because of carrier screening, today the incidence of Tay-Sachs is *lower* among Ashkenazi Jews than in other groups.

In contrast to screening, genetic testing, or clinical genetic testing, as it is sometimes called, refers to a procedure performed on an individual because of

that individual's risk factors. For example, if a woman has a history of breast cancer and/or ovarian cancer in her family, she may opt to be tested for the mutations or alterations in the genes BRCA1 or BRCA2 (short for breast cancer 1 and breast cancer 2) involved in many hereditary cases of breast and ovarian cancer. (Only 5–10 percent of breast and/or ovarian cancer is hereditary; most cases of breast or ovarian cancer are not the result of genetic mutations.) Women with an altered BRCA1 or BRCA2 gene are three to seven times more likely to develop breast cancer than women who do not have these mutations.

How should we regard the prenatal test for Down syndrome: as genetic testing or genetic screening? Many geneticists think that the distinction is very important because the purposes are different. Screening is done to decide where best to target public health programs aimed at reducing the incidence of disease in the group as a whole, whereas genetic testing is done to help individuals make personal medical (and other) decisions, including reproductive decisions. If the purpose of testing pregnant women for Down syndrome is to reduce the numbers of people in the population with Down syndrome, it is considered genetic screening. If, on the other hand, its purpose is to increase "reproductive autonomy," by giving the woman (or couple) information that she might consider relevant in deciding whether to terminate the pregnancy, it seems more plausible to call it genetic testing. The line between the two in the case of prenatal genetic diagnosis is a very fine one, because when a prenatal test is offered to all pregnant women, it is not based on individual risk factors. Partly because the line is fine, and partly because the distinction—at least in the context of prenatal testing—does not seem to have significant ethical implications, Norman Fost (1992) says that he does not find the distinction between testing and screening to be a particularly useful one. Instead of deciding whether a procedure is testing or screening, we should focus on which procedures should be performed and the constraints, such as informed consent, necessary to make them ethical. Fost writes:

> All screening programs involve performing a test on individuals. If the program is voluntary, then at least minimal standards for consent are implied and the issues overlap substantially with what is called testing. Conversely, some forms of testing are so widespread as

to constitute a standard of practice and have become de facto screening programs. The central question is what ethical principles and policies should guide proposals to perform a test on an asymptomatic individual or population of individuals. (Fost 1992, 2813)

At the present time, many genetic defects can be detected prenatally, through amniocentesis or chorionic villus sampling, but most cannot be corrected. Thus, testing cannot usually be done for the purpose of treating the fetus *in utero,* but it can be used by the prospective parents to prepare for the birth of an affected child. More commonly, prenatal genetic tests are used as the basis for selective abortion. That is, most of the time, the tests are reassuring—they do not reveal a genetic anomaly in the fetus. However, when they do, 85–90 percent of the time, the woman (or couple) decides to terminate the pregnancy. Clearly, the prospective parents' views on the morality of abortion are relevant to their attitudes toward prenatal testing. Other relevant factors include their attitudes toward disability, and which traits they consider serious enough to test for. The American Medical Association's Council on Ethical and Judicial Affairs (1994) says that a misuse of prenatal genetic testing would be "to ensure that children possess certain characteristics that should be irrelevant in an egalitarian society," and gives sex selection as a prime example. The council acknowledges the potential for discrimination, even when prenatal testing is used only to avoid genetic disease, because this might increase negative attitudes toward disabled individuals. Nevertheless, the council maintains that the use of genetic technology to avoid the birth of a child with a genetic disorder is in accordance with the physician's therapeutic role, although abortion or discard based on nondisease traits would be inappropriate.

In the first selection in Section 1, "Prenatal Diagnosis and Selective Abortion: A Challenge to Practice and Policy," Adrienne Asch argues that the medical paradigm contains a profound misunderstanding of disability. Most people with disabilities are healthy, not sick, and the problems they face stem not from the disability itself, but from discriminatory social arrangements. A public health approach, according to Asch, should not be focused on testing to prevent the births of children who will have disabilities, but rather on changing social arrangements so that all children, whatever their abilities, can reach their full

potential. In "Disability Prenatal Testing, and Selective Abortion," Bonnie Steinbock argues that the desirable goal of enabling all children to reach their full potential is compatible with another desirable public health goal: the prevention of disability. Steinbock maintains that expectant parents may reasonably wish to prevent the birth of a child with a serious disability, and it is legitimate for them to do this by aborting the pregnancy. This is because she views abortion as a form of prevention, something Asch denies. Another issue that divides them is the implications of the choice to abort a wanted child because of certain expected characteristics of that child. Asch sees this choice as inconsistent with the right ideal of parenting, which involves accepting one's children as they are. By contrast, Steinbock thinks that, while this is the correct ideal of parenting, this is not relevant to prenatal testing, since in her view one does not become a parent until after the child is born. Of course, the success of Steinbock's argument depends on how one views the moral status of the fetus and the morality of abortion. Interestingly, Asch does not regard abortion as itself morally wrong. Indeed, elsewhere (Asch 1988) she explicitly distinguishes between an abortion to avoid becoming a mother, which she regards as morally permissible, and abortion to avoid having a child with a disability, which she finds at least morally problematic, if not clearly wrong. The reader will have to decide whether her position against prenatal testing is consistent with her generally pro-choice view on abortion.

Preimplantation genetic diagnosis (PGD) may seem morally less problematic than prenatal testing and abortion, because affected embryos are discarded at a very early stage in their development, and before a pregnancy has been instantiated. However, as Jeffrey R. Botkin points out in "Ethical Issues and Practical Problems in Preimplantation Genetic Diagnosis," for those who view the fertilized human egg to be of equal moral status with the late-gestation fetus (and indeed any born human being), PGD is worse than abortion, since it involves a greater loss of human life. PGD also has the disadvantage of requiring the creation of embryos through IVF, with all the attendant risk and expense of that procedure. Furthermore, most clinicians recommend that PGD be followed up with prenatal diagnosis, which means that the abortion decision may still have to be faced.

All of these considerations make PGD less attractive as a method of prenatal diagnosis than it might at first appear. Botkin also considers the disability critique, acknowledging that "If prenatal diagnosis and PGD specifically were to have a significantly negative effect on the millions of disabled individuals in society, this would be a powerful argument for limiting or discouraging its use, at least for less than serious medical conditions." However, he does not think that it would have this effect. Despite the use of prenatal diagnosis for several decades, individuals with disabilities have never had more social support than they have today. Of greater concern, from Botkin's perspective, is the use of PGD to select against minor conditions or for desirable characteristics.

In the last selection in Section 1, "Using Preimplantation Genetic Diagnosis to Save a Sibling: The Story of Molly and Adam Nash," Bonnie Steinbock presents a case study in which PGD was used not simply to avoid having a child with a lethal genetic disease, but also to provide a tissue match for an existing child. Such children are sometimes referred to as "savior siblings." Does creating a savior sibling treat the created child as a source of "spare parts," and thus violate the Kantian dictum against treating others merely as means to our ends? Steinbock argues that this depends on whether the child will be loved and cherished for his own sake, regardless of the reasons for creating him in the first place. Her view has been echoed by a carefully circumscribed decision in 2005 by the Human Fertilization and Embryology Authority (HFEA) in the United Kingdom (where such decisions are regulated in a way that they are not in the United States) to allow a couple, Raj and Shahana Hashmi, to use PGD to conceive a child who would be both disease-free and a tissue match for their six-year-old son, Zain, who suffers from a potentially lethal disease, beta thalassemia (a blood disorder). The Hashmis hoped to use the baby's umbilical cord blood to provide Zain with the blood transfusions he regularly needed.

Although the HFEA permitted the use of PGD to save a child's life, some would reject this because of the potential for misuse. Will screening embryos for tissue type lead to screening for other characteristics, such as gender, height, or even intelligence? Is this the kind of choice prospective parents should have? And if not, are the dangers of the misuse of PGD sufficient to deny people the ability to use PGD to save an existing child?

Section 2 examines the ethics of stem cell research, and the cloning of human embryos for such research (known both as therapeutic cloning and cloning-for-biomedical-research). Human embryonic stem cells—hES cells—have enormous medical potential because they have the ability to develop into virtually any tissue in the body. In theory, they could be used to replace damaged cells in conditions such as Parkinson's disease and diabetes. Other diseases that have been mentioned as benefiting from human embryonic stem cell research (hESCR) include Alzheimer's, osteoporosis, macular degeneration, cancer, heart disease, and spinal cord injury. Nonembryonic stem cells (sometimes called, misleadingly, "adult" stem cells) also have medical applications. Indeed, bone marrow transplants are a form of adult stem cell therapy. However, most scientists believe that embryonic stem cells are more malleable than nonembryonic stem cells and thus hold even more medical promise.

Embryonic stem cells are derived from the inner cell mass of very early embryos (technically called blastocysts), comprised of between 100 to 200 cells, at roughly five to nine days after the embryo begins dividing. Blastocysts can be created by IVF (see Part 4), either specifically for research purposes, or as a by-product of infertility treatment, and then donated by couples who no longer need them for reproductive purposes. Another source of embryos from which to derive stem cells is somatic cell nuclear transfer (SCNT), or cloning. Stem cells derived from cloned embryos might someday have unique medical advantages, because the embryo could be cloned from the patient's own cells. Presumably this would avoid the problems of rejection that plague transplantation today.

The technique for cloning embryos is the same whether they are to be used for reproductive or research purposes. That is, the DNA is removed from a somatic cell and placed into an egg cell from which the nucleus containing its DNA has been removed. Fusion of the somatic cell's nucleus and the enucleated egg cell can be performed chemically, or more often by electrical stimulus. The cell begins to divide and grow, just as a fertilized egg would. It turns out to be relatively difficult to clone human embryos. In 2004, a Korean team led by Dr. Hwang Woo-suk claimed to have cloned the first human embryo. In 2005, it was discovered that he had fabricated his results. This scandal resulted in a two-year moratorium on cloning research in Korea. (In 2007, the government of South Korea announced that it plans to let scientists conduct experiments with cloned human embryos beginning in 2008.) However, human embryos have been cloned for research purposes elsewhere, for example, at the University of Newcastle. In November 2007, researchers in Oregon reported being able to extract stem cells from cloned embryos. The method is expected to work in humans as well. Nevertheless, most scientists agree that we are years away from treatments or cures from hESCR.

The ethical problem with hESCR comes from the fact that (at least at present) the derivation of hES cells destroys the embryo, making such research both politically controversial (in the United States anyway) and morally unacceptable to those who regard human embryos as human subjects, who may not be harmed or killed in biomedical research. Another development in November 2007 was the report that scientists in Japan and the United States had succeeded in reprogramming human somatic cells to pluripotent stem cells that exhibit the essential characteristics of embryonic stem cells. Some think that these "induced pluripotent stem cells" (IPSCs) will put an end to the morally controversial hESCR. However, it is a bit too soon to declare the controversy at an end. We do not yet know if IPSCs can replace ESCs, or if either will yield therapies. For this reason, scientists will want to keep working on both fronts. In the first selection in Section 2, "Embryo Ethics—The Moral Logic of Stem-Cell Research," Michael J. Sandel, a professor of government at Harvard University and a member of the President's Council on Bioethics, defends embryonic stem cell research. He considers, and rejects, the objection that human embryos must have the same moral status as any one of us, because each of us started out life as an embryo. This argument is flawed, he says, because human embryos differ from human beings in morally significant ways. In particular, embryos lack any form of consciousness or sentience. At the stage at which stem cells are derived, they lack even a rudimentary nervous system, necessary for the possibility of experiencing anything. In response, in "Acorns and Embryos" Robert P. George and Patrick Lee maintain that this

does not show that born human beings and nascent human embryos differ in kind. Sandel's argument works, they maintain, only if he disregards the key proposition asserted by opponents of embryo-killing: that all human beings, irrespective of age, size, stage of development, or condition of dependency, possess equal and intrinsic dignity on the basis of their humanity, and not any accidental characteristics.

Some of those inclined to support embryonic stem cell research because of its great medical potential maintain that an additional reason in favor of such research is that embryos left over from infertility treatment would ultimately be discarded anyway. Why not allow couples who do not need their embryos anymore to donate them for worthy scientific and medical research instead of having them destroyed? If this argument is used, then there is a fundamental moral difference between "spare" or "leftover" embryos and embryos specifically "created" for research purposes (whether by IVF or SCNT). Sandel rejects this claim on the ground that embryos created for infertility treatment are also destroyed, namely, the ones couples no longer need for reproductive purposes. If it is permissible to create and destroy embryos for the sake of treating infertility, it would seem equally permissible to create and destroy embryos for the sake of treating other (and more serious) diseases. In the third selection, "Surplus Embryos, Nonreproductive Cloning, and the Intend/Foresee Distinction," William FitzPatrick argues that Sandel is mistaken about the moral significance of the "spare/created" distinction. What makes embryos that are left over from infertility treatment and then discarded different from embryos that are created for research that will destroy them is the distinction between outcomes that are intended as opposed to those that are merely foreseen. This distinction is deeply embedded in Catholic moral thought, especially in the doctrine of double effect, in deontological ethics generally, and in commonsense morality. Not everyone accepts its moral significance; consequentialists, for example, deny that it has moral force. FitzPatrick maintains that the distinction between intending and foreseeing is a real moral distinction, with real moral implications, but he does not think that it always has overriding weight. In particular, he argues that it does not justify opposing cloning-for-biomedical-research.

REFERENCES

Asch, A. 1988. Reproductive technology and disability. In *Reproductive laws for the 1990s*, eds. S. Cohen and N. Taub, 69–124. Clifton, NJ: Humana Press.

Conrad, P. 2005. The shifting engines of medicalization. *Journal of Health and Social Behavior* 46:3–14.

Council on Ethical and Judicial Affairs, American Medical Association. 1994. Ethical issues related to prenatal genetic testing. *Archives of Family Medicine*, 3:633–642.

Fost, N. 1992. Ethical implications of screening asymptomatic individuals. *FASEB Journal* 6:2813–2817.

PRENATAL GENETIC TESTING

PRENATAL DIAGNOSIS AND SELECTIVE ABORTION: A CHALLENGE TO PRACTICE AND POLICY

Adrienne Asch

Although sex selection might ameliorate the situation of some individuals, it lowers the status of women in general and only perpetuates the situation that gave rise to it. . . . If we believe that sexual equality is necessary for a just society, then we should oppose sex selection.

Wertz and Fletcher[1](pp242–243)

The very motivation for seeking an "origin" of homosexuality reveals homophobia. Moreover, such research may lead to prenatal tests that claim to predict for homosexuality. For homosexual people who live in countries with no legal protections these dangers are particularly serious.

Schuklenk et al.[2](p6)

The tenor of the preceding statements may spark relatively little comment in the world of health policy, the medical profession, or the readers of this journal, because many recognize the dangers of using the technology of prenatal testing followed by selective abortion for the characteristic of fetal sex. Similarly, the medical and psychiatric professions, and the world of public health, have aided in the civil rights struggle of gays and lesbians by insisting that homosexuality is not a disease. Consequently, many readers would concur with those who question the motives behind searching for the causes of homosexuality that might lead scientists to develop a prenatal test for that characteristic. Many in our society, however, have no such misgivings about prenatal

From *American Journal of Public Health* 89, no. 11 (November 1999): 1649–1657. Reprinted with permission from the American Public Health Association.

Editors' note: Some text and author's notes have been cut. Students who want to read the article in its entirety should consult the original.

testing for characteristics regarded as genetic or chromosomal diseases, abnormalities, or disabilities:

> Attitudes toward congenital disability per se have not changed markedly. Both premodern as well as contemporary societies have regarded disability as undesirable and to be avoided. Not only have parents recognized the birth of a disabled child as a potentially divisive, destructive force in the family unit, but the larger society has seen disability as unfortunate (p 89). . . . Our society still does not countenance the elimination of diseased/disabled people; but it does urge the termination of diseased/disabled fetuses. The urging is not explicit, but implicit (p 90).[3]

Writing in the *American Journal of Human Genetics* about screening programs for cystic fibrosis, A. L. Beaudet acknowledged the tension between the goals of enhancing reproductive choice and preventing the births of children who would have disabilities:

> Although some would argue that the success of the program should be judged solely by the effectiveness of the educational programs (i.e., whether screenees understood the information), it is clear that prevention of [cystic fibrosis] is also, at some level, a measure of a screening program, since few would advocate expanding the substantial resources involved if very few families wish to avoid the disease.[4(p603)]

Prenatal tests designed to detect the condition of the fetus include ultrasound, maternal serum α-fetoprotein screening, chorionic villus sampling, and amniocentesis. Some (ultrasound screenings) are routinely performed regardless of the mother's age and provide information that she may use to guide her care throughout pregnancy; others, such as chorionic villus sampling or amniocentesis, do not influence the woman's care during pregnancy but provide information intended to help her decide whether to continue the pregnancy if fetal impairment is detected. Amniocentesis, the test that detects the greatest variety of fetal impairments, is typically offered to women who will be 35 years or older at the time they are due to deliver, but recently commentators have urged that the age threshold be removed and that the test be available to women regardless of age. Such testing is increasingly considered a standard component of prenatal care for women whose insurance covers these procedures, including women using publicly financed clinics in some jurisdictions.

These tests, which are widely accepted in the field of bioethics and by clinicians, public health professionals, and the general public, have nonetheless occasioned some apprehension and concern among students of women's reproductive experiences, who find that women do not uniformly welcome the expectation that they will undergo prenatal testing or the prospect of making decisions depending on the test results. Less often discussed by clinicians is the view, expressed by a growing number of individuals, that the technology is itself based on erroneous assumptions about the adverse impact of disability on life. Argument from this perspective focuses on what is communicated about societal and familial acceptance of diversity in general and disability in particular. Like other women-centered critiques of prenatal testing, this article assumes a pro-choice perspective but suggests that unreflective uses of testing could diminish, rather than expand, women's choices. Like critiques stemming from concerns about the continued acceptance of human differences within the society and the family, this critique challenges the view of disability that lies behind social endorsement of such testing and the conviction that women will, or should, end their pregnancies if they discover that the fetus has a disabling trait.

If public health frowns on efforts to select for or against girls or boys and would oppose future efforts to select for or against those who would have a particular sexual orientation, but promotes people's efforts to avoid having children who would have disabilities, it is because medicine and public health view disability as extremely different from and worse than these other forms of human variation. At first blush this view may strike one as self-evident. To challenge it might even appear to be questioning our professional mission. Characteristics such as chronic illnesses and disabilities (discussed together throughout this article) do not resemble traits such as sex, sexual orientation, or race, because the latter are not in themselves perceived as inimical to a rewarding life. Disability is thought to be just that—to be incompatible with life satisfaction. When public health considers matters of sex, sexual orientation, or race, it examines how factors in social and economic life pose obstacles to health and to health care, and it champions actions to improve the well-being of those disadvantaged by the discrimination that attends minority status. By contrast, public health fights to eradicate disease and disability or to treat, ameliorate, or cure these when they occur. For medicine and public health, disease and disability is the problem to solve, and so it appears natural to use prenatal testing and abortion as one more means of minimizing the incidence of disability.

In the remainder of this article I argue, first, that most of the problems associated with having a disability stem from discriminatory social arrangements that are changeable, just as much of what has in the past made the lives of women or gays difficult has been the set of social arrangements they have faced (and which they have begun to dismantle). After discussing ways in which the characteristic of disability resembles and differs from other characteristics, I discuss why I believe the technology of prenatal testing followed by selective abortion is unique among means of preventing or ameliorating disability, and why it offends many people who are untroubled by other disease prevention and health promotion activities. I conclude by recommending ways in which health practitioners and policymakers could offer this technology so that it promotes genuine reproductive choice and helps families and society to flourish.

CONTRASTING MEDICAL AND SOCIAL PARADIGMS OF DISABILITY

The definitions of terms such as "health," "normality," and "disability" are not clear, objective, and universal across time and place. Individual physical characteristics are evaluated with reference to a standard of normality, health, and what some commentators term "species-typical functioning." These commentators point out that within a society at a particular time, there is a shared perception of what is typical physical functioning and role performance for a girl or boy, woman or man. Boorse's definition of an undesirable departure from species-typicality focuses on the functioning of the person rather than the cause of the problem: "[A] condition of a part or process in an organism is pathological when the ability of the part or process to perform one or more of its species-typical biological functions

falls below some central range of the statistical distribution for that ability."[5(p370)] Daniels writes, "Impairments of normal species functioning reduce the range of opportunity open to the individual in which he may construct his plan of life or conception of the good."[6 (p27)]

Chronic illness, traumatic injury, and congenital disability may indeed occasion departures from "species-typical functioning," and thus these conditions do constitute differences from both a statistical average and a desired norm of well-being. Certainly society prizes some characteristics, such as intelligence, athleticism, and musical or artistic skill, and rewards people with more than the statistical norm of these attributes; I will return to this point later. Norms on many health-related attributes change over time; as the life span for people in the United States and Canada increases, conditions that often lead to death before 40 years of age (e.g., cystic fibrosis) may become even more dreaded than they are today. The expectation that males will be taller than females and that adults will stand more than 5 feet in height leads to a perception that departures from these norms are not only unusual but undesirable and unhealthy. Not surprisingly, professionals who have committed themselves to preventing illness and injury or to ameliorating and curing people of illnesses and injuries, are especially attuned to the problems and hardships that affect the lives of their patients. Such professionals, aware of the physical pain or weakness and the psychological and social disruption caused by acute illness or sudden injury, devote their lives to easing the problems that these events impose.

What many scholars, policymakers, and activists in the area of disability contend is that medically oriented understandings of the impact of disability on life contain 2 erroneous assumptions with serious adverse consequences: first, that the life of a person with a chronic illness or disability is forever disrupted, as one's life might be temporarily disrupted as a result of a back spasm, an episode of pneumonia, or a broken leg; second, that if a disabled person experiences isolation, powerlessness, unemployment, poverty, or low social status, these are inevitable consequences of biological limitation. Body, psyche, and social life do change immediately following an occurrence of disease, accident, or injury, and medicine, public health, and bioethics all correctly appreciate the psychological and physical vulnerability of patients and their families and friends during immediate medical crises. These professions fail people with disabilities, however, by concluding that because there may never be full physical recovery there is never a regrouping of physical, cognitive, and psychological resources with which to participate in a rewarding life. Chronic illness and disability are not equivalent to acute illness or sudden injury, in which an active disease process or unexpected change in physical function disrupts life's routines. Most people with conditions such as spina bifida, achondroplasia, Down syndrome, and many other mobility and sensory impairments perceive themselves as healthy, not sick, and describe their conditions as givens of their lives—the equipment with which they meet the world. The same is true for people with chronic conditions such as cystic fibrosis, diabetes, hemophilia, and muscular dystrophy. These conditions include intermittent flare-ups requiring medical care and adjustments in daily living, but they do not render the person as unhealthy as most of the public—and members of the health profession—imagine. . . .

The second way in which medicine, bioethics, and public health typically err is in viewing all problems that occur to people with disabilities as attributable to the condition itself, rather than to external factors. When ethicists, public health professionals, and policymakers discuss the importance of health care, urge accident prevention, or promote healthy lifestyles, they do so because they perceive a certain level of health not only as intrinsically desirable but as a prerequisite for an acceptable life. One commentator describes such a consensual view of types of life in terms of a "normal opportunity range": "The normal opportunity range for a given society is the array of life plans reasonable persons in it are likely to construct for themselves.[7(p33)] Health care includes that which is intended to "maintain, restore, or provide functional equivalents where possible, to normal species functioning.[8(p32)]

The paradigm of medicine concludes that the gaps in education, employment, and income that persist between adults with disabilities and those without disabilities are inevitable because the impairment precludes study or limits work. The alternative paradigm, which views people with disabilities in social, minority-group terms, examines how societal arrangements—rules, laws, means of communication, characteristics of buildings and transit systems, the typical 8-hour workday—exclude some people from participating in school, work, civic, or social life. This newer paradigm is expressed by enactment of the Individuals with Disabilities Education Act and the Americans with Disabilities Act and is behind the drive to ensure that employed disabled people will keep their access to health care through Medicaid or Medicare. This paradigm—still more accepted by people outside medicine, public health, and bioethics than by those within these fields—questions whether there is an inevitable, unmodifiable gap between people with disabilities and people without disabilities. Learning that in 1999, nine years after the passage of laws to end employment discrimination, millions of people with disabilities are still out of the work force, despite their readiness to work;[9] the social paradigm asks what remaining institutional factors bar people from the goal of productive work. Ethical and policy questions arise in regard to the connection that does or should exist between health and the range of opportunities open to people in the population. . . .

The Americans with Disabilities Act, signed into law in 1990, is a ringing indictment of the nation's history with regard to people with disabilities:

> Congress finds that . . . (3) discrimination against individuals with disabilities persists in such critical areas as employment, . . . education, recreation, . . . health services, ... and access to public services; (7) individuals with disabilities are a discrete and insular minority who have been faced with restrictions and limitations, subjected to a history of purposeful unequal treatment, and relegated to a position of political powerlessness in our society, based on characteristics that are beyond the control of such individuals and resulting from stereotypic assumptions not truly indicative of the individual ability of such individuals to participate in, and contribute to, society.[10]

Eight years after the passage of the Americans with Disabilities Act, disabled people reported some improvements in access to public facilities and that things are getting better in some areas of life, but major gaps between the disabled and the nondisabled still exist in income, employment, and social participation. To dramatically underscore the prevalence of social stigma and discrimination: "fewer than half (45%) of adults with disabilities say that people generally treat them as an equal after they learn they have a disability."[11]

It is estimated that 54 million people in the United States have disabilities, of which impairments of mobility, hearing, vision, and learning; arthritis; cystic fibrosis; diabetes; heart conditions; and back problems are some of the most well-known.[12] Thus, in discussing discrimination, stigma, and unequal treatment for people with disabilities, we are considering a population that is larger than the known gay and lesbian population or the African American population. These numbers take on new significance when we assess the rationale behind prenatal diagnosis and selective abortion as a desirable strategy to deal with disability.

Prenatal Diagnosis for Disability Prevention

If some forms of disability prevention are legitimate medical and public health activities, and if people with disabilities use the health system to improve and maintain their own health, there is an acknowledgment that the characteristic of disability may not be desirable. Although many within the disability rights movement challenge prenatal diagnosis as a means of disability prevention, no one objects to public health efforts to clean up the environment, encourage seat-belt use, reduce tobacco and alcohol consumption, and provide prenatal care to all pregnant women. All these activities deal with the health of existing human beings (or fetuses expected to come to term) and seek to ensure their well-being. What differentiates prenatal testing followed by abortion from other forms of disability prevention and medical treatment is that prenatal testing followed by abortion is intended not to prevent the disability or illness of a born or future human being but to prevent the birth of a human being who will have one of these undesired characteristics. In reminding proponents of the Human Genome Project that gene therapy will not soon be able to cure disability, James Watson declared,

> [W]e place most of our hopes for genetics on the use of antenatal diagnostic procedures, which increasingly will let us know whether a fetus is carrying a mutant gene that will seriously proscribe its eventual develop-

ment into a functional human being. By terminating such pregnancies, the threat of horrific disease genes contributing to blight many family's prospects for future success can be erased. [13(p19)]

But Watson errs in assuming that tragedy is inevitable for the child or for the family. When physicians, public health experts, and bioethicists promote prenatal diagnosis to prevent future disability, they let disability become the only relevant characteristic and suggest that it is such a problematic characteristic that people eagerly awaiting a new baby should terminate the pregnancy and "try again" for a healthy child. Professionals fail to recognize that along with whatever impairment may be diagnosed come all the characteristics of any other future child. The health professions suggest that once a prospective parent knows of the likely disability of a future child, there is nothing else to know or imagine about who the child might become: disability subverts parental dreams.

The focus of my concern here is not on the decision made by the pregnant woman or by the woman and her partner. I focus on the view of life with disability that is communicated by society's efforts to develop prenatal testing and urge it on every pregnant woman. If public health espouses goals of social justice and equality for people with disabilities, as it has worked to improve the status of women, gays and lesbians, and members of racial and ethnic minorities, it should reconsider whether it wishes to continue endorsing the technology of prenatal diagnosis. If there is an unshakable commitment to the technology in the name of reproductive choice, public health should work with practitioners to change the way in which information about impairments detected in the fetus is delivered.

Rationales for Prenatal Testing

The medical professions justify prenatal diagnosis and selective abortion on the grounds of the *costs* of childhood disability—the costs to the child, to the family, and to the society. Some proponents of the Human Genome Project from the fields of science and bioethics argue that in a world of limited resources, we can reduce disability-related expenditures if all diagnoses of fetal impairment are followed by abortion.

On both empirical and moral grounds, endorsing prenatal diagnosis for societal reasons is dangerous. Only a small fraction of total disability can now be detected prenatally, and even if future technology enables the detection of predisposition to diabetes, forms of depression, Alzheimer [sic] disease, heart disease, arthritis, or back problems—all more prevalent in the population than many of the currently detectable conditions—we will never manage to detect and prevent most disability. Rates of disability increase markedly with age, and the gains in life span guarantee that most people will deal with disability in themselves or someone close to them. Laws and services to support people with disabilities will still be necessary, unless society chooses a campaign of eliminating disabled people in addition to preventing the births of those who would be disabled. Thus, there is small cost-saving in money or in human resources to be achieved by even the vigorous determination to test every pregnant woman and abort every fetus found to exhibit disabling traits.

My moral opposition to prenatal testing and selective abortion flows from the conviction that life with disability is worthwhile and the belief that a just society must appreciate and nurture the lives of all people, whatever the endowments they receive in the natural lottery. I hold these beliefs because—as I show throughout this article—there is abundant evidence that people with disabilities can thrive even in this less than welcoming society. Moreover, people with disabilities do not merely take from others, they contribute as well—to families, to friends, to the economy. They contribute neither in spite of nor because of their disabilities, but because along with their disabilities come other characteristics of personality, talent, and humanity that render people with disabilities full members of the human and moral community.

IMPLICATIONS FOR PEOPLE WITH DISABILITIES

Implications for children and adults with disabilities, and for their families, warrant more consideration. Several prominent bioethicists claim that to knowingly bring into the world a child who will live with an impairment (whether it be a "withered arm," cystic fibrosis, deafness, or Down syndrome) is unfair to the child because it deprives the child of the "right to

an open future" by limiting some options. Green's words represent a significant strand of professional thinking: "In the absence of adequate justifying reasons, a child is morally wronged when he/she is knowingly, deliberately, or negligently brought into being with a health status likely to result in significantly greater disability or suffering, or significantly reduced life options relative to the other children with whom he/she will grow up."[14(p10)] Green is not alone in his view that it is irresponsible to bring a child into the world with a disability.

The biology of disability can affect people's lives, and not every feature of life with a disability is socially determined or medicated. People with cystic fibrosis cannot now expect to live to age 70. People with type 1 diabetes can expect to have to use insulin and to have to think carefully and continuously about what and how much they eat and about their rest and exercise, perhaps more than typical sedentary people who are casual about the nutritional content of their food. People who use a wheelchair for mobility will not climb mountains; people with the intellectual disabilities of Down syndrome or fragile X chromosome are not likely to read this article and engage in debate about its merits and shortcomings. Yet, as disability scholars point out, such limitations do not preclude a whole class of experiences, but only certain instances in which these experiences might occur. People who move through the world in wheelchairs may not be able to climb mountains, but they can and do participate in other athletic activities that are challenging and exhilarating and call for stamina, alertness, and teamwork. Similarly, people who have Down syndrome or fragile X chromosome are able to have other experiences of thinking hard about important questions and making distinctions and decisions. Thus, they exercise capacities for reflection and judgment, even if not in the rarified world of abstract verbal argument (P. Ferguson, e-mail, March 5, 1999).

The child who will have a disability may have fewer options for the so-called open future that philosophers and parents dream of for children. Yet I suspect that disability precludes far fewer life possibilities than members of the bioethics community claim. That many people with disabilities find their lives satisfying has been documented. For example, more than half of people with spinal cord injury (paraplegia) reported feeling more positively about themselves since becoming disabled. Similarly,

Canadian teenagers who had been extremely-low-birthweight infants were compared with nondisabled teens and found to resemble them in terms of their own subjective ratings of quality of life. "Adolescents who were [extremely-low-birthweight] infants suffer from a greater burden of morbidity, and rate their health-related quality of life as significantly lower than control teenagers. Nevertheless, the vast majority of the [extremely-low-birthweight] respondents view their health-related quality of life as quite satisfactory and are difficult to distinguish from controls."[15(p453)]

Interestingly, professionals faced with such information often dismiss it and insist that happy disabled people are the exceptions.[16] . . .

. . . The 1998 survey of disabled people in the United States conducted by Louis Harris Associates found gaps in education, employment, income, and social participation between people with disabilities and people without disabilities and noted that fewer disabled than nondisabled people were "extremely satisfied" with their lives. The reasons for dissatisfaction did not stem from anything inherent in the impairments; they stemmed from disparities in attainments and activities that are not inevitable in a society that takes into account the needs of one sixth of its members.[17] . . .

For children whose disabling conditions do not cause early degeneration, intractable pain, and early death, life offers a host of interactions with the physical and social world in which people can be involved to their and others' satisfaction. Autobiographical writings and family narratives testify eloquently to the rich lives and the even richer futures that are possible for people with disabilities today. . . .

Nonetheless, I do not deny that disability can entail physical pain, psychic anguish, and social isolation—even if much of the psychological and social pain can be attributed to human cruelty rather than to biological givens. In order to imagine bringing a child with a disability into the world when abortion is possible, prospective parents must be able to imagine saying to a child, "I wanted you enough and believed enough in who you could be that I felt you could have a life you would appreciate even with the difficulties your disability causes." If parents and siblings, family members and friends can genuinely love and enjoy the child for who he or she is and not lament what he or she is not; if child

care centers, schools, and youth groups routinely include disabled children; if television programs, children's books, and toys take children with disabilities into account by including them naturally in programs and products, the child may not live with the anguish and isolation that have marred life for generations of disabled children.

IMPLICATIONS FOR FAMILY LIFE

Many who are willing to concede that people with disabilities could have lives they themselves would enjoy nonetheless argue that the cost to families of raising them justifies abortion. Women are seen to carry the greatest load for the least return in caring for such a child. Proponents of using the technology to avoid the births of children with disabilities insist that the disabled child epitomizes what women have fought to change about their lives as mothers: unending labor, the sacrifice of their work and other adult interests, loss of time and attention for the other children in the family as they juggle resources to give this disabled child the best available support, and uncertain recompense in terms of the mother's relationship with the child. . . .

Assuming for a moment that there are "extra burdens" associated with certain aspects of raising children with disabilities, consider the "extra burdens" associated with raising other children: those with extraordinary (above statistical norm) aptitude for athletics, art, music, or mathematics. In a book on gifted children, Ellen Winner writes,

> [A]ll the family's energy becomes focused on this child. . . . Families focus in two ways on the gifted child's development: either one or both parents spend a great deal of time stimulating and teaching the child themselves, or parents make sacrifices so that the child gets high-level training from the best available teachers. In both cases, family life is totally arranged around the child's needs. Parents channel their interests into their child's talent area and become enormously invested in their child's progress.[18(p187)]

Parents, professionals working with the family, and the larger society all value the gift of the violin prodigy, the talent of the future Olympic figure skater, the aptitude of a child who excels in science and who might one day discover the cure for cancer. They perceive that all the extra work and rearrangement associated with raising such children will provide what people seek in parenthood: the opportunity to give ourselves to a new being who starts out with the best we can give, who will enrich us, gladden others, contribute to the world, and make us proud.

If professionals and parents believed that children with disabilities could indeed provide their parents many of the same satisfactions as any other child in terms of stimulation, love, companionship, pride, and pleasure in influencing the growth and development of another, they might reexamine their belief that in psychological, material, and social terms, the burdens of raising disabled children outweigh the benefits. A vast array of literature, both parental narrative and social science quantitative and qualitative research, powerfully testifies to the rewards—typical and atypical—of raising children with many of the conditions for which prenatal testing is considered de rigeur and abortion is expected (Down syndrome, hemophilia, cystic fibrosis, to name only some). Yet bioethics, public health, and genetics remain woefully—scandalously—oblivious, ignorant, or dismissive of any information that challenges the conviction that disability dooms families. . . .

The literature on how disability affects family life is, to be sure, replete with discussions of stress; anger at unsupportive members of the helping professions; distress caused by hostility from extended family, neighbors, and strangers; and frustration that many disability-related expenses are not covered by health insurance. And it is a literature that increasingly tries to distinguish why—under what conditions—some families of disabled children founder and others thrive. Contrary to the beliefs still much abroad in medicine, bioethics, and public health, recent literature does not suggest that, on balance, families raising children who have disabilities experience more stress and disruption than any other family.

IMPLICATIONS FOR PROFESSIONAL PRACTICE

Reporting in 1997 on a 5-year study of how families affected by cystic fibrosis and sickle cell anemia viewed genetic testing technologies, Duster and Beeson learned to their surprise that the closer the relationship between the family member and the affected individual, the more uncomfortable the family member was with the technology.

[The] closer people are to someone with genetic disease the more problematic and usually unacceptable genetic testing is as a strategy for dealing with the issues. The experience of emotional closeness to someone with a genetic disease reduces, rather than increases, the acceptability of selective abortion. A close relationship with an affected person appears to make it more difficult to evaluate the meaning or worth of that person's existence solely in terms of their genetic disease. Family members consistently affirm the value of the person's life in spite of the disorders, and see value for their family in their experiences with (and) of this member, and in meeting the challenges the disease poses.[19(p43)]

This finding is consistent with other reports that parents of children with disabilities generally reject the idea of prenatal testing and abortion of subsequent fetuses, even if those fetuses are found to carry the same disabling trait.

Professionals charged with developing technologies, offering tests, and interpreting results should assess their current assumptions and practice on the basis of the literature on disability and family life generally and data about how such families perceive selective abortion. Of the many implications of such data, the first is that familiarity with disability as one characteristic of a child one loves changes the meaning of disability for parents contemplating a subsequent birth. The disability, instead of being the child's sole, or most salient, characteristic, becomes only one of the child's characteristics, along with appearance, aptitudes, temperament, interests, and quirks. The typical woman or couple discussing prenatal testing and possible pregnancy termination knows very little about the conditions for which testing is available, much less what these conditions might mean for the daily life of the child and the family. People who do not already have a child with a disability and who are contemplating prenatal testing must learn considerably more than the names of some typical impairments and the odds of their child's having one.

To provide ethical and responsible clinical care for anyone concerned about reproduction, professionals themselves must know far more than they now do about life with disability; they must convey more information, and different information, than they now typically provide. Shown a film about the lives of families raising children with Down syndrome, nurses and genetic counselors—but not parents—described the film as unrealistic and too positive a portrayal of family life. Whether the clinician is a genetics professional or (as is increasingly the case) an obstetrician promoting prenatal diagnosis as routine care for pregnant women, the tone, timing, and content of the counseling process cry out for drastic overhaul. . . .

Until their own education is revamped, obstetricians, midwives, nurses, and genetics professionals cannot properly counsel prospective parents. With broader exposure themselves, they would be far more likely to engage in discussions with their patients that would avoid problems such as those noted by Lippmann and Wilfond in a survey of genetic counselors. These researchers found that counselors provided far more positive information about Down syndrome and cystic fibrosis to parents already raising children diagnosed with those conditions than they did to prospective parents deciding whether to continue pregnancies in which the fetus had been found to have the condition. . . .

. . . I call for change to ensure that everyone obtaining testing or seeking information about genetic or prenatally diagnosable disability receives sufficient information about predictable difficulties, supports, and life events associated with a disabling condition to enable them to consider how a child's disability would fit into their own hopes for parenthood. Such information for all prospective parents should include, at a minimum, a detailed description of the biological, cognitive, or psychological impairments associated with specific disabilities, and what those impairments imply for day-to-day functioning; a discussion of the laws governing education, entitlements to family support services, access to buildings and transportation, and financial assistance to disabled children and their families; and literature by family members of disabled children and by disabled people themselves.

If prenatal testing indicates a disabling condition in the fetus, the following disability-specific information should be given to the prospective parents: information about services to benefit children with specific disabilities in a particular area, and about which of these a child and family are likely to need immediately after birth; contact information for a parent-group representative; and contact information for a member of a disability rights group or independent living center. In addition, the parents should be offered a visit with both a child and family and an adult living with the diagnosed disability.

Although some prospective parents will reject some or all of this information and these contacts, responsible practice that is concerned with genuine informed decision making and true reproductive choice must include access to this information, timed so that prospective parents can assimilate general ideas about life with disability before testing and obtain particular disability-relevant information if they discover that their fetus carries a disabling trait. These ideas may appear unrealistic or unfeasible, but a growing number of diverse voices support similar versions of these reforms to encourage wise decision making. Statements by Little People of America, the National Down Syndrome Congress, the National Institutes of Health workshop, and the Hastings Center Project on Prenatal Testing for Genetic Disability all urge versions of these changes in the process of helping people make childbearing decisions.

These proposals may be startling in the context of counseling for genetically transmitted or prenatally diagnosable disability, but they resonate with the recent discussion about childbearing for women infected with the HIV virus:

> The primary task of the provider would be to engage the client in a meaningful discussion of the implications of having a child and of not having a child for herself, for the client's family and for the child who would be born. . . . Providers would assist clients in examining what childbearing means to them. . . . Providers also would assist clients in gaining an understanding of the factual information relevant to decisions about childbearing . . . however, the conversation would cover a range of topics that go far beyond what can be understood as the relevant *medical* facts, and the direction of the conversation would vary depending on each person's life circumstances and priorities [emphasis added].[20(pp453-454)]

. . . Along with others who have expressed growing concern about needed reforms in the conduct of prenatal testing and counseling, I urge a serious conversation between prospective parents and clinicians about what the parents seek in childrearing and how a disabling condition in general or a specific type of impairment would affect their hopes and expectations for the rewards of parenthood. For some people, any mobility, sensory, cognitive, or health impairment may indeed lead to disappointment of parental hopes; for others, it may be far easier to imagine incorporating disability into family life without believing that the rest of their lives will be blighted.

Ideally, such discussions will include mention of the fact that every child inevitably differs from parental dreams, and that successful parenting requires a mix of shaping and influencing children and ruefully appreciating the ways they pick and choose from what parents offer, sometimes rejecting tastes, activities, or values dear to the parents. If prospective parents cannot envision appreciating the child who will depart in particular, known ways from the parents' fantasy, are they truly ready to raise would-be athletes when they hate sports, classical violinists when they delight in the Grateful Dead? Testing and abortion guarantee little about the child and the life parents create and nurture, and all parents and children will be harmed by inflated notions of what parenting in an age of genetic knowledge can bring in terms of fulfilled expectations.

Public health professionals must do more than they have been doing to change the climate in which prenatal tests are offered. Think about what people would say if prenatal clinics contained pamphlets telling poor women or African American women that they should consider refraining from childbearing because their children could be similarly poor and could endure discrimination or because they could be less healthy and more likely to find themselves imprisoned than members of the middle class or than Whites. Public health is committed to ending such inequities, not to endorsing them, tolerating them, or asking prospective parents to live with them. Yet the current promotion of prenatal testing condones just such an approach to life with disability.

Practitioners and policymakers can increase women's and couples' reproductive choice through testing and counseling, and they can expend energy and resources on changing the society in which families consider raising disabled children. If families that include children with disabilities now spend more money and ingenuity on after-school care for those children because they are denied entrance into existing programs attended by their peers and siblings, public health can join with others to ensure that existing programs include *all* children. The principle of education for all, which is reforming public education for disabled children, must spread to incorporate those same children into the network of services and supports that parents count on for other children. Such programs, like other institutions, must change to fit the people who exist in the world, not claim that some people should not exist because society is not prepared for them. We can fight to reform insurance practices that deny reimbursement for diabetes test strips; special diets for people with disabilities; household modifications that give disabled children freedom to explore their environment; and modifications of equipment, games, and toys that enable disabled children to participate in activities comparable to those of their peers. Public health can fight to end the catch-22 that removes subsidies for life-sustaining personal assistance services once disabled people enter the workforce, a policy that acts as a powerful disincentive to productivity and needlessly perpetuates poverty and dependence. . . .

Despite the strides of the past few decades, our current society is far from the ideal . . . toward which the disability community strives. Medicine, bioethics, and public health can put their efforts toward promoting such a society; with such efforts, disability could become nearly as easy to incorporate into the familial and social landscape as the other differences these professions respect and affirm as ordinary parts of the human condition. Given that more than 50 million people in the US population have disabling traits and that prenatal tests may become increasingly available to detect more of them, we are confronting the fact that tests may soon be available for characteristics that we have until now considered inevitable facts of human life, such as heart disease.

In order to make testing and selecting for or against disability consonant with improving life for those who will inevitably be born with or acquire disabilities, our clinical and policy establishments must communicate that it is as acceptable to live with a disability as it is to live without one and that society will support and appreciate everyone with the inevitable variety of traits. We can assure prospective parents that they and their future child will be welcomed whether or not the child has a disability. If that professional message is conveyed, more prospective parents may envision that their lives can be rewarding, whatever the characteristics of the child they are raising. When our professions can envision such communication and the reality of incorporation and appreciation of people with disabilities, prenatal technology can help people to make decisions without implying that only one decision is right. If the child with a disability is not a problem for the world, and the world is not a problem for the child, perhaps we can diminish our desire for prenatal testing and selective abortion and can comfortably welcome and support children of all characteristics.

REFERENCES

1. Wertz DC, Fletcher JC. Sex selection through prenatal diagnosis. In: Holmes HB, Purdy LM, eds. *Feminist Perspectives in Medical Ethics.* Bloomington: Indiana University Press; 1992:240–253.
2. Schuklenk U, Stein E, Kerin J, Byne W. The ethics of genetic research on sexual orientation. *Hastings Center Rep.* 1997;27(4):6–13.
3. Retsinas J. Impact of prenatal technology on attitudes toward disabled infants. In: Wertz D. *Research in the Sociology of Healthcare.* Westport, Conn: JAI Press; 1991:75–102.
4. Beaudet AL. Carrier screening for cystic fibrosis. *Am J Hum Genet* 1990;47:603–605.
5. Boorse C. Concepts of health. In: Van de Veer D, Regan T, eds. *Health Care Ethics.* Philadelphia, Pa: Temple University Press; 1987:359–393.
6. Daniels NL. *Just Health Care: Studies in Philosophy and Health Policy.* Cambridge, England: Cambridge University Press; 1985.
7. Ibid.
8. Ibid.
9. National Organization on Disability's 1998 Harris Survey of Americans With Disabilities. Available at: http://www.nod.org/press.html #poll. Accessed August 29, 1999.
10. Americans with Disabilities Act (Pub L No. 101–336, 1990, § 2).
11. National Organization.
12. Ibid.
13. Watson JD. President's essay: genes and politics. *Annual Report Cold Springs Harbor.* 1996:1–20.
14. Green R. Prenatal autonomy and the obligation not to harm one's child genetically. *J Law Med Ethics.* 1996; 25(1):5–16.
15. Saigal S, Feeny D, Rosenbaum P, Furlong W, Burrows E, Stoskopf B. Self-perceived health status and health-related quality of life of extremely low-birth-weight infants at adolescence. *JAMA.* 1996;276:453–459.
16. Tyson JE, Broyles RS. Progress in assessing the long-term outcome of extremely low-birth-weight infants. *JAMA.* 1996;276:492–493.
17. National Organization.
18. Winner E. *Gifted Children: Myths and Realities.* New York, NY: Basic Books; 1996.
19. Duster T, Beeson D. *Pathways and Barriers to Genetic Testing and Screening: Molecular Genetics Meets the "High-Risk" Family.* Final report. Washington, DC: US Dept of Energy; October 1997.
20. Faden RR, Kass NE, Acuff KL, et al. HIV infection and childbearing: a proposal for public policy and clinical practice. In: Faden R, Kass N, eds. *HIV, AIDS and Childbearing: Public Policy. Private Lives.* New York, NY: Oxford University Press; 1996:447–461.

DISABILITY, PRENATAL TESTING, AND SELECTIVE ABORTION

Bonnie Steinbock

When Bob Dole addressed the international convention of B'nai B'rith a few years ago, he said that, as a member of a minority group himself—the disabled—he understands the wrong of discrimination. Some listeners were offended by this comparison. A professor of theology at Georgetown University was quoted in *The New York Times* as saying, "Most Jews today don't regard being Jewish as a handicap. They regard it as a privilege; it gives them roots and depth and a mission."

But some disabled people would argue that they do not regard their disabling condition as a handicap. It is not their medical condition that puts limits on what they can do, but rather the way in which society is organized. Some would go farther, arguing that disability makes one part of a community or culture, and that identification with that culture is as important to identity as being a member of a race or ethnic group. Erik Parens has characterized the position this way:

> Some people in the disability-rights community argue that so-called disabilities are forms of variation, which ought to be affirmed in the same way that most liberals want to affirm any other form of variation (such as being female or black).

Let us call this the "forms of variation" argument. Parens goes on to draw out an implication of this view for what physicians call "abortion for fetal indications":

> Some people in the disability-rights community argue that just as most liberals deplore sex selection (at least

in part) on the grounds that it exacerbates discrimination against women, so should they deplore other sorts of selective abortion on similar grounds. While we can accept that being a woman in this culture can be disadvantageous (can in its way be "disabling"), we think that we ought to change the culture, not aggressively pursue the elimination of female fetuses. According to this line, having a "traditional disability" is like being a woman: the disadvantages it brings are largely socially constructed; we should change how the culture treats people with disabilities, not try to eliminate fetuses with "disabling" traits.[1]

Let us call this view "the disability perspective on abortion."[2] The disability perspective on abortion is independent of the form of variation argument: it is possible to reject the form of variation argument while still holding the disability perspective on abortion. It is also important to note that the opposition to aborting fetuses likely to have a disability is not derived from a generally "pro-life" perspective. Some of the most passionate advocates of the disability perspective on abortion are generally "pro-choice." However, they regard abortion for "fetal indications" as discriminatory and pernicious in a way that abortion for other reasons is not.

Needless to say, the disability perspective on abortion is not a mainstream view. For most people who regard abortion as justifiable, a serious disabling condition[3] in the fetus is regarded as one of the strongest reasons for terminating a pregnancy, far stronger than reasons like inability to afford a child, having to drop out of school, not wanting to marry the father, and so forth. Even among those who are almost always opposed to abortion, a severe disability in the fetus, like rape and incest, is often regarded as justifying abortion. The disability perspective challenges this popular view, and therefore must be addressed.

In this paper, I will discuss five separate, though related, issues:

1. Whether so-called disabilities are neutral forms of variation.

2. Whether disabilities are best seen as medical problems or whether they are largely socially constructed.

3. Whether attempts to reduce the incidence of disability are generally morally acceptable.

4. Whether certain means of reducing the incidence of disability, in particular, prenatal testing and selective abortion, are morally acceptable.

5. Whether there is moral importance in the distinction between selective abortion and therapeutic interventions to prevent a person from developing a disabling condition.

Clearly these issues are related. If disabilities are merely forms of variation, like sex or skin color, then it is hard to see the justification for reducing them by abortion or any other means. If disabilities are not intrinsically handicapping, but become handicaps only due to societal arrangements, then removing the obstacles would seem preferable to preventing the incidence of disabilities. But though related, these are not all the same question. It is important to distinguish them, since individuals may agree on some of these issues but not on others.

In Section I, I consider the idea that disabilities are forms of variation. While the motivation for this idea is understandable—centuries of discrimination against people with disabilities—I argue that it is not a plausible position, nor is it intrinsic to a disability rights perspective. In Section II, I consider the claim that disabilities are socially constructed. I argue that while this claim has a great deal of truth to it, disability imposes real limitations, not all of which can be overcome through changing social institutions and attitudes.

If the argument in Section II is correct, then it follows that measures to prevent disability are in principle morally acceptable, indeed, desirable. At the same time, measures intended to prevent disability may not be justified, on all sorts of grounds, including ineffectiveness, cost, and stigmatization. Section III looks at a few examples of preventive measures, to illustrate some of the factors that are relevant to an assessment of prevention programs.

Section IV considers specifically prenatal testing and selective abortion as a means of preventing disability. I discuss Adrienne Asch's view that, while abortion is morally acceptable to prevent the birth of *any* child, it is morally unacceptable to prevent the birth of a *particular* child, because of some characteristic the child will have, such as sex or disability. I argue that the "any-particular" distinction does not have the moral force Asch claims, and that if abortion is a morally permissible means of avoiding other unwanted consequences (having a child too young, having to give up school or a job, etc.), it is also morally permissible to avoid the birth of a child with a serious disability.

I. ARE DISABILITIES "FORMS OF VARIATION"?

The claim that disabilities are just forms of variation presumably means something like the following. Most people get around by using their legs to walk. But some people use a wheelchair. Not worse, just different. Most people communicate by hearing voices and speaking. But some people use sign language to communicate. Not worse, just different.

On the face of it, this is a surprising claim. With other deviations from normal functioning, there's no claim that these are just "forms of variation." If I get laryngitis and cannot talk, I don't regard my inability to speak as just different, nor will anyone call me "differently abled." Why should laryngitis be considered a medical problem, but mental retardation, paralysis, blindness, deafness, etc. be just forms of variation?

Perhaps the distinction between ill health and disability is that it is possible to have a disability (be mentally retarded, blind, deaf, paralyzed) and be perfectly healthy. On this view, laryngitis is not just a form of variation because it is a kind of ill health. Mental retardation, on the other hand, is not a form of ill health, because mentally retarded people can be healthy. So their mental retardation is not a health issue or medical problem but just a form of variation.

However, the fact that one can be mentally retarded or blind or deaf and healthy does not show that these conditions are not medical, much less that they are just forms of variation. For long-term medical conditions like high blood pressure, diabetes, and susceptibility to migraines are also compatible with good health. You can be healthy and have high blood pressure, which you control with medication.

Why is there no group insisting that their blood pressure is just a form of variation, indeed, that the very term "high" blood pressure is offensive? Clearly it is because people with high blood pressure are not usually subjected to discrimination and stigmatization. This suggests that the problem with the "medical model" is not that it sees a health problem where none exists, but rather the problem lies in the discrimination and stigmatization that people with disabilities have experienced over the centuries. Discrimination against people with disabilities is uncontroversially bad. It is a separate question whether the medical model in general, and prenatal testing and selective abortion in particular, either lead to or manifest discrimination against people with disabilities. I will return to this issue.

For now, however, let us return to the claim that disabilities are just "forms of variation." If we compare disability with a paradigm of "form of variation"—language—we see a significant difference: the absence of a norm. All human groups speak some language, but no language is "the norm." By contrast, a human being beyond infancy who cannot speak any language is a deviation from the norm; he or she lacks normal human abilities.

Sometimes the term "normal" itself is considered offensive, as if the claim that an individual lacks "normal" human capacities, like sight, hearing, and reasoning power was insulting. There is nothing in principle objectionable about reference to what is normal. We speak of a "normal" body temperature, and this is useful in determining whether someone is sick and needs medical attention. It's only an average and you can be perfectly healthy with a body temperature of 96 or 99. But if you have 104, you're sick, and may need medical attention. Similarly, parents are told what is "normal" for a two-month-old, a six-month-old, a nine-month-old baby. There can be wide variations of ability and temperament within normal variation. But if your six-month-old never smiles or your nine-month-old cannot sit up, this indicates not merely difference, but a problem, a reason to check with the pediatrician.

In light of its initial implausibility, why would anyone put forward the idea that disabilities are just "forms of variation"? The answer is that this is supposed to counter all-too-prevalent stereotypical thinking about disability as inherently bad, inherently disadvantageous, inherently a problem. According to disability rights activists, this stereotypical thinking stems from an unthinking superiority on the part of the (temporarily) abled. As Anita Silvers writes:

> So habitual are our feelings of superiority to individuals with disabilities that we may automatically acquiescence in the . . . . equating of disability with disadvantage. However, even though an impairment is no advantage, it does not follow that to be impaired or disabled is to be disadvantaged *per se*. For disadvantage is relative to both context and end. A specific impairment need have no natural or necessary deleterious impact on a life.

However, Silvers appears to equivocate between something's being a *disadvantage* and its being *disadvantageous on balance*. Consider the example she gives of Itzhak Perlman. Due to polio as a child, Perlman walks with braces and canes. Is this a disadvantage? Surely it is. It limits his mobility, and makes walking slow and cumbersome. It also means that he can leave the stage and return for a bow, as is customary, only with difficulty. Perlman handles this disability with great charm and good humor. In a concert I attended in London, he walked off the stage and returned, to tumultuous applause, for one encore; after that, he remained seated, saying to the audience, waving his hand in the direction of the wings, "Now I have gone off and come back on again."

Not being able to walk easily is certainly *a disadvantage*. But is Perlman disadvantaged *on balance* due to his disability? Surely not; we should all be so disadvantaged. To be sure, there are careers that are not open to him (boxer, mountaineer), but so what? His disability has not interfered with his being a great musician. So, on balance, Perlman is not disadvantaged; but at the same time, his disability is a disadvantage, and probably one he would prefer not to have.

There are times when a disability is not a disadvantage. Someone who is blind is unlikely to be drafted and therefore may survive a war. The fact that a disability can be under unusual circumstances advantageous is consistent with its being ordinarily a disadvantage. However, some disabilities may have their own positive advantages, even under ordinary circumstances. For example, many deaf people find they can concentrate better because they are not distracted by noise. One woman, when asked by her daughter if she would want cochlear implants, said, "Heavens, no! Why would I want all that noise?" A professor of animal behavior claims that her autism enables her to understand animals in a way that non-autistic people cannot. (She uses this skill to design slaughter houses that prevent panic among the cattle.) In 1997, the newspapers reported the story of an autistic boy who became lost while swimming in Turtle Creek in Florida. His parents believe it is possible that he survived the horrors of the swamp not in spite of his autism, but because of it. His autism makes him impervious to fear and panic, and helps him to focus totally on the situation at hand.

Clearly, there are some advantages linked to disability. Nevertheless, disabilities are not generally advantageous, not something to be hoped for; indeed, they are to be avoided, if possible. They are not merely neutral forms of variation.

II. ARE DISABILITIES SOCIALLY CONSTRUCTED?

It may be objected that while having a disability is usually disadvantageous (hence, the term "disability"), nevertheless the disadvantage derives from the ways in which society responds to disability. That is, it is not the physical condition which is disabling, but rather the limitations imposed.

The World Health Organization differentiates between impairment, disability, and handicap is ways useful to this discussion:

An *impairment* is an abnormality or loss of any physiological or anatomical structure or function.

Disability refers to the consequences of an impairment, that is, any restriction or lack of ability to perform an activity in the manner or within the range considered appropriate for nonimpaired persons.

A *handicap* is the social disadvantage that results from an impairment or a disability.

Thus, paralysis of the legs (perhaps resulting from polio or spina bifida) is the impairment; the inability to walk is the disability; but it is "the social consequences of that disability—the refusal of employers to hire the disabled person . . . that renders him or her handicapped."

A disability becomes a handicap due to the choices of individuals and organizations. Handicaps are the result of social choices; they are not part of the "fabric of the universe." Because they are chosen, they can be changed.

Harlan Hahn contrasts the medical approach that focuses on functional impairments or the economic approach that emphasizes vocational limitations with a new *socio-political* approach which regards the fundamental restrictions of a disability as located in the surroundings that people encounter rather than within the disabled individual. Whether a disability becomes a handicap depends on many factors, including its prevalence and the attitudes of the nondisabled. Scheer and Groce use the example of hereditary deafness on Martha's Vineyard. The percentage of people born deaf was so great that the hearing residents found it advantageous to learn sign language, much as people who live near the U.S.-Mexico border find it advantageous to be bilingual in English and Spanish. They write:

Unlike modern industrial societies, where the inability of the deaf to communicate effectively with the hearing population and the ignorance of the hearing population about the capabilities of deaf individuals limit the degree to which they can integrate into the larger population, in the Vineyard there were no barriers to overcome. Accordingly, Vineyarders who were born deaf were not considered handicapped. They were able and, in fact, expected to work, marry, hold public office, vote, and participate in all social events, in exactly the same manner as did their hearing family, friends, and neighbors. Deaf island residents were well integrated into community life, with a strong cultural tradition at least 300 years old to support their inclusion. In this island community, what to us today would be considered a substantial handicap was reframed as a normal human variation. As one woman stated, the difference between the hearing and the deaf was "like if you had brown eyes and I had blue ones."

The example of deaf people on Martha's Vineyard is instructive in showing how something that might be a disability or even a handicapping condition in one context is not perceived as such in another. But the conclusion that all disability lies solely or even primarily in the environment is surely too strong. Not every disability can be overcome by social adaptation. As Wertz and Fletcher point out:

> Much of the literature on effects of prenatal diagnosis on attitudes toward people with disabilities regards all disabilities as a generic class and treats them as if equal. This is not a realistic approach. Most physical and some mental disabilities can be overcome with social support and changes in the physical environment. Some mental and neurologic disabilities, however, require lifetime care and overwhelm the parents' lives. Such disabilities may never be overcome even with massive economic and social support.

The motivation behind the claim that disability is just a form of variation is laudable: to end discrimination and make the larger community recognize that people with disabilities are people like the rest of us, with their own talents, abilities, and limitations. Disability rights activists have performed a much needed service in making the larger community aware that most people with disabilities find their lives rewarding and worthwhile. They do not wish they were dead, or that they had never been born. A disability rights perspective also forces us to recognize the extent to which socially constructed barriers, rather than natural conditions, prevent equal opportunity. At the same time, the claim that disability is completely, or mostly, a social construction is surely an exaggeration. Society can do a great deal to offer opportunities to people with disabilities, but not all disabilities can be overcome. Someone who is severely mentally retarded may have a life worth living, but cannot go to college, hold a job, or raise children. This is not a matter of social prejudice but of reality. This is acknowledged even by disability rights advocates like Adrienne Asch, who writes:

> Not all problems of disability are socially created and, thus, theoretically remediable. . . . The inability to move without mechanical aid, to see, to hear, or to learn is not inherently neutral. Disability itself limits some options. Listening to the radio for someone who is deaf, looking at paintings for someone who is blind, walking upstairs for someone who is quadriplegic, or reading abstract articles for someone who is intellectually disabled are precluded by impairment alone. . . . It is not irrational to hope that children and adults will live as long as possible without health problems or diminished human capacities.

III.   ASSESSING THE MORALITY OF VARIOUS MEANS OF PREVENTING DISABILITY

If Asch is right that many, if not all, disabilities are not inherently neutral, that they limit people's lives in undesirable ways, then prevention of disability is, in itself, desirable. While some disability activists might contest even this claim, most would agree that prevention of disability is a good thing. Disagreement arises about the way in which disability is prevented. Many disability activists draw a sharp distinction between actions that prevent individuals from becoming disabled and actions that prevent individuals who would be disabled from coming into existence, such as prenatal testing and selective abortion. The former category includes, for example, putting iodine in salt to prevent mental retardation or enriching flour with folic acid to reduce the incidence of neural tube disorders. Such measures are not viewed as intrinsically morally problematic, although they might not be justified from a public health perspective if the cost or risks were high. For example, too much folic acid can be bad for elderly people. This might be a reason to provide pregnant women with folic acid supplements, rather than putting folic acid into a food everyone will eat.

Other noncontroversial forms of preventing disability include efforts to get women to avoid certain behaviors during pregnancy, such as smoking and drinking alcohol. Cigarette smoking in pregnant women has been shown to increase the risk of miscarriage, stillbirth, prematurity, and low birthweight. Premature and low birth-weight babies are more likely to die during infancy than full-term and normal birth-weight babies, and are at greater risk of developing neurological problems. Heavy and prolonged alcohol consumption (at least 5.0 ounces of absolute alcohol a day) during pregnancy, especially binge drinking, has been demonstrated to cause fetal alcohol syndrome (FAS), which usually results in neurological damage causing mental retardation, emotional problems, or learning disabilities. Even less heavy drinking (1.5 oz. of alcohol a day) during pregnancy has been found by some researchers to triple the risk of subnormal I.Q. Because the risks to the fetus and subsequently born child are serious, and the impact of refraining from smoking or drinking during pregnancy is not deleterious to the pregnant woman (in fact, it is better for her health, as well as her baby's), virtually everyone agrees that educational and noncoercive methods of getting women to avoid tobacco and alcohol during pregnancy are morally acceptable, indeed, morally desirable, methods of preventing disability.

IV. ARE PRENATAL TESTING AND SELECTIVE ABORTION MORALLY ACCEPTABLE WAYS OF PREVENTING DISABILITY?[4]

The disability perspective holds that prenatal testing for disability is as destructively discriminatory as sex selection. It maintains that the view that "fetal indications" justify abortion (or embryo discard) stems from the ignorant and prejudiced belief that having a disability makes life unbearable, and that those who are disabled are "better off unborn." Moreover, since prenatal screening cannot prevent all disability, e.g., disabilities caused during or after birth, an attitude of inclusion is better than an attitude of removal. Furthermore, prenatal screening leads parents to expect a "perfect baby." It increases intolerance of imperfection, and thus increases discriminatory attitudes toward disability.

Adrienne Asch is one writer who finds abortion for "fetal indications" profoundly troubling. This is not because she regards fetuses as persons and abortion as seriously morally wrong. Her view is that abortion is morally acceptable if the woman does not want to become a mother. However, she distinguishes between abortion to prevent having a child (any child) and abortion to prevent having *this* child. Why, Asch asks, would someone who wants to be a mother reject this pregnancy and this (future) child because of one thing about that child: that is, that he or she will have, or is likely to have, a disability? She believes that such rejection is likely to stem from inaccurate and prejudiced ideas about what it is like to have a disability or to parent a child with a disability.

Asch considers aborting to avoid having a child with a disability morally on a par with abortion to avoid having a child of the "wrong" sex. It embodies the view that there is something undesirable about being a person with a disability; so undesirable that it is better that such people do not get born. George Annas agrees that this is the rationale for prenatal testing, but does not think that this makes such testing wrong. This is because he thinks that prenatal testing is used only to prevent the births of individuals whose lives would be so awful that they are better off not being born. He writes:

> Historically, prenatal screening has been used to find life-threatening or severely debilitating disease where a reasonable argument can be made that actually the fetus is better off dead than living a, usually, short life.

But this is simply false. Prenatal testing has not been, and is not today, used only or even primarily to detect life-threatening, extremely severe fetal anomalies. One of the most common reasons for screening women over 35 in the U.S. is to detect trisomy 21 (Down syndrome). Down syndrome is not a fatal disease; many people with Down's live into their fifties and sixties. Moreover, it is compatible with a good quality of life, with appropriate medical treatment and educational opportunities. It is simply not true that someone who has Down syndrome would be better off dead or unborn.

What, then, should we say about most prenatal testing, which is used to screen for conditions that are serious but compatible with a life worth living? Should we say that such screening is wrong, comparable to screening for sex?[5] I do not think we need to concede this. There is another way to defend prenatal screening, one that does not require the fiction that it is used only to prevent the births of children whose lives will be so awful that they are better off unborn. Prenatal screening, along with abortion and embryo selection, can be seen as a form of prevention. It enables prospective parents to prevent an outcome they reasonably want to avoid: the birth of a child who will be sick or have a serious disability.

Admittedly, abortion prevents this outcome by terminating a pregnancy, by killing a fetus. In this respect, it differs from giving the pregnant woman folic acid, which does not kill, but rather promotes healthy development in, the fetus. Obviously, if fetuses have the same moral status as born children, then this difference is crucial. It is permissible to reduce the incidence [of] disability by keeping people healthy; it is not permissible to reduce the incidence of disability by killing people with disabilities. But if embryos and fetuses are *not* people (something a pro-choicer like Asch concedes), then the impermissibility of killing *people* to prevent or reduce the incidence of disability is irrelevant to the permissibility of abortion or embryo selection.

At the same time, most people find the termination of a wanted pregnancy troubling. Having an abortion at 16 weeks, after an amniocentesis that reveals a serious, but not life-threatening, condition in the fetus, is not psychologically comparable to taking a folic acid supplement during pregnancy, and probably is not morally identical either. Even if fetuses are not people and do not have full moral status, they are potential people with some claim to our moral attention and concern, a claim that grows stronger as the fetus grows and develops. Most abortions for fetal indications take place in the second or even third trimester, when the fetus has many of the characteristics of a newborn, including human form, perhaps sentience, and some brain activity in the neocortex. All of these developments may incline us to extend the protection granted newborns to the late-gestation fetus.[6] For late abortions to be morally justifiable, the reason for having the abortion must be serious. In my view, abortion for fetal indications meets this requirement. It is reasonable for parents to wish to avoid having a child with a serious disability, like spina bifida or Down syndrome or cystic fibrosis, because these conditions may involve undesirable events, such as pain, repeated hospitalizations and operations, paralysis, a shortened life span, limited educational and job opportunities, limited independence, and so forth. This is not to say that everyone with a serious disability *will* experience these difficulties, only that they may, and that these are problems parents reasonably wish their children not to have. If abortion is permissible at all, it is permissible to avoid such outcomes, or the risk of such outcomes.

Asch rejects the idea that prenatal testing and abortion (or embryo selection) can be viewed as "prevention." She writes:

> What differentiates ending pregnancy after learning of impairment from striving to avoid impairment before life has begun is this: At the point one ends such a pregnancy, one is indicating that one cannot accept and welcome the opportunity to nurture a life that will have a potential set of characteristics—impairments perceived as deficits and problems.

This suggests that there is something morally deficient in not being able to accept and welcome the opportunity to nurture a child with disabilities, a suggestion I want to rebut. First, the impairments may not merely be *perceived* as creating problems. This may be a realistic assessment of the situation. We do no one, not disabled individuals, not women, not families, a service by minimizing the physical, mental, and emotional burdens that may result from parenting children with disabilities.

Wertz and Fletcher outline some of these burdens in a discussion of the probable impact of having a mentally retarded child. First, most of the care of the child tends to fall on the mother. Since most people with mental retardation live at home, she may have to stop working and adopt motherhood as her primary identification. She may have this role for the rest of her life. "It is not uncommon for parents in their eighties to be caring for children with Down syndrome who are in their fifties." These are not trivial burdens, and the desire to avoid them does not indicate a character flaw, any more than wanting to avoid an hiatus in one's education or career. Whether a woman wants to terminate a pregnancy to avoid the burdens that come with being a mother, or whether she wants to terminate a pregnancy to avoid the burdens that come with being the mother of *this* child, the rationale for the abortion is the same: the avoidance of burdens that she finds unacceptable.

Asch points out that prospective parents cannot protect themselves from all burdens. A child may become disabled during or after birth. If a woman is unwilling to expend the extra effort to parent a child with a disability, how good a parent will she be? But even if we agree that a good parent will be willing to undergo burdens and sacrifices for a child, it doesn't follow that it is impermissible to try to avoid such sacrifices and burdens before becoming a parent. From a pro-choice perspective at least, a fetus is not a child and a pregnant woman is not yet a mother. Therefore, she does not have the same obligations to her fetus as she would to a born child.

In my view, a pregnant woman still has a choice whether or not to continue her pregnancy. She may change her mind because her circumstances change (e.g., the couple divorces). Although the pregnancy was wanted, she may not want to become a mother if this means being a single parent. Similarly, she may prefer to terminate a wanted pregnancy, because she wants a healthy, non-disabled child. Terminating the pregnancy gives her and her husband the chance to try again.

We can all agree that prospective parents should be fully informed about the problems and challenges they are likely to face, and that the decision to terminate should not be based on fear or ignorance. However, we can also recognize that parenthood itself is a very difficult job, even raising children without disabilities. If a woman or couple prefer not to accept the burdens and challenges that go with raising a child with special needs, that is a morally acceptable choice, and not one for which they need feel guilty or inadequate as prospective parents.

The Discrimination Argument

Another argument from the disability community focuses on the symbolic meaning of prenatal testing and its implications for people with disabilities. Sometimes this is expressed by saying that prenatal testing "sends a message" that "we don't want any more of your kind." Prenatal testing is seen, on this view, as a public statement that the lives of the disabled are worth less than those of the able-bodied. As John Robertson characterizes the view, "In short, it engenders or reinforces public perceptions that the disabled should not exist, making intolerance and discrimination toward them more likely."

This is a powerful charge and one that needs to be taken seriously. If prenatal testing actually causes harm to disabled people by increasing discrimination or reducing opportunities, that is a strong policy reason against prenatal testing. Even if prenatal testing does not cause tangible harm to discreet individuals, but only makes a symbolic statement that the lives of disabled people are worth less, that is a reason to be troubled by prenatal testing.

However, I do not think that the argument is persuasive. From the fact that a couple wants to avoid the birth of a child with a disability, it just does not follow that they value less the lives of existing people with disabilities, any more than taking folic acid to avoid spina bifida indicates a devaluing of the lives of people with spina bifida. The wish to avoid having a child with disabilities

does not imply that if that outcome should occur, the child will be unwanted, rejected, or loved less. There is no inconsistency in thinking, "If I have a child who has a disability, or becomes ill, or has special needs, I will love and care for that child; but this is an outcome I would much prefer to avoid." Allen Buchanan illustrates this point with a thought experiment:

> Suppose God tells a couple: "I'll make a child for you. You can have a child that has limited opportunities due to a physical or cognitive defect or one who does not. Which do you choose?" Surely, if the couple says they wish to have a child without defects, this need not mean that they devalue persons with disabilities, or that they would not love and cherish their child if it were disabled. Choosing to have God make a child who does not have defects does not in itself in any way betray negative judgments or attitudes about the value of individuals with defects.

Disability activists have a laudable goal: to change society so that it is welcoming and accepting of people with disabilities. However, there is no reason why society cannot both attempt to prevent disability and to provide for the needs of those who are disabled. As a matter of fact, the rise of prenatal screening has coincided with more progressive attitudes toward the inclusion of people with disabilities, as evidenced in the United States by the passage of the Americans with Disabilities Act.

V.   CONCLUSION

Prejudice and discrimination against people with disabilities is no more acceptable than racial or gender prejudice and discrimination. The socio-political model can help nondisabled (or temporarily-abled) individuals see how the world might be changed to make it more accessible to those with disabilities. The result might be a greater willingness on the part of prospective parents to accept the risk of having a child with a serious disability, and might reduce the desire for prenatal testing.

On the other hand, it might not. Some couples will prefer not to have a child with a serious disability, no matter how wonderful the social services, no matter how inclusive the society. In my view, this is a perfectly acceptable attitude, one that does not impugn their ability to be good parents. Nor does this attitude imply a devaluing of the lives of existing people with disabilities, any more than programs to vaccinate children against polio or ensure that pregnant women get enough folic acid. There is no conflict between respecting the rights of people with disabilities, and respecting the rights of women to make their own informed decisions about whether to have prenatal testing, and if they have it, how to respond to the results of that testing.

NOTES

1. Letter to the author.
2. In calling this "the disability perspective on abortion," I do not mean to suggest that all people with disabilities embrace this view, or even that all people who are disability rights advocates take this view. At a meeting of the Society for Disability Studies (SDS), I heard one woman speak in favor of prenatal testing on the ground that it would not benefit a child with a disability to be born to parents who felt unwilling or unable to cope with raising such a child. Nevertheless, I think that the more prevalent view among disability activists is that abortion to prevent the birth of a person with disabilities is morally wrong, comparable to abortion for sex selection.
3. I limit myself in this paper to "serious disabilities," leaving aside the question of abortion for trivial conditions. People will differ on what they consider a "serious" disability and I do not attempt to define the term. In general, I consider a disability serious if most people would make strenuous efforts to prevent its occurrence.
4. Some of the material in this section comes from my paper, "Preimplantation Genetic Diagnosis and Embryo Selection," in Justine Burley and John Harris, eds., *A Companion to Genetics: Philosophy and the Genetic Revolution* (Blackwell Publishers, 1999).
5. While most people find sex selection generally morally problematic, there might be situations in which screening for sex would be morally permissible. Some genetic diseases affect only one sex, so it is reasonable to screen for sex to avoid having a child with the disease. In addition, there may be cultures in which being female *is* a disability. Ideally, those cultures should change, but until they do, I do not think it would be wrong for a woman to screen for sex, rather than undergo multiple pregnancies which might be damaging to her own health until she produces the required male child. Moreover, bringing female children into the world knowing they will be deprived of food and medical care is not necessarily a strike for feminism.
6. See Nancy Rhoden, "Trimesters and Technology: Revamping *Roe v. Wade*," *Yale Law Journal* 95:4 (1986), 639–697, for a good explanation of the moral significance of late-gestation.

ETHICAL ISSUES AND PRACTICAL PROBLEMS IN PREIMPLANTATION GENETIC DIAGNOSIS

Jeffrey R. Botkin

Preimplantation genetic diagnosis (PGD) is a new method of prenatal diagnosis that is developing from a union of in vitro fertilization (IVF) technology and molecular biology. Briefly stated, PGD involves the creation of several embryos in vitro from the eggs and sperm of an interested couple. The embryos are permitted to develop to a 6-to-10-cell stage, at which point one of the embryonic cells is removed from each embryo and the cellular DNA is analyzed for chromosomal abnormalities or genetic mutations. An embryo or several embryos found to be free of genetic abnormalities are subsequently transferred to the woman's uterus for gestation. Embryos found to carry a genetic abnormality are discarded or frozen. Extra normal embryos may be frozen for future transfer or donation to another couple.

From *Journal of Law, Medicine & Ethics* 26 (1998): 17–28. Reprinted by permission of the American Society of Law, Medicine & Ethics. Copyright © 2006, all rights reserved.

Editors' note: Some text and all author's notes have been cut. Students who want to follow up on sources should consult the original article.

The rationale for this approach to prenatal diagnosis is straight-forward: "Preimplantation diagnosis for some couples at risk of transmitting inherited disorders to their children is an alternative to prenatal diagnosis and recurrent abortion." But, as with other forms of prenatal diagnosis, the use of PGD need not be restricted to couples at high risk for inherited disorders. No doubt, continued developments in molecular biology will permit a detailed genetic analysis of a potential child for a wide range of conditions, susceptibilities and, perhaps, behavioral tendencies before gestation even begins.

As an alternative to an existing clinical practice, the ethics of PGD can be considered in reference to prenatal diagnosis using better established techniques such as amniocentesis and chorionic villus sampling (CVS)—hereafter termed "traditional" prenatal diagnosis. Because PGD does not involve abortion it has been offered as a less morally problematic alternative to prenatal diagnosis. I will argue that PGD does circumvent the problem of abortion, but it raises an interesting array of other practical and ethical issues. A primary conclusion is that PGD will not provide a solution to some of the most serious ethical concerns in prenatal diagnosis.

The emphasis of this discussion will be on the ethically relevant distinctions between PGD and traditional prenatal diagnostic techniques, and I will not develop in detail the many ethical issues involved with prenatal diagnosis in general. I also will not address the ethical issues raised by storage of embryos or the potential use of normal or abnormal embryos for research purposes—both of which are relevant to PGD.

IS THERE A DEMAND FOR PGD?

As a backdrop to the discussion of this technology, we should consider the extent to which PGD might be utilized as an alternative to traditional prenatal diagnosis. Utilization will depend as much, or more, on the complexity of the procedures as it will on its perceived ethical advantages. The basic notions of placing eggs and sperm in a dish, testing the resulting embryos and transferring the healthy ones to a receptive uterus are, in principle, quite simple and elegant. Yet the retrieval of multiple eggs, the growing of embryos, the complexities of

their analysis, and the subsequent induction of an initially fragile pregnancy require remarkable dedication by a couple and collaboration of a small army of physicians, scientists, and technicians. Willy Lissens et al. describe PGD:

> Preimplantation diagnosis is . . . a procedure requiring the multidisciplinary collaboration of a clinical IVF unit, a laboratory IVF unit with micromanipulation facilities, a molecular biology and cytogenetics laboratory, and a clinical genetics unit. Most centres still consider [PGD] an experimental method and request and advise follow-up prenatal diagnosis in cases of pregnancy.

But this orchestrated creation is not a one-shot deal for most couples—two or more cycles of egg retrieval, testing, and implantation usually are required to establish a successful pregnancy. For any individual couple, PGD involves months of time, multiple drugs, invasive procedures, a team of subspecialists at a center for reproductive medicine, and it requires the will to endure the failures of implantation or the loss of early pregnancies. Once a pregnancy is established, subsequent traditional prenatal diagnosis is still recommended to check the accuracy of the process.

Related to the complexity and physical burdens and risks of the procedures are their costs. PGD remains experimental, meaning there is no established set of services provided, and there is yet to emerge a literature on its associated costs. However, there is literature on the cost of IVF for infertile couples. In a 1994 article, Peter Neumann et al. estimate that the total direct and indirect cost of IVF per cycle of egg retrieval ranges from $67,000 for the first cycle to $114,000 for the sixth cycle. In a 1997 publication, Bradley Van Voorhis et al. calculate the cost per delivery of IVF in 71 couples to be $43,000 per delivery of an infant. Assuming PGD is on the same order of magnitude, it is an extraordinarily expensive intervention. It is likely that customers for PGD will have to pay for this service out-of-pocket because it is unlikely that insurance carriers or government funding agencies will cover these costs given the nonessential nature of this intervention, the cheaper alternatives, and the controversial nature of prenatal diagnosis in general. Currently, 85 percent of the costs of IVF are not covered by insurance in the United States. Many individuals using PGD to date have their costs covered by the experimental programs developing the technology.

The market demand for PGD will depend on several factors: (1) the number of people interested in prenatal diagnosis; (2) the proportion of those interested who would strongly desire to avoid abortion; and (3) the proportion of those reluctant to consider abortion who would be willing to meet the monetary and nonmonetary costs of PGD procedures. Remarkably, despite these apparent constraints on its appeal, Yuri Verlinski notes that most experimental PGD cycles at present are being done for maternal age–related chromosomal aneuploidy (trisomy 21, trisomy 18, and so forth). For many or most of these older couples, PGD probably is being used as an adjunct to IVF for infertility. PGD by older women outside the context of infertility is an unlikely market due to two considerations. First, the risk of bearing a child with a chromosomal aneuploidy for, say, a forty-year-old women, is approximately 2.5 percent. Second, the efficiency of IVF declines significantly with age. Richard Legro et al. summarize the literature, which indicates that the pregnancy rate per cycle is 5 percent or less in women over forty years of age. Assuming future costs will not be covered by experimental programs or insurance, it is unlikely that many older mothers will be willing to undergo multiple interventions at high cost to address a modest risk that can otherwise be addressed through CVS or amniocentesis (or, perhaps, through adoption). To be more specific, how many women would spend $40,000 for a procedure with a 5 percent success rate to ensure an outcome that would occur 97.5 percent of the time anyhow? Traditional prenatal diagnosis, counseling, and pregnancy termination would avoid the same outcome at a cost of under $3,000, and this full expense would occur only if a pregnancy is achieved and a fetus with an abnormality is detected.

Further, for a number of genetic conditions, there has been a marked ambivalence about the use of prenatal diagnosis in some populations—cystic fibrosis (CF) and sickle cell disease are notable examples because they are the most common genetic conditions in Caucasians and African Americans, respectively. In 1991, a prospective trial of population screening for sickle cell disease found that less than half of those couples identified as at risk pursued prenatal diagnosis. Further, for those couples who pursued prenatal diagnosis and learned of an affected fetus, a termination rate of 39 percent was documented in a 1987 survey of U.S. and Canadian centers performing prenatal diagnosis for sickle cell disease. If these attitudes remain prevalent in the African American community, utilization of PGD for sickle cell disease is likely to be unusual. The ability to do prenatal testing for CF in recent years is being met with limited interest in the United States on the part of at-risk families. The reluctance of many at-risk couples to use prenatal diagnosis and to terminate pregnancies for these conditions is due, in part, to a reluctance to abort a pregnancy—precisely the issue addressed by PGD. But this ambivalence about selective termination is more complex than this one issue of a reluctance to abort per se. Additional dimensions include cultural attitudes about the use of prenatal diagnosis in general, the presence of other options, such as having no more children, and concerns about what abortion may imply for the value of the life of an existing affected child.

These limitations suggest that PGD in the *commercial* market will be a boutique service for the foreseeable future, even if the efficiency rates increase considerably. It is questionable whether many couples will believe that the added benefits of PGD will justify its costs and other burdens. This raises the broader question of whether the development of this extraordinary technology is born more of consumer demand for an alternative to prenatal diagnosis, or more of a technical fascination with the manipulation of human life, albeit for justifiable reasons. The relevance of this question comes, in part, from wondering how we will respond if we build it and they do not come. There will be other uses for PGD, beyond that for serious genetic disabilities, that may emerge as attractive if this powerful technology has limited use for its currently designated purpose. Alternative [sic] uses, such as for genetic enhancement, will be discussed below.

THE PURPOSE OF PGD

Despite reasons to question the future demand for this technology, there is at least a clarity of purpose for PGD compared with more established prenatal diagnostic techniques. The literature on traditional prenatal diagnosis offers a variety of potential purposes for these interventions. One purpose is to reduce the risk of bearing a child with an unwanted genetic condition or congenital malformation. This purpose is the same for PGD, although this purpose must be clearly focused and understood by clients. With all prenatal diagnostic approaches, the reduction in risk applies only to the conditions being evaluated by the technology. PGD does not guarantee that the child will be free of genetic or congenital conditions (a "perfect" baby), only that the child will be free of conditions for which testing is done. Two points are relevant here. First, the current literature is reassuring that the use of PGD does not appear to cause an increase in the risk [of] congenital malformation in the resulting child—a reasonable concern because the procedure removes a substantial portion of the mass of the developing embryo. Joe Simpson and Inge Liebaers reviewed the literature in 1996 and report that pregnancy outcome data suggest that the prevalence of congenital malformation in infants following IVF with or without micromanipulation is about 3 to 4 percent, that is, the same as that in the general population. So although PGD does not appear to increase the overall risk, it does not decrease it below the general population level. Of course, it is important to emphasize that reduction of risk to the population level may look quite good to couples at high risk of bearing a child with a specific genetic condition.

The point here is that couples undergoing PGD should have the clear understanding that the child retains the same base-line risk of a congenital abnormality as children in the general population. More specifically, PGD is not useful for predicting congenital malformations or diseases that do not have an identified genetic basis. For couples who will not consider abortion, PGD alone will not reduce the risk of bearing a child with conditions such as spina bifida, anencephaly, encephalocele, omphalocele, hypoplastic left heart, bladder extrophy, renal agenesis, or many other conditions, because these malformations often do not have their origins in single-gene defects or in detectable chromosomal aberrations. It is interesting to note that Asangla Ao et al. report that more than 50 percent of the couples who underwent PGD for CF in their series did not want additional prenatal diagnostic evaluations of the fetus beyond routine ultrasound. Such decisions

may be quite reasonable, as long as the couples understand the limitations of PGD technology.

Another purpose often mentioned for prenatal diagnosis is simply to provide couples with information about the pregnancy. This is a more neutral goal for prenatal diagnostic services consistent with the nondirective tradition of genetic counseling. Because this goal appears less problematic than goals that entail abortion, it may be promoted in patient information materials or in physician-patient encounters. Nancy Press and Carol Browner's work demonstrates how issues surrounding pregnancy termination were not explicitly mentioned in materials and initial encounters in the alpha-fetoprotein screening program in California. Many women did not understand that the principal implication of a decision to be screened was a decision about abortion if an affected child was detected. At the public policy level, it remains a challenge to decide whether prenatal screening programs are a success when at-risk couples are identified and informed of the risk, or whether success requires a significant reduction in the number of affected children born to screened couples. In the prospective screening trial for hemoglobinopathies noted above, 18,907 women were screened to identify 810 carrier women, leading to one pregnancy termination (for hemoglobin H disease). The women generally were grateful for the information—a success. Nevertheless, the limited use of the information by the women indicates that the program was largely a failure in terms of reducing the incidence of serious hemoglobinopathies—at least for the pregnancies followed in the study.

These clinical and policy problems associated with trying to provide neutral information as a purpose for prenatal diagnosis are not relevant to PGD. It would make little sense to go through IVF procedures and genetic analyses only to be nondirective about which embryos to place in the uterus. The purpose of PGD is not simply to inform couples about the genetic nature of their embryos. The explicit purpose is also to transfer healthy embryos and to discard those destined to be affected. Once a couple has chosen PGD, nondirectiveness is no longer relevant.

Similarly, a third purpose often claimed for prenatal diagnosis is that it permits parents to prepare for the birth of an affected child. Several scholars question whether emotional preparation by parents can be effective prior to actually holding and experiencing the child. Nevertheless, the claim is plausible, particularly for conditions requiring immediate surgical interventions that would be facilitated by delivery at a tertiary center. In any case, this purpose for prenatal diagnosis is not relevant to PGD. Embryo diagnosis would not be necessary or appropriate as a mechanism to prepare for the birth of an affected child. . . .

ETHICAL ISSUES

An initial set of ethical issues to consider are ones that are shared by other forms of prenatal diagnosis and selective termination. These include the destruction of prenatal life, defining the appropriate uses of the technology, the broader social effects of prenatal diagnosis for those with disabilities, allocation of resource issues, and informed consent concerns. PGD presents some new and interesting ethical concerns in each of these familiar domains. Following this discussion, I turn briefly to two new issues that are raised by PGD alone: germ-line gene therapy and genetic enhancement.

Destruction of Prenatal Life

The advantage of PGD over traditional prenatal diagnosis hinges largely on the ethical distinction between discarding an affected embryo and aborting an affected fetus. The range of positions on the moral status of prenatal life will be familiar to most readers. The conservative position, consistent with the position taken by the Catholic church, is that all prenatal life post-fertilization is of full and equal moral status to that of all other persons. Under this conception, no distinction exists between discarding an embryo and aborting a fetus—both are morally unacceptable. The opposite position, characterized by the arguments of Michael Tooley, is the claim that moral status is conferred by cognitive traits that are probably lacking in newborns, and clearly absent in fetuses and embryos. Under this conception, fetuses and embryos are equal in their lack of significant moral standing. However, the majority of scholars and official bodies who have addressed the issue have adopted positions within

a broad center ground. These positions are similar in that they maintain that all prenatal human life should be afforded a special moral status, but a moral status that is not equal to that of a full-fledged person. Further, these views typically hold that the relative moral status is influenced by the developmental status of the embryo or fetus. Some commentators argue that development is a seamless continuum, therefore, the moral status of the embryo and fetus increases incrementally with development. However, the predominant set of arguments confer moral status based on the achievement of certain milestones in the developmental process that have moral significance. Developmental milestones that have been promoted as conferring increased (although not necessarily full) moral status for the developing human include formation of the primitive streak at 14 days, "quickening" at about 18 weeks, development of "brain life" at about 20 to 22 weeks, a sapient or sentient state emerging at about 22 to 24 weeks, and viability at 23 to 24 weeks of gestation. As Carson Strong notes, this developmental conception of moral status is in agreement with widely held moral intuitions that intrauterine devices are morally acceptable even though they destroy the preimplantation embryo, that early abortion is better than late abortion, and that infanticide is wrong. The recent partial birth abortion debate also illustrates the heightened ethical concern over pregnancy termination as the fetus approaches term.

The National Institutes of Health's Human Embryo Research Panel in 1994, in its review of the moral status of the embryo, observed that only the conservative position attributed personhood and full moral status to the preimplantation embryo. Other philosophical positions, the panel concluded, accord the preembryo either limited or no moral status. The panel preferred not to adopt any single criterion as determinative of the moral status of the embryo but rather what it called a "pluralistic approach."

> As gestation continues, the further development of human form, the onset of a heartbeat, the development of the nervous system leading to brain activity and with this at least some of the physical basis for future sentience, relational presence to the mother, and capacity for independent existence all counsel toward according an increasing degree of protectability.

Broad recognition of this pluralistic approach in our society provides solid support for the claim that the fetus has greater moral standing than the preimplantation embryo does. A preference by individual couples for discarding embryos versus terminating a fetus is ethically justified through reference to this widely accepted social standard. Therefore, PGD is ethically acceptable on this basis as a method of prenatal diagnosis and selective termination. Conversely, however, given the debatable nature of the moral status of prenatal life and the burdens and expense of PGD, it obviously cannot be claimed that PGD is ethically *obligatory*, as a method of prenatal diagnosis in contrast to more traditional methods.

One further point on the moral status of the preimplantation embryo deserves emphasis. For those who hold the conservative position, PGD will be seen as *more* ethically problematic than traditional prenatal diagnosis. PGD requires the creation of numerous embryos for each live birth produced. In a recent report by Ao et al., twelve couples utilized PGD to screen for CF. The couples produced 137 embryos, of which 26 were transferred to a woman's uterus and 5 births resulted. The loss of prenatal life was substantially greater through PGD than would have resulted had the twelve at-risk couples pursued traditional prenatal diagnosis and selective termination. Clearly, PGD does not resolve the ethical concerns in prenatal diagnosis for many who have fundamental objections to abortion—indeed, it makes the situation considerably worse.

Setting Limits on the Use of PGD

In general, there is social support for prenatal diagnosis for so-called "serious" conditions, including conditions like Tay Sachs disease, spina bifida, CF, sickle cell disease, hemophilia, muscular dystrophy, and a number of others. There is also a general conviction that prenatal diagnosis and abortion for "trivial" or minor conditions is ethically troubling, although a number of professionals and commentators could permit such use of prenatal diagnosis based on a respect for parental autonomy in reproductive matters. Gender selection is often used as an extreme example of selective abortion for frivolous reasons. Nevertheless, the majority of U.S. geneticists surveyed by Dorothy Wertz and John Fletcher

in 1985 would either perform prenatal diagnosis for a couple who did not want a fifth daughter or refer them to a colleague who would. Therefore, with traditional prenatal diagnosis, a conflict in social values arises between a reluctance to validate termination of a fetus for less than a serious medical condition and a desire to respect parental autonomy in this most intimate of enterprises.

This fundamental problem with traditional prenatal diagnosis will be exacerbated by the rapid increase in genetic tests for a wide range of conditions, including late-onset conditions, conditions with a limited impact on health, and, possibly, behavioral or physical characteristics that fall within the normal range. This is not to suggest that genes play a predominant role in complex human behaviors and characteristics. Increasingly, it could be found that, for all but the simplest genetic conditions, dozens or hundreds of genes interact with each other and with thousands of biochemical and environmental agents over extended periods of time to produce the phenotype. Such complexity could frustrate any meaningful predictions based on genetic tests alone. Richard Strohman argues that much of the contemporary interest in genetic testing will collapse as our overly deterministic genetic paradigm progressively fails. Nevertheless, we only may need a popular *perception* of genetic determinism, fueled by creative marketing and weak regulation, to move poorly predictive tests from the lab into the clinic.

If indeed, an extensive battery of genetic tests become available for prenatal diagnosis, what tests should be offered to couples and what tests should professionals provide on request? Should we draw a line, indicating which tests should and should not be provided by an ethical practitioner? Several general positions on the "line-drawing" question are beginning to emerge. John Robertson concedes the morally problematic nature of prenatal diagnosis for "minor" conditions, but argues that our respect for procreative liberty should be paramount, at least until some definitive harm is demonstrated from unfettered use. Robertson places no limits on the parents' ability to obtain prenatal testing for any condition. Strong advocates use of prenatal diagnosis for all diseases or susceptibilities to diseases, but not for nondisease conditions. Strong's analysis places a heavy emphasis on the value of nondirectiveness in prenatal diagnostic services, suggesting that line drawing between disease categories undermines this important value. In contrast, Stephen Post, Peter Whitehouse, and I have argued that minor and late-onset conditions do not justify testing. Angus Clark supports prenatal diagnosis only for the most serious conditions. Adrienne Asch, although deeply troubled by the termination of embryos and fetuses for disabling conditions, believes that a policy of line drawing would be enormously detrimental to those in the disabled community who fall below the line. She, therefore, opposes line drawing, but would couple prenatal diagnosis with better education, emphasizing a fuller understanding of life's prospects with a disabled child. The Institute of Medicine has taken the position that "prenatal diagnosis not be used for minor conditions or characteristics." These positions illustrate a balancing of a number of considerations, including the moral status of the embryo and fetus, the limits of professional authority; the limits, if any, of our respect for parental autonomy, and the impact of individuals with disabilities on the family and society. Also to be considered in this dilemma is the impact of prenatal diagnosis on those who live with disabilities and the impact of broad choice on the parent-child relationship. Much more work needs to be done on this line-drawing question for prenatal diagnosis in general to achieve some resolution at a societal level.

PGD will serve to complicate this dilemma by reducing the concern over one significant element in the equation—abortion. The technology, by its very design, offers each couple a range of choices in offspring. Choice in offspring through PGD is not contingent on abortion. Whether to transfer an affected embryo is not a dilemma with PGD, because this is its explicit purpose; but other more subtle choices are made possible by the technology. Imagine a couple who has 8 embryos in vitro, 2 of which are homozygous for CF, 2 are heterozygous, and 4 are neither carriers nor affected (termed *homozygous normal*). At the request of the parents, the embryos are sexed and three of the four homozygous normal embryos are female and both of the heterozygous embryos are male. The couple desires a son, so the homozygous normal male embryo is split—one-half (now a viable embryo itself) is implanted and the other is cryopreserved along with the other unaffected embryos.

Is there a problem with this scenario? No embryos have been destroyed on the basis of gender and the couple fulfills its wishes. Does this form of gender selection strike us as less problematic than gender selection by abortion? After all, the couple has quite a few embryos from which to choose—a primary choice has been made to discard the affected embryos, but why not choose the specific one to be implanted on the basis of secondary characteristics? By producing a number of embryos with each cycle and by eliminating the moral hurdle of abortion in the selection of offspring, PGD facilitates a broad range of possibilities for selecting the biologic characteristics of children.

If we are entering an age of genetic testing for a wide range of conditions, the extensive analysis of potential children may be a popular application. One example of a particularly interesting development is the chip technology in which tens of thousands of DNA fragments are imbedded in a glass slide that is used to analyze a target DNA sample. It is anticipated that these chips will enable a DNA sample to be evaluated for tens of thousands or hundreds of thousands of mutations or alleles. Backed by a powerful computer, it may be possible to correlate the results of such a DNA analysis with complex physical or psychological traits in individuals. For example, assuming intelligence has some genetic components, correlating a DNA chip analysis of, say, 100,000 random coding sites in the genome with traditional IQ scores may reveal patterns of results that are associated with higher or lower IQ scores in healthy individuals. Note that such a "test" can function with no true knowledge about the genetic influences on IQ. The same kind of testing might be used for any physical or psychological characteristic for which there are objective measures and any meaningful genetic contributions. As noted, these tests need not be very predictive to be adopted by some couples who want the very best that their sperm, eggs, and money can provide.

If such genetic tests are perceived as useful for predicting the physical and psychological characteristics of future children, some couples may pursue PGD for no other reason than to select their ideal embryo. This could well be a growth industry in the coming century for couples who can afford it.

For those who are uneasy with this notion, the challenge is to articulate the ethical problem with this approach to child bearing when abortion is no longer a concern (and assuming one does not hold the conservative position with respect to the moral weight of embryo destruction). One consistent criticism of prenatal diagnosis is the message of rejection that it sends to people with disabilities. It is feared that prenatal diagnosis will lead to heightened intolerance of disability as forces are marshaled to eliminate those embryos and fetuses with disabilities rather than to develop a society in which the disabled can live as welcomed partners. If prenatal diagnosis and PGD specifically were to have a significantly negative effect on the millions of disabled individuals in society, this would be a powerful argument for limiting or discouraging its use, at least for less than serious medical conditions.

The speculative nature of this concern, both in terms of whether people will use PGD or traditional prenatal diagnosis for a broad range of conditions, and whether such use will produce additional discrimination for the disabled, makes this concern difficult to weigh as a moral issue. There is no evidence of this kind of effect to date on a broad scale, despite the use of prenatal diagnosis for several decades. In contrast, individuals with disabilities have never had *more* social support than they do today, as reflected in the sentiment and substance of the Americans with Disabilities Act. Certainly, more social support is still due, but a generally improved social stature for the disabled has occurred in recent decades in parallel with the development and use of prenatal diagnostic techniques. Changes in technology, economics, and attitudes could adversely change the situation for the disabled in the future, but current experience indicates that society can simultaneously promote respect and opportunity for the disabled while enabling couples to prevent the birth of a disabled child through prenatal diagnosis.

However, distinctions may be made in the future between those disabled from genetic conditions that are detectable prenatally and the majority of the disabled who have limitations from a broad range of other causes (injury, stroke, infection, and so forth). Given the potential power of PGD to select the genetic characteristics of future children, it could promote societal expectations of "perfectibility" in children, thus fostering a more narrow intolerance of those disabled from genetic and congenital etiolo-

gies and, perhaps, of the parents who choose to have such a child. This is a serious concern that deserves scrutiny and persistent efforts to combat discriminatory attitudes toward the disabled.

It is likely, however, that broad changes in social attitudes concerning perfectibility and disability will be affected more by prenatal diagnostic techniques that may have much greater appeal than will PGD. For example, techniques that will enable the isolation of fetal cells from maternal blood samples early in pregnancy, in conjunction with medications to terminate early pregnancies privately and relatively painlessly, are more likely to have widespread utilization than PGD. There are even developments that may enable the determination of fetal sex through a maternal urine test. I suspect that any new approaches that make prenatal diagnosis accurate and selective termination substantially easier early in pregnancy would be widely adopted. For whatever benefits this technology may bring, widespread use could significantly reduce societal tolerance for "less than perfect" babies.

A second concern raised by the use of PGD to select against minor conditions (or for desirable characteristics) is the potential effect such control might have on the parent-child relationship. As noted, PGD facilitates the selection of children, as compared with traditional prenatal diagnosis, because it offers a range of choices with each set of embryos produced rather than the single choice of accepting or terminating an established pregnancy.

The most compelling argument from my perspective as a pediatrician is the adverse effect detailed selection may have on the parent-child relationship, whether by PGD or traditional prenatal diagnosis. Parents always have had hopes and expectations at the birth of a child, but these are layered on the knowledge that children will grow up and in directions over which they ultimately will have little control. We have all lived through our own parents' expectations and we all understand how supportive and damaging these can be. What would it mean for parents to have very specific expectations for a child based in prenatal testing and selection?

From the age of nine months onward when an infant begins to crawl, her project becomes increasingly one of independence. Her parents' project, in contrast, is one of control, indoctrination, and education to protect, to prepare, to bypass the mistakes made by others (often their own), and to fulfill their own conception of a life of value. This tension between the child's striving for independence and the parents' need for nurturing is fundamental to the parent-child relationship. Ultimately, we establish ourselves as independent—often to be quite different from what our parents had in mind. But remarkably, there need be no love lost in this clash of projects, although there sometimes is. For the most part, we continue to love our children (and our parents) as they are.

What influence could PGD technology have on this most important relationship? How might the knowledge that a child was deliberately selected for her biological characteristics affect how an individual regards her parents, how her parents regard her, and how she regards herself? Could the selection enhance the expectations of parents and alter the child's self-perception of strengths and weaknesses? Would children be strongly channeled in directions of the parents' choosing? To what extent would children resent such an intrusion on their own autonomy? Oscar Wilde observed: "Children begin by loving their parents. After a time they judge them. Rarely, if ever, do they forgive them." I suspect that the greater the power parents have over the biological nature of their children, the more this observation will hold true. This is not because the child would be directly harmed by the biological selection, but because the selection may well come with a stifling set of expectations. The question is whether the child's future autonomy—her right to an "open future"—will be sacrificed through a uncompromising respect for parental liberty in reproductive decisions.

My purpose here is to outline ethical concerns over the unfettered use of PGD that extend beyond the destruction of embryos alone. These concerns over the parent-child relationship are quite speculative and there is certainly no data as yet to support or refute these possibilities. Nevertheless, the fundamental importance of the parent-child relationship suggests that a burden of justification must rest with parents or professionals who would use PGD for the selection of offspring for characteristics other than significant health conditions. Parental desires to use technology in the fine-grained selection of children must be justified through claims of legitimate interest.

Parents traditionally have had only a *prima facie* right to liberty in reproductive decisions—not an absolute right in the face of potential countervailing harms. . . .

Why would parents want to select the biological characteristics of their children, beyond a selection against conditions causing significant disability? Is there a convincing rationale for such an intervention? If the claim is that such selections ultimately will make the resulting children happier with their lives, then the credibility of this claim can be challenged. Each of us can point to a number of biological characteristics that have influenced our lives favorably and unfavorably, but this provides little evidence for what characteristics our children will find beneficial or harmful in their lives as they unfold in very different ways, times, and places. Do we know which biological characteristics promote a contented life? If we were to look in detail at a list of genetic characteristics of a set of infants, would we presume to predict which children would experience the most fulfilling lives, by whatever definition we choose? We probably do have a list of traits that would make our children more *competitive* in contemporary society, but success in competition and contentment are two very different things. There is less moral force to the claim that parents should be supported in their efforts to gain competitive advantage for their children, particularly when competitive advantage remains possible through traditional means such as education, wealth, and hard work. . . .

It is essential that the appropriate uses and misuses of this technology be debated and defined. This is perhaps the greatest ethical challenge raised by PGD. At present, concerns over the impact on those with disabilities and the impact on the parent-child relationship suggest a limited use of PGD (and other prenatal diagnostic approaches) for significant health concerns. (This conclusion does not necessitate legal prohibitions on some uses of the technology, only the development of standards for which tests should be offered and/or provided by the ethical practitioner.) PGD avoids the problem of abortion, but it heightens more subtle and longer-term concerns over the limits of parental control over the biological nature of their children. . . .

ISSUES UNIQUE TO PGD:
GERM-LINE GENE THERAPY
AND GENETIC ENHANCEMENT

PGD could be a component of two controversial interventions that are not relevant to traditional prenatal diagnosis: germ-line gene therapy and genetic enhancement. The ability to manipulate the in vitro embryo will greatly facilitate the insertion of genetic material, either to treat a medical condition or, potentially, to enhance its genetic characteristics. Such gene therapy is germ-line therapy because the genetic insertion into an individual embryonic cell (or zygote), which is then grown as a separate embryo, would result in the transformation of all of the cells in the resulting individual, including the gametes. PGD could be used prior to and after insertion of genetic material in order first to identify a suitable embryo and then to evaluate the success of the genetic transfer.

Germ-line gene therapy has been the subject of a growing volume of literature, even though gene therapy in general has proven to be much more difficult than originally hoped. Leroy Walters and Judy Palmer outline eight arguments from the literature against germ-line gene therapy. The most compelling, at least for this purpose, is that the emergence of PGD has virtually eliminated the *need* for germ-line therapy. For many medical conditions in which genetic mutations produce structural or developmental abnormalities from early in gestation, successful therapy and prevention will require that the genetic material be inserted into the gamete(s) of the parents or into the early embryo. In this circumstance, the gene therapy becomes germ-line as a by-product of the primary therapeutic intent. However, in the foreseeable future, the difficulty of reliably introducing a stable, functional genetic element into in vivo human eggs and sperm will be very difficult to surmount. In contrast, the possibility of introducing functional genes into an in vitro zygote or embryo seems quite reasonable in the foreseeable future.

The basic question is why a couple would bother to treat an affected embryo with gene therapy when they could simply discard any affected embryos and transfer the ones destined to be healthy. Because embryos have little moral stature, there is no mandate to rescue

them with gene therapy. Further, the failure of the gene therapy protocol would result in miscarriage or a choice over abortion later in the pregnancy, both highly undesirable in comparison with discarding the affected embryo in the first place. The only rational reasons to undertake gene therapy in an embryo would be (1) if a couple were opposed to discarding or freezing embryos, in which case PGD technology is unlikely to be attractive at the outset, or (2) if a couple were both homozygous for a recessive condition, say, a couple both of whom had sickle cell disease. This latter possibility hardly seems a solid basis for the development of an experimental gene therapy intervention for human embryos, particularly if gene therapy were developed to where somatic gene therapy could treat the affected children.

The only plausible reason to insert genetic material into embryos would be for genetic enhancement. PGD to select the best embryo followed by insertion of advantageous genetic material would be the most logical method to produce genetic enhancement. The ethics of genetic enhancement is complex and beyond the scope of this paper. Suffice it to say that, in my view, some forms of genetic enhancement may be justifiable, in principle. An enhancement of the immune system to assist in fighting infectious diseases and/or to reduce the risk of cancer or autoimmune diseases may be an example of a justifiable intervention. Enhancement of other characteristics like intelligence or physical stature or coordination, assuming such things will ever be possible, are much more problematic. In any case, enhancement created through embryo manipulation (including PGD) rather than enhancement of fetuses or children brings no new concerns to the debate, other than those created by potential differences in risk or efficacy. Research in PGD could facilitate the development of genetic enhancement, so it is imperative that we clearly articulate the appropriate uses of the technology.

CONCLUSIONS

First, PGD is ethically permissible for its primary purpose, that is, to offer couples at high risk of bearing a child with a significant genetic condition the opportunity to have a healthy child without resorting to selective abortion.

Second, PGD currently is inefficient, burdensome, and expensive. When the costs are not being subsidized by research protocols, few couples are likely to find PGD attractive for its primary purpose.

Third, as with other forms of prenatal diagnosis, socially sanctioned uses need to be defined through broad social discourse. The option to avoid aborting a fetus through PGD does not justify the selection of embryos for less than serious genetic conditions. The definition of *serious* in this context needs much more work. . . .

And, [fourth], PGD provides a logical avenue for genetic enhancement, but ethical concerns over enhancement possibilities do not invalidate PGD for its contemporary use.

PGD provides a new opportunity for couples who desire prenatal diagnosis, but who want to avoid abortion of an affected fetus. Yet the potential power of this technology to manipulate human embryos raises a host of new concerns about the nature of the parent-child relationship and the limits of our biological control over succeeding generations. It remains to be determined whether this is a good trade of ethical concerns.

USING PREIMPLANTATION GENETIC DIAGNOSIS TO SAVE A SIBLING: THE STORY OF MOLLY AND ADAM NASH[1]

Bonnie Steinbock

Molly Nash was born on July 4, 1994 with multiple birth defects due to Fanconi anemia, a deadly genetic disease that causes bone marrow failure, eventually resulting in leukemia and other forms of cancer. Her best chance for survival was a bone marrow transplant from a perfectly matched sibling donor. Lisa and Jack Nash had considered having another child, not as a source of bone marrow but because they very much wanted another child. They had decided against it because there was a one-in-four chance that the infant would have the same illness as Molly, and aborting an affected fetus was not an option Mrs. Nash would consider. Then they learned about preimplantation genetic diagnosis (PGD), which would enable them to screen embryos for the disease, and implant only the healthy ones. Moreover, the embryos could also be tested to find which ones shared Molly's tissue type. The baby would be not only disease-free, but could also provide bone marrow to Molly. Moreover, because blood cells saved from the baby's umbilical cord and placenta could be used, there would be no need to

extract the bone marrow from the baby's body, a procedure which is both painful and carries some risk.

The odds of producing an embryo that is disease-free, a perfect match, and capable of initiating a pregnancy are daunting. In January 1999, Lisa Nash produced 12 eggs, 2 of which were healthy matches. She became pregnant, but miscarried. In June she produced only four eggs, one of which was a match, but she did not become pregnant. In September, she produced eight eggs, only one of which was a healthy match, but again she did not become pregnant. Molly was getting sicker and her physician recommended proceeding with a transplant from a nonrelated donor, although the odds that such a transplant would work were virtually nil. The Nashes decided to try a different IVF clinic, one known for being more aggressive. Lisa's hormone regimen was changed and in December 1999, 24 eggs were retrieved. Only one was a match, but this time she became pregnant. She was confined to bed to prevent a miscarriage. On August 29, 2000, after 52 hours of labor (Lisa resisted a cesarean section because more cord blood could be collected during a vaginal birth), Adam Nash was delivered by C-section. In October 2000, doctors at Fairview-University Hospital in Minneapolis, which specializes in bone marrow transplants for children with Fanconi anemia, successfully transferred tissue from Adam's umbilical cord into Molly's body. Molly, by all accounts, is doing very well. She is back at school, or rather a visiting teacher, who must wear a mask during lessons, comes to her home. She takes ballet lessons. Her transplant did not cure her of Fanconi anemia, but merely prevented her developing leukemia. She is likely to suffer Fanconi's other complications, particularly cancers of the mouth and neck, but that is far off in the future.

Adam Nash was not unique in being conceived to save a sibling. Ten years earlier, another couple, Abe and Mary Ayala, decided to have Abe's vasectomy reversed, in the hopes that Mary would become pregnant with a child who could be a bone marrow donor for their daughter, Anissa, aged 17, who had been diagnosed with leukemia. Surprisingly, the reversal worked and Mary, aged 42, became pregnant. Moreover, the baby, Marissa Eve, born on April 3, 1990, turned out to be a compatible donor. At the time, the reaction from medical ethicists was generally negative. Philip Boyle, an associate at the Hastings Center, said, "It's troublesome, to say the least. It's outrageous that people would go to this length." Alexander Capron, professor of law and medicine at the University of Southern California, suggested that having a baby to save another child was ethically unacceptable because it violated the Kantian principle that persons are never to be used solely as a means to another person's ends. Others, however, challenged the view that Marissa was being used as a means only, or that she was not given the respect due to persons. The crucial thing, they argued, was that her parents and siblings intended to love the new addition to the family as much as her older brother and sister, whether or not she could donate bone marrow. The risk to Marissa was minimal; indeed, if Anissa already had a baby sister with compatible marrow, no one would have questioned using the infant as a donor. Why should the moral situation be different if the choice is to create a child in the hopes that she will be a donor?

Unlike the Ayalas, who thought they had completed their family, the Nashes wanted another child. When they were told that the same technique that could prevent the birth of a child with Fanconi might also identify a compatible donor for Molly, they jumped at the chance. As Mrs. Nash put it, "You could say it was an added perk to have Adam be the right bone marrow type, which would not hurt him in the least and would save Molly's life. We didn't have to think twice about it."[2]

Are there ethical objections to what the Nashes did? Some oppose PGD even for its ordinary use, to prevent the birth of a child with a serious disability.[3] Others do not oppose PGD in principle, but think that it should not be used to save the lives of existing children. One concern is that the parents of fatally ill children will be unable to refuse to go through IVF if it is presented as their only chance for saving their child. Furthermore, not every story of a Fanconi child has the happy ending afforded the Nash family. Some women go through cycle after cycle of IVF, only to fail to produce a compatible embryo, or to suffer repeated miscarriages.[4] It may be argued that this is not a choice that doctors should offer desperate parents, given that the odds of success are relatively low. At the same time, many women choose to undergo the rigors of IVF to have babies. If it is not unethical to give them this choice, is it unethical to give them the chance to save their child's life, if they are fully informed about the burdens and risks, and the odds of success?

Some ethicists object to the idea of having a baby for "spare parts." Clearly it would be wrong to create a baby for spare parts if that would be harmful to the child. One could not create a baby for his heart or lungs or even kidney. In what sense has Adam Nash been harmed? He owes his very existence to the fact that he was a perfect match for Molly. Of course, many embryos were discarded and this is considered immoral by those who view preimplantation embryos as tiny children. This, however, is not an objection to using PGD to create donors, but to PGD generally, and indeed to all of IVF.

Finally, many are profoundly disturbed by the possibility of "having babies to spec," of choosing who will be born based on their genetic characteristics. "If we can screen an embryo for tissue type, won't we one day screen for eye color or intelligence?"[5] Some ethicists fear that the use of PGD to get compatible donors today will lead to a world in which parents will be able to select their children's physical, mental, and emotional traits. From one perspective, PGD offers parents of desperately ill children the hope of a miracle. From another, it opens the door to "genetic engineering" and a new eugenics.

NOTES

1. Much of the factual material in this case study comes from Lisa Belkin, "The Made-to-Order Savior," *The New York Times Magazine*, July 1, 2001.

2. Denise Grady, "Son Conceived to Provide Blood Cells for Daughter," *The New York Times*, October 4, 2000, A24.

3. See Adrienne Asch, "Prenatal Diagnosis and Selective Abortion: A Challenge to Practice and Policy," *American Journal of Public Health*, Vol. 89, no. 11 (November 1999): 1649–1657. In this volume, pp. 675–685. Though Asch does not specifically discuss PGD, her objections to selective abortion extend to embryo selection and discard as well.

4. See Belkin, *op. cit.*

5. *Ibid.*

THERAPEUTIC CLONING AND STEM CELL RESEARCH

EMBRYO ETHICS—THE MORAL LOGIC OF STEM-CELL RESEARCH

Michael J. Sandel

At first glance, the case for federal funding of embryonic stem-cell research seems too obvious to need defending. Why should the government refuse to support research that holds promise for the treatment and cure of devastating conditions such as Parkinson's disease, Alzheimer's disease, diabetes, and spinal cord injury? Critics of stem-cell research offer two main objections: some hold that despite its worthy ends, stem-cell research is wrong because it involves the destruction of human embryos; others worry that even if research on embryos is not wrong in itself, it will open the way to a slippery slope of dehumanizing practices, such as embryo farms, cloned babies, the use of fetuses for spare parts, and the commodification of human life.

Neither objection is ultimately persuasive, though each raises questions that proponents of stem-cell research should take seriously. Consider the first objection. Those who make it begin by arguing, rightly, that biomedical ethics is not only about ends but also about means; even research that achieves great good is unjustified if it comes at the price of violating fundamental human rights. For example, the ghoulish experiments of Nazi doctors would not be morally justified even if they resulted in discoveries that alleviated human suffering.

Few would dispute the idea that respect for human dignity imposes certain moral constraints on medical research. The question is whether the destruction of human embryos in stem-cell research amounts to the killing of human beings. The "embryo objection" insists that it does. For those who adhere to this view, extracting stem cells from a blastocyst is morally equivalent to yanking organs from a baby to save other people's lives.

From *New England Journal of Medicine* 351, no. 3 (July 15, 2004): 207–209. Copyright © 2004 Massachusetts Medical Society. All rights reserved.

Some base this conclusion on the religious belief that ensoulment occurs at conception. Others try to defend it without recourse to religion, by the following line of reasoning: Each of us began life as an embryo. If our lives are worthy of respect, and hence inviolable, simply by virtue of our humanity, one would be mistaken to think that at some younger age or earlier stage of development we were not worthy of respect. Unless we can point to a definitive moment in the passage from conception to birth that marks the emergence of the human person, this argument claims, we must regard embryos as possessing the same inviolability as fully developed human beings.

But this argument is flawed. The fact that every person began life as an embryo does not prove that embryos are persons. Consider an analogy: although every oak tree was once an acorn, it does not follow that acorns are oak trees, or that I should treat the loss of an acorn eaten by a squirrel in my front yard as the same kind of loss as the death of an oak tree felled by a storm. Despite their developmental continuity, acorns and oak trees are different kinds of things. So are human embryos and human beings. Sentient creatures make claims on us that nonsentient ones do not; beings capable of experience and consciousness make higher claims still. Human life develops by degrees.

Those who view embryos as persons often assume that the only alternative is to treat them with moral indifference. But one need not regard the embryo as a full human being in order to accord it a certain respect. To regard an embryo as a mere thing, open to any use we desire or devise, does, it seems to me, miss its significance as potential human life. Few would favor the wanton destruction of embryos or the use of embryos for the purpose of developing a new line of cosmetics. Personhood is not the only warrant for respect. For example, we consider it an act of disrespect when a hiker carves his initials in an ancient sequoia—not because we regard the sequoia as a person, but because we regard it as a natural wonder worthy of appreciation and awe. To respect the old-growth forest does not mean that no tree may ever be felled or harvested for human purposes. Respecting the forest may be consistent with using it. But the purposes should be weighty and appropriate to the wondrous nature of the thing.

The notion that an embryo in a petri dish has the same moral status as a person can be challenged on further grounds. Perhaps the best way to see its implausibility is to play out its full implications. First, if harvesting stem cells from a blastocyst were truly on a par with harvesting organs from a baby, then the morally responsible policy would be to ban it, not merely deny it federal funding. If some doctors made a practice of killing children to get organs for transplantation, no one would take the position that the infanticide should be ineligible for federal funding but allowed to continue in the private sector. If we were persuaded that embryonic stem-cell research were tantamount to infanticide, we would not only ban it but treat it as a grisly form of murder and subject scientists who performed it to criminal punishment.

Second, viewing the embryo as a person rules out not only stem-cell research, but all fertility treatments that involve the creation and discarding of excess embryos. In order to increase pregnancy rates and spare women the ordeal of repeated attempts, most in vitro fertilization clinics create more fertilized eggs than are ultimately implanted. Excess embryos are typically frozen indefinitely or discarded. (A small number are donated for stem-cell research.) But if it is immoral to sacrifice embryos for the sake of curing or treating devastating diseases, it is also immoral to sacrifice them for the sake of treating infertility.

Third, defenders of in vitro fertilization point out that embryo loss in assisted reproduction is less frequent than in natural pregnancy, in which more than half of all fertilized eggs either fail to implant or are otherwise lost. This fact highlights a further difficulty with the view that equates embryos and persons. If natural procreation entails the loss of some embryos for every successful birth, perhaps we should worry less about the loss of embryos that occurs in vitro fertilization and stem-cell research. Those who view embryos as persons might reply that high infant mortality would not justify infanticide. But the way we respond to the natural loss of embryos suggests that we do not regard this event as the moral or religious equivalent of the death of infants. Even those religious traditions that are the most solicitous of nascent human life do not mandate the same burial rituals and mourning rites for the loss of an embryo as for the death of a child. Moreover, if the embryo loss that accompanies natural procreation were the moral equivalent of infant death, then pregnancy would have to be regarded as a public health crisis of epidemic proportions; alleviating natural embryo loss would be a more urgent moral cause than abortion, in vitro fertilization, and stem-cell research combined.

Even critics of stem-cell research hesitate to embrace the full implications of the embryo objection. President George W. Bush has prohibited federal funding for research on embryonic stem-cell lines derived after August 9, 2001, but has not sought to ban such research, nor has he called on scientists to desist from it. And as the stem-cell debate heats up in Congress, even outspoken opponents of embryo research have not mounted a national campaign to ban in vitro fertilization or to prohibit fertility clinics from creating and discarding excess embryos. This does not mean that their positions are unprincipled—only that their positions cannot rest on the principle that embryos are inviolable.

What else could justify restricting federal funding for stem-cell research? It might be the worry, mentioned above, that embryo research will lead down a slippery slope of exploitation and abuse. This objection raises legitimate concerns, but curtailing stem-cell research is the wrong way to address them. Congress can stave off the slippery slope by enacting sensible regulations, beginning with a simple ban on human reproductive cloning. Following the approach adopted by the United Kingdom, Congress might also require that research embryos not be allowed to develop beyond 14 days, restrict the commodification of embryos and gametes, and establish a stem-cell bank to prevent proprietary interests from monopolizing access to stem-cell lines. Regulations such as these could save us from slouching toward a brave new world as we seek to redeem the great biomedical promise of our time.

ACORNS AND EMBRYOS

Robert P. George and Patrick Lee

The prestigious *New England Journal of Medicine (NEJM)* recently invited two members of the President's Council on Bioethics to reflect on the ethics of using embryonic stem cells in biomedical research. Paul McHugh, a professor of psychiatry at Johns Hopkins University, explained his opposition to the destruction of human embryos created by the union of gametes, but sought to distinguish such embryos

From Robert P. George and Patrick Lee, "Acorns and Embryos," *The New Atlantis*, no. 7 (Fall 2004/Winter 2005): 90–100. Copyright © 2005, Ethics and Public Policy Center. See www.TheNewAtlantis.com for more information.

from what he dubbed "clonotes": that is, embryos brought into being by cloning (a process known technically as "somatic cell nuclear transfer" or SCNT). He argued that human "clonotes" are not really human embryos, and thus do not enjoy the high moral status of embryos brought into being by ordinary sexual intercourse or by the process of in vitro fertilization (IVF). These "clonotes," McHugh argued, may be legitimately destroyed for purposes of stem cell harvesting, so long as they are destroyed before the fourteenth day of their development. Michael Sandel, a professor of political theory at Harvard University, defended the killing of human embryos in biomedical research without regard to the method by which such embryos are brought into being. In his view, human embryos, whether produced by union of sperm and egg or by somatic cell nuclear transfer, are not entitled to the moral immunity against direct attack that is enjoyed by human beings at later developmental stages.

Both McHugh and Sandel are leading figures in the embryo research debate, and the arguments they put forward are made frequently by others seeking moral grounds for engaging in the destruction of human embryos. But these arguments do not withstand critical examination. In our view, human beings in the embryonic stage are entitled to the same immunity from attack that is enjoyed by human beings at later developmental stages, and it is irrelevant whether these embryonic human beings came into existence by sexual union, in vitro fertilization, or somatic cell nuclear transfer.

THE BASIC DISPUTE

Part of the problem we face is the way the issue has been framed by the editors of the *New England Journal of Medicine* and many others who have waded into the debate. Absent the appropriate framing of the issue, there is little likelihood of generating an illuminating public discussion.

If we were to contemplate killing mentally retarded infants to obtain transplantable organs, no one would characterize the resulting controversy as a debate "about organ transplantation." The dispute would properly be characterized as a debate about the ethics of killing retarded children to harvest their vital organs. The issue could not be resolved by considering how many gravely ill non-retarded people could be saved by extracting a heart, two kidneys, and a liver from each retarded child. The threshold question would be whether it is unjust to relegate a certain class of human beings—the retarded—to the status of objects that can be killed and dissected to benefit others.

By the same token, we should not be speaking in terms of a debate "about embryonic stem cell research." No one would object to the use of embryonic stem cells in biomedical research or therapy if they could be harvested without killing or harming the embryos from whom they were obtained. Nor would anyone object to using such cells if they could

be obtained from embryos lost in spontaneous abortions. The point of controversy is the ethics of deliberately destroying human embryos for the purpose of harvesting their stem cells. The threshold question is whether it is unjust to kill members of a certain class of human beings—those in the embryonic stage of development—to benefit others.

But are human embryos human beings?

Indeed they are, and contemporary human embryology and developmental biology leave no significant room for doubt about it. The adult human being reading these words was, at an earlier stage of his or her life, an adolescent, and before that an infant. At still earlier stages he or she was a fetus and before that an embryo. In the infant, fetal, and embryonic stages, each of us was then what we are now, namely, a whole living member of the species *Homo sapiens*. Each of us developed by a gradual, unified, and self-directed process from the embryonic into and through the fetal, infant, child, and adolescent stages of human development, and into adulthood, with his or her determinateness, unity, and identity fully intact. Although none of us was ever a sperm cell or an ovum—the sperm and ovum from whose union we emerged were genetically and functionally parts of other human beings—each of us was once an embryo, just as we were once infants, children, and adolescents. In referring to "the embryo," then, we are referring not to something distinct from the human being that each of us is, but rather to a certain stage in the development of each human being—like saying "the teenager" or "the five-year old."

Some scientists and philosophers who agree with us about the status of human embryos as human beings nevertheless believe (mistakenly, in our view) that killing embryos in biomedical research can be justified. Some defend embryo-killing on utilitarian grounds, by asserting that killing a few thousand embryos today will help millions of suffering patients in the future. Others argue that no wrong is done in destroying "spare" IVF embryos that would otherwise be permanently frozen or discarded. There are, however, scholars who are prepared to deny that human embryos are human beings. Michael Sandel does just that in his *NEJM* article. He defends embryo-killing in biomedical research on the ground that human embryos and human beings are different *kinds* of entities.

A DIFFERENCE IN KIND?

At the core of Sandel's argument is an analogy:

> although every oak tree was once an acorn, it does not follow that acorns are oak trees, or that I should treat the loss of an acorn eaten by a squirrel in my front yard as the same kind of loss as the death of an oak tree felled by a storm. Despite their developmental continuity, acorns and oak trees are different kinds of things.

Sandel maintains that, by analogy, embryos are different in *kind* from human beings. But this argument cannot survive scrutiny.

As Sandel himself implicitly concedes, *we value human beings precisely because of the kind of entities they are.* (That is why he has staked his entire argument on the proposition that human embryos are different *in kind* from human beings.) Indeed, that is why we consider all human beings to be equal in basic dignity and human rights. By contrast, we value oak trees because of certain accidental attributes they have, such as their magnificence, their special beauty, or a certain grandeur that has taken perhaps seventy-five or a hundred years to achieve. If oak trees *were* valuable in virtue of the *kind* of entity they are, then it *would* follow that it is just as unfortunate to lose an acorn as an oak tree (though our emotional reaction to the two different kinds of loss might, for a variety of possible reasons, nevertheless differ). Sandel's purported analogy works only if he disregards the key proposition asserted by opponents of embryo-killing: that all human beings, irrespective of age, size, stage of development, or condition of dependency, possess equal and intrinsic dignity by virtue of *what* (i.e., *the kind* of entity) they are, not in virtue of any accidental characteristics, which can come and go, and which are present in human beings in varying degrees. Oak trees and acorns are not equally valuable, because the basis for their value is not *what* they are but precisely those accidental characteristics by which oak trees differ from acorns. We value the ugly, decaying oak tree less than the magnificent, still flourishing one; and we value the mature, magnificent oak more than the small, still growing one. But we would never say the same about human beings.

Sandel's argument begins to go awry with his choice of analogates. The acorn is analogous to the embryo and the oak tree (he says) is analogous to the "human being." But in view of the developmental continuity that Sandel rightly concedes, surely the proper analogate of the oak tree is the mature human being, i.e., *the adult.* Of course, Sandel's analogy has its force because we really do feel a sense of loss when a *mature* oak is felled. But while it is true that we do not feel the same sense of loss at the destruction of an acorn, *it is also true that we do not feel the same sense of loss at the destruction of an oak sapling.* (Indeed, our reaction to the destruction of a sapling is much more like our reaction to the destruction of an acorn than it is like our reaction to the destruction of a mature oak.) But clearly the oak tree does not differ *in kind* from the oak sapling. This shows that we value oak trees not because of the kind of entity they are, but rather because of their magnificence. Neither acorns nor saplings are magnificent, so we do not experience a sense of loss when they are destroyed.

But the basis for our valuing human beings is profoundly different. We do not believe that especially magnificent human beings—such as Michael Jordan or Albert Einstein—are of greater inherent worth and dignity than human beings who are physically frail or mentally impaired. We would not tolerate the killing of a retarded child or a person suffering from, say, brain cancer in order to harvest transplantable organs to save Jordan or Einstein.

And we do not tolerate the killing of infants, which on Sandel's analogy would be analogous to the oak saplings at whose destruction we feel no particular sense of loss. Managers of oak forests freely kill saplings, just as they might destroy acorns, to ensure the health of the more mature trees. No one regrets this, or gives it a second thought. This is precisely because we do not value members of the oak species—as we value human beings—because of the kind of entity they are. If we did value oaks for the kind of entity they are, and not for their magnificence, then we would likely feel a sense of loss at the destruction of saplings, and it would be reasonable to feel a similar sense of loss at the destruction of acorns. Conversely, if we valued human beings in a way analogous to that in which we value oak trees, then we would have no reason to object to killing human infants or even mature human beings who were severely "defective."

In sum, Sandel's defense of embryo-killings on the basis of an analogy between embryos and acorns collapses the moment one brings into focus the profound difference between the basis on which we value oak trees and the basis on which we ascribe intrinsic value and dignity to human beings. His analogy only makes sense if we reject the principle that all human beings possess equal moral worth—a principle that we assume Sandel wishes to uphold, not reject.

TAKING CONTINUITY SERIOUSLY

Sandel's argument also relies on an equivocation of the terms "oak tree" and "human being." Of course, as Sandel says, acorns are not oak trees—*if* by "oak tree" one means a *mature* member of the oak species. By the same token, a sapling is not an "oak tree" if *that* is what one means (nor, by the same reasoning, is an infant a human being). But if by "oak tree" (or "oak") one means simply any member of the *species,* then an acorn (or a sapling) *is* an oak tree—they are identical *substances,* differing only in maturity or stage of natural development.

Similarly, no one claims that embryos are *mature* human beings, that is, adults. But human embryos *are* human beings, that is, complete, though immature, members of the human species. Embryos are human individuals at an early stage of their development, just as adolescents, toddlers, infants, and fetuses are human individuals at various developmental stages. So to say, as Sandel does, that embryos and human beings are different *kinds* of things is true only if one focuses exclusively on the accidental characteristics—size, degree of development, and so on. But the central question is, precisely, should we focus only on the accidental characteristics by which embryonic human beings differ from mature human beings, or should we recognize their essential nature (that is, *what they are*)?

Sandel's claim that human embryos are not human beings, or not "full human beings," or merely "potential human life," simply cannot be squared with the facts of human embryogenesis and developmental biology. Briefly, modern embryology shows the following: (1) The embryo is from the start *distinct* from any cell of the mother or the father, for it is growing in its own distinct direction and its growth is internally directed to its own survival and maturation. (2) The embryo is *human,*

since it has the genetic constitution and epigenetic primordia characteristic of human beings. (3) Most importantly, the embryo is a *complete* or *whole* organism, though immature. From conception onward, the human embryo is fully programmed, and has the active disposition, to develop himself or herself to the next mature stage of a human being. And unless prevented by disease, violence, or a hostile environment, the embryo will actually do so, despite possibly significant variation in its circumstances (i.e., in the mother's womb). None of the changes that occur to the embryo after fertilization, for as long as he or she survives, generates a new direction of growth. Rather, *all* of the changes (for example those involving nutrition and environment) either facilitate or retard the internally directed growth of this persisting individual.

THE NATURE OF PERSONS

Perhaps with these facts in mind, Sandel sometimes seems to consider that though human embryos are human beings as a matter of biological fact (for example, he says that an oak tree was once an acorn, which, by analogy, would mean that more mature human beings were once embryos), they are not *persons.* According to this position, which has been famously promoted by Peter Singer and Ronald Dworkin, although we were once human embryos, we were not persons at that time and were not entitled to the respect and protection against lethal violence due to persons. And when did we become persons? Sandel, like Singer and Dworkin, says that the important difference between human embryos and human persons is that persons are not only sentient but "capable of experience and consciousness," and therefore "make higher claims" on us than beings who lack such capacities.

But personhood is *not* an accidental characteristic, that is, a characteristic which one acquires at some point after he exists and may lose at another point. One is a human person by being a living member of the human community, a member of the human species. It is true that many people cannot immediately exercise the rational capacities characteristic of members of the species—such as the elderly person with dementia whose rational powers are gone forever, or the comatose person whose rational powers may or may not return, or infants, fetuses, and embryos whose rational powers are still developing. But such individuals are still morally valuable persons, at least to those who value all human beings equally. They are still members of the human community. Being a person is not a result of acquired accidental attributes; rather, it is being a certain type of individual, an individual with a rational *nature*. And human beings are individuals with a rational nature at every stage of their existence. We come into being as individuals with a rational nature, and we do not cease being such individuals until we cease to be (by dying). We did not acquire a rational nature by achieving sentience or the immediately exercisable capacity for rational inquiry and deliberation. We were individuals with a rational nature even during the early childhood, infant, fetal, and embryonic stages of our lives. If we are persons *now*, we were persons *then*. We were never "human nonpersons."

THE IMPLICATIONS OF EQUALITY

Sandel's final argument is that holding that a human embryo is a person has logical implications that either no one accepts or that are simply unacceptable. Those who hold that human embryos are persons, Sandel says, should be in favor of a total ban on the destruction of human embryos for research, not just a prohibition on federal funding. And they should be opposed to any fertility treatments that involve the creation and discarding of "excess" embryos. To this we reply that we *are* opposed to those practices—we are opposed to *all* dissecting or deliberate discarding of living human embryos. It is worth pointing out, though, that federal funding for the killing or discarding of human embryos (the matter now being debated) is worse than the failure to provide equal protection of the law to a class of human beings (the larger issue). If the government funds embryo destruction, then it is forcing us to participate, as members of the political community, in the killing of human beings. And while we would surely support a national ban on the deliberate destruction of any human embryo, we also seek to uphold those limits that can be preserved at present, while making the fundamental moral arguments about why additional limits are

needed, and why other promising areas of research (like adult stem cells) should be pursued as morally desirable alternatives. It is better to prohibit the federal funding of embryo destruction than to prohibit nothing at all, even if it would be better still to prohibit the act of embryo destruction itself.

Sandel also points to the frequent occurrence of early spontaneous abortions, claiming that "more than half of all fertilized eggs either fail to implant or are otherwise lost." He then says that "the way we respond to the natural loss of embryos suggests that we do not regard this event as the moral or religious equivalent of the death of infants." There are, he points out, few burial rituals or mourning rites for the loss of an embryo. As a factual matter, Sandel somewhat exaggerates the rate of early pregnancy loss, with leading embryologists estimating a loss rate of roughly 45 to 50 percent. Moreover, as almost all authorities in human embryology note, many of these unsuccessful pregnancies are really due to incomplete or defective fertilizations, and so in many cases, what is lost is not actually a human embryo. (To be a complete human organism, a human being, the entity must have the epigenetic primordia for a functioning brain and nervous system, which may be lacking as a result of a severe chromosomal defect.) But even if Sandel had the facts right, his argument here does not hold up. The absence of formal burial rites and (in many cases) intense mourning for the embryo who dies is explained by numerous considerations having nothing to do with whether human beings in the embryonic stage of development possess human dignity or intrinsic worth. Chief among these is the fact that people have not had the opportunity to bond emotionally with the human being who is lost at an early stage of development. As to the way we respond to miscarriages, Sandel is mistaken to assume it is uniform. Many people, women in particular, very often *do* grieve intensely when a miscarriage occurs, even when it is early in pregnancy.

In any event, someone's status as a human being possessing dignity and intrinsic worth in no way depends on whether anyone would grieve for him or her after death. Emotional responses are notoriously limited in their capacity to function as sources of moral knowledge. The real question is whether human embryos are human beings, as we contend, or whether they are different *in kind* from human beings, as Sandel attempts to show by his analogy with acorns and oak trees. His argument succeeds only if the analogy holds. But the analogy fails dramatically. The dignity of human beings is *intrinsic* to the kind of entity we are; it does not depend on accidental attributes like size, skin color, age, or IQ. The value we accord to oak trees is *conditional*; it depends precisely on those accidental attributes, like size and beauty, that make some oaks more remarkable and thus more valuable than others. And so we object to killing human infants (though we experience no great feeling of loss at the destruction of saplings), and we should object to killing human embryos (though we feel no sense of loss at the trampling of acorns).

THE CLONOTE AND THE SHEEP

But what about the claims of Paul McHugh? Is there a morally relevant difference between blastocysts that come into being by the union of gametes and those that are produced by somatic cell nuclear transfer? Even if human embryos are nothing other than embryonic human beings, as we argue and McHugh agrees, are "clonotes" something other than human embryos?

Here is McHugh's argument in his own words:

> I argue that in vitro fertilization entails the begetting of a new human being right from its start as a zygote and that we should use it to produce babies rather than cells or tissues to be harvested for purposes dictated by other human beings. In contrast, SCNT is a biologic manufacturing process that we may use to produce cells but should not use to produce babies.

The trouble with this argument is that the "cells" he seeks from SCNT are derived by creating and destroying a cloned human embryo. And the "clonote" and the embryo, despite the different processes by which they come into being, are indistinguishable in their essential nature. What McHugh rightly says about the in vitro fertilization process, namely, that it "creates a new human being right from its start as a zygote," is also true of the entity produced by somatic cell nuclear transfer. All the biological characteristics of the embryo are to be found in the "clonote." Indeed, there is no point in inventing a new word. As the vast majority of people on both sides of the ethical debate understand perfectly well, what somatic cell nuclear transfer produces is a cloned *embryo*.

McHugh says that his "distinction rests on the origin of cells in SCNT, not on the process's vaunted potential for producing a living replica (clone) of the donor, as with Dolly the sheep." But, of course, Dolly the sheep began her life as an embryonic sheep. She did not skip the embryonic stage. In this respect, she was indistinguishable from other sheep. Similarly, a human adult brought into existence by somatic cell nuclear transfer would begin his life as a human embryo. The potential he fulfilled—namely, the potential to develop from the embryonic into and through the fetal, infant, child, and adolescent stages, and into adulthood—would be the potential he possessed from the embryonic stage forward. (Indeed, it is inaccurate to say that the embryonic Dolly had the "potential" to be a living replica of the sheep from which she was cloned. From the embryonic stage forward she *was* a living replica of that sheep.) Just as the life of a new human being conceived by sexual union develops by a gradual and gapless process during which the developing human never changes from one kind of entity into another, so too the life of a human being produced by somatic cell nuclear transfer would unfold without what philosophers call "substantial change" (i.e., a change from one kind of entity into another). In the life of such a being, there would be no point from the embryonic stage forward at which one could say that the developing being changed from a nonhuman entity into a human being. From the point at which SCNT succeeded in producing a distinct, self-integrating organism, a new human being existed.

McHugh attempts to support his position with an argument in the form of a *reductio ad absurdum*: "if one used the notion of 'potential' to protect cells developed through SCNT because with further manipulation they might become a living clone, then every somatic cell would deserve some protection because it has the potential to follow the same path." But this argument fails. Somatic cells that may be used in cloning are analogous not to embryos, but to gametes. Functionally, they are parts of other human beings. They are not distinct, complete, self-integrating organisms. They are not living members of the species *Homo sapiens*. Embryos—however produced—are.

In fact, McHugh's own argument is vulnerable to a *reductio ad absurdum*: if a "clonote" is not an embryonic member of the species of the animal from which it is cloned, then even in the adult stage the cloned entity cannot be a member of that species. By this reasoning, Dolly was in fact *not* a sheep, and the child, and later adult, who began life as a "clonote" would *not* be a human being. But that is absurd.

McHugh has one more argument. Relying on testimony given by Rudolf Jaenisch at the July 24, 2003 meeting of the President's Council on Bioethics, McHugh asserts that "SCNT performed with primate cells produces embryos with such severe epigenetic problems that they cannot survive to birth." The first thing to notice about this assertion is that it concedes that the entities produced by SCNT are, in fact, embryos, albeit severely disabled ones. More importantly, Jaenisch's testimony does nothing to prove that disabled or "defective" embryos lack moral worth. As we mentioned above, in some cases reproduction fails because fertilization is incomplete, and in such a case there is a growth (for example, a complete hydatidiform mole) but there is not a human embryo. But if SCNT is successful then it generates a distinct organism with the full genetic program and active disposition to develop itself in accord with that program (even if it also has a defect which will cause its early death). There are newborn infants who, as a result of genetic diseases, are destined to die in a matter of days or even hours. This fact does not alter their status as human beings. It would be scandalous to suppose that it authorizes us to treat afflicted children as impersonal collections of organs available for transplantation and research.

Human beings may be severely afflicted at any developmental stage, from the embryonic to the adult. All of us will eventually die, and many of us will die as a result of factors in our genetic makeup from the point at which we came into being. From the moral viewpoint, the certainty of death—whether in ninety years or nine minutes—does not alter our inherent dignity or relieve others of the obligation to respect our lives. That someone will soon die, no matter what we do, is never a license for killing him. That the human being whose death is imminent happens to be at an earlier rather than later stage of development is morally irrelevant. Cloned human embryos are still embryonic human beings, and the fact that this particular way of initiating human life (SCNT) might harm human life does not give us a license to destroy cloned embryos or a reason to pretend that these living organisms are mere artifacts.

MORAL NORMS AND MODERN MEDICINE

Like Michael Sandel and Paul McHugh, we desire to see biomedical science advance towards therapies and cures for diseases. Our objection is not to embryonic stem cell research as such, but to the killing of embryonic human beings to harvest their stem cells. We support research using stem cells that can be obtained harmlessly from bone marrow, fat, and other non-embryonic sources. The day may well come—and come soon—when it is possible to obtain embryonic stem cells without killing embryos. It is likely that at some point in the future scientists will be able to reprogam adult cells back to the embryonic stage. Even sooner, it may be possible to create non-embryonic entities, analogous to complete hydatidiform moles and teratomas, from which embryonic-type stem cells may be obtained. When that day comes, we will enthusiastically support research using these cells. Now and always, though, we believe that biomedical science must remain faithful to the moral norm against killing in the cause of healing. To fail in fidelity to this norm is to undermine the moral foundations of the very enterprise of biomedical science. We must not allow our desire for scientific advancements, and even for therapies and cures, to cloud our judgments as to what human embryos are and what it means for us deliberately to kill them.

SURPLUS EMBRYOS, NONREPRODUCTIVE CLONING, AND THE INTEND/FORESEE DISTINCTION

William FitzPatrick

One interesting view to emerge from the stem cell debate is that while it is sometimes permissible to use human embryos for stem cell derivation, it is wrong to create them just for this purpose. Public figures such as Senator Bill Frist and Dr. Charles Krauthammer have endorsed this view in calling for a ban on cloning-for-biomedical-research while at the same time accepting both the practice that gives rise to surplus embryos in U.S. fertility clinics, and the use of those surplus embryos for medical research or therapy. They reject cloning-for-biomedical-research because, unlike the other practices, it involves creating embryos with the intention of destroying them for medical use. This, they believe, exploits embryos in a way that the other practices do not.

Some, however, have attacked this hybrid position on the grounds that if concerns about exploitation arise for cloning-for-biomedical-research, then the very same concerns arise equally for the other practices. Michael Sandel (who serves with Krauthammer on the President's Council on Bioethics) asks: "If the creation and sacrifice of spare embryos in infertility treatment is morally acceptable, why isn't the creation and sacrifice of embryos for stem cell research also acceptable? After all, both practices serve worthy ends, and curing diseases like Parkinson's, Alzheimer's, and diabetes is at least as important as enabling infertile couples to have genetically related children."[1] He goes on to suggest that there is no difference with respect to the implicit attitude toward embryos:

> Opponents of research cloning cannot . . . endorse the creation and use of excess embryos from fertility clinics and at the same time complain that creating embryos

for regenerative medicine is exploitative. If cloning for stem cell research violates the respect the embryo is due, then . . . so do in vitro fertilization [IVF] procedures that create and discard excess embryos. . . . [T]he moral arguments for research cloning and for research on leftover embryos stand or fall together.[2]

He thus concludes that "if cloning-for-biomedical-research is morally wrong, then so is all embryonic stem cell research, and so is any version of IVF that creates and discards excess embryos.[3]

There are really two questions here. One is whether the claim that there is something specially problematic about creating embryos just for medical use is truly groundless in the way Sandel claims—a distinction without a moral difference. The other is whether that moral difference, if it can be defended, is sufficiently important to justify adopting a hybrid position such as Senator Frist's and opposing cloning-for-biomedical-research even while accepting the other practices.

I will argue that Sandel is mistaken on the first question: proponents of the hybrid position have identified a genuine moral difference, which can be explained and justified in terms of a distinction between outcomes that are intended and those that are merely foreseen (though as we will see, this use of the intend/foresee distinction differs from its more familiar application in the doctrine of double effect). This is the topic of the next section. I will then try to put to rest an important objection to this kind of use of the intend/foresee distinction, an objection that has led Sandel and others to miss the moral significance of the role of intention here.

Then I will take up the second question above, which turns out ultimately to be of greater importance. Even if the argument so far is accepted and the special moral concern over cloning-for-biomedical-research is legitimate, I will argue, it is not morally overriding in the end. It is a real moral concern, with some real moral implications, and it needs to be honestly faced and recognized, but it does not warrant

From *Hastings Center Report* 33, no. 3 (2003): 29–36. Reprinted by permission of The Hastings Center.

Editors' note: Some author's notes have been cut. Students who want to follow up on sources should consult the original article.

opposing cloning-for-biomedical-research (henceforth just "research cloning"), all things considered—at least not for those who already accept current IVF practices and research on surplus embryos.

THE INTEND/FORESEE DISTINCTION

Let us take up Sandel's question: "If the creation and sacrifice of spare embryos in infertility treatment is morally acceptable, why isn't the creation and sacrifice of embryos for stem cell research also acceptable?" Without yet trying to settle whether the latter is acceptable, all things considered, we can give a plausible reason for thinking it is at least *more* problematic. While U.S. fertility clinics create multiple embryos *foreseeing* that some will probably not be needed and will thus be discarded or donated for research, the *purpose* for which they are created is simply to maximize the chances of achieving a successful pregnancy. Every embryo is created in the pursuit of this goal, rather than with any intention of discarding it or of using it for purposes detrimental to its own welfare. As several members of the President's Council point out:

> In the eyes of those who create IVF embryos to produce a child, *every embryo,* at the moment of its creation, is a *potential child.* Even though more eggs are fertilized than will be transferred to a woman [in a given cycle], each embryo is brought into being as an end in itself, not simply as a means to other ends. Precisely because one cannot tell which IVF embryo is going to reach the blastocyst stage, implant itself in the uterine wall, and develop into a child, the embryo "wastage" in IVF is more analogous to the embryo wastage in natural sexual intercourse practice by a couple trying to get pregnant than it is to the creation and use of embryos that requires (without exception) their destruction.[4]

By contrast, what many find objectionable about research cloning (or any other deliberate creation of embryos specifically for research or therapy) is that an embryo is being created with a view to its destruction for our own use. The intention to destroy it is involved in the very act of creating it.

It is one thing to make use of leftover embryos that were created for reproductive purposes, on the grounds that by the time they have turned out not to be needed for those purposes after all, the consideration of their moral status is outweighed by the interests of medical research or therapy. It is quite another thing to bring them into being from the start with a strategic and opportunistic eye toward their destruction for our own purposes, which are entirely external to their welfare. The latter seems to involve a distinct kind of exploitative attitude, reflecting the thought that an embryo is something whose entire significance may be characterized by the external purposes for which we brought it into existence—the clearest possible case of treating something as a "mere means." Even if an embryo is not yet a human being, it is plainly at least *the first stages of a human-organism-under-construction,* and it arguably disrespects the dignity of human life to treat such an entity with the same sort of opportunistic attitude with which one might plant and grow a tree for wood.

This is not to deny that it is often possible to respect what one destroys. It has been pointed out, for example, that certain cultural attitudes and practices surrounding hunting enabled Native Americans to feel and to show respect and even reverence for the animals they killed; similarly, the Japanese practice of Mizuko Kuyo provides a context for the experience and demonstration of respect for an aborted human fetus. But cloning is a matter not merely of destroying something, but of bringing it into being in the first place only to destroy it.

The farming of animals would be a better analogy here. Now one could plausibly argue that meaningful respect may be shown to farmed animals through their humane treatment. The problem is that there is no analogue to humane treatment in the manufacturing and destroying of an embryo, which means that the opportunity for showing respect will effectively be limited to avoiding wastefulness or gratuitous disrespect. This minimal form of respect may be enough if one is using only existing surplus embryos for research, but it is hard to see how it can remove the special exploitative attitude associated with a practice such as research cloning. The claim that one is properly respecting a human embryo and taking on an "attitude of regret and loss" toward it will tend to ring hollow when put forth even as one sets about creating another for the very same treatment.

A related problem with the comparison to Native American hunting practices or to Mizuko Kuyo is that there is no similarly rich background of shared cultural beliefs, attitudes, and rituals that would give real content to a researcher's "respect" for a blastocyst in a lab. The hunter's giving a conciliatory speech to the animal he kills, for example, would have given content to his respect for it, making possible a relation to the animal through which that respect could be experienced and manifested. But as no analog to this exists in the lab, the opportunities for showing respect will be very limited—so limited that it's doubtful they can neutralize the sense that the attitude toward human embryos created for research is inherently exploitative.

So one may reasonably agree with Frist and Krauthammer at least that research cloning involves a kind of disrespect and exploitation of human life over and above anything involved in practices such as IVF and the use of surplus IVF embryos for research, even though the latter practices may also ultimately involve the destructive use of embryos. To frame the point in terms of the intend/foresee distinction while IVF doctors foresee that probably not all of the embryos they create for reproduction will wind up being needed, leaving some to be discarded or donated for research, they do not create embryos with the intention of destructively using them; nor do the researchers who derive stem cells from surplus IVF embryos. Only in the case of research cloning are we creating embryos with such an intention, exhibiting the distinctively exploitative and opportunistic attitude bound up with such a practice.

Even those who end up supporting research cloning should start by acknowledging this difference. They should rest their defense of the research on what they say about the moral weight of the difference (which I take up below), rather than on a denial that there is a relevant moral difference at all between research cloning and the other practices.

IS THE DISTINCTION PLAUSIBLE?

The appeal to the intend/foresee distinction will meet with resistance from many in ethics who argue that its application is arbitrary, so that if it applies where proponents wish to apply it, then it can be equally exploited by those on the other side, thus "proving too much." For example, someone might argue that the distinction, deployed above against research cloning, can be equally used to

cast cloning in a favorable light. All that is strictly *intended,* one might claim, is the curing of disease, while the destruction of the embryo is a *foreseen but unintended side-effect* of the process, just like the discarding of spare embryos by IVF doctors; we create the embryo not with the intent of destroying it, but only with the intent of curing disease.

This objection involves several confusions. First, it is true that all that is intended as an *end* is curing disease. But the intended *means* to that end is to harvest stem cells from the embryo we have created, by disaggregating it, and this is as relevant as the end. The embryo is being created with the intent of using it in a way that plainly destroys it.

Now someone who wishes to press the objection will at this point suggest that while this is true, we needn't thereby intend the *harm* itself. We intend to harvest stem cells from the embryo, by disaggregating it, but the harm is merely foreseen and not intended; the harm per se is not, after all, germane to our purposes. In fact, it is regretted: we just want the stem cells. According to this objection, then, we're just intending to get stem cells, not to harm the embryo: the intend/foresee distinction can ironically be used to show that cloning is actually no more problematic than the other practices, since it turns out that embryos are not after all being created with the intent of harming them.

As Philippa Foot once noted, however, such a line of thought would "make nonsense of [the intend/foresee distinction] from the beginning,"[5] The harm in question cannot plausibly be treated as a merely foreseen but unintended side effect, as if we could "simply bring it about that [we] intend *this* and not *that* by an inner act of 'directing [our] intention'."[6] In the case of research cloning, the relation between what is clearly aimed at—the embryo's being disaggregated to get stem cells—and the purported side effect—the embryo's being destroyed or killed—is "too close" to allow for an intelligible application of the intend/foresee distinction.

We can elucidate this intuitive but vague notion of excessive closeness as follows: the relation in this case is not merely a *causal* relation between distinct things, such that one might conceivably aim at the one without aiming at the other, but is instead a *constitutive* relation. This is what makes the two things too intimately connected to speak of aiming at the one without aiming at the other.

Consider a case to which the intend/foresee distinction clearly applies. The case is a favorite of philosophers. In turning a runaway trolley off of a crowded track onto a less crowded side track to minimize casualties, one plainly does not intend the subsequent death of the person stuck on the side track, either as an end or as a means; one's end is to save the many people straight ahead, and the intended means is to divert the trolley away from them. The very presence of the person on the side track is entirely incidental to one's purposes, and her death is not in any sense being used as a means to accomplish the aim of getting the trolley turned away from the crowd, although it is a foreseen side effect of doing so.[7] (Note that my concern here is simply with illustrating the intend/foresee distinction, and we may avoid deciding whether the distinction is necessary for justifying the act.)

This appeal to the intend/foresee distinction, however, depends on the fact that the relation between (1) the trolley's being diverted away from the crowd, and (2) a person's subsequently being killed down the side track, is merely a causal relation: the trolley's being diverted leads to her being killed, but it isn't itself constitutive of her being killed. This is true even though *the agent's turning the trolley* is plausibly identical to *the agent's killing the person*, which is a different point about the identity of an act. (It's not as if I first turned the trolley and then later did something else that was the killing; rather, the various effects of my single action become incorporated as further descriptions of what I did.) Our interest is instead in the relations between states of affairs, and we can clearly distinguish between *the trolley's being diverted* and various distinct results of this, such as *a person's being killed* down the side-track. This is what gives us the conceptual space to speak, without sophistry, of aiming at the one but not at the other—even if the death of the one was foreseen with virtual certainty (we might even imagine that she was tied to the track). The applicability of the intend/foresee distinction does not generally depend on the thought that the harm was merely likely and not inevitable; what matters is the causal and intentional structure of the case.

By contrast, consider another well-worn example also discussed by Foot, involving a large man stuck in the exit of a cave, trapping fellow explorers inside: if they blow him to bits with some handy dynamite, can they say that all they intended was to clear the exit so that they could get out, and that his death was an unfortunate side effect, foreseen but unintended. Surely not: their intended means of clearing the exit was to blow him to bits, and one can't intend a man's being blown to bits and then claim that his death was unintended simply because it wasn't his death *as such* that one wanted. *His being blown up* is not a *cause* of *his being killed* (as a trolley's being diverted is a cause of someone's being killed when it rolls over her): rather, his being blown up *constitutes* his being killed—both of these, of course, being caused by the detonation of the dynamite. And the point is that the constitutive relation between his being blown up and his being killed is too intimate to allow for the intend/foresee distinction: we cannot pry the two effects apart, so as to aim at the man's being blown up without aiming at his being killed.

Foot notes that the same point will apply to a craniotomy abortion: if we aim at crushing a fetus's skull as a means of removing the fetus in an emergency and saving the woman, we cannot then claim that its being harmed or killed was merely a foreseen but unintended side effect (although this is not to say that the act cannot be justified on other grounds).[8] Again, the relation between the skull's being crushed and the fetus' being harmed or killed is too intimate to allow for such a claim: the skull's being crushed, which is plainly aimed at, constitutes the fetus' being harmed or killed. Where the relation between the two states of affairs is a constitutive one, there is simply no conceptual room to speak of aiming at the one without aiming at the other. The structure of this case is entirely different from that of the trolley case and its crushed victim: there, the victim's being crushed is not aimed at as a means, as in the craniotomy case, but just the turning of the trolley away from the crowd, so there is not the same problem of aiming at something too intimately related to the harm to avoid thereby aiming at the harm.

A few brief clarifications and qualifications are necessary before returning to the case of stem cell derivation. First, I have claimed that where one state of affairs is constitutive of another, an agent cannot aim at the first without thereby aiming at the second. But this applies only where one is aware of this relation. If someone really didn't understand the biological significance of crushing a fetus's skull, he might intelligibly say that he aimed at the skull's being crushed without aiming at the fetus's being injured or killed. But barring such radical ignorance, there is no room for the intend/foresee distinction in such cases.

Second, it is true that the constitutive relations we have been considering are logically contingent, so that it is logically possible for the man's parts to reassemble miraculously after he is blown out of the cave, and so on. But this is irrelevant to my account. The claim of constitution is not about logical necessity; it's about the actual relations between certain states of affairs: it is a matter of fact that a man's being blown to bits constitutes his being killed, just as it is a matter of fact that a trolley's being turned is merely causally productive of someone's being killed down the side track. This factual difference in relations is all we need for the relevant points about intention.

One last qualification: I mean the thesis in question to apply only to cases where this constitutive relation is a matter of natural fact, as in all of the examples so far considered. It is much less clear that the thesis applies to cases where the constitutive relation is just a matter of convention. For example, a university might stipulate that a student who receives an "F" in any class is thereby ineligible for financial aid. Here, the university has stipulated that having an "F" constitutes ineligibility for financial aid; nonetheless, it may be possible for a professor to intend that a student receive an "F" (because he failed the course) without thereby intending that he be rendered ineligible for financial aid, even if the professor clearly foresees this. Even if that is right, however, a plausible explanation is just that the conventional nature of the relation brings in someone else's agency, and this creates space for the intend/foresee distinction. There is a sense in which the professor can legitimately say: "I am simply giving you the grade you deserve for my class, and the rest is *someone else's doing*, which I would prevent if I could." It would be sophistry to try to say something parallel in the cave or craniotomy cases, to claim that I am simply blowing the man up or crushing the fetus' skull and the rest is someone else's (the universe's?) doing.

To return, then, to stem cell derivation. The point I want to make is that harvesting embryonic stem cells is clearly more like the craniotomy or cave case than it is like the trolley case, and the relation in question is natural rather than merely conventional. The means we here aim at and employ in pursuit of curing disease involves isolating the inner cell mass of a five-day-old embryo by "removing" the trophectoderm (the rest of the blastocyst), which is done by cutting it away with microsurgery or breaking it down through immunosurgery. Like the crushing of the fetus's skull or the blowing up of the man in the cave, this procedure does not merely *cause* some distinct harm but *constitutes* the destruction of the embryo. We therefore cannot say we're aiming at the embryo's being disaggregated but not at its being destroyed, or that its destruction is a merely foreseen but unintended side effect of our action.

This point about relations does not itself distinguish between deriving stem cells from cloned embryos and deriving them from surplus IVF embryos—the destruction of embryos is aimed at in both cases. What sets the two cases apart is that only the former involves *creating* embryos with the intent of destroying them; in the other cases, we at most create embryos foreseeing the possibility that they will not be needed for reproductive purposes and will instead be discarded or destroyed. The point about relations serves only to undermine the objection that the intend/foresee distinction proves too much: since the intention in research cloning is to create an embryo for stem cell derivation, and since we cannot after all treat the harm to the embryo in that process as a merely foreseen but unintended side effect, we cannot avoid the conclusion that such cloning involves creating an embryo with the intent of destroying it.

HOW IMPORTANT IS THE DISTINCTION?

Yet even if the argument so far is sound, we may still wonder whether the special moral concern about research cloning is of sufficient importance that we ought to oppose the practice. There are, of course, other reasons why one might be specially concerned with cloning—such as the possibility that cloning technology might be appropriated by those who wish to use it for reproductive purposes, or the potential for exploiting the women who provided the many eggs needed to make the procedure clinically useful (especially if a lot of money were offered for the eggs). But I will set these issues aside now—along with the important empirical debates over how the benefits of research cloning might compare with alternatives—in order to focus on this question: how does the possibility of advancing medicine stack up against the fact that research cloning involves a distinctly exploitative attitude toward embryos? Is the latter important enough to justify opposing research cloning despite the substantial hopes we have at least good reason to attach to it?

There are serious reasons for doubt here, at least for those—such as Frist and Krauthammer—who independently accept IVF and the medical use of surplus IVF embryos. Even if there is something specially exploitative about research cloning, we must remember what sort of entity we're dealing with. The embryo whose exploitation we are worrying about is something that is at the same time viewed—at least by those who already accept IVF—as possessing a moral status low enough to justify foreseeably sacrificing embryos by the tens of thousands in IVF treatment, and deliberately destroying spares for research. This is an entity that most people view as lacking anything close to the moral status of a person. There may be legitimate moral concerns over its exploitation in the course of research cloning, but it is unclear why they should be thought strong enough to override the strong considerations of potential medical benefit on the other side—as they would if we were talking about the exploitation of a person. It seems deeply inconsistent for us to be so repulsed by the exploitation involved in cloning as to oppose it despite its plausible promise of benefits to countless patients, while at the same time holding the exploited entities in low enough regard as to find IVF practices unexceptionable.

I believe that this thought is what lies behind Sandel's rejection of the hybrid position taken by Frist and others, but it is better to bring it out as we have here, rather than by arguing mistakenly that there is no legitimate moral distinction between the different kinds of case—that they are all equally exploitative or disrespectful, and that intent does not matter. Research cloning (or, for that matter, naturally producing embryos for research) appears to be exploitative and disrespectful in a way that the other practices are not, and we need to recognize that point. After taking account of that, we can then go on properly to argue that this consideration, while it may have some implications about continuing to search for better alternatives to cloning, lacks sufficient moral weight to warrant opposing cloning in the end.

The opponent of cloning might reply that we have been placing too much emphasis on the moral status of the embryo itself. The concern about exploitation and disrespect is not limited to fair treatment of the embryo for its own sake, but has perhaps even more to do with worries about the broader social ramifications of adopting the attitudes involved in such treatment. As some members of the President's Council on Bioethics have argued. "To engage in cloning-for-biomedical-research requires the irreversible crossing of a very significant moral boundary: the creation of human life expressly and exclusively for the purpose of its use in research, research that necessarily involves its deliberate destruction"; and this boundary crossing threatens to "coarsen our moral sensibilities."[9]

There are at least two kinds of concern here. First, there is a specific practical worry (emphasized by Krauthammer) about a slippery slope leading from the crossing of this moral barrier to the blurring of others that are more significant. Nearly everyone now views with horror the prospect of cloning a human embryo and then growing it *past* the blastocyst stage, perhaps to the fetal stage, and then harvesting already differentiated tissues from it for transplant. We feel this way even though such a practice might eliminate the burden of developing complex techniques for directing the differentiation of embryonic stem cells for therapeutic purposes. But will it perhaps become easier for us to accept such a practice once we get used to the idea that it is okay to start human lives going with a view simply to exploiting them? Even if this kind of treatment could be justified when it involves only a blastocyst, the worry is that this will lead to a moral numbing that will make it hard for us as a society to resist predictable utilitarian arguments for going a step further, to fetuses.

The burden for resisting such a development would rest on arguments for the moral difference between a five-day-old blastocyst and a fetus, making it okay to create the former, but not the latter, just for medical use. And while there may indeed be sound arguments along such lines, it would perhaps be naïve to assume that such subtle philosophical arguments will be sufficient to guide our attitudes and to maintain a moral barrier in practice. The way to avoid such a slippery slope, according to this line of thought, is to dig in our heels at the earlier moral barrier, drawing a principled line at the *kind* of exploitation involved in cloning. By maintaining a moral barrier against this kind of exploitation of human life, we will have a more secure foothold than can be found once we cross that threshold and have to rely merely on arguments about *degree* (that is, about the significance of the exploited entity's degree of development) in stopping the slide.

Second, there is a more general worry that as a result of our being so blatantly opportunistic with regard to the first stages of developing human lives, we will grow to have less respect for the dignity of human life in general. Can our attitude toward very young children, for example, remain unaffected by such exploitative attitudes toward the first stages of human lives? Can we even continue to think of ourselves in the same way, given that we all had our origins in precisely the kind of entity we are now regarding in such an exploitative light?

Each of these worries can be answered. The first worry is the practical concern that crossing the barrier against creating embryos for medical purposes will set us on a slippery slope toward doing the same with fetuses—the assumption being that without this barrier in place we would come to find the extension unproblematic. But this assumption loses plausibility when we consider the wider context. Even those who condone a wide range of abortions have nearly universally found the idea of harmful research on fetuses—for *whatever* purposes they may have been created—to be morally beyond the pale. We have no difficulty maintaining a barrier against the harmful opportunistic use of a fetus, for which the technology has long been available, even when we are prepared to accept its being killed in a decision to abort it—witness federal policy that prohibits experimentation even on fetuses that are scheduled for abortion. We seem to have a stable awareness of a strong moral constraint not only against creating a fetus for medical exploitation, but even against any

harmful *use* of a fetus—a barrier that has withstood decades of legally protected abortion. But if we can maintain this barrier for fetuses even in light of the practice of abortion, why think that a practice such as research cloning—taking place, like most medical research, behind the scenes and mainly out of public view—will somehow undermine it?

Indeed, those who take Senator Frist's position already accept the opportunistic use of some embryos, which we reject for any fetuses, and yet they do not worry about a slippery slope there. So if we can cross the first moral barrier, making medical use of surplus IVF embryos, without sliding down the slope, then it is doubtful that crossing the next barrier and deliberately creating embryos for medical use will send us sliding toward the harmful exploitation of fetuses—something we have already long rejected quite apart from questions about their origins.

The second concern also loses much of its initial plausibility upon reflection. Whose attitudes, exactly, are supposed to be eroded? On the one hand, many people already place embryos in a very different moral category from persons, viewing them as having a moral status that falls far short of full personhood. Why, then, should these people come to have less respect for the intrinsic dignity of persons merely because they accept the exploitation of *embryos* in cloning? To take an analogy (and it is only an analogy): our acceptance of the exploitation of farm animals for labor or milk, at least under humane conditions, need not erode our respect for fellow human beings, because while farm animals are fellow sentient beings they are not widely viewed as having the same kind and degree of moral status that human beings have. We put them in a different category, and so our treating them in ways we would never treat fellow human beings need not coarsen our attitudes toward the latter (though certain kinds of treatment might). Likewise, as long as we view embryos as belonging to a distinct class with respect to moral status, rather than as being fellow persons or fellow human beings, it is not clear why their exploitation could not be similarly isolated rather than infecting our general moral attitude toward all of human life.

But some people regard embryos as persons: will the practice of non-reproductive cloning tend to erode *their* moral attitudes? Again, probably not. Such practices will strike people in this position as morally outrageous—clashing sharply with their belief that all human beings are ends in themselves, given their categorization of embryos as human beings. This is a problem in the political sphere, to which we might add the worry that the use of embryonic stem cell research, even apart from cloning, is likely to produce a "crisis of conscience" among patients who hold such views, comparable to that caused by the fact that "some widely used vaccines were cultured in human fetal tissue from induced abortions," which has led some to reject such vaccines for themselves or their children. But these are obviously not the problems that opponents of research cloning worry about. The question was whether there is a danger of a morally problematic shift in attitude that should be of serious concern even to those who accept IVF and stem cell research on surplus embryos. That case has not been made compellingly.

ACCEPTING WHAT IS INAPPROPRIATE

I have argued that cloning-for-biomedical-research raises special moral problems, but that these concerns should not ultimately lead us to oppose it, at least until we have clear evidence of less problematic, equally effective, and comparably accessible alternatives. Even if we accept this, however, we should recognize that we do so not because cloning is morally benign, but because we have judged certain powerful considerations to outweigh the moral problems with it.

The model to apply here is that of a deontological constraint that has been overridden by sufficiently compelling special considerations, as where one is justified in breaking a promise in order to attend to a crisis. We may act contrary to the usual moral constraint in such a case, but the moral value embodied by the constraint does not simply vanish. We must acknowledge that the situation is still morally problematic. In the promise-breaking case, an apology will normally be in order, and sometimes even some

sort of compensation, even though one's action was justified. In the case of cloning, the point will be that despite the all-things-considered justification of proceeding, we are taking what remains an *intrinsically inappropriate* attitude toward the beginning stages of human life. This consideration may ultimately be outweighed by others, but it retains some force, which means that the situation is not one we should allow ourselves to grow too comfortable with. In particular, it means that we should continue actively to pursue alternatives—such as the use of adult multipotent stem cells—even as we move forward with cloning-for-biomedical-research with a view to making it unnecessary in the end.

REFERENCES

1. M. J. Sandel, "The Anti-Cloning Conundrum," Editorial for *The New York Times*, 28 May 2002, A-19.
2. Ibid.
3. See Sandel's personal statement in *Human Cloning and Human Dignity: An Ethical Inquiry.*
4. Ibid., ch. 6, section 4.
5. P. Foot, "The Problem of Abortion and the Doctrine of the Double Effect," reprinted in *Killing and Letting Die*, ed. B. Steinbock and A. Norcross (N.Y.: Fordham University Press, 1994), 266–79, at 268–9. Foot was responding to Hatt's claim that the harm to the fetus in a craniotomy abortion might be treated as a foreseen but unintended side-effect of the procedure, no less than in the case of an emergency hysterectomy performed on a pregnant woman—a claim reiterated by Bennett in Morality and Consequences, 105–109.
6. G.E.M. Anscombe, "Medalist's Address: Action, Intention and 'Double Effect'," in *The Doctrine of Double Effect,* ed. P.A. Woodward (Notre Dame: University of Notre Dame Press, 2001), 50–66, at 63.
7. Foot, 270. For a good discussion of the further questions about the nature of the justification in this case, see J.J. Thomson, "The Trolley Problem," in *Rights, Restitution and Risk: Essays in Moral Theory* (Cambridge, Harvard University Press, 1986).
8. Foot, 268.
9. *Human Cloning and Human Dignity: An Ethical Inquiry,* Executive Summary.

RECOMMENDED SUPPLEMENTARY READING

PRENATAL GENETIC TESTING

Andre, Judith, Leonard M. Fleck, and Tom Tomlinson. "On Being Genetically 'Irresponsible'." *Kennedy Institute of Ethics Journal* 10 (2000): 129–146.

Annas, George J. "Noninvasive Prenatal Diagnostic Technology: Medical, Market; or Regulatory Model?" *Annals of the New York Academy of Sciences* 731 (1994): 262–268.

_____. "Prenatal Screening: Professional Standards and the Limits of Parental Choice." *Obstetrics and Gynecology* 75, no. 5 (1990): 328–329.

Bartels, Dianne M. et al. *Prescribing Our Future: Ethical Challenges in Genetic Counseling.* New York: Aldine de Gruyter, 1993.

Bernhardt, Barbara A. "Empirical Evidence That Genetic Counseling Is Directive: Where Do We Go from Here?" *American Journal of Human Genetics* 60 (1997): 17–20.

Brock, Dan. "The Non-Identity Problem and Genetic Harms—The Case of Wrongful Handicaps." *Bioethics* 9, no. 2 (1995): 269–276.

Bromage, D. T. "Prenatal Diagnosis and Selective Abortion: A Result of the Cultural Turn?" *Medical Humanities* 32, no. 1 (June 2006): 38–42.

Buchanan, Allen. "Choosing Who Will Be Disabled: Genetic Manipulation and the Morality of Inclusion." *Social Philosophy and Policy* 13, no. 2 (1996): 18–46.

Chadwick, Ruth, Darren Shickle, Henk ten Have, and Urban Wiesing, eds. *The Ethics of Genetic Screening.* Dordrecht, The Netherlands: Kluwer Academic, 1999.

Chipman, P. "The Moral Implications of Prenatal Genetic Testing." *Penn Bioethics Journal* 2, no. 2 (Spring 2006): 13–16.

Cohen, Cynthia B. "The Morality of Knowingly Conceiving Children with Serious Conditions: An Expanded "Wrongful Life" Standard." In *Contingent Future Persons,* edited by Nick Fotion and Jan C. Heller. Dordrecht, The Netherlands: Kluwer Academic, 1997.

Cohen, Cynthia B., and Elizabeth L. McCloskey, eds. "Genetic Testing." Special issue, *Kennedy Institute of Ethics Journal* 8, no. 2 (June 1998): 111–200.

Davis, Dena. "Genetic Dilemmas and the Child's Right to an Open Future." *Hastings Center Report* (March–April 1997): 7–15.

Feinberg, Joel. "Wrongful Life and the Counterfactual Element in Harming." *Social Philosophy & Policy* 4:1 (1987): 174.

Fost, Norman. "Ethical Implications of Screening Asymptomatic Individuals." *FASEB Journal* 6 (1992): 2813–2817.

Glover, Jonathan. "Future People, Disability and Screening." In *Justice Between Age Groups and Generations,* edited by Peter Laslett and James Fishkin. New Haven, CT: Yale University Press, 1992.

Kaji, Eugene H., and Jeffrey M. Leiden. "Gene and Stem Cell Therapies." *JAMA* 285 (February 7, 2001): 545–550.

Kodish, Eric D. "Testing Children for Cancer Genes: The Rule of Earliest Onset." *Journal of Pediatrics* 135 (1999): 390–395.

Lancaster, Johnathan M., Roger W. Wiseman, and Andrew Berchuck. "An Inevitable Dilemma: Prenatal Testing for Mutations in the BRCA1 Breast-Ovarian Cancer Susceptibility Gene." *Obstetrics and Gynecology* 87 (1996): 306–309.

Lawson, K. L., and R. A. Pierson. "Maternal Decisions Regarding Prenatal Diagnosis: Rational Choices or Sensible Decisions?" *Journal of Obstetrics and Gynaecology Canada* 29, no. 3 (March 2007): 240–246.

Lippman, Abby. "Prenatal Genetic Testing and Screening: Constructing Needs and Reinforcing Inequities." *American Journal of Law and Medicine* 17 (1991): 15–50.

McGee, Glenn. *The Perfect Baby: A Pragmatic Approach to Genetics.* Lanham, MD: Rowman & Littlefield, 1997.

Murphy, Timothy. "Abortion and the Ethics of Genetic Sexual Orientation Research." *Cambridge Quarterly of Healthcare Ethics* 4 (1995): 340–350.

New York State Task Force on Life and the Law. *Genetic Testing and Screening in the Age of Genomic Medicine.* November 2000.

Parens, Erik, and Adrienne Asch, eds. *Prenatal Testing and Disability Rights (Hastings Center Studies in Ethics).* Washington DC: Georgetown University Press, 2000.

President's Commission for the Study of Ethical Problems in Medicine and Biomedical and Behavioral Research. *Screening and Counseling for Genetic Conditions: The Ethical, Social, and Legal Implications of Genetic Screening, Counseling, and Education Programs.* Washington, DC: U.S. Government Printing Office, 1983.

Robertson, John A. "Ethical and Legal Issues in Preimplantation Genetic Screening." *Fertility and Sterility* 57 (1992): 1–11.

_____. "Genetic Selection of Offspring Characteristics." *Boston University Law Review* 76 (1996): 421–482.

Rothenberg, Karen H., and Elizabeth J. Thomson, eds. *Women & Prenatal Testing: Facing the Challenges of Genetic Technology.* Columbus: Ohio State University Press, 1994.

Savulescu, J. "Procreative Beneficence: Why We Should Select the Best Children." *Bioethics* 15 nos. 5–6 (2001): 413–426.

Schuklenk, Udo, Edward Stein, Jacinta Kerin, and William Byne. "The Ethics of Genetic Research on Sexual Orientation." *Hastings Center Report* 27, no. 4 (July–August 1997): 6–13.

Scott, R. "Prenatal Testing, Reproductive Autonomy, and Disability Interests." *Cambridge Quarterly of Healthcare Ethics* 14, no. 1 (Winter 2005): 65–82.

Stein, Edward. "Choosing the Sexual Orientation of Children." *Bioethics* 12, no. 1 (1998).

Warren, Mary Anne. *Gendercide: The Implications of Sex Selection.* Totowa, NJ: Rowman and Allenheld, 1985.

Wertz, Dorothy C., and John C. Fletcher. "A Critique of Some Feminist Challenges to Prenatal Diagnosis." *Journal of Women's Health* 2 (1993): 173–188.

_____. "Caught in the Middle Again: Professional Ethical Considerations in Genetic Testing for Health Risks." *Genetic Testing* 1, no. 3 (1997–1998): 189–200.

_____. "Concepts of Disease After the Human Genome Project." In *Ethical Issues in Health Care on the Frontiers of the Twenty-First Century,* edited by Stephen Wear, James J. Bono, Gerald Logue, and Adrianne McEvoy, 127–154, Dordrecht, The Netherlands: Kluwer Academic, 2000.

THERAPEUTIC CLONING AND STEM CELL RESEARCH

Doerflinger, Richard. "The Ethics of Funding Embryonic Stem Cell Research: A Catholic Viewpoint." *Kennedy Institute of Ethics Journal* 9, no. 2 (1999): 137–150.

Holland, Suzanne, Karen Lebacqz, and Laurie Zoloth, eds. *The Human Embryonic Stem Cell Debate.* Cambridge, MA: MIT Press, 2001.

Juengst, Eric, and Michael Fossel. "The Ethics of Embryonic Stem Cells—Now and Forever, Cells Without End." *JAMA* 284, no. 24 (December 27, 2000): 3180–3184.

McGee, Glenn, and Arthur Caplan. "The Ethics and Politics of Small Sacrifices in Stem Cell Research." *Kennedy Institute of Ethics Journal* 9 (1999): 151–158.

National Bioethics Advisory Commission. *Ethical Issues in Human Stem Cell Research,* vol 1–3. Rockville, MD: National Bioethics Advisory Commission, 2000.

Parens, Erik. "Ethics and Policy in Embryonic Stem Cell Research." *Kennedy Institute of Ethics Journal* 9 (1999): 109–136.

_____. "What Has the President Asked of NBAC? On the Ethics and Politics of Embryonic Stem Cell Research." In *Ethical Issues in Human Stem Cell Research,* National Bioethics Advisory Commission, vol. 2. Rockville, MD: National Bioethics Advisory Commission, 2000.

PART SIX

EXPERIMENTATION ON HUMAN SUBJECTS

Self-conscious scientific experimentation is a relatively new phenomenon in the long history of medicine. For centuries, the introduction of innovative medical procedures was regarded with suspicion. Anyone who deviated from the established norms of medical practice was likely to be regarded as an upstart medical heretic and could even be charged with the tort of negligence, or "malpractice." But the advent of properly scientific medicine in the nineteenth and twentieth centuries transformed controlled scientific investigation into the driving force behind the spectacular successes of modern medicine. With the impressive advances in medical care that have been generated by contemporary medical science, what previous centuries had regarded with fear and distrust has now become a scientific, and even an ethical, imperative.

But here, as elsewhere in the field of biomedicine, success has not been unalloyed: Ethical problems of the greatest magnitude have been posed by the methods of scientific medicine. With the development of ever more advanced research methods has come the ability to use the bodies of ordinary men and women as complex laboratories in which can be found the answers to questions of profound importance. At times, the zeal to unlock these mysteries has blinded researchers to the fact that these amazing engines of scientific progress are also individual people whose dignity and moral worth are equal to their own. In the worst of such cases, intolerable wrongs have been committed under the otherwise noble banner of medical science and regard for the welfare of future patients. The exposure of such cases to public scrutiny, and the controversies this exposure has engendered, have played a crucial role in shaping the development of research ethics in the United States.

Part 6 begins with some of the high-profile cases that have shaped the ethical response to, and regulation of, human-subjects research in the United States. The uproar over flagrant abuses of the rights of human subjects both abroad and at home led to the establishment of serious protections both at the national level, through the Food and Drug Administration, and at the local level, through institutional review boards (IRBs). This new era of biomedical research was defined by several important assumptions. It was assumed, for example, that participation in research was both risky and burdensome; that the maintenance of high ethical standards justified a slower rate of progress in finding effective medical interventions; and that populations that may be more vulnerable to exploitation—such as minority groups, women, and children—should be either shielded or excluded altogether from participation in research studies.

This view began to change in the 1980s, however, as it came under fire from a coalition of unlikely partners. One particularly effective force for change was composed of conservative libertarians and liberal AIDS activists who challenged the bureaucratic obstacles that hindered the public's access to innovative therapies. For conservatives, the lengthy review process that slowed the introduction of medical innovations represented a stumbling block to free enterprise, on the one hand, and to the liberty of consumers to make their own judgments about when they were ready to accept the risks associated with novel interventions, on the other. Alternatively, watching their family and friends die of AIDS while the nation's government and research establishment responded at glacial speed, a new generation of activists claimed that participation in research is a benefit and that it was unjustifiably paternalistic for governmental agencies to protect persons with AIDS from the very medical research that might stave off the death they were already facing from their disease. Soon, similar challenges were lodged by women whose exclusion from clinical trials was intended to safeguard their potential children from harmful effects of experimental agents and to protect pharmaceutical companies from lawsuits. While this exclusion may have been well intended, it was becoming clear that it had resulted in a gap in knowledge about how to diagnose and to treat common diseases in women. The legacy of this decade was the realization that protecting "vulnerable" groups from participating in research could have detrimental effects on the quality of the health care those groups received.

In the 1980s, the protectionism of previous decades gave way to an effort to include what were once perceived as vulnerable populations in research as a matter of health care equity. Although it is true that exclusion from medical research can have important social and individual consequences, it remains true that the ends of clinical research and the ends of therapeutic treatment often diverge. How can these ends be reconciled in an ethically and clinically responsible way? Under what circumstances is it acceptable to conduct clinical research? To Kantians, for instance, no research question is so important that it could justify treating persons as mere means to the ends of science—no matter how noble or important the objective. By what mechanisms, then, can we ensure that the dignity of individual subjects is properly respected

without compromising the integrity of important research? Is it ethical to enroll subjects in research who are not capable of giving free and fully informed consent, such as children, people with significant cognitive impairments, or institutionalized populations such as prisoners or elderly nursing home residents? Disparities in health and access to health care often track disparities in social and economic status. What role, if any, should research play in addressing health problems that are largely caused by circumstances of social and economic deprivation? Should different standards apply to research that crosses national boundaries if the social and economic circumstances of the target population are significantly different from those of the research sponsors?

BORN IN SCANDAL: THE ORIGINS OF U.S. RESEARCH ETHICS

At the end of World War II, the most gruesomely spectacular examples of unethical research were showcased at the trials of Nazi doctors at Nuremberg. During the war, physicians sympathetic to Nazi ideology conducted or participated in a range of medical experiments in which victims of the Nazi concentration camps were subjected to cruel, humiliating, and often lethal procedures in the name of medical research. At the Buchenwald camp, for example, homosexual men, Jews, Gypsies, and other prisoners were divided into study groups; subjects in the experimental arm were given an experimental vaccine against typhus and members of the control group were injected with typhus-infected blood. Nearly all of the unimmunized controls, and many who received the experimental vaccines, died as a result of the infections they contracted. At Revensbrück, bones were transplanted from one prisoner to another in order to study the regeneration of nerves, muscle, and bone. In other experiments, prisoners in the camps were shot in order to study the ballistics of bullets, starved in order to observe the physiology of malnutrition, or infected with gangrene so that the efficacy of different treatments could be studied.

In order to study the length of time that a downed pilot could survive in freezing water, Jewish and Russian prisoners were submerged in tubs of freezing water until they froze to death. Others were removed at various points and different methods for reviving them were tested, including the use of naked Jewish women who were forced to revive the near frozen subject with the warmth of their bare flesh. In order to study the effect of high altitude on pilots, camp prisoners were put into pressure chambers that subjected them to lethal extremes in atmospheric pressure. All the while researchers observed through a window, documenting the readouts of their instruments and the state of the agonized subject.

At the end of the war, twenty-three Nazi physicians and bureaucrats were placed on trial and sixteen were subsequently convicted of war crimes. Of these, seven were sentenced to death. In an effort to support and explicate the tribunal's judgment that the Nazi medical experiments were monstrosities masquerading as medical science, the judges enunciated a set of principles that would make explicit the ethical requirements for acceptable human-subjects research. The product of that effort, the Nuremberg Code, is the opening reading of Section 1.

In unambiguous and unqualified language the Nuremberg Code states as the first of its ten principles that:

> 1. The voluntary consent of the human subject is absolutely essential. This means that the person involved should have legal capacity to give consent; should be so situated as to be able to exercise free power of choice, without the intervention of any element of force, fraud, deceit, duress, over-reaching, or other ulterior form of constraint or coercion; and should have sufficient knowledge and comprehension of the elements of the subject matter involved as to enable him to make an understanding and enlightened decision.

Although the tribunal appeared to believe that the principles they articulated were already widely accepted by the medical and scientific community, one of the very reasons the trial of the Nazi doctors was so protracted was the ability of defense lawyers to show striking parallels to medical experiments that had been performed by American doctors. Far from merely codifying what was already common knowledge among allied medical researchers, the principles of the Nuremberg Code together set out stringent and revolutionary ethical constraints on human-subjects research.

In the immediate aftermath of World War II, the principles of the Nuremberg Code appear to have had little direct impact on the way public medical research was conducted in the United States. In part this was due to the fact that these principles had been enunciated in the context of the Nazi war crimes trials, and it was widely believed that the atrocities of the concentration camps had no parallel in civilized and scientifically sound medical research. Often what the Nazi doctors characterized as research had little or no scientific value and merely provided an excuse to brutalize people who were regarded as inferior. Additionally, however, it is precisely because the principles of the code were not widely accepted and the restrictions that they imposed were so severe that many researchers viewed them as applicable to monsters and mad men but not to legitimate medical researchers.

Until only fairly recently, when clinical research in the United States involved people who were already patients, the conduct of research was generally subsumed under the norms of the prevailing paternalistic model. This is poignantly illustrated in John D. Arras's case study "The Jewish Chronic Disease Hospital Case." Here, the validity of the research question and the quality of the research data were not an issue. Because previous studies had shown that people with cancer take longer to expel foreign cancer cells than do otherwise healthy people, Dr. Chester Southam and his colleagues wanted to measure the rate at which foreign cancer cells would be rejected from the bodies of people who were suffering from illnesses other then cancer. To do this, they injected foreign cancer cells into the skin of twenty-two debilitated residents of the Jewish Chronic Disease Hospital in Brooklyn, New York.

In order to ensure sufficient enrollment in their study, the researchers did not inform subjects of the nature of the injections—that they contained live cancer cells—because they wanted to avoid irrational fears about the word *cancer*. To the researchers, the importance of the research and the low probability of harm provided sufficient reason to justify the use of chronically debilitated hospital patients without further burdening them with irrational worries about contracting cancer. To members of the Board of Regents of the University of the State of New York, however, these considerations could not obviate the fact that the researchers subjected vulnerable individuals to nontherapeutic procedures without their informed consent, thereby violating the subjects' rights to control the disposition of their person and to be free from unwanted molestation.

This case thus represents the hub in which a range of important issues intersect. Here the research question is important and the risk of harm to participants very low. But should these considerations override the right of individuals to control their persons and safeguard their own bodily integrity? The trust that marks the foundation of the doctor–patient relationship is predicated on the idea that both parties are working toward the same goal—attending to the best interests of the patient. Is it ethical to exploit that trust for nontherapeutic purposes? Dr. Southam and his colleagues did not see their conduct as falling outside of the doctor–patient relationship, even though the reasons they offer to justify their conduct focus entirely on the importance of the research for society, since this research was not intended to benefit the individual subjects. Moreover, the fear and skepticism engendered by the revelation of such experiments has a corrosive effect on the very trust upon which they are predicated.

Additionally, the subjects of the research at the Jewish Chronic Disease Hospital were chronically ill, long-term residents of the facility whose compromised decisional capacity made them vulnerable targets. In contrast to the exhortations of the Nuremberg Code, the practice of using the most vulnerable as subjects of research has a long tradition in the United States. Consider the research that was conducted from 1956 to 1971 on the mentally retarded children housed at the Willowbrook State School in New York.

As described by David J. Rothman and Sheila M. Rothman in "The Willowbrook Hepatitis Studies," researchers at Willowbrook, led by Dr. Saul Krugman, intentionally infected children at the institution with hepatitis in the search for an effective vaccine. Here again, the quality of the data generated by the research was not in question, but the methods used were the subject of heated controversy. Hepatitis was one of a number of infectious diseases that spread easily through the unsanitary conditions of the overcrowded institution. After discovering that immunity could be generated by injections of gamma globulin, Krugman opened a separate unit at the school where children between three and eleven were divided into groups, some of whom were inoculated with gamma globulin and then fed live hepatitis virus while controls were merely fed the live virus.

As Saul Krugman (1986) argues in "The Willowbrook Hepatitis Studies Revisited: Ethical Aspects," the researchers reasoned that residents in the overcrowded institution would inevitably contract the virus on the ward and that the social will did not exist to clean up the unsanitary conditions responsible for the underlying problem. By infecting some children with a milder strain of the virus than the one they might contract on the ward, the researchers reasoned that the children themselves were better off for participating in the research and that the results of the research would provide invaluable results to future patients as well. Without the research, both the present children and future patients would have been worse off.

As Rothman notes, however, the consent form provided to parents painted a deceptively sanitized picture of the research carried out at Willowbrook, and the fact that participation in research was a condition for being admitted to the hospital exerted a coercive influence on parents. More important, however, is Rothman's skepticism about the claim that being infected with hepatitis could be seen as a benefit of participating in research. The retarded children of Willowbrook were under the care of the state and, as such, it was the state's responsibility to look after their welfare. Is it accurate to say that the children in the institution would *inevitably* be infected with the virus, given that the conditions through which the virus is spread *could have been ameliorated?* The school could have been closed or its conditions publicized in an effort to clean up the conditions that threatened residents and staff alike. At the very least, every resident could have been inoculated with gamma globulin in an effort to provide some positive benefit to all alike.

Critics of the Willowbrook studies argue that where a harm can be avoided, and the failure for preventing harm is someone's fault, that person or those persons are at least partly causally and morally responsible for the harm's occurring. Additionally, they worry about using the unsanitary conditions at Willowbrook as a laboratory because it creates a disincentive to undertake any actions that might disturb the laboratory environment. If this sounds incredible, consider what is perhaps the most profound case in unethical research in United States history. As recounted by historian Allan M. Brandt in "Racism and Research: The Case of the Tuskegee Syphilis Study," this project involved the systematic deception and abuse of poor African American men from 1932 to 1972. Undertaken in part to determine the effects of untreated syphilis in this population, the study recruited its 400 subjects by lying to them outright about providing treatment for "bad blood." As Brandt observes, "deceit was integral to the study." In addition to this flagrant disregard for the principles of veracity and informed consent, the Tuskegee researchers, drawn largely from the U.S. Public Health Service, also withheld all medical treatments that were considered standard therapy for syphilis at the time, including penicillin when it became widely available at the end of World War II. There can be no doubt that this failure to treat led to the premature deaths of many subjects, their spouses and sexual partners, and their children.

Brandt concludes that "the Tuskegee study revealed more about the pathology of racism than it did about the pathology of syphilis; more about the nature of scientific inquiry than the nature of the disease process." Like many of the Nazi experiments judged at Nuremberg, the revelation of the Tuskegee study shocked the public. In both cases: (1) the experiments were scientifically pointless or redundant; (2) their design was shoddy, precluding meaningful results; (3) subjects were either coerced or deceived into participating; and (4) research subjects were drawn from socially deprived groups.

Although the Tuskegee syphilis study was initiated before World War II, it was not until the summer of 1997 that President Clinton finally apologized on behalf of the United States to a handful of aged survivors and their relatives. In spite of this long overdue gesture of repentance and reconciliation, much damage had already been done both to the human beings involved in the study and to the fabric of trust between the enterprise of medical science and the African American community.

By the time the details of the Tuskegee syphilis study came to light in 1972, broader social reform movements were already scrutinizing the prevailing norms of American medicine. In 1974 the National Commission for the Protection of Human Subjects of Biomedical and Behavioral Research was formed

and given the task of identifying the basic principles that ought to govern ethically responsible human-subjects research. After four years of study they produced what has come to be known as "The Belmont Report." This seminal document has played a fundamental role in shaping contemporary ethical and regulatory standards for acceptable research.

The Belmont Report begins by distinguishing the practice of medicine from clinical research. Here, the principal difference lies in the ends around which the physician/researcher's activities are coordinated. In treatment, the goal is to enhance the well-being of an individual patient, whereas in medical research the primary goal is to generate generalizable knowledge. While these goals can support and enhance one another, they can also diverge and come into conflict. Next, the report articulates the general ethical principles that ought to govern medical research: respect for persons, beneficence, and justice. In order to illustrate the implications of these general principles for actual practice, they suggest mechanisms for ensuring that these requirements are met. Respect for persons requires the voluntary and informed consent of the subject. Beneficence requires a favorable assessment of the risks and benefits involved in research, and justice requires that equitable procedures for selecting subjects be employed so that vulnerable populations do not bear disproportionate burdens of research.

THE ETHICS OF RANDOMIZED CLINICAL TRIALS

The Hippocratic tradition and recent codes of medical ethics speak clearly and emphatically concerning the physician's duty to individual patients. The tradition has emphasized the physician's covenantal duty of undivided loyalty to the patient, as opposed to what Paul Ramsey has called "that celebrated non-patient—the future of medical science." This traditional duty of exclusive personal care for the individual patient is expressed in a number of applicable codes. For example, the AMA Principles of Medical Ethics state, "Physicians should merit the confidence of patients entrusted to their care, rendering to each a full measure of service and devotion," while the AMA's Ethical Guidelines for Clinical Investigation declare, "In conducting clinical investigation, the investigator should demonstrate the same concern and caution for the welfare, safety, and comfort of the person involved as is required of a physician who is furnishing medical care to a patient independent of any clinical investigation."

This traditional posture of undivided loyalty to the patient-subject was easy to maintain when clear-cut distinctions could be made between "therapeutic" and "nontherapeutic" experimentation—that is, between trials performed primarily for the benefit of patient-subjects and those designed primarily for the purpose of gaining valuable knowledge for future patients. Although this distinction is still useful in some contexts, the boundaries between these different kinds of experimentation have become blurred in the conduct of modern biomedical research.

Physicians plausibly maintain that they have a *moral obligation* to employ the most effective means for combating disease and disability, regardless of the time-honored status of standard procedures, many of which often turn out to be quite useless or even harmful. The duty, grounded in the physician's Hippocratic commitment to "do no harm," is expressed in Section 3 of the AMA Principles of Medical Ethics, which states that "a physician should practice a method of healing founded on a scientific basis." The vexing ethical problem posed by this kind of clinical research is that it places the physician's traditional duty of personal care in direct opposition to his or her duty to practice scientific medicine. Whereas the horrors of Nuremberg and Tuskegee invited spontaneous moral outrage, the dilemmas posed by research today demand nuanced ethical reflection and creative thinking about experimental design.

One of the most problematic features of scientific research design is the common practice of "randomizing" patients—that is, assigning them by chance—to one of several competing treatments or to a control group receiving no treatment. Section 2 begins with a discussion of three case studies of morally troubling randomizations, presented by Maurie Markman, a prominent cancer researcher. According to the advocates of so-called randomized clinical trials (RCTs), there are both scientific and ethical advantages to assigning research subjects to treatment groups by chance. By eliminating bias in the selection and care of patient-subjects, randomization helps generate scientifically reliable data that will enable future

patients to receive better care. Indeed, some defenders of RCTs claim that this disciplined procedure is *more ethical* than introducing new procedures on the informal basis of clinical impressions and historical comparisons.

The critics of RCTs, including Dr. Markman, are less sanguine about the prospects of reconciling the imperatives of hard science with the physician's duty to provide personal care. Samuel Hellman and Deborah S. Hellman, in "Of Mice but Not Men: Problems of the Randomized Clinical Trial," object to the fact that in an RCT, the individual's therapy is determined not simply by an investigation into his or her physical needs and personal values, but also by consideration of the needs of the experimental design. Randomization for the sake of future patients, they claim, thus supersedes the individualized treatment of present patients. Does this not amount to a sacrifice of the individual for the sake of society at large? Samuel and Deborah Hellman conclude that it does, and they therefore condemn RCTs for violating the central tenet of Kantian ethics: that the personhood of the individual should not be submerged in utilitarian calculations of social benefit. The Hellmans urge the medical community to develop and use less morally problematic techniques for gaining reliable knowledge.

Defenders of RCTs attempt to counter these objections by noting that in order to be ethically justified, the two (or more) arms of study—for example, comparing two different drugs, or one drug against a placebo—must be in "equipoise." That is, the researchers must not have any scientifically sound reason for preferring one arm to another. But what is to count as "scientific soundness" here?

Some critics of RCTs argue that such studies are problematic if the researchers have formed a "treatment preference" either before or after the initiation of the trial. In one of his case studies, for example, Markman contends that a physician who has a strong opinion in favor of a new cancer drug, taxol, cannot ethically advise his or her patients about a trial comparing taxol to the standard treatment. According to this view, if researchers develop a "strong hunch" about the comparative effectiveness of a new drug, either at the beginning or in the midst of a trial, it is unethical to continue an RCT.

Benjamin Freedman, in "A Response to a Purported Ethical Difficulty with Randomized Clinical

Trials," claims that such worries are based on a flawed conception of equipoise. Instead of insisting that the evidence on behalf of two treatments be exactly balanced and that the researchers develop no treatment preferences throughout the duration of the trial—both seemingly impossible requirements—Freedman argues for a concept of equipoise based on the existence of honest, professional disagreement within the scientific community. So long as there exists a genuine dispute among clinicians, Freedman contends, RCTs are ethically permissible even if a particular physician has a decided preference for one treatment over others. Indeed, he adds, the original and overriding purpose of RCTs is to dispel precisely this kind of professional disagreement. Many a strong hunch has become standard practice in medicine, not by virtue of meeting rigorous scientific standards, but rather by dint of the investigator's passionate commitment, charisma, or professional standing. When this has happened, patients have often been subjected to unnecessary risk and harm for extended periods of time.

ETHICAL ISSUES IN INTERNATIONAL RESEARCH

The moral tension between ensuring access to important medical research while safeguarding the welfare of individual trial participants is particularly acute when we turn to internationally sponsored research in developing countries. Collaborative international research often poses special challenges to researchers because of differences in language, custom, and culture. In many cases, these differences converge in the context of informed consent. Members of a host population may speak a language different from that of the researchers. They may differ in their level of formal education or familiarity with Western medicine or science, and they may have different beliefs about the relative importance of individual, rather than collective decision making. In such cases, researchers must struggle to negotiate these differences in ways that are respectful of the host population without compromising their own commitments to ethically responsible human-subjects research.

Equally troubling are differences that are rooted not in culture and custom, but in social and economic

circumstance. Every day an estimated 1,600 children are infected with HIV and 90 percent of these infections occur in countries of the developing world. In economically and technologically developed countries such as the United States the rate of HIV infection passed from mothers to children can be dramatically reduced (from roughly 30 percent to 8 percent) by giving pregnant women several doses of the drug AZT during pregnancy and at birth, followed by the administration of the drug to the infants themselves after delivery. This particular regimen (called the "076 protocol") has been hailed as a major breakthrough and quickly became the accepted standard of medical practice throughout the United States. But what of the plight of the millions of HIV-infected women in foreign countries too poor to afford AZT for everyone? What can and should be done for them?

This question led health officials in Africa and Asia to join forces with researchers at the U.S. National Institutes of Health (NIH) and Centers for Disease Control and Prevention (CDC) in an effort to test a lower and less-expensive dose of AZT in pregnant women. A wide variety of studies, examining a wide variety of doses and drugs, were subsequently initiated throughout Africa. With few exceptions, however, these studies exhibited a very controversial design element: Almost all of them compared the new, less-expensive drug regimens against a placebo group. In effect, a set proportion of the women in each study intentionally received an inert substance, while their more fortunate counterparts received a lesser (experimental) amount of the active drug; meanwhile, the truly fortunate inhabitants of Europe and North America receive a standard dose that is known to effect a dramatic reduction in the rate of infection from mothers to children.

While agreeing with these researchers that the discovery of a less-expensive preventive treatment for HIV-infected pregnant women is an important goal, critics have charged them and their sponsoring institutions with exploiting the vulnerable people of impoverished, postcolonial societies in a manner reminiscent of the infamous Tuskegee study (Angell 1997). Peter Lurie and Sidney M. Wolfe in "Unethical Trials of Interventions to Reduce Perinatal Transmission of the Human Immunodeficiency Virus in Developing Countries" charge that the use of the placebo controls following the discovery of an effective treatment constitutes a blatant violation of human rights and codes of research ethics that would never have been contemplated, let alone implemented, in developed countries. They contend that researchers from developed countries should apply the same high ethical standards and norms of appropriate treatment that they observe at home while collaborating with their counterparts in poorer nations. If, as Benjamin Freedman would put it, protocol 076 has upset "clinical equipoise" in Boston, researchers in Zaire cannot pretend that it exists there merely because governments and drug companies have decided not to make an effective drug available. Lurie and Wolfe conclude that sufficient information about these new drugs and doses may be obtained by pitting them in trials against the standard dose of the 076 protocol.

In "AZT Trials and Tribulations," Robert A. Crouch and John D. Arras offer a more charitable evaluation of the short-course AZT trials. They begin by arguing that the design of these studies should be evaluated in light of the purpose of the proposed research and the requirements of sound trial design. Here, they present a cautious defense of the placebo-controlled design as the most reliable method for conducting research that is tailored to the specific circumstances of developing world populations. With these considerations in place, they then consider whether there might be other factors in virtue of which the subjects in such trials would be morally entitled to a higher standard of care than they currently receive—that is, nothing. Drawing on what they refer to as the "liberal consensus view" of justice in health care, they argue that there are no grounds for such an entitlement. Together, these considerations provide a powerful argument in support of the claim that it was ethically permissible to use placebo controls in the short-course AZT studies.

Crouch and Arras recognize that the short-course AZT trials may have been morally problematic for other reasons, in particular, because it was not clear that the local populations that participated in the research would receive an effective treatment after the completion of the trial. We will return to these worries in a moment. For now, it is important to consider more carefully the relationship between the standard of care to which participants in clinical research are entitled, the demands of sound trial design, and the economic background conditions that limit the health care options of developing world populations.

In "The Ambiguity and the Exigency: Clarifying 'Standard of Care' Arguments in International Research," Alex John London takes a detailed look at the standard of care to which participants in international trials are entitled. He begins by arguing that the widespread focus on the question of whether the standard of care ought to be "local" or "global" is less important than the more fundamental question of whether the standard ought to be "de facto" or "de jure." Whereas de facto standards are set by the level of care that is *actually* available in the relevant population, the de jure standard is set by what the expert medical community knows to be effective for treating the relevant illness in the relevant population. He then argues that a de jure standard is the most ethically and scientifically defensible standard, and in doing so he links the standard of care to the requirement that clinical trials begin in and be designed to disturb equipoise.

Perhaps most importantly, London stresses that what we know about the effectiveness of possible interventions within a population cannot be separated from the issue of whether the interventions in question can be implemented and sustained over time within the relevant community (see London 2001). As a result, he argues that it is possible that equipoise would not exist between two interventions in a wealthy, developed nation with a robust health care infrastructure, but that it would exist in a developing country with only a rudimentary health care infrastructure. He also argues, however, that in addition to the existence of equipoise, researchers need to provide reasons for thinking that running a clinical trial will be a responsible means of meeting the health care needs of the population in question rather than attempting to ameliorate the conditions that cause equipoise to exist in their community when it does not exist in others.

In "Research in Developing Countries: Taking 'Benefit' Seriously," Leonard H. Glanz, George J. Annas, Michael A. Grodin, and Wendy K. Mariner take up in detail the requirement that medical research must be responsive to the needs of the host population. They note that the purpose of research is to gather generalizable data, not to treat large numbers of people, and that research will not provide a real benefit to host populations unless the resources are committed to make the fruits of that research reasonably available. As a result, they argue that before internationally sponsored research like the short-course AZT trials is approved, funding agreements must be in place to ensure that members of the host population will in fact be provided with an effective treatment developed out of the research. Making such funding agreements a condition for the approval of international research has met with resistance from many who view the proposal as a serious impediment to potentially valuable research. After all, such funding commitments are not required for domestic research and many worry that governmental and nongovernmental funding sources will refuse to commit significant resources to a treatment program without reliable data on the effectiveness of the proposed interventions.

In "Fair Benefits for Research in Developing Countries" the participants in the 2001 Conference on Ethical Aspects of Research in Developing Countries argue that the position endorsed by Glanz and colleagues is ethically misguided. In their view, it fails to provide sufficient benefit to host communities, it fails to protect sufficiently against exploitation, and it is overly restrictive of important clinical research.

To begin with, the conference participants argue that requiring pretrial agreements to make the fruits of any successful intervention reasonably available to host community members would prohibit some research from going forward. This is because the ability to establish such pretrial agreements will be limited since the therapeutic merits of the study intervention have yet to be ascertained. Additionally, they argue that this condition applies only to phase III studies—large clinical trials that seek to evaluate the effectiveness of medical interventions. It is not clear how to apply this standard to smaller phase I or II trials—smaller trials that study only the safety of an intervention in humans or that seek to ascertain a safe dosage range—since these trials do not usually provide sufficient evidence about the therapeutic merits of an intervention to warrant its use in clinical practice.

Finally, they argue that requiring reasonable availability is overly restrictive of the autonomy of host communities in that it forces them to accept a certain kind of benefit in exchange for participating in clinical research. But, there may be other benefits,

such as assistance with sanitation, infrastructure improvements, education, or access to ancillary medical care, that host communities would prefer instead. Allowing host communities greater flexibility in choosing what benefits they think would be acceptable in return for participating in clinical research would allow researchers to guarantee that host communities benefit, even when the results of the clinical trial are negative. After all, most study interventions turn out to be ineffective or positively harmful. In such cases there is nothing to make reasonably available to host communities.

The conference participants therefore propose to allow host communities to bargain with researchers and research sponsors for a wider range of benefits in exchange for hosting a research initiative. The centerpiece of their proposal is an approach through which community members and researchers engage in a "collaborative partnership" to ascertain what benefits would best serve the needs of the host community. Among the ethical conditions that must be obtained in order for clinical research to be ethical, they argue, is that the resulting package of benefits must be fair. That is, it must provide host community members with sufficient benefits that the research does not turn out to be exploitative.

The participants have a fairly local view of what constitutes exploitation. They hold that A exploits B when B receives an unfair level of benefit from the interaction with A. Exploitation is thus a property of localized exchanges between discrete parties. By relying on collaborative partnership and the requirement of "fair benefits," the participants argue that their framework would ensure that host communities are not made worse off by research and that they receive sufficient ancillary benefits to make the research worthwhile.

In evaluating the disagreement between proponents of the fair benefits approach and proponents of the reasonable availability approach, it is worth considering several important issues. First, what do these views presuppose about the relationship between clinical research and the massive, unmet health needs of those in the developing world? This question is of particular importance in light of what is referred to as the 10/90 gap: the statistic that 90 percent of global research dollars are spent in the service of research that targets diseases or conditions that affect only 10 percent of the world's population.

Second, to what extent can these local questions in research ethics be adequately addressed without taking a stand on the questions raised in Part 2, Section 4 concerning the question of whether affluent members of developed countries have a special moral obligation to aid the global poor? Does either of these positions presuppose a particular answer to this question?

RESEARCH ON CHILDREN

As we saw earlier, by the 1980s it was becoming clear that unmitigated protectionist attitudes toward vulnerable populations threatened to create, or to further exacerbate, significant disparities in medical knowledge about the distinctive health care needs of those populations. In some cases, however, the drive to ensure health care equity among these groups is in tension with the need to ensure that genuinely vulnerable individuals are not exploited for the benefit of future subjects. In Section 4 we examine a population in which this tension is particularly acute, children.

The vast majority of drugs prescribed to children in the United States has not been specifically evaluated for use in pediatric populations. Pediatricians prescribe these drugs by extrapolating information about dosage and effects that has been gained from trials in adults. In a 1997 report, the FDA listed the following ten drugs that are prescribed to children on an outpatient basis over five million times a year despite inadequate pediatric drug labeling:

> Albuterol inhalation solution for nebulization for treatment of asthma (prescribed 1,626,000 times to pediatric patients under 12);
> Phenergan for treatment of allergic reactions (prescribed 663,000 times to pediatric patients under 2); ampicillin injections for treatment of infection (prescribed 639,000 times to pediatric patients under 12);
> Auralgan otic solution for treatment of ear pain (prescribed 600,000 times to pediatric patients under 16);
> Lotrisone cream for treatment of topical infections (prescribed 325,000 times to pediatric patients under 12);
> Prozac for treatment of depression and obsessive compulsive disorder (prescribed 349,000 times to pediatric patients under 16, including 3,000 times to infants under 1);

> Intal for treatment of asthma (solution prescribed 109,000 times to pediatric patients under 2; aerosol prescribed 399,000 times to pediatric patients under 5);
> Zoloft for treatment of depression (prescribed 248,000 times to pediatric patients under 16);
> Ritalin for treatment of attention deficit disorders and narcolepsy (prescribed 226,000 times to pediatric patients under 6);
> Alupent for treatment of asthma (184,000 times to pediatric patients under 6). (Food and Drug Administration 1997)

In response to such findings, since 1994, federal agencies like the FDA and the NIH and the U.S. Congress have initiated policy changes aimed at increasing the inclusion of pediatric populations in medical research. These changes require pediatric populations to be included in federally funded research and in the evaluation of new drugs, unless researchers or their sponsors can provide a justification for their exclusion.

When new pharmaceuticals are not tested in pediatric populations under controlled conditions, children are exposed to greater risks than their adult counterparts when they receive these drugs in a clinical setting. Nevertheless, as we have seen, the ends of treatment and the ends of research can diverge, and expanding the mandate to include children in research means that more healthy children will be asked to participate in research that does not hold out the prospect of direct benefit to the individual child. Furthermore, unlike their adult counterparts, children are not capable of giving informed consent to participate in medical research. Instead, the task of looking after their welfare is entrusted to their parents or legal guardian. Under what circumstances is it permissible to enroll an individual child in a clinical trial in which there is little or no prospect of a direct benefit to that child?

In "Children and 'Minimal Risk' Research: The Kennedy-Krieger Lead Paint Study," Alex John London explores a recent case in which some of these issues were cast into stark relief. In order to quantify the effectiveness of several different methods for removing or controlling lead paint in low-income inner city housing units, researchers from the Johns Hopkins–affiliated Kennedy Krieger Institute (KKI) conducted a study in which families with small children were recruited to live in, or encouraged to remain living in, homes that received varying degrees of lead abatement. Although many of these units were not as safe as newly constructed suburban homes, they were probably significantly safer than alternative low-income housing that had not received any degree of lead removal or containment. To researchers from the KKI, this study provided a benefit to the individual participants, as well as to the group of impoverished inner city families whose poverty often restricts them to poor quality housing.

Others have taken a less sanguine view of this case. The Maryland Court of Appeals was skeptical about the claim that exposure to known levels of lead dust could constitute a benefit to study participants. They were also critical of the trial's informed consent process, and they went so far as to argue that in Maryland a parent, appropriate relative, or other applicable surrogate, cannot consent to the participation of a child or other person under legal disability in nontherapeutic research or studies in which there is *any risk* of injury or damage to the health of the subject. While it is unlikely that this ruling will change the legal requirement for conducting pediatric research, the court's reaction to this case enunciates a standard for nontherapeutic pediatric research that found its most ardent proponent in the theologian and ethicist Paul Ramsey.

In his popular and influential book *The Patient as Person*, Ramsey (2002) argued that parents violate the trust in which they hold the interests and welfare of their children if they attempt to consent for the child's participation in research that does not hold out the prospect of a direct benefit to the child. Ramsey was an early and vocal critic of the hepatitis studies at the Willowbrook State School and a staunch defender of the idea that the free and fully informed consent of research participants is a necessary condition for ethical research. In this respect, for Ramsey, the first principle of the Nuremberg Code had gotten it right; he thus viewed nontherapeutic research on children as abrogating the parents' most basic and profound duty.

In "Research on Children and the Scope of Responsible Parenthood," Thomas H. Murray confronts Ramsey's challenge head on. He begins by describing another controversial case of pediatric medical research, the NIH-sponsored trials of artificial human growth hormone in children. In this study, children were randomized either to an investigational arm that would receive between 600 and 1,100 injections of artificial human growth hormone over a seven-year period or to a control group that would receive the same number of injections of saline solution. Although Murray is sensitive to some of the potentially problematic assumptions in which this trial was predicated, he nevertheless argues that enrolling a child in this study would not necessarily fall outside the boundaries of responsible parenthood. Murray is dubious of the attempt to funnel all acceptable parental decisions through the condition of informed consent, and he notes that responsible parents often involve their children in activities that further worthwhile goals but which also pose some degree of risk to their children without the promise of direct benefit. He therefore defends the permissibility of enrolling children into research that poses only a minor increment over minimal risk on the ground that exposing one's children to such risks in the pursuit of a worthwhile goal is perfectly consistent with the trust in which parents hold the interest and welfare of their children.

In making this move, however, we are forced to grapple with one of the thornier issues raised by the Kennedy-Krieger lead paint study. In the federal regulations governing human-subjects research in the United States, it is considered acceptable to subject children to a minor increment over minimal risk, where *minimal risk* is defined as "the probability and magnitude of harm or discomfort anticipated in the research are not greater in and of themselves than those ordinarily encountered in daily life or during the performance of routine physical or psychological examinations or tests." As the KKI lead paint study illustrates, however, children in different areas may experience different degrees of risk in their daily lives. How are we to set the baseline against which risks are to be measured in a clinical trial?

This standard is the focus of "In Loco Parentis: Minimal Risk as an Ethical Threshold for Research upon Children," by Benjamin Freedman, Abraham Fuks, and Charles Weijer. These authors argue that although it is not possible to give a precise quantification of this standard, minimal risks are the ones to which we are exposed all the time. They thus suggest that the more uncertainty there is about whether a particular case meets this standard, the more likely it is that it does not. If norms differ across communities about the level of risk to which it is acceptable to expose children, they appear to endorse what they call a "both-and" approach in which the standards of both communities are applied. While this standard may remain fuzzy around the edges, they argue that it is clear enough to assist in the case by case examination of particular clinical trials.

REFERENCES

Angell, Marcia. 1997. The ethics of clinical research in the third world. *New England Journal of Medicine* 337 (12): 847–849.

Food and Drug Administration. 1997. Regulations requiring manufacturers to assess the safety and effectiveness of new drugs and biological products in pediatric patients. http://www.fda.gov/cder/guidance/pedrule.htm.

Krugman, S. 1986. The Willowbrook hepatitis studies revisited: Ethical aspects. *Reviews of Infectious Diseases* 8, no. 1 (January–February): 157–162.

London, Alex John. 2001. Equipoise and international human-subjects research. *Bioethics* 15 (4): 312–332.

Ramsey, Paul. 2002. *The patient as person: Explorations in medical ethics.* New Haven, CT: Yale University Press.

BORN IN SCANDAL: THE ORIGINS OF U.S. RESEARCH ETHICS

THE NUREMBERG CODE

(1) The voluntary consent of the human subject is absolutely essential.

This means that the person involved should have legal capacity to give consent; should be so situated as to be able to exercise free power of choice, without the intervention of any element of force, fraud, deceit, duress, over-reaching, or other ulterior form of constraint or coercion; and should have sufficient knowledge and comprehension of the elements of the subject matter involved as to enable him to make an understanding and enlightened decision. This latter element requires that before the acceptance of an affirmative decision by the experimental subject there should be made known to him the nature, duration, and purpose of the experiment; the method and means by which it is to be conducted; all inconveniences and hazards reasonably to be expected; and the effects upon his health or person which may possibly come from his participation in the experiment.

The duty and responsibility for ascertaining the quality of the consent rests upon each individual who initiates, directs or engages in the experiment. It is a personal duty and responsibility which may not be delegated to another with impunity.

(2) The experiment should be such as to yield fruitful results for the good of society, unprocurable by other methods or means of study, and not random and unnecessary in nature.

(3) The experiment should be so designed and based on the results of animal experimentation and a knowledge of the natural history of the disease or other problem under study that the anticipated results will justify the performance of the experiment.

(4) The experiment should be so conducted as to avoid all unnecessary physical and mental suffering and injury.

(5) No experiment should be conducted where there is an *a priori* reason to believe that death or disabling injury will occur; except, perhaps, in those experiments where the experimental physicians also serve as subjects.

From "Permissible Medical Experiments," *Trials of War Criminals before the Nuernberg Military Tribunals under Control Council Law No. 10: Nuernberg, October 1946–April 1949* (Washington: U.S. Government Printing Office, n.d., vol. 2), 181–182.

(6) The degree of risk to be taken should never exceed that determined by the humanitarian importance of the problem to be solved by the experiment.

(7) Proper preparations should be made and adequate facilities provided to protect the experimental subject against even remote possibilities of injury, disability, or death.

(8) The experiment should be conducted only by scientifically qualified persons. The highest degree of skill and care should be required through all stages of the experiment of those who conduct or engage in the experiment.

(9) During the course of the experiment the human subject should be at liberty to bring the experiment to an end if he has reached the physical or mental state where continuation of the experiment seems to him to be impossible.

(10) During the course of the experiment the scientist in charge must be prepared to terminate the experiment at any stage, if he has probable cause to believe, in the exercise of the good faith, superior skill and careful judgment required of him that a continuation of the experiment is likely to result in injury, disability, or death to the experimental subject.

THE JEWISH CHRONIC DISEASE HOSPITAL CASE

John D. Arras

During the summer of 1963, Chester M. Southam and Deogracias B. Custodio together injected live, cultured cancer cells into the bodies of 22 debilitated patients at the Jewish Chronic Disease Hospital (JCDH) in Brooklyn, New York. Custodio, a Philippine-born, unlicensed medical resident at JCDH, was participating in a medical experiment designed by Southam, a distinguished physician-researcher at the Sloan-Kettering Institute for Cancer Research, an attending physician at Memorial Hospital in New York City, and associate professor of medicine at Cornell University Medical College. The purpose of the research was to determine whether the previously established immune deficiency of cancer patients was caused by their cancer or, alternatively, by their debilitated condition. Southam thus looked to a group of noncancerous but highly debilitated elderly patients who might bear out his guiding hypothesis that cancer, not old age, was the cause of the previously witnessed

immune deficiency. Importantly, he believed on the basis of long experience that the injection of cultured cancer cells posed no risk to these patients, and that all of the cells would eventually be rejected by their immune systems. Although Southam's professional credentials were impeccable, and although his work was deemed by his peers to be of the utmost scientific importance, the JCDH experiment soon erupted in a major public controversy. Critics denounced Southam's methods as being morally comparable to those of the Nazi physicians tried at Nuremburg, while his defenders countered that he was a distinguished physician-researcher, and by all accounts an honorable man, who merely had the bad luck to be caught in the shifting rip tides of history.

Curiously, although the JCDH case has gone down in history as one of the most important milestones in the development of contemporary ethical and regulatory approaches to biomedical research, the case is not nearly as well known as similar scandals, such as the Tuskegee syphilis study or the Willowbrook hepatitis experiments (see Chapters 7 and 8). And although the JCDH case is almost always briefly mentioned in published litanies of important research scandals, including Henry Beecher's landmark study

From *Oxford Textbook of Research Ethics*, edited by Ezekiel Emanuel et al. New York: Oxford University Press, forthcoming 2007. Reprinted by permission of Oxford University Press.

of medical science run amok,[1] it has never been the exclusive subject of any full-length scholarly paper, let alone a book. (It has, however, been the focus of two very helpful short papers in recent years, on which I have been happy to draw.[2])

I.   BASIC CHRONOLOGY

Southam's research project focused on the relationship between the body's immune system and cancer. Beginning in 1954, Southam had performed numerous studies on more than 300 cancer patients at Memorial Hospital and on hundreds of healthy prison volunteers at the Ohio State Penitentiary. Southam had noticed that cancer patients exhibit a delayed immunological response to injected cancer cells. He had chosen cultured cancer cells for these experiments because they possessed the necessary uniformity, reproducibility, comparability, and growth potential to cause a measurable reaction in patients. Whereas the immune systems of healthy volunteers would normally reject such foreign tissue completely and promptly in roughly four to six weeks, it took cancer patients much longer, often 12 weeks or longer, to finally reject the injected cells. Southam worried about a gap in his data. Was the delayed immune response in cancer patients due to their cancer, or was it due instead to the fact that most such patients were elderly, debilitated, and chronically ill? In order to fill this gap in knowledge, Southam proposed to repeat his immunological study on a group of noncancerous but elderly and debilitated patients. He hypothesized that this study population would reject the injected material at the same rate as normal, healthy volunteers. He hoped that studies such as this would ultimately lead to progress in our ability to boost the human immune system's defenses against cancer, but he was also aware of possible applications in the area of transplant immunology. This, then, was important research.

To test his hypothesis, Southam contacted Emanuel Mandel, who was then director of the department of medicine at the JCDH. Eager to affiliate his modest hospital with the work of a famous doctor at a prestigious medical institution, Mandel immediately agreed to provide the requisite number of chronically ill patients for Southam's study. Like many of the studies criticized in Henry Beecher's famous whistle blowing exposé in the *New England Journal of Medicine*, this project was to be funded by eminently respectable sources, including the American Cancer Society and the U.S. Public Health Service. At their first meeting to discuss the study, Southam explained to Mandel that his proposal was not related to the care and treatment of patients; that it was, in other words, a pure example of "nontherapeutic" research. Southam also informed Mandel that it would not be necessary to obtain the written informed consent of patients at JCDH, since these immunological studies had become "routine" at Memorial Hospital. He also noted that there was no need to inform these elderly patients that the injected material consisted of live, cultured cancer cells, because that would be of "no consequence" to them. On the basis of his considerable prior experience of such studies with patients and prisoners, which easily included more than 600 subjects, Southam was convinced that the injection of cultured cancer cells from another person posed no discernible risk of transmitting cancer. In his opinion, it would simply be a question of when, not whether, such injected cells would eventually be rejected by the patients' immune systems. Since in his view the subjects would not be placed at risk by his study, Southam saw no need to inform them specifically that live cancer cells would be injected into their bodies. The whole point of using cancer cells had to do with their special properties within the context of his research project; no one, he opined, was actually at risk of getting cancer.

Prior to initiating the study at JCDH, Mandel hit a snag. He had asked three young staff physicians at the hospital—Avir Kagan, David Leichter, and Perry Fersko—to help with the injections of live cancer cells into the hospital's debilitated patients. All three had refused to cooperate on the ground that, in their view, informed consent could not be obtained from the potential subjects that Mandel and Southam had in mind for the study. Undeterred, Mandel and

---

1. Henry Beecher, "Ethics and Clinical Research," *New England Journal of Medicine* 274 (1966): 1354–60.

2. Beth Aviva Preminger, "The Case of Chester M. Southam: Research Ethics and the Limits of Professional Responsibility," *The Pharos* 65:2 (Spring 2002): 4–9; and Barron H. Lerner, "Sins of Omission—Cancer Research without Informed Consent," *New England Journal of Medicine* 351:7 (August 12, 2004): 628–630.

Southam forged ahead, eventually settling upon the unlicensed and comparatively vulnerable house officer, Custodio, to help with the injections.

On July 16, 1963, Custodio, Southam, and Mandel met at the JCDH to initiate the study. Custodio and Mandel had already selected the 22 chronically ill patients to be asked to participate. Southam demonstrated the injection procedure on the first three patients, and then Custodio proceeded to inject the remaining 19 with two separate doses of tissue-cultured cells. According to Southam and Custodio, each patient was told that the injections were being given to test their immune capacity—there was no mention of research—and that a small nodule would likely form at the site of the injections but would eventually disappear. In the investigators' view, this constituted sufficient "oral consent" to participate in the study. At the end of just two hours, 22 elderly and debilitated patients on six floors of two separate hospital buildings had received injections, and this first crucial phase of the research was complete.[3] With the passage of a few weeks, Southam's hypothesis would be fully vindicated: With the exception of patients who had died shortly after receiving their injections, all of the JCDH patients rejected the foreign tissue as completely and at the same rate as the prior group of physically healthy individuals. The gap in the data was thus filled: It was cancer, not debilitation and chronic illness, that was responsible for the impaired immune reaction of Southam's patients at Memorial Hospital. None of the JCDH patients, moreover, experienced any long lasting physical harms attributable to the study.

II.   THE BATTLE WITHIN JCDH

News of the Southam-Mandel study spread quickly along the corridors of the JCDH. Samuel Rosenfeld, chief of medicine at the Blumberg Pavilion of JCDH for the previous seven years, was outraged both by the nature of the study, which he regarded as immoral and illegal, and by the fact that he had not even been consulted about it.[4] The three young

physicians who had rebuffed Southam and Mandel—Kagan, Fersko, and Leichter—fearing that their silence might be construed as condoning the research, resigned en bloc on August 27, 1963, less than six weeks after the injections.[5] All three were Jewish; Leichter was a Holocaust survivor, and the other two had lost many family members to Nazi violence during the catastrophe of World War II. Each subsequently attributed his negative response to this study to a visceral revulsion at the thought of using such debilitated and helpless patients in experiments without their consent. None had had any training in ethics or law during their medical studies, and Kagan subsequently admitted that none of them had even heard of the Nuremberg Code.[6]

In order to quiet the gathering storm, authorities at the JCDH assembled the hospital's Grievance Committee on Sept. 7, 1963. After hearing testimony from the hospital's executive director, Solomon Siegel, and Southam, the Committee judged that the resignations of Kagan, Fersko, and Leichter were "irresponsible" and should therefore be accepted by the hospital. The Committee then fully and enthusiastically endorsed the scientific and medical importance of Southam's research and concluded that the allegations of the three young doctors and of the medical director, Rosenfeld, against Mandel and Southam were baseless.[7] Later that month, the JCDH's Board of Directors approved the Grievance Committee's report, and four months later the hospital's Research Committee approved the continuation of Southam's study at the JCDH, but only on the condition that he obtain the written consent of all subjects in the study.

Growing increasingly desperate, the three young doctors turned to William A. Hyman, an internationally recognized lawyer who had helped to found JCDH in 1926 and had sat on its Board ever since. Hyman had many reasons to be furious with his fellow Board members and with the medical authorities at the hospital, who, in his view, had aided, abetted, and then whitewashed this sordid story of human experimentation. One reason for his

---

3. John Lear, "Do We Need New Rules for Experiments on People?", *Saturday Review* 49 (February 5, 1966): 68.

4. Jay Katz, with Alexander Morgan Capron and Eleanor Swift Glass, eds., *Experimentation with Human Beings* (New York: Russell Sage Foundation, 1972): 15.

5. Katz, *Experimentation with Human Beings,* 14; Preminger, 6, 8.

6. Preminger, 6.

7. Katz, 32.

fury was, however, based upon the erroneous belief that the purpose of Southam's research was to determine whether cancer could be induced by the injection of live cancer cells.[8] Against the backdrop of this factual misunderstanding, it's no wonder that Hyman promptly accused Southam, Mandel, and Custodio of acting like Nazi doctors: "I don't want Nazi concentration camps in America. I don't want Nazi practices of using human beings as experimental guinea pigs."[9]

Fearing that the JCDH could be subject to legal liability for providing Southam with patients for his experiment, Hyman, in his capacity as Board member, sought the minutes of the Grievance Committee meeting of Sept. 9, 1963, as well as the medical records of all the patients enlisted in the study. Rebuffed by the hospital authorities and ignored by the New York State Department of Education, Hyman then took his case to the Supreme Court of Brooklyn (a terminological oddity, since this is the *lowest* level of judicial review in New York State), where he argued that, as a member of the JCDH Board of Directors, he had a legal right and responsibility to inspect committee minutes and patient records in response to allegations of wrongdoing and threats of potential legal liability. It is important to note at this point in the story that Hyman's quixotic legal quest was actually directed at a very narrowly focused topic. His case, *Hyman vs. Jewish Chronic Disease Hospital*,[10] was not an investigation into the substantive moral or legal issues raised by Southam's research. That would come later. The case was, rather, focused exclusively on the narrowly construed procedural question bearing on a Board member's right to see certain documents and patients' countervailing rights to the privacy of their medical records. Hyman's procedural claims were ultimately vindicated at the level of the state's highest court,[11] but the real significance of his legal odyssey lay elsewhere. Although the New York State Department of Education, whose Board of

Regents controlled medical licensure, had dithered and effectively ignored Hyman's original allegations, it was finally drawn into this case by the high public visibility and news accounts of the legal proceedings in Brooklyn. The Grievance Committee of the Board of Regents would henceforth provide the crucible for the ethical and legal implications of Southam's research at the JCDH.

III. ARGUMENTS IN THE CASE OF CHESTER SOUTHAM

In its 1965 inquiry into the JCDH case, the Grievance Committee of the Board of Regents focused on two major issues: the assessment of risk and the quality of informed consent. Southam offered strong arguments on both fronts, at least when viewed in the context of social and medical assumptions of the time.

The Inquiry into Risk

With regard to the presence or absence of risk in this study, Southam argued that the injection of cultured cancer cells from an extraneous source into the human body posed no appreciable risk. His 10 years of prior experience with more than 600 subjects—including cancer patients at Memorial Hospital in New York and healthy prison volunteers in Ohio—had led him to conclude that "it is biologically and medically impossible to induce cancer by this means."[12] The Regents concurred in this conclusion. As reported in the *New York Times*, the Regents established to their own satisfaction that prior to the JCDH study in July 1963, "medical opinion was unanimous that the patients were running no risk of contracting cancer and hence need not be cautioned that there was any such risk."[13]

Medical opinion at the time was not, however, entirely unanimous on the question of risk, as it hardly ever is on any question worthy of public debate. One reputable physician, Bernard Pisani, past president of the Medical Society of the County of New York and director of obstetrics and gynecology at St. Vincent's Hospital, testified during the

---

8. Katz, *Experimentation with Human Beings,* 11.

9. S. Raab, "Fear of Nazi tactics drives lawyer in cancer-test quiz," *World Telegram Sun* (January 23, 1964). Quoted in Preminger, 7.

10. 42 Misc.2d 427, 248 N.Y.S.2d 245 (Sup.Ct. 1964).

11. Katz, *Experimentation with Human Beings,* 41.

12. Ibid., 27.

13. *New York Times* (January 22, 1964): 38.

Supreme Court hearing that "the known hazards of such experiments include growth of nodules and tumors and may result in metastases of cancer if the patient does not reject these cells."[14] In addition, according to a recent account based upon an interview with Kagan many years after the fact, "Kagan, Leichter, and Fersko . . . disagreed with Southam's contention that the injections posed no risk to the patients involved."[15]

Another reason to doubt Southam's unequivocal denial of any risk in this experiment is the fact that in one of his own previous studies, the injected cancer cells had migrated 10 inches up the arm of a subject from the injection site to a nearby lymph node. The patient in question had died shortly thereafter, but there was some speculation at the time that, had the patient lived, cancer cells that had migrated that far might then have been subsequently disseminated throughout the body via the lymphatic system. Although Southam claimed that the cells would not have traveled beyond the lymph node if the patient had lived, he admitted that he could not settle the matter with a "statement based on fact."[16]

But perhaps the most telling and unintentionally humorous admission that Southam made regarding the possibility of risk came during his cross examination before the Board of Regents. Mr. Calanese, an attorney for the Regents, was quizzing Southam about an apparent contradiction in an article based upon an interview with him in the journal, *Science*.[17] While emphasizing Southam's confidence that there was "no theoretical likelihood" that the injections of live cancer cells would cause cancer, the article also noted Southam's unwillingness to inject himself or his colleagues. Calanese then quoted the following line from the interview: "But, let's face it, there are relatively few skilled cancer researchers, and it seemed stupid to take even the little risk." To which Southam responded: "I deny the quote. I am sure I didn't say, 'Let's face it.'"[18] In retrospect, we can

grant Southam the objective truth of the proposition that those live cancer cells posed zero appreciable risk to the residents of the JCDH. But we can also question his assertion that any right-minded physician *at the time* would have corroborated this claim. This doubt, plus Southam's own admission that the injections posed "little risk"—which suggests at least *some* risk—to himself and his staff, leads me to conclude that the doctor was being somewhat disingenuous and misleading in his outright denials of risk. Even if he believed that the likelihood of those injections causing cancer was vanishingly small, it is not obvious, even judging by the louche standards of informed consent operative at the time, that Southam did not owe these elderly residents of the JCDH some mention of the possibility of risk.

Informed Consent and Professional Norms

The historical importance and personal poignancy of Southam's story are both due in large measure to the fact that his case played out against a backdrop of changing societal and professional mores with regard to the physician-patient relationship. Southam was obviously brought up and trained within a system of medical education that was deeply and pervasively paternalistic. In those days, there were no "strangers at the bedside,"[19] no Institutional Review Boards, lawyers, bioethicists, patient advocates, or hospital risk managers to second guess the experienced judgments of physicians. Although the nascent doctrine of informed consent was beginning to percolate through the medical and research establishments, at the time of the JCDH case in 1963 most physician-researchers believed that obtaining the subject's consent was a matter of individual professional discretion. If one were doing research on healthy subjects in nontherapeutic experiments, then one might well ask for the subjects' written informed consent, as Southam did in his trials with state prisoners in Ohio. But research on sick patients was another matter, and here researchers were more likely to cloak themselves in the mantle of the traditional ethic governing relationships between

14. Katz, *Experimentation with Human Beings*, 33.

15. Preminger, 6.

16. Katz, *Experimentation with Human Beings*, 35–37.

17. Chester M. Southam, Alice E. Moore, and Cornelius P. Rhoads, "Homotransplantation of Human Cell Lines," *Science* (1957): 158–160.

18. Katz, *Experimentation with Human Beings*, 49.

19. David Rothman, *Strangers at the Bedside: A History of How Law and Bioethics Transformed Medical Decision Making*, 2nd ed. (New York: Aldine, 2003).

patients and physicians. In the clinical setting, truthful information regarding risks was regarded less as an ethical or legal matter and more as a matter of therapeutics. If the risks were small, physicians would likely conclude that informed consent was not necessary, especially if they believed that the information in question would upset or depress the patient. But if the risks were great, or if physicians needed the patient to be informed in order to better collaborate on recovery, then information would be "medically indicated." According to this paternalistic physician ethic, information regarding risks was viewed as essentially one more tool in the physician's black bag. Truth-telling was a matter of individual physician discretion, and the relevant yardstick for disclosure was the perceived benefit or harm of disclosing information bearing on the patient's medical condition. Even though medical researchers were primarily interested in producing knowledge rather than in the traditional physician's goal of advancing the best interests of particular patients, they felt free to avail themselves of this traditional physician ethic in their research.

Against the background of this professional practice, Southam's duty seemed clear. The risk of injecting cancer cells into the bodies of frail, elderly patients was, in his view, infinitesimally small, perhaps even non-existent. Were he to announce to these patients that he was about to inject them with *live cancer cells,* such a disclosure would have advanced no legitimate medical purpose while only serving to make the elderly residents very upset and anxious. In those days, physicians tended to avoid the dreaded word "cancer" when talking to their patients, preferring instead to speak cryptically of "nodes," "cysts," or "growths."[20] It was standard medical practice to envelop patients in a conspiracy of silence in order to shield them from information that was perceived to be alarming, depressing, or otherwise harmful.[21] Contrary to Board member Hyman's misguided allegation, Southam was not trying to determine if cancer could be induced through the injection of live, foreign

cancer cells; his choice of live, cultured cancer cells was dictated solely by methodological and comparative purposes. So, since using the word "cancer" was irrelevant to the actual state of affairs, since there was little to no risk, and since the dreaded word would only serve needlessly to alarm patients, Southam believed disclosure of the cells' derivation to be medically "contraindicated." In reaching this conclusion, Southam insisted that he was merely acting in the "best tradition of responsible clinical practice."[22] It is important to note that the notion of medical relevance advanced here by Southam was purportedly "objective" and scientific rather than subjective, and that the arbiter of what counts as medically relevant, objective information was, in his view, the physician (who also just happens to be a researcher), not the individual patient-subject.

Southam's paternalistic view of researchers' obligations to subjects was confirmed by a parade of distinguished witnesses on his behalf before the tribunal of the Board of Regents. High ranking medical officers and practitioners at such prestigious institutions as Memorial Hospital, Cornell University, West Virginia Medical Center, the University of Pennsylvania, and the Roswell Park Memorial Institute of Buffalo, New York, a cancer research center, all expressed their complete agreement with Southam's central contentions: specifically that his research was of high scientific and social merit; that there was no appreciable risk to subjects; that informed consent was a matter for individual physician discretion; that disclosure of information should be "titrated" according to the level of risk posed by research; that the word "cancer" was generally avoided so as not to upset patients, and would in any case not accurately and objectively represent the true nature of the injected materials; and, finally, that Southam's conduct towards the subjects in the JCDH trial was in complete conformity with the prevailing standards of medical practice. As one of Southam's lawyers remarked at the time, "If the whole profession is doing it, how can you call it 'unprofessional conduct'?"[23]

Even journalists chimed in on behalf of the beleaguered Southam. At a time when the authority of the

---

20. Donald Oken, "What to Tell Cancer Patients: A Study of Medical Attitudes," *Journal of the American Medical Association* 175 (1961): 1120–28.

21. Jay Katz, *The Silent World of Doctor and Patient* (New York: Free Press, 1984).

---

22. Katz, *Experimentation with Human Beings,* 38.

23. Ibid., 64.

legal and medical professions was still largely unchallenged, the press tended to echo the larger society's unbridled enthusiasm for medical progress while ignoring, if not denigrating, what we today would call the rights of patients and research subjects. Thus, journalist Earl Ubell, writing in the *New York Herald Tribune*, conjured images of "enormous pay-offs" from Southam's research, including a possible vaccine against cancer, in dismissing the controversy over the JCDH case as a mere "brouhaha." He concluded, "It would be a shame if a squabble over who-told-what-to-whom should destroy a thrilling lead in cancer research."[24]

IV.   THE JUDGMENT OF THE NEW YORK STATE BOARD OF REGENTS

The ultimate arbiters of professional medical norms in New York, the State Board of Regents, did not view Southam's case as a mere squabble over who-told-what-to-whom. On the contrary, the Board summoned Southam before its Grievance Committee as it heard evidence and eventually passed judgment on whether his license to practice medicine should be revoked. The Regents considered two related charges: (1) that Southam was guilty of fraud or deceit in the practice of medicine, and (2) that he was guilty of unprofessional conduct. The first charge focused on Southam's alleged failure to obtain informed consent from the patients at the JCDH, while the second implied that violating patient-subjects' rights of informed consent constituted a violation of professional norms.

Consent at the JCDH

The charge bearing on informed consent had two distinct components: the competency of the research subjects and the extent of information disclosure. Before discussing the adequacy of consent obtained at JCDH on these two indicia, let us recall what transpired on that day in the summer of 1963. Twenty-two residents were selected for this experiment. All were frail elderly residents of a long-term care hospital

and many were Holocaust survivors whose primary language was Yiddish. Following Southam's initial demonstration of the injection procedure on the first three subjects, Custodio proceeded during the next two hours to obtain "consent" from the remaining 19 residents in two separate buildings and to inject them all with the cancer cells. None of the residents was told the purpose of the injections or that they were about to participate in a research project having nothing to do with their own health and well-being. Each was told, however, that they were about to receive an injection designed to test their immune capacity, and that soon a nodule would form that would go away in a short time.

The first question, then, is whether all of these frail, debilitated elderly were "competent" to make an informed decision whether or not to hold out their arms to Southam and Custodio—that is, were they of "sound mind," capable of understanding complex medical information and coming to a decision on whether or not to participate? The evidence and testimony on this question were mixed. Custodio testified that all the patients were fully competent to make their own decisions, and that he had no trouble communicating with any of them. On the other hand, Samuel Rosenfeld, chief of medicine at the Blumberg Pavilion of the JCDH for many years, testified that many of the 18 patients injected on his ward were mentally incapable of giving consent.[25] Mendel Jacobi, the consultant pathologist at JCDH, added considerable specificity to this charge through an examination of the charts of five of the 22 patients. He painted the following picture: Chart No. K-14397 described a 67-year-old patient with "poor cerebration" who had been in a depressive state for a year. Chart No. 2290 showed a 63-year-old patient with advanced Parkinson's disease, low mentality, and lack of insight and judgment. Patient No. 8183 had a history of depressive psychosis and had been diagnosed at JCDH as suffering from dementia praecox and unsound judgment. And the chart of patient No. 3762 recorded a diagnosis of postencephalitic Parkinson's, difficulty in communicating, constant falling, suicidal ideation, and considerable sedation throughout the years. While it's at least theoretically conceivable that each one of

---

24. Ibid., 40.

25. Ibid., 15.

these debilitated patients was lucid during their brief interview with Custodio on that summer day, Saul Heller, one of the Regents who heard testimony and rendered a judgment in the case, concluded that under such conditions these debilitated patients could not possibly have understood such complex matters in a mere one- to five-minute encounter.[26]

The Regents' deliberations on the nature and extent of disclosure required for genuine consent were of far greater philosophical, legal and historic importance than their findings on the issue of competency; indeed, the Board's deliberations on this subject take us to the heart of the matter. Whereas Mandel, Custodio, and Southam were entirely satisfied with the amount of information disclosed to the residents, the Regents concluded that the patients' consent was woefully inadequate. In the first place, none of the residents was told that they were about to participate in a research project. The Regents reasoned that in order for consent to be valid, it had to be informed; and for consent to be adequately informed, subjects had to understand that they were being asked to participate in nontherapeutic research. For all these patients knew, the good doctors in white coats were merely running routine tests on their immune responses; they had every reason to think that the nature of the impending injections was entirely therapeutic and had nothing to do with research. A mere signature, mere verbal assent, or, worse yet, the resigned nod of a confused patient's head, were not enough. In the Regents' judgment, "[d]eliberate nondisclosure of the material fact [i.e., that the injections were done for research purposes] is no different from deliberate misrepresentation of such a fact."[27] They concluded that such misrepresentation constituted a serious deception and fraud perpetrated upon the JCDH subjects.

Secondly, the Regents were genuinely scandalized by Southam's deliberate omission of the word "cancer." Gauging his duties to research subjects through the lens of a paternalistic medical ethic, Southam had claimed that disclosure of the nature of the cells would have been both medically, objectively irrelevant and needlessly upsetting to frail, elderly patients. The Regents concluded, by contrast, that

physician-researchers had a legal duty to disclose all information "material" to a patient-subject's decision whether or not to participate. In contrast to Southam's belief that any negative reaction on the part of potential subjects to the word "cancer" would have been irrational, the Regents held that "any fact which might influence the giving or withholding of consent is material," whether or not physicians might consider such influence to be irrational. The bottom line for the Regents was that *the decision is the patient's to make*, not the physician's.[28] The patient's subjectivity (or at least that of a "reasonable person") was henceforth to be the touchstone of researchers' duty of disclosure, not physicians' estimates of objective truth. In taking this step, the Regents explicitly repudiated the entrenched paternalism of the traditional Hippocratic ethic in the domain of research on which Southam and his supporters had relied.

In response to Southam's additional claim that withholding the word "cancer" was dictated by a genuine concern for patients' well-being—a concern in keeping with "the best tradition of responsible clinical practice"—the Regents pointed out the obvious fact that in this particular case there was no pre-existing doctor-patient relationship. Southam may well have professed a concern to shield these patients from any undue emotional distress during a time when doctors often shielded patients from bad news, particularly about cancer; but they were not *his* patients. He was essentially an interloper at the JCDH who had never previously met the 22 injected residents, let alone had a longstanding professional relationship with them. The Regents concluded that, at least with regard to the kind of nontherapeutic research involved at the JCDH, Southam, Custodio, and Mandel were acting primarily as researchers who also just happened to be physicians. They thus had no right to help themselves to the wide ranging discretion normally allowed at that time to physicians charged with pursuing the best interests of their patients.

Viewing the charges against them through the lens of traditional (paternalistic) medical ethics, Custodio, Mandel, and Southam had focused narrowly on the question of physical harm. They contended

---

26. Ibid., 57.
27. Ibid., 61.

28. Ibid., 60.

that in the absence of a serious risk of harm, failure to disclose the experimental nature of the injections or the true nature of the cells injected could not possibly constitute a valid reason to reproach their behavior. As we currently say with good humor in the rough and tumble world of U.S. professional basketball, "No harm, no foul." The Regents concluded, however, that Southam and colleagues, while not physically harming anyone, had robbed the JCDH residents of their "basic human right" to make their own decisions whether or not to participate in research.[29] In the language of the law of torts, under which violations of informed consent would soon be subsumed,[30] Southam's failure adequately to inform his subjects constituted a "dignitary insult" and a legal wrong, quite apart from the question whether anyone was physically harmed.

After considering and sharply rejecting all of Southam's and Mandel's justifications for withholding vital information bearing on the nature, rationale, and conduct of the JCDH trial, the Board of Regents issued its final verdict in the case: Both physicians were guilty of fraud, deceit, and unprofessional conduct in the practice of medicine. They had allowed their zeal for research to override "the basic rights and immunities of a human person."[31] Having rendered their verdict, the Regents then considered the nature and severity of the punishment for the physicians' misdeeds. Fifteen of the 17 members of the Regents' Grievance Committee, meeting on June 10, 1965, voted for censure and reprimand, while the remaining two members, apparently believing that being dragged before that tribunal was punishment enough, voted for no further action. In its final action in this case, the Board voted to suspend the medical licenses of both Southam and Mandel for one year, a stinging rebuke especially to Southam, who was at the time a grandee of the New York and national communities of cancer researchers. The Regents softened this punishment considerably, however, by staying the license suspensions on the condition that the physicians stayed out of trouble for the next year, during which time they would remain on probation.

V.   DÉNOUEMENT

Events subsequent to the resolution of the JCDH case proved just as freighted with ambiguity as the evidence presented before the Regents' tribunal. Kagan and Fersko, two of the three courageous young residents who had refused to cooperate, were rewarded for their efforts with exclusion from the American College of Physicians. As Preminger reports, their exclusion was doubtless prompted by their refusal to cooperate in the experiment and their subsequent "irresponsible" resignations from the staff of the JCDH. They appealed, and their exclusion was eventually reversed on the ground that their "overreaction" to Southam's experiment was excusable in light of their families' "Holocaust situations."[32] These all-too-rare profiles in courage were thus trivialized by the governors of the American College of Physicians, reduced to the status of merely exculpatory psychological pathology. The three dissenters had refused to cooperate in wrongdoing, apparently, not because of any allegiance to an ethical principle or the "basic rights of the human person," but rather because Mandel's proposal had triggered their memories of the Holocaust, which, in turn, caused their "irresponsible" behavior.

William Hyman, the founding Board member of the JCDH whose protracted lawsuit to view the subjects' charts eventually brought the Regents into the case, was refused perfunctory re-election to the hospital's Board of Trustees in 1966. Even though he had won his narrowly focused lawsuit, and even though the larger issues for which he fought were eventually vindicated by the Regents, his fellow trustees of the JCDH expelled him from the Board of a hospital he helped to found.

But the most remarkable historical irony was reserved for Southam himself. Having been publicly humiliated by an inquisition before the New York State Board of Regents; having been found guilty of fraud, deceit, and the unprofessional conduct of medicine, and having had his medical license suspended and been placed on probation, as his lawyer put it, like some "low-brow scoundrel," Chester M. Southam was elected president of the American Association for Cancer Research in 1968.[33]

---

29. Ibid., 62.

30. Katz, *The Silent World of Doctor and Patient*.

31. Katz, *Experimentation with Human Beings*, 63.

32. Preminger, 8.

33. Katz, *Experimentation with Human Beings*, 65.

Although his case both reflected and helped to bring about profound changes in the ethos and rules governing biomedical research, those changes had not yet percolated down into the rank and file of the research community, which still clung to its paternalistic ways and duly rewarded Southam with one of its greatest honors. In most researchers' view, apparently, the JCDH case was nothing more than a mere "brouhaha," a mere "squabble over who-told-what-to-whom." For them, there were no lessons to be learned, but as we know now, history was on the side of Hyman and the brave young residents. The days of untrammeled physician discretion in research ethics were numbered, and strangers were indeed gathering at the bedside. It would not be long before the revelations at Tuskegee would explode once and for all any lingering doubts about the desirability and necessity of imposing strict rules on the practice of biomedical research.

THE WILLOWBROOK HEPATITIS STUDIES

David J. Rothman and Sheila M. Rothman

The attempt to bar Willowbrook's hepatitis carriers from the public schools had a special irony to it, for from 1956 through 1971, researchers fed live viruses to children in Willowbrook in order to study the disease and attempt to create a vaccine against it.

The head of the team was Saul Krugman. In appearance, he borders on the colorless, but controversy surrounds him. Krugman's research at Willowbrook brought him fame and power. He has chaired national committees on hepatitis, directed huge federally funded projects, been the subject of laudatory editorials in the *Journal of the American Medical Association,* and won the John Russell Award of the Markle Foundation (which read, in part: "In all his work Dr. Krugman proceeded quietly and cautiously. . . . He has zealously guarded the rights and sensibilities of patients and their families. . . . Dr. Krugman has provided an example of how [good clinical research] should be done"). Yet in April 1972, when Dr. Krugman received a prize from the American College of Physicians, a line of police surrounded the podium while 150 protesters denounced his research as grossly unethical.

Saul Krugman's interest in infectious diseases began when, as a physician with the armed forces in the South Pacific, he treated many patients who contracted malaria or jungle parasites. Upon discharge, Krugman took a residency at New York's public hospital for infectious diseases, Willard Parker, which in several ways prepared him to work at Willowbrook. Krugman recalled entering a pavilion where some sixty children lay one next to the other "with every complication of measles—encephalitis, pneumonia, everything. I could go to another area and see dozens of children with diphtheria. . . . Every summer the Parker Hospital would admit at least 50 and sometimes more than 100 children with paralytic poliomyelitis."

In such a setting, Krugman became convinced that even the most diligent efforts at treatment were not likely to bring benefits. "Therapeutics," he once remarked, "was a slender reed in those days." Rather, the goal had to be prevention, which to Krugman meant not cleaning up a water supply or sewer system, but finding vaccines.

In 1947, Krugman moved to Bellevue Hospital and joined the NYU faculty, and in 1954 he became consulting physician to the newly opened Willowbrook facility. He immediately conducted an epidemiological survey, which disclosed an amazing variety of infectious diseases: measles, hepatitis, respiratory infections, shigella, and assorted intestinal parasites.

If Willowbrook was a hell for its residents, it could be a paradise for a researcher. On these

From *The Willowbrook Wars,* by David J. Rothman and Sheila Rothman. New York: Harper and Row, 1984:260–267. Reprinted by permission of HarperCollins Publishers.

disease-ridden wards, the line between treatment and experimentation seemed to vanish. A researcher could select his disease and enjoy substantial freedom to experiment, believing that he was serving both society and the residents.

Events in 1960 confirmed the validity of these presumptions for Krugman. Every two years or so, New York City experienced a measles epidemic, and new admissions to Willowbrook invariably brought in the disease. The results were usually disastrous, with hundreds of cases and fatality rates as high as 10 percent. At the start of 1960, Dr. John Enders, working in Boston, had succeeded in growing measles virus in culture and had managed to attenuate it to the point where it might be an effective vaccine. Krugman wanted to run trial tests at Willowbrook. The disease struck there so often and so hard that findings could be obtained quickly; and if the vaccine offered protection, the Willowbrook residents would obviously benefit. Krugman contacted Enders, received twenty samples of the limited number of doses available, and vaccinated the residents of one ward.

A measles epidemic soon struck at Willowbrook, but no one among the vaccinated children contracted the disease. "Willowbrook's children," observed Dr. Krugman, "enabled us to acquire in a short time solid information about Dr. Enders's vaccine." By 1963, before the vaccine was officially licensed, 90 percent of Willowbrook's residents had been inoculated, and measles was never again a threat. The use of an experimental vaccine at Willowbrook, Krugman concluded, "was obviously beneficial to the children."

The measles study was a sideshow at Willowbrook. It was hepatitis that held center stage. Soon after completing his initial epidemiological survey, Dr. Krugman decided to explore this widespread but little understood disease. Its symptoms had been recognized for centuries, but not until World War II did medical researchers suspect that the disease was infectious and occurred in two varieties: the short, thirty-day-incubation type that we now label hepatitis A and commonly associate with eating contaminated shellfish; and the long, ninety-day-incubation type that we now label hepatitis B and commonly associate with blood transfusions. Beyond these simple categories, little was known about causes, cure, or prevention.

In this vacuum Dr. Krugman began his experiments. Between 1953 and 1957, Willowbrook had had about 350 cases of hepatitis among the residents and 76 among the staff; in 1955 alone (the year before his research began), the disease rate was 25 per thousand among the residents, 40 per thousand among the staff. (In New York State, the rate was 25 per *one hundred thousand* of the population.) And these figures included only the observable, acute cases of patients with jaundice; the number of milder, subclinical cases was still greater. To Dr. Krugman, these conditions called for an active research strategy. Scientists had not yet found a nonhuman host for the virus or succeeded in growing it in a laboratory culture. Thus experiments would have to be carried out on live subjects, and what better subjects than the Willowbrook children? The high rate of contagion in the institution meant that they were bound to get the disease and the effectiveness of intervention could be measured almost immediately.

Krugman's experiments had a logic, a simplicity, and, one would dare to add, an elegance about them. His initial project was to determine whether injections of gamma globulin, that part of the blood plasma which is rich in antibodies, protected recipients against hepatitis. The literature suggested that gamma globulin offered temporary, "passive" immunity; the antibodies in the fluid would be able to counteract the disease for some six weeks. The critical question was whether injections of gamma globulin in the presence of the virus would lead recipients to produce their own antibodies, thereby acquiring permanent immunity that would last for years.

The team first administered varying doses of gamma globulin to one group of new admissions to Willowbrook and withheld it from another. Then, eight to ten months later, it tallied the numbers from each group who had contracted the illness. The results were clear: of 1,812 residents who had been inoculated, only two cases of hepatitis occurred (a rate of 1.7 per 1,000); of the 1,771 residents who were not inoculated, forty-one contracted the disease (22.5 per 1,000). Thus Krugman confirmed that gamma globulin did protect against hepatitis and the finding "pointed the way to the practical method for the control of infectious hepatitis at this institution."

But had the gamma globulin injection stimulated active immunity? Those inoculated were protected against the disease for almost a year, but no one understood how this protection was acquired or how long it would last. Had the gamma globulin first provided a passive immunity, which then turned active when recipients came in contact with the live virus from other residents? Could permanent active immunity be acquired by injecting patients with gamma globulin and live virus at the same time?

To answer these questions, Krugman opened a separate unit on the Willowbrook grounds. Staffed by its own personnel, it admitted children between the ages of three and eleven, directly from their own homes; when their role in the research was completed, weeks or months later, they moved onto the general wards. The experiments typically involved injecting some of the unit residents with gamma globulin and feeding them the live hepatitis virus (obtained from the feces of Willowbrook hepatitis patients). At the same time, other unit residents served as "controls"; they were fed the live virus without the benefit of gamma globulin, to ascertain that the virus was actually "live," capable of transmitting the disease, and to measure the different responses. Then Krugman would calculate how many of those who had received both gamma globulin and live virus, as compared with controls, initially came down with hepatitis; six or nine or twelve months later, he would again feed both groups another dose of live virus and measure how many of those who had earlier received the gamma globulin contracted the disease as against those who had not.

As is often the case in scientific research, Dr. Krugman's most important observation came by chance. In keeping track of the hepatitis rates in the institution, he noted that 4 to 8 percent of those who contracted hepatitis went on to suffer a second attack within a year. The second attack might possibly have been caused by a very heavy exposure to the virus, which overwhelmed the immunity the body had built up after the first attack. But Dr. Krugman believed that the etiology of the disease was more complicated than researchers had recognized. The repeat attack indicated that more than one type of virus could be causing hepatitis.

To investigate this "very attractive hypothesis," Dr. Krugman in 1964 started a new series of experiments, and within three years he helped to clarify the distinction between hepatitis A and B. In this round, the Krugman team admitted new Willowbrook residents to its special unit and fed them a dose of pooled Willowbrook virus, that is, a mixture that came from a large number of hepatitis victims and, therefore, contained all the hepatitis viruses within the institution. In short order, these First Trial subjects contracted the disease and recovered from it. The team then reinfected these children with the same pooled virus in a Second Trial, and a number of them again contracted the disease. In the course of these procedures, the team drew a sample of blood from one of the boys during his first illness (and labeled it MS-1), and then another sample from him in his second illness (labeled MS-2). Next, the researchers admitted a new group of fourteen children to the unit and infected these Third Trial subjects with the MS-1 virus. Within thirty-one to thirty-eight days, all but one came down with hepatitis. Simultaneously, the team admitted still another fourteen children to the unit, and injected this Fourth Trial group with the MS-2 virus. Within forty-one to sixty-nine days, all but two contracted the illness. Now the stage was set for the final procedure. The team gave all the hepatitis victims in the third (MS-1) group and fourth (MS-2) group the MS-1 virus. It turned out that not one child in the Third Trial group came down with hepatitis a second time; six of the eight children in the Fourth Trial group again contracted the disease.

With these findings in hand, Krugman announced that hepatitis was caused by at least two distinct viruses. There was hepatitis A, MS-1, of short incubation and highly contagious (all of the controls who lived with the Third Trial group but were not fed the virus directly came down with the disease). And there was hepatitis B, MS-2, of long incubation and lower contagion (only two of the five controls living with the Fourth Trial group caught the disease). In short, the Krugman research established the distinctive features of two strains of hepatitis.

The findings met with acclaim, and Krugman was praised not only for his results but for his methods. The *Journal of the American Medical Association* credited Krugman's "judicious use of human beings"; Franz Inglefinger, later the editor of the *New England Journal of Medicine,* went further: "By being allowed to participate in a carefully supervised study and by receiving the most expert attention available for a disease of basically unknown nature, the patients themselves benefited. . . . How much better to have a patient with hepatitis, accidentally or deliberately acquired, under the guidance of a Krugman than under the care of a [rights-minded] zealot."

Underlying these attempts at justification, and those that Krugman himself made, was the notion that the Willowbrook experiments were, in the words of Claude Bernard, the nineteenth-century French physician who was among the first to address the ethics of research, "experiments in nature." Researchers who studied the course and spread of a disease that had no known antidote were acting ethically, for no intervention on their part could have altered the outcome. But how could feeding live hepatitis viruses to children be considered the equivalent of observing a disease? Krugman's answer was that if he had not infected the children, they still would have contracted hepatitis. Had he never come to Willowbrook, the likelihood was overwhelming that entering residents would have suffered the disease. Thus his feeding them the virus did not really change anything and was an experiment in nature. Krugman also noted that he had obtained permission from the parents of all his subjects, and he had signed consent forms to prove it.

Many parents of children accepted at Willowbrook but still awaiting actual admission—a wait that could last for several years—did receive the following letter from Dr. H. H. Berman, then Willowbrook's director:

November 15, 1958

Dear Mrs. ———:

We are studying the possibility of preventing epidemics of hepatitis on a new principle. Virus is introduced and gamma globulin given later to some, so that either no attack or only a mild attack of hepatitis is expected to follow. This may give the children immunity against this disease for life. We should like to give your child this new form of prevention with the hope that it will afford protection.

Permission form is enclosed for your consideration. If you wish to have your child given the benefit of this new preventive, will you so signify by signing the form.

Almost every phrase in this particular letter encourages parents to commit their children to the unit. The team is "studying" hepatitis, not doing research. The virus "is introduced," in the passive voice, rather than the team's being said to feed the child a live virus. Gamma globulin is given "to some," but the letter does not explicitly state that it is withheld from others. "No attack" or a "mild attack" of the disease "is expected to follow," but absent gamma globulin, a claim of "no attack" was false and left unsaid was that in some cases the attack would not be mild. Finally, the letter twice described introducing the live virus as a "new form of prevention," but feeding a child hepatitis hardly amounted to prevention. In truth, the goal of the experiment was to *create*, not deliver, a new form of protection.

To send such a letter over the signature of Willowbrook's director appeared coercive. These parents wanted to please the man who would be in charge of their child. Moreover, an especially raw form of coercion may have occasionally intruded. When overcrowding at Willowbrook forced a close in regular admissions, an escape hatch was left— admission via Krugman's unit. A parent wanting to institutionalize a retarded child had a choice: Sign the form or forgo the placement.

What of Krugman's contention that his research was an experiment in nature? The claim ignores the fact that the underlying problem was not ignorance about a disease but an unwillingness to alter the social environment. Had Krugman wished to, he could have insisted that hygienic measures be introduced to decrease the spread of the virus. Should the facility resist carrying out the necessary cleanup, he might have asked the Department of Health to close the place down as a health hazard, which it surely was. Furthermore, Krugman had at hand an antidote of some efficacy. His own findings demonstrated that gamma globulin provided some protection, and yet he infected control groups with the virus and withheld the serum from them in order to fulfill the requirements of his research design.

Finally, to introduce one more irony to this account: While Krugman was trying to discover the etiology of hepatitis at Willowbrook, Dr. Baruch Blumberg was actually solving the puzzle in his laboratory, without conducting experiments on humans. In the course of his research on the body's immunological reaction to transfused blood, Blumberg observed that a strange band occurred when he mixed a vial of blood drawn from a hemophiliac with that drawn from an Australian aborigine.

Labeling the band the Australia antigen, he investigated its properties; like a detective on the trail of a culprit, he followed several false leads and then the true one, discovering that the Australia antigen was the infective agent in hepatitis B. His first published report appeared in 1967 and Krugman confirmed the finding (the Australia antigen was in the blood of the MS-2 children but not the MS-1 children). Thus those with a utilitarian bent, who might be prepared to give Krugman leeway with his means because his ends were important, will have to consider that, however accidentally, we would have learned almost everything we needed to know about hepatitis B in the laboratory.

RACISM AND RESEARCH: THE CASE OF THE TUSKEGEE SYPHILIS STUDY

Allan M. Brandt

In 1932 the U.S. Public Health Service (USPHS) initiated an experiment in Macon County, Alabama, to determine the natural course of untreated, latent syphilis in black males. The test comprised 400 syphilitic men, as well as 200 uninfected men who served as controls. The first published report of the study appeared in 1936 with subsequent papers issued every four to six years, through the 1960s. When penicillin became widely available by the early 1950s as the preferred treatment for syphilis, the men did not receive therapy. In fact on several occasions, the USPHS actually sought to prevent treatment. Moreover, a committee at the federally operated Center for Disease Control decided in 1969 that the study should be continued. Only in 1972, when accounts of the study first appeared in the national press, did the Department of Health, Education and Welfare halt the experiment. At that time seventy-four of the test subjects were still alive; at least twenty-eight, but perhaps more than 100, had died directly from advanced syphilitic lesions.[1] In August 1972, HEW appointed an investigatory panel which issued a report the following year. The panel found the study to have been "ethically unjustified," and argued that penicillin should have been provided to the men.[2]

This article attempts to place the Tuskegee Study in a historical context and to assess its ethical implications. Despite the media attention which the study received, the HEW *Final Report,* and the criticism expressed by several professional organizations, the experiment has been largely misunderstood. The most basic questions of *how* the study was undertaken in the first place and *why* it continued for forty years were never addressed by the HEW investigation. Moreover, the panel misconstrued the nature of the experiment, failing to consult important documents available at the National Archives which bear significantly on its ethical assessment. Only by examining the specific ways in which values are engaged in scientific research can the study be understood.

RACISM AND MEDICAL OPINION

A brief review of the prevailing scientific thought regarding race and heredity in the early twentieth century is fundamental for an understanding of the Tuskegee Study. By the turn of the century, Darwinism had provided a new rationale for American racism. Essentially primitive peoples, it was argued, could not be assimilated into a complex, white civilization. Scientists speculated that in the struggle for survival the Negro in America was doomed. Particularly prone to disease, vice, and crime, black Americans could not be helped by education or

From *Hastings Center Report* 8, no. 6 (December 1978): 21–29. Reprinted by permission of The Hastings Center.

Editors' note: Many author's notes have been cut. Students who want to follow up on sources should consult the original article.

philanthropy. Social Darwinists analyzed census data to predict the virtual extinction of the Negro in the twentieth century, for they believed the Negro race in America was in the throes of a degenerative evolutionary process.

The medical profession supported these findings of late nineteenth- and early twentieth-century anthropologists, ethnologists, and biologists. Physicians studying the effects of emancipation on health concluded almost universally that freedom had caused the mental, moral, and physical deterioration of the black population. They substantiated this argument by citing examples in the comparitive [sic] anatomy of the black and white races. As Dr. W. T. English wrote: "A careful inspection reveals the body of the negro a mass of minor defects and imperfections from the crown of the head to the soles of the feet. . . ."[3] Cranial structures, wide nasal apertures, receding chins, projecting jaws, all typed the Negro as the lowest species in the Darwinian hierarchy.

Interest in racial differences centered on the sexual nature of blacks. The Negro, doctors explained, possessed an excessive sexual desire, which threatened the very foundations of white society. As one physician noted in the *Journal of the American Medical Association*, "The negro springs from a southern race, and as such his sexual appetite is strong; all of his environments stimulate this appetite, and as a general rule his emotional type of religion certainly does not decrease it." Doctors reported a complete lack of morality on the part of blacks:

> Virtue in the negro race is like angels' visits—few and far between. In a practice of sixteen years I have never examined a virgin negro over fourteen years of age.[4]

A particularly ominous feature of this overzealous sexuality, doctors argued, was the black males' desire for white women. "A perversion from which most races are exempt," wrote Dr. English, "prompts the negro's inclination towards white women, whereas other races incline towards females of their own."[5] Though English estimated the "gray matter of the negro brain" to be at least a thousand years behind that of the white races, his genital organs were overdeveloped. As Dr. William Lee Howard noted:

> The attacks on defenseless white women are evidences of racial instincts that are about as amenable to ethical culture as is the inherent odor of the race. . . . When education will reduce the size of the negro's penis as

well as bring about the sensitiveness of the terminal fibers which exist in the Caucasian, then will it also be able to prevent the African's birthright to sexual madness and excess.[6]

One southern medical journal proposed "Castration Instead of Lynching," as retribution for black sexual crimes. "An impressive trial by a ghost-like kuklux klan [sic] and a 'ghost' physician or surgeon to perform the operation would make it an event the 'patient' would never forget," noted the editorial.[7]

According to these physicians, lust and immorality, unstable families, and reversion to barbaric tendencies made blacks especially prone to venereal diseases. One doctor estimated that over 50 percent of all Negroes over the age of twenty-five were syphilitic.[8] Virtually free of disease as slaves, they were now overwhelmed by it, according to informed medical opinion. Moreover, doctors believed that treatment for venereal disease among blacks was impossible, particularly because in its latent stage the symptoms of syphilis become quiescent. As Dr. Thomas W. Murrell wrote:

> They come for treatment at the beginning and at the end. When there are visible manifestations or when they are harried by pain, they readily come, for as a race they are not averse to physic; but tell them not, though they look well and feel well, that they are still diseased. Here ignorance rates science a fool. . . .[9]

Even the best educated black, according to Murrell, could not be convinced to seek treatment for syphilis. Venereal disease, according to some doctors, threatened the future of the race. The medical profession attributed the low birth rate among blacks to the high prevalence of venereal disease which caused stillbirths and miscarriages. Moreover, the high rates of syphilis were thought to lead to increased insanity and crime. One doctor writing at the turn of the century estimated that the number of insane Negroes had increased thirteen-fold since the end of the Civil War. Dr. Murrell's conclusion echoed the most informed anthropological and ethnological data:

> So the scourge sweeps among them. Those that are treated are only half cured and the effort to assimilate a complex civilization driving their diseased minds until the results are criminal records. Perhaps here, in conjunction with tuberculosis, will be the end of the negro problem. Disease will accomplish what man cannot do.[10]

This particular configuration of ideas formed the core of medical opinion concerning blacks, sex, and disease in the early twentieth century. Doctors generally discounted socioeconomic explanations of the state of black health, arguing that better medical care could not alter the evolutionary scheme. These assumptions provide the backdrop for examining the Tuskegee Syphilis Study.

THE ORIGINS OF THE EXPERIMENT

In 1929, under a grant from the Julius Rosenwald Fund, the USPHS conducted studies in the rural South to determine the prevalence of syphilis among blacks and explore the possibilities for mass treatment. The USPHS found Macon County, Alabama, in which the town of Tuskegee is located, to have the highest syphilis rate of the six counties surveyed. The Rosenwald Study concluded that mass treatment could be successfully implemented among rural blacks.[11] Although it is doubtful that the necessary funds would have been allocated even in the best economic conditions, after the economy collapsed in 1929, the findings were ignored. It is, however, ironic that the Tuskegee Study came to be based on findings of the Rosenwald Study that demonstrated the possibilities of mass treatment.

Three years later, in 1932, Dr. Taliaferro Clark, Chief of the USPHS Venereal Disease Division and author of the Rosenwald Study report, decided that conditions in Macon County merited renewed attention. Clark believed the high prevalence of syphilis offered an "unusual opportunity" for observation. From its inception, the USPHS regarded the Tuskegee Study as a classic "study in nature,"* rather than an experiment.[12] As long as syphilis was so prevalent in Macon and most of the blacks went untreated

throughout life, it seemed only natural to Clark that it would be valuable to observe the consequences. He described it as a "ready-made situation." Surgeon General H. S. Cumming wrote to R. R. Moton, Director of the Tuskegee Institute:

> The recent syphilis control demonstration carried out in Macon County, with the financial assistance of the Julius Rosenwald Fund, revealed the presence of an unusually high rate in this county and, what is more remarkable, the fact that 99 per cent of this group was entirely without previous treatment. This combination, together with the expected cooperation of your hospital, offers an unparalleled opportunity for carrying on this piece of scientific research which probably cannot be duplicated anywhere else in the world.

Although no formal protocol appears to have been written, several letters of Clark and Cumming suggest what the USPHS hoped to find. Clark indicated that it would be important to see how disease affected the daily lives of the men:

> The results of these studies of case records suggest the desirability of making a further study of the effect of untreated syphilis on the human economy among people now living and engaged in their daily pursuits.

It also seems that the USPHS believed the experiment might demonstrate that antisyphilitic treatment was unnecessary. As Cumming noted: "It is expected the results of this study may have a marked bearing on the treatment, or conversely the non-necessity of treatment, of cases of latent syphilis."

The immediate source of Cumming's hypothesis appears to have been the famous Oslo Study of untreated syphilis. Between 1890 and 1910, Professor C. Boeck, the chief of the Oslo Venereal Clinic, withheld treatment from almost two thousand patients infected with syphilis. He was convinced that therapies then available, primarily mercurial ointment, were of no value. When arsenic therapy became widely available by 1910, after Paul Ehrlich's historic discovery of "606," the study was abandoned. E. Bruusgaard, Boeck's successor, conducted a follow-up study of 473 of the untreated patients from 1925 to 1927. He found that 27.9 percent of these patients had undergone a "spontaneous cure," and now manifested no symptoms of the disease. Moreover, he estimated that as many as 70 percent of all syphilitics went through life without inconvenience from the disease.[13] His study,

---

*In 1865, Claude Bernard, the famous French physiologist, outlined the distinction between a "study in nature" and experimentation. A study in nature required simple observation, an essentially passive act, while experimentation demanded intervention which altered the original condition. The Tuskegee Study was thus clearly not a study in nature. The very act of diagnosis altered the original condition. "It is on this very possibility of acting or not acting on a body," wrote Bernard, "that the distinction will exclusively rest between sciences called sciences of observation and sciences called experimental."

however, clearly acknowledged the dangers of untreated syphilis for the remaining 30 percent.

Thus every major textbook of syphilis at the time of the Tuskegee Study's inception strongly advocated treating syphilis even in its latent stages, which follow the initial inflammatory reaction. In discussing the Oslo Study, Dr. J. E. Moore, one of the nation's leading venereologists wrote, "This summary of Bruusgaard's study is by no means intended to suggest that syphilis be allowed to pass untreated."[14] If a complete cure could not be effected, at least the most devastating effects of the disease could be avoided. Although the standard therapies of the time, arsenical compounds and bismuth injection, involved certain dangers because of their toxicity, the alternatives were much worse. As the Oslo Study had shown, untreated syphilis could lead to cardiovascular disease, insanity, and premature death.[15] Moore wrote in his 1933 textbook:

> Though it imposes a slight though measurable risk of its own, treatment markedly diminishes the risk from syphilis. In latent syphilis, as I shall show, the probability of progression, relapse, or death is reduced from a probable 25-30 percent without treatment to about 5 percent with it; and the gravity of the relapse if it occurs, is markedly diminished.[16]

"Another compelling reason for treatment," noted Moore, "exists in the fact that every patient with latent syphilis may be, and perhaps is, infectious for others."[17] In 1932, the year in which the Tuskegee Study began, the USPHS sponsored and published a paper by Moore and six other syphilis experts that strongly argued for treating latent syphilis.

The Oslo Study, therefore, could not have provided justification for the USPHS to undertake a study that did not entail treatment. Rather, the suppositions that conditions in Tuskegee existed "naturally" and that the men would not be treated anyway provided the experiment's rationale. In turn, these two assumptions rested on the prevailing medical attitudes concerning blacks, sex, and disease. For example, Clark explained the prevalence of venereal disease in Macon County by emphasizing promiscuity among blacks:

> This state of affairs is due to the paucity of doctors, rather low intelligence of the Negro population in this section, depressed economic conditions, and the very common promiscuous sex relations of this population

group which not only contribute to the spread of syphilis but also contribute to the prevailing indifference with regard to treatment.

In fact, Moore, who had written so persuasively in favor of treating latent syphilis, suggested that existing knowledge did not apply to Negroes. Although he had called the Oslo Study "a never-to-be-repeated human experiment," he served as an expert consultant to the Tuskegee Study:

> I think that such a study as you have contemplated would be of immense value. It will be necessary of course in the consideration of the results to evaluate the special factors introduced by a selection of the material from negro males. Syphilis in the negro is in many respects almost a different disease from syphilis in the white.

Dr. O. C. Wenger, chief of the federally operated venereal disease clinic at Hot Springs, Arkansas, praised Moore's judgment, adding, "This study will emphasize those differences." On another occasion he advised Clark, "We must remember we are dealing with a group of people who are illiterate, have no conception of time, and whose personal history is always indefinite."

The doctors who devised and directed the Tuskegee Study accepted the mainstream assumptions regarding blacks and venereal disease. The premise that blacks, promiscuous and lustful, would not seek or continue treatment, shaped the study. A test of untreated syphilis seemed "natural" because the USPHS presumed the men would never be treated; the Tuskegee Study made that a self-fulfilling prophecy.

SELECTING THE SUBJECTS

Clark sent Dr. Raymond Vonderlehr to Tuskegee in September 1932 to assemble a sample of men with latent syphilis for the experiment. The basic design of the study called for the selection of syphilitic black males between the ages of twenty-five and sixty, a thorough physical examination including x-rays, and finally, a spinal tap to determine the incidence of neuro-syphilis. They had no intention of providing any treatment for the infected men.[18] The USPHS originally scheduled the whole experiment to last six months; it seemed to be both a simple and inexpensive project.

The task of collecting the sample, however, proved to be more difficult than the USPHS had supposed. Vonderlehr canvassed the largely illiterate, poverty-stricken population of sharecroppers and tenant farmers in search of test subjects. If his circulars requested only men over twenty-five to attend his clinics, none would appear, suspecting he was conducting draft physicals. Therefore, he was forced to test large numbers of women and men who did not fit the experiment's specifications. This involved considerable expense since the USPHS had promised the Macon County Board of Health that it would treat those who were infected, but not included in the study. Clark wrote to Vonderlehr about the situation: "It never once occurred to me that we would be called upon to treat a large part of the county as return for the privilege of making this study. . . . I am anxious to keep the expenditures for treatment down to the lowest possible point because it is the one item of expenditure in connection with the study most difficult to defend despite our knowledge of the need therefor." Vonderlehr responded: "If we could find from 100 to 200 cases . . . we would not have to do another Wassermann on useless individuals . . ."

Significantly, the attempt to develop the sample contradicted the prediction the USPHS had made initially regarding the prevalence of the disease in Macon County. Overall rates of syphilis fell well below expectations; as opposed to the USPHS projection of 35 percent, 20 percent of those tested were actually diseased. Moreover, those who had sought and received previous treatment far exceeded the expectations of the USPHS. Clark noted in a letter to Vonderlehr:

> I find your report of March 6th quite interesting but regret the necessity of Wassermanning [*sic*] . . . such a large number of individuals in order to uncover this relatively limited number of untreated cases.

Further difficulties arose in enlisting the subjects to participate in the experiment, to be "Wassermanned," and to return for a subsequent series of examinations. Vonderlehr found that only the offer of treatment elicited the cooperation of the men. They were told they were ill and were promised free care. Offered therapy, they became willing subjects.[19] The USPHS did not tell the men that they were participants in an experiment; on the contrary, the subjects believed they were being treated for "bad blood"—the rural

South's colloquialism for syphilis. They thought they were participating in a public health demonstration similar to the one that had been conducted by the Julius Rosenwald Fund in Tuskegee several years earlier. In the end, the men were so eager for medical care that the number of defaulters in the experiment proved to be insignificant.

To preserve the subjects' interest, Vonderlehr gave most of the men mercurial ointment, a noneffective drug, while some of the younger men apparently received inadequate dosages of neoarsphenamine. This required Vonderlehr to write frequently to Clark requesting supplies. He feared the experiment would fail if the men were not offered treatment.

> It is desirable and essential if the study is to be a success to maintain the interest of each of the cases examined by me through to the time when the spinal puncture can be completed. Expenditure of several hundred dollars for drugs for these men would be well worth while if their interest and cooperation would be maintained in so doing. . . . It is my desire to keep the main purpose of the work from the negroes in the county and continue their interest in treatment. That is what the vast majority wants and the examination seems relatively unimportant to them in comparison. It would probably cause the entire experiment to collapse if the clinics were stopped before the work is completed.

On another occasion he explained:

> Dozens of patients have been sent away without treatment during the past two weeks and it would have been impossible to continue without the free distribution of drugs because of the unfavorable impression made on the negro.

The readiness of the test subjects to participate of course contradicted the notion that blacks would not seek or continue therapy.

The final procedure of the experiment was to be a spinal tap to test for neuro-syphilis. The USPHS presented this purely diagnostic exam, which often entails considerable pain and complications, to the men as a "special treatment." Clark explained to Moore:

> We have not yet commenced the spinal punctures. This operation will be deferred to the last in order not to unduly disturb our field work by any adverse reports by the patients subjected to spinal puncture because of some disagreeable sensations following this procedure. These negroes are very ignorant and easily influenced by things that would be of minor significance in a more intelligent group.

The letter to the subjects announcing the spinal tap read:

> Some time ago you were given a thorough examination and since that time we hope you have gotten a great deal of treatment for bad blood. You will now be given your last chance to get a second examination. This examination is a very special one and after it is finished you will be given a special treatment if it is believed you are in a condition to stand it. . . .
>   REMEMBER THIS IS YOUR LAST CHANCE FOR SPECIAL FREE TREATMENT. BE SURE TO MEET THE NURSE.[20]

The HEW investigation did not uncover this crucial fact: the men participated in the study under the guise of treatment.

Despite the fact that their assumption regarding prevalence and black attitudes toward treatment had proved wrong, the USPHS decided in the summer of 1933 to continue the study. Once again, it seemed only "natural" to pursue the research since the sample already existed, and with a depressed economy, the cost of treatment appeared prohibitive—although there is no indication it was ever considered. Vonderlehr first suggested extending the study in letters to Clark and Wenger:

> At the end of this project we shall have a considerable number of cases presenting various complications of syphilis, who have received only mercury and may still be considered untreated in the modern sense of therapy. Should these cases be followed over a period of from five to ten years many interesting facts could be learned regarding the course and complications of untreated syphilis.

"As I see it," responded Wenger, "we have no further interest in these patients until they die." Apparently, the physicians engaged in the experiment believed that only autopsies could scientifically confirm the findings of the study. Surgeon General Cumming explained this in a letter to R. R. Moton, requesting the continued cooperation of the Tuskegee Institute Hospital:

> This study which was predominantly clinical in character points to the frequent occurrence of severe complications involving the various vital organs of the body and indicates that syphilis as a disease does a great deal of damage. Since clinical observations are not considered final in the medical world, it is our desire to continue observation on the cases selected for the recent study and if possible to bring a percentage of these cases to autopsy so that pathological confirmation may be made of the disease processes.

Bringing the men to autopsy required the USPHS to devise a further series of deceptions and inducements. Wenger warned Vonderlehr that the men must not realize that they would be autopsied:

> There is one danger in the latter plan and that is if the colored population become aware that accepting free hospital care means a post-mortem, every darkey will leave Macon County and it will hurt [Dr. Eugene] Dibble's hospital.

"Naturally," responded Vonderlehr, "it is not my intention to let it be generally known that the main object of the present activities is the bringing of the men to necropsy." The subjects' trust in the USPHS made the plan viable. The USPHS gave Dr. Dibble, the Director of the Tuskegee Institute Hospital, an interim appointment to the Public Health Service. As Wenger noted:

> One thing is certain. The only way we are going to get post-mortems is to have the demise take place in Dibble's hospital and when these colored folks are told that Doctor Dibble is now a Government doctor too they will have more confidence.*

---

*The degree of black cooperation in conducting the study remains unclear and would be impossible to properly assess in an article of this length. It seems certain that some members of the Tuskegee Institute staff such as R. R. Moton and Eugene Dibble understood the nature of the experiment and gave their support to it. There is, however, evidence that some blacks who assisted the USPHS physicians were not aware of the deceptive nature of the experiment. Dr. Joshua Williams, an intern at the John A. Andrew Memorial Hospital (Tuskegee Institute) in 1932, assisted Vonderlehr in taking blood samples of the test subjects. In 1973 he told the HEW panel: "I know we thought it was merely a service group organized to help the people in the area. We didn't know it was a research project at all at the time." (See, "Transcript of Proceedings," Tuskegee Syphillis Study Ad Hoc Advisory Panel, February 23, 1973, Unpublished typescript. National Library of Medicine, Bethesda, Maryland.) It is also apparent that Eunice Rivers, the black nurse who had primary responsibility for maintaining contact with the men over the forty years, did not fully understand the dangers of the experiment. In any event, black involvement in the study in no way mitigates the racial assumption of the experiment, but rather, demonstrates their power.

After the USPHS approved the continuation of the experiment in 1933, Vonderlehr decided that it would be necessary to select a group of healthy, uninfected men to serve as controls. Vonderlehr, who had succeeded Clark as Chief of the Venereal Disease Division, sent Dr. J. R. Heller to Tuskegee to gather the control group. Heller distributed drugs (noneffective) to these men, which suggests that they also believed they were undergoing treatment. Control subjects who became syphilitic were simply transferred to the test group—a strikingly inept violation of standard research procedure.[21]

The USPHS offered several inducements to maintain contact and to procure the continued cooperation of the men. Eunice Rivers, a black nurse, was hired to follow their health and to secure approval for autopsies. She gave the men noneffective medicines— "spring tonic" and aspirin—as well as transportation and hot meals on the days of their examinations.[22] More important, Nurse Rivers provided continuity to the project over the entire forty-year period. By supplying "medicals," the USPHS was able to continue to deceive the participants, who believed that they were receiving therapy from the government doctors. Deceit was integral to the study. When the test subjects complained about spinal taps one doctor wrote:

> They simply do not like spinal punctures. A few of those who were tapped are enthusiastic over the results but to most, the suggestion causes violent shaking of the head; others claim they were robbed of their procreative powers (regardless of the fact that I claim it stimulates them).

Letters to the subjects announcing an impending USPHS visit to Tuskegee explained: "[The doctor] wants to make a special examination to find out how you have been feeling and whether the treatment has improved your health." In fact, after the first six months of the study, the USPHS had furnished no treatment whatsoever.

Finally, because it proved difficult to persuade the men to come to the hospital when they became severely ill, the USPHS promised to cover their burial expenses. The Milbank Memorial Fund provided approximately $50 per man for this purpose beginning in 1935. This was a particularly strong inducement as funeral rites constituted an important component of the cultural life of rural blacks. One report of the study concluded, "Without this suasion it would, we believe, have been impossible to secure the cooperation of the group and their families."

Reports of the study's findings, which appeared regularly in the medical press beginning in 1936, consistently cited the ravages of untreated syphilis. The first paper, read at the 1936 American Medical Association annual meeting, found "that syphilis in this period [latency] tends to greatly increase the frequency of manifestations of cardiovascular disease." Only 16 percent of the subjects gave no sign of morbidity as opposed to 61 percent of the controls. Ten years later, a report noted coldly, "The fact that nearly twice as large a proportion of the syphilitic individuals as of the control group has died is a very striking one." Life expectancy, concluded the doctors, is reduced by about 20 percent.

A 1955 article found that slightly more than 30 percent of the test group autopsied had died *directly* from advanced syphilitic lesions of either the cardiovascular or the central nervous system.[23] Another published account stated, "Review of those still living reveals that an appreciable number have late complications of syphilis which probably will result, for some at least, in contributing materially to the ultimate cause of death."[24] In 1950, Dr. Wenger had concluded, "We now know, where we could only surmise before, that we have contributed to their ailments and shortened their lives." As black physician Vernal Cave, a member of the HEW panel, later wrote, "They proved a point, then proved a point, then proved a point."

During the forty years of the experiment the USPHS had sought on several occasions to ensure that the subjects did not receive treatment from other sources. To this end, Vonderlehr met with groups of local black doctors in 1934, to ask their cooperation in not treating the men. Lists of subjects were distributed to Macon County physicians along with letters requesting them to refer these men back to the USPHS if they sought care. The USPHS warned the Alabama Health Department not to treat the test subjects when they took a mobile VD unit into Tuskegee in the early 1940s. In 1941, the Army drafted several subjects and told them to begin antisyphilitic treatment immediately. The USPHS supplied the draft board with a list of 256 names they desired to have excluded from treatment, and the board complied.

In spite of these efforts, by the early 1950s many of the men had secured some treatment on their own. By 1952, almost 30 percent of the test subjects had received some penicillin, although only 7.5 percent had received what could be considered adequate doses.[25] Vonderlehr wrote to one of the participating physicians, "I hope that the availability of antibiotics has not interfered too much with this project." A report published in 1955 considered whether the treatment that some of the men had obtained had "defeated" the study. The article attempted to explain the relatively low exposure to penicillin in an age of antibiotics, suggesting as a reason: "the stoicism of these men as a group; they still regard hospitals and medicines with suspicion and prefer an occasional dose of time-honored herbs or tonics to modern drugs." The authors failed to note that the men believed they were already under the care of the government doctors and thus saw no need to seek treatment elsewhere. Any treatment which the men might have received, concluded the report, had been insufficient to compromise the experiment.

When the USPHS evaluated the status of the study in the 1960s they continued to rationalize the racial aspects of the experiment. For example, the minutes of a 1965 meeting at the Center for Disease Control recorded:

> Racial issue was mentioned briefly. Will not affect the study. Any questions can be handled by saying these people were at the point that therapy would no longer help them. They are getting better medical care than they would under any other circumstances.

A group of physicians met again at the CDC in 1969 to decide whether or not to terminate the study. Although one doctor argued that the study should be stopped and the men treated, the consensus was to continue. Dr. J. Lawton Smith remarked, "You will never have another study like this; take advantage of it." A memo prepared by Dr. James B. Lucas, Assistant Chief of the Venereal Disease Branch, stated: "Nothing learned will prevent, find, or cure a single case of infectious syphilis or bring us closer to our basic mission of controlling venereal disease in the United States." He concluded, however, that the study should be continued "along its present lines." When the first accounts of the experiment appeared in the national press in July 1972, data were still being collected and autopsies performed.

THE HEW FINAL REPORT

HEW finally formed the Tuskegee Syphilis Study Ad Hoc Advisory Panel on August 28, 1972, in response to criticism that the press descriptions of the experiment had triggered. The panel, composed of nine members, five of them black, concentrated on two issues. First, was the study justified in 1932 and had the men given their informed consent? Second, should penicillin have been provided when it became available in the early 1950s? The panel was also charged with determining if the study should be terminated and assessing current policies regarding experimentation with human subjects. The group issued their report in June 1973.

FROM THE HEW FINAL REPORT (1973)

1. In retrospect, the Public Health Service Study of Untreated Syphilis in the Male Negro in Macon County, Alabama, was ethically unjustified in 1932. The judgment made in 1973 about the conduct of the study in 1932 is made with the advantage of hindsight acutely sharpened over some forty years, concerning an activity in a different age with different social standards. Nevertheless, one fundamental ethical rule is that a person should not be subjected to avoidable risk of death or physical harm unless he freely and intelligently consents. There is no evidence that such consent was obtained from the participants in this study.

2. Because of the paucity of information available today on the manner in which the study was conceived, designed and sustained, a scientific justification for a short term demonstration study cannot be ruled out. However, the conduct of the longitudinal study as initially reported in 1936 and through the years is judged to be scientifically unsound and its results are disproportionately meager compared with known risk to human subjects involved. . . .

By focusing on the issues of penicillin therapy and informed consent, the *Final Report* and the investigation betrayed a basic misunderstanding of the experiment's purposes and design. The HEW report implied that the failure to provide penicillin constituted the study's major ethical misjudgment; implicit was the assumption that no adequate therapy existed prior to penicillin. Nonetheless medical authorities firmly believed in the efficacy of arsenotherapy for treating syphilis at the time of the experiment's inception in 1932. The panel further failed to recognize that the entire study had been predicated on nontreatment. Provision of effective medication would have violated the rationale of the experiment—to study the natural course of the disease until death. On several occasions, in fact, the USPHS had prevented the men from receiving proper treatment. Indeed, there is no evidence that the USPHS ever considered providing penicillin.

The other focus of the *Final Report*—informed consent—also served to obscure the historical facts of the experiment. In light of the deceptions and exploitations which the experiment perpetrated, it is an understatement to declare, as the *Report* did, that the experiment was "ethically unjustified," because it failed to obtain informed consent from the subjects. The *Final Report's* statement, "Submitting voluntarily is not informed consent," indicated that the panel believed that the men had volunteered *for the experiment*.[26] The records in the National Archives make clear that the men did not submit voluntarily to an experiment; they were told and they believed that they were getting free treatment from expert government doctors for a serious disease. The failure of the HEW *Final Report* to expose this critical fact—that the USPHS lied to the subjects—calls into question the thoroughness and credibility of their investigation.

Failure to place the study in a historical context also made it impossible for the investigation to deal with the essentially racist nature of the experiment. The panel treated the study as an aberration, well-intentioned but misguided.[27] Moreover, concern that the *Final Report* might be viewed as a critique of human experimentation in general seems to have severely limited the scope of the inquiry. The *Final Report* is quick to remind the reader on two occasions: "The position of the Panel must not be construed to be a general repudiation of scientific research with human subjects."[28] The Report assures us that a better designed experiment could have been justified:

> It is possible that a scientific study in 1932 of untreated syphilis, properly conceived with a clear protocol and conducted with suitable subjects who fully understood the implications of their involvement, might have been justified in the prepenicillin era. This is especially true when one considers the uncertain nature of the results of treatment of late latent syphilis and the highly toxic nature of therapeutic agents then available.[29]

This statement is questionable in view of the proven dangers of untreated syphilis known in 1932.

Since the publication of the HEW *Final Report*, a defense of the Tuskegee Study has emerged. These arguments, most clearly articulated by Dr. R. H. Kampmeier in the *Southern Medical Journal*, center on the limited knowledge of effective therapy for latent syphilis when the experiment began. Kampmeier argues that by 1950, penicillin would have been of no value for these men.[30] Others have suggested that the men were fortunate to have been spared the highly toxic treatments of the earlier period. Moreover, even these contemporary defenses assume that the men never would have been treated anyway. As Dr. Charles Barnett of Stanford University wrote in 1974, "The lack of treatment was not contrived by the USPHS but was an established fact of which they proposed to take advantage."[31] Several doctors who participated in the study continued to justify the experiment. Dr. J. R. Heller, who on one occasion had referred to the test subjects as the "Ethiopian population," told reporters in 1972:

> I don't see why they should be shocked or horrified. There was no racial side to this. It just happened to be in a black community. I feel this was a perfectly straightforward study, perfectly ethical, with controls. Part of our mission as physicians is to find out what happens to individuals with disease and without disease.[32]

These apologies, as well as the HEW *Final Report*, ignore many of the essential ethical issues which the study poses. The Tuskegee Study reveals the persistence of beliefs within the medical profession about the nature of blacks, sex, and disease—beliefs that had tragic repercussions long after their alleged "scientific" bases were known to be incorrect. Most strikingly, the entire health of a community was jeopardized by leaving a communicable disease untreated.[33] There can be little doubt that the Tuskegee researchers regarded their subjects as less than human.[34] As a result, the ethical canons of experimenting on human subjects were completely disregarded.

The study also raises significant questions about professional self-regulation and scientific bureaucracy. Once the USPHS decided to extend the experiment in the summer of 1933, it was unlikely that the test would be halted short of the men's deaths. The experiment was widely reported for forty years without evoking any significant protest within the medical community. Nor did any bureaucratic mechanism exist within the government for the periodic reassessment of the Tuskegee experiment's ethics and scientific value. The USPHS sent physicians to Tuskegee every several years to check on the study's progress, but never subjected the morality or usefulness of the experiment to serious scrutiny. Only the press accounts of 1972 finally punctured the continued rationalizations of the USPHS and brought the study to an end. Even the HEW investigation was compromised by fear that it would be considered a threat to future human experimentation.

In retrospect the Tuskegee Study revealed more about the pathology of racism than it did about the pathology of syphilis; more about the nature of scientific inquiry than the nature of the disease process. The injustice committed by the experiment went well beyond the facts outlined in the press and the HEW *Final Report*. The degree of deception and damages have been seriously underestimated. As this history of the study suggests, the notion that science is a value-free discipline must be rejected. The need for greater vigilance in assessing the specific ways in which social values and attitudes affect professional behavior is clearly indicated.

NOTES

1. The best general account of the study is James Jones, *Bad Blood*, 2nd ed. (New York: The Free Press, 1993).

2. *Final Report* of the Tuskegee Syphilis Study Ad Hoc Advisory Panel, Department of Health, Education, and Welfare (Washington, D.C.: GPO, 1973). (Hereafter, HEW *Final Report*).

3. W. T. English, "The Negro Problem from the Physician's Point of View," *Atlanta Journal-Record of Medicine* 5 (October 1903), 461.

4. Daniel David Quillian. "Racial Peculiarities: A Cause of the Prevalence of Syphilis in Negroes," *American Journal of Dermatology and Genito-Urinary Diseases* 10 (July 1906), p. 277.

5. English, p. 463.

6. William Lee Howard. "The Negro as a Distinct Ethnic Factor in Civilization," *Medicine* (Detroit) 9 (June 1903), 424.

7. "Castration Instead of Lynching," *Atlanta Journal-Record of Medicine* 8 (October 1906), 457.

8. Searle Harris, "The Future of the Negro from the Standpoint of the Southern Physician." *Alabama Medical Journal* 14 (January 1902), 62.

9. Thomas W. Murrell, "Syphilis in the Negro: Its Bearing on the Race Problem," *American Journal of Dermatology and Genito-Urinary Diseases* 10 (August 1906), 307.

10. Murrell, "Syphilis in the Negro; Its Bearing on the Race Problem," p. 307.

11. Taliaferro Clark, *The Control of Syphilis in Southern Rural Areas* (Chicago: Julius Rosenwald Fund, 1932), 53–58. Approximately 35 percent of the inhabitants of Macon County who were examined were found to be syphilitic.

12. See Claude Bernard, *An Introduction to the Study of Experimental Medicine* (New York: Dover, 1865, 1957), pp. 5–26.

13. The best discussion of the Boeck-Bruusgaard data is E. Gurney Clark and Niels Danbolt, "The Oslo Study of the Natural History of Untreated Syphilis," *Journal of Chronic Diseases* 2 (September 1955), 311–44.

14. Joseph Earl Moore, *The Modern Treatment of Syphilis* (Baltimore: Charles C. Thomas, 1933), p. 24.

15. Moore, pp. 231–47.

16. Moore, p. 237.

17. Moore, p. 236.

18. As Clark wrote: "You will observe that our plan has nothing to do with treatment. It is purely a diagnostic procedure carried out to determine what has happened to the syphilitic Negro who has had no treatment." Clark to Paul A. O'Leary, September 27, 1932, NA-WNRC.

19. Vonderlehr later explained: The reason treatment was given to many of these men was twofold: First, when the study was started in the fall of 1932, no plans had been made for its continuation and a few of the patients were treated before we fully realized the need for continuing the project on a permanent basis. Second it was difficult to hold the interest of the group of Negroes in Macon County unless some treatment was given." Vonderlehr to Austin V. Diebert, December 5, 1938, Tuskegee Syphilis Study Ad Hoc Advisory Panel Papers, Box 1, National Library of Medicine, Bethesda, Maryland (Hereafter, TSS-NLM). This collection contains the materials assembled by the HEW investigation in 1972.

20. Macon County Health Department, "Letter to Subjects," n.d., NA-WNRC.

21. Austin V. Diebert and Martha C. Bruyere, "Untreated Syphilis in the Male Negro, III," *Venereal Disease Information* 27 (December 1946), 301–14.

22. Eunice Rivers, Stanley Schuman, Lloyd Simpson, Sidney Olansky, "Twenty-Years of Followup Experience In a Long-Range Medical Study," *Public Health Reports* 68 (April 1953), 391–95. In this article Nurse Rivers explains her role in the experiment. She wrote: "Because of the low educational status of the majority of the patients, it was impossible to appeal to them from a purely scientific approach. Therefore, various methods were used to maintain their interest. Free medicines,

burial assistance or insurance (the project being referred to as 'Miss Rivers' Lodge'), free hot meals on the days of examination, transportation to and from the hospital, and an opportunity to stop in town on the return trip to shop or visit with friends on the streets all helped. In spite of these attractions, there were some who refused their examinations because they were not sick and did not see that they were being benefited." (p. 393).

23. Jesse J. Peters, James H. Peers, Sidney Olansky, John C. Cutler, and Geraldine Gleeson, "Untreated Syphilis in the Male Negro: Pathologic Findings in Syphilitic and Non-Syphilitic Patients," *Journal of Chronic Diseases* 1 (February 1955), 127–48.

24. Sidney Olansky, Stanley H. Schuman, Jesse J. Peters, C. A. Smith, and Dorothy S. Rambo, "Untreated Syphilis in the Male Negro, X. Twenty Years of Clinical Observation of Untreated Syphilitic and Presumably Nonsyphilitic Groups," *Journal of Chronic Diseases* 4 (August 1956), 184.

25. Stanley H. Schuman, Sidney Olansky, Eunice Rivers, C. A. Smith, and Dorothy S. Rambo, "Untreated Syphilis in the Male Negro: Background and Current Status of Patients in the Tuskegee Study," *Journal of Chronic Diseases* 2 (November 1955), 550–53.

26. HEW *Final Report*, p. 7.

27. The notable exception is Jay Katz's eloquent "Reservations About the Panel Report on Charge 1," HEW *Final Report*, pp. 14–15.

28. HEW *Final Report*, pp. 8, 12.

29. HEW *Final Report*, pp. 8, 12.

30. See R. H. Kampmeier, "The Tuskegee Study of Untreated Syphilis," *Southern Medical Journal* 65 (October 1972), 1247–51; and "'Final Report on the 'Tuskegee Syphilis Study,'" *Southern Medical Journal* 67 (November 1974), 1349–53.

31. Quoted in "Debate Revives on the PHS Study," *Medical World News* (April 19, 1974), p. 37.

32. Heller to Vonderlehr, November 28, 1933, quoted in *Medical Tribune* (August 23, 1972), p. 14.

33. Although it is now known that syphilis is rarely infectious after its early phase, at the time of the study's inception latent syphilis was thought to be communicable. The fact that members of the control group were placed in the test group when they became syphilitic proves that at least some infectious men were denied treatment.

34. When the subjects are drawn from minority groups, especially those with which the researcher cannot identify, basic human rights may be compromised. Hans Jonas has clearly explicated the problem in his "Philosophical Reflections on Experimentation," *Daedalus* 98 (Spring 1969), 234–37. As Jonas writes: "If the properties we adduced as the particular qualifications of the members of the scientific fraternity itself are taken as general criteria of selection, then one should look for additional subjects where a maximum of identification, understanding, and spontaneity can be expected—that is, among the most highly motivated, the most highly educated, and the least 'captive' members of the community."

THE BELMONT REPORT: ETHICAL PRINCIPLES AND GUIDELINES FOR THE PROTECTION OF HUMAN SUBJECTS OF RESEARCH

April 18, 1979

The National Commission for the Protection of Human Subjects of Biomedical and Behavioral Research

ETHICAL PRINCIPLES AND GUIDELINES FOR RESEARCH INVOLVING HUMAN SUBJECTS

Scientific research has produced substantial social benefits. It has also posed some troubling ethical questions. Public attention was drawn to these questions by reported abuses of human subjects in biomedical experiments, especially during the Second World War. During the Nuremberg War Crime Trials, the Nuremberg code was drafted as a set of standards for judging physicians and scientists who had conducted biomedical experiments on concentration camp prisoners. This code became the prototype of many later codes intended to assure that research involving human subjects would be carried out in an ethical manner.

The codes consist of rules, some general, others specific, that guide the investigators or the reviewers of research in their work. Such rules often are inadequate to cover complex situations; at times they come into conflict, and they are frequently difficult to interpret or apply. Broader ethical principles will provide a basis on which specific rules may be formulated, criticized and interpreted.

Three principles, or general prescriptive judgments, that are relevant to research involving human subjects are identified in this statement. Other principles may also be relevant. These three are comprehensive, however, and are stated at a level of generalization that should assist scientists, subjects, reviewers and interested citizens to understand the ethical issues inherent in research involving

human subjects. These principles cannot always be applied so as to resolve beyond dispute particular ethical problems. The objective is to provide an analytical framework that will guide the resolution of ethical problems arising from research involving human subjects.

This statement consists of a distinction between research and practice, a discussion of the three basic ethical principles.

PART A: BOUNDARIES BETWEEN PRACTICE & RESEARCH

It is important to distinguish between biomedical and behavioral research, on the one hand, and the practice of accepted therapy on the other, in order to know what activities ought to undergo review for the protection of human subjects of research. The distinction between research and practice is blurred partly because both often occur together (as in research designed to evaluate a therapy) and partly because notable departures from standard practice are often called "experimental" when the terms "experimental" and "research" are not carefully defined.

For the most part, the term "practice" refers to interventions that are designed solely to enhance the well-being of an individual patient or client and that have a reasonable expectation of success. The purpose of medical or behavioral practice is to provide diagnosis, preventive treatment or therapy to particular individuals.[1] By contrast, the term "research" designates an activity designed to test an hypothesis, permit conclusions to be drawn, and thereby to develop or contribute to generalizable knowledge (expressed, for example, in theories, principles, and statements of relationships). Research is usually described in a formal protocol that sets forth an objective and a set of procedures designed to reach that objective.

From http://ohrp.osophs.dhhs.gov/humansubjects/guidance/belmont.htm.22 October2001.

Editors' note: Some author's notes have been cut. Students who want to follow up on sources should consult the original article.

When a clinician departs in a significant way from standard or accepted practice, the innovation does not, in and of itself, constitute research. The fact that a procedure is "experimental," in the sense of new, untested or different, does not automatically place it in the category of research. Radically new procedures of this description should, however, be made the object of formal research at an early stage in order to determine whether they are safe and effective. Thus, it is the responsibility of medical practice committees, for example, to insist that a major innovation be incorporated into a formal research project.

Research and practice may be carried on together when research is designed to evaluate the safety and efficacy of a therapy. This need not cause any confusion regarding whether or not the activity requires review; the general rule is that if there is any element of research in an activity, that activity should undergo review for the protection of human subjects.

PART B: BASIC ETHICAL PRINCIPLES

The expression "basic ethical principles" refers to those general judgments that serve as a basic justification for the many particular ethical prescriptions and evaluations of human actions. Three basic principles, among those generally accepted in our cultural tradition, are particularly relevant to the ethics of research involving human subjects: the principles of respect [for] persons, beneficence and justice.

1. Respect for Persons Respect for persons incorporates at least two ethical convictions: first, that individuals should be treated as autonomous agents, and second, that persons with diminished autonomy are entitled to protection. The principle of respect for persons thus divides into two separate moral requirements: the requirement to acknowledge autonomy and the requirement to protect those with diminished autonomy.

An autonomous person is an individual capable of deliberation about personal goals and of acting under the direction of such deliberation. To respect autonomy is to give weight to autonomous persons' considered opinions and choices while refraining from obstructing their actions unless they are clearly detrimental to others. To show lack of respect for an autonomous agent is to repudiate that person's considered judgments, to deny an individual the freedom to act on those considered judgments, or to withhold information necessary to make a considered judgment, when there are no compelling reasons to do so.

However, not every human being is capable of self-determination. The capacity for self-determination matures during an individual's life, and some individuals lose this capacity wholly or in part because of illness, mental disability, or circumstances that severely restrict liberty. Respect for the immature and the incapacitated may require protecting them as they mature or while they are incapacitated.

Some persons are in need of extensive protection, even to the point of excluding them from activities which may harm them; other persons require little protection beyond making sure they undertake activities freely and with awareness of possible adverse consequence. The extent of protection afforded should depend upon the risk of harm and the likelihood of benefit. The judgment that any individual lacks autonomy should be periodically reevaluated and will vary in different situations.

In most cases of research involving human subjects, respect for persons demands that subjects enter into the research voluntarily and with adequate information. In some situations, however, application of the principle is not obvious. The involvement of prisoners as subjects of research provides an instructive example. On the one hand, it would seem that the principle of respect for persons requires that prisoners not be deprived of the opportunity to volunteer for research. On the other hand, under prison conditions they may be subtly coerced or unduly influenced to engage in research activities for which they would not otherwise volunteer. Respect for persons would then dictate that prisoners be protected. Whether to allow prisoners to "volunteer" or to "protect" them presents a dilemma. Respecting persons, in most hard cases, is often a matter of balancing competing claims urged by the principle of respect itself.

2. Beneficence Persons are treated in an ethical manner not only by respecting their decisions and protecting them from harm, but also by making efforts to secure their well-being. Such treatment falls under the principle of beneficence. The term "beneficence" is often understood to cover acts of kindness or charity that go beyond strict obligation. In this document, beneficence is understood in a stronger sense, as an obligation. Two general rules have been formulated as complementary expressions of beneficent actions in this sense: (1) do not harm and (2) maximize possible benefits and minimize possible harms.

The Hippocratic maxim "do no harm" has long been a fundamental principle of medical ethics. Claude Bernard extended it to the realm of research, saying that one should not injure one person regardless of the benefits that might come to others. However, even avoiding harm requires learning what is harmful; and, in the process of obtaining this information, persons may be exposed to risk of harm. Further, the Hippocratic Oath requires physicians to benefit their patients "according to their best judgment." Learning what will in fact benefit may require exposing persons to risk. The problem posed by these imperatives is to decide when it is justifiable to seek certain benefits despite the risks involved, and when the benefits should be foregone because of the risks.

The obligations of beneficence affect both individual investigators and society at large, because they extend both to particular research projects and to the entire enterprise of research. In the case of particular projects, investigators and members of their institutions are obliged to give forethought to the maximization of benefits and the reduction of risk that might occur from the research investigation. In the case of scientific research in general, members of the larger society are obliged to recognize the longer term benefits and risks that may result from the improvement of knowledge and from the development of novel medical, psychotherapeutic, and social procedures.

The principle of beneficence often occupies a well-defined justifying role in many areas of research involving human subjects. An example is found in research involving children. Effective ways of treating childhood diseases and fostering healthy development are benefits that serve to justify research involving children—even when individual research subjects are not direct beneficiaries. Research also makes it possible to avoid the harm that may result from the application of previously accepted routine practices that on closer investigation turn out to be dangerous. But the role of the principle of beneficence is not always so unambiguous. A difficult ethical problem remains, for example, about research that presents more than minimal risk without immediate prospect of direct benefit to the children involved. Some have argued that such research is inadmissible, while others have pointed out that this limit would rule out much research promising great benefit to children in the future. Here again, as with all hard cases, the different claims covered by the principle of beneficence may come into conflict and force difficult choices.

3. Justice   Who ought to receive the benefits of research and bear its burdens? This is a question of justice, in the sense of "fairness in distribution" or "what is deserved." An injustice occurs when some benefit to which a person is entitled is denied without good reason or when some burden is imposed unduly. Another way of conceiving the principle of justice is that equals ought to be treated equally. However, this statement requires explication. Who is equal and who is unequal? What considerations justify departure from equal distribution? Almost all commentators allow that distinctions based on experience, age, deprivation, competence, merit and position do sometimes constitute criteria justifying differential treatment for certain purposes. It is necessary, then, to explain in what respects people should be treated equally. There are several widely accepted formulations of just ways to distribute burdens and benefits. Each formulation mentions some relevant property on the basis of which burdens and benefits should be distributed. These formulations are (1) to each person an equal share, (2) to each person according to individual need, (3) to each person according to individual effort, (4) to each person according to societal contribution, and (5) to each person according to merit.

Questions of justice have long been associated with social practices such as punishment, taxation and political representation. Until recently these questions have not generally been associated with scientific research. However, they are foreshadowed even in the earliest reflections on the ethics of research involving human subjects. For example, during the 19th and early 20th centuries the burdens of serving as research subjects fell largely upon poor ward patients, while the benefits of improved medical care flowed primarily to private patients. Subsequently, the exploitation of unwilling prisoners as research subjects in Nazi concentration camps was condemned as a particularly flagrant injustice. In this country, in the 1940's the Tuskegee syphilis study used disadvantaged, rural black men to study the untreated course of a disease that is by no means confined to that population. These subjects were deprived of demonstrably effective treatment in order not to interrupt the project, long after such treatment became generally available.

Against this historical background, it can be seen how conceptions of justice are relevant to research involving human subjects. For example, the selection of research subjects needs to be scrutinized in order to determine whether some classes (e.g., welfare patients, particular racial and ethnic minorities, or persons confined to institutions) are being systematically selected simply because of their easy availability, their compromised position, or their manipulability, rather than for reasons directly related to the problem being studied. Finally, whenever research supported by public funds leads to the development of therapeutic devices and procedures, justice demands both that these not provide advantages only to those who can afford them and that such research should not unduly involve persons from groups unlikely to be among the beneficiaries of subsequent applications of the research.

PART C: APPLICATIONS

Applications of the general principles to the conduct of research leads to consideration of the following requirements: informed consent, risk/benefit assessment, and the selection of subjects of research.

1. Informed Consent Respect for persons requires that subjects, to the degree that they are capable, be given the opportunity to choose what shall or shall not happen to them. This opportunity is provided when adequate standards for informed consent are satisfied.

While the importance of informed consent is unquestioned, controversy prevails over the nature and possibility of an informed consent. Nonetheless, there is widespread agreement that the consent process can be analyzed as containing three elements: information, comprehension and voluntariness.

Information Most codes of research establish specific items for disclosure intended to assure that subjects are given sufficient information. These items generally include: the research procedure, their purposes, risks and anticipated benefits, alternative procedures (where therapy is involved), and a statement offering the subject the opportunity to ask questions and to withdraw at any time from the research. Additional items have been proposed, including how subjects are selected, the person responsible for the research, etc.

However, a simple listing of items does not answer the question of what the standard should be for judging how much and what sort of information should be provided. One standard frequently invoked in medical practice, namely the information commonly provided by practitioners in the field or in the locale, is inadequate since research takes place precisely when a common understanding does not exist. Another standard, currently popular in malpractice law, requires the practitioner to reveal the information that reasonable persons would wish to know in order to make a decision regarding their care. This, too, seems insufficient since the research subject, being in essence a volunteer, may wish to know considerably more about risks gratuitously undertaken than do patients who deliver themselves into the hand of a clinician for needed care. It may be that a standard of "the reasonable volunteer" should be proposed: the extent and nature of information should be such that persons, knowing that the procedure is neither necessary for their care nor perhaps fully understood, can decide whether they wish to participate in the furthering of knowledge. Even when some direct benefit to them is anticipated, the subjects should understand clearly the range of risk and the voluntary nature of participation.

A special problem of consent arises where informing subjects of some pertinent aspect of the research is likely to impair the validity of the research. In many cases, it is sufficient to indicate to subjects that they are being invited to participate in research of which some features will not be revealed until the research is concluded. In all cases of research involving incomplete disclosure, such research is justified only if it is clear that (1) incomplete disclosure is truly necessary to accomplish the goals of the research, (2) there are no undisclosed risks to subjects that are more than minimal, and (3) there is an adequate plan for debriefing subjects, when appropriate, and for dissemination of research results to them. Information about risks should never be withheld for the purpose of eliciting the cooperation of subjects, and truthful answers should always be given to direct questions about the research. Care should be taken to distinguish cases in which disclosure would destroy or invalidate the research from cases in which disclosure would simply [in]convenience the investigator.

Comprehension The manner and context in which information is conveyed is as important as the information itself. For example, presenting information in a disorganized and rapid fashion, allowing too little time for consideration or curtailing opportunities for questioning, all may adversely affect a subject's ability to make an informed choice.

Because the subject's ability to understand is a function of intelligence, rationality, maturity and language, it is necessary to adapt the presentation of the information to the subject's capacities. Investigators are responsible for ascertaining that the subject has comprehended the information. While there is always an obligation to ascertain that the information about risk to subjects is complete and adequately comprehended, when the risks are more serious, that obligation increases. On occasion, it may be suitable to give some oral or written tests of comprehension.

Special provision may need to be made when comprehension is severely limited—for example, by conditions of immaturity or mental disability. Each class of subjects that one might consider as incompetent (e.g., infants and young children, mentally disabled patients, the terminally ill and the comatose) should be considered on its own terms. Even for these persons, however, respect requires giving them the opportunity to choose to the extent they are able, whether or not to participate in research. The objections of these subjects to involvement should be honored, unless the research entails providing them a therapy unavailable elsewhere. Respect for persons also requires seeking the permission of other parties in order to protect the subjects from harm. Such persons are thus respected both by acknowledging their own wishes and by the use of third parties to protect them from harm.

The third parties chosen should be those who are most likely to understand the incompetent subject's situation and to act in that person's best interest.

The person authorized to act on behalf of the subject should be given an opportunity to observe the research as it proceeds in order to be able to withdraw the subject from the research, if such action appears in the subject's best interest.

Voluntariness An agreement to participate in research constitutes a valid consent only if voluntarily given. This element of informed consent requires conditions free of coercion and undue influence. Coercion occurs when an overt threat of harm is intentionally presented by one person to another in order to obtain compliance. Undue influence, by contrast, occurs through an offer of an excessive, unwarranted, inappropriate or improper reward or other overture in order to obtain compliance. Also, inducements that would ordinarily be acceptable may become undue influences if the subject is especially vulnerable.

Unjustifiable pressures usually occur when persons in positions of authority or commanding influence—especially where possible sanctions are involved—urge a course of action for a subject. A continuum of such influencing factors exists, however, and it is impossible to state precisely where justifiable persuasion ends and undue influence begins. But undue influence would include actions such as manipulating a person's choice through the controlling influence of a close relative and threatening to withdraw health services to which an individual would otherwise be entitled.

2. Assessment of Risks and Benefits The assessment of risks and benefits requires a careful arrangement of relevant data, including, in some cases, alternative ways of obtaining the benefits sought in the research. Thus, the assessment presents both an opportunity and a responsibility to gather systematic and comprehensive information about proposed research. For the investigator, it is a means to examine whether the proposed research is properly designed. For a review committee, it is a method for determining whether the risks that will be presented to subjects are justified. For prospective subjects, the assessment will assist the determination whether or not to participate.

The Nature and Scope of Risks and Benefits The requirement that research be justified on the basis of a favorable risk/benefit assessment bears a close relation to the principle of beneficence, just as the moral requirement that informed consent be obtained is derived primarily from the principle of respect for persons. The term "risk" refers to a possibility that harm may occur. However, when expressions such as "small risk" or "high risk" are used, they usually refer (often ambiguously) both to the chance (probability) of experiencing a harm and the severity (magnitude) of the envisioned harm.

The term "benefit" is used in the research context to refer to something of positive value related to health or welfare. Unlike, "risk," "benefit" is not a term that expresses probabilities. Risk is properly contrasted to probability of benefits, and benefits are properly contrasted with harms rather than risks of harm. Accordingly, so-called risk/benefit assessments are concerned with the probabilities and magnitudes of possible harm and anticipated benefits. Many kinds of possible harms and benefits need to be taken into account. There are, for example, risks of psychological harm, physical harm, legal harm, social harm and economic harm and the corresponding benefits. While the most likely types of harms to research subjects are those of psychological or physical pain or injury, other possible kinds should not be overlooked.

Risks and benefits of research may affect the individual subjects, the families of the individual subjects, and society at large (or special groups of subjects in society). Previous codes and federal regulations have required that risks to subjects be outweighed by the sum of both the anticipated benefit to the subject, if any, and the anticipated benefit to society in the form of knowledge to be gained from the research. In balancing these different elements, the risks and benefits affecting the immediate research subject will normally carry special weight. On the other hand, interests other than those of the subject may on some occasions be sufficient by themselves to justify the risks involved in the research, so long as the subjects' rights have been protected. Beneficence thus requires that we protect against risk of harm to subjects and also that we be concerned about the loss of the substantial benefits that might be gained from research.

The Systematic Assessment of Risks and Benefits

It is commonly said that benefits and risks must be "balanced" and shown to be "in a favorable ratio."

The metaphorical character of these terms draws attention to the difficulty of making precise judgments. Only on rare occasions will quantitative techniques be available for the scrutiny of research protocols. However, the idea of systematic, nonarbitrary analysis of risks and benefits should be emulated insofar as possible. This ideal requires those making decisions about the justifiability of research to be thorough in the accumulation and assessment of information about all aspects of the research, and to consider alternatives systematically. This procedure renders the assessment of research more rigorous and precise, while making communication between review board members and investigators less subject to misinterpretation, misinformation and conflicting judgments. Thus, there should first be a determination of the validity of the presuppositions of the research; then the nature, probability and magnitude of risk should be distinguished with as much clarity as possible. The method of ascertaining risks should be explicit, especially where there is no alternative to the use of such vague categories as small or slight risk. It should also be determined whether an investigator's estimates of the probability of harm or benefits are reasonable, as judged by known facts or other available studies.

Finally, assessment of the justifiability of research should reflect at least the following considerations: (i) Brutal or inhumane treatment of human subjects is never morally justified. (ii) Risks should be reduced to those necessary to achieve the research objective. It should be determined whether it is in fact necessary to use human subjects at all. Risk can perhaps never be entirely eliminated, but it can often be reduced by careful attention to alternative procedures. (iii) When research involves significant risk of serious impairment, review committees should be extraordinarily insistent on the justification of the risk (looking usually to the likelihood of benefit to the subject—or, in some rare cases, to the manifest voluntariness of the participation). (iv) When vulnerable populations are involved in research, the appropriateness of involving them should itself be demonstrated. A number of variables go into such judgments, including the nature and degree of risk, the condition of the particular population involved, and the nature and level of the anticipated benefits. (v) Relevant risks and benefits must be thoroughly arrayed in documents and procedures used in the informed consent process.

3. Selection of Subjects Just as the principle of respect for persons finds expression in the requirements for consent, and the principle of beneficence in risk/benefit assessment, the principle of justice gives rise to moral requirements that there be fair procedures and outcomes in the selection of research subjects.

Justice is relevant to the selection of subjects of research at two levels: the social and the individual. Individual justice in the selection of subjects would require that researchers exhibit fairness: thus, they should not offer potentially beneficial research only to some patients who are in their favor or select only "undesirable" persons for risky research. Social justice requires that distinction be drawn between classes of subjects that ought, and ought not, to participate in any particular kind of research, based on the ability of members of that class to bear burdens and on the appropriateness of placing further burdens on already burdened persons. Thus, it can be considered a matter of social justice that there is an order of preference in the selection of classes of subjects (e.g., adults before children) and that some classes of potential subjects (e.g., the institutionalized mentally infirm or prisoners) may be involved as research subjects, if at all, only on certain conditions.

Injustice may appear in the selection of subjects, even if individual subjects are selected fairly by investigators and treated fairly in the course of research. Thus injustice arises from social, racial, sexual and cultural biases institutionalized in society. Thus, even if individual researchers are treating their research subjects fairly, and even if IRBs are taking care to assure that subjects are selected fairly within a particular institution, unjust social patterns may nevertheless appear in the overall distribution of the burdens and benefits of research. Although individual institutions or investigators may not be able to resolve a problem that is pervasive in their social setting, they can consider distributive justice in selecting research subjects.

Some populations, especially institutionalized ones, are already burdened in many ways by their infirmities and environments. When research is proposed that involves risks and does not include a therapeutic component, other less burdened classes of persons should be called upon first to accept these risks of research, except where the research is directly related to the specific conditions of the class involved. Also, even though public funds for research may often flow in the same directions as public funds for health care, it seems unfair that populations dependent on public health care constitute a pool of preferred research subjects if more advantaged populations are likely to be the recipients of the benefits.

One special instance of injustice results from the involvement of vulnerable subjects. Certain groups, such as racial minorities, the economically disadvantaged, the very sick, and the institutionalized may continually be sought as research subjects, owing to their ready availability in settings where research is conducted. Given their dependent status and their frequently compromised capacity for free consent, they should be protected against the danger of being involved in research solely for administrative convenience, or because they are easy to manipulate as a result of their illness or socioeconomic condition.

NOTE

1. Although practice usually involves interventions designed solely to enhance the well-being of a particular individual, interventions are sometimes applied to one individual for the enhancement of the well-being of another (e.g., blood donation, skin grafts, organ transplants) or an intervention may have the dual purpose of enhancing the well-being of a particular individual, and, at the same time, providing some benefit to others (e.g., vaccination, which protects both the person who is vaccinated and society generally). The fact that some forms of practice have elements other than immediate benefit to the individual receiving an intervention, however, should not confuse the general distinction between research and practice. Even when a procedure applied in practice may benefit some other person, it remains an intervention designed to enhance the well-being of a particular individual or groups of individuals; thus, it is practice and need not be reviewed as research.

THE ETHICS OF RANDOMIZED CLINICAL TRIALS

ETHICAL DIFFICULTIES WITH RANDOMIZED CLINICAL TRIALS INVOLVING CANCER PATIENTS: EXAMPLES FROM THE FIELD OF GYNECOLOGIC ONCOLOGY

Maurie Markman

In a recent issue of the *New England Journal of Medicine*, two prominent clinical investigators took opposite sides in a debate on the need for and the ethics of randomized clinical trials.[1] The basic argument in support of randomized clinical trials is that in the absence of such studies it is not possible to be certain that a new drug or clinical intervention is actually beneficial to patients with a particular disease or condition, compared either to a "standard" (accepted or approved) therapeutic strategy or to no treatment at all (an untreated control population). The major argument against the performance of randomized clinical trials is that the individual physician's principal ethical responsibility is to the *individual patient* that he or she is treating, and *not* to future patients who may benefit from the potentially important information gained through a well-designed and well-conducted randomized trial. If one accepts this argument, a physician should only recommend that an individual patient participate in a randomized trial if he or she is convinced that neither one of the treatment programs is superior based on previous data available in the medical literature. If it is the *physician's best judgment*—based on his or her interpretation of this data, personal experience, and knowledge of the individual patient's specific medical condition—that one regimen would be preferred over the other(s), then the physician should not recommend that the patient participate in this trial, no matter how important the information gained may be to society.

Physicians working with cancer patients have frequently been able to avoid the difficult ethical dilemma presented above, as experimental (not FDA-approved) antineoplastic agents have traditionally

From *Journal of Clinical Ethics* 3, no. 3 (Fall 1992): 193–195. Copyright © 1992 by the *Journal of Clinical Ethics*. All rights reserved. Reprinted with permission.

only been available to patients who are willing to participate in a clinical trial. Drug development of new agents has followed a logical sequence: toxicity/dose finding studies (phase 1), followed by single-arm efficacy trials in specific disease settings (phase 2), followed by randomized trials to define the "true benefit" of the new therapy (phase 3). In the toxicity studies, the major goal of the treatment is to define the appropriate dose that produces acceptable toxicity, while in the efficacy studies, the aim is to determine if the agent is effective in a particular disease setting. Thus, the physician who believes, based on previously reported clinical data (usually from phase-2 drug trials), that a new drug is potentially superior to the standard therapy would have no choice but to recommend that the patient participate in the trial. In this way, the patient would have a 50 percent chance of receiving the new therapy (and a 50 percent chance of being placed in the control group), compared to a 0 percent chance if he or she does not participate in the study.

We are currently witnessing this process with the new antineoplastic agent, taxol. The drug, which has a unique mechanism of cytotoxic activity, has recently been demonstrated to cause temporary regression of tumor in approximately 20 to 30 percent of patients with advanced ovarian cancer who have previously failed standard therapy for their disease.[2] At the present time, there is absolutely no evidence that the drug is curative when used in the advanced refractory disease setting, and most responses last less than six to nine months. However, the response rate observed in this particular patient population is superior to what has been demonstrated with other commercially available drugs.

Interest in, and praise for, the effectiveness of taxol has spread far beyond the confines of medical meetings and the peer-reviewed medical literature. This is partly due to the fact that the agent is a natural product, and obtaining sufficient quantities of the drug requires the sacrifice of a large number of endangered trees in the Pacific Northwest. A number of scientists and biomedical companies, as well as the National Cancer Institute, are actively seeking to find new sources of taxol so as to make the drug more widely available to patients with ovarian cancer and other malignancies.

Currently, the Gynecologic Oncology Group, a national multi-institutional cooperative group

devoted to the study of cancers involving gynecologic organs, is conducting a randomized trial of a standard chemotherapy regimen (without taxol) compared to a program that includes taxol, in patients with ovarian cancer who have not previously received chemotherapy. This is an important trial, as it should determine what role, if any, taxol should play in the initial management of a patient with advanced ovarian cancer.

A physician hoping to give a patient taxol, in the belief that a regimen that includes this drug may be superior to the current standard regimen, would have to attempt to enter the patient into this randomized trial. But what if the drug, still considered an experimental agent, were made more widely available from the National Cancer Institute? Would a physician who wanted a woman with ovarian cancer to receive taxol be justified in placing the individual on a randomized trial when there were other methods to obtain the drug without randomization? Or, as is frequently asked of cancer specialists when they discuss treatment options with patients, would they recommend this trial to their wife, sister, or mother? This question, perhaps the most difficult one addressed to oncologists concerning experimental clinical trials, gets to the fundamental core of the issue: Is the physician acting *solely* in the best interest of the patient, or are other considerations (such as the scientific or societal need to know whether one treatment program is superior) playing a role in the doctor's deliberations?

A second example of the physician's dilemma over whether to recommend that a patient participate in a randomized trial—one that is more complex, as it does not involve the use of experimental drugs whose access can be controlled—concerns the current status of chemotherapy for advanced metastatic cancer of the uterus (endometrial cancer). Unfortunately, chemotherapy has only demonstrated limited activity in this disease, with partial responses of short durations being observed in approximately 20 percent of treated patients.

Recently, clinical investigators at the Mayo Clinic reported the results of a nonrandomized trial of a combination chemotherapy regimen in twenty-five patients with advanced cancer of the uterus that employed four commercially available cytotoxic agents.[3] The investigators observed a 60 percent objective response rate, and the authors of the report concluded that the regimen "is highly active in advanced endometrial carcinoma and results in improved survival compared to literature controls."[4] The Mayo Clinic investigators are noted for the quality of their work. In addition, they are generally conservative in the interpretation of their own data. Thus, the results of this trial are quite interesting and encouraging. However, this was a nonrandomized trial, and it is possible that unintentional selection bias may have accounted for the results observed. The only method available to determine definitively if the more toxic, multidrug combination regimen is superior in efficacy to a standard single-agent program would be to conduct a randomized clinical trial.

One can be fairly certain that a randomized trial comparing these two treatment programs will be forthcoming. Should patients be entered into such a trial? Again, the ethical issue for the individual physician comes down to how he or she interprets the results of this investigative program compared to a standard chemotherapy regimen in cancer of the uterus. If the physician cannot accept the results as providing reasonable evidence for superiority of the newer regimen over standard therapy, then he or she is justified in entering patients into such a trial. But if the physician believes that the results suggest increased efficacy with acceptable toxicity, it is difficult to agree with the argument that the physician is acting in the *patient's* best interest if he recommends entry into the randomized trial. The question must be asked again: If this were your wife, mother, or sister, what would you recommend?

A final example illustrates the potential for serious ethical conflict between the importance of obtaining information to define management options for future patients with malignancy, and the critical need to safeguard the patient's best interest. Standard treatment of patients with advanced cancer of the ovary involves an attempt to remove surgically as much tumor as possible from the abdominal cavity (tumor "debulking") prior to the institution of chemotherapy.[5] This is a unique management strategy. In almost all other malignancies, surgery is employed in the initial management of the disease only when it is believed possible that all macroscopic tumor can be removed. However, in patients with ovarian cancer, this surgery is a standard management strategy, even though physicians know that the approach cannot cure patients with disease disseminated throughout

the abdominal cavity. What, then, is the justification for this therapeutic strategy?

Multiple retrospective and prospective studies have demonstrated that patients with ovarian cancer who start chemotherapy after surgical resection with small-volume residual disease respond better to the chemotherapy and survive longer than patients with large-volume residual disease.[6] This has led to the conclusion that the surgical removal of tumor increases the effectiveness of chemotherapy, presumably resulting from improved blood supply and delivery of the cytotoxic drug to the remaining tumor, or removal of a large portion of cells that may be resistant to the effects of the anticancer agents. However, this hypothesis has *never* been tested in a randomized trial. It is certainly possible that the surgeon's ability to remove bulky intraabdominal tumor and leave the patient with small-volume residual disease may simply select patients who would have done well with chemotherapy even if surgery were not performed. Perhaps the factors that permit invasiveness and interfere with a surgeon's ability to debulk tumor are the same factors that lead to a tumor having an enhanced ability to develop drug-resistant cells rapidly and escape the effects of the antineoplastic agents.

Thus, the only way to answer this important biological and clinical question would be to randomize women with ovarian cancer *who would otherwise be able to undergo debulking surgery* either to have the procedure performed or to start the treatment program with chemotherapy but without surgery. In this way, the role of a major surgical procedure could be evaluated definitively. Unfortunately, the conduct of such a trial leads to serious ethical difficulties. A woman who is randomized to debulking surgery, followed by chemotherapy, will be receiving standard therapy, and her ultimate clinical outcome will be unaffected by the conduct of the trial. However, a woman randomized to receive chemotherapy without surgery cannot be given such a guarantee. While that patient may experience less morbidity by not undergoing the debulking surgery, there is no reason to believe her ultimate outcome will be favorably influenced by participating in this trial. And if it is subsequently determined that surgery does, in fact, play an important role in the management of this condition, *her* survival may have been compromised by participating in the study. Clinical science may have benefited greatly from the conduct of this study, but individual patients may have paid dearly for their participation. Thus, unless another method can be found to address the question of the role of debulking surgery in patients with cancer of the ovary, this procedure must remain a major part of the management of individuals with the disease.

In this article, I have attempted to present examples of the ethical difficulties with randomized clinical trials experienced by physicians caring for real patients with malignant disease. Above all, the physician's responsibility is to the individual patient, and the need to increase knowledge to improve the lot of future patients must always take second place.

NOTES

1. S. Hellman and D. Hellman, "Of Mice but Not Men: Problems of the Randomized Clinical Trial," *New England*

Journal of Medicine 324 (1991): 1585–89; E. Passamani, "Clinical Trials: Are They Ethical?" *New England Journal of Medicine* 324 (1991): 1589–92.

2. W.P. McGuire, E.K. Rowinsky, N.B. Rosenshein, *et al.,* "Taxol: A Unique Antineoplastic Agent with Significant Activity in Advanced Ovarian Epithelial Neoplasms," *Annals of Internal Medicine* 111 (1989): 273–79.

3. H.J. Long, R.M. Langdon, and H.S. Wieand, "Phase II Trial of Methotrexate, Vinblastine, Doxorubicin, and Cisplatin in Women with Advanced Endometrial Carcinoma," *Proceedings of the American Society of Clinical Oncology* 10 (1991): 184.

4. *Ibid.*

5. R.C. Young, Z. Fuks, and W.J. Hoskins, "Cancer of the Ovary," in *Cancer: Principles and Practice of Oncology,* ed. V.T. DeVita, Jr., S. Hellman, and S.A. Rosenberg (Philadelphia: J.B. Lippincott, 1989), 1162–96.

6. *Ibid.*

OF MICE BUT NOT MEN: PROBLEMS OF THE RANDOMIZED CLINICAL TRIAL

Samuel Hellman and Deborah S. Hellman

As medicine has become increasingly scientific and less accepting of unsupported opinion or proof by anecdote, the randomized controlled clinical trial has become the standard technique for changing diagnostic or therapeutic methods. The use of this technique creates an ethical dilemma.[1,2] Researchers participating in such studies are required to modify their ethical commitments to individual patients and do serious damage to the concept of the physician as a practicing, empathetic professional who is primarily concerned with each patient as an individual. Researchers using a randomized clinical trial can be described as physician-scientists, a term that expresses the tension between the two roles.

From *New England Journal of Medicine* 324, no. 22 (May 30, 1991): 1589–1592. Copyright © 1991, Massachusetts Medical Society. All rights reserved. Used with permission.

The physician, by entering into a relationship with an individual patient, assumes certain obligations, including the commitment always to act in the patient's best interests. As Leon Kass has rightly maintained, "the physician must produce unswervingly the virtues of loyalty and fidelity to his patient."[3] Though the ethical requirements of this relationship have been modified by legal obligations to report wounds of a suspicious nature and certain infectious diseases, these obligations in no way conflict with the central ethical obligation to act in the best interests of the patient medically. Instead, certain nonmedical interests of the patient are preempted by other social concerns.

The role of the scientist is quite different. The clinical scientist is concerned with answering questions—i.e., determining the validity of formally constructed hypotheses. Such scientific information, it is presumed, will benefit humanity in general.

The clinical scientist's role has been well described by Dr. Anthony Fauci, director of the National Institute of Allergy and Infectious Diseases, who states the goals of the randomized clinical trial in these words: "It's not to deliver therapy. It's to answer a scientific question so that the drug can be available for everybody once you've established safety and efficacy."[4] The demands of such a study can conflict in a number of ways with the physician's duty to minister to patients. The study may create a false dichotomy in the physician's opinions; according to the premise of the randomized clinical trial, the physician may only know or not know whether a proposed course of treatment represents an improvement; no middle position is permitted. What the physician thinks, suspects, believes, or has a hunch about is assigned to the "not knowing" category, because knowing is defined on the basis of an arbitrary but accepted statistical test performed in a randomized clinical trial. Thus, little credence is given to information gained beforehand in other ways or to information accrued during the trial but without the required statistical degree of assurance that a difference is not due to chance. The randomized clinical trial also prevents the treatment technique from being modified on the basis of the growing knowledge of the physicians during their participation in the trial. Moreover, it limits access to the data as they are collected until specific milestones are achieved. This prevents physicians from profiting not only from their individual experience, but also from the collective experience of the other participants.

The randomized clinical trial requires doctors to act simultaneously as physicians and as scientists. This puts them in a difficult and sometimes untenable ethical position. The conflicting moral demands arising from the use of the randomized clinical trial reflect the classic conflict between rights-based moral theories and utilitarian ones. The first of these, which depend on the moral theory of Immanuel Kant (and seen more recently in neo-Kantian philosophers, such as John Rawls[5]), asserts that human beings, by virtue of their unique capacity for rational thought, are bearers of dignity. As such, they ought not to be treated merely as means to an end; rather, they must always be treated as ends in themselves. Utilitarianism, by contrast, defines what is right as the greatest good for the greatest number—that is, as social utility.

This view, articulated by Jeremy Bentham and John Stuart Mill, requires that pleasures (understood broadly, to include such pleasures as health and well-being) and pains be added together. The morally correct act is the act that produces the most pleasure and the least pain overall.

A classic objection to the utilitarian position is that according to that theory, the distribution of pleasures and pains is of no moral consequence. This element of the theory severely restricts physicians from being utilitarians, or at least from following the theory's dictates. Physicians must care very deeply about the distribution of pain and pleasure, for they have entered into a relationship with one or a number of individual patients. They cannot be indifferent to whether it is these patients or others that suffer for the general benefit of society. Even though society might gain from the suffering of a few, and even though the doctor might believe that such a benefit is worth a given patient's suffering (i.e., that utilitarianism is right in the particular case), the ethical obligation created by the covenant between doctor and patient requires the doctor to see the interests of the individual patient as primary and compelling. In essence, the doctor-patient relationship requires doctors to see their patients as bearers of rights who cannot be merely used for the greater good of humanity.

As Fauci has suggested,[6] the randomized clinical trial routinely asks physicians to sacrifice the interests of their particular patients for the sake of the study and that of the information that it will make available for the benefit of society. This practice is ethically problematic. Consider first the initial formulation of a trial. In particular, consider the case of a disease for which there is no satisfactory therapy— for example, advanced cancer or the acquired immunodeficiency syndrome (AIDS). A new agent that promises more effectiveness is the subject of the study. The control group must be given either an unsatisfactory treatment or a placebo. Even though the therapeutic value of the new agent is unproved, if physicians think that it has promise, are they acting in the best interests of their patients in allowing them to be randomly assigned to the control group? Is persisting in such an assignment consistent with the specific commitments taken on in the doctor-patient relationship? As a result of interactions with patients with AIDS and their advocates, Merigan[7] recently suggested modifications in the design of clinical trials that attempt to deal with the unsatisfactory treatment given to the control group. The view of such activists has been expressed by Rebecca Pringle Smith of Community Research Initiative in New York: "Even if you have a supply of compliant martyrs, trials must have some ethical validity."[8]

If the physician has no opinion about whether the new treatment is acceptable, then random assignment is ethically acceptable, but such lack of enthusiasm for the new treatment does not augur well for either the patient or the study. Alternatively, the treatment may show promise of beneficial results but also present a risk of undesirable complications. When the physician believes that the severity and likelihood of harm and good are evenly balanced, randomization may be ethically acceptable. If the physician has no preference for either treatment (is in a state of equipoise[9,10]), then randomization is acceptable. If, however, he or she believes that the new treatment may be either more or less successful or more or less toxic, the use of randomization is not consistent with fidelity to the patient.

The argument usually used to justify randomization is that it provides, in essence, a critique of the usefulness of the physician's beliefs and opinions, those that have not yet been validated by a randomized clinical trial. As the argument goes, these not-yet-validated beliefs are as likely to be wrong as right. Although physicians are ethically required to provide their patients with the best available treatment, there simply is no best treatment yet known.

The reply to this argument takes two forms. First, and most important, even if this view of the reliability of a physician's opinions is accurate, the ethical constraints of an individual doctor's relationship with a particular patient require the doctor to provide individual care. Although physicians must take pains to make clear the speculative nature of their views, they cannot withhold these views from the patient. The patient asks from the doctor both knowledge and judgment. The relationship established between them rightfully allows patients to ask for the judgment of their particular physicians, not merely that of the medical profession in general. Second, it may not be true, in fact, that the not-yet-validated beliefs of physicians are as likely to be wrong as right. The greater certainty obtained with a randomized clinical trial is beneficial, but that does not mean that a lesser degree of certainty is without value. Physicians can acquire knowledge through methods other than the randomized clinical trial. Such knowledge, acquired over time and less formally than is required in a randomized clinical trial, may be of great value to a patient.

Even if it is ethically acceptable to begin a study, one often forms an opinion during its course— especially in studies that are impossible to conduct in a truly double-blinded fashion—that makes it ethically problematic to continue. The inability to remain blinded usually occurs in studies of cancer or AIDS, for example, because the therapy is associated by nature with serious side effects. Trials attempt to restrict the physician's access to the data in order to prevent such unblinding. Such restrictions should make physicians eschew the trial, since their ability to act in the patient's best interests will be limited. Even supporters of randomized clinical trials, such as Merigan, agree that interim findings should be presented to patients to ensure that no one receives what seems an inferior treatment.[11] Once physicians have formed a view about the new treatment, can they continue randomization? If random assignment is stopped, the study may be lost and the participation of the previous patients wasted. However, if physicians continue the randomization when they have a definite opinion about the efficacy of the experimental drug, they are not acting in accordance with the requirements of the doctor-patient relationship. Furthermore, as their opinion becomes more firm, stopping the randomization may not be enough. Physicians may be ethically required to treat the patients formerly placed in the control group with the therapy that now seems probably effective. To do so would be faithful to the obligations created by the doctor-patient relationship, but it would destroy the study.

To resolve this dilemma, one might suggest that the patient has abrogated the rights implicit in a doctor-patient relationship by signing an informed-consent form. We argue that such rights cannot be waived or abrogated. They are inalienable. The right to be treated as an individual deserving the physician's best judgment and care, rather than to be used as a means to determine the best treatment for others, is inherent in every person. This right, based on the concept of dignity, cannot be waived. What of altruism, then? Is it not the patient's right to make a sacrifice for the general good? This question must be considered from both positions—that of the patient and that of the physician. Although patients may decide to waive this right, it is not consistent with the role of a physician to ask that they do so. In asking, the doctor acts as a scientist instead. The physician's role here is to propose what he or she believes is best medically for the specific patient, not to suggest participation in a study from which the patient cannot gain. Because the opportunity to help future patients is of potential value to a patient, some would say physicians should not deny it. Although this point has merit, it offers so many opportunities for abuse that we are extremely uncomfortable about accepting it. The responsibilities of physicians are much clearer; they are to minister to the current patient.

Moreover, even if patients could waive this right, it is questionable whether those with terminal illness would be truly able to give voluntary informed consent. Such patients are extremely dependent on both their physicians and the health care system. Aware of this dependence, physicians must not ask for consent, for in such cases the very asking breaches the doctor-patient relationship. Anxious to please their physicians, patients may have difficulty refusing to participate in the trial the physicians describe. The patients may perceive their refusal as damaging to the relationship, whether or not it is so. Such perceptions of coercion affect the decision. Informed-consent forms are difficult to understand, especially for patients under the stress of serious illness for which there is no satisfactory treatment. The forms are usually lengthy, somewhat legalistic, complicated, and confusing, and they hardly bespeak the compassion expected of the medical profession. It is important to remember that those who have studied the doctor-patient relationship have emphasized its empathetic nature.

> [The] relationship between doctor and patient partakes of a peculiar intimacy. It presupposes on the part of the physician not only knowledge of his fellow men but sympathy. . . . This aspect of the practice of medicine has been designated as the art; yet I wonder whether it should not, most properly, be called the essence.[12]

How is such a view of the relationship consonant with random assignment and informed consent? The Physician's Oath of the World Medical Association affirms the primacy of the deontologic view of patients' rights: "Concern for the interests of the subject must always prevail over the interests of science and society."[13]

Furthermore, a single study is often not considered sufficient. Before a new form of therapy is generally accepted, confirmatory trials must be conducted. How can one conduct such trials ethically unless one is convinced that the first trial was in error? The ethical problems we have discussed are only exacerbated when a completed randomized clinical trial indicates that a given treatment is preferable. Even if the physician believes the initial trial was in error, the physician must indicate to the patient the full results of that trial.

The most common reply to the ethical arguments has been that the alternative is to return to the physician's intuition, to anecdotes, or to both as the basis of medical opinion. We all accept the dangers of such a practice. The argument states that we must therefore accept randomized, controlled clinical trials regardless of their ethical problems because of the great social benefit they make possible, and we salve our conscience with the knowledge that informed consent has been given. This returns us to the conflict between patients' rights and social utility. Some would argue that this tension can be resolved by placing a relative value on each. If the patient's right that is being compromised is not a fundamental right and the social gain is very great, then the study might be justified. When the right is fundamental, however, no amount of social gain, or almost none, will justify its sacrifice. Consider, for example, the experiments on humans done by physicians under the Nazi regime. All would agree that these are unacceptable regardless of the value of the scientific information gained. Some people go so far as to say that no use should be made of the results of those experiments because of the clearly unethical manner in which the data were collected. This extreme example may not seem relevant, but we believe that in its hyperbole it clarifies the fallacy of a utilitarian approach to the physician's relationship with the patient. To consider the utilitarian gain is consistent neither with the physician's role nor with the patient's rights.

It is fallacious to suggest that only the randomized clinical trial can provide valid information or that all information acquired by this technique is valid.

Such experimental methods are intended to reduce error and bias and therefore reduce the uncertainty of the result. Uncertainty cannot be eliminated, however. The scientific method is based on increasing probabilities and increasingly refined approximations of truth.[14] Although the randomized clinical trial contributes to these ends, it is neither unique nor perfect. Other techniques may also be useful.[15]

Randomized trials often place physicians in the ethically intolerable position of choosing between the good of the patient and that of society. We urge that such situations be avoided and that other techniques of acquiring clinical information be adopted. For example, concerning trials of treatments for AIDS, Byar et al.[16] have said that "some traditional approaches to the clinical-trials process may be unnecessarily rigid and unsuitable for this disease." In this case, AIDS is not what is so different; rather, the difference is in the presence of AIDS activists, articulate spokespersons for the ethical problems created by the application of the randomized clinical trial to terminal illnesses. Such arguments are equally applicable to advanced cancer and other serious illnesses. Byar et al. agree that there are even circumstances in which uncontrolled clinical trials may be justified: when there is no effective treatment to use as a control, when the prognosis is uniformly poor, and when there is a reasonable expectation of benefit without excessive toxicity. These conditions are usually found in clinical trials of advanced cancer.

The purpose of the randomized clinical trial is to avoid the problems of observer bias and patient selection. It seems to us that techniques might be developed to deal with these issues in other ways. Randomized clinical trials deal with them in a cumbersome and heavy-handed manner, by requiring large numbers of patients in the hope that random assignment will balance the heterogeneous distribution of patients into the different groups. By observing known characteristics of patients, such as age and sex, and distributing them equally between groups, it is thought that unknown factors important in determining outcomes will also be distributed equally. Surely, other techniques can be developed to deal with both observer bias and patient selection. Prospective studies without randomization, but with the evaluation of patients by uninvolved third parties, should remove observer bias. Similar methods have been suggested by Royall.[17] Prospective

matched-pair analysis, in which patients are treated in a manner consistent with their physician's views, ought to help ensure equivalence between the groups and thus mitigate the effect of patient selection, at least with regard to known covariates. With regard to unknown covariates, the security would rest, as in randomized trials, in the enrollment of large numbers of patients and in confirmatory studies. This method would not pose ethical difficulties, since patients would receive the treatment recommended by their physician. They would be included in the study by independent observers matching patients with respect to known characteristics, a process that would not affect patient care and that could be performed independently any number of times.

This brief discussion of alternatives to randomized clinical trials is sketchy and incomplete. We wish only to point out that there may be satisfactory alternatives, not to describe and evaluate them completely. Even if randomized clinical trials were much better than any alternative, however, the ethical dilemmas they present may put their use at variance with the primary obligations of the physician. In this regard, Angell cautions, "If this commitment to the patient is attenuated, even for so good a cause as benefits to future patients, the implicit assumptions of the doctor-patient relationship are violated."[18] The risk of such attenuation by the randomized trial is great. The AIDS activists have brought this dramatically to the attention of the academic medical community. Techniques appropriate to the laboratory may not be applicable to humans. We must develop and use alternative methods for acquiring clinical knowledge.

NOTES

1. Hellman S. Randomized clinical trials and the doctor-patient relationship: an ethical dilemma. *Cancer Clin Trials* 1979; 2:189–93.
2. *Idem*. A doctor's dilemma: the doctor-patient relationship in clinical investigation. In: Proceedings of the Fourth National Conference on Human Values and Cancer, New York, March 15–17, 1984. New York: American Cancer Society, 1984:144–6.
3. Kass LR. *Toward a more natural science: biology and human affairs*. New York: Free Press, 1985:196.
4. Palca J. AIDS drug trials enter new age. *Science* 1989; 246:19–21.

5. Rawls J. *A theory of justice.* Cambridge, Mass.: Belknap Press of Harvard University Press, 1971:183–92, 446–52.

6. Palca, AIDS drug trials.

7. Merigan TC. You *can* teach an old dog new tricks—how AIDS trials are pioneering new strategies. *N Engl J Med* 1990; 323: 1341–3.

8. Ibid.

9. Freedman B. Equipoise and the ethics of clinical research. *N Engl J Med* 1987; 317:141–5.

10. Singer PA, Lantos JD, Whitington PF, Broelsch CE, Siegler M. Equipoise and the ethics of segmental liver transplantation. *Clin Res* 1988; 36:539–45.

11. Merigan, You *can* teach.

12. Longcope WT. Methods and medicine. *Bull Johns Hopkins Hosp* 1932; 50:4–20.

13. Report on medical ethics. *World Med Assoc Bull* 1949; 1:109, 111.

14. Popper K. The problem of induction. In: Miller D, ed., *Popper selections.* Princeton, N.J.: Princeton University Press, 1985: 101–17.

15. Royall RM. Ethics and statistics in randomized clinical trials. *Stat Sci* 1991; 6(1):52–62.

16. Byar DP, Schoenfeld DA, Green SB, et al. Design considerations for AIDS trials. *N Engl J Med* 1990; 323: 1343–8.

17. Royall, Ethics and statistics.

18. Angell M. Patients' preferences in randomized clinical trials. *N Engl J Med* 1984; 310:1385–7.

A RESPONSE TO A PURPORTED ETHICAL DIFFICULTY WITH RANDOMIZED CLINICAL TRIALS INVOLVING CANCER PATIENTS

Benjamin Freedman

In recent years, for a variety of reasons, the mainstay of clinical investigation—the randomized controlled clinical trial (RCT)—has increasingly come under attack. Since Charles Fried's influential monograph,[1] the opponents of controlled trials have claimed the moral high ground. They claim to perceive a conflict between the medical and scientific duties of the physician-investigator, and between the conduct of the trial and a patient's rights. Samuel and Deborah Hellman write, for example, that "the randomized clinical trial routinely asks physicians to sacrifice the interests of their particular patients for the sake of the study and that of the information that it will make available for the benefit of society."[2] Maurie Markman's attraction to this point of view is clear when he writes that "the individual physician's principal ethical responsibility is to the *individual*

patient that he or she is treating, and *not* to future patients [emphases in original]." In the interests of returning Markman to the fold, I will concentrate on resolving this central challenge to the ethics of RCTs.

It is unfortunately true that the most common responses from pro-trialists, by revealing fundamental misunderstandings of basic ethical concepts, do not inspire confidence in the ethics of human research as it is currently conducted. Proponents of clinical trials will commonly begin their apologia by citing benefits derived from trials—by validating the safety and efficacy of new treatments, and, at least as important, by discrediting accepted forms of treatment. So far so good. But they often go on to argue that there is a need to balance the rights of subjects against the needs of society. By this tactic, the proponents of clinical trials have implicitly morally surrendered, for to admit that something is a right is to admit that it represents a domain of action protected from the claims or interests of other individuals or of society itself. A liberal society has rightly learned to look askance at claims that rights of individuals

From *Journal of Clinical Ethics* 3, no. 3 (Fall 1992): 231–234. Copyright © 1992 by the *Journal of Clinical Ethics.* All rights reserved. Reprinted by permission.

need to yield to the demands of the collective. Patients' claims, then, because of their nature as rights, supersede the requirements of the collectivity.

Sometimes, indeed, the surrender is explicit. At the conclusion of a symposium on the ethics of research on human subjects, Sir Colin Dollery, a major figure in clinical trials, complained to the speaker: "You assume a dominant role for ethics—I think to the point of arrogance. Ethical judgments will be of little value unless the scientific innovations about which they are made . . . are useful."[3] But it is the nature of ethical judgments that they are, indeed, "dominant" as normative or accepted guides to action. One may say, "I know that X is the ethical thing to do, but I won't X." That expresses no logical contradiction, but simply weakness of will. But it is, by contrast, plainly contradictory to admit that X is ethical, yet to deny or doubt that one ought to X.

Closer examination and finer distinctions reveal, however, that the conflict between patients' rights and social interests is not at all at issue in controlled clinical trials. There is no need for proponents of clinical trials to concede the moral high ground.

What is the patient right that is compromised by clinical trials? The fear most common to patients who are hesitant about enrolling is that they would not receive the best care, that their right to treatment would be sacrificed in the interests of science. This presumes, of course, that the patient has a right to treatment. Such a right must in reason be grounded in patient need (a patient who is not ill has no right to treatment) and in medical knowledge and capability (a patient with an incurable illness has rights to be cared for, but no right to be cured).

That granted, we need to specify the kind of treatment to which a patient might reasonably claim a right. It was in this connection that I introduced the concept of *clinical equipoise* as critical to understanding the ethics of clinical trials.[4] Clinical equipoise is a situation in which there exists (or is pending) an honest disagreement in the expert clinical community regarding the comparative merits of two or more forms of treatment for a given condition. To be ethical, a controlled clinical trial must begin and be conducted in a continuing state of clinical equipoise—as between the arms of the study—and must, moreover, offer some reasonable hope that the successful conclusion of the trial will disturb

equipoise (that is, resolve the controversy in the expert clinical community).

This theory presumes that a right to a specific medical treatment must be grounded in a professional judgment, which is concretized in the term *clinical equipoise*. A patient who has rights to medical treatment has rights restricted to, though not necessarily exhaustive of, those treatments that are understood by the medical community to be appropriate for his condition. A patient may eccentrically claim some good from a physician that is not recognized by the medical community as appropriate treatment. A physician may even grant this claim; but in so doing, he must realize that he has not provided medical treatment itself. Contrariwise, by failing to fulfill this request, the physician has not failed to satisfy the patient's right to medical treatment.

Provided that a comparative trial is ethical, therefore, it begins in a state of clinical equipoise. For that reason, by definition, nobody enrolling in the trial is denied his or her right to medical treatment, for no medical consensus for or against the treatment assignment exists.

(The modern climate requires that I introduce two simple caveats. First, I am ignoring economic and political factors that go into the grounding of a right to treatment. This is easy enough for one in Canada to write, but may be difficult for someone in the United States to read. Second, when speaking of treatment that is recognized to be condition-appropriate by the medical community, I mean to include only those judgments grounded in medical knowledge rather than social judgments. I would hope to avoid the current bioethical muddle over "medical futility," but if my claims need to be translated into terms appropriate to that controversy, "physiological futility" is close but not identical to what I mean by "inappropriate." For simplicity's sake, the best model to have in mind is the common patient demand for antibiotic treatment of an illness diagnosed as viral.)

Two errors are commonly committed in connection with the concept of clinical equipoise. The first mistake is in thinking that clinical equipoise (or its disturbance) relates to a single endpoint of a trial—commonly, efficacy. As a function of expert clinical judgment, clinical equipoise must incorporate all of the many factors that go into favoring one regimen over its competitors. Treatment *A* may be favored over *B* because it is more effective; or, because it is almost as effective but considerably less toxic; or, because it is easier to administer, allowing, for example, treatment on an outpatient basis; or, because patients are more compliant with it; and so forth.

Just as equipoise may be based upon any one or a combination of these or other factors, it may be disturbed in the same way. Markman's second example, which discusses the efficacy of a multidrug combination chemotherapy regimen, seems vulnerable to this objection. Even were the results of the Mayo trial convincing with regard to the efficacy of this approach, it has not disturbed clinical equipoise in its favor unless other issues, such as toxicity, have been resolved as well. It is well worth pointing out that the endpoints of trials, particularly in cancer treatment, are far too narrow to disturb clinical equipoise in and of themselves, but they are necessary steps along a seriatim path. For that matter, in ignoring the compendious judgment involved in ascertaining equipoise, some studies spuriously claim that all of their arms are in equipoise on the basis of one variable (such as five-year survival rates), when they are clearly out of equipoise because of other factors (such as differences in pain and disfigurement).

The second mistake occurs in identifying clinical equipoise with an individual physician's point of indifference between two treatments. Citing the article in which I developed the concept and another article applying it, for example, the Hellmans write, "If the physician has no preference for either treatment (is in a state of equipoise), then randomization is acceptable."[5] But an individual physician is not the arbiter of appropriate or acceptable medical practice.

There are numerous occasions outside of clinical trials where outsiders need to determine whether the treatment provided was appropriate to the patient's condition. Regulators, as well as third-party payers— private or governmental—need to answer the question, as do health planners and administrators of health-care facilities. Disciplinary bodies of professional associations, and, most tellingly, courts judging allegations of malpractice, have to ascertain this as well. It is never the case that the judgment of an individual physician concerning whether a treatment is condition-appropriate (that is, whether it belongs within the therapeutic armamentarium) is sufficient. In all of these instances, however varied might be their rules of investigation and procedure, the ultimate question is: Does the expert professional community accept this treatment as appropriate for this condition? Since clinical equipoise and its disturbance applies to putative medical treatments for given conditions, this is a matter that is determined legally, morally, and reasonably by that medical community with the recognized relevant expertise.

Markman may have fallen into this error, writing repeatedly of the judgment of the treating or enrolling physician (and, in the first page, of the responsibility of "the individual physician") with respect to the clinical trial. There is, however, another way of looking at this. Whereas the status of a putative treatment within the medical armamentarium must be settled by the medical *community*, the application of that judgment *vis-à-vis* a given patient is, of course, the judgment (and the responsibility) of the *individual physician*. This individual clinical judgment must be exercised when enrolling a subject, rather than subjugated to the judgment of those who constructed the trial. Indeed, many studies will list this as a criterion of exclusion: "Those subjects who, in the judgment of the accruing physician, would be put at undue risk by participating."

Another point: the Hellmans write of a physician's duty in treating a patient to employ what he "thinks, suspects, believes, or has a hunch about."[6] This is clearly overstated as a duty: why not add to the list the physician's hopes, fantasies, fond but dotty beliefs, and illusions? Yet patients do choose physicians, in part, because of trust in their tacit knowledge and inchoate judgment, and not merely their sapient grasp of the current medical consensus. It would be a disservice to patients for a physician to see his or her role simply as a vehicle for transmitting the wisdom received from the expert medical community in all cases (though when a departure is made, this is done at the legal peril of the doctor!).

But what follows from this inalienable duty of the treating physician? Not as much as the opponents of trials would have us believe. A physician certainly has the right to refuse to participate in a trial that he believes places some participants at a medical disadvantage. Moreover, if he or she is convinced of that, he or she has a *duty* to abstain from participating. But that only speaks to the physician, and does not necessarily affect the patient. What opponents of trials forget is that the patient—the subject—is the ultimate decision maker—in fact, in law, and in ethics. In at least some cases, the fact that there is an open trial for which a patient meets the eligibility criteria needs to be disclosed as one medical alternative, to satisfy ethical norms of informed consent. A physician with convictions that the trial will put subjects at undue risk should inform the prospective subject of that conviction and the reasons for it, and may well recommend to the subject to decline participation. It will then be up to the patient whether to seek enrollment via another physician.

Most commonly at issue, though, is a physician's preference rather than conviction. In such cases, it is perfectly ethical—and becomingly modest—for a physician to participate in a trial, setting aside private misgivings based upon anecdote as overbalanced by the medical literature.

Finally, something should be said about the underlying philosophical buttress on which antitrialists rely. Following Kant, the Hellmans argue that the underlying issue is that persons "ought not to be treated merely as means to an end; rather, they must always be treated as ends in themselves."[7] Clinical trials, however, are designed to yield reliable data and to ground scientifically valid inferences. In that sense, the treatments and examinations that a subject of a clinical trial undergoes are means to a scientific end, rather than interventions done solely for the subject's own benefit.

But the Kantian formulation is notoriously rigoristic, and implausible in the form cited. We treat others as means all the time, in order to achieve ends the others do not share, and are so treated in return. When buying a carton of milk or leaving a message, I am treating the cashier or secretary as means to an end they do not share. Were this unvarnished principle to hold, all but purely altruistic transactions would be ethically deficient. Clinical trials would be in very good (and, indeed, very bad) company. Those who follow the Kantian view are not concerned about treating another as a means, but rather about treating someone in a way that contradicts the other's personhood itself—that is, in

a way that denies the fact that the person is not simply a means but is also an end. A paradigm case is when I treat someone in a way that serves my ends but, at the same time, is contrary to the other's best interests. It is true that a subject's participation in a clinical trial serves scientific ends, but what has not been shown is that it is contrary to the best interests of the subject. In cases where the two equipoise conditions are satisfied, this cannot be shown.

However, in some cases we are uncertain about whether an intervention will serve the best interests of the other, and so we ask that person. That is one reason for requiring informed consent to studies. There is another. By obtaining the consent of the other party to treat him as an end to one's own means, in effect, an identity of ends between both parties has been created. Applying this amended Kantian dictum, then, we should ask: Is there anything about clinical trials that necessarily implies that subjects are treated contrary to their personhood? And the answer is, of course, no—provided a proper consent has been obtained.

There remain many hard questions to ask about the ethics of controlled clinical studies. Many talents will be needed to address those questions and to reform current practice. Since those questions will only be asked by those who understand that such studies rest upon a sound ethical foundation, I am hopeful that Markman and others will reconsider their misgivings.

NOTES

1. C. Fried, *Medical Experimentation: Personal Integrity and Social Policy* (New York: Elsevier, 1974).
2. S. Hellman and D.S. Hellman, "Of Mice but Not Men," *New England Journal of Medicine* 324 (1991): 1585–89, at 1586.
3. Comment by Sir Colin Dollery in discussion following H.-M. Sass, "Ethics of Drug Research and Drug Development," *Arzneimittel Forschung/Drug Research* 39 (II), Number 8a (1989): 1041–48, at 1048.
4. B. Freedman, "Equipoise and the Ethics of Clinical Research," *New England Journal of Medicine* 317 (1987): 141–45.
5. Hellman and Hellman, "Of Mice," 1586.
6. *Ibid.*
7. *Ibid.*

ETHICAL ISSUES IN INTERNATIONAL RESEARCH

UNETHICAL TRIALS OF INTERVENTIONS TO REDUCE PERINATAL TRANSMISSION OF THE HUMAN IMMUNODEFICIENCY VIRUS IN DEVELOPING COUNTRIES

Peter Lurie and Sidney M. Wolfe

It has been almost three years since the *Journal*[1] published the results of AIDS Clinical Trials Group (ACTG) Study 076, the first randomized, controlled trial in which an intervention was proved to reduce the incidence of human immunodeficiency virus (HIV) infection. The antiretroviral drug zidovudine, administered orally to HIV-positive pregnant women in the United States and France, administered to the newborn infants, reduced the incidence of HIV infection by two thirds.[2] The regimen can save the life of one of every seven infants born to HIV infected women.

Because of these findings, the study was terminated at the first interim analysis and within two months after the results had been announced, the Public Health Service had convened a meeting and concluded that the ACTG 076 regimen should be recommended for all HIV-positive pregnant women without substantial prior exposure to zidovudine and should be considered for other HIV-positive pregnant women on a case-by-case basis.[3] The standard of care for HIV-positive pregnant women thus became the ACTG 076 regimen.

In the United States, three recent studies of clinical practice report that the use of the ACTG 076 regimen is associated with decreases of 50 percent or more in perinatal HIV transmission.[4-6] But in developing countries, especially in Asia and sub-Saharan Africa, where it is projected that by the year 2000, 6 million pregnant women will be infected with HIV,[7] the potential of the ACTG 076 regimen remains unrealized primarily because of the drug's exorbitant cost in most countries.

From *New England Journal of Medicine* 337 (September 18, 1997): 853–856. Copyright © 1997 Massachusetts Medical Society. All rights reserved. Used with permission.

Clearly, a regimen that is less expensive than ACTG 076 but as effective is desirable, in both developing and industrialized countries. But there has been uncertainty about what research design to use in the search for a less expensive regimen. In June 1994, the World Health Organization (WHO) convened a group in Geneva to assess the agenda for research on perinatal HIV transmission in the wake of ACTG 076. The group, which included no ethicists, concluded, "Placebo-controlled trials offer the best option for a rapid and scientifically valid assessment of alternative antiretroviral drug regimens to prevent [perinatal] transmission of HIV.[8] This unpublished document has been widely cited as justification for subsequent trials in developing countries. In our view, most of these trials are unethical and will lead to hundreds of preventable HIV infections in infants.

Primarily on the basis of documents obtained from the Centers for Disease Control and Prevention (CDC), we have identified 18 randomized, controlled trials of interventions to prevent perinatal HIV transmission that either began to enroll patients after the ACTG 076 study was completed or have not yet begun to enroll patients. The studies are designed to evaluate a variety of interventions: antiretroviral drugs such as zidovudine (usually in regimens that are less expensive or complex than the ACTG 076 regimen), vitamin A and its derivatives, intrapartum vaginal washing, and HIV immune globulin, a form of immunotherapy. These trials involve a total of more than 17,000 women.

In the two studies being performed in the United States, the patients in all the study groups have unrestricted access to zidovudine or other antiretroviral drugs. In 15 of the 16 trials in developing countries, however, some or all of the patients are not provided with antiretroviral drugs. Nine of the 15 studies being conducted outside the United States are funded by the U.S. government through the CDC or the National Institutes of Health (NIH), 5 are funded by other governments, and 1 is funded by the United Nations AIDS Program. The studies are being conducted in Côte d'Ivoire, Uganda, Tanzania, South Africa, Malawi, Thailand, Ethiopia, Burkina Faso, Zimbabwe, Kenya, and the Dominican Republic. These 15 studies clearly violate recent guidelines designed specifically to address ethical issues pertaining to studies in developing countries.

According to these guidelines, "The ethical standards applied should be no less exacting than they would be in the case of research carried out in [the sponsoring] country."[9] In addition, U.S. regulations governing studies performed with federal funds domestically or abroad specify that research procedures must "not unnecessarily expose subjects to risk."[10]

The 16th study is noteworthy both as a model of an ethically conducted study attempting to identify less expensive antiretroviral regimens and as an indication of how strong the placebo-controlled trial orthodoxy is. In 1994, Marc Lallemant, a researcher at the Harvard School of Public Health, applied for NIH funding for an equivalency study in Thailand in which three shorter zidovudine regimens were to be compared with a regimen similar to that used in the ACTG 076 study. An equivalency study is typically conducted when a particular regimen has already been proved effective and one is interested in determining whether a second regimen is about as effective but less toxic or expensive.[11] The NIH study section repeatedly put pressure on Lallemant and the Harvard School of Public Health to conduct a placebo-controlled trial instead, prompting the director of Harvard's human subjects committee to reply, "The conduct of a placebo controlled trial for [zidovudine] in pregnant women in Thailand would be unethical and unacceptable, since an active-controlled trial is feasible."[12] The NIH eventually relented, and the study is now under way. Since the nine studies of antiretroviral drugs have attracted the most attention, we focus on them in this article.

ASKING THE WRONG RESEARCH QUESTION

There are numerous areas of agreement between those conducting or defending these placebo-controlled studies in developing countries and those opposing such trials. The two sides agree that perinatal HIV transmission is a grave problem meriting concerted international attention; that the ACTG 076 trial was a major breakthrough in perinatal HIV prevention; that there is a role for research on this topic in developing countries; that identifying less expensive, similarly effective interventions would be of enormous benefit, given the limited resources for medical care in most developing countries; and that randomized studies can help identify such interventions.

The sole point of disagreement is the best comparison group to use in assessing the effectiveness of less-expensive interventions once an effective intervention has been identified. The researchers conducting the placebo-controlled trials assert that such trials represent the only appropriate research design, implying that they answer the question, "Is the shorter regimen better than nothing?" We take the more optimistic view that, given the finding of ACTG 076 and other clinical information, researchers are quite capable of designing a shorter antiretroviral regimen that is approximately as effective as the ACTG 076 regimen. The proposal for the Harvard study in Thailand states the research question clearly: "Can we reduce the duration of prophylactic [zidovudine] treatment without increasing the risk of perinatal transmission of HIV, that is, without compromising the demonstrated efficacy of the standard ACTG 076 [zidovudine] regimen?"[13] We believe that such equivalency studies of alternative antiretroviral regimens will provide even more useful results than placebo-controlled trials, without the deaths of hundreds of newborns that are inevitable if placebo groups are used.

At a recent congressional hearing on research ethics, NIH director Harold Varmus was asked how the Department of Health and Human Services could be funding both a placebo-controlled trial (through the CDC) and a non-placebo-controlled equivalency study (through the NIH) in Thailand. Dr. Varmus conceded that placebo-controlled studies are "not the only way to achieve results."[14] If the research can be satisfactorily conducted in more than one way, why not select the approach that minimizes loss of life?

INADEQUATE ANALYSIS OF DATA FROM ACTG 076 AND OTHER SOURCES

The NIH, CDC, WHO, and the researchers conducting the studies we consider unethical argue that differences in the duration and route of administration of antiretroviral agents in the shorter regimens, as compared with the ACTG 076 regimen, justify the use of a placebo group.[15–18] Given that ACTG 076 was a well-conducted, randomized, controlled trial, it is disturbing that the rich data available from the study were not adequately used by the group assembled by WHO in June 1994, which recommended placebo-controlled trials after ACTG 076, or by the investigators of the 15 studies we consider unethical.

In fact, the ACTG 076 investigators conducted a subgroup analysis to identify an appropriate period for prepartum administration of zidovudine. The approximate median duration of prepartum treatment was 12 weeks. In a comparison of treatment for 12 weeks or less (average, 7) with treatment for more than 12 weeks (average, 17), there was no univariate association between the duration of treatment and its effect in reducing perinatal HIV transmission ($P = 0.99$) (Gelber R: personal communication). This analysis is somewhat limited by the number of infected infants and its post hoc nature. However, when combined with information such as the fact that in non–breast-feeding populations an estimated 65 percent of cases of perinatal HIV infection are transmitted during delivery and 95 percent of the remaining cases are transmitted within two months of delivery,[19] the analysis *suggests* that the shorter regimens may be equally effective. This finding should have been explored in later studies by randomly assigning women to longer or shorter treatment regimens.

What about the argument that the use of the oral route for intrapartum administration of zidovudine in the present trials (as opposed to the intravenous route in ACTG 076) justifies the use of a placebo? In its protocols for its two studies in Thailand and Côte d'Ivoire, the CDC acknowledged that previous "pharmacokinetic modeling data suggest that [zidovudine] serum levels obtained with this [oral] dose will be similar to levels obtained with an intravenous infusion."[20]

Thus, on the basis of the ACTG 076 data, knowledge about the timing of perinatal transmission, and pharmacokinetic data, the researchers should have had every reason to believe that well-designed shorter regimens would be more effective than placebo. These findings seriously disturb the equipoise (uncertainty over the likely study result) necessary to justify a placebo-controlled trial on ethical grounds.[21]

DEFINING PLACEBO AS THE STANDARD OF CARE IN DEVELOPING COUNTRIES

Some officials and researchers have defended the use of placebo-controlled studies in developing countries by arguing that the subjects are treated at least according to the standard of care in these countries, which consists of unproven regimens or no treatment at all. This assertion reveals a fundamental misunderstanding of the concept of the standard of care. In developing countries, the standard of care (in this case, not providing zidovudine to HIV-positive pregnant women) is not based on a consideration of alternative treatments or previous clinical data, but is instead an economically determined policy of governments that cannot afford the prices set by drug companies. We agree with the Council for International Organizations of Medical Sciences that researchers working in developing countries have an ethical responsibility to provide treatment that conforms to the standard of care in the sponsoring country, when possible.[22] An exception would be a standard of care that required an exorbitant expenditure, such as the cost of building a coronary care unit. Since zidovudine is usually made available free of charge by the manufacturer for use in clinical trials, excessive cost is not a factor in this case. Acceptance of a standard of care that does not conform to the standard in the sponsoring country results in a double standard in research. Such a double standard, which permits research designs that are unacceptable in the sponsoring country, creates an incentive to use as research subjects those with the least access to health care.

What are the potential implications of accepting such a double standard? Researchers might inject live malaria parasites into HIV-positive subjects in China in order to study the effect on the progression of HIV infection, even though the study protocol had been rejected in the United States and Mexico. Or researchers might randomly assign malnourished San (bushmen) to receive vitamin-fortified or standard bread. One might also justify trials of HIV vaccines in which the subjects were not provided with condoms or state-of-the-art counseling about safe sex by arguing that they are not customarily provided in the developing countries in question. These are not simply hypothetical worst-case

scenarios; the first two studies have already been performed,[23–24] and the third has been proposed and criticized.[25]

Annas and Grodin recently commented on the characterization and justification of placebos as a standard of care: "'Nothing' is a description of what happens; 'standard of care' is a normative standard of effective medical treatment, whether or not it is provided to a particular community."[26]

JUSTIFYING PLACEBO-CONTROLLED TRIALS BY CLAIMING THEY ARE MORE RAPID

Researchers have also sought to justify placebo-controlled trials by arguing that they require fewer subjects than equivalency studies and can therefore be completed more rapidly. Because equivalency studies are simply concerned with excluding alternative interventions that fall below some preestablished level of efficacy (as opposed to establishing which intervention is superior), it is customary to use one-sided statistical testing in such studies.[27] The numbers of women needed for a placebo-controlled trial and an equivalency study are similar.[28] In a placebo-controlled trial of a short course of zidovudine, with rates of perinatal HIV transmission of 25 percent in the placebo group and 15 percent in the zidovudine group, an alpha level of 0.05 (two-sided), and a beta level of 0.2, 500 subjects would be needed. An equivalency study with a transmission rate of 10 percent in the group receiving the ACTG 076 regimen, a difference in efficacy of 6 percent (above the 10 percent), an alpha level of 0.05 (one-sided), and a beta level of 0.2 would require 620 subjects (McCarthy W: personal communication).

TOWARD A SINGLE INTERNATIONAL STANDARD OF ETHICAL RESEARCH

Researchers assume greater ethical responsibilities when they enroll subjects in clinical studies, a precept acknowledged by Varmus recently when he insisted that all subjects in an NIH-sponsored needle-exchange trial be offered hepatitis B vaccine.[29] Residents of impoverished, postcolonial countries, the majority of whom are people of color, must be protected from potential exploitation in research.

Otherwise, the abominable state of health care in these countries can be used to justify studies that could never pass ethical muster in the sponsoring country.

With the increasing globalization of trade, government research dollars becoming scarce, and more attention being paid to the hazards posed by "emerging infections" to the residents of industrialized countries, it is likely that studies in developing countries will increase. It is time to develop standards of research that preclude the kinds of double standards evident in these trials. In an editorial published nine years ago in the *Journal*, Marcia Angell stated, "Human subjects in any part of the world should be protected by an irreducible set of ethical standards."[30] Tragically, for the hundreds of infants who have needlessly contracted HIV infection in the perinatal-transmission studies that have already been completed, any such protection will have come too late.

REFERENCES

1. Conner EM, Sperling RS, Gelber R, et al. Reduction of maternal–infant transmission of immunodeficiency virus type 1 with zidovudine treatment. N Engl J Med 1994;331:1173–80.
2. Sperling KS, Shapiro DE, Coombs RW, et al. Maternal viral load, zidovudine treatment, and the risk of transmission of human immunodeficiency virus type 1 from mother to infant. N Engl J Med 1996;33i:1621–9.
3. Recommendations of the U.S. Public Health Service Task Force on the use of zidovudine to reduce perinatal transmission of human immunodeficiency virus. MMWR Morb Mortal Wkly Rep 1994;43(RR-11):1–20.
4. Fiscus SA, Adimora AA, Schoenbach VJ, et al. Perinatal HIV infection and the effect of zidovudine therapy on transmission in rural and urban counties. JAMA 1996; 275;1483–8.
5. Cooper E, Diaz C, Pitt J, et al. Impact of ACTG 076: use of zidovudine during pregnancy and changes in the rate of HIV vertical transmission. In: Program and abstracts of the Third Conference on Retroviruses and Opportunistic Infections, Washington, D.C., January 28–February 1, 1996. Washington, D.C.: Infectious Diseases Society of America, 1996:57.
6. Simonds RJ, Nesheim, Matheson P. et al. Declining mother to child HIV transmission following perinatal ZDV recommendations. Presented at the 11th International Conference on AIDS, Vancouver, Canada, July 7–12, 1996. abstract.
7. Scarlatti C, Paediatric HIV infection. Lancet 1996; 348:863–8.
8. Recommendations from the meeting on mother-to-infant transmission of HIV by use of antiretrovirals, Geneva, World Health Organization, June 23–25, 1994.
9. World Health Organization. International ethical guidelines for biomedical research involving human subjects. Geneva: Council for International Organizations of Medical Sciences, 1993.
10. 45 CFR 46.111(a)(1).
11. Testing equivalence of two binomial proportions. In: Machin D, Campbell MJ. Statistical tables for the design of clinical trials. Oxford, England: Blackwell Scientific, 1987:35–53.
12. Brennan TA, Letter to Gilbert Meier. NIH Division of Research Ethics, December 28, 1994.
13. Lallemant M, Vithayasai V. A short ZDV course to prevent perinatal HIV in Thailand. Boston: Harvard School of Public Health, April 28, 1995.
14. Varmus H. Testimony before the Subcommittee on Human Resources, Committee on Government Reform and Oversight, U.S. House of Representatives, May 8, 1997.
15. Draft talking points: responding to Public Citizen press conference. Press release of the National Institutes of Health, April 22, 1997.
16. Questions and answers: CDC studies of AZT to prevent mother-to-child HIV transmission in developing countries. Press release of the Centers for Disease Control and Prevention, Atlanta. (undated document.)
17. Questions and answers on the UNAIDS sponsored trials for the prevention of mother-to-child transmission: background brief to assist in responding to issues raised by the public and the media. Press release of the United Nations AIDS Program. (undated document.)
18. Halsey NA, Meinert CL, Ruff AJ., et al. Letter to Harold Varmus, Director of National Institutes of Health. Baltimore: Johns Hopkins University, May 6, 1997.
19. Wiktor SZ, Ehounou E. A randomized placebo-controlled intervention study to evaluate the safety and effectiveness of oral zidovudine administered in late pregnancy to reduce the incidence of mother-to-child transmission of HIV-1 in Abidjan, Côte D'Ivoire. Atlanta: Centers for Disease Control and Prevention. (undated document.)
20. Rouzioux C, Costagliola D, Burgard M, et al. Timing of mother-to-child HIV-1 transmission depends on maternal status. AIDS 1993; 7: Suppl 2: S49-S52.
21. Freedman B. Equipoise and the ethics of clinical research. N Engl J Med 1987; 317:141–5.
22. World Health Organization, International ethical guidelines.
23. Heimlich HJ, Chen XP, Xiao BQ et al. CD4 response in HIV-positive patients treated with malaria therapy.

Presented at the 11th International Conference on AIDS, Vancouver, B.C., July 7–12, 1996. abstract.

24. Bishop WB, Laubscher I, Labadarios D, Rehder P. Louw ME, Fellingham SA. Effect of vitamin-enriched bread on the vitamin status of an isolated rural community—a controlled clinical trial. S Afr Med J 1996;86: Suppl:458–62.

25. Lurie P, Bishaw M, Chesney MA, et al. Ethical, behavioral, and social aspects of HIV vaccine trials in developing countries. JAMA 1994;271:295–301.

26. Annas G, Grodin M. An apology is not enough. Boston Globe. May 18, 1997:C1–C2.

27. Ibid.

28. Freedman B, Weijer C, Glass KC. Placebo orthodoxy in clinical research. I. Empirical and methodological myths. J Law Med Ethics 1996; 24:243–51.

29. Varmus H. Comments at the meeting of the Advisory Committee to the Director of the National Institutes of Health, December 12, 1996.

30. Angell M. Ethical imperialism? Ethics in international collaborative clinical research. N Engl J Med 1988; 319:1061–3.

AZT TRIALS AND TRIBULATIONS

Robert A. Crouch and John D. Arras

With the successful completion of a placebo-controlled trial of zidovudine (AZT) in pregnant women in Thailand—a study designed to determine the safety and efficacy of a short course of AZT in the prevention of maternal-infant HIV transmission—the Centers for Disease Control and Prevention [has] announced the suspension or modification of all similar trials involving placebos elsewhere in the world. The CDC has claimed victory, asserting that its hotly contested placebo-driven methodology has been vindicated by the study's impressive results. But the critics of this controversial research remain unmoved. For them, the moral of the CDC/Thailand study is a rueful "Better late than never." Both sides can agree on one thing, however: they are glad it's over.

But our society and research communities in fact have yet to definitively resolve some crucial questions posed by these studies. Are placebo-controlled trials justified in the developing world when a proven treatment already exists in developed countries? Must the same ethical standards be used to judge research conducted at home or abroad, in Rochester or Rwanda? We must try to come to terms with these crucial questions bearing on the ethical conduct of international trials because they will soon recur, either in the form of studies on AIDS vaccines, the effects of breastfeeding on HIV transmission, or any number of other pressing issues on the horizon of biomedical research.

THE CONTROVERSY: ARE PLACEBO-CONTROLLED TRIALS JUSTIFIED?

While HIV-infected women and their newborns in industrialized nations can look forward to receiving the AIDS Clinical Trials Group (ACTG) 076 study treatment, the largest public health burden associated with perinatal HIV transmission is to be found in the developing world, where the vast majority of the approximately 1,000 babies born HIV-infected each day reside. Given such grim facts, it is imperative that an alternative safe and effective therapy be established for use in the developing world, where, it has been argued, the intensive 076 protocol could not realistically be implemented. First, the regimen of

From *Hastings Center Report* 28, no. 6 (1998): 26–34. Reprinted by permission of The Hastings Center.

Editors' note: Most authors' notes have been cut. Students who want to follow up on sources should consult the original article.

antenatal, intrapartum, and neonatal AZT requires that women present to the clinic early in their pregnancy for HIV testing and counseling; that they follow the rigorous 076 protocol, which includes five pills per day for at least twelve weeks, and intravenous administration of AZT during delivery; and that the neonates follow a six-week, four-times-per-day, oral AZT regimen, during which time the women are required to abstain from breastfeeding. Unfortunately, however, pregnant women in many developing world settings do not turn up for prenatal care until very late in their pregnancy if indeed at all; many health care clinics in such locales are not equipped to administer intravenous AZT or, generally, to deliver the fastidious care required by the treatment protocol; and, finally, almost all women in the developing world breastfeed because of the established health benefits for their children and the prohibitive expense of baby formula, thus making adherence to the treatment protocol all but impossible. Second, the 076 regimen has been variously estimated to cost as much as $1,000 to $1,500, but certainly no less than $800 per mother and infant—a sum that makes it unaffordable for most of the developing world.

Consequently, U.S. researchers, in cooperation with researchers and public health officials in eleven developing world nations, designed and planned to carry out clinical trials that would compare a shorter, less intensive regimen of AZT to placebo, in the hope of demonstrating that the short course AZT was safe and effective in preventing perinatal HIV transmission in local populations, and that it would be affordable to most developing nations. Though these goals are laudable and endorsed by all, the proposed means to achieve them have engendered fierce criticism, as well as analogies to the infamous Tuskegee syphilis study, from those who believe that the planned means to achieve these results—in particular, the inclusion of a placebo arm in the studies—are unethical.

Three main lines of argument are advanced against the ethical permissibility of the clinical trials planned for the developing world. First, as Peter Lurie and Sidney Wolfe argue, the main point of conflict revolves around the choice of an appropriate comparison group. As against the study designers, Lurie and Wolfe claim that the short course AZT should be compared not to placebo, but rather to the 076 regimen itself, because an equivalency study will yield "even more useful results than placebo-controlled trials, without the deaths of hundreds of newborns that are inevitable if placebo groups are used."[1]

Second, according to Lurie and Wolfe, a subgroup analysis within the 076 protocol indicates that short course AZT (treatment no longer than twelve weeks) is as effective as long course AZT (treatment longer than twelve weeks), suggesting an affirmative answer to the research question implied by the placebo-controlled design—"Is the shorter regimen better than nothing?"—and thereby rendering the studies unnecessary and, thus, unethical.[2]

Finally, as Lurie and Wolfe and Marcia Angell have stated, Western researchers in the studies are shirking their duties to their research subjects on two accounts. First, as set out in the Declaration of Helsinki (Article II.3), all research subjects, including those in the control group, should be assured of the "best proven diagnostic and therapeutic method."[3] Thus in conditions of genuine uncertainty as to the comparative merits of the two AZT regimens, enrolled subjects have a right to, and researchers a correlative duty to provide, either the short course AZT or the 076 regimen, thereby making the use of a placebo arm in the international studies unethical. Second, Lurie and Wolfe interpret guideline 15 of the *International Ethical Guidelines for Biomedical Research Involving Human Subjects* promulgated by the Council for International Organizations of Medical Sciences (CIOMS) as mandating that researchers have "an ethical responsibility to provide treatment that conforms to the standard of care in the sponsoring country, when possible."[4] Since this standard of care would include access to AZT for all participants, to rest the justification for the placebo-controlled design on the fact that the standard of care in most developing world countries consists of no treatment is to fail to recognize a prior duty and to endorse a potentially dangerous double standard for research.

CLARIFYING THE ISSUES

It is well established that for a clinical trial to be ethical, a state of genuine uncertainty as to the comparative merits of the treatments under study must exist within the expert clinical community. Given the uncertainty regarding the study treatments—in other words, given that a state of clinical equipoise exists—trials must be conducted with the aim of removing this uncertainty. The aim of the study must be to disturb equipoise and, thus, alter clinical practice. This means, *inter alia,* that conduct of a clinical trial requires that the "compendious effect of a treatment, a portmanteau measure including all the elements that contribute to the acceptance of a drug within clinical practice," rather than one discrete measure of a treatment's effect should be the focus of the research.[5] And, because clinical trials are responsive to and centrally concerned with the realities of clinical practice, it is crucial for the clinical trialists to take the study context into account when designing and conducting such studies. Recognition of these considerations has several consequences for this discussion.

Given the widespread poverty and lack of resources endemic to much of the developing world, to be understood properly the proposed trials must be analyzed within a framework of extreme fiscal scarcity. Within such a framework, clinical trialists should be concerned with a compendious evaluation of the AZT regimen's effects: reduction of HIV transmission, safety, ease of administration, and, importantly, cost.

In these studies, therefore, the question is not merely whether short course AZT is better than nothing. Rather, the study question is whether the shorter AZT regimen is safe in these populations, and, if so, whether the demonstrated efficacy is large enough, as compared to the placebo group, to make it affordable to the governments in question. For government officials in the developing world to make sound public health policy decisions regarding a treatment to reduce perinatal HIV transmission, trials must demonstrate that AZT is safe for women and their infants and offer convincing evidence about the treatment difference that exists between short course AZT and placebo.

Unanswered questions about the safety of AZT for populations among whom anemia is prevalent, as is well documented among pregnant women in Africa, and whose immune status is compromised by malnutrition argue against use of the 076 regimen as a control arm in these efficacy studies, as

does the real possibility that zidovudine-resistant HIV variants may develop in the mother and be passed on to the fetus.

Further, the use of the 076 regimen (or, indeed, another less intensive AZT regimen) as a comparison would yield less informative results because there is ample evidence to suggest that the mother-to-infant HIV transmission rate is highly variable within the developing world (as well as between developed and developing worlds) and that determinants of this variation are not fully understood and hence cannot easily be predicted. Thus part of the information to be gleaned from a placebo-controlled study is the background rate of perinatal HIV transmission in a particular population, which will give researchers a more definite baseline against which to assess AZT efficacy.

This leaves us with the final charge raised by critics of the trials: that it is simply unjust for researchers to operate according to a double standard with regard to the developed and developing worlds. There are two distinct issues here: Are the subjects in placebo-controlled trials morally entitled to more than nothing? And, are these trials unjust because they exploit poor, deprived, developing world subjects largely for the benefit of the more affluent populations of sponsoring countries?

THE CLAIM OF ENTITLEMENT

The critics of placebo-controlled AZT studies assume, either implicitly or explicitly, that all research subjects are morally entitled to receive the prevailing standard of care in more developed countries. One possible source of such an entitlement would be a theory of health care justice as applied to the host countries in question. Importantly, this approach does not rely on any special research-related features of the situation. Although there are many competing theories of equitable access to health care, the account we present here for illustrative purposes embodies several elements common to a variety of leading theories. According to what we will call "the liberal consensus view," justice is equivalent to the kind and amounts of health care that informed, rational, and prudent individuals would choose for themselves against a background entitlement to a fair share of their society's resources. Realizing that they have a limited but fair amount of resources to spend on health care—and that they have many competing needs both within the health care sphere and in such areas as education, housing, employment, and leisure—individuals would no doubt abandon their usual "spare no cost" attitude toward health care in favor of a much more discriminating, cost effective approach. Would they opt for a good, solid basic package of health care benefits? Most likely. Would they pay thousands of extra dollars to insure continuing care for years in a persistent vegetative state? Surely not. According to the liberal consensus view, then, health care justice simply is what such real or hypothetical persons would choose against a backdrop of basic equity.

Applying the liberal consensus view to the situation of individuals in developing countries, we must first ask whether their present standard of living would qualify as a fair share of societal resources. If their present shares were deemed to constitute a reasonably just baseline situation, the citizens of most, if not all, developing countries would clearly not choose to purchase and thus would have no right to expensive antiretroviral therapies. Given the extreme shortages of goods, services, infrastructure, and personnel across a wide spectrum of basic needs, individuals and governments would realize that they simply don't have the money to invest in such treatments, and that the meager amount of money that they do control would be better spent on cheaper, more effective interventions that could reach many more people and save many more lives. Instead of the 076 protocol at $800 per person—or even the CDC/Thailand protocol at $50—in a country that currently spends $5 per person per year on health care, they might favor more modest public health measures, such as improved nutrition or water systems. According to this analysis, research subjects randomized to placebos in the recent short course trials were not deprived of anything to which they were already justly entitled.

It is highly debatable, however, whether the current holdings of citizens in most developing countries satisfy the condition of background fairness required by the liberal consensus view. Agreeing with Judith Shklar's perceptive observation that it is always "easier to see misfortune rather than injustice

in the afflictions of other people,"[6] we are loathe to conclude that the current plight of these impoverished peoples is unfortunate but not unjust. Their misery must be due in no small measure to the flagrantly unjust behavior of the former colonial powers, which plundered their natural resources and subjugated their peoples; in many subsequent cases to the rapacious behavior of their home-grown military dictators, who treated their country's natural resources as their own private stock; and more recently to global economic policies that often stifle economic growth under huge debt-servicing policies. In a more just world, the citizens of the developing world would have a more equitable share of their country's resources, and the colonial powers and the generals would have a lot less. Recalculating their social and economic baseline to reflect the demands of compensatory justice, would these people have a just claim to expensive antiretroviral therapy, a claim denied by placebo-driven AIDS trials?

Although we support any and all efforts to narrow the huge economic gap separating developing from more developed countries, we doubt that even taking past injustices into account would yield a moral entitlement to expensive antiretroviral treatments. In the first place, many of these countries are so poor and underdeveloped that even the best efforts at compensatory redistribution would not take them very far. Under the rosiest of estimates, such countries might be able to afford the $50 CDC/Thailand protocol, but certainly not the hugely expensive 076 regimen.

Second, even if compensatory redistribution were required by justice, it will usually be impossible to tell who owes what kind and amount of compensation to whom, and there are currently no authoritative international bodies that could legitimately adjudicate such compensatory claims. As a result, the citizens of these impoverished countries may indeed have a moral right to a better standard of living, but this is almost certainly a claim that will go unredeemed for the foreseeable future. Hence the desirability and feasibility of choosing to pay for expensive antiretroviral therapies must be gauged against the backdrop of their present, admittedly unjust, baseline.

Third, claiming and *per impossibile* securing such a right would surely generate new injustices, as more numerous people with equally pressing needs would be passed over in favor of HIV-infected pregnant women and their children. The families of children and adults dying from diarrhea, malnutrition, and malaria could reasonably claim a higher priority on public funds. Their numbers are greater and it would cost far less to mount effective preventive programs in such areas.

Perhaps most importantly, the plausibility of a claimed right to antiretroviral treatment fundamentally depends upon the successful completion of the contested placebo-controlled trials. Even if we assume that the potential subjects' current baseline situation is unjust, any set of more just holdings will perforce be limited, they will have many competing (and expensive) needs, and they will thus be extremely sensitive to the opportunity costs of spending money on expensive AIDS therapies rather than on less expensive and more cost-effective lifesaving interventions. To tell whether they would reasonably choose to spend large sums of money on AIDS therapies, reliable scientific data on their costs, risks, and benefits must first be accumulated so that reasonable and prudent investment comparisons might be made. Thus until we know just how safe and effective the short course of AZT is in these host countries, it makes little sense to say that people there independently have a right to it.

A second approach to justifying an entitlement would focus not on theories of health care justice, but rather on certain role-specific duties of researchers. Whether or not potential subjects have a preexisting right to antiretroviral therapies, it might be claimed that researchers have a duty to provide it to them based upon their special relationship. One might claim, for example, that participating subjects assume additional burdens by participating in a drug trial and are therefore owed special treatment. Or one could argue that researchers have special fiduciary responsibilities for all those who are placed in their care, responsibilities that include providing all subjects in the control group with the highest standard of care in the world (that is, with the 076 protocol).

Although both of these arguments contain a large grain of truth, neither succeeds in justifying a claim to the 076 protocol for subjects in the control group. Even if subjects do assume additional burdens by participating in a trial, they also become eligible for important benefits not normally available off study,

especially if they end up receiving a safe and efficacious active drug. And even if they end up in the placebo group, they will probably receive better basic medical care than would have been available to them otherwise. Moreover, there are other more realistic ways of compensating them for burdens incurred, especially when this proposed method of compensation would have the undesirable effect of preventing researchers from answering the most meaningful questions that motivated the research in the first place.

This last point is crucial for determining the scope of researchers' fiduciary responsibilities to subjects entrusted to their care. Although researchers undeniably have such role-specific duties, we doubt that they would include enticements to kinds and amounts of health care services that, first, are unavailable elsewhere in the host country and to which its citizens have no independent right of access, and second, would arguably preclude the timely and successful completion of desperately needed clinical trials. As we argued above, the point of running a clinical trial is to disturb equipoise and thereby potentially change clinical practice. Researchers must therefore show that the proposed short course AZT intervention is both safe and sufficiently effective to warrant large-scale investments on the part of host governments, developed nations, and pharmaceutical companies. In the absence of reliable information on the background vertical HIV transmission rate—information that can only be gained via a placebo group—researchers will be unable to meet this burden of demonstration. Neither the assumption of special burdens nor the enhanced fiduciary responsibilities of researchers for their subjects can ground an entitlement to the best treatment available anywhere. . . .

REFERENCES

1. Peter Lurie and Sidney M. Wolfe, "Unethical Trials of Interventions to Reduce Perinatal Transmission of the Human Immunodeficiency Virus in Developing Countries," *NEJM* 337 (1997): 853–56, at 854.
2. Lurie and Wolfe, "Unethical Trials"; Sidney M. Wolfe and Peter Lurie, letter to Donna Shalala, Secretary of Health and Human Services, 23 October 1997.
3. Wolfe and Lurie, letter to Donna Shalala; Marcia Angell, "The Ethics of Clinical Research in the Third World," *NEJM* 337 (1997): 847–49.

4. Lurie and Wolfe, "Unethical Trials," p. 855.

5. Benjamin Freedman, "Placebo-Controlled Trials and the Logic of Clinical Purpose," *IRB: A Review of Human Subjects Research* 12, no. 6 (1990): 1–6, at 5.

6. Judith N. Shklar, *The Faces of Injustice* (New Haven: Yale University Press, 1990), p. 15.

THE AMBIGUITY AND THE EXIGENCY: CLARIFYING "STANDARD OF CARE" ARGUMENTS IN INTERNATIONAL RESEARCH

Alex John London

I.   INTRODUCTION

For some time now, the medical and bioethics communities have been struggling with a number of difficult and sometimes divisive issues concerning the ethics of international research. Many of these issues were raised in the recent controversy over the decision to use placebo control groups in clinical trials designed to test the efficacy of a short-course of zidovudine (AZT) for the prevention of maternal-infant HIV infection in sixteen countries in sub-Saharan Africa, Southeast Asia, and the Caribbean. The studies, sponsored by the National Institutes of Health (NIH) and the Centers for Disease Control and Prevention (CDC), became the topic of a heated debate when a pair of articles published in the *New England Journal of Medicine* (Angell, 1997; Lurie and Wolfe, 1997) charged that the use of a placebo control group made them unethical. Even though subsequent studies involving placebos were either suspended or modified after the completion of a CDC-sponsored study in Thailand, the controversy has continued and the ethical and scientific debate has intensified. Now, however, the dispute surrounding some of these issues could have far-reaching implications for the whole of international human

From *Journal of Medicine and Philosophy* 25, no. 4(2000): 379–397. Reprinted with permission.

Editors' note: All author's endnotes have been cut. Students who want to follow up on sources should consult the original article.

subjects research. Plans are underway to revise key guidelines governing the ethical conduct of international medical research, and several of the most controversial issues at the heart of the short-course AZT trials are playing a central role in the debate over some of the proposed revisions.

Rather than attempting a wholesale appraisal of the diverse and complex array of issues involved in this debate, the present paper will focus instead on one prominent, and highly controversial, issue. From the outset of the controversy over the short-course AZT studies, both proponents and critics of the placebo-controlled design supported their positions with what I will call the 'standard of care' argument. Critics argued that the placebo driven trial design was unethical, at least in part, because it failed to provide the current standard of care to all members of the clinical trial. In support of their position they pointed to article II.3 of the Declaration of Helsinki which states that "In any medical study, every patient—including those of a control group, if any—should be assured of the best proven diagnostic and therapeutic method." They also pointed to the fact that in technologically developed countries such as France and the U.S., the standard treatment used for preventing the transmission of HIV from seropositive pregnant women to their infant children, known as the AIDS Clinical Trials Group (ACTG) regimen 076, had been shown to cut maternal-infant HIV transmission rates by more than half. To adopt a standard of care for developing nations that falls below the standard of care in the sponsoring countries, it was argued, was to adopt an unacceptable double standard in international research.

Proponents of the placebo design countered by pointing out that the 076 protocol was unavailable in the countries that would host the short-course trials because, at $800 per dose, it far outstripped the $10 average per-capita health budgets of the developing countries in which the trials had been proposed. As a result, they argued, the standard of care that governs the citizens of those countries is no treatment at all. Because they believed that the local standard of care was the most relevant, they concluded that the placebo design was not unethical. Now, current proposals would amend the Declaration of Helsinki so as to reflect this view. Instead of requiring that subjects receive the "best proven diagnostic and therapeutic method," one proposed revision would require only that subjects "not be denied access to the best proven diagnostic, prophylactic, or therapeutic method that would otherwise be available to him or her."

In what follows, I will argue that this debate has been complicated by some unrecognized ambiguities in the notion of a standard of care. In particular, I will argue that this concept is ambiguous along two different axes, with the result that there are at least four possible standard of care arguments that must be clearly distinguished. Without a clear map of the normative terrain it has been difficult to assess the implications of opposing standard of care arguments, to recognize important differences in their supporting rationales, and even to locate the crux of the disagreement in some instances. The goal of this discussion, therefore, is to disambiguate the concept of a standard of care and to make the areas of genuine disagreement among different standards salient. This kind of conceptual cartography is fundamentally important for assessing the relevance and validity of the arguments in question and I will argue that it highlights important ways in which one of these arguments in particular may be more complex than it originally appears.

Because the goal of this paper is to provide a careful examination of the concept of a standard of care and the normative arguments that it supports, it does not attempt to provide an overall evaluation of the short-course AZT studies. As a result, it also will not present an overall evaluation of the importance

of standard of care arguments relative to these broader concerns. This is important because it may be the case that there are other issues raised by these trials that carry sufficient moral weight to trump the standard of care argument. Before we can know whether this is so, however, we need to carry out the necessary conceptual and ethical analysis of the standard of care arguments that will enable this larger conversation to proceed more carefully, and hopefully, more fruitfully as well.

II. WHAT IS (ARE) THE STANDARD OF CARE ARGUMENT(S)?

In order to tease out some important ambiguities in the concept of a standard of care, it will be helpful to look carefully at one prominent way in which the debate over the standard of care has been framed. Consider the following claims:

> When Helsinki calls for the "best proven therapeutic method" does it mean [A] the best therapy available anywhere in the world? Or does it mean [B] the standard that prevails in the country in which the trial is conducted? Helsinki is not clear about this. But I think that [1] a careful analysis of this document and its history suggests that the best proven therapy standard was intended primarily as a standard of medical practice. A consideration of that conclusion yields a second conclusion: that [2] the best proven therapy standard must necessarily mean the standard that prevails in the country in which the clinical trial is carried out (Levine, R.J., 1998, p. 6; letters and numbers added).

In part, interpretations A and B differ over what I will call the question of the *relevant reference point.* Emphasizing this disagreement makes it appear as though the dispute hinges on the question of whose medical practice constitutes the relevant medical practice. Interpretation A holds that the relevant standard of care is the one determined by the best therapeutic methods available anywhere in the world. Call this the *global* reference point. Interpretation B holds that the relevant standard of care is determined by the standard that prevails in the country in which the trial is conducted. Call this the *local* reference point. So understood, the sides of this debate are divided into proponents of a local standard of care and critics who champion a global standard of care.

Framing the debate as a question of the relevant reference point, however, effectively obscures a more fundamental and largely unarticulated source of disagreement. To see this, consider a crucial assumption that lies behind the following argument. It is sometimes claimed that (1) because the content of the standard of care is fixed by the local reference point and (2) because the prevailing treatment for preventing maternal-infant HIV transmission in the countries where the short-course AZT trials were conducted was no treatment at all, that (3) the use of a placebo does not fall below the established standard of care. It is important to see, however, that in order for (3) to follow from (1) and (2), we have to do more than simply adopt the local reference point for the standard of care. For the argument to be valid it must also employ what I will call a *de facto* interpretation of the concept of the standard of care. Let me explain.

Let's grant the claim that the standard of care is intended to be a standard of medical practice. The above argument tacitly assumes a *de facto* interpretation of the standard of care according to which the standards of medical practice for a community are set by the actual medical practices of that community. It is only under this interpretation that the use of a placebo does not fall below the standard of care in countries where there is no effective treatment for maternal-infant transmission of HIV. For the sake of clarity, the argument from the *local de facto* interpretation of the standard of care can be stated as follows:

(A) 1. It is unethical to conduct a clinical trial in which some subjects receive a level of care that falls below the established standard of care.
2. The established standard of care is to be determined by the local *de facto* practices of the host community.
3. In the countries where the short-course AZT trials were conducted the local *de facto* clinical practice for preventing maternal-infant HIV transmission was no treatment at all.
4. The use of a placebo control group in these countries does not fall below the established standard of care.
5. Therefore, the use of a placebo control group is not unethical on the ground that it fails to provide the established standard of care.

If we assume that the crux of the debate hinges on the question of the relevant reference point then we must also assume that critics of this argument accept the *de facto* interpretation but opt instead for a more global reference point. So understood, they would be making a *global de facto* argument:

(B) 1. It is unethical to conduct a clinical trial in which some subjects receive a level of care that falls below the established standard of care.
2. The established standard of care is to be determined by the broader *de facto* practices of the sponsoring nations.
3. The *de facto* clinical practice for preventing maternal-infant HIV transmission in the countries of the developed world sponsoring the short-course AZT trials is the 076 protocol.
4. The use of a placebo control group in the countries where short-course AZT trials were proposed falls below the established standard in the developed world.
5. Therefore, the use of a placebo control group is unethical on the ground that it fails to provide the established standard of care.

This may represent a common way of framing the debate over the standard of care, but it obscures the fact that the *de facto* interpretation of the standard is itself highly contentious. As a result, it fails to capture a more fundamental area of disagreement. If we return to the language of the Declaration of Helsinki, for example, we see that it speaks of providing the best *proven* diagnostic and therapeutic interventions. This seems to indicate that the idea of a standard of care is what I will call a *de jure* standard in that it is set, not by what physicians in some locality actually do, but by the judgment of experts in the medical community as to which diagnostic and therapeutic practices have proven most effective against the illness in question. This is the interpretation embraced by Marcia Angell when she argues that the investigators conducting a trial "would be guilty of knowingly giving inferior treatment to some participants of the trial," unless subjects in the control group "receive the best known treatment." For critics like Angell, the question of the relevant reference point is irrelevant because adopting the *de jure* interpretation of the standard of care allows them to argue that a placebo control is unjustified even relative to the local point of reference. To see how this might be so, consider the argument from the *local de jure* standard of care:

(C) 1. It is unethical to conduct a clinical trial in which some subjects receive a level of care that falls below the established standard of care.
   2. The established standard of care is to be determined by the judgment of medical experts in the host community as to which diagnostic and therapeutic interventions have been proven most effective.
   3. Medical experts in the relevant host communities know the 076 protocol has been shown to cut the maternal-infant HIV transmission rate by more than half in developed nations such as the United States.
   4. The use of a placebo control group in the developing countries where the short-course AZT trials were proposed falls below the established standard in those very countries.
   5. Therefore, the use of a placebo control group is unethical on the ground that it fails to provide the established standard of care.

A global version of this argument can be constructed by substituting the following for premise C2:

(D) 2. The established standard of care is to be determined by the judgment of medical experts in some larger medical community as to which diagnostic and therapeutic interventions have been proven most effective.

Below, I will suggest that this argument is more complex than even its proponents may realize and that its implications have yet to be clearly explored. For the moment, however, I simply want to note that the choice of reference points does not affect the conclusion of the argument. As a result, it looks like the real crux of the dispute may hinge, not on the question of the relevant reference point, but on the way we interpret the standard of medical practice that is embodied in the standard of care: is it a *de facto* or a *de jure* standard?

When the crux of the argument is understood this way, it becomes absolutely essential not to confuse the argument from the global *de facto* standard (B) with the argument from the local *de jure* standard (C). In part, this is because arguments (B) and (C) themselves differ over the question of the relevant reference point. As a result, objections that tell against the use of a global reference point may carry weight against argument (B) and not militate against—and may even support—argument (C). Furthermore, given that these arguments embody different conceptions of the standard of care, each of which has a substantially different supporting rationale, we must not assume that they will have the same implications for the conduct of international research. In the following section I will suggest that a failure to differentiate arguments (B) and (C) may have led to the acceptance of a false dilemma: either we accept the local *de facto* standard of care or we accept a higher standard that rules out altogether the international research that could be most important for populations of the developing world. In order to appreciate this, however, and to evaluate the merits of the local *de facto* and local *de jure* arguments, it will be necessary to look more carefully at the differences between the *de facto* and *de jure* interpretations of the standard of care.

III.   THE LOCAL *DE FACTO* STANDARD OF CARE

One fairly simple reason that we might be inclined to accept the local *de facto* standard of care is that it appears to be more reasonable than the global *de facto* standard. Consider, for instance, some of the problems with the latter argument (B). On its face it appears to place arbitrary restrictions on important international research. Critics can easily question why the practices of some wealthy, technologically developed groups with sophisticated and well-entrenched healthcare infrastructures should also govern people who live under conditions of extreme fiscal scarcity, without a robust healthcare infrastructure, under different cultural and social conditions. Isn't this arbitrary? Might it not be ethical, rather than social or cultural, imperialism?

In contrast, proponents of the narrow *de facto* argument (A) argue that it will foster the research that will ultimately lead to the kinds of interventions that will best address the healthcare concerns of developing populations. The local *status quo* frames the appropriate clinical question and enables us to design a study that will demonstrate the effectiveness of an intervention when compared to the current treatment situation (in the case of the short-course trials, nothing) (Levine, R. J., 1998, p. 7). This difference in the treatment situation is what makes it permissible to conduct a placebo-controlled trial in a developing country when it could not be conducted ethically in the U.S. Furthermore, it is argued, the use of a placebo does not deny subjects of developing countries care that they would otherwise receive, since they aren't currently receiving any beneficial care, and it does not inflict new or additional health burdens on research subjects. In fact, it is likely that in many cases research subjects would receive a net benefit from participating in this kind of research since they would probably receive routine health care, otherwise unavailable, as a part of the clinical trial.

When the alternative is the global *de facto* argument (B), we may be inclined to support the local *de facto* argument (A) simply out of the desire to help developing countries conduct the research that will answer the healthcare questions that best address their substantial and urgent healthcare needs. This way of thinking, however, may also keep us from recognizing the substantial shortcomings of the local *de facto* standard of care. For many, the most appealing aspect of this standard of care is the fact that it allows us to design clinical trials that will answer the right experimental questions. In the case of the short-course AZT trials, for instance, the relevant question was not how a short-course of AZT compared to the 076 regimen but how much better it would be than nothing. Unfortunately, however, it is precisely because the *status quo* is what sets research into motion that it cannot also function as an independent test of the moral acceptability of a clinical trial. Let me be clear about what this means. The research questions that are relevant to a particular community are, to a large degree, a function of the needs of the people in that community relative to the level of healthcare they actually receive. It is also true that acceptable clinical trials should produce results that will be relevant to a community's healthcare needs. But it doesn't follow from this that all research that would be relevant to a community's healthcare needs is morally acceptable research.

Relevance, elegance, efficiency, these are all virtues that morally acceptable trials should possess. But not all relevant, elegant, and efficient trials are morally acceptable.

It is important to recognize, therefore, that the local *de facto* standard of care does not receive independent support from the claim that subjects who would not receive medical care outside of a clinical trial are not denied care when they are given a placebo. Rather than providing independent support for the *de facto* standard of care, this is simply an alternative formulation of the very standard in question. As a result, the truth of this claim itself presupposes the truth of the argument from the local *de facto* standard of care. Those who reject the latter argument would rightly reject this claim on the grounds that it simply assumes the conclusion that is in dispute. This means that proponents of a different standard of care could make an equally valid claim that subjects of medical research *are* being denied medical care to which they are entitled if, for example, they do not receive the same level of care that the researchers or their sponsoring agencies normally provide to people with their condition. I will return to this point in a moment.

For now, consider some of problems that argument (A) faces in its own right. For example, the scope of this argument is more comprehensive than its proponents may be willing to accept. In particular, we want to know whether there are non-arbitrary reasons for keeping this argument, and its supporting rationale, from applying to sub-groups within established political borders. After all, if the standard of care is set by a community's *de facto* medical practices, and if the actual practices of doctors differ within ethnic, cultural, or economic subgroups, shouldn't those subgroups be governed by different standards of care in research? This is a powerful and potentially damning objection, because most proponents of the placebo design appear to believe that it would be genuinely unethical to conduct short-course AZT trials with a placebo control in the U.S. If this objection cannot be met, it would mean that the members of marginalized or oppressed subgroups, even within a developed nation like the U.S., would be governed by a lower standard of care in medical research than their wealthier counterparts precisely because they have been socially and economically marginalized or oppressed. This, however, is antithetical to the very idea of ethically sound human subjects research. As a result, anyone who is inclined to accept this argument takes on the increased burden of providing nonarbitrary reasons for limiting its scope of applicability.

This is also a powerful objection because it highlights the degree to which the narrow *de facto* standard of care appears to be out of step with the rationale for protecting human subjects in research within the U.S. This way of formulating the standard of care trades on the assumption that the level of care research subjects receive should be determined by factors that are extrinsic to the researcher/subject relationship. Another way of putting this is to say that, on this view, the terms of the researcher/subject relationship are to be determined by circumstances that are largely independent of the existence of that relationship. In order to know what standard of care subjects are entitled to, researchers, on this view, have to look at the circumstances in which those subjects live. In order to know whether subjects in Tanzania should be subject to the same standards of care as subjects in Tucson, we have to look at the socioeconomic circumstances in which they live. Traditionally, however, the debate about the protections that human research subjects should receive has been formulated largely in terms of problems that are inherent to the nature of medical research and the researcher/subject relationship. Socio-economic factors were important but largely because they marked out vulnerable populations where an increased sensitivity to issues of exploitation and competence was warranted. As such, Lurie and Wolfe (1997) were right to argue that this interpretation of the standard of care marks a change in the way research protections are conceived—a double standard for medical research.

Not only is this a different standard, it is a dangerous standard because it fails to take account of the context in which a community's *de facto* medical practices originate. By simply elevating the status quo to the level of a normative standard it does not distinguish between situations of scarcity that are the result of exploitation, force or fraud and those that are not. This leaves it open to exploitation and the danger of being manipulated in unscrupulous ways, on the international level by the economic or military interference of an outside group on the availability of medicines, medical personnel, or medical training within a particular nation, and on an *intra*-national

level by these same activities on the part of dominant power groups.

The fact that argument (A) unreflectively embraces the status quo may sometimes be overlooked because of an ambiguity in the notion of a 'practice.' As it has come to be used by some (communitarians, for example), a practice is a norm-governed activity in which people engage, in part at least, for the sake of goods that are internal to the practice. On this view, a practice is an activity through which people pursue certain goods and understand themselves, their community, and perhaps their larger world. Because practices of this kind can play an integral part in the identity of individuals or communities, they may deserve special protections or carry special normative weight. However, the *de facto* 'practice' of physicians in Thailand, for example, is not such a practice. Thai physicians understand that they are unable to effectively prevent maternal-infant transmission of HIV and are themselves calling for the international help required to change this. As Lurie and Wolfe rightly point out, "In developing countries, the standard of care . . . is not based on a consideration of alternative treatments or previous clinical data, but is instead an economically determined policy of governments that cannot afford the prices set by drug companies" (1997, p. 855). So we must be careful not to confuse this kind of *de facto* practice with the more normatively weighty sense of "practice" favored by communitarians.

IV.   THE LOCAL *DE JURE* STANDARD OF CARE

When the crux of the debate over the standard of care is framed, not as a question of the relevant reference point, but as hinging on the choice between the local *de facto* and local *de jure* interpretations, many of these problems with argument (A) become salient. For the proponents of a *de jure* standard, the local *de facto* standard is formulated in response to the wrong question. The latter standard answers the question of what research subjects may be entitled to outside of the research context, what they would be entitled to if research were not taking place (with the dubious assumption that their current situation is unfortunate and not unjust). But this is not what is at issue. What is at issue is what subjects are entitled to within the context of research itself, given the nature of scientific research and the fact that the researchers studying them have the knowledge and training—and often work for governments or institutions with the resource—to prevent some of the harms they encounter as a result of their vast, unmet healthcare needs. It may be true that the use of analogies with past research scandals has not generally helped to advance the present debate, but critics of this position are right to point out that this idea—that research subjects are only entitled to what they would otherwise receive outside of the research context and that researchers are under no independent obligation to prevent outcomes that would occur outside of the research context anyway—was also used to support the studies at Tuskegee and Willowbrook. It may also be true that the proposed short-course trials were crucially different from these scandalous studies. But this point only highlights the need for those who defend the former studies to reject a moral justification that would also license the latter. After all, the claim that roughly the same states of affairs would likely have obtained even if no research had been conducted does not obviate the fact that, in the actual case, the state of affairs that actually obtains is at least partially a product of the explicit choices and activities of specific individuals and agencies.

For this reason, the *de jure* standard is founded upon the researchers' obligation to ensure that subjects of clinical trials are not knowingly exposed to foreseeable and preventable harms. Clinical trials are not the products of natural events or inevitable processes; they are the result of deliberation and choice on the part of actual individuals and agencies. The *de jure* requirement that researchers provide the treatment that has been shown to be most effective against the relevant illness is itself a corollary of the requirement that equipoise exist in order for a clinical trial to be morally permissible.

Clinical equipoise exists when there is genuine uncertainty among experts as to whether a proposed intervention is as good as or better than the current, known beneficial treatment for the illness at issue (Freedman, 1987 and 1990). A trial of a short course of AZT that used a placebo control group within the United States would be unethical because the 076 protocol has been shown to cut maternal-infant HIV transmission rates by more than half. In order for clinical equipoise to exist, the short course would

have to be tried against the 076 regimen *and* there would have to be reason to believe that the short-course of AZT might be equally or more effective than its established counterpart.

By linking the standard of care to the knowledge and abilities of researchers, argument (C) highlights the fact that medical research is a human activity, the terms of which are fundamentally shaped by human agency and choice. The fundamental goal of medical research is not to provide health care but to gather medical knowledge which, it is hoped, will result in the development or perfection of interventions that will benefit future patients. Because the design of a trial is the result of the exercise of such agency and choice, the researchers and agencies that sponsor clinical trials are responsible for the ramifications that trial designs have on the welfare of the people who submit themselves to scientific study. The requirement that clinical equipoise obtain is essential to the conduct of acceptable medical research because it ensures that researchers do not undertake trials in which the welfare of some individuals is knowingly sacrificed in exchange for knowledge, and, ultimately, the welfare of future patients. By providing the *de jure* standard of care, researchers and their sponsoring agencies ensure that the subjects of clinical research are not exploited, even for what we can all agree is a noble end.

Now that the rationale for the *de jure* standard is clear, it remains to elucidate the implications of this standard for international medical research. I suggested above that, to some degree, support for the local *de facto* interpretation may be rooted in the perception that a higher standard of care would place unduly stringent restrictions on the use of placebos in international research. Although this may be true for the global *de facto* standard, is it true for the local *de jure* standard as well?

V. THE COMPLEXITY OF THE *DE JURE* FRAMEWORK

I want to suggest that the local *de jure* standard of care does not yield as unequivocal a restriction on the use of placebo controls as one might think and that answering this question will be more complicated than it may first appear. In particular, because this standard is built around the concept of clinical equipoise, the severity of the restriction that it does yield will depend in large part on the nature of the conception of clinical equipoise that we embrace. This is an important claim, because it points to a way in which we might formulate the debate over the moral legitimacy of the use of placebo controls in international research from within the framework of the local *de jure* standard of care itself. In order to see how this is so, and why it might be desirable, let me explain how some placebo controls might be justified according to the local *de jure* standard of care.

In her original article in the *New England Journal of Medicine,* Marcia Angell argued for what I am calling a *de jure* standard of care. However, it is not clear how sweeping a restriction she takes this standard to yield. At one point, for instance, she says that "only when there is no known effective treatment is it ethical to compare a potential new treatment with a placebo" (1997, p. 847). This has encouraged some to frame the debate as a question of what I call the local *de facto* standard versus the best therapy available anywhere in the world (e.g., Levine, R.J., 1998, p. 6). But Angell's claim can be interpreted in two different ways:

I1. Only when there is no known effective treatment for illness *x* anywhere in the world is it ethical to compare a potential new treatment with a placebo.
I2. Only when there is no known effective treatment anywhere in the world for illness *x* within a population *p* is it ethical to compare a potential new treatment with a placebo in population *p*.

Although the local *de facto* standard is often contrasted with interpretation I1—the more restrictive standard—this interpretation is itself out of step with the rationale of the *de jure* conception of the standard of care. The reason is simply that such substantial differences between treatment populations can exist as to warrant genuine and credible doubts in the medical community about whether a treatment that is effective in one population will be effective in another. As a result, interpretation I2 most accurately reflects the *de jure* standard of care. It yields a more reasonable and defensible standard because it recognizes that the same standard can yield different conclusions if it is applied the same way in sufficiently different contexts. It is also less

restrictive than its critics, and perhaps its proponents, may recognize.

Exactly how restrictive I2 is, however, will depend on our conception of clinical equipoise. If we embrace a narrow conception of clinical equipoise according to which effectiveness is measured solely by the brute biological impact of an intervention on the illness in question relative to some end point, then the resulting standard of care will likely permit the use of a placebo only in cases where the biological differences between populations are substantial enough to cast credible doubt on the intervention's ability to function effectively in the trial population.

If we subscribe to a more robust concept of clinical equipoise, however, the ability to effect beneficial healthcare outcomes within a population will be measured as a product of a wider range of factors. For instance, Freedman (1990) has argued that the attractiveness of a drug in comparison to its alternatives should always be determined by a "compendious measure of a drug's net therapeutic advantage" (p. 2). Here, however, the concept of "net therapeutic advantage" is conceived of as a "*portmanteau* measure including all the elements that contribute to the acceptance of a drug within clinical practice" (p. 5). In addition to concerns about relative toxicity, this sort of robust conception of clinical equipoise will include factors such as ease of administration and availability. Some recent commentators have argued for the importance of relying on this conception of clinical equipoise when evaluating the short-course AZT trials (Crouch and Arras, 1998, p. 27). But their arguments have mainly emphasized the fact that doing so enables researchers to design trials that will change clinical practice. This is an important point, but one which also supports the local *de facto* standard of care and whose implications I criticized above. What needs to be stressed, instead, is that the rationale for including such broader factors in our concept of clinical equipoise can be supported by the epistemological concerns central to the *de jure* standard of care itself. The reason is that in order to know whether a treatment will be effective within a specific population we need to know whether it can be successfully administered in that context. This, however, will likely depend on a variety of social, cultural, and economic factors.

Consider, for instance, a treatment protocol that required frequent and prolonged hospital stays.

Such a protocol might fail to have a significant health impact in a nomadic population if compliance required what members of that population viewed as unacceptable changes to their way of life. The same might be true for a highly diffuse and largely immobile population with few hospitals if the travel that would be required for compliance required unacceptable social or economic sacrifices. Likewise, consider the case of an illness that can only be treated by a surgical procedure that requires sophisticated equipment, an extended intensive care stay, and frequent, sophisticated follow up treatments. This procedure is the *de jure* standard of care in wealthy nations with well-established, high-tech healthcare infrastructures, because it can be safely and effectively administered in such a setting. In a country that lacks this kind of setting it may be practically impossible to establish the conditions under which it could be effectively implemented even for a small group of people.

These examples are put forth as suggestive instances of cases in which equipoise could exist in one population even though it is disturbed in more developed nations, for other than purely biological reasons. The point of sketching them is to suggest that, in instances such as these, a *prima facie* case can be made—on the very grounds that support the *de jure* standard of care—for the legitimacy of a placebo control when testing a more portable intervention (assuming that one does not already exist). This kind of argument does not rest solely on the need to design a clinical trial that will provide a clear answer to a clinical question, although it ensures that all morally acceptable trials will have this feature. Nor does it rest on the claim that the subjects of such trials are not denied care that they would not otherwise receive. Instead, it rests on the claim that it may be ethically permissible to answer this particular question with a placebo-controlled trial because, in doing so, researchers would not knowingly be denying subjects *care that has proven effective for their illness in their population.*

As I said earlier, the implications of this position are far from clear and it may in fact raise more questions than it answers. For my present purposes, it is sufficient simply to note (a) that there are compelling reasons to treat equipoise as a broad measure of a treatment's effectiveness, and (b) that as we broaden our measure of an intervention's effectiveness the use of a placebo control may become acceptable in a wider variety of situations. Unlike the global *de facto* argument, this standard pays greater attention to substantive differences in social, cultural, and economic contexts and their impact on the permissibility of international research. Unlike the local *de facto* argument, however, it would prohibit the use of a placebo control in cases of international research where an intervention is known to be effective (where effectiveness is broadly construed) for illness *x* in population *p*, even if it is not currently available in population *p*.

Nevertheless, difficult questions would need to be resolved in order to make this a workable standard. We still need to know, for example, which social, cultural, and economic factors should bear on the question of equipoise and how much weight different factors should be afforded. For instance, what if we had a safe, effective, easily administered treatment that was simply so expensive that it could not be reasonably supplied to significant numbers of a developing population? Should this fact alone be sufficient to establish equipoise in the relevant population? What should we do in situations where the *de jure* standard in one population can be administered to members of the control group in another population, even though it could not be made available to members of the larger population?

Those who are familiar with the debate over the short course AZT trials will recognize many of these questions. The fact that they can be raised from within the framework of the local *de jure* argument testifies to its complexity. I believe that it also testifies to the fact that we can retain some of the most substantive areas of genuine dispute over the standards that should govern international research even if we agree that the local *de facto* standard of care is a bad, if not a perfidious, standard. In itself this is an important point because it may help us to reorient the current debate in a way that makes the actual lines of dispute salient. Not only might this allow both sides to agree on the values that structure the problem and then to recognize the operative areas of genuine dispute, it might make it possible to find a way towards building a more stable and sustainable consensus on these issues.

One thing that we can say, even from this admittedly terse sketch, is that relocating the debate within the context of the local *de jure* standard of care will provide a more coherent framework for relating technical questions that concern the conduct of specific clinical trials to ethical issues that arise at a broader social and political level. At the trial level, for instance, this standard requires researchers to ensure that their choice of trial design does not allow some participants to suffer harms that could be foreseen and prevented with reasonable care. At the policy level, however, this standard requires researchers, their sponsoring agencies, and relevant political bodies to ensure that conducting a clinical trial represents a responsible means of addressing the healthcare priorities of the population in question. In cases where equipoise exists in one country but not in another we will have to consider whether equally or more profound healthcare outcomes could be achieved, perhaps with the imposition of fewer burdens, by altering some of the conditions that cause equipoise to exist in the one case when it does not exist in the other. In other words, not only is it necessary that morally acceptable clinical trials be effective and efficient, it must also be the case that conducting a clinical trial represents the most effective and efficient means of addressing the healthcare needs of a particular population.

The short course AZT trials have generated a lengthy and trenchant debate because they are open to reasonable challenges on a variety of fronts at both of these levels. As a result, I agree with those who remind us that tough cases generally make bad policy. The local *de facto* standard of care may be attractive for the way it promises a simple solution to this complex debate, but this simplicity is purchased at the price of important ethical principles. I have tried to argue that the local *de jure* standard of care may not yield as simple a solution as either its proponents or its critics may think, but that this is itself an exciting discovery. The possibility that both sides of this debate may be able to articulate their concerns within a shared framework holds out the possibility of moving beyond the present state of affairs in which the proponents of different standards of care appear only to be entrenching and fortifying their positions. I hope that the present study is sufficient to show that the work it will take to explore the complexities of the *de jure* standard, and its implications for the short-course AZT studies and future international research, is important, and remains to be done.

REFERENCES

Angell, M. (1997). 'The ethics of clinical research in the third world,' *New England Journal of Medicine* 337, 847–849.

Crouch, R.A. and J.D. Arras (1998). 'AZT trials and tribulations,' *Hastings Center Report* 28, 26–34.

Freedman, B. (1990). 'Placebo-controlled trials and the logic of clinical purpose,' *IRB: A Review of Human Subjects Research* 12, 1–6.

Freedman, B. (1987). 'Equipoise and the ethics of clinical research,' *New England Journal of Medicine* 317, 141–145.

Levine, R.J. (1999). 'The need to revise the Declaration of Helsinki,' *New England Journal of Medicine* 341, 531–534.

Levine, R.J. (1998). 'The "best proven therapeutic method" standard in clinical trials in technologically developing countries,' *IRB: A Review of Human Subjects Research* 20, 5–9.

Lurie, P. and S.M. Wolfe (1997). 'Unethical trials of interventions to reduce perinatal transmission of the Human Immunodeficiency Virus in developing countries,' *New England Journal of Medicine* 337, 853–856.

RESEARCH IN DEVELOPING COUNTRIES: TAKING "BENEFIT" SERIOUSLY

Leonard H. Glantz, George J. Annas, Michael A. Grodin, and Wendy K. Mariner

An April 1998 *New York Times Magazine* article described Ronald Munger's efforts to obtain blood samples from a group of extremely impoverished people in the Philippine island of Cebu.[1] Munger sought the blood to study whether there was a genetic cause for this group's unusually high incidence of cleft lip and palate. One of many obstacles to the research project was the need to obtain the cooperation of the local health officer. It was not clear to Munger, or the reader, whether the health officer had a bona fide interest in protecting the populace or was looking for a bribe. The health officer asked Munger a few perfunctory questions about informed consent and the study's ethical review in the United States, which Munger answered. Munger also explained the benefits that mothers and children would derive from participating in the research. The mothers would learn their blood types (which they apparently desired) and whether they were anemic. If they were anemic, they would be given iron pills. Lunch would be served, and raffles arranged so that families could win simple toys and other small items.

Munger told the health officer that if his hypotheses were correct, the research would benefit the population of Cebu: if the research shows that increased folate and vitamin B6 reduces the risk of cleft lip and palate, families could reduce the risk of facial deformities in their future offspring. The reporter noted that the health officer "laughs aloud at the suggestion that much of what is being discovered in American laboratories will make it back to Cebu any time soon." Reflecting on his experience with another simple intervention, iodized salt, the health officer said that when salt was iodized, the price rose threefold

"so those who need it couldn't afford it and those who didn't need it are the only ones who could afford it."

The simple blood collecting mission to Cebu illustrates almost all the issues presented by research in developing countries. First is the threshold question of the goal of the research and its importance to the population represented by the research subjects. Next is the quality of informed consent including whether the potential subjects thought that participation in the research was related to free surgical care that was offered in the same facility (although it clearly was not) and whether one could adequately explain genetic hypotheses to an uneducated populace. Finally, there is the question whether the population from which subjects were drawn could benefit from the research. This research intervention is very low risk—the collection of 10 drops of blood from affected people and their family members. The risk of job or insurance discrimination that genetic research poses in this country did not exist for the Cebu population; ironically, they were protected from the risk of economic discrimination by the profound poverty in which they lived.

Even this simple study raises the most fundamental question: "Why is it acceptable for researchers in developed countries to use citizens of developing countries as research subjects?" A cautionary approach to permitting research with human subjects in underdeveloped countries has been recommended because of the risk of their inadvertent or deliberate exploitation by researchers from developed countries. This cautionary approach generally is invoked when researchers propose to use what are considered "vulnerable populations," such as prisoners and children, as research subjects. Vulnerable populations are those that are less able to protect themselves, either because they are not capable of making their own decisions or because they are particularly susceptible to mistreatment. For example, children may be incapable of giving informed

From *Hastings Center Report* 28, no. 6 (1998): 38–42. Reprinted by permission of The Hastings Center.

Editors' note: Some authors' notes have been cut. Students who want to follow up on sources should consult the original article.

consent or of standing up to adult authority, while prisoners are especially vulnerable to being coerced into becoming subjects. Citizens of developing countries are often in vulnerable situations because of their lack of political power, lack of education, unfamiliarity with medical interventions, extreme poverty, or dire need for health care and nutrition. It is the dire need of these populations that may make them both appropriate subjects of research and especially vulnerable to exploitation. This combination of need and vulnerability has led to the development of guidelines for the use of citizens of developing countries as research subjects.

CIOMS GUIDELINES

In 1992, the Council for International Organizations of Medical Sciences (CIOMS), in collaboration with the World Health Organization, published guidelines for the appropriate use of research subjects from "underdeveloped communities."

Like other human research codes, the CIOMS guidelines combine the protection of subjects' rights with protection of their welfare; as subjects become less able to protect their own rights (and therefore become more vulnerable), researchers and reviewers must increase their efforts to protect the welfare of subjects. Perhaps the most important statement in these guidelines is what appears to be the injunction against using subjects in developing countries if the research could be carried out reasonably well in developed countries. Commentary to guideline 8 notes, for example, that there are diseases that rarely or never occur in economically developed countries, and that prevention and treatment research therefore needs to be conducted in the countries at risk for those diseases. The conclusion to be drawn from the substance of these guidelines is that in order for research to be ethically conducted, it must offer the potential of actual benefit to the inhabitants of that developing country.

In order for underdeveloped communities to derive potential benefit from research, they must have access to the fruits of such research. The CIOMS commentary to guideline 8 states that, "as a general rule, the sponsoring agency should ensure that, at the completion of successful testing, any product developed *will* be made reasonably available to

inhabitants of the underdeveloped community in which the research was carried out: exceptions to this general requirement should be justified, and agreed to by all concerned parties before the research is begun." This statement is directed at minimizing exploitation of the underdeveloped community that provides the research subjects. If developed countries use inhabitants of underdeveloped countries to create new products that would be beneficial to both the developed and the underdeveloped country, but the underdeveloped country cannot gain access to the product because of expense, then the subjects in the underdeveloped countries have been grossly exploited. As written, however, this CIOMS guideline is not strong or specific enough to prevent exploitation. Exemplifying this problem are recent short course zidovudine (AZT) studies in Africa that were approved and conducted despite the existence of the CIOMS guidelines.

THE AFRICAN MATERNAL-FETAL HIV TRANSMISSION STUDIES

The goal of the short course AZT studies was to see if lower doses of the drug AZT than those used in the United States could reduce the rate of maternal-child transmission of HIV. It was well established that doses of AZT that cost $800 (not taking into account screening and other related costs) reduced maternal-fetal transmission of HIV by as much as two-thirds in the United States. If the developed countries had been willing to subsidize the cost of this regimen in Africa, no additional research would have been needed. But because many African countries could not afford this expense, the decision was made to attempt to see if lower (and therefore cheaper) doses would prevent maternal-fetal HIV transmission. Several impoverished countries were chosen as research sites. The justification for conducting research in those countries was not that they suffered from a disease that did not afflict people in developed countries, and not because no treatment existed, but because their impoverishment made an existing therapy unavailable to them (as long as developed countries refused to subsidize the costs).

The issue, as always, is to determine the ethical acceptability of the proposed research *before* it is conducted. In a case like this, where the researchable problem exists *solely* because of economic reasons, the research hypothesis must contain an economic component. The research question should be formulated as follows:

1. We know that a given regimen of AZT will reduce the rate of maternal-child transmission of HIV.
2. Maternal-child transmission of HIV in many African countries is a serious problem but the effective AZT regimen is not available because it is too expensive.
3. If an effective AZT regimen costs $X, then it will be made available in the country in which it is to be studied.
4. Therefore, we will conduct trials in certain African countries to see if $X worth of AZT will effectively reduce maternal-child transmission of HIV in those countries.

The most important part of the development of this research question is number 3. Without knowing what dollar amount X actually represents, it is impossible to formulate a research question that can lead to any benefit to the citizens of the country in which the research is to be conducted. There is no way to determine what $X represents in the absence of committed funding. Therefore, an essential prerequisite to designing ethical research in underdeveloped countries is identifying the source and amount of funding for providing the fruits of the research to the people of the developing country in which it is to be studied as a condition of the research being approved.

If a study found, for example, that $50 worth of AZT has the same effect as $800 worth of AZT, it would greatly benefit the developed world. Developed countries, which currently spend $800 per case on drugs alone, could pay substantially less for this preventive measure, and, because the research was conducted elsewhere, none of their citizens would have been put at any risk. At the same time, if the underdeveloped country could not afford to spend $50 any more than it could spend $800, then it could not possibly derive information that would be of any benefit to its population. This is the definition of exploitation.[2]

It is only now that an effort is being made to determine how to raise the money to actually provide AZT to prevent maternal-child HIV transmission

(as well as the other costly services that go with the appropriate administration of the drug) to the impoverished African countries that provided the human subjects. These efforts began after parallel studies conducted in Thailand reported that lower doses of AZT reduced maternal-fetal transmission of HIV. The Thai government had committed to providing the AZT before its trials began. In the African trials, however, no one "ensured" that at the completion of successful testing the product would be made reasonably available, thereby violating the CIOMS guidelines. The guidelines say that there can be exceptions to this general requirement, but that exceptions must be "justified" and "agreed to by all concerned parties." It is not clear to whom the exception must be "justified" or on what grounds. Moreover, if the "concerned parties" are the sponsor and/or the investigator and the host country, they may not adequately represent the interests of the research subjects. The fact that representatives of the research community and officials of the host countries agree to exploit the population does not make the research any less exploitive.

RULES FOR ETHICAL RESEARCH IN DEVELOPING COUNTRIES

We believe the standards for research in developing countries should include the following.

There should be a rebuttable presumption that researchers from developed countries will not conduct research in developing countries unless it can be shown that a direct benefit *will* be bestowed upon the residents of that country if the research proves to be successful. The person or entities proposing to conduct the study must demonstrate that there is a realistic plan, which includes identified funding, to provide the newly proven intervention to the population from which the potential pool of research subjects is to be recruited. In the absence of a realistic plan and identified funding, the population from which the research subjects will be drawn cannot derive benefit from the research. Therefore, the benefits cannot outweigh the risks, because there are, and will be, no benefits. Only by having committed funding and a plan to make a successful intervention available can it be determined that there will be sufficient benefit to justify conducting research on the target population. The distribution plan must be realistic. Where the health care infrastructure is so undeveloped that it would be impossible to deliver the intervention even if it were free, research would be unjustified in the absence of a plan to improve that country's health care delivery capabilities.

Some might argue that this standard is too strict and that it would reduce the amount of research that could be conducted in certain countries. The answer, of course, is that if the benefits of the research are not made available to the inhabitants of that country, they have lost nothing by the lack of such research. Others might argue that research in underdeveloped countries is justified if it might benefit the individual research subjects, even if it will not benefit anyone else in the population. However, research is, by definition, designed to create generalizable knowledge, and is legitimate in a developing country only if its purpose is to create generalizable knowledge that will benefit the citizens of that country. If the research only has the potential to benefit the limited number of individuals who participate in the study, it cannot offer the benefit to the underdeveloped country that legitimizes the use of its citizens as research subjects. It should be emphasized that research whose goal is to prevent or treat large populations is fundamentally public health research, and public health research makes no sense (and thus should not be done) if its benefits are limited to the small population of research subjects.

It might be argued that there is no requirement that such a plan be devised prior to conducting research in the United States, and, therefore, that by adopting such a requirement we would be imposing a higher standard for research conducted in developing countries than we do for research conducted in the United States.

This argument only further demonstrates the differences between wealthy and poor countries. The reality in the United States is that regardless of the very significant gaps in insurance and Medicaid coverage and the health care discrepancies between the rich and poor, medical interventions are relatively widely available, especially when compared to developing countries. Upon the successful completion of the research that demonstrated the effectiveness of the 076 regimen in reducing maternal-child transmission, the primary beneficiaries of this new preventive intervention in the United States were poor women and their newborns. Unlike the United States, absent a plan to pay for a new intervention and lacking the infrastructure to deliver an intervention, it is virtually guaranteed that the intervention will not be generally available in a developing country.

The more accurate analogy to the African AIDS trials would be if investigators proposed the 076 protocol in the United States knowing that only poor women would be recruited as research subjects and that, if successful, the intervention would not be made generally available to poor women. Such research would be clearly unethical. Not only would this be a gross violation of the ethical principle of distributive justice, it would be a violation of the regulatory obligation of the equitable selection of subjects.

A further objection is that one cannot always trust what a government or another potential funder promises. What is to prevent the promisor from reneging? The answer is, nothing. One can try to expose the funder to embarrassment and other pressures that might cause it to live up to the promise upon which researchers and subjects relied. However, the potential unethical behavior in the future by the funder is no excuse for not having a realistic plan at the outset. Furthermore, if we take this obligation seriously, this should only occur once per funder. After reneging once, they cannot be relied upon again to justify research in the future.

An additional objection to our position is that it will restrict access to new interventions because once a new intervention is developed, the price will come down and therefore the intervention will become available to the people of the impoverished country. The answer is to ask those who control the pricing of interventions if this will be the case in any particular instance. One could have asked Glaxo if it would reduce its price once it was shown that lower doses of AZT were effective. If the answer is yes, one can proceed. If the answer is no, or "we have not decided," there seems to be no justification to proceed if the current price would significantly restrict availability. There is nothing magical about pricing. Pricing is in the absolute control of manufacturers and there is no need to guess or speculate about what will happen to price. Indeed, this objection to our argument would justify conducting the full 076 trial itself in developing countries. The price *might* come down enough so that determining the efficacy of short course AZT regimens might not be needed at all. Such speculation should not be sufficient to put subjects at risk.

Finally, it might be argued that there are diseases that only affect people in developing countries for which there are no effective treatments, but that the treatments that might be discovered could be expensive. The argument continues that it is not right to fail to develop treatments that could benefit some affected people because it will not be available to most affected people. This objection raises quite a different issue from the one addressed in this article. The impetus for such research is the absence of effective treatment and not the absence of economic resources. We have discussed research intended to determine whether effective but unaffordable interventions would work if used in lower, less expensive dosages. The researchable issue arises from an economic circumstance. The only way such research could offer any benefit is by "curing" the economic problem by establishing that the less expensive form of the intervention will be affordable and available. Absent knowledge of financial resources, one might well be creating a new unaffordable, and therefore useless, intervention. In contrast, in the case in which one is developing a new intervention, not because of poverty; but because no known effective intervention exists, and the disease is prevalent in a particular geographic area, the issue is quite different. In such a case one is not conducting research to try to "cure" the effects of poverty but rather because of the need to create new knowledge to treat a currently untreatable disease. However, even this case may raise problems similar to the ones addressed here. If one were to try to develop an intervention for such a condition and chose research subjects from impoverished segments of a society, knowing that only the richest segment of that society could benefit from that intervention, such subject selection would be unethical for many of the reasons we have discussed.

Our proposal to require researchers and their funders to develop realistic plans to make their interventions available to the relevant population of the developing country in which the research is proposed should not be controversial. It is well accepted in principle not only by groups like CIOMS, but by the funders of many of the African HIV trials, including the Centers for Disease Control and Prevention and the National Institutes of Health. The principle is often honored in the breach, however. Research funders who hope that their studies will yield beneficial knowledge may neglect the steps necessary to ensure that the benefits will be made available. Ethical codes have not been sufficiently specific or enforceable to protect research subjects from exploitation. It is essential to replace vague promises with realistic plans that must be reviewed and approved before the research commences.

In at least one other instance it has been suggested that economic issues be addressed in the review of proposed research projects. The U.S. National Research Council's Committee on Human Genome Diversity recommended that "Arrangements regarding financial interests in the products or outcomes of the research should be negotiated *as part of the original project review* and informed-consent process."[3]

It is essential that the wealthier countries of the world use their resources, both financial and technological, to help resolve the health problems that afflict the poor of the world. Doing so will undoubtedly require research. But research is a means to solving health problems, not an end in itself. The goal must be to create interventions that will benefit the people of the countries in which the research is conducted. They will benefit only if the knowledge gained produces interventions that are affordable and accessible. This needs to be determined as a condition of approval before research is conducted so that limited research funds are not wasted, and research subjects are not drawn from populations that will not be able to benefit from the research.

REFERENCES

1. Lisa Belkin, "The Clues Are in the Blood," *New York Times Magazine,* 26 April 1998.
2. The per capita health care expenditures of most of the African countries involved in mother-to-child HIV transmission prevention trials range from $5 to $22 U.S. *World Bank Sector Strategy Health Nutrition and Population,* 1997.
3. Committee on Human Genetic Diversity, *Evaluating Human Genetic Diversity* (Washington, D.C.: National Academy Press, 1997), pp. 55–68.

FAIR BENEFITS FOR RESEARCH IN DEVELOPING COUNTRIES

Participants in the 2001 Conference on Ethical Aspects of Research in Developing Countries

Collaborative, multinational clinical research, especially between developed and developing countries, has been the subject of controversy. Much of this attention has focused on the standard of care used in randomized trials. Much less discussed, but probably more important in terms of its impact on health, is the claim that, in order to avoid exploitation, interventions proven safe and effective through research in developing countries should be made "reasonably available" in those countries.

This claim was first emphasized by the Council for International Organizations of Medical Sciences: "As a general rule, the sponsoring agency should agree in advance of the research that any product developed through such research will be made reasonably available to the inhabitants of the host community or country at the completion of successful testing"[1] The reasonable availability requirement has received broad support, with disagreement focusing on two elements. First, how strong or explicit should the commitment to provide the drug or vaccine be at the initiation of the research study? Some suggest that advanced discussions without assurances are sufficient, while others require advance guarantees that include identifiable funding and distribution networks. Second, to whom must the drugs and vaccines be made available? Should the commitment extend only to the participants in the study, the community from which participants have been recruited, the entire country, or the region of the world? Although these disagreements have ethical and practical implications, there is a deeper question about whether reasonable availability is necessary, or the best way, to avoid exploitation in developing countries.

What constitutes exploitation? A exploits B when B receives an unfair level of benefits as a result of

From *SCIENCE* 298 (December 13, 2002): 2133–2134. Reprinted by permission.

Editors' note: Some notes have been cut. Students who want to follow up on sources should consult the original article.

B's interactions with A. The fairness of the benefits B receives depends on the burdens that B bears as a result of the interaction, and the benefits that A and others receive as a result of B's participation. Fairness is the crucial aspect, not equality of benefits. Although being vulnerable may increase the chances for exploitation, it is neither necessary nor sufficient for exploitation.

The potential for clinical research to exploit populations is not a major concern in developed countries since there are processes, albeit haphazard and imperfect, for ensuring that interventions proven effective are introduced into the health-care system and benefit the general population. In contrast, target populations in developing countries often lack access to regular health care, political power, and an understanding of research. They may be exposed to the risks of research, while access to the benefits of new, effective drugs and vaccines goes predominantly to people in developed countries and the profits go to the biopharmaceutical industry. This situation fails to provide fair benefits and thus constitutes the paradigm of exploitation.

By focusing on a particular type of benefit, the reasonable availability requirement fails to avoid exploitation in many cases. First, and most importantly, the ethical concern embedded in exploitation is about the amount or level of benefits received and not the type of benefits. Reasonable availability fails to ensure a fair share of benefits; for instance, it may provide for too little benefit when risks are high or benefits to the sponsors great. Moreover, it applies only to phase III research that leads to an effective intervention; it is inapplicable to phase I and II and unsuccessful phase III studies. Consequently, reasonable availability fails to protect against the potential of exploitation in a great deal of research conducted in developing countries. Furthermore, reasonable availability embodies a narrow concept of benefits. It does not consider other potential benefits of research in developing countries, including training of health-care or research personnel, construction of health-care facilities and other physical infrastructure, and provision of public health measures and health services beyond those required as part of the research trial. Finally, insisting on reasonable availability precludes the community's deciding which benefits it prefers.

Reasonable availability should not be imposed as an absolute ethical requirement for research in developing countries without affirmation by the countries themselves. The authors,[2] who are from developed countries and African developing countries, have proposed an alternative to reasonable availability to avoid exploitation in developing countries: Fair Benefits. This framework would supplement the usual conditions for ethical conduct of research trials, such as independent review by an institutional review board or research ethics committee and individual informed consent. In particular, Fair Benefits relies on three widely accepted ethical conditions. First, the research must address a health problem of the developing country population, although, as with HIV/AIDS, it could also be relevant to other populations. Second, the research objectives, not vulnerability of the population, must provide a strong justification for conducting the research in this population. For instance, the population may have a high incidence of the disease being studied or high transmission rates of infection necessary to evaluate a vaccine. Third, the research must pose few risks to the participants, or the benefits to them clearly must outweigh the risks.

The Fair Benefits framework requires satisfaction of the following three additional fundamental principles to protect developing communities from exploitation.

FAIR BENEFITS

In assessing whether studies offer a fair level of benefits, the population could consider benefits from both the conduct and results of research. Among potential benefits to research participants are additional diagnostic tests, distribution of medications and vaccinations, and emergency evacuation services. Research might also provide collateral health services to members of the population not enrolled in the research, such as determining disease prevalence and drug resistance patterns, or providing interventions such as antibiotics for respiratory infections or the digging of boreholes for

---

THE FAIR BENEFITS FRAMEWORK*

Fair Benefits

Benefits to Participants During the Research
Improvements to health and health care
Collateral health services unnecessary for research study

Benefits to Population During the Research
Collateral health services unnecessary for research study
Public health measures
Employment and economic activity

Benefits to Population After the Research
Reasonable availability of effective intervention
Research and medical care capacity development
Public health measures
Long-term research collaboration
Sharing of financial rewards from research results

Collaborative Partnership

Community involvement at all stages
Free, uncoerced decision-making by population bearing the burdens of the research

Transparency

Central, publicly accessible repository of benefits agreements
Process of community consultations

*It is not necessary to provide each benefit.

---

clean water. Conducting research usually entails the benefits of employment and enhanced economic activity for the population as well.

Reasonable availability of a safe and effective intervention may provide an important benefit for the population after the completion of some research trials. Alternatively, other postresearch benefits might include capacity development, such as enhancing health-care or research facilities, providing critical equipment, other physical infrastructure such as roads or vehicles, training of health-care and research staff, and training of individuals in research ethics.

Furthermore, any single research trial could be an isolated endeavor or form part of a long-term collaboration between the population and the researchers. Long-term collaboration embodies engagement with and a commitment to the population; it can also provide the population with long-term training, employment, investment, and additional research on other health issues. Finally, profits from direct sales of proven interventions or from intellectual property rights can be shared with the developing country. It is not necessary to provide each of these benefits; the ethical imperative is for a fair level of benefits overall—not an equal level.

COLLABORATIVE PARTNERSHIP

Collaborative partnership means that researchers must engage the population in developing, evaluating, and benefiting from the research. Currently, there is no shared, international standard of fairness. In part this is because of conflicting conceptions of international distributive justice. Ultimately, the determination of whether the benefits are fair and worth the risks cannot be entrusted to people outside the population, no matter how well intentioned. They may be ill-informed about the health, social, and economic context and are unlikely to appreciate the importance of the proposed benefits to the host community. The relevant population for the Fair Benefits framework is the community that is involved with the researchers, bears the burdens of the research, and would be the potential victims of exploitation. There is no justification for including an entire region or every citizen of a country in the distribution of benefits and decision-making, unless the whole region or country is involved in the research study. To avoid exploitation, it is the village, tribe, neighborhood, or province whose members are approached for enrollment, whose health-care personnel are recruited to staff the research teams, whose physical facilities and social networks are utilized to conduct the study who must receive the benefits from research and determine what constitutes a fair level of benefits.

The population's decision about whether research is worthwhile and fair must be free and uncoerced. Practically, this means that a decision not to participate in the proposed research is a realistic alternative. Deciding if a population can really refuse will not

be easy. Nonetheless, proceeding with a research trial requires that the population in which it is to be conducted genuinely supports it.

TRANSPARENCY

The lack of an international standard for fairness and the disparity in bargaining power between populations and researchers in developing countries and sponsors and researchers from developed countries means that even in the presence of collaborative partnership, the community might agree to an unfair level of benefits. The Fair Benefits framework can be used to catalog the array of benefits that are provided in different research studies (see Table, this page). An independent body, such as the World Health Organization, could establish a central and publicly accessible repository of all the formal and informal benefit agreements of previous studies. This repository would allow populations, researchers, and others to make independent and transparent comparisons of the level of the benefits provided in particular studies to ensure their fairness.

To further facilitate transparency, this body should develop a program of community consultations that actively informs the communities, researchers, and others in developing countries likely to participate in research about previously negotiated agreements. These consultations would also provide forums in which all interested parties could deliberate on the fairness of the agreements. Over time, such a central repository and the community consultations would generate a collection of critically evaluated benefits agreements that would become a kind of "case law" generating shared standards of fair benefits.

REFERENCES AND NOTES

1. *International Ethical Guidelines for Biomedical Research Involving Human Subjects* [Council for International Organizations of Medical Science (CIOMS), Geneva, 1993], guidelines 8 and 15.
2. Meeting held 26 to 28 March 2001 in Blantyre, Malawi. It was cosponsored by the Department of Clinical Bioethics and NIAID of the NIH (USA) and the University of Malawi College of Medicine. Author affiliations at www.sciencemag.org/cgi/content/full/298/5601/2133/DC1

RESEARCH ON CHILDREN

CHILDREN AND "MINIMAL RISK" RESEARCH: THE KENNEDY-KRIEGER LEAD PAINT STUDY

Alex John London

In 1993 the Kennedy Krieger Institute (KKI), a Johns Hopkins affiliated children's hospital and research center, received a $200,000 grant from the U.S. Environmental Protection Agency to study the short and long-term efficacy of several different strategies for removing or containing lead-paint in residential housing units in Baltimore City. For researchers at the prestigious research center, the grant represented an important step in the KKI's ongoing fight to encourage a more proactive approach to preventing lead poisoning in children. In August of 2001, however, less than a decade after the study's inception, the Maryland Court of Appeals would compare the study to some of the darkest and most troubling abuses of human subjects in history, including the Tuskegee Syphilis Study and the typhus experiments at Buchenwald concentration camp during World War II.[1]

Unlike many industrialized nations that banned lead paint for interior use at the dawn of the twentieth century, it was not until 1978 that the U.S. outlawed its use. As a result, even in early 1990's it was estimated that 35–40% of children from low-income inner-city neighborhoods nationwide had dangerous levels of lead in their blood, compared to only 5% of non-Hispanic white children living outside of city centers. In some urban areas the prevalence of lead paint in low-income housing was particularly high. Researchers from the KKI estimated that as many as 95% of the low-income housing units in Baltimore's inner-city neighborhoods were contaminated with lead paint and the number of children from those neighborhoods with elevated blood lead levels was estimated to be as high as two thirds. Children are at special risk for lead poisoning because their high rate of hand-to-mouth activity

---

1. *Erika Grimes* v. *Kennedy Krieger Institute, Inc. Myron Higgins, a minor, etc., et al.* v. *Kennedy Krieger Institute, Inc.* No.

128, No. 129 Court Appeals of Maryland, 2001 Md. August 16, 2001, Filed.

increases the likelihood that they will ingest the lead-contaminated dust generated by deteriorating paints. When lead is absorbed into their bodies it can adversely affect their cognitive development, behavior, and growth. In fact, extremely high levels of lead can precipitate seizures, coma, and even death.

Safely removing lead paint from home interiors poses special challenges. In the late 1980's researchers at the KKI helped to show that traditional methods of removing lead paint—burning or scraping it off—actually generated large amounts of contaminated dust, thereby exacerbating the hazard for the children who would occupy those homes. New methods of abatement would have to be developed that would provide safer methods of removing or containing the hazard posed by the poisonous paint. In addition, in urban settings where affordable low-income housing is at a premium, the cost of removing lead from rental units frequently exceeds the value of the properties themselves. When faced with the financial burdens of abating what are often only marginally profitable properties in the first place, many landlords chose simply to close their properties and leave them unoccupied. In 1990 the Department of Housing and Urban Development estimated the cost of complete lead abatement nationwide at roughly $500 billion.

Prior to the 1993 study, researchers at the KKI had shown that several more economical strategies for removing or controlling lead paint could effectively reduce the amount of lead-contaminated dust in empty houses. In order to know whether these strategies would translate into a similar reduction of lead poisoning in children, researchers wanted to measure the effectiveness of these strategies in terms of their impact on the blood lead levels of children who would occupy such units. The 1993 study would therefore measure lead levels in household dust and in the blood of children residing in housing units involved in the study.

The study included 75 housing units that were divided into five groups. Group I houses received a minimal level of repair and maintenance costing approximately $1,650. Group II houses received a greater level of repair and maintenance costing approximately $3,500. Repair and maintenance in Group III houses was more extensive and cost between $6,000 and $7,000. The study also included two control groups. Group IV properties consisted of

houses that had been fully abated by the city under a local government program. Because of the extent of this previous abatement, these properties received no additional repair or maintenance. Finally, Group V properties were modern units constructed after 1980 in which it could reasonably be assumed that no lead paints had been used.

Researchers from the KKI worked with landlords to obtain grants and loans to fund these repairs. In many cases the properties were already occupied by families prior to the inception of the study, but when properties were vacant, landlords were encouraged to rent to families with small children. In all cases, researchers were looking for families with healthy children between 5 and 48 months old who did not have plans to leave the properties before the study was completed. Parents were asked to sign consent forms in which they were informed that the purpose of the study was to measure the effectiveness of repairs that were intended to reduce, but not to completely remove, the lead exposure in their home. In return for their participation they received small payments of $5 and $15 and they were told that the KKI would provide them with the results of the periodic blood lead testing.

To the researchers conducting the study, this was a win-win situation.[2] Every property in the study had received what they believed was a significant level of lead abatement and, as a result, the families residing in those properties faced lower risks than they would have experienced if they had lived in comparable properties that had not been so repaired. Additionally, the data generated by this study would provide valuable information about the efficacy of more affordable measures of reducing and controlling lead exposure for reducing child lead poisoning. If successful, these measures would offer significant and affordable means of reducing a widespread public health hazard that disproportionately affects the poorest and most vulnerable populations of children in the United States.

Some of the families that participated in the study had different views. Two families in particular

---

2. See the "Lead-Based Paint Study Fact Sheet" published on the Johns Hopkins School of Medicine web page at: http://www.hopkinsmedicine.org/press/2001/SEPTEMBER/leadfactsheet.htm

brought law suits against the KKI alleging that their respective children were poisoned, or were at least exposed to the risk of being poisoned, by lead dust due to the negligence of the KKI researchers. They also alleged that they were not fully informed of the risks of the research and that the KKI failed to warn them in a timely manner of the children's exposure to the known presence of lead. In August of 2001 the Maryland Court of Appeals unanimously overturned a lower court decision that would have barred the suits from going forward. Six of the seven judges signed on to an opinion that offered a sweeping indictment of the lead paint study.

Writing for these six judges, Judge Dale R. Cathell criticized the basic design of the study:

> Otherwise healthy children, in our view, should not be enticed into living in, or remaining in, potentially lead-tainted housing and intentionally subjected to a research program, which contemplates the probability, or even the possibility, of lead poisoning or even the accumulation of lower levels of lead in blood, in order for the extent of the contamination of the children's blood to be used by scientific researchers to assess the success of lead paint or lead dust abatement measures (p. 7).

To the court, the language of the consent form did not provide a clear and complete explanation that the purpose of the study was to measure the efficacy of the abatement procedures by measuring the extent to which the children's blood was being contaminated. As a result, it was not clear that the parents understood that the very design of the research presupposed the accumulation of lead in their children's blood.

The extent to which the families that participated in this study understood its design and purpose is a question that was disputed before the court. Judge Cathell was clear, however, that in the court's view "parents, whether improperly enticed by trinkets, food stamps, money or other items, have no more right to intentionally and unnecessarily place children in potentially hazardous nontherapeutic research surroundings, than do researchers. In such cases, parental consent, no matter how informed, is insufficient" (p. 7). In fact, the majority went even further, stating that, "We hold that in Maryland a parent, appropriate relative, or other applicable surrogate, cannot consent to the participation of a child

or other person under legal disability in nontherapeutic research or studies in which there is any risk of injury or damage to the health of the subject" (pp. 89–90).

As a result of this decision, the substantive legal issues raised by these lawsuits will be argued before a trial court. But many observers were surprised by the scope and severity of the Appeals Court opinion. In the estimation of the court, the KKI lead paint study was similar to research abuses of the past in which vulnerable populations were knowingly subjected to harmful or poisonous substances, not for some direct benefit to themselves, but in order to generate generalizable scientific data. Those who agree with the court will argue that children from low-income inner-city families are already disadvantaged in ways that their more affluent middle- and upper-class counterparts are not. The high prevalence of lead in their living quarters, and the significant threat it poses to their mental and physical health, is simply one particularly visible way in which the opportunity range of these children is unfairly limited by their poverty. Why should the fact that poverty consigns many of these children to toxic housing conditions justify providing them with less stringent research protections than would be extended to children from more affluent and socially mobile families? Does their poverty and lower-income social status make the lead to which they were exposed in this study less toxic, or the risks to their health less profound or important?

In defense of this study, the KKI has argued that the methods they employed "were then believed to be the best practices within high-risk housing" and that the interventions and follow up provided by the study "were greater than those children would have received without the Study and likely would not have occurred without the Study." They estimate that the lead reduction measures implemented in these properties improved them by approximately 80% over all other existing housing alternatives in these neighborhoods. They also note that "The Court was silent with respect to the obligations of various levels of government that tolerated the evidence of lead paint for decades, and a society that does not offer realistic options for low income families to move out of high risk neighborhoods." Relative to the thousands of families living in nonabated houses, the subjects of this study could reasonably be said to have benefited by their participation. Furthermore, one reason for the inaction of the public and private sectors in the face of this pervasive public health hazard is a reluctance to pay the high cost of lead abatement procedures whose relative merits over less expensive alternatives have not been clearly quantified. From this point of view, the KKI can be seen as a well-intentioned agent of social reform seeking to provide clear data on effective means of curbing a public health problem that will otherwise persist and continue to damage the lives of innocent lower-income inner-city children.

In ruling that parents and guardians cannot consent to the participation of children in research that poses *any* degree of risk, the Maryland Court of Appeals enunciated an ideal for research protections that could threaten the permissibility of important pediatric research. Is this standard too high? The current federal regulations permit research on children that is a minor increment over minimal risk, where minimal risk is defined as "the probability and magnitude of harm or discomfort anticipated in the research are not greater in and of themselves than those ordinarily encountered in daily life or during the performance of routine physical or psychological examinations or tests." Would the KKI lead paint study be permissible in high-risk neighborhoods of Baltimore City, but not in newer, wealthier suburbs, because the inner-city children are exposed to higher risks of lead poisoning in their daily lives whereas their suburban counterparts are not?

Even after the legal questions raised by this case are settled, other ethical issues will likely remain. In particular, this case raises troubling questions about the role of research into health problems that are due, in large part, to social and economic inequalities between populations. When the ultimate goal is to get local and federal agencies to spend the money it will take to alleviate the lead hazards in low-income neighborhoods, is it permissible to conduct research in which the protections afforded to subjects fall below standards that are enjoyed by wealthier members of society? Should the way a trial is designed be determined by whether or not the social will exists to spend significant amounts of money to improve the housing conditions of largely low-income inner-city populations? Is there a guarantee that the social will exists to spend smaller, but

still significant amounts of money to reduce, but not eliminate such hazards? Should it be required before such research can begin that there be an agreement in place guaranteeing that some money will be spent to implement an effective lead abatement strategy in the places where research is conducted? In criticizing the design of this study are critics washing their hands of the larger public health and social justice issues that the researchers were hoping this study would address?

While the Court of Appeals compared the KKI study to the infamous Tuskegee Syphilis Study, the above questions suggest that a more instructive comparison might be the internationally sponsored short-course AZT trials that were conducted in developing countries in collaboration with entities from the developed world [see Part 6, Section 3]. In both cases the proposed research was designed to be responsive to a health problem that disproportionately affects one population, but not some others. Furthermore, in both cases a major reason for this difference is economic. Many developing countries cannot afford the full course of AZT—known as the 076 protocol—that is the current standard of care in the developed world. In response, researchers designed a study to find a shorter and more economical regimen of AZT that would offer some significant, but not optimal, protection against mother-to-child transmission of HIV. Similarly, many low-income inner-city families cannot afford to pay for complete lead abatement or to move to safer, but more expensive, housing. In response, researchers from the KKI designed a study to quantify the efficacy of several affordable methods of removing or controlling lead paint exposure in low-income housing units without removing the hazard completely. Is this a fair comparison? Does it make a difference to the moral evaluation of these studies that many of the countries that hosted the short-course AZT trials are themselves technologically and economically underdeveloped whereas the United States is one of, if not the, wealthiest and most technologically advanced nation in the world?

As medical research is deployed to alleviate health problems that are rooted in economic disparities between populations, the line between studying an illness or disease and exploiting economic deprivations is blurred. As more is learned about the social determinants of health and the impact of social inequalities on health status, the more pressing these issues will become. One of the challenges posed by the Kennedy Krieger lead paint study, and the short-course AZT studies, is to find a framework for evaluating clinical research that is responsive to these realities, and to the important moral principles they bring into conflict.

RESEARCH ON CHILDREN AND THE SCOPE OF RESPONSIBLE PARENTHOOD

Thomas H. Murray

The voluntary consent of the human subject is absolutely essential.
—The Nuremberg Code

To attempt to consent for a child to be made an experimental subject is to treat a child as not a child. . . . If the grounds for this are alleged to be the presumptive or implied consent of the child, that must simply be characterized as a violent and false presumption.
—Paul Ramsey, *The Patient as Person*

Consent is the heart of the matter.
—Richard McCormick, "Proxy Consent in the Experimentation Situation"

What obligations do parents have to their children? On the whole, bioethics has not grappled with the nuances of parental obligations and duties. Sometimes its treatment of issues even seems to lack common sense. Part of the problem has been that bioethicists have considered mostly life-or-death decisions. But sometimes we create our own difficulty by the way we frame the problem. Nowhere has this been more true than in discussions of research on children, in which a history of morally abominable research, mostly on adults, led to the

problem—and solution—being framed in terms that were simply irrelevant to children.

When the tools we have at hand are poorly suited for the job, the work is more difficult and the result inferior. We have some useful distinctions for understanding the ethics of research on children. But we have also been stuck with some downright clumsy contraptions. The problems become inescapable when we try to make sense of a morally complex proposal, like one to study the impact of human growth hormone on children with short stature.

A CONTROVERSIAL STUDY OF GROWTH HORMONE

Our bodies produce human growth hormone, or hGH, as part of the normal processes of growth. Children whose bodies cannot produce it do not grow as do other children. Unless they receive hGH somehow, they will become adults with extremely short stature. In a society that values height, those children can suffer severe disadvantages and discrimination.

But not all short children lack hGH. Height is like many other natural characteristics: people vary in how much of it they have. A few are very tall or very short; some are a bit taller or shorter than average; most are near the average. Some of the children who are much shorter than average have no discernible lack of hGH. Nor do they have any of the other signs that often accompany dwarfism caused by the absence of hGH. They are short, in all likelihood, because their parents are short, just as other

From *The Worth of a Child*, by Thomas H. Murray. Berkeley: University of California Press, 1996: 70–95, 194–195. Copyright © 1996 University of California Press. Reprinted with permission.

Editors' note: Most author's notes have been cut. Students who want to follow up on sources should consult the original article.

children are well muscled because their parents are well muscled.

The quandary is this: short stature is a problem for children and adults not merely when it is a disease. In a world constructed for adults of a particular height range, being short enough (or, for that matter, tall enough) to fill outside the range is like having a disability. The world is harder to navigate when you are the "wrong" size. There is nothing intrinsically wrong with being substantially shorter or taller than average; the world could be made to fit a broader range of sizes. But for now at least it is not. And so extreme short stature can be a disability.

For most short children, the problem takes another form. Parents understand that short stature can make life tougher for their child; children can be very cruel to those who look or act "different." Furthermore, the adult world is "heightist." Tall people get many advantages, just by virtue of their height. Most parents want to give their children whatever advantages they can. If they can make a short child taller, why not? Many parents seem to have reasoned this way, because many have sought growth hormone for their children who are not lacking it but who are nonetheless short

The increasing use of hGH for children who are not hGH-deficient prompted the National Institutes of Health (NIH) to approve a research project to study the effects of hGH injections on such children. The study raised enough questions that NIH asked a special panel to consider its ethical acceptability.

The study was originally planned to include eighty children ages nine through fifteen with normal levels of hGH but well below average height for their age. Each child receives three injections a week for as long as seven years. The study has a control group. Children in that group are treated exactly like the children in the experimental group, except that the injections they receive—600 to 1,100 over the life of the study—contain no hGH. Let me put that another way: None of the children in this study were ill. Some of them will receive as many as one thousand or more injections of a potent hormone; the others will get the same number of shots of salt water.

The special panel concluded that this study was acceptable. The panel's reasoning clung closely to the language of the regulations governing research on children. There are problems with the panel's strategy. A good ethical result is unlikely if the

regulations lack a sound moral foundation. When we lack vigorous moral concepts for analyzing problems, we are tempted to take refuge in legalisms. A look at the moral debate at the time the regulations were written reveals that they were built on a flawed effort to understand the ethics of research with children.

THE NATIONAL COMMISSION AND THE NUREMBERG CODE

Research on children covers a lot of moral ground. When a child has a grave disease and there is no good standard treatment, the child's only hope may be an experimental therapy. The novel therapy might carry its own substantial risks. But if previous research indicates that the experimental treatment is promising, and there is no solid alternative, then involvement of that child in research makes good moral sense. What makes the case persuasive is the hope that the particular child may benefit.

The ethics of research become more complex as the possibility of benefit to each of the children involved in the research becomes murkier. There are moral complexities, to be sure, when parents are asked to allow an experimental therapy to be used on their child who is suffering from disease. In most relevant respects, though, such a decision is not that different from other choices parents must make about treatment for their ill child. The uncertainty involved in experimental treatments is greater, of course, but we can never eliminate uncertainty. The crucial question in acceding to either standard or experimental treatment is the same: Will this benefit my child?

Another class of research studies has been more controversial: so-called nontherapeutic research, or in plainer language, research intended to gain knowledge but not to benefit its subjects directly. For example, the parents of a healthy, normal newborn might be asked to allow their child to serve as a control subject in a study of the physiology of some awful disease that strikes other babies. Perhaps the researchers want to monitor your baby's blood pressure more carefully than would otherwise be done for a healthy newborn; perhaps they want to draw an extra drop of blood from a heel prick, or a sample of blood from a vein; or perhaps in a study of infant heart disease, they want to insert a catheter through your baby's artery and into the heart, where they can measure changes in pressures and gas concentrations while they administer powerful drugs. It does not require much sophistication in ethics or science to notice great differences between the last experiment and the others. What would moral common sense say about these proposed studies?

If we were assured that there was no risk of harm or discomfort in the first proposed study—more frequent monitoring of blood pressure—indeed that the baby would not even notice it, then we might well agree to allow our newborn to participate in the study. Even if we refused, it is difficult to see what criticisms could be made of parents who did agree. Parents who allow their children to be observed in this manner do not seem to be failing in any important parental duty.

At the other extreme, we would be highly suspicious if parents consented to exposing their healthy babies to the pain and risk of having catheters threaded into their hearts and given powerful drugs, all with no conceivable benefit to their child. We might suspect that the parents did not understand what was to be done to their babies, or were so blinded by awe or gratitude that they were powerless to refuse; or, if they did understand the risks, that they were lousy parents who were not protecting their infant from a completely unnecessary risk of grave harm.

Such were the issues facing the members of the National Commission for the Protection of the Human Subjects of Biomedical and Behavioral Research when they developed their recommendations regarding the ethics of research on children. Should parents be prohibited from consenting to any research that held no hope of benefiting their children? Or should such research be permitted, with restrictions and safeguards?

As with any reasonably complex issue, many morally relevant questions arise. The ones of greatest interest to us are the nature and scope of parents' obligations to their children and in particular whether parents are ever justified in allowing their child to be used to benefit the community. Must we always refuse to expose our children to any risks or discomforts except when they might benefit our child? In the absence of any substantial risk or discomfort, do we wrong our children by allowing them to be used for others' benefit?

What makes this controversy particularly interesting for bioethics is that the most forceful, convincing argument was for banning all nontherapeutic research. Nonetheless, the commission adopted a more moderate stance allowing nontherapeutic research of children if the risks approximated those encountered in daily life and if parents consented. The commission accepted this policy even though the arguments supporting it were notably weaker than the arguments favoring a complete ban on such research. Paul Ramsey, a brilliant, acerbic, and relentless Protestant theologian championed a ban. Richard McCormick, equally brilliant, gave the most thorough defense of the moderate view. Their exchange over this issue illuminates the moral obligations of parents toward their children, even as it exemplifies the dangers of moral reasoning that fails to give full weight to context—in this case, both the historical context that shaped discussions of the ethics of research with human beings and the social context of parent-child relationships.

Ramsey opened his discussion by citing in full a classic text in bioethics, the first article of what has come to be known as the Nuremberg Code. The first sentence of the article is the key: "The voluntary consent of the human subject is absolutely essential." The second sentence is also worth citing in full: "This means that the person involved should have legal capacity to give consent; should be so situated as to be able to exercise free power of choice, without the intervention of any element of force, fraud, deceit, duress, overreaching, or other ulterior form of constraint or coercion; and should have sufficient knowledge and comprehension of the elements of the subject matter as to enable him to make an understanding and enlightened decision."[1] The remainder of the article discusses the sort of information a subject should be given.

If we take the Nuremberg Code seriously—if we accept this first article as a firm moral rule governing research—the implications for research on children are straightforward: there will be none. If the consent of the subject is "absolutely essential" and if this requires that the person "have legal capacity to give consent" and be able to reach "an understanding and enlightened decision," all infants and young children are disqualified along with all youth below the age of legal consent and all adults with significant mental impairments.

Note that this blanket prohibition makes no distinction between research intended to help the child—an innovative therapy, for example—and the nontherapeutic research that troubled the commission. If we followed strictly the Nuremberg Code, all medical experiments on children would be banned, including all studies of promising treatments for children dying from diseases like leukemia and brain cancer. This defies moral common sense. What prompted the drafters of the Nuremberg Code to make such a stark and unqualified declaration?

The Nuremberg Tribunal's task was to try people accused of war crimes. Confronted with overwhelming evidence of astoundingly cruel, almost unimaginable treatment of human beings in the name of science, the tribunal had to articulate a set of standards by which to judge the abominable conduct of the accused who came before it. Grave evil had been done. The catalog of horrors was long and gruesome: prisoners left naked in freezing weather, or immersed in near-freezing water until they lost consciousness or died; wounds inflicted, then exacerbated with glass fragments or dirt to simulate battle injuries; prisoners infected with typhus, some even used as human viral cultures; the list goes on.

Faced with such an unconscionable register of horrors inflicted on people who were captives in the first place and never given any choice whether to participate, there is little wonder why the Nuremberg judges adopted voluntary consent as a clear and ringing first principle. When dealing with unmitigated evil, subtlety and nuance are less important than firmness and clarity. They might have reasoned this way: the Nazi experiments were morally atrocious because they inflicted terrible harms on unconsenting victims; no reasonable person would ever consent to such treatment; insisting that no person be used without his or her voluntary consent prevents the evils of coercion and of excessively risky or harmful experiments; therefore, a policy of voluntary consent will prevent morally monstrous research, like the Nazi experiments, from occurring in the future.

The judges at Nuremberg were not formulating timeless and detailed rules to govern all scientific research. They needed a set of principles for a specific task—trying war criminals for their barbarous treatment of prisoners in what was called, often very loosely, "science." The principles they articulated, the Nuremberg Code, served their purposes

very well. In putting it this way, I intend no criticism of the court. To the contrary, I believe they showed admirable wisdom in formulating moral standards for research that would become the starting point for all later efforts. We should not fault them for failing to answer questions they were not asked, questions such as, what to do about children or others incapable of giving consent, or whether it makes a morally important difference if the research may or may not be intended to benefit the subject. Later bodies could deal with such questions. The Nuremberg court's emphasis on consent, though, would color all subsequent efforts to understand the ethics of research with human subjects.

By the time the national commission deliberated on the ethics of research with children, a new distinction and a new concept had entered the discussion. The distinction was between research intended to benefit the subject and research with no such intention—what are commonly referred to as therapeutic research and nontherapeutic research. The concept was proxy consent, that is, consent by someone other than the subject who, presumably, knows what the subject would have wanted or has the subject's best interests at heart. Much ink and even a little (symbolic) blood has been spilled by bioethicists arguing over the meanings and significance of these two ideas. I have no desire to add to the deluge of words. What I want to do is to show how readily even the most perceptive thinker can become bewitched by ethical abstractions and how appreciating moral common sense and social context can, in the best sense, disenchant. To do that, though, we must revisit the debate in some detail.

PAUL RAMSEY AND THE RESPONSIBILITIES OF PARENTHOOD

In his influential book *The Patient as Person*, Paul Ramsey began with a chapter on the ethics of research with children. Contrasting research on humans with research on animals, Ramsey asserts, "Any human being is more than a patient or experimental subject; he is a *personal* subject—every bit as much a man as the physician-investigator." He then links consent to the fidelity that should characterize relationships between persons: "The principle of an informed consent is the *canon of loyalty* joining men together in medical practice and investigation." Though his language and metaphors are drawn from theology rather than law, his debt to the Nuremberg judges seems clear. Ramsey, though, is fully aware of the quandary created by Nuremberg: how to justify therapeutic research with children. Should children's inability to give a mature and understanding consent deprive them of experimental treatments that might help them? Ramsey articulates a principle that he never abandons: "From consent as a canon of loyalty in medical practice it follows that children, who cannot give a mature and informed consent, . . . should not be made the subjects of medical experimentation unless . . . it is reasonable to believe that [the experimental therapy] may further *the patient's own recovery.*"

Ramsey is suspicious of the idea of "proxy" consent. Certainly, it is necessary at times for someone to decide, on a child's behalf, whether to administer some treatment that might benefit the child. Ramsey is adamant about what such proxy consent could not be: "To attempt to consent for a child to be made an experimental subject is to treat a child as not a child. It is to treat him as if he were an adult person who has consented to become a joint adventurer in the common cause of medical research. If the grounds for this are alleged to be the presumptive or implied consent of the child, that must simply be characterized as a violent and false presumption." The parents' duty is to safeguard their child's welfare, to be their child's protector. But the parent's consent on behalf of the child is not morally equivalent to an adult's consent on his or her own behalf. An adult can consent to participate in a risky experiment, but, Ramsey claims, "no parent is morally competent to consent that his child shall be submitted to hazardous or other experiments having no diagnostic or therapeutic significance for the child himself."

Ramsey is correct that consent has a different moral significance when it comes from the person directly affected, rather than from another presuming to speak for that person. Consent is an extremely powerful moral warrant, particularly in a liberal secular society that gives enormous moral weight to individuals and their preferences. Why are you riding Emily's bike? She said it was OK. What right do you have to demand money from me? Because we have a contract. I paint your house; you pay me $2,000. It is not much of an exaggeration to say that

for some persons, inducting a few moral theorists, consent functions as a universal moral solvent, dissolving all moral dilemmas; as long as there is consent, no further moral justification is needed. Not everyone believes this. Outside of a few doctrinaire libertarians, debates over the appropriate scope and limits of individual liberty are taken very seriously. Are contracts for surrogate motherhood legitimate expressions of individual liberty? Should we be permitted to sell our babies? Our kidneys?

Ramsey's argument is that however potent you think consent is in justifying particular actions, children are incapable of consent. Fictions such as "proxy" consent can only disguise that fact. When consent is a necessary condition for something being morally acceptable—as the Nuremberg Code suggests is true for medical research—it would always be morally wrong to perform that action without genuine consent. Children cannot consent to participate in research. Therefore, without some other compelling moral justification, children cannot be subjects in research. What other justification is possible? Pursuing the child's own welfare. Thus therapeutic research for children can be justified; nontherapeutic research on children cannot.

Ramsey's suspicion of proxy consent contrasts with his enthusiastic embrace of the distinction between research that does and does not benefit the child. He sees this as decisive: "What is at stake here is the covenantal obligations of parents to children—the protection with which a child should be surrounded, and the meaning and duties of parenthood. . . . The issue here is the wrong of making a human being subject." As always, Ramsey chooses his concepts with care: children made the subject of research with no benefit to themselves are wronged even if no harm comes to them. The analogous concept in a law is a battery, an unconsented touching, and Ramsey explicitly pursues the parallel.

Here is where Ramsey runs into difficulties. Because he makes consent a moral fulcrum, he is compelled to defend the proposition that all research on children, however innocuous, that is not done with the hope of benefiting its child-subjects, is immoral and violates "the meaning and duties of parenthood." Our task would be easier if we could consult an authoritative list of parental duties. Lacking such a list, Ramsey employs several strategies to persuade us that parental duties include the obligation to protect our children from nontherapeutic research, even riskless research. He appeals to our ideals of parenthood: "A parent's decisive concern," he writes, "is for the care and protection of the child, to whom he owes the highest fiduciary loyalty, even when he also appreciates the benefits to come to others from the investigation and might submit his own person to experiment in order to obtain them." He expresses skepticism that there could be a scientific experiment that did not exceed "the ordinary risks of daily living." He echoes Kant in stating that "fidelity to a human child also includes never treating him as a means only, but always also as an end." He launches the rhetorical equivalent of a nuclear weapon by suggesting, in a somewhat opaque passage, that research even with "no *discernible* risks . . . imposed on subjects for the sake of supposable or actual good to come" puts us "back with the Nazis." Finally, he acknowledges that the problem is "the *use* of children in research, in which the risks are minimal or 'negligible,' but still not in their behalf medically. It is hard to see how this can be an expression of parental care (or of the state's care *in loco parentis*), or anything other than a violation of the nature and meaning of the responsibilities of parenthood as a covenant among the generations of men."

Is permitting one's child to be a subject in a scientific study where the risks are minimal or negligible "a violation of the nature and meaning of the responsibilities of parenthood"? A frightfully strong and austere conclusion: Could there be some flaw in Ramsey's reasoning? The best contemporary effort to find such a flaw, Richard McCormick's defense of minimally risky research on children, was at best only a partial success.

RICHARD MCCORMICK AND "VICARIOUS CONSENT"

McCormick, a Roman Catholic theologian, agrees with Ramsey that "consent is the heart of the matter."[2] But he points out that we take parents' consent to their children's medical treatment to be morally justifiable: Why cannot parental consent work as well in justifying the involvement of children in research? Saying as Ramsey does that it would amount to treating the child as an object does not provide an answer.

McCormick employs the concept of "vicarious consent" which, he says, is a close relative of proxy consent. Vicarious consent, he argues, "is morally valid precisely insofar as it is a reasonable presumption of the child's wishes, a construction of what the child would wish could he consent for himself." Many children are too young to express their wishes; we are loath to accept a young child's wishes in any event, unless we believe that honoring a particular one would not be opposed to the child's best interest. McCormick asserts that a sound understanding of what a child would wish requires asking, "Why *would* the child so wish?" His answer: "[The child] would choose he were capable of choice because he *ought* to do so."

By now McCormick's difficulties are obvious. He has made consent the moral centerpiece of his case and is trying to rescue the moral authority of parental consent by equating what a child *would* want with what it *ought* to want. McCormick is not completely lost for intellectual resources to buttress his case. He calls on natural law theory, a position closely associated with Catholic theology. Focusing on the values and goods that constitute or promote our flourishing as humans, McCormick claims that two assertions account for our willingness to allow parents to consent to therapy for their children: "(a) that there are certain values . . . definitive of our good and flourishing, hence values that we *ought* to choose and support if we want to become and stay human, and that therefore these are good also for the child; and (b) that these 'ought' judgments, at least in their more general formulations, are a common patronage available to all men, and hence form the basis on which policies can be built."

Another big step remains. McCormick needs to make a plausible case that the child—say, an infant whom researchers want to enroll in a study of pulmonary physiology—*ought* to want to volunteer for it. He argues: "To pursue the good that is human life means not only to choose and support this value in one's own case, but also in the case of others when the opportunity arises. . . . [T]he individual *ought* also to take into account, realize, make efforts in behalf of the lives of others also, for we are social beings and, the goods that define our growth and invite to it are goods that reside also in others." So infants and children *ought* to want to help others by, for example, participating as research subjects.

McCormick tries to clinch the argument thus: "To share in the general effort and burden of health maintenance and disease control is part of our flourishing and growth as humans. To the extent that it is good for all of us to share this burden, we all *ought* to do so. And to the extent that we *ought* to do so, it is a reasonable construction or presumption of our to say that we would do so." He then concludes: "The reasonableness of this presumption validates vicarious consent."

McCormick has traveled a long way from the sort of infants and children of my acquaintance, most of whom recognize a sharp distinction between what they *should* do (in the eyes of their parents at least) and what they would or want to do. I accept that a crucial part of a parent's job is to help their children understand what they ought to do, and to develop a conscience and motivation that helps them want to do what they should do. In other words, bringing *should* and *would* into closer conjunction is one of the principal tasks of parenthood. The move from "ought" to "would" is an interminable battle fought between parents and children as well as within every person's psyche. Far from the "reasonable construction or presumption of our wishes" that McCormick optimistically maintains, presuming that a child want what it *would* want what it *should* want imputes capacities and preferences that most young children flatly lack.

CONSENT, PARENTAL DUTIES, AND THE ETHICS OF RESEARCH

In contrast to this awkward theoretical effort to rescue the concept of consent as a moral justification for nontherapeutic research on children, McCormick's practical conclusions seem eminently reasonable and wise. If the scientific experiments are "well designed," "cannot succeed unless children are used," and "contain no discernible risk or undue discomfort for the child," then McCormick believes "parental consent to this type of invasion can be justified."

Here is our quandary. On the one hand, we have an incisive, comprehensive analysis—Ramsey's—that reaches what seems to be an unreasonable conclusion: that no research on children which does not have direct benefit of its subjects as an aim is ethically justified. Ramsey's analysis would rule out the

most innocuous research on children that might be hugely beneficial to other children. On the other hand, we have a nuanced but strained and unconvincing analysis—McCormick's—that reaches what seem to be very sensible conclusions. McCormick would permit nontherapeutic research on children under very strict circumstances, including no discernible risks, with parental consent.

The problem, I believe, is the shared way in which they formulated the problem. For both Ramsey and McCormick, the issue was the ethics of consent. Recall McCormick agreeing with Ramsey that "consent is the heart of the matter." The social and historical context helps us understand why this particular formulation of the ethics of nontherapeutic research with children suggested itself to both scholars. The horrifying history of Nazi experimentation, the primacy and availability of consent as a moral warrant for participating in research, and the focus on medical experimentation with its propensity for dramatic risks and bodily invasions combined to make consent look like *the* moral solution to unethical human experimentation. The fact that consent could be applied to children at best metaphorically did not deter scholars and researchers from trying to beat it into a shape that might justify research with children, as did McCormick, or writing it off—at least for nontherapeutic research—as a "false and violent presumption" as did Ramsey.

Consent, of course, is not the entirety of the ethics of research even with fully competent adult volunteers. The research must be competent, have some reasonable goal, impose no greater risks than are necessary, and protect subjects' confidentiality, among other considerations. In one of the episodes in Woody Allen's movie *Everything You Always Wanted to Know about Sex but Were Afraid to Ask,* a mad scientist appears. He brings Woody and his companion into the laboratory where he shows them his great experiment: he explains that he is exchanging the brains of a lesbian and a telephone repairman. Even if his two subjects had consented to this experiment (a point not clarified in the movie) it would still be unethical because, well, it's nuts. Even a competent experiment that exposed its subjects to more risk than necessary, or to great risk when there was no corresponding benefit to them such as cure of their disease, would be unethical. Consent may be a crucial concept in the ethics of research, but it is not the whole story. It must be a much smaller part of the story when the subjects of the research cannot give consent—children, for example.

If consent is not the entire, perhaps not even the most important, consideration in the ethics of experimentation with children, then Ramsey's and McCormick's formulation of the problem is defective. Rather than try to hammer consent into a shape that accommodates all of our ethical concerns about the involvement of children in research, we can reformulate the question. Let us ask under what circumstances, if any, parents are morally permitted to enroll their children in nontherapeutic research.

We will not expect to find the answer in any reshaped metaphor of consent. And we should not be embarrassed by that. Yes, it would be wrong to impose research on unconsenting adults. It would be wrong even if it caused them no harm; much worse if, like the Nazi experiments, it heartlessly tortured and killed. It is equally wrong to harm children in the name of research. Relying on parental consent is an important, if imperfect, bulwark against abuse; but it does not have the same moral status as an adult volunteer's consent to participate.

Both Ramsey and McCormick saw that the content of parents' obligations to their children was crucial. Ramsey simply failed to go beyond dismissive pronouncements. Recall what he wrote about parents who would permit their children to participate in minimally risky research: "It is hard to see how this can be an expression of parental care or anything other than a violation of the nature and meaning of the responsibilities of parenthood." There have been countless occasions when I have rebuked myself for failing to fulfill my responsibilities as a parent. I cannot say that having any of my children participate in riskless research would rank high among them. McCormick tried to stuff the huge and ungainly octopus of parental obligations into a sack labeled "vicarious consent: it was an awkward fit at best. He became entangled in the metaphor; his effort to cut his way out with natural law theory strained common sense.

If Ramsey and McCormick became prisoners to their framing of the problem, leaving themselves with, respectively, an extreme solution and an ill-fitting one, can our reframing do any better? When a problem does not yield to a head-on confrontation, a useful strategy is to try to capture its crucial features

but move them into a different context. If the context of research raises inescapable echoes of Nuremberg, but our problem is what parents may or may not do with their children that is not directly to their child's benefit, let us look for analogous choices that parents face.

Your next door neighbors have been out of work for a year since the factory closed. They are good hardworking people and fine neighbors, but they are in terrible financial trouble at the moment. Their new baby has been sleeping in a dresser drawer since she came home four weeks ago, but she must move to a crib as soon as possible. They do not have one and cannot afford to buy one. Your two-year-old son will be ready to give up his crib in another six months. It is a bit early to move him into a youth bed: there is always the chance that he might fall out of it in his sleep, or get out of bed at night, wander around the house, and hurt himself. You weigh your neighbors' need and the small risks to your son, and you offer to lend them the crib.

Have you done the right thing?

Your generosity and compassion for your neighbors exposes your child to some slight risks—at the most, probably a small bump on the head. Ramsey's understanding of parenthood, with his exclusive focus on protecting children from any threats to their physical safety, implies that lending the crib would be morally unacceptable, "a violation of the nature and meaning of the responsibilities of parenthood." Surely that is too harsh a judgment. The ethics of neighborliness and charity may not strictly oblige you to lend the crib, but generosity such as this should be valued and is certainly morally permitted. We could jiggle the circumstances of the case to steer judgments toward the obligatory or the prohibited: if the risk to your own child was trivial and the benefit to your neighbors was life-saving or otherwise monumental, we would be more likely to conclude that a genuine moral obligation existed; if the risk to your child became substantial without major benefit to your neighbors (if, for example, the object to be lent was a gate preventing a dangerous tumble down a steep staircase), we would judge it a morally prohibited action, a violation of parental duties to safeguard one's child. The particular factors of the case always do and properly should affect our moral judgments. In the original version it seems fair to say that "what those parents did was morally permitted, despite the fact that it added an iota to the risks facing their own child. Under some circumstances, parents are morally permitted to do things that do not take protection of their own child's safety as the preeminent concern. Some people might argue that this case is different from volunteering your child for research. Our relations with our near neighbors are more intimate, the moral obligations more stringent, than those characterizing the relationship between parents and children, on the one hand, and researchers and those who might someday benefit from the research, on the other. Fair enough. Consider another case.

It is 4 P.M. on a Christmas Eve. Your baby has been cranky today, but has finally fallen asleep. You look forward to her and her parents (that is, you and your spouse) having a couple of peaceful hours. The phone rings. It is the director of the Christmas pageant at the church you visited for the first time last Sunday to see if it was the sort of place you and your family would like to attend regularly. One visit was not sufficient for you to make up your mind, but you had left your name and phone number with the friendly usher who had approached you and admired your baby. Back to the phone call: the pageant director (who also happened to be the amiable usher) is desperate and flattering: the infant who was to have played the part of Baby Jesus has chicken pox. (This actually happened to my wife in a pageant she coordinated.) Your lovely baby would be the perfect replacement. All the adults and children attending the pageant would be *sooo* disappointed if they had to substitute a doll for a live infant. Would you be willing to bring your darling to church in half an hour?

Some parents would probably decline, preferring to let their baby sleep and to enjoy the quiet themselves. I cannot see how they can be said to have any moral obligation to do this favor for these strangers. Other parents would accede, some happily, some reluctantly but moved by the prospective disappointment of the pageant's audience. Do the parents who disturb their baby's slumber to benefit these strangers violate their parental duties? The facts, as always, are important. Their baby may be unhappy for awhile, but she may find the colors of the costumes interesting. In all likelihood, she will go back to sleep soon afterward, only a little the worse for wear. The pageant will be successful and the audience gratified.

What we must decide is whether the parents are morally permitted to donate their infant's services to the pageant or whether they are morally forbidden to do so. This does not strike me as a terrible moral quandary. Of course, the parents may bring their baby to church that afternoon if they wish. The child suffers no great hardship from it, and some people derive a little good—enjoyment at the spectacle, perhaps a little religious edification, and, most of all, delight in watching the unalloyed joy of the children present. Even though there may be no direct benefit for their child, bringing her to the pageant falls well within the compass of permissible moral discretion. It also reminds us that no impenetrable barricade separates moral relationships within families from the moral world outside. We have special and strong moral obligations to those closest to us; but attending to our familial obligations does not mean ignoring all moral interests and relationships outside the family that might in any way, however insignificantly, affect the interests of those within the family circle. This would not merely put the family first but would put the family above everything else—a dangerously shortsighted view of moral life.

In both of these hypothetical cases parents accept some risk, discomfort, or inconvenience for their child, with no direct benefit for that child. Yet in neither case does it seem that the parents have acted immorally or irresponsibly toward their children. The accusation that they have treated their child as a means rather than an end makes no sense. Neither does any claim that they have violated their sacred parental duty.

Two points about parents' moral obligations to children emerge from these analogies. First, protecting a child's physical safety may be very important but is not the entirety of our moral obligations to our children; risks, especially very small ones, may be accepted in the service of other goods and values. Second, the goods and values that may justify accepting risks to our children can include those of other persons and need not always be limited to our child's immediate well-being.

Turn our conclusions on their head for a moment. Imagine a parent who took Ramsey's comments about parental responsibilities with respect to research and generalized them to the whole of parenthood. This parent would refuse to do anything that did not directly benefit the child, citing all the while a parent's moral duty. We have probably all known overprotective parents, but this case might reach new heights—or, rather, depths. The best description of this parental style is "smothering." Those of us with a more cynical bent might suspect that the parent is using purported parental duties as an excuse for avoiding other moral obligations, perhaps out of miserliness or laziness. At best, we would say that they show a lack of proportion or perspective in their moral judgments, that they suffer from an affliction that might be called moral myopia.

At no point in this discussion of parental duties outside the realm of research have we needed to invoke some fictitious or metaphorical notion of the child's own consent to analyze what the parent is permitted morally to do. If the debate over using children in nontherapeutic research has been bewitched by consent, a little disenchantment can be liberating. Consent *is* crucially important when it is genuinely possible—with competent adults. But different problems call for different analyses more suited to their particular circumstances. Children cannot consent; why try to understand the ethics of research with children through the concept of consent? If parental obligations are central as both Ramsey and McCormick acknowledge, then look directly at those obligations.

The cursory look we have taken suggests that involving children in activities that impose no significant hazards on those children but that may contribute substantially to other goods and values even though the child may not benefit directly is well within the circle of morally permissible parental discretion. Nontherapeutic research, when the risks are truly minimal and the benefits to others potentially substantial, is just that kind of activity.

Whether any particular study satisfies the criterion of minimal risk depends on the particulars of the study. Monitoring a baby's blood pressure, if it involved no invasiveness or discomfort, seems to qualify, as would a quick heel prick for a drop of blood. There might be some disagreement about taking repeated vials of blood by venipuncture: the risks are tiny, but the needle will sting. Threading catheters into the heart and injecting powerful drugs, though, is clearly well beyond what any responsible parent should allow: the pain and discomfort are substantial, the risks real and potentially catastrophic.

Where the risks are minimal and the study is competent and potentially significant, parents are permitted morally, but not obliged, to allow their child to participate: not because the child would consent or should consent—consent being an ill-fitting metaphor in this case—but because such participation does not violate the parents' duties to their offspring and because it enhances other goods and values prized by the community.

GROWTH HORMONE FOR SHORT STATURE REVISITED

Should the National Institutes of Health sponsor a study that gives as many as 1,100 injections to children whose only "deviation" from normal is that they are short? We must consider two separate questions here. First, do parents who enroll their children in this experiment exceed the limits of parental discretion? Second, is it good, morally sound, public policy to encourage such an experiment?

Why would parents permit their children to participate in the study? The only plausible answer is that parents want to protect their children from the cruelty and discrimination experienced by people of short stature. Parents do all sorts of things to try to spare their children from pain or to give them whatever advantages they can provide. A drug that might make their child a little taller could be seen as just another measure parents take to help their children.

When a child's body cannot make a substance necessary for normal growth, development, or function, we say that the child suffers from a disease. Administering a drug that compensates for the missing substance is a benefit for that child, if it does more good than harm. A child who suffers from diabetes cannot make insulin. Responsible parents of such children do their best to promote their children's health by watching their diet, monitoring their blood sugar, and ensuring that they receive appropriate doses of insulin. Children who are short but who have no deficiency of hGH do not have a disease—unless we declare that all those who differ substantially from average on any human characteristic are similarly "diseased." So they are not like children with diabetes, for whom treatment with a drug is justified. A reason that justifies giving a potent drug to your child is that the child has a serious disease for which the drug is an effective treatment. Because short children with normal hGH do not have a disease, we need another good reason for giving them a drug. Perhaps hGH benefits children with short stature.

Unfortunately, the evidence that hGH actually benefits such children is scanty. Growth hormone does appear to accelerate growth, but what matters most to these children and their parents is the child's final adult height. Here the evidence is equivocal: despite the acceleration in growth velocity, the children may stop growing sooner and end up no taller as adults. Let us say that several years worth of hGH injections did add two or three inches to adult height. What sort of benefit is that?

If growth hormone does in fact increase the adult height of children with short stature, then the benefit is far different from the benefit a child with diabetes derives from insulin. A diabetic child's health and life are threatened by the inability to make insulin. A short child who makes normal hGH is not ill and does not suffer from any dire physiological imbalance. Short children with normal hGH are not in any special danger from disease. Growth hormone for such children is not a treatment for any physiological disease, and there is no particular medical benefit from it. But, it is true, being a bit taller for such children could mean that they will suffer fewer cruelties at the hands of other children and less discrimination as adults.

The benefit is entirely social. If it works at all, growth hormone in such cases works by blunting the impact of social prejudice against short people, not by dealing with the roots of prejudice. Those roots are left untouched. Instead, the use of growth hormone for children of short stature tacitly accepts heightism. Parents who seek it for their children understandably want to spare them from discrimination. But as their children benefit, other children, whose parents perhaps cannot afford the tens of thousands of dollars a year needed to pay for hGH, continue to bear the burden of discrimination. Indeed, as those who are fortunate enough to be able to afford hGH climb closer to average height, those left behind will stand out as even more "different."

Imagine that we discovered a possible "treatment" for another form of social prejudice—a hormone that reduces the amount of melanin in the skin. If it worked, giving it to children would cause

them to have a lighter hue. It might diminish the amount of racial discrimination they will face by making them appear less different from the light-skinned majority. Does it make sense to deal with racial prejudice by trying to obliterate physical differences? Should we encourage biomedical fixes for complex social problems? Or would we be wiser to deal with the roots of prejudice?

Even if we were able to lay aside our concerns about justice and the sources of discrimination, to defend this research we need to consider the risks to the children involved and weigh them against the potential benefits. We can divide both risks and benefits into two categories: physical and psychological. The most obvious physical harms are the 600 to 1,100 injections each child in the study will receive. Half of the children will get hGH in their shots, half will receive nothing more than sterile salt water.

Consider first the children receiving the saltwater placebo. Other than the pain of the shots and the very remote chance of infection or other complications, the study exposes them to no other significant physical risks. But a thousand-plus injections is not a trivial matter. Anyone who can recall how as a child you regarded the prospect of a *single* injection will not dismiss lightly an experiment designed to give as many as 1,100 to each participant.

The physical benefits to such children are much less clear. They will receive a three-day workup by the researchers and regular follow-up by experts. This intensive medical scrutiny might uncover subtleties that normal health care did not. If that happened—and no one can say how likely it is—then children in the placebo group might benefit. Another possible benefit for the children receiving growth hormone is a so-called placebo effect. Sometimes people who receive a presumed inactive treatment nonetheless do better than those who receive nothing at all. In this study, finding a placebo effect would mean that the children injected with saline solution grew taller than they otherwise would have. The possibility of such a placebo effect was the primary reason offered by the experimenters for injecting salt water into half of the children. I know that the mind and body interact in often mysterious ways. But I must say that the likelihood that saline injections will make kids grow taller seems about as likely as pixie dust allowing them to fly. In any event, it seems fair to say that the likelihood of children in the control group benefiting by an increase in their adult height is remote. On purely physical grounds, then, the study brings more harms than benefits to the children in the control group.

To be fair, we should also look at the balance of psychological benefits and risks. The committee convened by the NIH identified two kinds of potential psychological benefits: "the possible gratification of participating in an important study" and "information that may later be useful to one as a parent."[3] I don't mean to downplay the satisfaction gained by doing something important that can aid others in distress. But these hypothetical psychological benefits are awfully insubstantial compared to the psychological risks.

Children learn what is important about them according to how we treat them. They can learn that their short stature is just one, relatively insignificant, aspect of who they are that pales in importance compared to their wit or expressiveness, the warmth of their smile, or any of hundreds of other details of character and appearance. Or children can learn that their short stature is such a grievous deficiency that it justifies hundreds of injections, regular visits to the doctor, great worry, and, for many, tens of thousands of dollars. Children, that is, can learn that their short stature is a central defining characteristic of their identity—one in which they will assuredly, even with hGH, come up short. The children who receive placebo injections will get this message just as surely as the children getting the drug. Unless salt water *is* a kind of pixie dust, these children will be no taller for all of the hundreds of injections they endure. But they will have learned that their short stature is a severe and crucial deficiency.

The children who receive hGH face a slightly different array of risks and benefits. A leading authority on pediatric endocrinology lists several possible hazards, including diabetes, hypertension, and abnormal growth of both soft and bony tissues, and reports that some children developed leukemia after treatment with hGH. Nevertheless, most experts appear to believe that hGH is reasonably safe. The significant hazards are either rare or unproved. The physical benefit, of course, would be an increase in adult height. But in what sense is increased height a benefit? Being short is not a physical illness, and being taller is not its cure. The point of trying to make children taller is to diminish psychological distress and social discrimination. Increasing height is

the means, not the end. The important balance will be between the psychological and social risks and benefits.

If children who receive hGH gain a few inches in adult height, and if that gain diminishes the discrimination they experience at the hands of others, and if the intense focus on their short stature is more than offset by their pride at being less short than anticipated, then they may benefit on the whole. Of course, some, perhaps most, of the children who receive hGH will be no taller for their trouble. Even when the treatment is effective, the increase in height in unlikely to be dramatic. For a boy of 5'3" or a girl of 4'10½" a gain of even three inches will not bring them up to average height for their sex. Previous studies found that children with demonstrable hGH deficiency expected greater height gains than hGH treatment could deliver. The children, as well as their parents, experienced disappointment and a sense of failure. Nor were they any happier about themselves.[4] At best, the evidence that a child would benefit significantly from hGH treatment is equivocal. We do not know whether there will be any increase in final height. Even children who gain a few inches may find little comfort. They will still be shorter than average. Their self-confidence may be blighted by their failure to grow as tall as they and their parents thought was so vitally important.

Under the circumstances, do parents who enroll their children in this experiment exceed the limits of parental discretion? The most likely motive for a parent is the hope that his or her child might indeed be one of the fortunate few who would benefit from participating. I say "fortunate few" because the children would have to be lucky in three ways. They would have to be among those participants randomly assigned to receive hGH rather than saline solution. They would have to be one of the as yet unknown proportion of those receiving hGH who become significantly taller. And they would have to experience less discrimination and develop a more robust sense of self by virtue of that gain in height. The odds are not favorable. But then neither are the odds that any particular child will benefit significantly from music lessons. I suspect that most parents who enroll their children in music lessons hope that the child's latent musical gifts will blossom, that he or she will learn habits of dedication and lessons about the relationship of hard work and success that will last a lifetime, and that their perfected talent will provoke respect, if not awe, among their peers. I have no idea what the actual numbers are of children who reap such marvelous fruits from their musical experience compared to those for whom it becomes mainly an exercise in parent-child conflict. But it would not surprise me if the ratio of success to failure was roughly comparable to the ratio for children enrolled in this experiment—substantially less than half.

If we take the optimistic view about physical risks—that the serious ones are fanciful and the pain of the injections tolerable—and an equally optimistic view about the likelihood of social and psychological benefit, then we can draw a rough analogy between enrolling one's child in this experiment or in music lessons. The psychological risks are probably much greater in the experiment, but then so is the concern to spare your child from discrimination and damage to self-esteem.

I do not believe we can say that parents who enroll their children in this experiment clearly violate their obligations to their children. They hope that their children will benefit from participating, even if the benefit does not so clearly fall into the realm of the "therapeutic." I would have to say the same about the parents of dark-skinned children who wanted to spare them from discrimination by placing them in a (nonexistent and hypothetical) study of a skin-lightening hormone that was no more physically risky than hGH. On the other side, parents who choose not to use hGH for their short-stature children also act as responsible parents. They may look at the pain and risks involved and decide that it is more important to stress their child's strengths. (I would say exactly the same about parents who chose to emphasize their children's abilities and accomplishments as well as pride in their ethnic history rather than attempting to change the color of their skin.)

Deciding that parents do not choose wrongly by choosing either way is not the end of the story. We need to address the second question: Is it good, morally sound, public policy to encourage such an experiment? There are many reasons to say no. First, at least half [and] probably more than half of the children in the study are likely to be harmed more than helped by it. Second, if the study showed

that some non-hGH-deficient children grew a few more inches, parents of other short children would have an additional incentive to seek growth hormone for their kids. Since their children are not ill, insurers would resist paying for such an expensive treatment, just as they oppose paying for certain kinds of cosmetic surgery. If insurers resisted successfully but hGH was still available to those who could afford it, then savvy, wealthy parents could get it for their children as just another of the advantages that money can buy. Nor would there be any reason to limit it to short children. If you can buy a few inches, and height confers a competitive advantage, then parents of average and tall children might also want to give their kids a leg up, so to speak. To the advantages of wealth would be added one more—enhanced height.

We do have options. We could adopt the egalitarian approach and make hGH available to all children at public expense. Unfortunately, this would do nothing to defeat heightism. Although average height would rise, there would still be a wide range with plenty of children at the lower end of the curve. Indeed, with a premium placed on height, discrimination against the relatively shorter might intensify. A few groups would benefit. Pediatric endocrinologists would be kept very busy. Investors in the drug companies that manufacture hGH would become wealthy. And a few others would profit, for example, fabric makers, because everyone would need larger sizes. On the whole, though, we would be worse off. Many mere children would get hundreds of shots, more of our national resources would go into making hGH, and discrimination against the relatively shorter would be reinforced rather than diminished. Not a pretty picture.

Perhaps the best result would be proof that growth hormone does nothing for short children who are not hGH-deficient. Parents would then have no reason to give it to their children, and the ugly scenarios would not have to be played out.

There are, and have been, other possibilities for controlling the nontherapeutic use of human growth hormone. The companies that make hGH could require that it be given only to children with medically demonstrable hGH deficiency. That is unlikely to happen. Companies want to sell more, not less, of their products. Indeed, the NIH experiment has corporate sponsorship. More plausibly, pediatricians could take a professional stand that firmly opposes hGH treatment for children not clearly suffering from disease or at great risk of disability. To their credit, pediatric professional societies have urged caution in the use of hGH. Nonetheless, persistent parents can usually find a physician willing to prescribe hGH for their child (who will, incidentally, probably be male, as were approximately 90 percent of the children enrolled in the NIH study). Firmer stands with tighter professional self-regulation is probably our best strategy for now.

HONORING THE WORTH
OF A CHILD IN RESEARCH

How should we honor the worth of children in research? We should, of course, protect them from needless harm. We do that in at least two ways: by requiring researchers to demonstrate that the research is important and the risks minimal and by respecting parents' authority to protect and guide their children. We also honor children's moral worth by acknowledging that young children are not just tiny adults when it comes to the moral weight we should give to their consent. Young children's consent does not protect them from harm as well as an adult's consent. To say that a young child consented to participate in an extremely risky nontherapeutic study would never excuse our subjecting them to such unjustified risks.

A better acknowledgment of children's moral worth would be to see participation in nontherapeutic research as one of a class of activities in which parents and children are asked to contribute to the community's well-being and that involve minimal risks to the children. We honor children's worth here by protecting them from overzealous researchers and awestruck or uncaring parents and by recognizing that good rearing of children does not mean a phobic shielding from all imaginable dangers, but rather a sense of proportion that includes acting responsibly toward one's community.

Perhaps because the moral foundation for research on children has been so vague, even well-intentioned people trying to make sense of a proposal like the NIH study of growth hormone for children of short stature may take refuge in tenuous readings of regulations rather than ask the two questions I believe we need to ask: Do parents who enroll their children in this experiment exceed the moral limits of parental discretion? Is it good, morally sound, public policy to encourage such an experiment?

A preliminary look at the limits of parental discretion suggests that parents act within the bounds of good parenting when they consent to a wide range of research protocols for their children, including research likely to benefit their child but also research that might benefit others without being unduly risky to their children. Parents who enroll their children in the NIH growth hormone study are probing the boundaries of parental discretion. Many people might feel that they have stepped over that boundary. Even with a tentative yes to the question whether parents are morally permitted to enroll their children in such a study, the second question remains.

What may be permissible for individual parents may not be wise for us as a community. Encouraging hormonal treatment for social discrimination muddies the line between disease and disadvantage and prompts us to look for medical solutions for social problems. If hGH works in children with normal growth hormone levels, then we must make hard choices. If we permit parents to obtain hGH for their nondeficient children, we would face two equally unpalatable scenarios. We could either heap another, physically distinctive, inequality on top of the other inequalities wealth can buy. Or we could engage in a futile and expensive orgy of competition after which there would be the same number of winners and losers as before.

The most sensible course is to restrict this powerful drug to occasions when it treats disease. Professionals could accomplish this by self-regulation, bolstered, if needed, by laws to discourage the proliferation of hGH treatment for nontherapeutic uses. We should not thwart parents who want to do what is right for their children. But as a community we must recognize that there are situations, like arms races, when the effect of each individual party pursuing self-advantage makes everyone, collectively, worse off. We do not need an experiment on growth hormone for healthy children to show us that.

NOTES

1. Cited in Paul Ramsey, *The Patient as Person* (New Haven: Yale University Press, 1970), 1.
2. Richard A. McCormick, "Proxy Consent in the Experimentation Situation," *Perspectives in Biology and Medicine* 18, no. 1 (Autumn 1974): 9.
3. National Institutes of Health, *Report of the NIH Human Growth Hormone Protocol Review Committee*, 2 October 1992, 13.

4. Diane Rotnem, Donald J. Cohen, Raymond Hintz, and Myron Genel, "Psychological Sequelae of Relative 'Treatment Failure' for Children Receiving Human Growth Hormone Replacement," *Journal of the American Academy of Child Psychiatry* 18 (1979): 505–520.

IN LOCO PARENTIS: MINIMAL RISK AS AN ETHICAL THRESHOLD FOR RESEARCH UPON CHILDREN

Benjamin Freedman, Abraham Fuks, and Charles Weijer

While respect for rights is the hallmark of a liberal society, responsibility toward vulnerable persons unable to care for themselves or even speak on their own behalf is the mark of a humane society. And within the broad field of social ethics, bioethics in particular must focus upon such responsibilities: to the very old and very young, those muted or rendered incoherent by illness. Yet delineating the nature of that responsibility has proven to be among the most vexing problems bioethics has faced.

Agreement in principle upon the touchstone of responsibility toward the incompetent is elusive. Should we act in their best interests, or as they would have directed us to act? More difficult still is the application of such a standard, as when we attempt to describe what is required by the best interests of a particular handicapped newborn. Most difficult, perhaps, is the application of a standard under conditions of risk and uncertainty, when our ethical calculus, ill-grounded as it is, is put to work on shifting and statistically ill-defined values.

From *Hastings Center Report* 23, no. 2 (1993): 13–19. Reprinted by permission of The Hastings Center.

Editors' note: Some text and most authors' notes have been cut. Students who want to read the article in its entirely should consult the original.

The ethics of clinical research in children seems tailor-made for addressing these moral quandaries. Is it ever ethical to expose children to risks associated with research? If it is, what are the ethical limits to such risk? How can a specific threshold to research risk be formulated, justified, and applied? These questions have preoccupied pediatric researchers and others for many years. Recent revisions of United States regulations regarding research with human subjects and the formulation of a "common rule" applying to all federal departments involved with human research make it necessary to examine these questions.

The new definition provided in the "common rule" states, "'Minimal risk' means that the probability and magnitude of harm or discomfort anticipated in the research are not greater in and of themselves than those ordinarily encountered in daily life, or during the performance of routine physical or psychological examinations or tests. Finding that a research study poses only 'minimal risk' has some important procedural consequences for review. In this paper, though, we will focus upon another role: 'Minimal risk' is the concept used in American regulation to serve as an anchoring measure of allowable risk (or—the other side of the coin—relative safety) in clinical research. The critical threshold of risk that may not be surpassed (short of special federal approval) is in fact one level higher: 'minor increment over minimal risk.' However, since the rule offers no independent definition or specification of 'minor increment,' attention must first be focused upon its anchor, 'minimal risk.' . . .

THE UBIQUITY OF RESEARCH RISK

In any ethical consideration of research, the question of the allowable maximum of research risk must inevitably arise. Every activity poses some risks to its participants, and research is no exception to this rule. Risk, commonly expressed as the magnitude of some harm multiplied by the probability of its occurrence, can never be eliminated. . . . Absolute safety can therefore never be guaranteed to participants in clinical research.

Ethics requires that clinical trials comparing two forms of treatment begin with an honest null hypothesis, a state of clinical equipoise—uncertainty in the expert clinical community concerning the comparative merits and disadvantages of each trial arm. As current United States regulations put it, a trial comparing, for example. standard therapy with a nonvalidated intervention may only be approved if "the risk is justified by the anticipated benefit to the subjects" and "the relation of the anticipated benefit to the risk is at least as favorable to the subjects as that presented by available alternative approaches." When this condition is satisfied, some will feel that while one trial arm may involve more *uncertainty* than another, no arm is *riskier* than any other.

However, comparative trials raise their own problems of specific research risk. Once the trial's arms are established to be in clinical equipoise, a second stage of analyzing research risks proceeds. Now those interventions that have no therapeutic warrant, but that are required to answer the trial's scientific question, are separated from the treatment interventions. The risks associated with those interventions required purely for research purposes are tabulated and added separately. Their sum represents the incremental research risk of the study. . . .

The doctrine of informed consent to research constitutes one major response to the ethical challenge of research risks. Competent subjects with the capacity of understanding research risks and benefits, by consenting to serve as research subjects, voluntarily assume these risks. As the legal maxim states, *Volenti non fit injuria* (One who has agreed to an activity is not wronged by it). Conceivably the same justification applies to research upon persons who have while competent executed a valid advance directive permitting specified forms of research to be performed upon them when their competency should lapse. This stratagem, the research analogue to treatment's 'living will,' may in the future serve an important role in research upon Alzheimer's dementia.

But no such solution is available on behalf of incompetent subjects who were never competent—most importantly, infants and small children but also those suffering from congenital intellectual handicaps. Unless safety is understood in a relative sense, permitting some small risk that falls below a specified threshold, these incompetent persons could never be permitted to participate in clinical research—a situation that would in the long run leave them 'therapeutic orphans' and for that reason at even greater risk.

THE MEANING AND USE OF 'MINIMAL RISK'

What does 'minimal risk' mean in the medical literature? How is it understood by clinical investigators? How is it defined within the regulations, and what role does it play in ethically evaluating research upon children? As we will see, a purely definitional approach without reference to the ethical purpose underlying the threshold, is incapable of capturing anything significant by the term.

Which procedures are said in the medical literature to impose no more than minimal risk? Such highly invasive maneuvers as splenectomy, transthoracic enucleation of esophageal leiomyomas and pancreatic biopsies are all described as "of minimal risk." This characterization, on the surface so surprising, is nonetheless justifiable given the necessity for the procedure in the patient populations in question and the risks associated with alternative intentions. Clearly, the term cannot be defined without specifying a context: minimal risk to what end, from whose point of view; and under which situations? On a semantic level, 'minimal risk' is relational, context-dependent. To understand its meaning in the research context, we must examine that specific usage.

Even if we restrict the context to research interventions upon children, though, and even if we restrict our inquiry to investigators, significant disagreement remains. Janofsky and Starfield surveyed chairpersons of pediatric departments and directors of pediatric clinical research units in the United States to elicit their understanding of 'minimal risk,' 'minor increment over minimal risk,' and 'more than minor increment over minimal risk.'[1] (Recall that 'minor increment over minimal risk' is the critical threshold, determining whether a study could be approved by a local committee or would require approval by a special federal panel.) Respondents were asked to classify common research procedures as administered to pediatric subjects of different ages.

The results demonstrated serious disagreements among respondents: 14 percent thought tympanocentesis (puncturing of the ear drum) posed minimal risk or less, 46 percent classified this as a minor increment over minimal risk, and 40 percent thought it more than a minor increase. Expressed in practical terms, 40 percent thought research requiring tympanocentesis was impermissible, despite the importance of the research, without the approval of a federally authorized panel of ethics experts in addition to the approval of the parents. (With regard to a population of research subjects aged one to four years, respondents came close to the three-way mathematical maximum of dissension: 34% thought it minimally risky, 31% a minor increment, 35% more than a minor increment.) While these are extreme examples, substantial scatter across the categories was the rule rather than the exception throughout the study.

It does not seem, therefore, that 'minimal risk' or the other thresholds it anchors may be clarified by examination of sense or signification within the medical literature, nor by usage of the community of clinical investigators. There appears to be no natural or uniform understanding of 'minimal risk' upon which we can draw. If that is the case we are left with only the definition of 'minimal risk' provided in the regulations: the risk of daily life or that encountered in routine physical or psychological examinations. Although other interpretations are possible, this definition seems to set the risks of daily life as the baseline and the risks of routine examinations as an example of the risks of everyday life most similar to the kinds of interventions found in research

studies—routine immunizations, developmental testing, and the obtaining of urine and blood specimens. An intervention's satisfaction of the minimal risk standard can therefore be demonstrated in one of two ways: directly, by showing that it falls within the definition; or indirectly, by showing that it is relevantly similar to other interventions known to fall within the definition.

But how is the definition itself to be interpreted? What is meant. by 'the risks of everyday life'? As Kopelman notes, the risks of everyday life may be understood in several different ways; for example, it may refer to all the risks any person might encounter or those that all of us encounter. She rightly rejects the first possibility. The fact that some people commonly face very high risks (parachuting, firefighting) could not justify allowing a similar level of risk in research upon children. The second characterization is much more restrictive, constituting a lowest common denominator of risk. Kopelman criticizes this interpretation of the risks of everyday life as follows:

> This interpretation assumes that we know the kinds of risks we all encounter and their probability and magnitude. Neither is obvious. Most of us drive cars, walk across busy streets, and fly in airplanes. Are these the everyday risks the definition refers to? How do we determine what risks are encountered routinely by all of us and estimate the probability and magnitude of these risks?[2]

In the passage two distinct claims are made, one concerning the difficulty in *identifying* the risks of everyday life, the difficulty in *quantifying* them. The first difficulty, though, is clearly exaggerated. While there will always be exceptions, within any given society daily life will present the bulk of its citizens with ordinary hazards at home, at work, at play, and in transit, crossing the street or taking a bath. It is not hard to identify this set of common social risks. We are, by definition, each acquainted with them; and, almost by definition, if we are unsure whether they belong within the set of common risks then they don't.

On quantification Kopelman seems on firmer ground. While we all ride in cars, few of us know the likelihood of our being in a fatal accident. And it is certainly true that IRBs or other research ethics bodies typically consider whether a given proposal is acceptable without recourse to actuarial charts of the risks of daily living.

Indeed, Kopelman could have posed a far more fundamental challenge to the concept. As noted above, the critical threshold for allowable research risk in children is not 'minimal risk' itself; but rather, 'a minor increase over minimal risk.' What meaning attaches to the qualification minor increase that is not defined, specified, or characterized in any way within the regulations? If, as Kopelman believes, these thresholds are quantitative measures, verbal surrogates for numbers expressing the probability and magnitude of potential harms of everyday life, the question is unanswerable, This strongly suggests that an alternative, nonquantitative understanding of 'minimal risk' is intended. To understand that, we need to turn to the basic principles that underlie committee research review.

THE PURPOSE OF 'MINIMAL RISK'

A number of parties must concur in the judgment that a clinical study is ethically appropriate before that study will proceed. The first and probably most important decision-maker is the investigator, who must consider before developing a protocol whether the task may be ethically achieved, how risks may be minimized, how the study's goals and risks may be explained, and so forth. If the study is done upon competent persons, their consent represents another ethical decision node. If the subjects are young children the agreement of parents is required, as well as the assent of the child herself to the extent that she is capable of giving it.

What role does a research ethics committee play? The institution within which research proceeds, both in itself and as society's agent, has its own obligation to treat subjects in a trustworthy capacity. Research review by the ethics committee is a concrete expression of this institutional fiduciary responsibility. In addition, as investigators are sometimes overly enthusiastic or bold, committee review of the ethics of research serves in part as a fail-safe mechanism to curb inappropriate zeal. For example, in assessing any protocol, the IRB must determine that its risk-to-knowledge ratio is reasonable and that the scientific importance of the undertaking is proportional to the risks subjects will be undergoing. These issues should have been considered by the investigators; and usually they do that. Nonetheless, the research

committee is charged not to take that for granted, to serve as a backup in case the investigator has not competently discharged his or her personal and professional obligation. Again, it is the inalienable obligation of the investigators properly to inform subjects prior to their participation in a trial. The IRB, in reviewing the study's consent form, serves as a failsafe mechanism to ensure that the investigator's plan for informing subjects will satisfy ethical norms and the institution's own moral obligation to protect subjects.

The IRB plays the same backup role vis-à-vis parental (or guardian) approval of participation of a child (or other incompetent person) in research. Parents may be ignorant, apathetic, or merely inattentive. Cognizant of these and other possibilities, and of its own moral obligation to protect incompetent research subjects, the institution charges a review committee to act as surrogate for the scrupulous parent by filtering out those studies that would impose an unacceptable level of risk upon child participants. It is in this light that the threshold concept, 'minor increase over minimal risk,' needs to be understood. In applying this standard, the IRB is attempting to track those decisions that would be made by informed and scrupulous parents whose children are being invited to participate in research. This fail-safe measure does not ensure that parents will scrupulously evaluate studies; rather, it ensures that they will only have the opportunity to enroll a child in a study that could have passed such an evaluation.

Asking a parent to agree to the child's participation in research is asking for a decision for participation in a new situation, with new attendant risks. These decisions are not arrived at quantitatively, by calculating risks, but rather on a *categorial* basis. Consider another such choice. A child has been asked out to an overnight camping trip for the first time. The risks of the trip are not the risks of everyday life—it is a new experience. If the threshold of allowable risk never permitted anything other than the risks of everyday life, no new experiences could ever be enjoyed (something which itself in the not-very-long run would not be in the child's best interests). Rather, a mother asks herself, "Is the child ready for this? Should the child approach this by stages? *Are the risks sufficiently similar to those in my child's everyday life that I should allow this experience at this time?*" In discussions about whether to permit this involvement—with the mother resisting, and the child pressing—a certain logic may be discerned. Appealing to consistency, the child will say that he has been permitted, and successfully undergone, situations relevantly and roughly similar though not identical—while the parent will focus upon difference.

In other words, the parental decision to permit exposure to new risks is not itself governed by, but rather anchored to, the risks of everyday life. And this point is of course exactly mirrored in our understanding of the regulations, in which the upper threshold of research risk is not governed by, but anchored to, the concept of minimal risk. Almost by definition, exciting and important research ventures into the unknown. A prohibition on such research involvement would be to the long-term detriment of this child and other children, just as a prohibition on new experiences is harmful to children over the long term. Therefore, the limit is set as a 'minor increase over minimal risk.' This limit is not quantitative, but represents a categorical judgment that focuses upon the comparison of new experiences to those of everyday life. It is this form of discussion that needs to take place in research ethics committees considering the approval of research involving children.

JUSTIFYING AND APPLYING THE THRESHOLD

Because children and their situations differ, a judgment anchored to the risks of everyday life, whether arrived at by parent or IRB, must be made relative to the child's actual situation. A diabetic child's everyday life includes pinprick blood tests, and additional such tests required by a study protocol represent much less of a variation in that child's daily life than in the life of a healthy child. This relativistic understanding of minimal risk, held by the National Commission for the Protection of Human Subjects (with the exception of Commissioner Turtle), is in fact the current interpretation of the regulations.

We should also point out that by choosing the risks of everyday life as an anchor to an acceptable level of research risk, less net added risk is imposed upon the child than might be thought. The risks of research are to a degree substitutive, rather than additive: research risks are undergone, but the risks of alternative activities are forgone. Normal, healthy subjects of research would otherwise be pursuing their normally risky daily lives; and ill subjects who are not enrolled in research studies may nonetheless receive treatments and diagnostic tests under the rubric of therapy that are similar to those they would have experienced in research. Furthermore, although in principle any given level of risk associated with an activity can be reduced, there is substantial empirical evidence that past a certain point individuals cease efforts at risk reduction, and the efforts of third parties to reduce risk yield severely diminishing returns. When cars have more safety features built in, for example, people seem to feel free to drive in a riskier fashion. Insurance companies have long since identified the problem under the phrase "moral hazard": property owners who are insured against damage or theft take fewer contingencies. People do differ in their propensity to trade off safety for other goods, but by specifying a threshold at or near the risks of everyday life we approximate a lowest common denominator of risk, the level at which most reasonable people feel 'safe enough' so that their choices can be made without considering the small risk repercussions.

The concept, 'risks of everyday life,' has normative as well as descriptive force, reflecting a level of risk that is not simply accepted but is deemed socially acceptable. Without defining the scope of parental authority and discretion within the law, therefore, we may be reasonably certain that the risks of everyday life fall within those bounds. There is, however, no precise legal analogue to this level. Questions of child abuse deal with risks and harms far above this threshold; so does the question of parental refusal of medical treatment for a child on religious grounds. In some ways, the closest analogy arises in disputes over child custody, which consider and weigh the risks of a child's transferring to a new school, being exposed to (or shielded from) church teachings, and so on. But these cases inevitably are resolved on the relative basis of which parent is the better custodian rather than on the basis of whether parentally imposed risks fall beneath a threshold of acceptability.

One last aspect of the 'risks of everyday life' should be discussed: its flexibility, in conformity to time and circumstance. Kopelman sees this as a serious drawback: "the risks to children living in Belfast and Edinburgh are different; but we would not want to have this automatically influence what sort of research we think would be 'not too risky' for them."[3] In our understanding developed above, the example is inapt—parental concern in Belfast may not be less than in Edinburgh—but the point that standards diverge across cultures is true.

However, this flexibility of the threshold is to our minds an advantage. Any society's notion of what demands on children are allowable changes over time. The routine labor expectations of children fifty years ago are considered exploitative now, and those made one hundred years ago would now be actionable child abuse. The same is true of exposure to risk. Given the huge historical and geographical differences among cultures as to the degree to which children should be protected from risk or engaged in life's risky activities, only the most parochial would maintain that the currently prevailing view in Western Europe and North America is necessarily the one right approach. The ethical evaluation of research can and must insist upon the rigorous protection of subjects, but cannot in so doing lose all reference to common social norms. An ethics of research must be sufficiently flexible as to incorporate and accommodate cultural variance, as is done when 'the risks of everyday life' is used as a categorical anchor for research risk.

Intercultural variance does, however, raise a very distasteful possibility. A Western researcher, frustrated by restrictions upon his or her own research, might go shopping for a community whose children are sufficiently destitute and underprotected that even exposure to heinous risk falls within the expected daily routine. Exploiting their miserable conditions of life, this researcher would claim simply to be accommodating cultural differences.

This stratagem would be precluded by recognizing that research in these circumstances is governed not by cultural but by intercultural ethics. It follows from what we have said that because cultures differ in the degree of protection to which their children are entitled, a research project might be ethical in culture A and unethical in culture B. But when a researcher from culture B contemplates doing research upon children from culture A, the question is, Whose values should be controlling? Some students of intercultural research ethics have adopted a "both-and" approach: in cross-cultural research the norms of both groups A *and* B must be respected. Such a

requirement would eliminate, on ethical grounds, the prospect of a researcher's shopping for a useful risk pool.

The final question remaining is that of applying the standard. When is the aggregated risk of research interventions an increase above a minor increment over minimal risk? The status of many of the most common research interventions, for example, blood sampling, dietary restrictions and other measures listed by the National Commission is easily settled: they are associated with routine physical examinations and so are of minimal risk. Some other interventions not on that list because not associated with the risks of everyday life of healthy persons are minor interventions common to the lives of all ill children within the relevant class. In accepting the principle of commensurate risks, it follows that the form, and perhaps also the sum, of research risk for ill children may exceed that imposed upon their healthy counterparts. The question, Is this research risk sufficiently similar to their daily experience? could not receive the same answer in two groups whose daily experience of risk is so different as the healthy and the ill. On the other hand, some interventions—for example, liver biopsies—are so risky and unfamiliar that no colorable case could be made on their behalf.

What are the hard cases the threshold needs to address? One kind of problem is posed by the reiteration of minimally risky procedures for research purposes. One or two venipunctures are minimally risky; four, arguably so, but still not more than a minor increase over minimal risk. But what of five, ten, forty, or any number in between? Similarly, when testing a new treatment for meningitis it is acceptable to perform one lumbar puncture on a sick child to satisfy the protocol's scientific needs, but not five. Where is the break point? Another set of problems is posed by those procedures (arterial punctures performed upon healthy children, for example) that are qualitatively different from common procedures, although of low risk.

It is not to be expected that the threshold definition of minimal risk as the risk of everyday life will settle each of these questions in an unambiguous and nonarbitrary fashion. Neither this nor any other threshold definition is self-interpreting; each will require the exercise of judgment. But we can require that the threshold define the terms of the argument, the kinds of questions that will need to be posed in the committee's deliberations. This the threshold can do. The arguments will parallel those familiar to any parent considering allowing a child to undergo a new experience. The committee, acting *in loco parentis*, will need to debate whether the demarcated research intervention is similar to a common experience of this child, and whether the incremental research risks are similar to the risks this child or others like him runs on a routine basis. The debate takes place within a context recognizing that the committee owes a fiduciary duty to these subjects, and that this duty entails imposing upon a child no risks substantially above a socially defined minimum for any scientific end, however worthy.

If the above analysis is sound, it may shed light upon our broader responsibilities to children and other incompetent persons as well. All cases of medical intervention occur under conditions of relative uncertainty; because of patient variability treatment is always an experiment in nature. And so, in clinical treatment as well as research, those concerned with the care of the patient—doctors, nurses, members of the institution's ethics committee. among

others—may acknowledge their fiduciary responsibility to act *in loco parentis*. In doing so, we suggest, the same kinds of considerations we have raised for clinical research reappear. Risk is always present and seems more appropriately dealt with in categorical rather than quantitative fashion; the allowable limits of risk will always, ineluctably, rely upon a social consensus that varies over time and geographical setting. This consensus itself fuzzy at the edges, is better at identifying those numerous and varied acts contrary to a person's best interests than at defining the one course of action dictated by them.

REFERENCES

1. Jeffrey Janosky and Barbara Starfield, "Assessment of Risk in Research on Children," *Journal of Pediatrics* 98, no. 5 (1981): 842–846.
2. Loretta Kopelman, "Estimating Risk in Human Research," *Clinical Research* 29 (1981): 1–8, 4.
3. Loretta Kopelman, "When Is the Risk Minimal Enough for Children to Be Research Subjects?" in *Children and Health Care: Moral and Social Issues,* ed. Loretta Kopelman and John Moskop (Dordrecht: Kluwer, 1989), p. 91.

RECOMMENDED SUPPLEMENTARY READING

GENERAL WORKS

Annas, George P. *American Bioethics: Crossing Human Rights and Health Law Boundaries.* New York: Oxford University Press, 2004.

Brody, Baruch A. *Ethical Issues in Drug Testing, Approval, and Pricing: The Clot-Dissolving Drugs.* New York: Oxford University Press, 1995.

Childress, James F., Eric M. Meslin, and Harold T. Shapiro, eds. *Belmont Revisited: Ethical Principles for Research with Human Subjects.* Washington, DC: Georgetown University Press, 2007.

Dresser, Rebecca. *When Science Offers Salvation: Patient Advocacy and Research Ethics.* New York: Oxford University Press, 2001.

Foster, Claire. *The Ethics of Medical Research on Humans.* Cambridge: Cambridge University Press, 2001.

Gruskin, Sofia. *Perspectives on Health and Human Rights.* Oxford: Routledge, 2005.

IRB: A Review of Human Subjects Research. Hastings-on-Hudson, NY: Hastings Center (10 vols. per year).

Kahn, Jeffrey P., Anna C. Mastroianni, and Jeremy Sugarman, eds. *Beyond Consent: Seeking Justice in Research.* New York: Oxford University Press, 1998.

Katz, Jay, Alexander M. Capron, and Eleanor Swift Glass, eds. *Experimentation with Human Beings.* New York: Russell Sage Foundation, 1972.

Levine, Robert J. *Ethics and Regulation of Clinical Research.* 2nd ed. New Haven, CT: Yale University Press, 1988.

National Bioethics Advisory Commission. *Ethical and Policy Issues in Research Involving Human Participants.* Bethesda, MD: National Bioethics Advisory Commission, 2001.

Rothman, David J. *Strangers at the Bedside: A History of How Law and Bioethics Transformed Medical Decision Making.* New York: Basic Books, 1991.

Shamoo, Adil E., and David B. Resnik. *Responsible Conduct of Research.* New York: Oxford University Press, 2002.

Thompson, Andrew, and Norman J. Temple, eds. *Ethics, Medical Research, and Medicine: Commercialism Versus Environmentalism and Social Justice.* Boston: Kluwer Academic, 2001.

Vanderpool, Harold Y., ed. *The Ethics of Research Involving Human Subjects: Facing the 21st Century.* Frederick, MD: University Publishing Group, 1996.

Veatch, Robert. *The Patient as Partner: A Theory of Human Experimentation Ethics.* Bloomington: Indiana University Press, 1987.

BORN IN SCANDAL: THE ORIGINS OF U.S. RESEARCH ETHICS

American Philosophical Association. *Newsletter on Philosophy and Medicine* 5, no. 2 (Spring 2006): 4–24.

Annas, George J., and Michael A. Grodin, eds. *The Nazi Doctors and the Nuremberg Code: Human Rights in Human Experimentation.* New York: Oxford University Press, 1992.

Caplan, Arthur L., ed. *When Medicine Went Mad: Bioethics and the Holocaust.* Clifton, NJ: Humana Press, 1992.

Fairchild, Amy L., and Ronald Bayer. "The Uses and Abuses of Tuskegee." *Science* 284 (May 7, 1999): 919–921.

Human Radiation Experiments: Final Report of the Advisory Committee on Human Radiation Experiments. New York, Oxford University Press, 1996.

Jonas, Hans. "Philosophical Reflections on Experimenting with Human Subjects." In *Experimentation with Human Subjects,* edited by Paul Freund. New York: Braziller, 1970.

Jones, James. *Bad Blood: The Tuskegee Syphilis Experiment: A Tragedy of Race and Medicine.* Rev. ed. New York: Free Press, 1993.

Lasagna, Louis. "Some Ethical Problems in Clinical Investigation." In *Human Aspects of Biomedical Innovation,* edited by E. Medelsohn et al. Cambridge, MA: Harvard University Press, 1971.

Lederer, Susan E. *Subjected to Science: Human Experimentation in America Before the Second World War.* Baltimore: Johns Hopkins University Press, 1995.

Lifton, Robert Jay. *The Nazi Doctors: Medical Killing and the Psychology and Genocide.* New York: Basic Books, 1986.

Moreno, Jonathan D. *Undue Risk: Secret State Experiments on Humans.* New York: Routledge, 2001.

Reverby, Susan M., ed. *Tuskegee's Truths: Rethinking the Tuskegee Syphilis Study.* Chapel Hill: University of North Carolina Press, 2000.

Rothman, David J. "Were Tuskegee & Willowbrook 'Studies in Nature'?" *Hastings Center Report* 12, no. 2 (1982): 5–7.

Shuster, Evelyne. "Fifty Years Later: The Significance of the Nuremberg Code." *New England Journal of Medicine* 337, no. 20 (November 1997): 1436–1440.

Thomas, Stephen B., and Sandra Crouse Quinn. "The Tuskegee Syphilis Study, 1932 to 1972: Implications for HIV Education and AIDS Risk Education Programs in the Black Community." *American Journal of Public Health* 81, no. 11 (November 1991): 1498–1504.

"Trusting Science: Nuremberg and the Human Radiation Experiments." *Hastings Center Report* (syposium, September–October 1996).

"Twenty Years After: The Legacy of the Tuskegee Syphilis Study." *Hastings Center Report* (November–December 1992): 29ff.

THE ETHICS OF RANDOMIZED CLINICAL TRIALS

Appelbaum, Paul S. et al. "False Hopes and Best Data: Consent to Research and the Therapeutic Misconception." *Hastings Center Report* 17, no. 2 (April 1987): 20–24.

Brody, Baruch A. "Conflicts of Interests and the Validity of Clinical Trials." In *Conflicts of Interest,* edited by D. S. Shim and R. G. Spece. New York: Oxford University Press, 1993.

Christakis, Nicholas. "Ethics Are Local: Engaging Cross-Cultural Variation in the Ethics for Clinical Research." *Social Sciences in Medicine* 35, no. 9 (1992): 1079–1091.

Emanuel, Ezekiel J., Robert A. Crouch, John D. Arras, and Jonathan D. Moreno, eds. *Ethical and Regulatory Aspects of Clinical Research: Readings and Commentary.* Baltimore: Johns Hopkins University Press, 2003.

Freedman, Benjamin, Charles Weijer, and Kathleen C. Glass. "Placebo Orthodoxy in Clinical Research I: Empirical and Methodological Myths." *Journal of Law, Medicine Ethics* 24 (1996): 243–251.

———. "Placebo Orthodoxy in Clinical Research II: Ethical, Legal, and Regulatory Myths." *Journal of Law, Medicine Ethics* 24 (1996): 252–259.

Fried, Charles. *Medical Experimentation: Personal Integrity and Social Policy.* New York: American Elsevier, 1974.

Gifford, Fred. "Community-Equipoise and the Ethics of Randomized Clinical Trials." *Bioethics* 9, no. 2 (April 1995): 127–148.

———. "Freedman's 'Clinical Equipoise' and 'Sliding-Scale All Dimensions-Considered Equipoise." *Journal of Medicine and Philosophy* 25, no. 4. (August 2000): 399–427.

Kadane, Joseph B., ed. *Bayesian Methods and Ethics in a Clinical Trial Design.* New York: Wiley 1996.

Kopelman, Loretta. "Randomized Clinical Trials, Consent, and the Therapeutic Relationship." *Clinical Research* 31 (1983): 1–11.

Levine, Carol, Nancy N. Dubler, and Robert Levine. "Building a New Consensus: Ethical Principles and Policies for Clinical Research on HIV/AIDS." *IRB: A Review of Human Subjects Research* 13, nos. 1–2 (January–April 1991): 1–17.

Levine, Robert J. "Uncertainty in Clinical Research." *Law, Medicine and Health Care* 16, nos. 3–4 (Winter 1988): 174–182.

London, A. J. "Clinical Equipoise: Foundational Requirement or Fundamental Error." In *Oxford Handbook of Bioethics,* edited by Bonnie Steinbock. New York: Oxford University Press, 2007.

———. "Reasonable Risks in Clinical Research: A Critique and a Proposal for the Integrative Approach." *Statistics in Medicine* 25, no. 17 (2006): 2869–2885.

———. "Sham Surgery and Reasonable Risks." In *Cutting to the Core: Exploring the Ethics of Contested Surgeries,* edited by David Benatar. New York: Rowman & Littlefield, 2006.

———. "Threats to the Common Good: Biochemical Weapons and Human Subjects Research." *Hastings Center Report* 33, no. 5 (2003): 17–25.

Marquis, Don. "Leaving Therapy to Chance." *Hastings Center Report* 13, no. 4 (1983): 40–47.

Miller, Bruce. "Experimentation on Human Subjects: The Ethics of Random Clinical Trials." In *Health Care Ethics,* edited by Donald VanDeVeer and Tom Regan. Philadelphia: Temple University Press, 1987.

Miller, Franklin G., and Howard Brody. "What Makes Placebo-Controlled Trials Unethical?" *American Journal of Bioethics* 2, no. 2 (Spring 2002): 3–9.

Schaffner, Kenneth F., ed. "Ethical Issues in the Use of Clinical Controls." *Journal of Medicine and Philosophy* 1, no. 4 (November 1986).

Tannsjo, Torbjorn. "The Morality of Clinical Research—a Case Study." *Journal of Medicine and Philosophy* 19 (1994): 7–21.

Weijer, Charles. "The Ethical Analysis of Risk." *Journal of Law, Medicine & Ethics* 28 (2000): 344–361.

ETHICAL ISSUES IN INTERNATIONAL RESEARCH

Angell, Marcia. "The Ethics of Clinical Research in the Third World." *New England Journal of Medicine* 337, no. 12 (September 18, 1997): 847–849.

Annas, George J., and Michael A. Grodin. "Human Rights and Maternal-Fetal HIV Transmission Prevention Trials in Africa." *American Journal of Public Health* 88 (1998): 560–563.

Benetar, Soloman R. "Justice and Medical Research: A Global Perspective." *Bioethics* 15, no. 4 (August 2001): 333–340.

Benatar, Solomon R., and Peter A. Singer. "A New Look at International Research Ethics." *British Medical Journal* 321 (2000): 824–826.

Bhat, S. B., and T. T. Hegde, "Ethical International Research on Human Subjects Research in the Absence of Local Institutional Review Boards." *Journal of Medical Ethics* 32, no. 9 (September 2006): 535–536.

Brody, Baruch A. *The Ethics of Biomedical Research: An International Perspective.* New York: Oxford University Press, 1998.

Del Río, Carlos. "Is Ethical Research Feasible in Developed and Developing Countries?" *Bioethics* 12 (1998): 328–330.

De Zulueta, Paquita. "Randomized Placebo-Controlled Trials and HIV-Infected Pregnant Women in Developing Countries. Ethical Imperialism or Unethical Exploitation?" *Bioethics* 15, no. 4 (August 2001): 289–311.

Farrell, K. "Human Experimentation in Developing Countries: Improving International Practices by Identifying Vulnerable Populations and Allocating Fair Benefits." *Journal of Health Care Law Policy* 9, no. 1 (2006): 136–361.

Gbadegesin, S., and D. Wendley, "Protecting Communities in Health Research from Exploitation." *Bioethics* 20, no. 5 (September 2006): 248–253.

Grady, Christine. "Science in the Service of Healing." *Hastings Center Report* 28, no. 6 (1998): 34–38.

Hawkins, J. S. "Justice and Placebo Controls." *Social Theory and Practice* 23, no. 3 (July 2006): 467–496.

Ijsselmuiden, Carel B., and Ruth Faden. "Research and Informed Consent in Africa: Another Look." *New England Journal of Medicine* 326, no. 12 (March 19, 1992): 830–834.

Kelleher, F. "The Pharmaceutical Industry's Responsibility for Protecting Human Subjects of Clinical Trials in Developing Nations." *Columbia Journal of Law and Social Problems* 38, no. 1 (Fall 2004): 67–106.

King, Nancy M. P. "Experimental Treatment: Oxymoron or Aspiration?" *Hastings Center Report* (July–August 1995): 6–15.

Lavery, James V., Christine Grady, Elizabeth R. Wahl, and Ezekiel J. Emanuel, eds. *Ethical Issues in International Biomedical Research: A Casebook.* New York: Oxford University Press, 2007.

Levi, Jeffrey. "Unproven AIDS Therapies: The Food and Drug Administration and ddI." In *Biomedical Politics.* Washington, DC: Institute of Medicine, 1991:9–42.

Levine, Robert J. "The 'Best Proven Therapeutic Method' Standard in Clinical Trials in Technologically Developing Countries." *IRB: A Review of Human Subjects Research* 20, no. 1 (1998):5–9.

London, A. J. "Justice and the Human Development Approach to International Research." *Hastings Center Report* 35, no. 1 (2005): 24–37.

London, Alex John. "Equipoise and International Human-Subjects Research." *Bioethics* 15, no. 4 (August 2001): 312–332.

Luna, Florencia. "Is 'Best Proven' A Useless Criterion?" *Bioethics* 15, no. 4 (August 2001): 273–289.

Macklin, Ruth. "After Helsinki: Unresolved Issues in International Research." *Kennedy Institute of Ethics Journal* 11, no. 1 (March 2001): 17–36.

———. *Double Standards in Medical Research in Developing Countries (Cambridge Law, Medicine and Ethics).* Cambridge: Cambridge University Press, 2004.

National Bioethics Advisory Commission. *Ethical and Policy Issues in International Research: Clinical Trials in Developing Countries.* Bethesda, MD: National Bioethics Advisory Commission, 2001.

Resnik, David B. "The Ethics of HIV Research in Developing Nations." *Bioethics* 12 (1998): 286–306.

Schüklenk, Udo, and Richard Ashcroft. "International Research Ethics." *Bioethics* 14 (2000): 158–172.

Shamoo, Adil E., and Timothy J. Keay. "Ethical Concerns about Relapse Studies." *Cambridge Quarterly of Healthcare Ethics* 5 (1996): 373–386.

Varmus, Harold, and David Satcher. "Ethical Complexities of Conducting Research in Developing Countries." *New England Journal of Medicine* 337 (1997): 1003–1005.

Wendler, Dave. "Informed Consent, Exploitation and Whether It Is Possible to Conduct Human Subjects Research Without Either One." *Bioethics* 14, no. 4 (2000): 310–339.

RESEARCH ON CHILDREN

Glantz, Leonard H. "Research with Children." *American Journal of Law & Medicine* 24, nos. 2–3 (1998): 213–244.

Grodin, Michael A., and Leonard H. Glantz, eds. *Children as Research Subjects: Science, Ethics, and Law.* New York: Oxford University Press, 2006.

Kass, Nancy E. et al. "Harms of Excluding Pregnant Women from Clinical Research: The Case of HIV-Infected Pregnant Women." *Journal of Law, Medicine Ethics* 24, no. 1 (Spring 1996): 36–46.

Kopelman, Loretta M. "Children as Research Subjects: A Dilemma." *Journal of Medicine and Philosophy* 25, no. 6 (2000): 745–764.

Kopelman, Loretta M., and John C. Moskop, eds. *Children and Health Care: Moral and Social Issues* (Boston: Kluwer Academic, 1989).

PART SEVEN

EMERGING TECHNOLOGIES AND PERENNIAL ISSUES

In Parts 4 and 5, we examined some technologies currently in use, such as prenatal genetic testing, pre-implantation genetic diagnosis (PGD); some that are in their infancy, such as embryonic stem cell research, including therapeutic cloning; and some that may be developed in the future, such as reproductive cloning. In this Part, we take a look at some emerging technologies that have exciting—and disturbing—potential. It is important to think about such possibilities before they are realized because waiting until the technologies are perfected may leave us with insufficient time to control them, and to prevent abuse. It is better to start the ethical debate in advance, so that social, regulatory, and deeply personal decisions can be made with the benefit of extended discussion and analysis. At the same time, it is important not to get carried away about potential dangers. It is salutary to remember that nearly every advancement in medicine, from vaccination to blood donation to organ transplantation, has been initially regarded by some people as unnatural, dangerous and contrary to the will of God. Another reason for examining these emerging technologies are their implications for perennial debates, including the assessment of risks and benefits, autonomy and informed consent, free will and responsibility, blame and punishment, the relation of parents and children, inequality and fairness, and the value of human mastery over nature.

EMERGING TECHNOLOGIES

The topics in Section 1 include genetic enhancement, behavioral genetics, and neuroscience. Although genetic enhancement can be achieved through current methods, such as PGD and embryo discard or prenatal genetic testing and selective abortion, discussed in Part Five, this section considers the possibility of creating desirable traits in offspring through genetic interventions—"genetic engineering," as it is often called. Some day it might be possible to prevent or cure serious genetic disease by gene therapy: removing a deleterious mutation or splicing in a healthy gene. So far, gene therapy has had some successes, in particular with the treatment of severe combined immunodeficiency syndrome (SCIDS), and many failures (Cavazzana-Calvo et al 2004). It remains an experimental treatment that is currently being tested only for the treatment of diseases that have no other cures. Should gene therapy in born human beings become safe and effective, it might conceivably be used on embryos.

If gene therapy at the embryonic level were to become a real possibility, the next step might be genetic enhancement of embryos. Genetic enhancement would use the same techniques as gene therapy, not for the purpose of curing disease, but rather to alter traits such as shyness, aggressiveness, intelligence, musical talent, or athletic prowess. However, before we begin the debate about whether society should take social or legal steps to prohibit prospective parents from utilizing such technologies, we need to consider whether such precise control over behavioral traits is even feasible. In the first selection, "The Designer Baby Myth," Steven Pinker explains why he is skeptical about engineering babies with genes for desirable traits. It turns out that many inheritable traits are not the result of a single gene, but of a number of genes acting together, considerably complicating the prospect of genetic intervention. Moreover, whether these genes are activated and result in a behavior or behavioral disorder, also depends on environmental conditions. For example, schizophrenia is a disease that clearly has a genetic component and tends to run in families. However, many individuals who have no family history of the disease become schizophrenic, suggesting a strong environmental contribution, although what elements in the environment lead to the disease is still unknown. Several studies report a correlation between schizophrenia and in-utero exposure to influenza (Brown et al 2004). It is possible that there are genetic and environmental causes that operate independently to create schizophrenia, or that both must work together for the disease to develop. If this is true of disease, how much more likely is it to be true of complex traits, like intelligence or creativity. And even if scientists manage to discover all the genes and all the environmental factors necessary to produce a trait, there could be unforeseen and undesirable side effects from splicing in genes, making dubious the value of genetic intervention. Pinker gives the example of mice that were given extra copies of the NMDA receptor which is critical to learning and memory. They did learn mazes faster but they were also hypersensitive to pain. Furthermore, it is difficult to think of a trait that is purely good or purely bad. Consider aggressiveness. We don't want out children to be bullies, but aggressiveness is also a trait of leaders and CEOs. If these reasons are not sufficient to give most people pause, remember that genetic engineering would have to be combined with assisted reproduction to create an embryo outside the body in order to manipulate it. Those anxious to give their children a genetic edge (and that is all it would be, not a guarantee of a trait) would have to give up making babies the old-fashioned way, which is for most people part of the attraction.

The second selection in Section 1, "Applications of Behavioral Genetics: Outpacing the Science?" by Mark A. Rothstein, concerns behavioral genetics research: Research into the degree to which human traits and behaviors are due to genetic factors, as opposed to environmental factors. Rothstein explains the science of behavioral genetics and some recent scientific developments in the field, and then goes on to explain the economic and legal pressures that might lead to a misuse of preliminary studies in behavioral genetics. One problem is the unfortunate (though pervasive) tendency of the public to regard genetic causes as both more fundamental and immutable than environmental ones. This, combined with new knowledge about genetic factors, induces a kind of fatalistic despair in the public, a belief that the amelioration of bad environments is useless toward the end of reducing crime or improvement of education. It should be obvious that nothing is further from the truth.

Advances in behavioral genetics may also have important implications for our conceptions of legal and moral responsibility. It is becoming increasingly common for criminal defense attorneys to obtain a brain scan and, upon finding an abnormality, to claim that the defendant is not morally culpable (or as morally culpable) because his action was determined by a genetic predisposition or compulsion. Undoubtedly, the pretty pictures (that is, the brain scans) displayed in court rooms are new; but is the claim any different from the claim that the defendant's responsibility is mitigated because of horrific abuse or neglect in childhood? If such abuse occurred, surely that would be a reason to think that the defendant should be punished less severely, even if there was no obvious damage to the brain. By the same token, a brain abnormality all by itself is not an indication of diminished responsibility, since there could be thousands of people with similar brain scans who never committed crimes. Thus, it seems that behavioral genetics adds no support to "hard determinism," the view that all our behavior is determined because all our behavior is caused— unless one accepts the implausible suggestion that genetic causes are more real or privileged than environmental ones. Questions about freedom and responsibility cannot be settled by science; they are by their very nature both pragmatic and philosophical. They are pragmatic in that the impulse to blame and punish, central to the law, is probably impossible to eradicate. While behavioral genetics may shed new light on causes of behavior, fleshing out the causal story of certain behaviors in a new way (as in the discovery of the influence of the MAOA gene on the disposition toward violence, in the presence of moderate to severe abuse), it leaves untouched the underlying philosophical debate about whether we are free, and what this freedom means.

The last selection in Section 1, "Neuroethics" by Walter Glannon, examines ethical issues that arise from neuroimaging. The first is the implications for moral and criminal responsibility. Glannon notes that studies show that children with psychopathic tendencies have structural and functional abnormalities in their brains. As noted previously, there is a tendency to think that this counts as an excuse if they commit violent crimes. However, psychopaths do not completely lack the capacity to control their impulses. To the extent that they *could have done otherwise*—the perennial question in discussions of free will—it seems that they are responsible for their behavior, despite the abnormalities in their brains. As Glannon comments, ". . . brain images alone will not enable us to draw a clear distinction between responsibility and excuse."

A possible future use of brain scans will be to predict the risk of diseases, such as schizophrenia and Alzheimer's disease. Should brain scans turn out to be reliable predictors, this could be very beneficial to patients. Early pharmacological intervention could delay or prevent the onset of psychosis in patients with schizophrenia and slow memory loss in patients with Alzheimer's. However, it is not clear that brain scans, before symptoms appear, are reliable predictors of disease. Moreover, antipsychotic drugs often have significant long-term adverse effects. The risk of using these drugs thus must be weighed against the risk of not using them. Another ethical dilemma concerns healthy adolescents who served as controls in clinical trials whose brain scans show less gray matter than normal in the prefrontal cortex. This could be a risk factor for developing psychopathology. On the one hand, it seems that the researcher should give this information to them (or their parents who gave consent for them to participate). On the other hand, given uncertainty about whether the scans actually predict disease, the risk of causing undue anxiety, and perhaps even stigmatizing unnecessarily, there is an argument against providing this information. Glannon asks, "If the risk of developing psychopathology is uncertain, then would there be more harm than benefit in forming people of the results of brain scans?" Like the disclosure of misattributed paternity addressed in Part One, this issue demonstrates a conflict between autonomy and beneficence. Unlike DNA testing for paternity, however, there is

considerable uncertainty about what brain scans mean, which complicates the issue of disclosure further. One lesson from both situations is that the question of what might be revealed must be discussed with patients or subjects prior to the testing or the clinical trial, if there is to be genuinely informed consent.

Glannon then turns to psychosurgery and neurostimulation. Ever since *One Flew Over the Cuckoo's Nest* dramatized the horrors of lobotomy, the practice has been viewed with revulsion. Yet lobotomy can relieve symptoms of severe psychiatric illness when all else fails. How should the risks be weighed against the potential benefits? What should be the standard of informed consent when the condition itself militates against the capacity to consent? Electric shock or electroconvulsive therapy (ECT) might seem less drastic and thus more attractive than psychosurgery. The trouble with ECT and other techniques of neurostimulation is that their long-term effects are not known. ECT has been known to result in significant memory loss in some patients. Glannon concludes that more long-term studies are needed, and that the same strict experimental conditions should be applied to all forms of neurostimulation, regardless of the degree of invasiveness.

He ends the article with a discussion of enhancement, focusing on the drug modafinil. Originally approved for the treatment of narcolepsy, the drug has proved to increase alertness and decrease the need for sleep in normal patients, without having the potential for addiction to amphetamines and cocaine. However, there could be unwanted and unforeseen health risks to decreasing sleep. Chronically sleep-deprived people are at greater risk of hypertension, obesity, and diabetes. Moreover, chronic use of the drug could result in permanent changes in the brain. Thus, even a seemingly harmless drug used for enhancement purposes could have serious adverse effects. The same is true of drugs used to enhance memory or other cognitive abilities. Aside from these risks, enhancement raises questions about social inequality and unfairness, considered in Section 2.

ENHANCEMENT

Readers of the sixth edition will be familiar with the first two selections in Section 2. However, in the sixth edition, these articles were placed in the chapter Allocation, Social Justice, and Health Policy, because they raise the question of whether the distinction between the treatment of disease and the enhancement of what are otherwise normal abilities or characteristics should be the basis for allocating treatment. In this edition, we have moved these articles to a section on the ethics of enhancement, in recognition that enhancement itself presents ethical issues apart from allocation of scarce resources. In "Growth Hormone Therapy for the Disability of Short Stature," pediatrician David B. Allen challenges the relevance of the treatment/enhancement distinction as regards prescribing growth hormone for persons of short stature. Imagine two children each of very short stature, one whose condition is the result of having very short parents and the other who is diagnosed with growth hormone deficiency (GHD). GHD is recognized as a disease, as a deviation from normal human functioning, while just being very short is the result of bad luck in the genetic lottery. Both children suffer equally from being extremely short; both experience limitations in the range of opportunities available to them due to their height. Moreover, there are no disadvantages that come from a deficiency in growth hormone aside from the disadvantage of being way below normal height. In both cases, the children may, through their own temperaments and character, overcome the disadvantages of being short. (There are many examples of extremely short men and women who have been successful, from Martin Scorsese and Danny DeVito to Madeleine Albright and Dr. Ruth Westheimer.) It does not seem to matter morally what the etiology of the condition is, that is, in one case short stature is caused by disease and in the other case by ancestry and luck, when the suffering and limitations of opportunity are the same in both cases, so long as the condition can be successfully treated by injections of growth hormone.

In "The Genome Project, Individual Differences, and Just Health Care," Norman Daniels takes up the example of growth hormone for extremely short stature and attempts to defend the treatment/enhancement distinction. Daniels wants to resist what he views as a move toward "equalizing capabilities" because it vastly expands the range of deficiencies in need of correction, resulting in an unattainable social ideal that he fears will undermine the consensus on the importance of health care as traditionally

understood. In other words, we need a principle that will limit access to treatments, especially ones that are expensive, and the principle he adheres to is the distinction between normal and diseased. Daniels plants his feet firmly on the intuition that some health needs are more "urgent" than others and he argues that this intuition is captured by the idea that disease represents a deviation from normal species functioning. The goal of medicine is to restore individuals to the normal opportunity range that they would have enjoyed had they not been prevented from doing so by what is generally recognized as a disease or disability.

Daniels thus recognizes the point made by disability advocates that concepts of "disease" and "normality" are value laden and, perhaps, socially constructed (see Part 5, Section 1). The point of his argument is that, as our ability to control a broader range of our personal traits and characteristics expands, we need to ensure that the most urgent health needs are given priority. If we try to correct for every inequality between people, the cost will be prohibitive, and the result may be an even more inequitable health care system. Although the distinction between disease and enhancement may not map perfectly onto every example, Daniels argues that it is a better guideline for allocating health care resources than a pure subjective standard based on the importance that individuals ascribe to some perceived health need. Adhering to a subjective standard risks allowing the health care system to be hijacked by the delicate and the vain whose small breasts, balding head, or chubby chin is the source of profound anguish and personal shame. For Daniels, only a more objective standard rooted in a scientifically informed conception of normal species functioning will yield a conception of "urgency" that is in step with our deeper intuitions about the significance of health and the importance of health care. The case for prioritizing problems that can be addressed by medicine is indeed strong, as is the imperative to distinguish between genuine needs and mere wants. The question remains whether the correction of extremely short stature, a genuine need when caused by a lack of growth hormone, becomes a mere want when caused by genetic bad luck.

In the next article, "Genetic Interventions and the Ethics of Enhancement of Human Beings," Julian Savulescu argues that enhancement is not merely permissible but obligatory. He compares parents who have a child with stunning intellect but whose intellect can only be sustained with a special diet. To fail to provide the child with the special diet, allowing his intellect to fall to normal would be "clearly wrong," Savulescu says. But it would be equally wrong for parents of a normal child to fail to give their child a dietary supplement that would increase his intellect to stunning. The same holds true for other biological interventions. Other things being equal, we should enhance our children's physical, psychological or cognitive abilities.

It may be objected that this rests on a huge and unjustified assumption: That more is better. However, Savulescu is not arguing that it is always better to have more of a trait. Obviously, there will be limits to the advantage, for example, of increasing a child's height. At some point, being extremely tall becomes a disadvantage. Rather, Savulescu is saying that whatever amount of whatever trait is optimal, we should strive to give our children that amount, by whatever means we have at our disposal. It is precisely this to which Michael Sandel objects in "The Case Against Perfection." If we are ambivalent about Botox for sagging chins and furrowed brows, we are, he thinks, all the more troubled by genetic engineering for stronger bodies, sharper memories, greater intelligence, and happier moods. But why? Is there a rational basis for our concern? Sandel rejects many of the arguments usually given. For example, muscle enhancement may be rejected on grounds of fairness: A genetically enhanced athlete may be seen as having an unfair advantage over his unenhanced competitors. But this argument has a fatal flaw according to Sandel. Namely, that some athletes are better endowed genetically than others. From the standpoint of fairness, enhanced genetic differences are no worse than natural ones. The same is true for memory or intelligence. Moreover, if the objection is fairness, then the solution is making sure that everyone has access to enhancement. The real objection, Sandel says, has nothing to do with fair distribution of enhancement technology. Rather, the real objection is to the drive to mastery, the Promethean aspiration to remake nature.

Prometheus was the Titan who ignored Zeus's express desire and gave fire to mankind, and was, as a result, punished by having his liver eaten and regenerated every day by an eagle. In referring to "Promethean aspiration," Sandel evokes the sin of hubris, or excessive pride or arrogance. But wherein lies the sin of hubris? It could simply lie in the failure to acknowledge the limits of our knowledge. Any attempt to genetically engineer anything, whether corn or mosquitoes or a child, can have unforeseen, unwanted, and irreparable consequences. Consider the following example: Scientists have genetically engineered a species of mosquito that does not transmit malaria. Malaria is a terrible scourge of humanity, killing about two and a half million people each year, according to the World Health Organization (WHO). Spraying is not a perfect solution since the mosquitoes with mutations that enable them to survive reproduce and spread the mutation. Mosquito sleeping nets help to reduce transmission, but not all mosquito bites occur during sleep. Thus the development of a species of mosquito that does not infect people with malaria, and moreover, tends to drive out other species of mosquitoes that do transmit the disease, looks like a great benefit. But what if this new species would be a better vector for other diseases, such as encephalitis, West Nile virus, dengue fever, and yellow fever? It might be very difficult to know this in advance, and the results of such genetic engineering could be very bad indeed. In part, the difference between proponents and opponents of genetic enhancement may be in their levels of optimism about what we can predict and control.

However, Sandel has a deeper point. It is that "the drive to mastery misses and may even destroy . . . an appreciation of the gifted character of human powers and achievements." By this he means, in part, that parents ought to accept their children "as they come, not as objects of our design or products of our will or instruments of our ambition." While it is certainly permissible, and even admirable, for parents to seek the best for their children, this can be taken to unfortunate extremes. Sandel sees the desire to genetically enhance children as another example of the heavily managed, high-pressure child rearing—hyperparenting—that is unfortunately so common today. Genetic enhancement might not be any worse than sparing no expense or effort to get one's child into the "right" pre-school, so that he or she can go to the "right" elementary school, the "right" high school and ultimately the "best" college (or post-graduate school), but it is not any better. The push to excel has led to a great increase in pharmacological treatment of children for attention deficit disorders and hyperactivity. Even children who do not have attention deficit disorders can benefit from drugs like Ritalin, but do we really want to live in a world in which all children (and maybe adults) are on Ritalin?

Like Savulescu, Sandel rejects genetic exceptionalism. That is, it is not the genetic means of enhancement that he finds objectionable, but enhancement itself. Savulescu would undoubtedly agree that putting everyone on Ritalin would be undesirable, but he would maintain that this is because of the drug's potentially harmful side effects, which include weight loss due to decreased appetite, vomiting, abdominal pain (which can lead to malnutrition), nervousness, insomnia, increase in blood pressure, dizziness, heart palpitations, headaches, allergic skin rashes, toxic psychosis, drug dependence syndrome, and severe depression upon withdrawal. If Ritalin just improved memory and concentration, and did not have these side effects, why not give it to everyone? That's a pretty big "if," and might be enough to make most people skeptical of enhancement. However, it is clear that Sandel is not resting his case against enhancement on side effects alone. Rather, it is the desire for mastery and control over nature that is flawed, because it threatens our appreciation of life as a gift, with nothing to affirm or behold beyond our own will. Readers should consider whether Sandel's ideal of "giftedness" is irreducibly religious or whether, as Sandel maintains, "its resonance extends beyond religion" and can be made intelligible within a secular context.

We end Section 2 with a very brief defense by journalist Ronald Bailey of another aspect of enhancement, life-extension, or perhaps life-extension so long as it is accompanied with good health. Whereas some have argued that there is a "natural" life span, a "decently long and adequate life," beyond which we ought not to try to extend life (Callahan 1988), Bailey argues that our descendants will thank us for having engaged in research that will make longer and healthier lives possible.

FREE WILL AND RESPONSIBILITY

Section 3 looks more deeply at a topic touched on in Section 1: The implications of neuroscience for the age-old problem of free will and responsibility. In "Neurobiology, Neuroimaging, and Free Will," Walter

Glannon expands on the topic of neuroimaging, and whether structural and functional abnormalities in the brain are excuses for violent or criminal behavior. Glannon begins with a useful explanation of the traditional positions in the debate over free will. Defenders of determinism maintain that freedom is just an illusion because every event, including every human action, is caused. Defenders of an extreme version of free will insist that our actions are (sometimes at least) freely chosen, and therefore determinism is false. Defenders of compatibilism attempt to reconcile determinism as an accurate scientific picture of the world with our experience of ourselves as freely choosing between alternative courses of action. Compatibilism, which can be traced back to Aristotle, maintains that actions are free when they are performed without compulsion, coercion, or ignorance of the circumstances. Actions are not free, and a person can be excused from responsibility for his or her behavior, when any of these three conditions—compulsion, coercion, or ignorance—is present. However, it should be recognized that free will is often not an all-or-nothing capacity, but one that comes in degrees along a spectrum of control. Many cases of criminal or immoral behavior fall in a gray area between the two extremes of complete control and no control. As the technology develops and becomes more sophisticated, Glannon suggests, neuroimaging may one day be a helpful diagnostic tool, and one that contribute to our understanding of responsibility and excusing conditions. "But it should supplement, not supplant, existing moral and legal criteria of responsibility." Whatever causes are found to influence behavior, whether environmental or neurological, it remains a normative, not scientific, judgment what conditions exempt people from blame and punishment.

REFERENCES

Brown AS, Begg MD, Schaefer CA, et al. In-utero exposure to infection and schizophrenia in adult offspring. Program and abstracts of the American Psychiatric Association 2004 Annual Meeting; May 1–6, 2004; New York, NY. Symposium 13A.

Callahan, D. (1988) Aging and the ends of medicine. *Annals of the New York Academy of Sciences* 530: 125–133.

Cavazzana-Calvo, M, Thrasher T, and Mavillo, F. (2004) The future of gene therapy. *Nature* 427, 26 February: 779–81.

EMERGING TECHNOLOGIES

THE DESIGNER BABY MYTH

Steven Pinker

This year's 50th anniversary of the discovery of the structure of DNA has kindled many debates about the implications of that knowledge for the human condition. Arguably the most emotionally charged is the debate over the prospect of human genetic enhancement or "designer babies". It's only a matter of time, many say, before parents will improve their children's intelligence and personality by having suitable genes inserted into them shortly after conception.

A few commentators have welcomed genetic enhancement as just the latest step in the struggle to improve human life. Many more are appalled. They warn that it is a Faustian grab at divine powers that will never be used wisely by us mortals. They worry that it will spawn the ultimate inequality, a genetic caste system. In his book *Our Posthuman Future* (just released in paperback), the conservative thinker Francis Fukuyama warns that genetic enhancement will change human nature itself and corrode the notion of a common humanity that undergirds the social order. Bill McKibben, writing from the political left, raises similar concerns in his new jeremiad *Enough: Staying Human in an Engineered Age.*

Whether they welcome or decry it, almost everyone agrees that genetic enhancement is inevitable if research proceeds on its current course. In America, genetic enhancement is a major concern of the president's Council on Bioethics; its chairman, Leon Kass, and several of its members, including Fukuyama, are outspoken worriers.

As it happens, some kinds of genetic enhancement are already here. Anyone who has been turned down for a date has been a victim of the human drive to exert control over half the genes of one's future children. And it is already possible to test embryos conceived in vitro and select ones that are free of genetic defects such as cystic fibrosis.

From The Guardian Web site, http://www.guardian.co.uk/print/0,,4683679-111396,00.html (accessed January 6, 2007). Reprinted by permission of Steven Pinker.

But when it comes to direct genetic enhancement—engineering babies with genes for desirable traits—there are many reasons to be sceptical. Not only is genetic enhancement not inevitable, but it is not particularly likely in our lifetimes. This skepticism comes from three sources: the limits of futurology, the science of behavioural genetics, and human nature itself.

The history of the future should make us raise an eyebrow whenever the experts tell us how we will live 10, 20, or 50 years from now. Not long ago we were assured that by the turn of the century we would live in domed cities, commute by jet-pack, and clean our homes with nuclear-powered vacuum cleaners wielded by robot maids. More recently we were promised the paperless office, interactive television, the internet refrigerator, and the end of bricks-and-mortar retail. It's not just that these developments have not yet happened, many of them, like domed cities, never will happen. Even in mundane cases, technological progress is far from inexorable. Air travel, for example, is barely faster or more comfortable today than it was when commercial jets were introduced 50 years ago.

Why are technological predictions usually wrong? Many futurologists write as if current progress can be extrapolated indefinitely—the fallacy of climbing trees to get to the moon. They routinely underestimate the number of things that have to go right for a development to change our lives. It takes more than a single eureka!; it takes a large number of more boring discoveries, together with the psychological and sociological imponderables that make people adopt some invention en masse. Who could have predicted the videophones of the 1960s would sink like a stone while the text messaging of the 1990s would become a teenage craze?

Finally, futurologists tend to focus their fantasies on the benefits of a new technology, whereas actual users weigh both the benefits and the costs. Do you really want to install software upgrades on your refrigerator or reboot it when it crashes?

Many prognosticators assume that we are in the midst of discovering genes for talents such as mathematical giftedness, musical talent and athletic prowess. The reality is very different. The achilles heel of genetic enhancement will be the rarity of single genes with consistent beneficial effects.

Behavioural genetics has uncovered a paradox. We know that tens of thousands of genes working together have a large effect on the mind. Twin studies show that identical twins (who share all their genes) are more similar than fraternal twins (who share half their genes, among those that vary from person to person), who in turn are more similar than adopted siblings (who share even fewer of the varying genes). Adoption studies show that children tend to resemble their biological relatives in personality and intelligence more than they resemble their adopted relatives.

But these are effects of sharing an entire genome, or half of one. The effects of a single gene are much harder to show. Geneticists have failed to find single genes that consistently cause schizophrenia, autism or manic-depressive disorder, even though there is overwhelming evidence that these conditions are substantially heritable. And if we can't find a gene for schizophrenia, we're even less likely to find one for humour, musical talent, or likeability, because it's easier to disrupt a complex system with a single defective part than to improve it by adding a single beneficial one. The 1998 report of a gene that was correlated with a four-point advantage in IQ was recently withdrawn because it did not replicate in a larger sample—a common fate for putative single gene discoveries.

So don't hold your breath for the literary creativity gene or the musical talent gene. The human brain is not a bag of traits with one gene for each trait. Neural development is a staggeringly complex process guided by many genes interacting in feedback loops. The effect of one gene and the effect of a second gene don't produce the sum of their effects when they're simultaneously present. The pattern of expression of genes (when they are turned on or off by proteins and other signals) is as important as which genes are present.

Even when genes should be at their most predictable—in identical twins, who share all their genes, and hence all the interactions among their genes—we don't have foregone conclusions. Identical twins reared together (who share not only their genes but most of their environments) are imperfectly correlated in personality measures such as extroversion and neuroticism. The correlations, to be sure, are much larger than those for fraternal twins or unrelated people, but they are seldom greater than 50%. This tells us there is an enormous role for chance in the development of a human being.

It gets worse. Most genes have multiple effects, and evolution selects the ones that achieve the best compromise among the positive and the negative ones. Take the most famous candidate for genetic enhancement: the mice that were given extra copies of the NMDA receptor, which is critical to learning and memory. These poster mice did learn mazes more quickly, but they also turned out to be hypersensitive to pain. Closer to home, there is a candidate gene in humans that appears to be correlated with a 10-point boost in IQ. But it is also associated with a 10% chance of developing torsion dystonia, which can confine the sufferer to a wheelchair with uncontrollable muscle spasms.

This places steep ethical impediments to research on human enhancement. Even if some day it might be possible, could you get there from here? How can scientists try out different genes to enhance the minds of babies given that many of them could have terrible side effects?

Genetic enhancement faces another problem: most traits are desirable at intermediate values. Wallis Simpson said that you can't be too rich or too thin, but other traits don't work that way. Take aggressiveness. Parents don't want their children to be punching bags or doormats, but they also don't want Attila the Hun either. Most want their children to face life with confidence rather than sitting at home cowering in fear, but they don't want a reckless daredevil out of *Jackass*. So even if a gene had some consistent effect, whether the effect was desirable would depend on what the other tens of thousands of genes in that child were doing.

The third obstacle to re-engineering human nature comes from human nature itself. We are often told that it's only human for parents to give their children every possible advantage. Stereotypical yuppies who play Mozart to their pregnant bellies and bombard their newborns with flash cards would stop at nothing, it is said, to give their children the ultimate head start in life.

But while parents may have a strong desire to help their children, they have an even stronger desire "not to hurt" their children. Playing Mozart may not make a foetus smarter, but it probably won't make it

stupider or harm it in other ways. Not so for genetic enhancement. It is not obvious that even the most overinvested parent would accept a small risk of retardation in exchange for a moderate chance of improvement.

Another speed bump from human nature consists of people's intuitions about naturalness and contamination. People believe that living things have an essence that gives them their powers and which can be contaminated by pollutants. These intuitions have been powerful impediments to the acceptance of other technologies. Many people are repelled by genetically modified foods even though they have never been shown to be unsafe or harmful to the environment. If people are repulsed by genetically modified soybeans, would they really welcome genetically modified children?

Finally, anyone who has undergone in-vitro fertilisation knows that it is a decidedly unpleasant procedure, especially in comparison to sex. Infertile couples may choose the procedure as a last resort, and some kooks may choose it to have a child born under a certain astrological sign or for other frivolous reasons. But people who have the choice generally prefer to conceive their children the old-fashioned way.

It is misleading, then, to assume that parents will soon face the question, "Would you opt for a procedure that would give you a happier and more talented child?" When you put it like that, who would say no? The real question will be, "Would you opt for a traumatic and expensive procedure that might give you a slightly happier and more talented child, might give you a less happy, less talented child, might give you a deformed child, and probably would make no difference?" For genetic enhancement to "change human nature" not just a few but billions of people would have to answer yes.

My point is not that genetic enhancement is impossible, just that it is far from inevitable. And that has implications. Some bioethicists have called for impeding, or even criminalising, certain kinds of research in genetics and reproductive medicine, despite their promise of improvement in health and happiness. That is because the research, they say, will inevitably lead to designer babies. If genetic enhancement really were just around the corner, these proposals would have to be taken seriously. But if the prospect is very much in doubt, we can deal with the ethical conundrums if and when they arise. Rather than decrying our posthuman future, thinkers should acknowledge the frailty of technological predictions and should base policy recommendations on likelihoods rather than fantasies.

APPLICATIONS OF BEHAVIOURAL GENETICS: OUTPACING THE SCIENCE?

Mark A. Rothstein

The study of the role of heredity in human behaviour emerged at the end of the nineteenth century, and since then the resulting scientific data has been extremely controversial. Studies that claim to show a genetic basis of low intelligence and antisocial behaviour among immigrants to the United States from southern and eastern Europe in the early 1900s paved the way for restrictive immigration laws. The asserted genetic basis of immorality and mental defects was misused to enact eugenic sterilization laws in most of western Europe and many states of the United States at the beginning of the twentieth century. Behavioural genetics research was also misused to support Nazi claims of racial superiority (and non-Aryan inferiority), which had a direct and important role in the Holocaust.

As we contemplate the potential for misuse of new behavioural genetics research, it is important to recognize the crucial role that the media has in informing the public of new scientific discoveries. The public has traditionally shown a keen interest in behavioural genetics, and genetic explanations of human behaviours have always been popular in the mass media. Although scientific publications of new findings are usually properly controlled and qualified, descriptions of new research in the popular media are not always as constrained. As one journalist recently explained, "We science reporters occupy a humble niche in the vast news and entertainment industry [and we] must compete fiercely for editors' and readers' attention. The public is increasingly confronted with reports claiming that violence, happiness, impulsivity, religiosity, fidelity and other behaviours are 'hard wired' rather than being caused by many factors. Although the accuracy and effect of media reports of genetic discoveries have been debated in the literature, public confusion is an expected result.

Because many individuals and institutions might act on the basis of these misconceptions, popular misunderstanding of behavioural genetics is of great concern. In this article I summarize recent scientific developments in behavioural genetics, with emphasis on the genetics of mental disorders, aggression, addiction and personality. I discuss the economic and legal pressures that might lead to the misuse of preliminary studies in behavioural genetics. I then analyse the most probable settings for the use of behavioural genetic information—criminal law, education, employment and insurance. I conclude by considering the ethical and legal framework for applications of behavioural genetics.

SCIENTIFIC DEVELOPMENTS

The traditional tools of behavioural genetic research consist of animal studies, family studies (including adoption studies), twin studies, LINKAGE ANALYSIS and population studies. Although these studies have revealed a statistical correlation between genetic factors and certain behaviours, they can only predict in a probabilistic way the likelihood that individuals will show a particular behaviour. More recently,

From *Science and Society* 6 (October 2005): 793–797. Reprinted by permission of Nature Publishing Group.

Editors' note: All author's notes have been cut. Students who want to follow up on sources should consult the original article.

the application of genomics to behavioural genetics has been accelerated by the Human Genome Project, and could provide the means to individualize behavioural genetic assessments in the future. By analysing the genotype of an individual, scientists might be able to make more accurate predictions about the influence of genetic factors on that individual's behaviour.

Genomics—and associated fields such as proteomics, transcriptomics, metabolomics and pharmacogenomics—also holds great promise for understanding how the brain and CNS function. Emerging behavioural genetic insights could have an important role in the prevention and treatment of a wide range of behavioural and psychiatric disorders. These developments might also have a wider application for treating minor anxieties, addictions, phobias and adjustment problems that individuals routinely face in daily life.

Although scientists overwhelmingly agree that human behaviour is affected by genes that is largely as far as agreement on this subject goes. The range of behaviours that are influenced by genes, the effect of the environment on particular behaviours, the methodology for determining heritability, the plasticity of genetic predispositions and numerous other issues are still under debate. With only a few exceptions, behavioural genetics involves complex interactions of many genes and environmental factors. Furthermore, there is an important distinction between psychopathology and variation within normal bounds. Minor variations in personality and temperament are likely to be more difficult to link with genetic factors than well-characterized mental disorders, although there is no guarantee that even studies that deal with well-studied psychiatric illnesses will be successful. Bearing in mind these caveats, I provide a brief overview of areas of behavioural genetics in which links have been found between genetic components and behaviours that have implications for use in legal, commercial and educational settings.

Genes and Mental Disorders

Genetic influences on various mental diseases have been reported in the literature but have not been thoroughly characterized. Studies of depression, BIPOLAR DISORDER and schizophrenia have identified genetic loci or regions of genes associated with molecular pathways that lead to diagnosable psychiatric conditions. However, defects in many of these pathways result in various behavioural disorders with a range of severity and presentation, making it even more difficult to make definitive links. For example, there are two isoforms of monoamine oxidase (MAO) in humans—MAOA and MAOB—both of which are encoded on the X chromosome. MAO has an important role in metabolizing and modulating neurotransmitters that are essential for brain function. Mutations in the gene that encodes MAOA, although rare, are thought to be associated with certain pathologies and abnormal behaviours, including schizophrenia, bipolar disorder, Parkinson disease, alcoholism and nicotine addiction. Variation in MAOA activity has also been associated with depression, aggressiveness, impulsivity and other antisocial behaviours and psychopathologies.

In frequently cited research, investigators studied a large Dutch family, including several males with borderline mental retardation who showed abnormal and impulsive behaviours, including aggressive and violent behaviour, arson, exhibitionism, voyeurism, rape and attempted suicide. A complete deficiency of MAOA activity was found to be related to "abnormal aggressive behaviour in affected males." Other studies, including those with females and adolescents, confirmed the hypothesis that substantially reduced levels of MAOA activity correlate with higher levels of impulsivity, low socialization and vulnerability for criminal behaviour.

Genes and Aggressive Behaviour

Studies of the genetics of aggression have been increasingly used in criminal law and other areas, which are discussed below. Serotonin is an important neurotransmitter that has been linked to human aggression, and some of the receptor sites for serotonin have known genetic polymorphisms, which might underlie variations in aggressive behaviour. Serotonergic neurons, which are located primarily in the BRAINSTEM and project to almost every part of the CNS, have been implicated in many functions of the CNS, including sleep, arousal, feeding, motor activity, mood and stress resilience. Reduced levels of serotonin metabolites in the cerebrospinal fluid have been found in aggressive psychiatric patients,

impulsive violent men and victims of violent suicide. Other studies have shown that low levels of
these molecules were predictive of RECIDIVISM in violent offenders and arsonists, and they were strongly
associated with a family history of paternal violence
and alcoholism. Serotonin polymorphisms have also
been correlated with panic disorder, impulsivity and
poor behavioural control.

Dopamine, another neurotransmitter, has also
been shown to have an effect on behaviour. Six
dopamine receptors have been well characterized
so far. Dopamine release induces a 'reward cascade'
in the brain, which leads to feelings of well-being
and stress reduction. Preliminary studies have
shown a correlation between dopamine D3 receptor
polymorphisms and aggressive behaviour.

Genes and Addictions

Substantial genetic research has established correlations between certain genes and a propensity to
addictive behaviour, including gambling and the
use of alcohol, tobacco and various licit and illicit
substances. A polymorphism in the D2 receptor has
been associated with craving for a dopamine fix,
which is satisfied by ingesting alcohol, cocaine,
heroin, marijuana or nicotine. The genetic factors
that predispose to addictive behaviour, violence and
other antisocial behaviours can be interrelated for
several reasons. First, the genetic factors that have
been identified as having a causal role in addiction
also have causal roles in violent, aggressive or
impulsive behaviour. Second, even if these genotypes are not independently linked, merely being
addicted is often associated with these other behaviours. Last, the continuing need for large sums of
money to satisfy an addiction, which might be
partly caused by genetic factors, often causes individuals to engage in aggressive criminal activity.

Genes and Personality

If and when behavioural genetic screening begins it
will probably grow out of the desire to make an early
assessment of a psychopathology or to avoid commercial and other relationships with individuals that
are at an increased risk of antisocial behaviours. Nevertheless, research is also being carried out that relates

to the non-pathological dimension of behavioural
genetics. Researchers have studied, among other
things, the genetic influence on happiness, intelligence, novelty seeking, sexual orientation, shyness,
sociability and positive emotionality, and memory
skills. All these aspects of personality are important in
employment, education and other settings, which are
discussed below.

WHY RELY ON PRELIMINARY STUDIES?

As noted above, media reports that suggest determinative links between genotype and behaviour might
lead to the public's over-estimation of the role of
genes in human behaviour. Various entities with
financial interests in the behaviour of certain individuals might then attempt to use genetic information to
predict behaviour. For example, employers and
insurers might be liable for injuries caused by an
impulsive, aggressive or emotionally unstable individual. Many employers undoubtedly believe that
learning about potential employee's behavioural
proclivities could result in substantial savings.
Behavioural genetics might seem appealing because
it is more 'high tech' than the use of references that
relate to past behaviour, and it operates predictively,
rather than relying on phenotypic expression.

There is ample indication that some entities would
be willing to use new technologies despite the lack of
adequate scientific proof for their validity. For example—in an incident involving medical rather than
behavioural genetics—in early 2001 it was disclosed
that the Burlington Northern Santa Fe Railroad, the
second largest railroad in the United States, carried
out genetic testing without the knowledge or consent
of employees who had filed compensation claims for
CARPAL TUNNEL SYNDROME. A laboratory under contract
with the employer used a genetic test for a chromosomal deletion that is associated with HEREDITARY
NEUROPATHY WITH LIABILITY TO PRESSURE PALSIES, a rare
condition that might predict some forms of carpal tunnel syndrome. Scientists overwhelmingly asserted
that the use of this genetic test was improper and
inappropriate because it tested for a rare mutation that
was unlikely to have caused the disability of employees with known workplace exposures to repetitive
motion and vibration. The company quickly settled

BOX 1
Behavioural Genetics and the Death Penalty

Thirty-eight of the fifty states in the United States provide the death penalty for at least some types of serious crime. In these states, capital punishment is considered to be appropriate on the basis of the severity of the crime and the culpability of the defendant. In *Thompson v. Oklahoma*, 487 US 815 (1988), the US Supreme Court held that execution of individuals who were 15 years old or younger at the time of their crimes violated the ban on 'cruel and unusual punishment' contained in the Eighth Amendment to the US Constitution. In *Atkins v. Virginia*, 536 US 304 (2002), the Supreme Court held that it was unconstitutional to execute mentally retarded offenders on the basis of their diminished culpability.

Most recently, in *Roper v. Simmons*, 125 S. Ct. 1183 (2005), the Supreme Court held that it was unconstitutional to execute individuals who were under 18 years old at the time that they committed their crime. The decision in *Roper v. Simmons* was based largely on "evolving national and international standards of decency" and the consensus that children lack the emotional and mental maturity necessary for the most culpable criminal intent. FRIEND OF THE COURT briefs submitted on behalf of the defendant emphasized, among other things, that teenagers have "an underdeveloped sense of responsibility." Studies using modern neuroscience imagining techniques were offered to show that the brain does not mature until the age of 20–25 and therefore teenagers do not have fully developed frontal lobes that are capable of impulse control.

On the basis of this line of reasoning, it is possible that the Supreme Court will be asked to rule on a future defendant's argument that it is cruel and unusual punishment to execute an adult who does not suffer from mental retardation, but whose impulse control has been compromised by a genetic mutation. Such a case would call into question a bedrock assumption of Anglo-American jurisprudence: individuals are assumed to have free will in their actions and therefore are legally responsible for their conduct.

---

lawsuits that were based on the testing and promised not to repeat the genetic test. Because the railroad was willing to use an inappropriate genetic test in an attempt to identify predisposition to a physical condition, and in light of other unproven, non-genetic behavioural tests already in use, it can be assumed that other employers would be tempted to use unproven behavioural genetic tests.

The likelihood of preliminary behavioural genetic information being used in courts must be considered in light of the Anglo-American legal system. Each side in a legal case has its own lawyer, who has an ethical duty to assert all plausible claims on behalf of his (or her) client. The ethical mandate of zealous advocacy is especially applicable to defence lawyers in criminal cases, in which the conviction of a client could result in imprisonment or even execution (BOX 1). In 2003 the United States Supreme Court held that it was "ineffective assistance of counsel" for a defence lawyer to fail to

investigate the family history of a convicted client before sentencing occurred. In subsequent cases defendants have asserted that genetic predisposition to uncontrollably violent conduct and a family history of uncontrollably violent conduct should mitigate a sentence of death. Various unproven scientific hypotheses have been introduced in support of the defendants' claims.

SPECIFIC APPLICATIONS
Criminal Law

Genetic explanations of antisocial behaviour represent an important area of research and one of the earliest applications of behavioural genetics. Behavioural genetics could potentially be used in several ways—from the earliest stages of a criminal investigation through to almost every aspect of the criminal justice system.

DNA forensic techniques are used by law-enforcement agencies around the world. In the absence of a match between the evidence from a crime scene and the profiles stored in forensic DNA databases, DNA forensic profiling can be used for several purposes—to identify the gender of and make predictions about the race or ethnicity, health status, age, or physical characteristics of the sample source. Behavioural genetic forensic profiling might be increasingly used in law enforcement to predict the perpetrator's behavioural traits and psychiatric conditions, such as learning disabilities and personality traits.

Once a suspect is arrested and charged with a crime, behavioural genetic information could be presented at a bail hearing. Prosecutors might urge that bail should not be granted or should be set at a high amount because of the defendant's genetic predisposition to impulsivity (for example, risk of flight) or aggression (for example, risk of committing further crimes).

At trial, evidence of behavioural genetic variation within the normal range is unlikely to establish an independent basis for acquittal. More extreme deviations might be part of the scientific evidence used to support an insanity defence. Behavioural genetic evidence might also be used to claim that the defendant lacked the mental capacity to form the intent necessary to commit the crime. For example, on this basis a defendant charged with premeditated murder might be convicted of a lesser offence, such as manslaughter.

In many states in the United States it is common for convicted defendants to introduce evidence that relatives across many generations have engaged in violent criminal activities, that the defendant has inexplicably engaged in antisocial activities from a young age, or that the individual has been diagnosed with a neurogenetic disorder. This is then used to assert that defendants who commit crimes caused at least in part by a genetic predisposition or compulsion are not as morally culpable and do not deserve the harshest sentences. It is difficult to determine whether such arguments have had an effect on the sentences imposed, but the willingness of some courts to consider such evidence leaves open the possibility that behavioural genetics could be afforded greater weight in the future.

Behavioural genetic information could also be introduced in parole hearings. Ironically, the positions of the government and the inmate with respect to the behavioural genetic evidence are likely to be the opposite of their arguments at the trial. At a parole hearing, the government might attempt to use genetic predisposition as a basis for denying parole; the inmate might use the absence of genetic predisposition as a basis for release under the theory that he or she is less likely to commit another crime in the future.

Finally, many states in the United States have enacted 'sexual predator laws', which permit the indefinite confinement of individuals who have been convicted of multiple sex crimes against children and who are considered likely to commit further crimes if released. In theory, behavioural genetic evidence might be used to predict the likelihood of the individual committing future sex crimes.

As a scientific matter, it is difficult to determine the contribution of genetic factors in the criminal activities of any particular individual. When these scientific issues are considered by judges and juries with little or no scientific training, there is a risk that the general public will give too much credence to unproven scientific theories, thereby increasing the likelihood of faulty or premature application of behavioural genetic research.

Education

Behavioural genetic research has shed light on various traits and disorders that are relevant to education, ranging from preschool through to graduate and professional school. Behavioural genetic testing might help to diagnose or identify the cause of mental retardation or other impairments much earlier than current assessment methods. Among the conditions that give rise to identifiable neurodevelopmental and neuropsychiatric disabilities that have an impact on educational development are FRAGILE X SYNDROME, KLINEFELTER SYNDROME, TURNER SYNDROME and WILLIAMS SYNDROME. Researchers have also attempted to identify the genetic factors in autism.

Genetic factors also have an important role in learning disabilities, such as dyslexia and dyscalculia. Furthermore, genetic links have been identified for ATTENTION-DEFICIT HYPERACTIVITY DISORDER and emotional disorders. The genetic contribution to cognitive ability, memory skills and other measures of academic potential could also be applied in educational settings for classroom placement and curriculum development.

Educational programming for students with mental retardation is the area that is most likely to be affected by behavioural genetics. In the past, definitive diagnoses, helped by genetic test results, have been used for several educational purposes. These include student evaluation, assignment of special services and instruction, placement, curriculum development, and determination of appropriate discipline. As research in this field progresses, it is possible that behavioural genetic information could be used for a wider range of students to assess general academic potential and specialized talents.

The use of behavioural genetics by educational institutions raises two main concerns. First, school officials have little expertise in evaluating behavioural genetic technologies and deciding when and how to rely on genetic information. Schools also often lack the privacy safeguards needed to ensure that this sensitive information is not wrongfully disclosed. Second, there is a concern that behavioural genetic information will be given greater weight than it deserves in assessing complex phenotypes such as cognition. An unfortunate result could be to deny educational opportunities to many individuals, to the detriment of both the individuals and society. In most of the developed world, universal public education embodies meritocracy, vertical social mobility and social justice. Actions that limit opportunity, even on the basis of scientific considerations, might demand a social cost. For the near future at least, behavioural genetics is much more likely to be valuable in assessing learning disabilities (in which the influence of genetics is greater than that of the environment) than learning abilities (in which genetic influence is less than that of the environment). Socioeconomic status and other factors will further complicate this analysis.

Employment

Many employers spend substantial sums of money carrying out psychological, personality, intelligence and aptitude tests on applicants and employees. Although there have been questions raised concerning the appropriateness of many of these tests, the purpose of the testing is understandable. Inappropriate employee selection and job placement are expensive

for employers in terms of increased turnover, decreased morale, losses due to theft, lost productivity and damage to the employer's reputation. Furthermore, employers are concerned about potential legal liability resulting from the negligent or wilful misconduct of employees. Consequently, employers are especially careful in hiring employees for positions of trust, such as law-enforcement officers, day-care workers, teachers, transportation workers and employees who handle large sums of cash or valuables.

Some employers are willing to use hand-writing analysis, honesty questionnaires and other unproven measures. In the United States, polygraphs were widely used until 1988, when Congress banned their use for most private-sector employment. In the future, some employers almost certainly would be willing to use behavioural genetic testing, providing that the tests were not too expensive. Employers might attempt to identify individuals who are genetically predisposed to sexual predation, pathological gambling or poor impulse control. They might also seek to learn about genetic predisposition to shyness, assertiveness, ability to work under stress or other traits that are relevant to the position.

As with the use of behavioural genetics in educational settings, its inappropriate use in employment could result in the wrongful exclusion of individuals from important opportunities. Behavioural genetics might implicate various laws, including statutes that specifically prohibit genetic discrimination in employment and more general laws that prohibit discrimination based on physical or mental disability. Similar to criminal law, the use of behavioural genetics in employment law could challenge courts to understand the findings and limitations of new scientific discoveries and also to rule on the relative rights of employers and workers in hiring decisions.

Insurance

Behavioural genetic information could be used in establishing eligibility and setting rates for various insurance products. The most obvious use of behavioural genetics would be in private health insurance to predict which applicants for individually underwritten insurance might require mental health services for psychiatric conditions or addictions. Disability insurance companies might also want to

---

BOX 2

How a Lawsuit Could Spur the Growth of Behavioural Genetic Testing

---

As an indication of how behavioural genetic information of dubious scientific value could become more widely used, take the theoretical example of a publicized personal-injury lawsuit. Suppose a young boy at an overnight summer camp is seriously injured when he is hit in the head by a rock that is unexpectedly but deliberately thrown by another boy. The injured boy might have substantial medical bills and other expenses and might, through his parents, seek legal compensation. But [whom] should the boy sue? If neither the aggressor's parents nor the camp had any forewarning that such an attack might occur, it is doubtful that a lawsuit would be successful in charging negligent supervision or failure to control the child.

Behavioural genetics might indicate another legal theory. The injured child's lawyer might assert that had the camp required behavioural testing to be carried out, perhaps including behavioural genetic testing of all campers, it would have learned that the aggressor child had a particular genotype that the plaintiff's expert would testify confers a genetic predisposition to violent behaviour. Therefore, as the argument would go, if the camp had required behavioural genetic testing to be carried out, it would have refused to admit the child to camp and the injury would have been averted. In personal-injury cases, defendants, their lawyers and their insurers often attempt to calculate their legal exposure. If the odds of the plaintiff recovering on this theory are 5%, and the potential damages are US$3 million if the plaintiff wins, then the case would have a settlement value of at least $150,000, because the defendant would also save on legal fees. Accordingly, even a scientific explanation with questionable merit could support a substantial settlement.

If the defendants opt to settle and the case receives publicity, there might be a widespread misimpression that behavioural genetic screening has scientific support. Parents might start to demand testing before sending their children to camp, and insurers might pressure camps to adopt testing. Undoubtedly, commercial laboratories would attempt to promote even wider testing, including testing by boarding schools, dormitories and various residential workplaces, such as offshore oil rigs.

---

predict which applicants for insurance were at increased risk of temporary or permanent disability from behavioural health problems.

A less obvious, but possible future use of behavioural genetic information, at least in the United States, is in life insurance, where a genetic predisposition to risk-taking, novelty-seeking, depression or impulsivity could be considered a risk for premature mortality. In the United Kingdom and other countries, voluntary or mandatory restrictions have been applied to the use of genetic information in life-insurance underwriting. In addition, behavioural genetic traits might be considered to establish a high risk of claims being filed in the context of automobile, household or property insurance. Behavioural genetic screening could be used in an

attempt to avoid the liability caused by the intentional or negligent acts of mentally unstable individuals (BOX 2).

The use of behavioural genetic information in any insurance product raises two fundamental questions. First, how accurate is the scientific information on which actuarial predictions are based? Second, assuming that the predictions are accurate, what is the social role of private insurance? Does medical underwriting of the insurance product further societal interests, such as access to health care and financial security for families after the death of the primary bread-winner? Policy decisions that relate to behavioural genetics and insurance should be attuned to overall policies for the use of genetic information in insurance.

Glossary

- ATTENTION-DEFICIT HYPERACTIVITY DISORDER

  A persistent pattern of inattention and/or hyperactivity or impulsivity that is more frequently displayed and more severe than is typically observed in individuals that are at a comparable level of development.

- BIPOLAR DISORDER

  A mood disorder that is characterized by periodic swings between exaggerated elation and depression.

- BRAINSTEM

  A portion of the deep posterior part of the brain that consists of the midbrain, pons and medulla.

- CARPAL TUNNEL SYNDROME

  Compression of the median nerve as it passes through the carpal tunnel in the wrist, which is often caused by repetitive flexion and extension of the wrist.

- FRAGILE X SYNDROME

  X-linked mental retardation. It occurs in both genders, but with a higher frequency in males.

- FRIEND OF THE COURT

  An individual or group that has an interest in a case, but is not a party to it.

- HEREDITARY NEUROPATHY WITH LIABILITY TO PRESSURE PALSIES

  A disorder of the peripheral nerves that results in unusual sensitivity to touch, numbness and loss of muscle strength.

- KLINEFELTER SYNDROME

  A disorder in which males have an XXY-chromosomal constitution. It is associated with a predisposition to learning disabilities and other symptoms.

- LINKAGE ANALYSIS

  A method for tracking the transmission of genetic information across generations to identify the map location of genetic loci on the basis of co-inheritance of genetic markers and discernable phenotypes in families.

- RECIDIVISM

  The tendency to relapse into a behavioural condition, especially criminal behaviour.

- TURNER SYNDROME

  An aneuploidy disorder in which females have a single X-chromosome constitution. It is associated with a diminution in perceptual abilities.

- WILLIAMS SYNDROME

  A disorder that is caused by deletion in chromosome 7 resulting in mental retardation, aortic stenosis and other symptoms.

CONCLUSIONS

The Human Genome Project has led to greater public awareness of the role of genes in disease and behaviour, but it has also led to an increase in popular ideas of behavioural genetic determinism. Despite the preliminary or qualified nature of some associations between genes and behaviour, the applications of behavioural genetic information in everyday life will probably increase. The adversary legal system and the inclination of employers and other institutions to embrace new technologies in the absence of scientific proof of their efficacy are both likely to encourage the proliferation of behavioural genetic testing and genetic explanations of behaviour. This is supported by the economic incentives of insurers and other institutions to avoid commercial relations with individuals who are believed to be at an increased risk of costly behavioural problems. Although the type of scientific data and the reason for its possible use differ for each of the areas in which behavioural genetics might be applied, some common societal challenges emerge. First, there is great potential for misinterpreting and misusing behavioural genetic information, therefore researchers need to be careful in public pronouncements and should temper their enthusiasm for the potential implications of preliminary studies. Second, public and media education programmes need to devote more attention to behavioural genetics, including learning about past abuses and the scientific limitations of research findings. Third, commercial and social institutions need to deliberate carefully and consult with experts before applying behavioural genetics to avoid limiting opportunities for individuals or stigmatizing them. Fourth, because behavioural genetic information is extremely sensitive, those who hold such information must ensure that it is kept confidential. Unless these concerns are addressed there is a real risk that the legal and commercial applications of behavioural genetics will outpace the science to the detriment of us all.

Even assuming the validity of the research findings, behavioural genetics raises important ethical issues and societal challenges. Behavioural genetic information might call into question individual and social ideas of equality of opportunity, discrimination and personal responsibility. As we consider the legal and policy implications of behavioural genetics it is important to undertake further social scientific research on the effect of genetic explanations of behaviour on individuals and society.

NEUROETHICS

Walter Glannon

INTRODUCTION

Some of the most innovative and exciting work in contemporary medicine is being done in the clinical neurosciences of psychiatry, neurology, and neurosurgery. Advances in basic and clinical neuroscience during the last 25 years, combined with advances in radiology, have provided new insight into the relation between the human brain and mind. They have also contributed to a better understanding of the differences between normal and abnormal brain activity, as well as to the etiology and progression of diseases of the brain. The significance of these advances is illustrated by the fact psychiatric and neurological disorders affect roughly 400 million people globally. In June 2004, the *Journal of the American Medical Association* published results from the world's largest survey on mental health. From 1–5% of the populations of most countries surveyed have serious mental illness, much of it untreated or undertreated.

From Walter Glannon, "Neuroethics," *Bioethics* 20, no. 1 (2006): 37–52, Blackwell Publishers.

Editors' note: Most author's notes have been cut. Students who want to follow up on sources should consult the original article.

Neuroimaging in the form of computed tomography (CT), positron emission tomography (PET), single photon emission computed tomography (SPECT), magnetic resonance imaging (MRI), and functional magnetic resonance imaging (fMRI) can reveal the neurobiological bases of both normal mental activity and various psychopathologies. Brain scans may detect early signs of neurological and psychiatric disorders well before their characteristic symptoms appear. Psychosurgery can alleviate or even eliminate the symptoms of obsessive-compulsive disorder (OCD), severe depression, and other conditions that are refractory to all other treatments. Electrical and magnetic stimulation of the brain may relieve these symptoms in a noninvasive way. Stimulating electrodes implanted deep in the brain can enable people with motor disorders such as Parkinson's disease to regain some control of their body. Antidepressant and antipsychotic drugs may restore or regenerate neurons and neuronal connections disrupted or destroyed by depression and schizophrenia. It may even be possible to use psychotropic drugs to enhance normal cognition and mood.

But the ability to map, intervene in, and alter the neural correlates of the mind raises important ethical questions. Indeed, these questions are arguably weightier and more momentous than any other set of questions in any other area of bioethics. This is because techniques that target the brain can reveal and modify the source of the mind and affect personal identity, the will, and other aspects of our selves. The mind consists of interrelated cognitive, affective, and conative capacities, which include beliefs, desires, emotions, and volitions that are generated and sustained by the brain. These core features of the philosophy of mind overlap with the ethical notions of benefit and harm, since whether an action benefits or harms one depends on whether and how it affects one's mind. Our identities as persons, our experience of agency, and our first-person phenomenological experience as conscious beings consist in the unity and integrity of our mental states. Mapping or intervening in the brain can reveal and affect the nature and content of our minds and thus who we essentially are.

I will explore some of the ethical issues in five broad areas of clinical neuroscience: diagnostic neuroimaging, predictive neuroimaging, psychosurgery, neurostimulation, and cognitive and affective enhancement. There are other areas of neuroscience that raise additional ethical issues. But I will limit the discussion to the issues that are or will become the most prominent and controversial in this rapidly developing field.

DIAGNOSTIC NEUROIMAGING

The main purpose of CT, PET, SPECT, MRI, and fMRI scans in medicine has been and will continue to be to confirm a diagnosis based on behavioral symptoms and established clinical criteria. As more sophisticated and higher-resolution versions of this technology develop, pharmacological and surgical interventions will more precisely target damaged regions of the brain and thereby enable more effective treatments for neurological and psychiatric disorders. For example, more refined images of glucose metabolism in the prefrontal cortex may help psychiatrists to administer antidepressants that more directly affect serotonergic and noradrenergic receptors in the brain. This could at once relieve depressive symptoms and minimize adverse side effects. The potential therapeutic value of neuroimaging for this and related purposes is obvious. There are other potential uses of diagnostic brain imaging that are more ethically contentious, however.

Suppose that one person kills another in a fit of rage and is charged with second-degree murder. The offender claims that his action resulted from a violent impulse he could not control. He undergoes MRI and PET scans, which show structural damage and abnormal function in the prefrontal cortex of his brain. This brain region is the seat of executive functions regulating decisions and actions and is crucial for rational planning and impulse control. The offender and his defense lawyer argue that the brain damage undermined his capacity for moral reasoning and his ability to control his behavior. To be morally and legally responsible for one's behavior, one must have the capacity to control that behavior. Because the offender lacked this capacity, he could not be responsible for killing his victim and thus should be exonerated. Would this defense be convincing in a court of law? To answer this question, we need to look at empirical studies in brain science and what they indicate about the neurobiological basis of behavior.

Studies conducted by neurologist Antonio Damasio and colleagues have shown that lesions in the orbitofrontal cortex of the brain correlate with impulsive and antisocial behavior. Despite being intellectually unimpaired, individuals with damage to this region seem unable to conform to social and moral norms when they act. Adults and children who sustained this damage presented with a syndrome resembling psychopathy. Similarly, brain-imaging studies by psychologists Adrian Raine and Richard Davidson have also shown that some violent people have diminished activity in the prefrontal region of the brain. At the same time, these individuals have increased activity in the amygdala, the most important region of the limbic system that regulates emotions. Specifically, an overactive amygdala often correlates with heightened negative emotions such as fear and anger. PET and fMRI scans measure the rate of glucose uptake by brain cells. Diminished glucose metabolism is a marker for diminished functioning in regions such as the prefrontal cortex. Heightened glucose metabolism can be a marker for overactive functioning in limbic structures such as the amygdala. The studies by Damasio, Raine, and Davidson suggest that structural and functional abnormalities in the brain regions underlying the mental states leading to actions can undermine one's ability to control these states and actions.

The prefrontal cortex, amygdala, and other interacting brain regions constitute a complex neural circuit that control interacting cognitive and emotional systems. By generating and sustaining these systems, the brain generates and sustains the mind. This model of the mind is monistic rather than dualistic because it conceives of brain and mind as interdependent aspects of a human organism. Cognitive information processing in the prefrontal cortex regulates emotional processing in the limbic system. Emotional processing in the limbic system regulates planning, decision-making, and other cognitive and executive functions in the prefrontal cortex. Each of these brain regions modulates the other in a feedback loop. Normal functioning of these two interdependent systems ensures a healthy balance between cognition and emotion. Damage to either of these regions of the brain can disrupt this balance and cause a person to lose control of his motivational states and actions. Given the damage to his prefrontal cortex, the individual in my hypothetical case presumably would lack control of his emotions and impulses and would not be responsible for his behavior. But in many cases brain dysfunction by itself does not explain violent behavior or prove that a person cannot control his actions and cannot be responsible for them.

In the *Nicomachean Ethics,* Aristotle defends the default assumption that a person acts freely and is morally responsible for his behavior barring evidence of compulsion, coercion, or ignorance of the circumstances of action. The first two of these conditions are metaphysical, or freedom-relevant, while the third condition is epistemological, or knowledge-relevant. A person can be excused from responsibility for his behavior when any of these conditions is present. Impulsive violent behavior correlating with structural or functional brain abnormalities would appear to meet Aristotle's excusing conditions. Yet free will is often not an all-or-nothing capacity. Instead, it is a capacity that comes in degrees along a spectrum of control. At one end of the spectrum, persons are in complete control of their behavior and are completely responsible for what they do. At the other end of the spectrum, persons have no control of their behavior and should be completely excused from responsibility for what they do. Many cases involving violent criminal behavior fall in a gray area between the two extremes. Just as there

are degrees of control of behavior, so too there are degrees of responsibility for behavior.

There are differences between moral and legal responsibility. For example, strict liability has no equivalent in the moral domain. In general, though, both moral and legal conceptions of responsibility presuppose certain mental capacities. The Model Penal Code version of the Not Guilty By Reason of Insanity defense has cognitive and volitional components. According to the first component, a person is not guilty if he suffers from a mental illness causing him to be ignorant of what he is doing. According to the second component, a person is not guilty if he suffers from a mental illness causing him to lose control of his impulses. These same legal conditions apply to judgments about moral responsibility.

The degree of control one has over one's motivational states and actions is obviously influenced by the brain. But it can be influenced by factors in the social and physical environment as well. In addition, some people may put more mental effort than others into exercising the control they have over their behavior. Just because one displays weakness of will does not mean that one lacks free will. Except for cases of severe damage to regions of the brain directly regulating the capacity for moral reasoning and choice, how much control one has over one's behavior, and how responsible one is for it, will not be determined by measuring brain function or dysfunction alone.

Most brain-damaged people are not violent. So it is implausible to claim that structural and functional abnormalities in the brain always cause violent behavior. Nor does brain dysfunction constitute a sufficient reason to excuse people from responsibility for what they do. Perhaps the best illustration of this point is psychopathy. This is a disorder characterized by callousness, diminished capacity for empathy and remorse, and poor behavior controls. Impaired moral reasoning may be due to deficits in emotional processing or in arousal to fear-inducing stimuli. A deficit in the ability to feel remorse and empathy may explain why psychopaths fail to consider the interests of others when they act. A deficit in the ability to experience fear may explain why they act impulsively. In imaging studies similar to those conducted by Damasio, R.J.R. Blair has shown that children with psychopathic tendencies have structural and functional abnormalities in the orbitofrontal cortex and the amygdala. Interestingly, unlike violent individuals, psychopaths tend to have a hypoactive rather than hyperactive amygdala. Nevertheless, psychopaths do not completely lack the capacity to control their impulses. Moreover, although they act without concern for the needs and interests of others, they have some understanding of what it means to harm someone and that other people can be harmed by their actions. On this basis, psychopaths seem to have some control over their behavior and can be at least partly responsible for it. In these and other cases, brain images alone will not enable us to draw a clear distinction between responsibility and excuse.

Another difficulty with brain imaging is that regions other than the orbitofrontal cortex may play a role in cognitive processing. Focusing on this region alone may be an oversimplified way of explaining the link between the brain and behavior. An abnormality in this region does not necessarily mean that the balance between cognitive and emotional processing has been entirely disrupted. The parietal cortex may also play a role in maintaining this balance. Reasoning and executive functions are probably distributed across multiple regions of the cortex. Even the subcortical cerebellum appears to play a role in cognition in addition to regulating motor function. In a deeper sense, scans of the prefrontal cortex or other regions of the brain will not tell us *how* our actions are willed. They cannot explain how actions issue from intentions and decisions. Nor can they explain the phenomenology of free will, or why we *feel* in control (or out of control) of our actions. This is because the relation between the structure and function of the prefrontal cortex and our motivational states and actions is one of correlation rather than causation.

A similar problem besets those who would insist on using brain scans to test for damage to brain systems controlling declarative, or explicit, memory. This consists in the capacity for conscious recollection of specific facts and events. Negligent acts or omissions that result in harm to others may be due to damage or dysfunction in the network involving the hippocampus and neocortex that regulates memory retrieval. But a scan of one brain region will not decisively tell us whether a mother whose child dies from hyperthermia in an overheated car

was unable to remember leaving her in the car because of brain dysfunction, or whether she was able to remember but failed to exercise her capacity to do so. Several regions in the brain regulate the formation, storage, and retrieval of memory. Dysfunction in one region does not necessarily mean that other regions are also dysfunctional. There are redundancies in the brain. Some systems can compensate for others that have been damaged and can perform the same tasks.

The main reason for questioning the use of neuroimaging to make ethical or legal judgments is that it involves a move from empirical claims about the brain to normative claims about how people ought to behave. Free will and responsibility are not primarily empirical but normative notions reflecting social conventions and expectations about how people can or should act. Although our understanding of free will and responsibility is informed to some extent by brain science, normative claims cannot be reduced to empirical ones. This is the principal reason why questions about control and responsibility cannot be answered by appeal to brain imaging alone. What complicates this problem is that brain-based measures of psychological traits have an illusory accuracy and objectivity. An fMRI scan showing anomalous brain function is not necessarily diagnostic, because it can be modulated by the experimental tasks taken to mimic actual functions in the scanner. There is also the potential for bias in the design of functional imaging experiments using brain-damaged patients, which can influence how data from these experiments are analyzed. If this bias can be eliminated, and if brain scans can be perfected, then we may have a more accurate picture of the link between the brain and the mind. This would minimize the risk of abuse of information about the brain. Yet, as American cognitive neuroscientist Martha Farah points out, 'for now, however, this is not the case, and there is the risk that juries, judges, parole boards, the immigration service and so on will weigh such measures too heavily in their decision-making.'[1] Even if functional neuroimaging is perfected, it will not necessarily translate into simple

1. M. Farah. Emerging Ethical Issues in Neuroscience. *Nat Neurosci* 2002; 5: 1127.

answers to normative questions such as when and to what degree people are responsible. These will always be influenced by social norms.

More sophisticated higher-resolution brain scans may enable researchers to identify features of the brain that play an important role in moral reasoning and the execution of intention in action. Moreover, they may enable researchers to distinguish between true and false memory and thus improve the science of lie detection. Ideally, the combination of this technology and established clinical criteria will contribute to a clearer distinction between complete responsibility, on the one hand, and excuse or mitigation, on the other. The information derived from functional neuroimaging will be a helpful tool indeed. But it should supplement, not supplant, existing criteria of responsibility and liability in the criminal justice system. Because it is still an imprecise science, it will be some time before diagnostic brain imaging is or should be used as evidence in criminal law, in the same way that DNA evidence is now used.

More ethically controversial is whether we should intervene in the neural circuitry or biochemistry of people whose structural and functional brain images display abnormalities that strongly correlate with violent behavior. Even if this intervention were done with the best of intentions, surgical manipulation of the brain as a form of forced behavior control would be morally objectionable to most people. Would we think the same way about pharmacological intervention that could restore normal cognitive processing in the prefrontal cortex and normal emotional processing in the amygdala? This would not be as objectionable as psychosurgery because it would not entail permanent modification of the brain. Nor would drug treatment be as invasive. Doses of selective serotonin reuptake inhibitors (SSRIs) might increase serotonin levels in the prefrontal cortex and in turn might decrease aggression by modulating a hyperactive amygdala. What if forced pharmacological intervention could modulate violent impulses and thereby prevent violent actions from being committed? Although they would not be as objectionable as psychosurgery, would there still be reasons against using pharmacological agents for this purpose?

The question is especially contentious in the case of children with severe abnormalities in the prefrontal cortex and no moral sensibility. A bleak future of psychopathy and violence may be written into their neurons. Unless they had structural or functional brain damage that was beyond repair, intervening pharmacologically at an early age to correct or ameliorate brain dysfunction might prevent a lifetime of criminal behavior. The personalities of these individuals would be altered, and they could not give informed consent to this intervention. But would this be morally objectionable if their pathological personalities entailed a high risk of harm to themselves and others? Even if one answered this question affirmatively, the prospect of personality change would have to be weighed against the prevention of harm that could result from the intervention. Philosopher Patricia Smith Churchland's views on this issue are instructive:

> Certainly, some kinds of direct intervention are morally objectionable. So much is easy. But *all* kinds? Even pharmacological? Is it possible that some forms of nervous-system intervention might be more humane than lifelong incarceration or death? I do not wish to propose specific guidelines to allow or disallow any form of direct intervention. Nevertheless, given what we now understand about the role of emotion in reason, perhaps the time has come to give such guidelines a calm and thorough reconsideration.[2]

PREDICTIVE NEUROIMAGING

Diagnostic and predictive brain scans involve very different patient populations. In recently published studies, brain scans of adolescents considered at high risk for schizophrenia showed structural and functional abnormalities in certain regions of their brains. The abnormalities became even more marked once they went on to develop psychotic symptoms and were diagnosed with schizophrenia. These subjects had less gray matter in the frontal and temporal lobes, as well as in the cingulate gyrus. Diminished gray matter in these brain regions is associated with the disrupted cognitive processing symptomatic of schizophrenia. Most significant about this study was that the images predicted this mental disorder before the subjects developed full-blown symptoms. This suggests the possibility of

---

2. Churchland, *op. cit.* note 7, pp. 235–236.

using structural MRI scans to predict later-onset neurological and psychiatric disorders. Schizophrenia is one of the most debilitating of these disorders. Once symptoms of cognitive impairment appear, brain images showing critical neurological markers could enable physicians to administer antipsychotic drugs that could better control the progression of the disease. Early pharmacological intervention might also prevent or delay the onset of psychosis. The earlier this and other mental disorders are treated, the better is their prognosis. This is especially important because of the rapidly changing neural circuitry in adolescents.

Imaging techniques can also show diminished glucose metabolism in the hippocampus. As noted, this is one of the brain regions that regulate memory. These techniques may be developed to the point where they can reveal a loss of cholinergic neurons in this and other brain regions. Brain scans can also display the first signs of amyloid plaques and neurofibrillary tangles. All of these are signature characteristics of Alzheimer's disease, which is by far the most common form of dementia. Significantly, brain scans already may reveal indicators of this disease years before memory loss and other symptoms appear. Neuroimaging may therefore enable neurologists to predict who will develop Alzheimer's. Periodic brain scans can reveal subtle changes in the brains of Alzheimer's patients as the disease progresses over time. The scans can enable neurologists to evaluate and monitor the effects of cholinesterase inhibitors such as donepezil on cholinergic neurons in the hippocampus. This drug can slow memory loss in the early stage of the disease by slowing the progression of atrophy in this region of the brain. Brain scans can also test the efficacy of nonsteroidal anti-inflammatory drugs, which have shown some promise in possibly preventing the neurodegenerative processes associated with Alzheimer's.

The combination of brain imaging and drug therapy can be especially beneficial to people with the mutation on the APOe4 allele of the gene coding for the beta-amyloid precursor protein. They have a high risk of developing Alzheimer's at around age 40. Knowing that there is a strong genetic component to this early-onset form of the disease provides a reason for using brain imaging to detect and monitor its early signs. A smaller number of cholinergic neurons might predict Alzheimer's and warrant

early pharmacological intervention, which might retard the progression of the disease. Similarly, brain scans can be used for adolescents with a high genetic risk of schizophrenia who display subtle cognitive symptoms of the disorder. Scans showing abnormalities in the frontal lobes, temporal lobes, and cingulate gyrus may predict schizophrenia and provide a reason for early pharmacological intervention as well.

It remains unclear which structural or functional brain abnormalities can accurately predict disorders before symptoms appear. Although there may be a correlation between earlier brain abnormalities and later cognitive abnormalities, this is not equivalent to a causal relation between them. Having less gray matter in the brain, for example, by itself does not necessarily mean that one will become psychotic. This can have ethical implications for those suspected of developing schizophrenia. Chronic use of antipsychotic drugs can result in tardive dyskinesia, a movement disorder associated with dopamine-blocking agents. A newer generation of these drugs that was introduced in the 1990s lacks some of these side effects. But like any psychotropic medications, these drugs may have other significant long-term adverse effects. Administering these drugs on predictive rather than definitive diagnostic grounds might mean that an iatrogenic disorder would result from treatment for a possible disorder that never would have developed. The risk of using these drugs must be weighed against the risk of not using them for those who are at high risk of developing schizophrenia.

In the case of Alzheimer's, should predictive neuroimaging be offered for a future neurological illness when no cure is available? The crux of the discussion should be whether such imaging offers benefits to those who undergo it. Currently, there is no clear benefit. Predictive neuroimaging would be beneficial if it led to cholinesterase inhibitor therapy that delayed the onset of Alzheimer's disease. Informing a person that scans of her brain showed early signs of the dread disease may harm her by causing anxiety about her future. This is analogous in many respects to predictive presymptomatic genetic testing for Huntington's disease. Yet knowing early on that one would subsequently develop Alzheimer's could enable one to plan one's future more prudently. Moreover, acetylcholine-boosting drugs might slow the memory loss and cognitive decline associated with this disease. This is more than what a person with predicted Huntington's disease can hope for, since there are presently no drugs that might even retard the progression of its symptoms. Nevertheless, the emotional fallout of information from predictive neuroimaging can be devastating, regardless of the condition in question.

Predictive neuroimaging is still in the experimental stage. Its applications are not yet proven. Clinical trials have been designed where subjects are separated into experimental and control arms. The first group includes people who are considered to have a significant risk of developing one of the disorders I have been discussing. The adolescents with early signs of schizophrenia in the study mentioned at the beginning of this section were in the experimental arm of that study. Risk is determined by family history or by the presence of a known genetic cause. Suppose that some of the controls in one of these trials are healthy but have brain scans showing less gray matter than normal in the prefrontal cortex. As we have seen, this feature of the brain may be a risk factor for developing psychopathology. What should the researcher do with these incidental findings? Should he tell the subjects, or the parents who consented to allow their children to participate in the trial, that their brains indicate a predisposition to psychopathology? Given the possibility that less gray matter may lead to mental illness, is the researcher obligated to disclose this information? Or is he obligated not to inform them, given the uncertainty about what the findings can predict and the likelihood of causing anxiety in the subjects or their parents? If the risk of developing psychopathology is uncertain, then would there be more harm than benefit in informing people of the results of brain scans?

It is crucial that the researcher inform subjects of the aim of a predictive neuroimaging clinical trial, what brain scans might reveal, and the uncertainty about what these findings might suggest for late-onset neurological and psychiatric conditions. The researcher is obligated to do this before the trial begins. Only in this way can subjects give valid informed consent to participate in such a trial. This applies both to those assigned to the experimental group and those assigned to the control group. Even in the best of circumstances, information about clinical trials can easily be misunderstood.

The problem is more acute in predictive neuroimaging because of people's general difficulty in assessing probability and risk, combined with the uncertainty surrounding the medical significance of structural and functional brain abnormalities. Researchers have an obligation to point out to subjects and patients that predictive brain scanning is not an exact science. This can minimize the risk of harm in interpreting the information derived from scans. It can help to prevent distress in individuals who might otherwise think that their brains were not so 'normal' after all.

How a subject interprets information about the brain, or how a researcher presents this information to the subject, are not the only problems with predictive brain scans. Analogous to genetic information indicating a predisposition to a disease, potential insurers or employers may use information from brain scans to discriminate against people seeking employment or medical insurance. With the exception of monogenic diseases, just because one is genetically predisposed to a disease does not mean that one will have that disease. Similarly, just because an asymptomatic individual has some structural or functional brain anomaly does not mean that this individual will develop a neurological or psychiatric illness. Unless there is a known causal connection between a brain scan and subsequent mental illness with a high risk of violent or otherwise harmful behavior, information about the brain should remain confidential and should not be disclosed or made available to third parties. In these days of managed care and the move toward electronic medical records, however, this standard for confidentiality is becoming increasingly difficult to ensure.

Predictive neuroimaging may become a useful tool in locating the first signs of neurological and psychiatric diseases. It could enable earlier pharmacological intervention to prevent or control the progression of these diseases. But what imaging can predict about future medical conditions is fraught with uncertainty and could lead to considerable abuse, discrimination, and harm. Accordingly, these brain scans should be used only to track nervous-system disorders with a known family history or genetic cause. Subjects in the control arm of a predictive imaging clinical trial should have the right to not have information about incidental brain findings disclosed to them. There should be general agreement within the research and clinical community about the medical rationale for and medical significance of these scans. This should reflect what is currently based on evidence, what might be possible, and what should be done in populations at risk. Indeed, whether and how this technology should be used must be framed and discussed as broader social questions. In the words of neuroscientist Joseph LeDoux:

> Such studies force us to confront ethical decisions as a society. How far should we go in using brain imaging to read minds, and how should we use the information we discover? It is testimony to the progress being made that these questions need to be asked.[3]

PSYCHOSURGERY

The Portuguese neurologist Egas Moniz coined the term 'psychosurgery' to describe the procedure of prefrontal leucotomy for the treatment of certain psychoses. The procedure consisted in injecting alcohol into the white matter of the frontal lobes. Moniz received the Nobel Prize for Medicine in 1949 for the 'therapeutic' value of leucotomy. But the most enthusiastic proponent and practitioner of psychosurgery was the American neurologist Walter Freeman, who performed some 3,500 frontal lobotomies in the United States in the 1940s and 1950s. This involved inserting an instrument through the skull just above the eyes and then swinging it back and forth to disconnect white matter tracts in the frontal lobes. Although lobotomies relieved some symptoms of severe psychiatric illnesses, they often resulted in severe neurological and psychological sequelae. These included seizures, significant personality changes, apathy, loss of social control, and in some cases death.

The notorious history of psychosurgery has generated revulsion in some people to the very thought of it. In spite of this, it continues to be practiced as a defensible medical treatment of last resort for OCD and severe depression and anxiety disorders that are refractory to all other treatments. Although it is relatively rare, most forms of psychosurgery are not experimental. More selective MRI-guided stereotactic techniques have improved the safety and efficacy of surgically intervening in the brain and ablating certain circuits or pathways. Nevertheless, the risk of permanent damage to brain circuits, and severe adverse psychological effects of this damage, cannot be ignored. It is precisely for this reason that psychosurgery remains an intervention of last resort.

Cingulotomy has been the surgical procedure of choice to treat severe OCD. A dysfunctional anterior cingulate gyrus has been implicated as the cause of patients' obsession with contamination and compulsion to wash their hands. This procedure may be used experimentally to treat intractable pain as well, since the anterior cingulate plays a role in modulating pain sensation and pain affect. In a cingulotomy, bilateral burr holes are drilled in the skull, and two small holes are then made in the cingulate. The goal is to alter the main pathway between the limbic system and the prefrontal cortex and thereby correct the imbalance between cognitive and emotional processing due to the dysfunctional cingulate. This same procedure has been performed on severely depressed patients as well. Subcaudate tractotomy and limbic leucotomy are similar procedures targeting different regions of the brain. They have been performed to treat severe anxiety disorders. As in cingulotomy, the goal of these procedures is to correct the dysfunctional region or system of the brain in order to restore normal cognitive and emotional functioning. Data from cingulotomies performed over the last 30 years at the Massachusetts General Hospital indicate that 30% of patients experienced significant improvement, while 60% experienced mild to moderate improvement.

Curing or relieving uncontrolled pathological obsessions, compulsions, anxiety and mood through psychosurgery is clearly an important therapeutic achievement. But for the patients who experience significant memory loss or personality change as a result of the procedure, the cure may come at the cost of their identities, their selves. In these metaphysical terms, the cure may seem worse than the disease. Some philosophers and neuroscientists equate personal identity and the self. Others treat them as related but different concepts. For the latter, the self pertains to the first-person phenomenological feel of conscious experience. Identity is a unity relation pertaining to the connectedness and continuity of

3. J. LeDoux, 2002. *The Synaptic Self: How Our Brains Become Who We Are.* New York: Viking: 221.

mental states over time. Core features of the self may be altered by neurological and psychiatric illness. Or they may be altered by psychosurgery to control or cure these illnesses. This alteration could occur if the surgery damaged the somatosensory system in the brain, which regulates one's orientation in space, or the temporal lobe, which regulates one's orientation in time. These changes would not necessarily undermine personal identity. Yet if the connections between memory of past experience and anticipation of future experience were severed as a result of surgical intervention in the brain, then the unity of these mental states over time would also be severed. The person after the surgery intuitively would be different from the person before the surgery. A good example of this is severe retrograde amnesia resulting from damage to the hippocampus and the temporal lobe. The loss of episodic memory can disrupt the psychological continuity that extends from the past to the present.

Some patients who have undergone unilateral temporal lobotomy to control the seizures in severe epilepsy have exhibited impaired fear conditioning after the surgery. This is due to damage to the amygdala, which regulates fear and other emotions. Excessive fear is often a symptom of depression and anxiety disorders. Antidepressant medication and psychotherapy are means of enabling patients to restore a balance between too much and too little fear. Brain surgery resulting in the loss of the capacity to fear can be more harmful to a patient than excessive fear. This capacity is necessary for survival, and losing it can make one unable to recognize and protect oneself from real threats. Despite the possibility of these serious side effects, when a neuropsychiatric disorder is so severe that it interferes with a person's ability to have a normal life, the potential benefits of psychosurgery appear to outweigh the risks. Yet it is because these risks may have significant medical, ethical, and metaphysical implications that psychosurgery is justified only to treat severe conditions.

Whether valid informed consent can be obtained from patients undergoing these procedures is another ethically contentious question. Although the fact that certain conditions do not respond to any other treatments would seem to justify psychosurgery, patients may agree to undergo such a procedure out of a desperate desire for relief from their symptoms. This desperation may impair their ability to rationally weigh the benefits against the risks. To be sure, there are other conditions in which patients have a desperate desire for relief from symptoms. What is distinctive about psychosurgery is that the dysfunctional region of the brain that is the target of the intervention is often the cause of the patient's impaired competence or incompetence. This suggests that there should be a higher threshold of consent for psychosurgery than for most, if not all, other procedures. Another reason for a higher threshold of consent for psychosurgery is that the procedure could have significant and permanent adverse effects on personality.

For these reasons, a careful psychological evaluation of the patient must be part of the selection of candidates for surgery. A family member or other person who knows the patient well should be part of the consent process, together with the patient. The problem of consent is especially acute in cases of severe depression, where the patient may have little or no capacity to consent. An appropriately designated surrogate acting in the best interests of the patient can consent to the treatment on the patient's behalf. This can be justified when the patient poses a significant risk of harm to himself or others. Proxy consent might also be justified when there is no risk of suicide or harm to others, but when the patient's quality of life is so poor that the potential benefit of surgery to the patient clearly outweighs the risk. This would apply to depression, anxiety, or OCD. Similar justification could be given for proxy consent on behalf of patients with brain tumors causing significant cognitive or affective impairment. Even in these cases, though, the potential neurological and psychological side effects of psychosurgery require that consent be a sustained deliberative process involving the neurosurgeon, the supporting medical team, the patient, and the surrogate.

Proxy consent for psychosurgery should be held to a higher standard than proxy consent for other procedures. In the light of the risk of serious changes to thought and behavior from psychosurgery, a group of neurosurgeons in Scotland recently formulated and defended 'a policy of not offering ablative neurosurgery for mental disorders to anyone who is incapable of providing sustained, informed consent'. Yet if a patient's condition is severe, does not respond to any other therapy, and the potential benefit of psychosurgery outweighs the potential harm, then proxy consent for this procedure can be justified. The requirement of consent would rule out forced psychosurgery even for therapeutic reasons.

NEUROSTIMULATION

Neurostimulation can be a medically and ethically preferable alternative to the brain lesioning in psychosurgery. This form of brain intervention is in its early stages and is still experimental. Neurostimulation often involves stimulating a dysfunctional area of the brain using implanted electrodes connected to a battery. Because the electrodes are usually implanted in subcortical regions deep in the brain, it has also been described as 'deep-brain stimulation' (DBS). This procedure has helped to restore coordinated movement in patients affected by the rigidity or tremors of Parkinson's disease. The same technology could also be used to prevent or treat epilepsy by inhibiting hyperactive neural circuits causing the seizures that are symptomatic of the disorder. A device implanted in the brain could automatically release a very low dose of an anti-epilepsy drug or deliver an electrical signal that could block seizures. In 2002, an ethics commission in France approved clinical trials using neurostimulation for OCD. In contrast to the lesioning in psychosurgery, neurostimulation has the advantage of being reversible. The electrodes can be removed and patients can control the function of the electrodes by switching them on or off. This also makes it easier to justify conducting blind controlled clinical trials and to obtain informed consent from research subjects.

Still, implantation and stimulation of electrodes in the brain must be precise. Implanting or stimulating one millimeter off target may cause unforeseeable adverse neurological sequelae. In these instances, a patient could develop seizures. Or the patient's emotional processing could be affected, causing the patient to become emotionally flat or even suicidal. Even when the target area is stimulated as intended, activating one brain circuit in isolation from other circuits that play a role in movement could adversely affect the patient's capacity for motor control. This could defeat the purpose for which the technique was designed. Accordingly, the commission overseeing the OCD study in France set strict experimental conditions for it. This included careful selection of subjects

(only those whose OCD was refractory to all other treatments), obtaining informed consent, and evaluation of results. Belgian neurosurgeon Bart Nuttin and colleagues drafted and published general ethical guidelines for the use of deep—brain stimulation to treat psychiatric illness in August 2002.[4]

Neurostimulation can be expanded to treat severe depression and anxiety disorders. In patients who fail to respond to antidepressant medication, stimulating the prefrontal cortex may help to modulate a hyperactive amygdala and restore the balance between cognitive and emotional processing. One recent study has shown that DBS modulated elevated activity in the subgenual cingulate region and produced some benefit in six patients with refractory depression. DBS can function as a 'pacemaker' for the brain in treating motor and mood disorders. The behavioral symptoms of affective and anxiety disorders are more subtle than those of Parkinson's or OCD, however. This complicates drawing a direct link between brain stimulation and behavior. Locating the organic cause or causes of mood and anxiety disorders is also more complicated. This is because the etiology of these disorders may include psychological factors such as beliefs and emotions that have a widely distributed neurological underpinning. These mental states may also be influenced by factors in the physical and social environment. So the efficacy of DBS as a treatment for a broad range of neurological and psychiatric disorders may be limited.

Electroconvulsive Therapy (ECT), Transcranial Magnetic Stimulation (TMS), and Vagus Nerve Stimulation (VNS) may seem more attractive as treatments for severe depression and other psychiatric disorders because they avoid surgical intervention in the brain altogether. In ECT, electrodes are applied to the head, and a series of electric shocks are delivered to the brain to induce seizures. The technique appears to restore the proper balance of neurotransmitters and neuronal connections in the pathway between the prefrontal cortex and limbic system. TMS also aims at restoring the cortical-limbic balance. It involves delivering a localized magnetic

4. B. Nuttin et al. Ethical Guidelines for Deep-Brain Stimulation. *Neurosurgery* 2002; 51: 519

pulse to the brain through the scalp by application of hand-held coils. VNS has been used to treat epilepsy, as well as severe depression and bipolar disorder. It involves stimulating the left vagus nerve in the neck with a series of electrical pulses. These pulses travel through a surgically implanted wire attached to a pulse generator in the chest. The vagus nerve has connections to the limbic structures and the thalamus, which play an important role in regulating affective states.

The fundamental problem with these techniques, as with the other techniques I have discussed, is that their long-term effects are not known. Despite being less invasive, ECT, TMS, and VNS may prove to be no more medically or ethically acceptable than the other procedures. ECT has been known to result in significant memory loss in some patients. TMS can excite only the cortex because the strength of the magnetic field falls off sharply beyond the distance of only a few centimeters. Yet dysfunction of both cortical and subcortical regions of the brain has been implicated in most psychiatric disorders. Also, the effects of TMS may be of only short duration. Clinical trials aiming to increase the depth and duration of TMS to treat depression are under way in the United States, though it remains to be seen whether these trials will achieve the desired effects. Like internal and external electrical stimulation, external magnetic stimulation of the brain may adversely affect circuits other than those targeted by the procedure. Neural stimulation can either excite or inhibit neurons. Some of these techniques involve both excitation of some neurons and inhibition of others. This can make it difficult to control the effects of stimulation. These effects also depend on the frequency used and on which areas of the brain are stimulated.

This does not mean that TMS and other procedures should be banned. Rather, more long-term studies are needed to adequately assess their benefits and risks. Given the uncertainty about the effects of these techniques, the same strict experimental conditions should be applied to all forms of neurostimulation, regardless of the degree of invasiveness. In addition, informed consent from patients or subjects, or from appropriate surrogates, must be obtained. This requires that the researcher explain the potential benefits and risks of these techniques and point out the uncertainty about these benefits

and risks. Finally, the medical uncertainty of these experiments indicates that they are ethically justifiable only when the neuropsychiatric conditions they are designed to treat are refractory to pharmacological or other proven treatments.

COGNITIVE AND AFFECTIVE ENHANCEMENT

Unlike techniques designed to monitor or treat neurological and psychiatric disorders, some drugs are being used to enhance normal cognition and mood. Perhaps the most intriguing of these drugs is modafinil. This drug was approved for the treatment of narcolepsy in 1998 and is now prescribed to treat sleep apnea and shift-work sleep disorder. All of these conditions are caused by dysregulated circadian rhythm/sleep-wake cycles in the central nervous system. Studies have shown that modafinil reduces daytime sleepiness among shift workers, reducing the incidence of motor vehicle accidents caused by people who otherwise would have fallen asleep at the wheel.

The benefits of modafinil are clear. But this drug is also being used to promote alertness in people with regular sleep-wake cycles. In fact, roughly 90% of prescriptions for the drug are for this and other off-label uses. Those taking the drug could have prolonged periods of alertness and could function at a sustained high cognitive level on much less sleep than is considered normal. Experiments involving B-2 Bomber and commercial airline pilots on transcontinental flights have shown that modafinil can keep them alert and engaged in mental activities despite sleep deprivation. In some respects, modafinil would function like methylphenidate (Ritalin) and other stimulants that can improve people's cognitive capacity for focusing attention on specific tasks. Would there be any medical or ethical reason to object to the use of this drug for cognitive enhancement?

Researchers believe that modafinil does not produce the hyperactive and addictive effects of stimulants like amphetamines and cocaine because of its selectivity in targeting the dopamine pathway that controls wakefulness and blocking the hypothalamus from promoting sleep. Yet sleep plays an important role in maintaining neural plasticity. Limiting sleep through pharmacological means could impair the brain's ability to adapt to changing environments or to adjust to injury. Moreover, people who are chronically sleep-deprived generally are at greater risk of hypertension, as well as metabolic disorders such as obesity and diabetes. More recent studies suggest that sleep is important for consolidation of newly acquired memories. Constant manipulation of the natural alertness system could have harmful consequences. The main issue with modafinil and other alertness-enhancing drugs is that their exact biochemical mechanisms and long-term effects are not known. Chronic use of these drugs could remodel synapses, alter neural circuits, and result in permanent changes in the brain. A sufficient number of longitudinal studies are needed to ascertain these effects and determine whether the benefits of the drugs outweigh the risks.

Another form of psychopharmacological enhancement involves drugs that would increase memory storage and expedite memory retrieval. These drugs most likely would target working memory, which enables us to perform cognitive tasks and executive functions like reasoning and decision-making. Working memory can be described as a short-term form of declarative memory. Declarative memory consists of semantic memory, which involves the ability to consciously recall concepts, facts, and numbers, and episodic memory, which involves the ability to consciously recall events. Declarative memory is distinct from procedural memory, which enables us to unconsciously perform such skills as riding a bicycle or driving a car. The prefrontal cortex regulates working memory. Drugs that are already under development aim to increase memory storage by acting on the transcription factor cyclic AMP (cAMP) and the protein it modulates, CREB (cyclic AMP response element binding protein). This protein is responsible for switching on and off the genes involved in memory formation and storage. Memory-enhancing 'smart drugs' would increase the supply of CREB inside neurons and thereby strengthen memory consolidation.

It is not clear that increasing the brain's ability to store memories would not impair its ability to retrieve these memories. This point is motivated by an evolutionary interpretation of memory. The limits we have in our capacity to remember only so many facts or events may be part of a natural design that is critical for our survival. Ideally, we would want to use drugs that both increased memory formation and storage and made memory retrieval

more efficient. But increased storage would not necessarily mean quicker retrieval. More facts stored in the brain might result in an overloaded working memory, which could impair the ability to execute cognitive tasks. It might also impair our ability to learn new things, which depends on a certain degree of forgetting.

These considerations suggest that there may be an optimal amount of CREB in our brains for memory. Too much CREB could result in an overproduction and oversupply of memory, which could result in our brains and minds becoming cluttered with memories of facts or events that served no purpose. If there is an optimal balance between remembering and forgetting, then it seems plausible to hypothesize that increased semantic memory storage and decreased forgetting could result in impaired semantic memory retrieval, as well as impaired ability to learn new things. Farah supports this point:

> We understand very little about the design constraints that were being satisfied in the process of creating a human brain. Therefore, we don't know which 'limitations' are there for a good reason . . . normal forgetting rates seem to be optimal for information retrieval.[5]

Farah further warns of 'hidden costs' of trying to enhance memory, and that evolutionary considerations should make us wary of the prospect of general cognitive enhancement as a 'free lunch'. We should be wary of making the inference that, if a certain amount of memory is good, then more memory is better.

There may be important social implications of drugs that enhanced alertness, attention, memory, or other cognitive capacities. Some might argue that cognitive enhancement should aim to reduce unfairness, but without eliminating beneficial options. The cognitive capacities that constitute intelligence are a competitive good that can give some people an advantage over others in gaining employment, income, wealth, and a higher level of wellbeing. If we could ensure universal access to drugs that enhanced cognitive capacities and intelligence, then

---

5. M. Farah. Emerging Ethical Issues in Neuroscience. *Nat Neurosci* 2002; 5: 1125. Also M. Farah et al. Neurocognitive Enhancement: What Can We Do and What Should We Do? *Nat Rev Neurosci* 2004; 5: 421–425.

presumably this would reduce social inequality and unfairness. It would give everyone an equal opportunity for access to the education and employment that would guarantee a moderate to high level of wellbeing for everyone. But this would not necessarily follow. Equal access to a competitive good, or to the means that would facilitate such access, would not imply equal outcomes from the use of these means.

Differing parental attitudes to competitive goods such as an elite education and lucrative jobs could mean substantial differences between children regarding how enhancement drugs would be utilized. Some parents would be more selective than others in sending their children to better schools or in arranging for private tutors. In these respects, equality in access to cognitive enhancement would not imply equality of achievement among children, adolescents, and adults. Furthermore, some adolescents and adults would use cognitive enhancement drugs to engage in trivial or even pathological tasks, such as gambling. Not everyone would use these drugs in a beneficial way. There would be inequality of outcomes of cognitive enhancement with respect to the competitive goods at issue. Any beneficial options of enhancement would probably come on top of existing social inequality and would more likely exacerbate than ameliorate it.

Cognitive enhancement must be distinguished from mood enhancement. The latter has been associated with exaggerated claims that many people use SSRIs to overcome shyness or to create a general feeling of wellbeing. These claims are due in part to Peter Kramer's popular 1993 book *Listening to Prozac,* which includes some discussion of using SSRIs such as Prozac to boost self-confidence and self-esteem. But this view makes light of the fact that the majority of the people who take these drugs do so because of the debilitating affective, cognitive, and physical symptoms of major depression.[6] The aim of these drugs is not to make people feel better about themselves, but to restore them to normal levels of mental and physical functioning. Some people may take these drugs to enhance mood; but most

do not. In fact, for those whose effective symptoms fail to meet criteria of major clinical depression, the positive effects of these drugs are minimal. American psychiatrist Greg Sullivan explains:

> If someone is pleased with the effects of an SSRI, that usually is an indication that the drug has had a significant impact on serious symptoms, including those caused by a chronic low-level depression (dysthymia) . . . But SSRIs are not 'happy pills', and people without significant mood or physical dysfunction do not generally get much benefit from them, certainly nothing that would make them sustain their use.[7]

Even if the risks of using psychopharmacology to enhance cognition or mood were minimal, the potential of these drugs to alter personality raises a metaphysical question. If one's cognitive ability or emotional capacity changed substantially, then would one retain one's identity and remain the same person, the same self? Or would one become a different person or self? If one's psychological connectedness and continuity were disrupted by these changes, then it is unclear *who* would have benefited from the drug intervention. The change could preclude a comparison of two states of affairs in which the same person existed, which would be necessary for there to be any benefit for that person. All of the issues raised in this section indicate the need for broad public discussion of the rationale for psychopharmacological enhancement. They also indicate the need for studies to determine the safety and efficacy of these interventions.

CONCLUSION

As brain imaging, psychosurgery, neurostimulation, and psychopharmacology become more refined and more available, researchers will become more able to map and modify the neural basis of the human mind and behavior. This will enable doctors to more accurately predict, prevent, diagnose, and treat neurological and psychiatric disorders. But the brain is by far the most complex and least understood organ in the human body. We still do not know precisely

---

6. Kramer's *Against Depression* is in many respects a sobering antidote to his earlier book. Peter Kramer. 2005. *Against Depression.* New York: Viking.

---

7. Cited in LeDoux, *op. cit.* note 3, p. 276.

how all of the different systems of the brain interact, or what a particular brain abnormality can predict about future psychopathology. Nor do we know precisely how intervening in these systems can affect the beliefs, desires, intentions, and emotions that constitute the human mind. The measures and interventions I have discussed have the potential to affect our minds and alter who we are in both positive and negative ways. Thus we need to carefully weigh the potential benefits against the potential harms of the different measures and interventions in clinical neuroscience.

Neuroscience is perhaps the fastest growing and most exciting area of medicine and biotechnology. Although it is in some respects still an emerging field, in other respects it is already being practiced in clinical and experimental settings. The ethical issues emerging from clinical neuroscience are as significant as those associated with stem-cell research, genetic testing, or any other area of bioethics. Acknowledging the differences between actual and possible applications of these techniques, we need to appreciate the dilemmas that already exist and those that will arise in the future. It is because neuroscience is developing at such a rapid pace and can affect us so directly and deeply that we should now be paying attention to and debating the important ethical issues arising from it.

ENHANCEMENT

GROWTH HORMONE THERAPY FOR THE DISABILITY OF SHORT STATURE

David B. Allen

INTRODUCTION AND CONCEPTUAL GUIDELINES

Limited availability of human growth hormone (GH) once provided a barrier to expanding its use beyond children who were unequivocally GH deficient (GHD). By necessity, strict arbitrary criteria were established to identify classic GHD children entitled to GH. Today, increased availability of recombinant DNA-derived GH has allowed investigation of its growth-promoting effect in short children who do not fit traditional definitions of GHD. Increased supply has created increased demand:

From *Access to Treatment With Human Growth Hormone: Medical, Ethical, and Social Issues.* Supplement to *Growth, Genetics, and Hormones* 8 (Suppl. 1, May 1992): 70–73. Reprinted with permission of the author and publisher.

Editors' note: All author's notes have been cut. Students who want to follow up on sources should consult the original article.

more than twice as many children received GH therapy in 1989 and 1990 than in 1985 and 1986 at an average annual cost per child of $10,000.

Advantages conferred by increased height in social, economic, professional, and political realms of Western society are well-documented. Stigmatization and discrimination are shared by *all* extremely short children, whether GHD or not. *If* GH is shown to have growth-promoting effects in non-GHD children and *if* treatment of such children can be accomplished without toxicity, then what ethical criteria should determine entitlement to long-term, invasive, and (currently) expensive therapy? Would it be justified to restrict access to GH based on the diagnosis of GHD? And whatever the indication for GH therapy, to what attained height should GH therapy be considered an entitlement?

Answering these questions requires rethinking of the medical indications for GH therapy. Toward the goal of achieving both controlled but fair access to GH, the following conceptual guidelines are proposed: (1) GH be viewed as a treatment for the disability of short stature (SS) and not for the diagnosis of GHD; (2) GH-responsiveness, not GHD, be the central criterion for GH treatment; and (3) entitlement to (and reimbursement for) GH therapy be guided by the degree of disability and the degree of GH-responsiveness rather than by a child's diagnosis.

THE CONTINUUM OF GROWTH HORMONE SECRETION: DISEASE, POTENTIAL, AND HANDICAP

The once clear boundary between GHD and GH sufficiency has become blurred. Traditional criteria for the diagnosis of GHD do not identify all children who are GH-responsive. A continuum of "inadequate" GH secretion likely spans classic and partially GHD children, children with delayed growth and puberty, and other poorly growing short children who pass provocative tests but still secrete less GH than their peers. Furthermore, GH *augmentation* therapy in short children with no detectable abnormalities of GH secretion increases growth velocity and, if given for sufficient time prior to puberty, may increase eventual adult height.

Arguments emphasizing proven GHD as the primary criterion for GH therapy are often rooted in notions of disease, handicap, or potential. The treatment of disease, "an abnormal condition of an organism that impairs normal physiologic functioning" (*American Heritage Dictionary*, 1985), is one function of medicine. One might argue that GH therapy be confined to those with the "disease" of GHD. Restoration of hormonal equilibrium by supplementing deficient or suppressing excessive levels of hormones is a justifiable, time-honored principle in endocrinology. The GHD child is viewed as more entitled to therapy because something has been taken away that needs to be restored. The American Academy of Pediatrics statement recommending GH therapy only for GHD children concludes with the old adage, "If it ain't broke, don't fix it." But what exactly is "broke" when it comes to SS and GH therapy? This view ignores both the likely, though yet unrecognized, physiologic "defects" that lead to genetic SS and its accompanying psychosocial impairment. Both GHD and non-GHD short children, if they have a disease at all, have the disease of SS.

If the legitimate function of medicine includes the alleviation of handicap, "a disadvantage or deficiency, especially a physical or mental disability that prevents or restricts normal achievement," then the short child's well-being is viewed in the context of his or her interaction with the environment. GH therapy is justified by recognition that extreme SS interferes with normal activities such as driving a car and reaching shelves, as well as competition for jobs, schools, incomes, and mates. After all, preventing handicapping SS is the primary impetus for treating GHD children. Other beneficial physiologic effects occur with GH therapy, but these are of secondary importance. Growth rate and final adult height are the measures by which we judge therapeutic success. Whether burdens associated with SS of a given degree qualify for designation as a handicap is not the central question. The point is that short children of equal height have the same handicap regardless of the cause.

The concept of potential is also invoked to distinguish treatment of GHD and non-GHD children. For some, a GHD child with parents of normal height is "meant," by virtue of genetic endowment, to be taller than the child with familial SS. He or she is entitled to treatment with GH until a height appropriate for the genetic endowment is attained. GH supplementation of the familial short child who appears to be GH-sufficient is "tampering with nature" and outside the proper province of medicine. But this analysis fails, since both children (given an equal height prognosis) are equally unlucky, one by virtue of having GHD and the other by virtue of having short parents. For both, attaining maximum adult height requires "tampering with nature" by providing exogenous GH.

EQUITABLE RESTRICTION OF GROWTH HORMONE THERAPY

While concepts of disease, handicap, and potential do not distinguish GHD from GH-responsive children with regard to entitlement to GH therapy, it does not follow that *all* GH-responsive short children are entitled to therapy. Resolving that question requires consideration of balancing benefits and risks and asking further questions about allocation of health-care resources.

Response to GH is not an "all or none" phenomenon. GHD children are likely to be *more* responsive than non-GHD children, justifying their preferential treatment as a class. Possible GH toxicity in non-GHD children, while apparently rare, still requires further study. Risks of psychosocial stigmatization also require careful consideration; short, otherwise normal children exposed to injections to promote growth may conclude (with some accuracy) that their bodies are unacceptable in the eyes of their parents and physicians. Statistically significant increments in final adult height may not actually improve psychosocial adaptation, failing a primary objective of GH therapy. Finally, unrestricted access to GH would shift the bell-shaped curve of height upward without changing the handicap for those at the lower percentiles in competing for social, professional, and athletic status.

Assuming that clinical trials of GH in non-GHD children show efficacy with acceptable risk, how might access to GH therapy be equitably restricted? First, the goals in treating SS must be clarified. If the goal is to achieve each child's maximum height potential, GH therapy would (ethically) need to be offered to any potentially responsive short child. Providing GH therapy only to those with documented GHD and treating them until maximal adult stature is reached would be unfair to equally short, non-GHD children who could grow with GH supplementation. On the other hand, if the goal is to alleviate the disability of extreme SS (from any cause), GH-responsive short children should have equal access to treatment until they reach a height no longer considered a handicap.

This latter goal, bringing short children into the normal opportunity range for height, coincides with society's duty to provide basic needs to its citizens. There is no duty to provide the *very best* opportunity for all, and an insistence on equal access to GH by those who have already achieved a normal final height compromises this goal. To improve opportunities for those truly disabled by height, GH must be selectively available to them. The challenge is to define this group, and to apply criteria of disability consistently in deciding when to commence and when to *discontinue therapy*. The diagnosis of GHD should not be rewarded with unlimited access to GH while access is denied to equally handicapped non-GHD but potentially GH-responsive children.

TOWARD RESPONSIBLE USE OF GROWTH HORMONE

Any definition of "handicapping height" would be arbitrary, but the difficulty in defining boundaries precisely should not be an obstacle to making distinctions. Decisions about treatment are always based on probability, not certainty. While current methods for height prediction remain suboptimal, *some* determination of a height considered a handicap needs to be made if GH allocation in the future is to be both controlled and fair.

Emphasizing degree of disability and GH-responsiveness as selection criteria for therapy equitably fulfills reasonable goals of growth-promoting therapy. Children disadvantaged by stature, regardless of pathogenesis, would be brought closer to or within the normal opportunity range for height. The attainment of maximum height potential would not be a valid treatment goal, and the use of GH to make normal-statured children taller would be opposed. The normal range of height would not be altered, but rather the disparity between percentiles—for example, between the 0.1th and 1st percentiles would be lessened. By restricting GH therapy to those seeking only to achieve the normal opportunity range for height, we would not exploit the perception that taller is better.

Widespread distribution of GH has been deterred in part by high drug prices and concern about toxicity. Assuming efficacy of GH in increasing final adult height, the relevant question is not how much should be spent on GHD versus non-GHD children but rather how should health-care resources be responsibly and fairly expended on the treatment of SS in general. Resources for this endeavor may in fact be limited, but treatment of severely SS individuals can still be approached with *consistency*. If our goal is to help (all) children attain a height closer to the normal opportunity range, the cause of the SS really should not matter. The central question about allocation of GH is this: To what maximum height should any GH-treated child be entitled to receive private or public support?

Moreover, the crisis in GH allocation will expand not with its failures but with its successes, and not as the cost of therapy rises but as it falls. These impediments, which may be resolved soon, have distracted attention from the issue of responsible use of GH. What we can do with GH therapy is not necessarily what we *should* do. We who prescribe GH should now ask how we would respond if families who do not require insurance reimbursement strongly request GH therapy. Without guidelines for restriction based arbitrarily on likely final adult height, access to treatment would increasingly reflect ability to pay, providing yet another societal advantage to those already well-off. Rather, a consistent goal of growth-promoting therapy should be to lessen the burden for those who are so short as to be handicapped; that is, to provide GH therapy to those disabled by height only until a height within the normal opportunity range is attained. Consideration of degree of disability, rather than diagnosis, both when commencing and when discontinuing

GH therapy, will most responsibly contain an expanding cohort of candidates for GH treatment.

The physician's duty to respond to the needs of each child does not necessarily extend to parental aspirations or hopes for the child. In an era of plentiful GH, child advocacy requires consideration of the needs of all children, bringing as many as possible into the normal opportunity range of height without deliberately trying to make some taller than others. The paradox of GH therapy is that no policy regarding its use will ever eliminate the 1st percentile. GH cannot replace parental love and nurturing of a child, regardless of the child's height. Prudent use of GH will recognize these limitations, encouraging physicians to respond to concerns about SS more often with counseling than with injections.

THE GENOME PROJECT, INDIVIDUAL DIFFERENCES, AND JUST HEALTH CARE

Norman Daniels

The mapping of the human genome is likely to have important implications for the just distribution of health care services. Some of these implications will be the result of the new medical technologies that will be developed once we learn more about the human genome. Despite their likely importance, I will not speculate about them in what follows, nor will I comment on the way they add to the burden we already have in deciding how to disseminate and ration new technologies under conditions of resource scarcity. Instead, I want to focus on the fact that the mapping of the genome will give us

From *Justice and the Human Genome Project*, edited by Timothy F. Murphy and Marc A. Lappé. Berkeley: University of California Press, 1994. Copyright © 1994 University of California Press. Edited and reprinted with permission.

Editors' note: Some text and author's notes have been cut. Students who want to read the article in its entirety should consult the original.

specific, new *information about individual variation.* This information can be used in good and bad, fair and unfair ways, and it raises, or rather refocuses, important questions about how we should distribute health care resources. . . .

. . . [C]an we defend the distinction between medical therapies that *treat* and those that *enhance* in the face of new genetic information that allows us to pinpoint the genetic contributors to traits we want to alter? Imagine, for example, that we will come to identify particular genes or patterns of genes that contribute to making people very short. (I say "imagine" advisedly, since all interesting traits are highly heterogeneous; in what follows, we indulge in some of the fanciful expectations advanced by human genome proponents.) These genes do not represent pathology of the usual sort; for example, they do not lead to growth hormone deficiency. But being able to look at the microstructure underlying the "normal" distribution of height may produce strong pressures to identify a new class of "bad genes" and to suggest that people who have those genes now have a claim on others to assist them in changing their traits. These questions thus have vast implications for resource allocation. . . . [T]hey also take us deep into political philosophy. What we are really asking is which inequalities among people give rise to claims on others and which are matters of individual responsibility. . . .

CAN WE RETAIN THE TREATMENT VERSUS ENHANCEMENT DISTINCTION?

We have social obligations to treat disease and disability because of their impact on opportunity, and so we should not accept the barriers to access that follow from standard underwriting practices. Are these obligations limited to treating disease and disability? Or does any condition that creates an inequality in opportunity for welfare or advantage among individuals give rise to claims on others? In rejecting the argument from actuarial fairness, we countered an attack from the right on our social obligations to treat disease and disability. I want to consider now an attack from the left on the way I have formulated these obligations. The attack rests on the view that our egalitarian concerns require us to eliminate inequalities among people that arise from many conditions other than disease and disability. In effect, it is a demand for a more radical version of equality of opportunity. In the context of health care, the attack takes the form of a challenge to the distinction between treatment and enhancement.

I suggested earlier that the genome project may provide us with information that will erode the distinction we often draw between uses of medical technology for treatment of disease and disability and uses that enhance human appearance or performance. This distinction is closely connected to the frequently used, but poorly understood, concept of "medical necessity." Many public and private insurance schemes in the United States (and Canada) claim to provide only medically necessary services: many services that involve only enhancement (such as "cosmetic" surgery) are thus excluded from coverage on these grounds. I shall suggest in what follows that the treatment versus enhancement distinction does have a moral justification, at least

relative to a *standard* way of thinking about equality of opportunity. The genetic information about human variation provided by the genome project may make that distinction seem more arbitrary, and to the extent that it does, it poses a challenge to the standard model and the use to which I have put it in thinking about justice and health care. Of course, this is not a conceptually novel threat; viewed from the perspective of the attack from the left, the distinction and the standard model it depends on already seem arbitrary. But the new information may heighten the appearance of moral arbitrariness, and that is the reason for discussing the issue here.

Many medical technologies, new and old, can alter people in ways they desire to be changed. When do we have a social obligation to ensure that such preferences are met? Do rights to health care include entitlements to have those preferences met, resources permitting? What should insurance cover?

The most inclusive answer to these questions would be that we have such obligations whenever someone desires to eliminate an unwanted physical or mental condition. This would allow "subjective" preferences to place enormous demands on resources, making everyone hostage to the extravagant tastes of everyone else. Since we generally do not believe it is medicine's task to make everyone equally happy, we reject this view and its implication that we should have to pay for liposuction or face lifts. Instead, we think obligations arise only when medical treatments address more important problems. The stance we thus take about medicine is compatible with rejecting, as Rawls and Dworkin do, a broad form of egalitarianism that would require us to ensure the equal welfare or happiness of all individuals.

A less inclusive answer would be that we have obligations to provide medical care whenever people desire to eliminate conditions that put them at some disadvantage. The notion of disadvantage is meant to be objective, including some forms of suffering as well as the competitive disadvantages that result from the lack of capabilities, such as marketable talents or skills. This view has some initial moral appeal when the disadvantages are not our fault or the (even unlucky) result of our prior choices. Our egalitarian inclinations may incline us to think we owe something toward eliminating them. If we adopt such a radical view—the left position I referred to earlier—we may have to assign medicine a much greater role as a social equalizer than we now assign it. At least currently, it is not medicine's task to make everyone an equal competitor, wherever possible eliminating all inequalities in the distribution of talents and skills or other capabilities.

A more modest answer, one that tends to match a wide range of our practices, including our insurance practices, is that we have obligations to provide services whenever someone desires that a medical *need* be met. Generally, this is taken to mean that the service involves *treatment of a disease or disability,* where disease and disability are seen as departures from species-typical normal functional organization or functioning. Characterizing medical need in this way implies a contrast between uses of medical services that *treat* disease (or disability) conditions and uses that merely *enhance* human performance or appearance. Enhancement does not meet a medical need even where the service may correct for a competitive disadvantage that does not result from prior choices. Accordingly, medicine has the role of making people *normal* competitors, not *equal* competitors; this role fits, I shall claim, with the standard model for thinking about equality of opportunity.

Despite its wide appeal, the distinction between treatment and enhancement may seem arbitrary in light of hard cases such as these:

> Johnny is a short 11-year-old boy with documented GH [growth hormone] deficiency resulting from a brain tumor. His parents are of average height. His predicted adult height without GH treatment is approximately 160 cm (5 feet 3 inches).
>
> Billy is a short 11-year-old boy with normal GH secretion according to current testing methods. However, his parents are extremely short, and he has a predicted adult height of 160 cm (5 feet 3 inches).[1]

These cases make the distinction seem arbitrary for several reasons. First, Johnny and Billy will suffer disadvantage equally if they are not treated. There is no reason to think the difference in the underlying causes of their shortness will lead people to treat them in ways that make one happier or more advantaged than the other. Second, although Johnny is short because of dysfunction whereas Billy is short because of his (normal) genotype, both are short through no choice or fault of their own. The shortness is in both cases the result of a biological "natural

lottery." Both thus seem to suffer undeserved disadvantages. Third, Billy's preference for greater height, just like Johnny's, is a preference that most people hold; it is not peculiar, idiosyncratic, or extravagant. Indeed, it is a response to a social prejudice, "heightism." The prejudice is what we should condemn, not the fact that they both form an "expensive taste" in reaction to it.

Cases such as these raise the following question: does the concept of disease underlying the treatment versus enhancement distinction force us to treat relevantly similar cases in dissimilar ways? Are we violating the old Aristotelian requirement that justice requires treating like cases similarly? Is dissimilar treatment unfair or unjust?

Despite the challenge of hard cases, the treatment versus enhancement distinction should play a role in deciding what obligations we have to provide medical services. To show that this distinction is not arbitrary from the viewpoint of justice, despite the hard cases, I shall argue that it fits better than do alternatives with what I call the *standard model* for thinking about equality of opportunity. Of course, the standard model may itself be indefensible, a point I will return to shortly. First, though, I want to show that the standard model helps specify a reasonable limit on the central task of health care.

Earlier I noted that disease and disability restrict the range of opportunities open to an individual. Health care services maintain, restore, and compensate for losses of function that result from disease and disability. They thus restore people to the range of capabilities they *could be expected to have had* without disease or disability, given their allotment of talents and skills. Our *standard model* for thinking about equality of opportunity thus depends on *taking as a given the fact that talents and skills and other capabilities are not distributed equally* among people. Some people are better at some things than others. Accordingly, we ensure people *fair* equality of opportunity if we judge them by their capabilities while ignoring "morally irrelevant" traits such as sex or race when we place people in schools, jobs, and offices. Often, however, we must correct for cases in which capabilities have been misdeveloped through racist, sexist, or other discriminatory practices. Similarly, by preventing or treating disease and disability, we can correct for impairment of the capabilities people would otherwise have.

The standard model does not call for eliminating differences in normal capabilities in general, let alone through medical enhancement.

This limitation of the standard model can appear arbitrary. As I noted earlier, our capabilities are themselves the result of a natural and social lottery, and we do not "deserve" them. We just are fortunate or unfortunate in having them. We can mitigate this underlying arbitrariness somewhat as follows. Those who are better endowed with marketable capabilities are likely to enjoy more goods such as income, wealth, and power. If we constrain inequalities in these goods so that those who are worst off do as well as possible, considering all alternatives, then social cooperation will work to the benefit of all. Still, this constraint does not eliminate all inequalities in the individual capabilities or in the resulting opportunities individuals enjoy, especially since we are enjoined to judge people by their capabilities and not by their "morally irrelevant" traits such as sex or race. If our egalitarian concerns require that we strive to give people equal capabilities, wherever technologically feasible, then we should not settle for mitigating the effects of the normal distribution of capabilities, as proponents of the standard model of equality of opportunity would have it. Rejecting the standard model pushes us toward equalizing all differences in capabilities; from that perspective, the distinction between treatment and enhancement has no point, at least where enhancement is aimed at equalizing capabilities.

Information from the genome project might make the distinction between disease (including genetic disease) and the normal distribution of capabilities seem more arbitrary. Suppose we learn that some particular pattern of genes explains the extreme shortness of Billy, the child who was not deficient in growth hormone. That is, we learn just which "losing numbers" in the natural lottery placed Billy in the bottom one percent of the normal distribution for height. Identifying these genes may then tempt us to think of them as "bad" ones: they lead to Billy's unhappiness or disadvantage in a "heightist" world. We will then be sorely tempted to think of them very much on the model of genetic defects or diseases, especially if they work through mechanisms that have some analogy to pathological defects. In other words, we will be tempted to medicalize what we have hitherto considered normal.

What, after all, allows us to treat the "bad genes" differently from genes that lead to growth hormone deficiency or to receptor insensitivity to growth hormone? If we can remedy the effects of these genes with growth hormone treatment or other treatments, including genetic tampering, we might think it quite arbitrary to maintain the treatment versus enhancement distinction.

I want to offer several points as a limited defense of the standard model and the treatment versus enhancement distinction. Both versions of equality of opportunity, the standard model and the more radical one that requires equalizing capabilities, seem to appeal to the same underlying intuition— that advantages and disadvantages resulting from the natural lottery are not themselves deserved. But they use the intuition differently. The standard model suggests we mitigate the effects of normally distributed capabilities through restrictions on other inequalities we allow. Since some inequality in capabilities is a fact of life, the task is to mitigate their effects while adopting principles that let everyone benefit from social cooperation. The criticism from the left rests far more weight on the underlying intuition: it says that wherever possible we must actually try to reduce variance in the distribution of capabilities, equalizing them wherever possible. I believe that the standard model better captures our actual concerns about equality than the more radical version. (Of course, our actual concerns may be too limited, so this is not a conclusive argument.)

Some supporting evidence for this point derives from our moral beliefs and practices concerning health care. We regard medical services as meeting *urgent needs* when they are aimed at restoring or maintaining "normal functioning." Our consensus about where to draw the line focuses on eliminating disease and disability. We already have many technologies that can enhance functioning for individuals, even giving them advantages (such as beauty or athletic performance) they previously did not have. But we generally resist assimilating these cases of enhancement to cases of treatment because we do not see them as meeting important needs. Although these enhancing services alter traits that may be the results of a natural lottery, they involve optimizing capabilities that are not departures from normal functional organization or functioning.

Of course, what makes the case of Billy and Johnny problematic is that they both suffer equal disadvantage as a result of the natural lottery (and social prejudice). But there is justification for adhering to a distinction that captures and sustains social agreement on important matters, even if the distinction seems arbitrary in isolated hard cases. The line between treatment and enhancement is generally uncontroversial and ascertainable through publicly accepted methods, such as those of the biomedical sciences. Being able to draw a line in this way allows us to refer counterfactually in a relatively clear and objective way to the range of opportunities a person *would have had* in the absence of disease and disability; it facilitates public agreement. Because of these virtues, not every hard case counts as a counterexample that warrants overturning the distinction.

The "equal capabilities" approach, bolstered by new information from the genome project, is likely to undermine agreement on the importance of meeting medical needs. According to it, we would now have many more such needs, for much of what we now take to be normal would become conditions in need of rectification. Since we are far less likely to think that it is "urgent" to correct the effects of these newly labeled "bad genes," shifting away from the standard model is likely to undermine consensus on the moral importance of health care.

Will it be possible to hold the line? Some relief may come from a more careful attempt to examine the distinction between genetic disease and normal variation. This may enable us to offer a theoretical justification, coming out of the biological sciences, for a baseline distinction. It is important to note that I am not trying to save the appeal to a natural baseline here because there is something magical or metaphysically basic about it. Nor am I violating Hume's injunction against deriving "ought" from "is." Rather, the natural baseline both facilitates and reflects moral agreement about the urgency of medical care. I also believe there is moral justification for

limiting in some ways the task involved in protecting equality of opportunity, otherwise it will be discredited as too demanding an ideal. If, however, no theoretical justification is forthcoming that lets us distinguish "bad" (or nonoptimal) genes from genetic disease, then we will have to give more complex justifications for drawing the line between cases in which we have obligations to provide services and those in which we do not. My claim is simply that it will be harder to reach consensus on these justifications without the ability to appeal to a natural baseline, however imperfectly drawn.

I have been offering reasons not to expand our goals in protecting equality of opportunity from the more limited ones of the standard model to the more encompassing one of equalizing capabilities. Nevertheless, our obligations to provide medical services need not derive solely from the concerns about equality of opportunity that I have argued are central. For example, I think we have compelling reasons for providing public funding of nontherapeutic abortions that go beyond their importance for preventive health care. Similarly, suppose an inexpensive treatment became available for improving cognitive capabilities in childhood; administering it would greatly enhance the results of education, close the gap between poor but "normal" students and others, and contribute greatly to social productivity. We might then have compelling reasons to seek enhancement in this way, even if they differ from our standard justification for the importance of health care. Of course, we already have excellent reasons for putting more resources into education, yet we do not, despite the fact that our failure to do so results in misdeveloped talents and skills along race and class lines. . . .

NOTE

1. D. B. Allen and N. C. Fost, "Growth Hormone Therapy for Short Stature: Panacea or Pandora's Box?" *Journal of Pediatrics* 117:1(1990): 16–21.

GENETIC INTERVENTIONS AND THE ETHICS OF ENHANCEMENT OF HUMAN BEINGS

Julian Savulescu

Should we use science and medical technology not just to prevent or treat disease, but to intervene at the most basic biological levels to improve biology and enhance people's lives? By 'enhance', I mean help them to live a longer and/or better life than normal. There are various ways in which we can enhance people but I want to focus on biological enhancement, especially genetic enhancement.

There has been considerable recent debate on the ethics of human enhancement. A number of prominent authors have been concerned about or critical of the use of technology to alter or enhance human beings, citing threats to human nature and dignity as one basis for these concerns. The President's Council Report entitled *Beyond Therapy* was strongly critical of human enhancement. Michael Sandel, in a widely discussed article, has suggested that the problem with genetic enhancement

> is in the hubris of the designing parents, in their drive to master the mystery of birth . . . it would disfigure the relation between parent and child, and deprive the parent of the humility and enlarged human sympathies that an openness to the unbidden can cultivate. . . . [T]he promise of mastery is flawed. It threatens to banish our appreciation of life as a gift, and to leave us with nothing to affirm or behold outside our own will. (Sandel 2004)

Frances Kamm has given a detailed rebuttal of Sandel's arguments, arguing that human enhancement is permissible. Nicholas Agar, in his book *Liberal Eugenics*, argues that enhancement should be permissible but not obligatory. He argues that what distinguishes liberal eugenics from the objectionable eugenic practices of the Nazis is that it is not based on a single conception of a desirable genome and that it is voluntary and not obligatory.

Editors' note: Most references have been cut. Students who want to follow up on sources should consult the original article.

In this chapter I will take a more provocative position. I want to argue that, far from its being merely permissible, we have a moral obligation or moral reason to enhance ourselves and our children. Indeed, we have the same kind of obligation as we have to treat and prevent disease. Not only *can* we enhance, we *should* enhance.

I will begin by considering the current interests in and possibilities of enhancement. I will then offer three arguments that we have very strong reasons to seek to enhance.

Tom Murray concludes 'Enhancement' by arguing that 'the ethics of enhancement must take into account the meaning and purpose of the activities being enhanced, their social context, and the other persons and institutions affected by them' (Murray, 2007: 514). Such caution is no doubt well grounded. But it should not blind us to the very large array of cases in which biological modification will improve the opportunities of an individual to lead a better life. In such cases, we have strong reasons to modify ourselves and our children. Indeed, to fail to do so would be wrong. Discussion of enhancement can be muddied by groundless fears and excessive caution and qualification. I will outline some ethical constraints on the pursuit of enhancement.

CURRENT INTEREST IN ENHANCEMENT

There is great public interest in enhancement of people. Women employ cosmetic surgery to make their noses smaller, their breasts larger, their teeth straighter and whiter, to make their cheekbones higher, their lips fuller, and to remove wrinkles and fat. Men, too, employ many of these measures, as well as pumping their bodies with steroids to increase muscle bulk. The beauty industry is testimony to the attraction of enhancement. Body art, such as painting and tattooing, and body modification, such as piercing, have, since time began, represented ways in which humans have attempted to express their creativity, values, and symbolic attachments through changing their bodies.

Modern professional sport is often said to be corrupted by widespread use of performance-enhancing drugs, such as human erythropoietin, anabolic steroids, and growth hormone. However, some effective performance enhancements are permitted in sport, such as the use of caffeine, glutamine, and creatine in diets, salbutamol, hypoxic air tents, and altitude training. Many people attempt to improve their cognitive powers through the use of nicotine, caffeine, and drugs like Ritalin and Modavigil.

Mood enhancement typifies modern society. People use psychological 'self-help', Prozac, recreational drugs, and alcohol to feel more relaxed, socialize better, and feel happier.

Even in the most private area of sexual relations, many want to be better. Around 34 percent of all men aged 40–70—around 20 million in the United States—have some erectile dysfunction, which is a part of normal ageing. There is a 12 percent decline in erectile function every decade normally. As a result, 20 million men worldwide use Viagra (Cheitlin *et al.* 1999).

More radical forms of biological enhancement appear possible. Even if all disease (heart disease, cancer, etc.) were cured, the average human lifespan would only be extended by twelve years. However, stem cell science has the potential to extend human lifespan radically further than this, by replacing ageing tissue with healthy tissue. We could live longer than the current maximum of 120 years.

But instead of the radical prolongation of length of life, I want to focus on the radical improvement in quality of life through biological manipulation. Some sceptics believe that this is not possible. They claim that it is our environment, or culture, that defines us, not genetics. But a quiet walk in the park demonstrates the power of a great genetic experiment: dog-breeding. It is obvious that different breeds of dog differ in temperament, intelligence, physical ability, and appearance. No matter what the turf, a Dobermann will tear a corgi to pieces. You can debilitate a Dobermann through neglect and abuse. And you can make him prettier with a bow. But you will never turn a chihuahua into a Dobermann through grooming, training, and affection. Dog breeds are all genetic—for over 10,000 years we have bred some 300–400 breeds of dog from early canids and wolves.

The St Bernard is known for its size, the greyhound for its speed, the bloodhound for its sense of smell. There are freaks, hard workers, vicious aggressors, docile pets, and ornamental varieties. These characteristics have been developed by a crude form of genetic selection—selective mating or breeding.

Today we have powerful scientific tools in animal husbandry: genetic testing, artificial reproduction, and cloning are all routinely used in the farming industry to create the best stock. Scientists are now starting to look at a wider range of complex behaviours. Changing the brain's reward centre genetically may be the key to changing behaviour.

Gene therapy has been used to turn lazy monkeys into workaholics by altering the reward centre in the brain. In another experiment, researchers used gene therapy to introduce a gene from the monogamous male prairie vole, a rodent that forms lifelong bonds with one mate, into the brain of the closely related but polygamous meadow vole. Genetically modified meadow voles became monogamous, behaving like prairie voles. This gene, which controls a part of the brain's reward centre different from that altered in the monkeys, is known as the vasopressin receptor gene. It may also be involved in human drug addiction.

Radical enhancements may come on the back of very respected research to prevent and treat disease. Scientists have created a rat model of the genetic disease Huntington's Chorea. This disease results in progressive rapid dementia at the age of about 40. Scientists found that rats engineered to develop Huntington's Chorea who were placed in a highly stimulating environment (of mazes, coloured rings, and balls) did not go on to develop the disease—their neurons remained intact. Remotivation therapy improves functioning in humans, suggesting that environmental stimulation in this genetic disease may affect brain biology at the molecular level (by altering neurotrophins). Prozac has also been shown to produce a beneficial effect in humans suffering from Huntington's Chorea. Neural stem cells have also been identified that could potentially be induced to proliferate and differentiate, mediated through nerve growth factors and other factors. We now know that a stimulating environment, drugs like Prozac, and nerve growth factors can affect nerve proliferation and connections—that is our brain's biology. These same interventions could, at least in theory, be used to increase the neuronal complement of normal brains and increase cognitive performance in normal individuals.

IQ has been steadily increasing since first measured, about twenty points per decade. This has been called the Flynn effect. Large environmental effects have been postulated to account for this effect. The capacity to increase IQ is significant. Direct biological enhancement could have an equal if not greater effect on increase in IQ.

But could biological enhancement of human beings really be possible? Selective mating has been occurring in humans ever since time began. Facial asymmetry can reflect genetic disorder. Smell can tell us whether our mate will produce the child with the best resistance to disease. We compete for partners in elaborate mating games and rituals of display that sort the best matches from the worst. As products of evolution, we select our mates, both rationally and instinctively, on the basis of their genetic fitness—their ability to survive and reproduce. Our (subconscious) goal is the success of our offspring.

With the tools of genetics, we can select offspring in a more reliable way. The power of genetics is growing. Embryos can now be tested not only for the presence of genetic disorder (including some forms of bowel and breast cancer), but also for less serious genetic abnormalities, such as dental abnormalities. Sex can be tested for too. Adult athletes have been genetically tested for the presence of the ACTN3 gene to identify potential for either sprint or endurance events. Research is going on in the field of behavioural genetics to understand the genetic basis of aggression and criminal behaviour, alcoholism, anxiety, antisocial personality disorder, maternal behaviour, homosexuality, and neuroticism.

While at present there are no genetic tests for these complex behaviours, if the results of recent animal studies into hard work and monogamy apply to humans, it may be possible in the future to change genetically how we are predisposed to behave. This raises a new question: Should we try to engineer better, happier people? While at present genetic technology is most efficient at selecting among different embryos, in the future it will be possible to genetically alter existing embryos, with considerable progress already being made to the use of this technology for permanent gene therapy for disease. There is no reason why such technology could not be used to alter non-disease genes in the future.

THE ETHICS OF ENHANCEMENT

We want to be happy people, not just healthy people.

I will now give three arguments in favour of enhancement and then consider several objections.

First Argument for Enhancement: Choosing Not to Enhance Is Wrong

Consider the case of the Neglectful Parents. The Neglectful Parents give birth to a child with a special condition. The child has a stunning intellect but requires a simple, readily available, cheap dietary supplement to sustain his intellect. But they neglect the diet of this child and this results in a child with a stunning intellect becoming normal. This is clearly wrong.

But now consider the case of the Lazy Parents. They have a child who has a normal intellect but if they introduced the same dietary supplement, the child's intellect would rise to the same level as the child of the Neglectful Parent. They can't be bothered with improving the child's diet so the child remains with a normal intellect. Failure to institute dietary supplementation means a normal child fails to achieve a stunning intellect. The inaction of the Lazy Parents is as wrong as the inaction of the Neglectful Parents. It has exactly the same consequence: a child exists who could have had a stunning intellect but is instead normal.

Some argue that it is not wrong to fail to bring about the best state of affairs. This may or may not be the case. But in these kinds of case, when there are no other relevant moral considerations, the failure to introduce a diet that sustains a more desirable state is as wrong as the failure to introduce a diet that brings about a more desirable state. The costs of inaction are the same, as are the parental obligations.

If we substitute 'biological intervention' for 'diet', we see that in order not to wrong our children, we should enhance them. Unless there is something special and optimal about our children's physical, psychological, or cognitive abilities, or something different about other biological interventions, it would be wrong not to enhance them.

Second Argument: Consistency

Some will object that, while we do have an obligation to institute better diets, biological interventions like genetic interventions are different from dietary supplementation. I will argue that there is no difference between these interventions.

In general, we accept environmental interventions to improve our children. Education, diet, and training are all used to make our children better people and increase their opportunities in life. We train children to be well behaved, cooperative, and intelligent. Indeed, researchers are looking at ways to make the environment more stimulating for young children to maximize their intellectual development. But in the study of the rat model of Huntington's Chorea, the stimulating environment acted to change the brain structure of the rats. The drug Prozac acted in just the same way. These environmental manipulations do not act mysteriously. They alter our biology.

The most striking example of this is a study of rats that were extensively mothered and rats that were not mothered. The mothered rats showed genetic changes (changes in the methylation of the DNA) that were passed on to the next generation. As Michael Meaney has observed, 'Early experience can actually modified protein–DNA interactions that regulate gene expression' (Society for Neuroscience 2004). More generally, environmental manipulations can profoundly affect biology. Maternal care and stress have been associated with abnormal brain (hippocampal) development, involving altered nerve growth factors and cognitive, psychological, and immune deficits later in life.

Some argue that genetic manipulations are different because they are irreversible. But environmental interventions can equally be irreversible. Child neglect or abuse can scar a person for life. It may be impossible to unlearn the skill of playing the piano or riding a bike, once learnt. One may be wobbly, but one is a novice only once. Just as the example of mothering of rats shows that environmental interventions can cause biological changes that are passed onto the next generation, so too can environmental interventions be irreversible, or very difficult to reverse, within one generation.

Why should we allow environmental manipulations that alter our biology but not direct biological manipulations? What is the moral difference between producing a smarter child by immersing that child in a stimulating environment, giving the child a drug, or directly altering the child's brain or genes?

One example of a drug that alters brain chemistry is Prozac, which is a serotonin reuptake inhibitor. Early in life it acts as a nerve growth factor, but it may also alter the brain early in life to make it more prone to stress and anxiety later in life by altering receptor development. People with a polymorphism that reduced their serotonin activity were more likely than others to become depressed in response to stressful experiences. Drugs like Prozac and maternal deprivation may have the same biological effects.

If the outcome is the same, why treat biological manipulation differently from environmental manipulation? Not only may a favourable environment improve a child's biology and increase a child's opportunities, so too may direct biological interventions. Couples should maximize the genetic opportunity of their children to lead a good life and a productive, cooperative social existence. There is no relevant moral difference between environmental and genetic intervention.

Third Argument: No Difference from Treating Disease

If we accept the treatment and prevention of disease, we should accept enhancement. The goodness of health is what drives a moral obligation to treat or prevent disease. But health is not what ultimately matters—health enables us to live well; disease prevents us from doing what we want and what is good. Health is instrumentally valuable—valuable as a resource that allows us to do what really matters, that is, lead a good life.

What constitutes a good life is a deep philosophical question. According to hedonistic theories, what is good is having pleasant experiences and being happy. According to desire fulfilment theories, and economics, what matters is having our preferences satisfied. According to objective theories, certain activities are good for people: developing deep personal relationships, developing talents, understanding oneself and the world, gaining knowledge, being a part of a family, and so on. We need not decide on which of these theories is correct in order to understand what is bad about ill health. Disease is important because it causes pain, is not what we want, and stops us engaging in those activities that giving meaning to life. Sometimes people trade health for well-being: mountain climbers take on risk to achieve, smokers sometimes believe that the pleasures outweigh the risks of smoking, and so on. Life is about managing risk to health and life to promote well-being.

Beneficence—the moral obligation to benefit people—provides a strong reason to enhance people in so far as the biological enhancement increases their chance of having a better life. But can biological enhancements increase people's opportunities for well-being? There are reasons to believe that they might.

Many of our biological and psychological characteristics profoundly affect how well our lives go. In the 1960s Walter Mischel conducted impulse control experiments in which 4-year-old children were left in a room with one marshmallow, after being told that if they did not eat the marshmallow, they could later have two. Some children would eat it as soon as the researcher left; others would use a variety of strategies to help control their behaviour and ignore the temptation of the single marshmallow. A decade later they reinterviewed the children and found that those who were better at delaying gratification had more friends, better academic performance, and more motivation to succeed. Whether the child had grabbed for the marshmallow had a much stronger bearing on their SAT scores than did their IQ.

Impulse control has also been linked to socio-economic control and avoiding conflict with the law. The problems of a hot and uncontrollable temper can be profound.

Shyness too can greatly restrict a life. I remember one newspaper story about a woman who blushed violet every time she went into a social situation. This led her to a hermitic, miserable existence. She eventually had the autonomic nerves to her face surgically cut. This revolutionized her life and had a greater effect on her **well-being than the treatment of many diseases.**

Buchanan and colleagues have discussed the value of 'all purpose goods'. These are traits that are valuable regardless of the kind of life a person chooses to live. They give us greater all-round capacities to live a vast array of lives. Examples include intelligence, memory, self-discipline, patience, empathy, a sense of humour, optimism, and just having a sunny temperament. All of these characteristics—sometimes described as virtues—may have some

biological and psychological basis capable of manipulation using technology.

Technology might even be used to improve our moral character. We certainly seek through good instruction and example, discipline, and other methods to make better children. It may be possible to alter biology to make people predisposed to be more moral by promoting empathy, imagination, sympathy, fairness, honesty, etc.

In so far as these characteristics have some genetic basis, genetic manipulation could benefit us. There is reason to believe that complex virtues like fair-mindedness may have a biological basis. In one famous experiment a monkey was trained to perform a task and rewarded with either a grape or a piece of cucumber. He preferred the grape. On one occasion he performed the task successfully and was given a piece of cucumber. He watched as another monkey who had not performed the task was given a grape and he became very angry. This shows that even monkeys have a sense of fairness and desert—or at least self-interest!

At the other end, there are characteristics that we believe do not make for a good and happy life. One Dutch family illustrates the extreme end of the spectrum. For over thirty years this family recognized that there were a disproportionate number of male family members who exhibited aggressive and criminal behaviour. This was characterized by aggressive outbursts resulting in arson, attempted rape, and exhibitionism. The behaviour was documented for almost forty years by an unaffected maternal grandfather, who could not understand why some of the men in his family appeared to be prone to this type of behaviour. Male relatives who did not display this aggressive behaviour did not express *any* type of abnormal behaviour. Unaffected males reported difficulty in understanding the behaviour of their brothers and cousins. Sisters of the males who demonstrated these extremely aggressive outbursts reported intense fear of their brothers. The behaviour did not appear to be related to environment and appeared consistently in different parts of the family, regardless of social context and degree of social contact. All affected males were also found to be mildly mentally retarded, with a typical IQ of about 85 (females had normal intelligence) (Brunner 1993a). When a family tree was constructed, the pattern of inheritance was clearly X-linked recessive. This means, roughly, that women can carry the gene without being affected; 50 percent of men at risk of inheriting the gene get the gene and are affected by the disease.

Genetic analysis suggested that the likely defective gene was a part of the X chromosome known as the monoamine oxidase region. This region codes for two enzymes that assist in the breakdown of neurotransmitters. Neurotransmitters are substances that play a key role in the conduction of nerve impulses in our brain. Enzymes like the monoamine oxidases are required to degrade the neurotransmitters after they have performed their desired task. It was suggested that the monoamine oxidase activity might be disturbed in the affected individuals. Urine analysis showed a higher than normal amount of neurotransmitters being excreted in the urine of affected males. These results were consistent with a reduction in the functioning of one of the enzymes (monoamine oxidase A).

How can such a mutation result in violent and antisocial behaviour? A deficiency of the enzyme results in a build-up of neurotransmitters. These abnormal levels of neurotransmitters result in excessive, and even violent, reactions to stress. This hypothesis was further supported by the finding that genetically modified mice that lack this enzyme are more aggressive.

This family is an extreme example of how genes can influence behaviour: it is the only family in which this mutation has been isolated. Most genetic contributions to behaviour will be weaker predispositions, but there may be some association between genes and behaviour that results in criminal and other antisocial behaviour.

How could information such as this be used? Some criminals have attempted a 'genetic defence' in the United States, stating that their genes caused them to commit the crime, but this has never succeeded. However, it is clear that couples should be allowed to test to select offspring who do not have the mutation that predisposes them to act in this way, and if interventions were available, it might be rational to correct it since children without the mutation have a good chance of a better life.

'Genes, Not Men, May Hold the Key to Female Pleasure' ran the title of one recent newspaper article (*The Age* 2005), which reported the results of a large study of female identical twins in Britain and Australia. It found that 'genes accounted for 31 percent of the chance of having an orgasm during intercourse and 51 percent during masturbation'. It concluded that the 'ability to gain sexual satisfaction is largely inherited' and went on to speculate that 'The genes involved could be linked to physical differences in sex organs and hormone levels or factors such as mood and anxiety.'

Our biology profoundly affects how our lives go. If we can increase sexual satisfaction by modifying biology, we should. Indeed, vast numbers of men attempt to do this already through the use of Viagra.

Summary: The Case for Enhancement

What matters is human well-being, not just treatment and prevention of disease. Our biology affects our opportunities to live well. The biological route to improvement is no different from the environmental. Biological manipulation to increase opportunity is ethical. If we have an obligation to treat and prevent disease, we have an obligation to try to manipulate these characteristics to give an individual the best opportunity of the best life.

HOW DO WE DECIDE?

If we are to enhance certain qualities, how should we decide which to choose? Eugenics was the movement early in the last century that aimed to use selective breeding to prevent degeneration of the gene pool by weeding out criminals, those with mental illness, and the poor, on the false belief that these conditions were simple genetic disorders. The eugenics movement had its inglorious peak when the Nazis moved beyond sterilization to extermination of the genetically unfit.

What was objectionable about the eugenics movement, besides its shoddy scientific basis, was that it involved the imposition of a state vision for a healthy population and aimed to achieve this through coercion. The movement was aimed not at what was good for individuals, but rather at what benefited society. Modern eugenics in the form of testing for disorders, such as Down syndrome, occurs very commonly but is acceptable because it is voluntary, gives couples a choice of what kind of child to have, and enables them to have a child with the greatest opportunity for a good life.

There are four possible ways in which our genes and biology will be decided:

1. nature or God;
2. 'experts' (philosophers, bioethicists, psychologists, scientists);
3. 'authorities' (government, doctors);
4. people themselves: liberty and autonomy.

It is a basic principle of liberal states like the United Kingdom that the state be 'neutral' to different conceptions of the good life. This means that we allow individuals to lead the life that they believe is best for themselves, implying respect for their personal autonomy or capacity for self-rule. The sole ground for interference is when that individual choice may harm others. Advice, persuasion, information, dialogue are permissible. But coercion and infringement of liberty are impermissible.

There are limits to what a liberal state should provide:

1. safety: the intervention should be reasonably safe;
2. harm to others: the intervention (like some manipulation that increases uncontrollable aggressiveness) should not result in harm. Such harm should not be direct or indirect, for example, by causing some unfair competitive advantage;
3. distributive justice: the interventions should be distributed according to principles of justice.

The situation is more complex with young children, embryos, and fetuses, who are incompetent. These human beings are not autonomous and cannot make choices themselves about whether a putative enhancement is a benefit or a harm. If a proposed intervention can be delayed until that human reaches maturity and can decide for himself or herself, then the intervention should be delayed. However, many genetic interventions will have to be performed very early in life if they are to have an effect. Decisions about such interventions should be left to parents, according to a principle of procreative liberty and autonomy. This states that parents have the freedom to choose when to have children, how many children to have, and arguably what kind of children to have.

Just as parents have wide scope to decide on the conditions of the upbringing of their children, including schooling and religious education, they should have similar freedom over their children's genes. Procreative autonomy or liberty should be extended to enhancement for two reasons. Firstly, reproduction: bearing and raising children is a very private matter. Parents must bear much of the burden of having children, and they have a legitimate stake in the nature of the child they must invest so much of their lives raising.

But there is a second reason. John Stuart Mill argued that when our actions only affect ourselves, we should be free to construct and act on our own conception of what is the best life for us. Mill was not a libertarian. He did not believe that such freedom is valuable solely for its own sake. He believed that freedom is important in order for people to discover for themselves what kind of life is best for themselves. It is only through 'experiments in living' that people discover what works for them and others come to see the richness and variety of lives that can be good. Mill strongly praised 'originality' and variety in choice as being essential to discovering which lives are best for human beings.

Importantly, Mill believed that some lives are worse than others. Famously, he said that it is better to be Socrates dissatisfied than a fool satisfied. He distinguished between 'higher pleasures' of 'feelings and imagination' and 'lower pleasures' of 'mere sensation' (Mill 1910: 7). He criticized 'apelike imitation', subjugation of oneself to custom and fashion, indifference to individuality, and lack of originality (1910: 119–20, 123). Nonetheless, he was the champion of people's right to live their lives as they choose.

I have said that it is important to give the freest rein possible to things that are not customary, in order that it may in time transpire which of them are fit to become customary. But independence of action and disregard of custom are not deserving of encouragement solely for the chance they afford for better modes of action, and customs more worthy of general adoption, to be discovered; nor is it only people of decided mental superiority who have a just claim to carry on their lives in their own way. There is no reason for all human existence to be constructed on some single or small number of patterns. If a person possesses a tolerable amount of common sense and experience, his own mode of designing his existence is the best, not because it is the best in itself, but because it is his own mode.

I believe that reproduction should be about having children with the best prospects. But to discover what are the best prospects, we must give individual couples the freedom to act on their own judgment of what constitutes a life with good prospects. 'Experiments in reproduction' are as important as 'experiments in living' (as long as they don't harm the children who are produced). For this reason, procreative freedom is important.

There is one important limit to procreative autonomy that is different from the limits to personal autonomy. The limits to procreative autonomy should be:

1. safety;
2. harm to others;
3. distributive justice;
4. *such that the parent's choices are based on a plausible conception of well-being and a better life for the child;*
5. *consistent with development of autonomy in the child and a reasonable range of future life plans.*

These last two limits are important. It makes for a higher standard of 'proof' that an intervention will be an enhancement because the parents are making choices for their child, not themselves. The critical question to ask in considering whether to alter some gene related to complex behaviour is: Would the change be better for the individual? Is it better for the individual to have a tendency to be lazy or hardworking, monogamous or polygamous? These questions are difficult to answer. While we might let adults choose to be monogamous or polygamous, we would not let parents decide on their child's predispositions unless we were reasonably clear that some trait was better for the child.

There will be cases where some intervention is plausibly in a child's interests: increased empathy with other people, better capacity to understand oneself and the world around, or improved memory. One quality is especially associated with socio-economic success and staying out of prison: impulse control. If it were possible to correct poor impulse control, we should correct it. Whether we should remove impulsiveness altogether is another question.

Joel Feinberg has described a child's right to an open future (Feinberg 1980). An open future is one in which a child has a reasonable range of possible lives to choose from and an opportunity to

choose what kind of person to be; that is, to develop autonomy. Some critics of enhancement have argued that genetic interventions are inconsistent with a child's right to an open future. Far from restricting a child's future, however, some biological interventions may increase the possible futures or at least their quality. It is hard to see how improved memory or empathy would restrict a child's future. Many worthwhile possibilities would be open. But it is true that parental choice should not restrict the development of autonomy or reasonable range of possible futures open to a child. In general, fewer enhancements will be permitted in children than in adults. Some interventions, however, may still be clearly enhancements for our children, and so just like vaccinations or other preventative health care.

OBJECTIONS

Playing God or Against Nature

This objection has various forms. Some people in society believe that children are a gift, of God or of nature, and that we should not interfere in human nature. Most people implicitly reject this view: we screen embryos and fetuses for diseases, even mild correctable disease. We interfere in nature or God's will when we vaccinate, provide pain relief to women in labour (despite objections of some earlier Christians that these practices thwarted God's will), and treat cancer. No one would object to the treatment of disability in a child if it were possible. Why, then, not treat the embryo with genetic therapy if that intervention is safe? This is no more thwarting God's will than giving antibiotics.

Another variant of this objection is that we are arrogant if we assume we could have sufficient knowledge to meddle with human nature. Some people object that we cannot know the complexity of the human system, which is like an unknowable magnificent symphony. To attempt to enhance one characteristic may have other unknown, unforeseen effects elsewhere in the system. We should not play God since, unlike God, we are not omnipotent or omniscient. We should be humble and recognize the limitations of our knowledge.

A related objection is that genes are pleiotropic—which means they have different effects in different environments. The gene or genes that predispose to manic depression may also be responsible for heightened creativity and productivity.

One response to both of these objections is to limit intervention, until our knowledge grows, to selecting between different embryos, and not intervening to enhance particular embryos or people. Since we would be choosing between complete systems on the basis of their type, we would not be interfering with the internal machinery. In this way, selection is less risky than enhancement.

But such a precaution could also be misplaced when considering biological interventions. When benefits are on offer, such objections remind us to refrain **from hubris and over-confidence. We must do adequate research before intervening.** And because the benefits may be fewer than when we treat or prevent disease, we may require the standards of safety to be higher than for medical interventions. But we must weigh the risks against the benefits. If confidence is justifiably high, and benefits outweigh harms, we should enhance.

Once technology affords us the power to enhance our own and our children's lives, to fail to do so would be to be responsible for the consequences. To fail to treat our children's diseases is to wrong them. To fail to prevent them from getting depression is to wrong them. To fail to improve their physical, musical, psychological, and other capacities is to wrong them, just as it would be to harm them if we gave them a toxic substance that stunted or reduced these capacities.

Another variant of the 'Playing God' objection is that there is a special value in the balance and diversity that natural variation affords, and enhancement will reduce this. But in so far as we are products of evolution, we are merely random chance variations of genetic traits selected for our capacity to survive long enough to reproduce. There is no design to evolution. Evolution selects genes, according to environment, that confer the greatest chance of survival and reproduction. Evolution would select a tribe that was highly fertile but suffered great pain the whole of their lives over another tribe that was less fertile but suffered less pain. Medicine has changed evolution: we can now select individuals who experience less pain and disease. The next stage of human evolution will be rational evolution, according to which we select children who not only have the greatest chance of surviving, reproducing, and being free of disease, but who have the greatest opportunities to have the best lives in their likely environment. Evolution was indifferent to how well our lives went; we are not. We want to retire, play golf, read, and watch our grandchildren have children.

'Enhancement' is a misnomer. It suggests luxury. But enhancement is no luxury. In so far as it promotes well-being, it is the very essence of what is necessary for a good human life. There is no moral reason to preserve some traits—such as uncontrollable aggressiveness, a sociopathic personality, or extreme deviousness. Tell the victim of rape and murder that we must preserve diversity and the natural balance.

Genetic Discrimination

Some people fear the creation of a two-tier society of the enhanced and the unenhanced, where the inferior, unenhanced are discriminated against and disadvantaged all through life.

We must remember that nature allots advantage and disadvantage with no gesture to fairness. Some are born terribly disadvantaged, destined to die after short and miserable lives. Some suffer great genetic disadvantage while others are born gifted, physically, musically, or intellectually. There is no secret that there are 'gifted' children naturally. Allowing choice to change our biology will, if anything, be more egalitarian, allowing the ungifted to approach the gifted. There is nothing fair about the natural lottery: allowing enhancement may be fairer.

But more importantly, how well the lives of those who are disadvantaged go depends not on whether enhancement is permitted, but on the social institutions we have in place to protect the least well off and provide everyone with a fair chance. People have disease and disability: egalitarian social institutions and laws against discrimination are designed to make sure everyone, regardless of natural inequality, has a decent chance of a decent life. This would be no different if enhancement were permitted. There is no necessary connection between enhancement and discrimination, just as there is no necessary connection between curing disability and discrimination against people with disability.

The Perfect Child, Sterility, and Loss of the Mystery of Life

If we engineered perfect children, this objection goes, the world would be a sterile, monotonous place where everyone was the same, and the mystery and surprise of life would be gone.

It is impossible to create perfect children. We can only attempt to create children with better opportunities of a better life. There will necessarily be difference. Even in the case of screening for disability, like Down syndrome, 10 percent of people choose not to abort a pregnancy known to be affected by Down syndrome. People value different things. There will never be complete convergence. Moreover, there will remain massive challenges for individuals to meet in their personal relationships and in the hurdles our unpredictable environment presents. There will remain much mystery and challenge—we will just be better able to deal with these. We will still have to work to achieve, but our achievements may have greater value.

Against Human Nature

One of the major objections to enhancement is that it is against human nature. Common alternative phrasings are that enhancement is tampering with our nature or an affront to human dignity. I believe that what separates us from other animals is our rationality, our capacity to make normative judgements and act on the basis of reasons. When we make decisions to improve our lives by biological and other manipulations, we express our rationality and express what is fundamentally important about our nature. And if those manipulations improve our capacity to make rational and normative judgements, they further improve what is fundamentally human. Far from being against the human spirit, such improvements express the human spirit. To be human is to be better.

Enhancements Are Self-Defeating

Another familiar objection to enhancement is that enhancements will have self-defeating or other adverse social effects. A typical example is increase in height. If height is socially desired, then everyone will try to enhance the height of their children at great cost to themselves and the environment (as taller people consume more resources), with no advantage in the end since there will be no relative gain.

If a purported manipulation does not improve well-being or opportunity, there is no argument in favour of it. In this case, the manipulation is not an enhancement. In other cases, such as enhancement of intelligence, the enhancement of one individual may increase that individual's opportunities only at the expense of another. So-called positional goods are goods only in a relative sense.

But many enhancements will have both positional and non-positional qualities. Intelligence is good not just because it allows an individual to be more competitive for complex jobs, but because it allows an individual to process information more rapidly in her own life, and to develop greater understanding of herself and others. These non-positional effects should not be ignored. Moreover, even in the case of so-called purely positional goods, such as height, there may be important non-positional values. It is better to be taller if you are a basketball player, but being tall is a disadvantage in balance sports such as gymnastics, skiing, and surfing.

Nonetheless, if there are significant social consequences of enhancement, this is of course a valid objection. But it is not particular to enhancement: there is an old question about how far individuals in society can pursue their own self-interest at a cost to others. It applies to education, health care, and virtually all areas of life.

Not all enhancements will be ethical. The critical issue is that the intervention is expected to bring about more benefits than harms to the individual. It must be safe and there must be a reasonable expectation of improvement. Some of the other features of ethical enhancements are summarized below.

What Is an Ethical Enhancement?

An ethical enhancement:

1. is in the person's interests;
2. is reasonably safe;
3. increases the opportunity to have the best life;
4. promotes or does not unreasonably restrict the range of possible lives open to that person;

5. does not unreasonably harm others directly through excessive costs in making it freely available;
6. does not place that individual at an unfair competitive advantage with respect to others, e.g. mind-reading;
7. is such that the person retains significant control or responsibility for her **achievements and self that cannot be wholly or directly attributed to the** enhancement;
8. does not unreasonably reinforce or increase unjust inequality and discrimination—economic inequality, racism.

What Is an Ethical Enhancement for a Child or Incompetent Human Being?

Such an ethical enhancement is all the above, but in addition:

1. the intervention cannot be delayed until the child can make its own decision;
2. the intervention is plausibly in the child's interests;
3. the intervention is compatible with the development of autonomy.

CONCLUSION

Enhancement is already occurring. In sport, human erythropoietin boosts red blood cells. Steroids and growth hormone improve muscle strength. Many people seek cognitive enhancement through nicotine, Ritalin, Modavigil, or caffeine. Prozac, recreational drugs, and alcohol all enhance mood. Viagra is used to improve sexual performance.

And of course mobile phones and aeroplanes are examples of external enhancing technologies. In the future, genetic technology, nanotechnology, and artificial intelligence may profoundly affect our capacities.

Will the future be better or just disease-free? We need to shift our frame of reference from health to life enhancement. What matters is how we live. Technology can now improve that. We have two options:

1. Intervention:
   - treating disease;
   - preventing disease;
   - supra-prevention of disease—preventing disease in a radically unprecedented way;
   - protection of well-being;
   - enhancement of well-being.
2. No intervention, and to remain in a state of nature—no treatment or prevention of disease, no technological enhancement.

I believe that to be human is to be better. Or, at least, to strive to be better. We should be here for a *good* time, not just a *long* time. Enhancement, far from being merely permissible, is something we should aspire to achieve.

REFERENCES

The Age (2005), 'Genes, Not Men, May Hold the Key to Female Pleasure', 9 June.

Brunner, H. G., Nelen, M., *et al.* (1993*a*), 'Abnormal Behaviour Associated with a Point Mutation in the Structural Gene for Monoamine Oxidase A', Science, 262/5133: 578–80.

Cheitlin, M. D., Hutter, A. M., *et al.* (1999), 'ACC/AHA Expert Consensus Document JACC: Use of Sildenafil (Viagra) in Patients with Cardiovascular Disease', *Journal of the American College of Cardiology*, 33/1: 273–82.

Feinberg, J. (1980), 'The Child's Right to an Open Future,' in W. Aiken and H. LaFollette (eds.), *Whose Child? Parental Rights, Parental Authority and State Power* (Totowa, NJ: Rowman and Littlefield), 124–53.

Mill, J. S. (1910), *On Liberty* (London: J. M. Dent).

Murray, T. (2007), 'Enhancement', in B. Steinbock (ed.), *The Oxford Handbook of Bioethics* (Oxford: Oxford University Press), 491–515.

Sandel, M. (2004), 'The Case Against Perfection,' *Atlantic Monthly* (Apr. 2004), 51–62.

Society for Neuroscience (2004), 'Early Life Stress Harms Mental Function and Immune System in Later Years According to New Research,' 26 Oct., <http://apu.sfn.org/content/AboutSFN1/NewsReleases/am2004_early.html>, accessed Feb. 2006.

THE CASE AGAINST PERFECTION: WHAT'S WRONG WITH DESIGNER CHILDREN, BIONIC ATHLETES, AND GENETIC ENGINEERING

Michael J. Sandel

Breakthroughs in genetics present us with a promise and a predicament. The promise is that we may soon be able to treat and prevent a host of debilitating diseases. The predicament is that our newfound genetic knowledge may also enable us to manipulate our own nature—to enhance our muscles, memories, and moods; to choose the sex, height, and other genetic traits of our children; to make ourselves "better than well." When science moves faster than moral understanding, as it does today, men and women struggle to articulate their unease. In liberal societies they reach first for the language of autonomy, fairness, and individual rights. But this part of our moral vocabulary is ill equipped to address the hardest questions posed by genetic engineering. The genomic revolution has induced a kind of moral vertigo.

Consider cloning. The birth of Dolly the cloned sheep, in 1997, brought a torrent of concern about the prospect of cloned human beings. There are good medical reasons to worry. Most scientists agree that cloning is unsafe, likely to produce offspring with serious abnormalities. (Dolly recently died a premature death.) But suppose technology improved to the point where clones were at no greater risk than naturally conceived offspring. Would human cloning still be objectionable? Should our hesitation be moral as well as medical? What, exactly, is wrong with creating a child who is a genetic twin of one parent, or of an older sibling who has tragically died—or, for that matter, of an admired scientist, sports star, or celebrity?

Some say cloning is wrong because it violates the right to autonomy: by choosing a child's genetic makeup in advance, parents deny the child's right to an open future. A similar objection can be raised against any form of bioengineering that allows

parents to select or reject genetic characteristics. According to this argument, genetic enhancements for musical talent, say, or athletic prowess, would point children toward particular choices, and so designer children would never be fully free.

At first glance the autonomy argument seems to capture what is troubling about human cloning and other forms of genetic engineering. It is not persuasive, for two reasons. First, it wrongly implies that absent a designing parent, children are free to choose their characteristics for themselves. But none of us chooses his genetic inheritance. The alternative to a cloned or genetically enhanced child is not one whose future is unbound by particular talents but one at the mercy of the genetic lottery.

Second, even if a concern for autonomy explains some of our worries about made-to-order children, it cannot explain our moral hesitation about people who seek genetic remedies or enhancements for themselves. Gene therapy on somatic (that is, non-reproductive) cells, such as muscle cells and brain cells, repairs or replaces defective genes. The moral quandary arises when people use such therapy not to cure a disease but to reach beyond health, to enhance their physical or cognitive capacities, to lift themselves above the norm.

Like cosmetic surgery, genetic enhancement employs medical means for nonmedical ends—ends unrelated to curing or preventing disease or repairing injury. But unlike cosmetic surgery, genetic enhancement is more than skin-deep. If we are ambivalent about surgery or Botox injections for sagging chins and furrowed brows, we are all the more troubled by genetic engineering for stronger bodies, sharper memories, greater intelligence, and happier moods. The question is whether we are right to be troubled, and if so, on what grounds.

In order to grapple with the ethics of enhancement, we need to confront questions largely lost from view—questions about the moral status of nature,

From *Atlantic Monthly* 293, no. 3 (April 2004). Reprinted by permission of Michael J. Sandel.

and about the proper stance of human beings toward the given world. Since these questions verge on theology, modern philosophers and political theorists tend to shrink from them. But our new powers of biotechnology make them unavoidable. To see why this is so, consider four examples already on the horizon: muscle enhancement, memory enhancement, growth-hormone treatment, and reproductive technologies that enable parents to choose the sex and some genetic traits of their children. In each case what began as an attempt to treat a disease or prevent a genetic disorder now beckons as an instrument of improvement and consumer choice.

MUSCLES

Everyone would welcome a gene therapy to alleviate muscular dystrophy and to reverse the debilitating muscle loss that comes with old age. But what if the same therapy were used to improve athletic performance? Researchers have developed a synthetic gene that, when injected into the muscle cells of mice, prevents and even reverses natural muscle deterioration. The gene not only repairs wasted or injured muscles but also strengthens healthy ones. This success bodes well for human applications. H. Lee Sweeney, of the University of Pennsylvania, who leads the research, hopes his discovery will cure the immobility that afflicts the elderly. But Sweeney's bulked-up mice have already attracted the attention of athletes seeking a competitive edge. Although the therapy is not yet approved for human use, the prospect of genetically enhanced weight lifters, home-run sluggers, linebackers, and sprinters is easy to imagine. The widespread use of steroids and other performance-improving drugs in professional sports suggests that many athletes will be eager to avail themselves of genetic enhancement.

Suppose for the sake of argument that muscle-enhancing gene therapy, unlike steroids, turned out to be safe—or at least no riskier than a rigorous weight-training regimen. Would there be a reason to ban its use in sports? There is something unsettling about the image of genetically altered athletes lifting SUVs or hitting 650-foot home runs or running a three-minute mile. But what, exactly, is troubling about it? Is it simply that we find such superhuman spectacles too bizarre to contemplate?

Or does our unease point to something of ethical significance?

It might be argued that a genetically enhanced athlete, like a drug-enhanced athlete, would have an unfair advantage over his unenhanced competitors. But the fairness argument against enhancement has a fatal flaw: it has always been the case that some athletes are better endowed genetically than others, and yet we do not consider this to undermine the fairness of competitive sports. From the standpoint of fairness, enhanced genetic differences would be no worse than natural ones, assuming they were safe and made available to all. If genetic enhancement in sports is morally objectionable, it must be for reasons other than fairness.

MEMORY

Genetic enhancement is possible for brains as well as brawn. In the mid-1990s scientists managed to manipulate a memory-linked gene in fruit flies, creating flies with photographic memories. More recently researchers have produced smart mice by inserting extra copies of a memory-related gene into mouse embryos. The altered mice learn more quickly and remember things longer than normal mice. The extra copies were programmed to remain active even in old age, and the improvement was passed on to offspring.

Human memory is more complicated, but biotech companies, including Memory Pharmaceuticals, are in hot pursuit of memory-enhancing drugs, or "cognition enhancers," for human beings. The obvious market for such drugs consists of those who suffer from Alzheimer's and other serious memory disorders. The companies also have their sights on a bigger market: the 81 million Americans over fifty, who are beginning to encounter the memory loss that comes naturally with age. A drug that reversed age-related memory loss would be a bonanza for the pharmaceutical industry: a Viagra for the brain. Such use would straddle the line between remedy and enhancement. Unlike a treatment for Alzheimer's, it would cure no disease; but insofar as it restored capacities a person once possessed, it would have a remedial aspect. It could also have purely nonmedical uses: for example, by a lawyer cramming to memorize facts for an upcoming trial, or by a business executive eager to learn Mandarin on the eve of his departure for Shanghai.

Some who worry about the ethics of cognitive enhancement point to the danger of creating two classes of human beings: those with access to enhancement technologies, and those who must make do with their natural capacities. And if the enhancements could be passed down the generations, the two classes might eventually become subspecies—the enhanced and the merely natural. But worry about access ignores the moral status of enhancement itself. Is the scenario troubling because the unenhanced poor would be denied the benefits of bioengineering, or because the enhanced affluent would somehow be dehumanized? As with muscles, so with memory: the fundamental question is not how to ensure equal access to enhancement but whether we should aspire to it in the first place.

HEIGHT

Pediatricians already struggle with the ethics of enhancement when confronted by parents who want to make their children taller. Since the 1980s human growth hormone has been approved for children with a hormone deficiency that makes them much shorter than average. But the treatment also increases the height of healthy children. Some parents of healthy children who are unhappy with their stature (typically boys) ask why it should make a difference whether a child is short because of a hormone deficiency or because his parents happen to be short. Whatever the cause, the social consequences are the same.

In the face of this argument some doctors began prescribing hormone treatments for children whose short stature was unrelated to any medical problem. By 1996 such "off-label" use accounted for 40 percent of human-growth-hormone prescriptions. Although it is legal to prescribe drugs for purposes not approved by the Food and Drug Administration, pharmaceutical companies cannot promote such use. Seeking to expand its market, Eli Lilly & Co. recently persuaded the FDA to approve its human growth hormone for healthy children whose projected adult height is in the bottom one percentile— under five feet three inches for boys and four feet

eleven inches for girls. This concession raises a large question about the ethics of enhancement: If hormone treatments need not be limited to those with hormone deficiencies, why should they be available only to very short children? Why shouldn't all shorter-than-average children be able to seek treatment? And what about a child of average height who wants to be taller so that he can make the basketball team?

Some oppose height enhancement on the grounds that it is collectively self-defeating; as some become taller, others become shorter relative to the norm. Except in Lake Wobegon, not every child can be above average. As the unenhanced began to feel shorter, they, too, might seek treatment, leading to a hormonal arms race that left everyone worse off, especially those who couldn't afford to buy their way up from shortness.

But the arms-race objection is not decisive on its own. Like the fairness objection to bioengineered muscles and memory, it leaves unexamined the attitudes and dispositions that prompt the drive for enhancement. If we were bothered only by the injustice of adding shortness to the problems of the poor, we could remedy that unfairness by publicly subsidizing height enhancements. As for the relative height deprivation suffered by innocent bystanders, we could compensate them by taxing those who buy their way to greater height. The real question is whether we want to live in a society where parents feel compelled to spend a fortune to make perfectly healthy kids a few inches taller.

SEX SELECTION

Perhaps the most inevitable nonmedical use of bioengineering is sex selection. For centuries parents have been trying to choose the sex of their children. Today biotech succeeds where folk remedies failed.

One technique for sex selection arose with prenatal tests using amniocentesis and ultrasound. These medical technologies were developed to detect genetic abnormalities such as spina bifida and Down syndrome. But they can also reveal the sex of the fetus—allowing for the abortion of a fetus of an undesired sex. Even among those who favor abortion rights, few advocate abortion simply because the parents do not want a girl. Nevertheless, in traditional societies with a powerful cultural preference for boys, this practice has become widespread.

Sex selection need not involve abortion, however. For couples undergoing *in vitro* fertilization (IVF), it is possible to choose the sex of the child before the fertilized egg is implanted in the womb. One method makes use of pre-implantation genetic diagnosis (PGD), a procedure developed to screen for genetic diseases. Several eggs are fertilized in a petri dish and grown to the eight-cell stage (about three days). At that point the embryos are tested to determine their sex. Those of the desired sex are implanted; the others are typically discarded. Although few couples are likely to undergo the difficulty and expense of IVF simply to choose the sex of their child, embryo screening is a highly reliable means of sex selection. And as our genetic knowledge increases, it may be possible to use PGD to cull embryos carrying undesired genes, such as those associated with obesity, height, and skin color. The science-fiction movie *Gattaca* depicts a future in which parents routinely screen embryos for sex, height, immunity to disease, and even IQ. There is something troubling about the *Gattaca* scenario, but it is not easy to identify what exactly is wrong with screening embryos to choose the sex of our children.

One line of objection draws on arguments familiar from the abortion debate. Those who believe that an embryo is a person reject embryo screening for the same reasons they reject abortion. If an eight-cell embryo growing in a petri dish is morally equivalent to a fully developed human being, then discarding it is no better than aborting a fetus, and both practices are equivalent to infanticide. Whatever its merits, however, this "pro-life" objection is not an argument against sex selection as such.

The latest technology poses the question of sex selection unclouded by the matter of an embryo's moral status. The Genetics & IVF Institute, a for-profit infertility clinic in Fairfax, Virginia, now offers a sperm-sorting technique that makes it possible to choose the sex of one's child before it is conceived. X-bearing sperm, which produce girls, carry more DNA than Y-bearing sperm, which produce boys; a device called a flow cytometer can separate them. The process, called MicroSort, has a high rate of success.

If sex selection by sperm sorting is objectionable, it must be for reasons that go beyond the debate about the moral status of the embryo. One such reason is that sex selection is an instrument of sex discrimination—typically against girls, as illustrated by the chilling sex ratios in India and China. Some speculate that societies with substantially more men than women will be less stable, more violent, and more prone to crime or war. These are legitimate worries—but the sperm-sorting company has a clever way of addressing them. If offers MicroSort only to couples who want to choose the sex of a child for purposes of "family balancing." Those with more sons than daughters may choose a girl, and vice versa. But customers may not use the technology to stock up on children of the same sex, or even to choose the sex of their firstborn child. (So far the majority of MicroSort clients have chosen girls.) Under restrictions of this kind, do any ethical issues remain that should give us pause?

The case of MicroSort helps us isolate the moral objections that would persist if muscle-enhancement, memory-enhancement, and height-enhancement technologies were safe and available to all.

It is commonly said that genetic enhancements undermine our humanity by threatening our capacity to act freely, to succeed by our own efforts, and to consider ourselves responsible—worthy of praise or blame—for the things we do and for the way we are. It is one thing to hit seventy home runs as the result of disciplined training and effort, and something else, something less, to hit them with the help of steroids or genetically enhanced muscles. Of course, the roles of effort and enhancement will be a matter of degree. But as the role of enhancement increases, our admiration for the achievement fades—or, rather, our admiration for the achievement shifts from the player to his pharmacist. This suggests that our moral response to enhancement is a response to the diminished agency of the person whose achievement is enhanced.

Though there is much to be said for this argument, I do not think the main problem with enhancement and genetic engineering is that they undermine effort and erode human agency. The deeper danger is that they represent a kind of hyperagency—a Promethean aspiration to remake nature, including human nature, to serve our purposes and satisfy our desires. The problem is not the drift to mechanism but the drive to mastery. And what the drive to mastery misses and may even destroy is an appreciation of the gifted character of human powers and achievements.

To acknowledge the giftedness of life is to recognize that our talents and powers are not wholly our own doing, despite the effort we expend to develop and to exercise them. It is also to recognize that not everything in the world is open to whatever use we may desire or devise. Appreciating the gifted quality of life constrains the Promethean project and conduces to a certain humility. It is in part a religious sensibility. But its resonance reaches beyond religion.

It is difficult to account for what we admire about human activity and achievement without drawing upon some version of this idea. Consider two types of athletic achievement. We appreciate players like Pete Rose, who are not blessed with great natural gifts but who manage, through striving, grit, and determination, to excel in their sport. But we also admire players like Joe DiMaggio, who display natural gifts with grace and effortlessness. Now, suppose we learned that both players took performance-enhancing drugs. Whose turn to drugs would we find more deeply disillusioning? Which aspect of the athletic ideal—effort or gift—would be more deeply offended?

Some might say effort: the problem with drugs is that they provide a shortcut, a way to win without striving. But striving is not the point of sports; excellence is. And excellence consists at least partly in the display of natural talents and gifts that are no doing of the athlete who possesses them. This is an uncomfortable fact for democratic societies. We want to believe that success, in sports and in life, is something we earn, not something we inherit. Natural gifts, and the admiration they inspire, embarrass the meritocratic faith; they cast doubt on the conviction that praise and rewards flow from effort alone. In the face of this embarrassment we inflate the moral significance of striving, and depreciate giftedness. This distortion can be seen, for example, in network-television coverage of the Olympics, which focuses less on the feats the athletes perform than on heartrending stories of the hardships they have overcome and the struggles they have waged to triumph over an injury or a difficult upbringing or political turmoil in their native land.

But effort isn't everything. No one believes that a mediocre basketball player who works and trains even harder than Michael Jordan deserves greater acclaim or a bigger contract. The real problem with genetically altered athletes is that they corrupt athletic competition as a human activity that honors the cultivation and display of natural talents. From this standpoint, enhancement can be seen as the ultimate expression of the ethic of effort and willfulness—a kind of high-tech striving. The ethic of willfulness and the biotechnological powers it now enlists are arrayed against the claims of giftedness.

Bioengineering and genetic enhancement threaten to dislodge it. To appreciate children as gifts is to accept them as they come, not as objects of our design or products of our will or instruments of our ambition. Parental love is not contingent on the talents and attributes a child happens to have. We choose our friends and spouses at least partly on the basis of qualities we find attractive. But we do not choose our children. Their qualities are unpredictable, and even the most conscientious parents cannot be held wholly responsible for the kind of children they have. That is why parenthood, more than other human relationships, teaches what the theologian William F. May calls an "openness to the unbidden."

May's resonant phrase helps us see that the deepest moral objection to enhancement lies less in the perfection it seeks than in the human disposition it expresses and promotes. The problem is not that parents usurp the autonomy of a child they design. The problem lies in the hubris of the designing parents, in their drive to master the mystery of birth. Even if this disposition did not make parents tyrants to their children, it would disfigure the relation between parent and child, and deprive the parent of the humility and enlarged human sympathies that an openness to the unbidden can cultivate.

To appreciate children as gifts or blessings is not, of course, to be passive in the face of illness or disease. Medical intervention to cure or prevent illness or restore the injured to health does not desecrate nature but honors it. Healing sickness or injury does not override a child's natural capacities but permits them to flourish.

Nor does the sense of life as a gift mean that parents must shrink from shaping and directing the development of their child. Just as athletes and artists have an obligation to cultivate their talents, so parents have an obligation to cultivate their children, to help them discover and develop their talents and gifts. As May points out, parents give their children two kinds of love: accepting love and transforming love. Accepting love affirms the being of the child, whereas transforming love seeks the wellbeing of the child. Each aspect corrects the excesses of the other, he writes: "Attachment becomes too quietistic if it slackens into mere acceptance of the child as he is." Parents have a duty to promote their children's excellence.

These days, however, overly ambitious parents are prone to get carried away with transforming love—promoting and demanding all manner of accomplishments from their children, seeking perfection. "Parents find it difficult to maintain an equilibrium between the two sides of love," May observes. "Accepting love, without transforming love, slides into indulgence and finally neglect. Transforming love, without accepting love, badgers and finally rejects." May finds in these competing impulses a parallel with modern science: it, too, engages us in beholding the given world, studying and savoring it, and also in molding the world, transforming and perfecting it.

The mandate to mold our children, to cultivate and improve them, complicates the case against enhancement. We usually admire parents who seek the best for their children, who spare no effort to help them achieve happiness and success. Some parents confer advantages on their children by enrolling them in expensive schools, hiring private tutors, sending them to tennis camp, providing them with piano lessons, ballet lessons, swimming lessons, SAT-prep courses, and so on. If it is permissible and even admirable for parents to help their children in these ways, why isn't it equally admirable for parents to use whatever genetic technologies may emerge (provided they are safe) to enhance their children's intelligence, musical ability, or athletic prowess?

The defenders of enhancement are right to this extent: improving children through genetic engineering is similar in spirit to the heavily managed, high-pressure child-rearing that is now common. But this similarity does not vindicate genetic enhancement. On the contrary, it highlights a problem with the trend toward hyperparenting. One conspicuous example of this trend is sports-crazed parents bent on making champions of their children. Another is the frenzied drive of overbearing parents to mold and manage their children's academic careers.

As the pressure for performance increases, so does the need to help distractible children concentrate on the task at hand. This may be why diagnoses of attention deficit and hyperactivity disorder have increased so sharply. Lawrence Diller, a pediatrician and the author of *Running on Ritalin*, estimates that five to six percent of American children under eighteen (a total of four to five million kids) are currently prescribed Ritalin, Adderall, and other stimulants, the treatment of choice for ADHD. (Stimulants counteract hyperactivity by making it easier to focus and sustain attention.) The number of Ritalin prescriptions for children and adolescents has tripled over the past decade, but not all users suffer from attention disorders or hyperactivity. High school and college students have learned that prescription stimulants improve concentration for those with normal attention spans, and some buy or borrow their classmates' drugs to enhance their performance on the SAT or other exams. Since stimulants work for both medical and nonmedical purposes, they raise the same moral questions posed by other technologies of enhancement.

However those questions are resolved, the debate reveals the cultural distance we have traveled since the debate over marijuana, LSD, and other drugs a generation ago. Unlike the drugs of the 1960s and 1970s, Ritalin and Adderall are not for checking out but for buckling down, not for beholding the world and taking it in but for molding the world and fitting in. We used to speak of nonmedical drug use as "recreational." That term no longer applies. The steroids and stimulants that figure in the enhancement debate are not a source of recreation but a bid for compliance—a way of answering a competitive society's demand to improve our performance and perfect our nature. This demand for performance and perfection animates the impulse to rail against the given. It is the deepest source of the moral trouble with enhancement.

Some see a clear line between genetic enhancement and other ways that people seek improvement in their children and themselves. Genetic manipulation seems somehow worse—more intrusive, more sinister—than other ways of enhancing performance and seeking success. But morally speaking, the difference is less significant than it seems. Bioengineering gives us reason to question the low-tech, high-pressure child-rearing practices we commonly accept. The hyperparenting familiar in our time represents an anxious excess of mastery and dominion that misses the sense of life as a gift. This draws it disturbingly close to eugenics.

The shadow of eugenics hangs over today's debates about genetic engineering and enhancement. Critics of genetic engineering argue that human cloning, enhancement, and the quest for designer children are nothing more than "privatized" or "free-market" eugenics. Defenders of enhancement reply that genetic choices freely made are not really eugenic—at least not in the pejorative sense. To remove the coercion, they argue, is to remove the very thing that makes eugenic policies repugnant.

Sorting out the lesson of eugenics is another way of wrestling with the ethics of enhancement. The Nazis gave eugenics a bad name. But what, precisely, was wrong with it? Was the old eugenics objectionable only insofar as it was coercive? Or is there something inherently wrong with resolve to deliberately design our progeny's traits?

James Watson, the biologist who, with Francis Crick, discovered the structure of DNA, sees nothing wrong with genetic engineering and enhancement, provided they are freely chosen rather than state-imposed. And yet Watson's language contains more than a whiff of the old eugenic sensibility. "If you really are stupid, I would call that a disease," he recently told *The Times* of London. "The lower 10 percent who really have difficulty, even in elementary school, what's the cause of it? A lot of people would like to say, 'Well, poverty, things like that.' It probably isn't. So I'd like to get rid of that, to help the lower 10 percent." A few years ago Watson stirred controversy by saying that if a gene for homosexuality were discovered, a woman should be free to abort a fetus that carried it. When his remark provoked an uproar, he replied that he was not singling out gays but asserting a principle: women should be free to abort fetuses for any reason of genetic preference—for example, if the child would be dyslexic, or lacking musical talent, or too short to play basketball.

Watson's scenarios are clearly objectionable to those for whom all abortion is an unspeakable crime. But for those who do not subscribe to the pro-life position, these scenarios raise a hard question: If it is morally troubling to contemplate abortion to avoid a gay child or a dyslexic one, doesn't this suggest that something is wrong with acting on any eugenic preference, even when no state coercion is involved?

Consider the market in eggs and sperm. The advent of artificial insemination allows prospective parents to shop for gametes with the genetic traits they desire in their offspring. It is a less predictable way to design children than cloning or pre-implantation genetic screening, but it offers a good example of a procreative practice in which the old eugenics meets the new consumerism. A few years ago some Ivy League newspapers ran an ad seeking an egg from a woman who was at least five ten inches tall and athletic, had no major family medical problems, and had a combined SAT score of 1400 or above. The ad offered $50,000 for an egg from a donor with these traits. More recently a Web site was launched claiming to auction eggs from fashion models whose photos appeared on the site, at starting bids of $15,000 to $150,000.

On what grounds, if any, is the egg market morally objectionable? Since no one is forced to buy or sell, it cannot be wrong for reasons of coercion. Some might worry that hefty prices would exploit poor women by presenting them with an offer they couldn't refuse. But the designer eggs that fetch the highest prices are likely to be sought from the privileged, not the poor. If the market for premium eggs gives us moral qualms, this, too, shows that concerns about eugenics are not put to rest by freedom of choice.

A tale of two sperm banks helps explain why. The Repository for Germinal Choice, one of America's first sperm banks, was not a commercial enterprise. It was opened in 1980 by Robert Graham, a philanthropist dedicated to improving the world's "germ plasm" and counteracting the rise of "retrograde humans." His plan was to collect the sperm of Nobel Prize-winning scientists and make it available to women of high intelligence, in hopes of breeding supersmart babies. But Graham had trouble persuading Nobel laureates to donate their sperm for his bizarre scheme, and so settled for sperm from young scientists of high promise. His sperm bank closed in 1999.

In contrast, California Cryobank, one of the world's leading sperm banks, is a for-profit company with no overt eugenic mission. Cappy Rothman, M.D., a co-founder of the firm, has nothing but disdain for Graham's eugenics, although the standards Cryobank imposes on the sperm it recruits are exacting. Cryobank has offices in Cambridge, Massachusetts, between Harvard and MIT, and in Palo Alto, California, near Stanford. It advertises for donors in campus newspapers (compensation up to $900 a month), and accepts less than five percent of the men who apply. Cryobank's marketing materials play up the prestigious source of its sperm. Its catalogue provides detailed information about the physical characteristics of each donor, along with his ethnic origin and college major. For an extra fee prospective customers can buy the results of a test that assesses the donor's temperament and character type. Rothman reports that Cryobank's ideal sperm donor is six feet tall, with brown eyes, blond hair, and dimples, and has a college degree—not because the company wants to propagate those traits, but because those are the traits his customers want: "If our customers wanted high school dropouts, we would give them high school dropouts."

Not everyone objects to marketing sperm. But anyone who is troubled by the eugenic aspect of the Nobel Prize sperm bank should be equally troubled by Cryobank, consumer-driven though it be. What, after all, is the moral difference between designing children according to an explicit eugenic purpose and designing children according to the dictates of the market? Whether the aim is to improve humanity's "germ plasm" or to cater to consumer preferences, both practices are eugenic insofar as both make children into products of deliberate design.

A number of political philosophers call for a new "liberal eugenics." They argue that a moral distinction can be drawn between the old eugenic policies and genetic enhancements that do not restrict the autonomy of the child. "While old-fashioned authoritarian eugenicists sought to produce citizens out of a single centrally designed mould," writes Nicholas Agar, "the distinguishing mark of the new liberal eugenics is state neutrality." Government may not tell parents what sort of children to design, and parents may engineer in their children only those traits that improve their capacities without biasing their choice of life plans. A recent text on genetics and justice, written by the bioethicists Allen Buchanan, Dan W. Brock, Norman Daniels, and Daniel Wikler, offers a similar view. The "bad reputation of eugenics," they write, is due to practices

that "might be avoidable in a future eugenic program." The problem with the old eugenics was that its burdens fell disproportionately on the weak and the poor, who were unjustly sterilized and segregated. But provided that the benefits and burdens of genetic improvement are fairly distributed, these bioethicists argue, eugenic measures are unobjectionable and may even be morally required.

The libertarian philosopher Robert Nozick proposed a "genetic supermarket" that would enable parents to order children by design without imposing a single design on the society as a whole: "This supermarket system has the great virtue that it involves no centralized decision fixing the future human type (s)."

Even the leading philosopher of American liberalism, John Rawls, in his classic *A Theory of Justice* (1971), offered a brief endorsement of noncoercive eugenics. Even in a society that agrees to share the benefits and burdens of the genetic lottery, it is "in the interest of each to have greater natural assets," Rawls wrote. "This enables him to pursue a preferred plan of life." The parties to the social contract "want to insure for their descendants the best genetic endowment (assuming their own to be fixed)." Eugenic policies are therefore not only permissible but required as a matter of justice. "Thus over time a society is to take steps at least to preserve the general level of natural abilities and to prevent the diffusion of serious defects."

But removing the coercion does not vindicate eugenics. The problem with eugenics and genetic engineering is that they represent the one-sided triumph of willfulness over giftedness, of dominion over reverence, of molding over beholding. Why, we may wonder, should we worry about this triumph? Why not shake off our unease about genetic enhancement as so much superstition? What would be lost if biotechnology dissolved our sense of giftedness?

From a religious standpoint the answer is clear: To believe that our talents and powers are wholly our own doing is to misunderstand our place in creation, to confuse our role with God's. Religion is not the only source of reasons to care about giftedness, however. The moral stakes can also be described in secular terms. If bioengineering made the myth of the "self-made man" come true, it would be difficult to view our talents as gifts for which we are indebted, rather than as achievements for which we are responsible. This would transform three key features of our moral landscape: humility, responsibility, and solidarity.

In a social world that prizes mastery and control, parenthood is a school for humility. That we care deeply about our children and yet cannot choose the kind we want teaches parents to be open to the unbidden. Such openness is a disposition worth affirming, not only within families but in the wider world as well. It invites us to abide the unexpected, to live with dissonance, to rein in the impulse to control. A *Gattaca*-like world in which parents became accustomed to specifying the sex and genetic traits of their children would be a world inhospitable to the unbidden, a gated community writ large. The awareness that our talents and abilities are not wholly our own doing restrains our tendency toward hubris.

Though some maintain that genetic enhancement erodes human agency by overriding effort, the real problem is the explosion, not the erosion, of responsibility. As humility gives way, responsibility expands to daunting proportions. We attribute less to chance and more to choice. Parents become responsible for choosing, or failing to choose, the right traits for their children. Athletes become responsible for acquiring, or failing to acquire, the talents that will help their teams win.

One of the blessings of seeing ourselves as creatures of nature, God, or fortune is that we are not wholly responsible for the way we are. The more we become masters of our genetic endowments, the greater the burden we bear for the talents we have and the way we perform. Today when a basketball player misses a rebound, his coach can blame him for being out of position. Tomorrow the coach may blame him for being too short. Even now the use of performance-enhancing drugs in professional sports is subtly transforming the expectations players have for one another; on some teams players who take the field free from amphetamines or other stimulants are criticized for "playing naked."

The more alive we are to the chanced nature of our lot, the more reason we have to share our fate with others. Consider insurance. Since people do not know whether or when various ills will befall them, they pool their risk by buying health insurance and life insurance. As life plays itself out, the healthy wind up subsidizing the unhealthy, and those who live to a ripe old age wind up subsidizing the families of those who die before their time. Even without a sense of mutual obligation, people pool their risks and resources and share one another's fate.

But insurance markets mimic solidarity only insofar as people do not know or control their own risk factors. Suppose genetic testing advanced to the point where it could reliably predict each person's medical future and life expectancy. Those confident of good health and long life would opt out of the pool, causing other people's premiums to skyrocket. The solidarity of insurance would disappear as those with good genes fled the actuarial company of those with bad ones.

The fear that insurance companies would use genetic data to assess risks and set premiums recently led the Senate to vote to prohibit genetic discrimination in health insurance. But the bigger danger, admittedly more speculative, is that genetic enhancement, if routinely practiced, would make it harder to foster the moral sentiments that social solidarity requires.

Why, after all, do the successful owe anything to the least-advantaged members of society? The best answer to this question leans heavily on the notion of giftedness. The natural talents that enable the successful to flourish are not their own doing but, rather, their good fortune—a result of the genetic lottery. If our genetic endowments are gifts, rather than achievements for which we can claim credit, it is a mistake and a conceit to assume that we are entitled to the full measure of the bounty they reap in a market economy. We therefore have an obligation to share this bounty with those who, through no fault of their own, lack comparable gifts.

A lively sense of the contingency of our gifts—a consciousness that none of us is wholly responsible for his or her success—saves a meritocratic society from sliding into the smug assumption that the rich are rich because they are more deserving than the poor. Without this, the successful would become even more likely than they are now to view themselves as self-made and self-sufficient, and hence wholly responsible for their success. Those at the bottom of society would be viewed not as disadvantaged, and thus worthy of a measure of compensation, but as simply unfit, and thus worthy of eugenic repair. The meritocracy, less chastened by chance, would become harder, less forgiving. As perfect genetic knowledge would end the simulacrum of solidarity in insurance markets, so perfect genetic control would erode the actual solidarity that arises when men and women reflect on the contingency of their talents and fortunes.

Thirty-five years ago Robert L. Sinsheimer, a molecular biologist at the California Institute of Technology, glimpsed the shape of things to come. In an article titled "The Prospect of Designed Genetic Change" he argued that freedom of choice would vindicate the new genetics, and set it apart from the discredited eugenics of old.

> To implement the older eugenics . . . would have required a massive social programme carried out over many generations. Such a programme could not have been initiated without the consent and co-operation of a major fraction of the population, and would have been continuously subject to social control. In contrast, the new eugenics could, at least in principle, be implemented on a quite individual basis, in one generation, and subject to no existing restrictions.

According to Sinsheimer, the new eugenics would be voluntary rather than coerced, and also more humane. Rather than segregating and eliminating the unfit, it would improve them. "The old eugenics would have required a continual selection for breeding of the fit, and a culling of the unfit," he wrote. "The new eugenics would permit in principle the conversion of all the unfit to the highest genetic level."

Sinsheimer's paean to genetic engineering caught the heady, Promethean self-image of the age. He wrote hopefully of rescuing "the losers in that chromosomal lottery that so firmly channels our human destinies," including not only those born with genetic defects but also "the 50,000,000 'normal' Americans with an IQ of less than 90." But he also saw that something bigger than improving on nature's "mindless, age-old throw of dice" was at stake. Implicit in technologies of genetic intervention was a more exalted place for human beings in the cosmos. "As we enlarge man's freedom, we diminish his constraints and that which he must accept as given," he wrote. Copernicus and Darwin had "demoted man from his bright glory at the focal point of the universe," but the new biology would restore his central role. In the mirror of our genetic knowledge we would see ourselves as more than a link in the chain of evolution: "We can be the agent of transition to a whole new pitch of evolution. This is a cosmic event."

There is something appealing, even intoxicating, about a vision of human freedom unfettered by the given. It may even be the case that the allure of that vision played a part in summoning the genomic age into being. It is often assumed that the powers of enhancement we now possess arose as an inadvertent by-product of biomedical progress—the genetic revolution came, so to speak, to cure disease, and stayed to tempt us with the prospect of enhancing our performance, designing our children, and perfecting our nature. That may have the story backwards. It is more plausible to view genetic engineering as the ultimate expression of our resolve to see ourselves astride the world, the masters of our nature. But that promise of mastery is flawed. It threatens to banish our appreciation of life as a gift, and to leave us with nothing to affirm or behold outside our own will.

ANYONE FOR TENNIS, AT THE AGE OF 150?

Ronald Bailey

By the end of this century, the typical European may attend a family reunion in which five generations are playing together. Great-great-great grandma, at 150 years old, will be as vital, with muscle tone as firm and supple, skin as elastic and glowing, as her 30-year-old great-great-granddaughter with whom she's playing tennis.

After the game, while enjoying a plate of vegetables filled with not only a solid day's worth of nutrients but medicines she needs to repair damage to her ageing cells, she'll be able to chat about some academic discipline she studied in the 1980s with as much acuity and memory as her 50-year-old great-grandson, who is studying it now.

The younger members of her extended family will have never caught a cold. From birth they will have been immune to most of the shocks to which human flesh has long been heir, such as diabetes and Parkinson's disease. Her grandson, who recently suffered a car accident, will be sporting new versions of the arm and lung that got damaged in the wreck. He'll be playing a game of football as skilled and energetic as anyone else there.

Aids and Sars [sic] will be horrific historical curiosities for the family to chat about over their plates of superfat farm-raised salmon. Surrounding them will be a world that's greener and cleaner, more abundant in natural vegetation, with less of an obvious human footprint, than the one we live in today. It will be a remarkably peaceful and pleasant world even beyond their health and wealth—antisocial tendencies and crippling depression will all be managed by individual choice through biotech pharmaceuticals and even genetic treatments.

This idyll is more than realistic, given reasonably expected breakthroughs and extensions of our knowledge of human, plant and animal biology, as well as mastery of the manipulation of these biologies to meet our needs and desires.

Although you would think most people would devoutly wish for this vision, an extraordinary coalition of left-wing and right-wing bioconservatives is resisting the biotechnological progress that could make it real. Forget Osama bin Laden and the so-called clash of civilisations. The defining political conflict of the 21st century will literally be the battle over life and death.

On one side stand the partisans of mortality. From the Left, the bioethicist Daniel Callahan declares: "There is no known social good coming from the conquest of death." On the Right, stands Leon Kass, former head of George Bush's Council on Bioethics, who insists: "The finitude of human life is a blessing for every human individual, whether he knows it or not."

Such people counsel humanity quietly to accept our morbid fate and go gently into that good night, as we and our ancestors always have. For example, both Kass and Callahan persuaded President Bush to impose strict limits on human embryonic stem-cell research. Kass strongly favoured the proposed UN treaty that would have imposed a global ban on therapeutic cloning to produce stem cells. The treaty, which was almost approved by the General Assembly in 2004, would have outlawed therapeutic cloning research being done in the UK, which Kass denounced as having transgressed a "moral boundary".

Opposing this influential alliance of bioconservatives stands the party of life, whose champions include Aubrey de Grey, a theoretical biogerontologist at Cambridge University, who rage against the dying of the light and yearn to extend the enjoyment of healthy life to as many people as possible for as long as possible.

This conflict is brewing because the rapid progress in biotechnology will utterly transform human life by the end of this century. By the middle of this century humanity may see 20 to 40-year leaps in average life spans; human bodies and minds enhanced by advanced drugs and other biotherapies; the conquest of most infectious and degenerative dis-

This article first appeared in *The Times* newspaper on April 8, 2006. Reprinted by permission of Ronald Bailey.

eases; and genetic science that allows parent to ensure that their children will have stronger immune systems, more athletic bodies and cleverer brains. Even the possibility of human immortality beckons.

Researchers are making progress on figuring out why our bodies age and are discovering pathways to prevent it. Companies such as Elixir, based in Boston, are hot on the trail of compounds called sirtuins that retard ageing in simple organisms and which they believe will work for people, too. Other researchers are pursuing techniques to renew and replace the tiny cellular powerplants called mitochondria that most gerontologists think are the cause of the damage that leads to ageing.

Stem-cell researchers are getting ever closer to working out how to create perfect transplants to replace and restore damaged tissues and organs. The Geron Corporation, for example, plans later this year to begin experiments using human embryonic stem cells to repair broken spinal cords. Amazingly fast progress is being made using RNA interference, which is a technology that can selectively turn genes on and off in our bodies.

Researchers recently reported that they can turn off the genes for producing "bad" cholesterol in monkeys. If this works for humans, and there seem to be plenty of reasons to believe it will, it could slash heart disease rates.

Since 1978, more than one million babies have been born using assisted reproduction techniques.

More than 5,000 healthy children have been born using pre-implantation genetic diagnosis in which embryos were tested for specific disease genes before they were implanted in their mother's wombs. By the middle of this century, technologies such as artificial human chromosomes will enable parents to endow their children with genes for good health, strong bodies and sharp minds. Instead of submitting to the tyranny of nature's lottery, which cruelly blights futures with sickness, stunted mental abilities and early death, parents will be able to open more possibilities for their children to lead flourishing lives.

Beyond human biology the possibilities are immense too. Plants and animals genetically enhanced to resist drought, insects and disease and to provide higher yields and improved nutrition will enable humanity to produce more food, fibre and fuel on less than half the land currently used for agriculture, allowing huge swaths of Earth to revert to nature.

The highest expression of human nature and dignity is to strive to overcome the limitations imposed on us by our genes, our evolution and our environment. Future generations will look back at the beginning of the 21st century with astonishment that some well-meaning and intelligent people actually wanted to stop biomedical research just to protect their cramped and limited vision of human nature. Our descendants will look back, I predict, and thank us for making their world of longer, healthier lives possible.

FREE WILL AND RESPONSIBILITY

NEUROBIOLOGY, NEUROIMAGING, AND FREE WILL

Walter Glannon

INTRODUCTION

Advances in the theoretical and clinical neurosciences have shed considerable light on the neurobiological correlates of our thought and behavior. In particular, brain imaging in the form of computed tomography (CT), magnetic resonance imaging (MRI), positron emission tomography (PET), and functional magnetic resonance imaging (fMRI) can display the structure and function of the brain regions that regulate our capacity for impulse control, reasoning, and decision-making. PET and fMRI scans are especially significant because they can display real-time brain function by measuring changes

in glucose metabolism and blood flow in specific brain regions. These techniques can measure activity in the cerebral cortex while subjects are engaged in cognitive tasks. They can also measure activity in subcortical areas associated with emotions when subjects are shown photos of people or events.

Although our motivational states may not be reducible to, or explained entirely in terms of, the physical properties of the brain, they are generated and sustained by the brain. Neuroimaging can reveal much of what goes on in the brain when we reason, choose, and act. It can also reveal neurobiological abnormalities that might explain impairment in the capacity to respond to prudential and moral reasons, form intentions, and execute intentions in decisions and actions. Insofar as this capacity is necessary for one to control one's behavior, and control of one's behavior is necessary for one to have free will and be responsible for what one does or fails to do, brain imaging may be a helpful tool in determining whether persons have free will and can be held morally and legally responsible for their

From Walter Glannon, "Neurobiology, Neuroimaging, and Free Will," *Midwest Studies in Philosophy* 29 (2005): 68–82, Blackwell Publishers.

Editors' note: Some author's notes have been cut. Students who want to read the article in its entirety should consult the original.

behavior. Depending on what imaging techniques show about the brain, and how we interpret these images, they could influence moral and legal judgments about culpability, blame, and excuse.

I will explore possible uses and examine actual uses of diagnostic brain imaging in cases where individuals have committed violent offenses or have been accused of culpable omissions. This will include discussion of whether structural or functional abnormalities in regions of the brain that regulate our ability to reason, choose, and act can excuse individuals with these abnormalities from responsibility for their actions. I will pay particular attention to what images of the brain might tell us about how much control people have over their thought and behavior, discussing whether empirical data from diagnostic neuroimaging could influence traditional criteria of free will and responsibility and lead to a better understanding of these concepts.

TRADITIONAL ACCOUNTS

Much of the historical and contemporary debate on free will has centered on the idea of alternative possibilities. Incompatibilists argue that free will requires the ability to do otherwise, which requires that alternative possible courses of choice and action be open to us. These alternative possibilities are incompatible with causal determinism, which says that laws of nature and events in the past jointly entail a unique future. This means that any action one performs at a particular time is the only action one could have performed at that time. But our deep-seated conviction that we are the ultimate authors of our actions who act freely in virtue of our ability to choose among alternative courses of action suggests that causal determinism is false. This is the libertarian version of incompatibilism, as distinct from the hard incompatibilist view we do not have free will because causal determinism is true. In contrast, compatibilists argue that free will does not require traditionally conceived alternative possibilities of choice and action. They generally hold that one acts freely and responsibly when one chooses and acts in accord with one's autonomous motivational states in the absence of coercion or compulsion. These motivational states are autonomous in

the sense that one generates them on one's own and identifies with them after a period of critical reflection. Any alternative possibilities are internal rather than external to the agent. They are a function of different combinations of an agent's desires, beliefs, intentions, decisions, and the different actions to which they can lead, not of states of affairs that an agent can only actualize in accord with natural laws and the past. In this regard, causal determinism is compatible with free will and responsibility.

This conception of free will is consistent with the evolutionary account of freedom recently defended by Daniel Dennett.[1] He claims that, as humans evolved, they developed the ability to speculate about the future, to consider possible threats that jeopardize their interests and plans, and to choose and act in ways that enable them to avoid these threats. The human brain has developed in a way that supports this mental ability. Dennett calls this "evitability," and it confers an evolutionary advantage on humans by promoting and enhancing their survival. This account is compatible with causal determinism because it says that the ability to plan, choose, and act in different ways is not threatened by laws of nature and events in the past.

The weaker, compatibilist account of free will that I have just outlined can be traced to Aristotle. In the *Nicomachean Ethics*, Aristotle presents the default assumption that a person acts freely (voluntarily) and is responsible for his behavior barring evidence of compulsion, coercion, or ignorance of the circumstances of action.[2] The first two of these conditions can be described as metaphysical, or freedom-relevant, conditions, while the third can be described as an epistemic, or knowledge-relevant, condition. On the Aristotelian model, free will in the broad sense requires that all of these negative

---

1. *Freedom Evolves* (New York: Viking, 2003). This work follows Dennett's earlier defense of compatibilism in *Elbow Room: The Varieties of Free Will Worth Wanting* (Cambridge, MA: MIT Press, 1984).

2. *The Complete Works of Aristotle*, Volume II, Book III, J. Barnes, trans. and ed. (Princeton: Princeton University Press, 1984). H. L. A. Hart proposes a similar default position in *Punishment and Responsibility* (Oxford: Clarendon Press, 1968).

conditions be met. Each condition is necessary but not sufficient; all of them are jointly necessary and sufficient for the freedom of thought and action required for one to be responsible. A more recent model formulates free will and responsibility in positive terms as the capacity to respond to reasons for or against certain actions. The reasons are not just prudential but also moral, in the sense that they involve social expectations about what we should or should not do in performing actions that can affect others. The idea of reasons-responsiveness as a necessary condition of free will and responsibility can be plausibly construed as an extension of Aristotle's account. This is because the capacity to respond appropriately to reasons presupposes the capacity for appropriate beliefs about the circumstances of action. It also presupposes the capacity to have or form desires, beliefs, and emotions, and to execute these motivational states by acting in an uncoerced and uncompelled way.

These conative, cognitive, and affective capacities are all necessary for one to be responsible for one's behavior. A person can be excused from responsibility for his behavior when any one of the three conditions—coercion, compulsion, ignorance—described by Aristotle is present. It is important to emphasize that I am describing a capacity-theoretic conception of free will and responsibility. It requires only that persons have the relevant mental capacities, not that they exercise them in every instance. Moreover, some people possess these capacities in varying degrees, suggesting that free will and responsibility may be matters of degree falling along a spectrum of control. The Aristotelian model can be helpful in framing the general question of whether individuals with abnormal brain features have impaired capacity for control of thought and behavior. This in turn will help to address the question of how free they are in acting and how responsible they can be for what they do or fail to do. Framed in this way, free will is not about causal determinism but rather the relation between the mind and the brain. I will present hypothetical and actual cases to generate intuitions about free will with respect to impulse control, psychopathy, and memory. The first set of cases can be framed in terms of the Aristotelian metaphysical condition, while the last case can be framed in terms of the Aristotelian epistemic condition. Analysis of some forms of diagnostic brain imaging can test our intuitions about what it means to be free and responsible agents.

IMPULSE CONTROL, PSYCHOPATHY, AND FORGETTING

Suppose that one person kills another in a fit of rage and is charged with second-degree murder. The offender claims that his action resulted from a violent impulse he could not control. Prosecution and defense agree that a brain scan could test the veracity of this claim. He agrees to undergo a PET scan, which shows abnormally low metabolic activity in the prefrontal cortex and abnormally high metabolic activity in the amygdala. The prefrontal cortex is the seat of executive functions and is crucial for rational planning and impulse control. The amygdala is the seat of emotional processing in the limbic system, which projects to the prefrontal cortex and interacts with it in modulating executive functions. The offender and his lawyer argue that his brain abnormality undermined his capacity for moral reasoning and impulse control at the time of the crime. To be morally and legally responsible for one's behavior, one must have the capacity to control that behavior, which includes the capacity to respond appropriately to reasons and to restrain impulses. Because the brain scan indicates that he lacked this capacity when he acted, he could not be responsible for killing his victim. He lacked free will and therefore should be excused on the basis of his brain abnormality.

Or suppose that a different person performs a similar act. His act does not result from a violent, uncontrolled impulse, but instead from lack of empathy for his victim and an inability to act in accord with social norms of behavior. An MRI scan shows reduced amygdaloid volume, a feature that has been associated with psychopathy, a disorder characterized by diminished or no capacity for empathy and remorse, as well as poor behavior controls. This individual also argues that his brain abnormality and associated psychopathy are beyond his control and that he too lacked free will when he acted. Accordingly, he should be excused from responsibility for his action.

Would either of these defenses hold up in a court of law? How do these cases test our intuitions about free will and responsibility for our motivational states and actions? To respond to these questions, we need to consider what neuroimaging studies indicate about the neurobiological basis of thought and behavior. Although it is not always clear why certain brain structures and systems are dysfunctional, brain imaging may yield important insights into explaining why dysfunction at the neural level can lead to disturbances at the mental and behavioral level.

Neuroimaging studies of violent offenders conducted by Adrian Raine and Richard Davidson have shown hyperactivity in the amygdala and diminished activity in the prefrontal cortex when compared with images of the same brain regions of normal subjects.[3] In contrast, brain images of individuals who display psychopathic behavior have shown a smaller and less active amygdala. Some images of psychopaths have shown intact functioning of the prefrontal cortex. Others have shown contrary indications. For example, Antonio Damasio and colleagues have found that lesions in the orbitofrontal cortex (OFC) correlate with impulsive and antisocial behavior.[4] Despite appearing cognitively intact, individuals with damage in this region of the brain seem unable to conform to social norms when they act. Adults and children who sustained this damage presented with a syndrome resembling psychopathy. More recently, R. J. R. Blair has obtained similar results from imaging studies on a similar

group of subjects.[5] Because the OFC receives extensive projections from and sends extensive projections to the amygdala, this might explain why the emotional deficiency of psychopaths impairs their ability to deliberate about and rationally choose between different possible courses of action. This ability is not simply one of cognition alone, but of cognition and emotion working together. In particular, the emotion of regret is critical to this counterfactual reasoning and is strongly associated with the feeling of responsibility. The OFC appears to be at the interface of emotion and cognition, mediating our capacity to experience regret and responsibility. Damage to the OFC can impair or undermine this combined emotional-cognitive capacity, thus suggesting that people with orbitofrontal cortical lesions might not be able to control their behavior and be morally and legally responsible for it.

Damage to the ventromedial frontal cortex can result in a similar type of psychopathology. Neuroimaging showing reduced metabolic activity in this region of the cortex, together with hyperactivity in the anterior cingulate (a subcortical structure in the limbic system), has been observed in a class of individuals displaying inappropriate social behavior and blunted responses to tear-inducing stimuli. Because of its interaction with the anterior cingulate, the ventromedial cortex regulates the emotions that color decision-making. This was the main brain area implicated in the well-known case of Phineas Gage. A metal projectile penetrated Gage's skull and resulted in extensive damage to the ventromedial cortex of his brain as a consequence of an explosion during construction on the Rutland & Burlington Railroad in Vermont in 1848. Gage lost

---

3. Adrian Raine et al., "Reduced Prefrontal Gray Matter Volume and Reduced Autonomic Activity in Antisocial Personality Disorder," *Archives of General Psychiatry* 57 (2002): 119–27. Richard Davidson et al., "Dysfunction in the Neural Circuitry of Emotion Regulation—A Possible Prelude to Violence," *Science* 289 (2000): 591–94.

4. A. Damasio, H. Damasio, S. Anderson et al., "Impairment of Social and Moral Behavior Related to Early Damage in Human Prefrontal Cortex," *Nature Neuroscience* 2 (1999): 1032–37. See also R. J. Dolan, "On the Neurology of Morals," *Nature Neuroscience* 2 (1999): 927–29, Joshua Greene et al., "The Neural Bases of Cognitive Conflict and Control in Moral Judgment," *Neuron* 44 (2004): 389–400, and Ekhonen Goldberg, *The Executive Brain: Frontal Lobes and the Civilized Mind* (New York: Oxford University Press, 2002).

5. R. J. R. Blair and L. Cipolotti, "Impaired Social Response Reversal: A Case of 'Acquired Sociopathy'," *Brain* 123 (2002): 1122–41, Blair, "Neurobiological Basis of Psychopathy," *British Journal of Psychiatry* 182 (2003): 5–7, and K. A. Kiel et al., "Limbic Abnormalities in Affective Processing by Criminal Psychopaths as Revealed by Functional Magnetic Resonance Imaging," *Biological Psychiatry* 50 (2001): 677–84. These disorders fall within a larger general framework of mental illness. Dennis Charney and Eric Nestler (eds.) provide such a framework in *Neurobiology of Mental Illness*, second edition (Oxford: Oxford University Press, 2004), as does the *Diagnostic and Statistical Manual of Mental Disorders*, fourth edition, Text Revision—DSM-IV-TR (Washington, D.C.: American Psychiatric Association, 2000).

his capacity to restrain his impulses, conform to social norms of behavior, and rationally deliberate and plan for the future. Because factors beyond his control caused him to lose this capacity, and hence his ability to control his behavior, one could say that he no longer had free will. The neurobiological basis of his decision-making was so damaged, and his mental capacity for making decisions was so flawed, that he was no longer able to function effectively as a social being.

Imaging studies of people with obsessive-compulsive disorder (OCD) suggest similar judgments about free will and responsibility for people with severe forms of this disorder. Studies using fMRI of people with OCD have shown reduced metabolic activity in the ventromedial cortex and increased activity in subcortical motor regions. These are manifestations of dysfunction in the orbitofrontal-subcortical circuit, whose member structures include the OFC, the caudate nucleus, globus pallidus, and thalamus, which plays a critical role in the processing of sensory input. People with OCD feel that they must do certain things, or that they must think certain thoughts, though they claim that they do not want to have these feelings and thoughts and often desperately try to fight them. One hypothesis for the disorder is that a "worry input" in the frontal lobes projects to the basal ganglia via the ventromedial cortex. The ganglia's reduced filter function impairs the sensory filtering function of the thalamus, producing abnormal sensory processing that disrupts other brain systems. Another hypothesis is that the obsessions and compulsions are due to a dysfunctional cingulate, which disrupts normal cognitive and emotional processing. This is the rationale for the psychosurgical procedure of cingulotomy to treat severe OCD. It involves altering the main pathway between the limbic system and the prefrontal cortex. The more general upshot is that, in severe cases at least, OCD impairs the cognitive and emotional processing necessary for one to choose and act freely.

All of the examples that I have presented thus far about impairment or loss of behavior control involve dysfunctional brain systems that previously functioned in a normal way. An argument for a lack of control of thought and behavior could also be given on the basis of immature development of the relevant structures and functions in the adolescent brain. In October 2004, the United States Supreme

Court began reviewing the case of Christopher Simmons (*Roper v. Simmons*). At 17, Simmons and a friend robbed a woman, tied her up with an electrical cable and duct tape, and then threw her over a bridge to her death. Simmons was convicted of first-degree murder and sentenced to death by a Missouri court in 1994. But the Missouri Supreme Court dropped the death sentence in 2003, resentencing him to life in prison without parole. The state of Missouri then appealed to have the death penalty reinstated. In March 2005, the U.S. Supreme Court ruled that it is unconstitutional to impose the death penalty on individuals like Simmons who were under 18 at the time of their crimes.

The main argument against execution in this case is that, when Simmons committed the crime, the frontal lobe of his brain was not yet mature. Presumably, this made him incapable of rational and moral decision-making and unable to restrain his impulse to kill. Because the frontal lobe is critical to the executive functions necessary to control thought and behavior, and because Simmons' frontal lobe was not yet fully developed, Simmons arguably was not capable of controlling his behavior and therefore was not responsible for his crime. This would seem to be enough to excuse him and overturn his conviction. MRI scans of children's and adolescents' brains show that the frontal lobe develops last of all brain regions and does not fully mature until around 21 years of age. Imaging studies involving these two groups generally indicate that different regions in a child's or adolescent's brain operate in a more localized way, with more activity in limbic areas associated with emotions such as fear and anger and less activity in the neocortex associate with reasoning. In contrast, adults have more distributed and collaborative interactions among different brain regions. While these interactions in the adult brain promote greater impulse control, the absence or immature development of these interactions makes impulse control more difficult for children and adolescents. Another explanation for the difference in the capacity for impulse and general behavior control between these age groups is that adults have more experience confronting situations requiring rational deliberation and decision-making. This enables them to cultivate strategies of choice and action that promote their short- and long-term best interests.

Consider now a case involving memory lapse that could meet the Aristotelian epistemic condition of excuse.[6] Carrie Engholm was a hospital administrator. She drove to work one morning with her young son and daughter in the back of her van. She was not accustomed to taking her daughter with her in the morning, however, and after dropping off her son at day care drove to work, forgetting that her daughter was in the van. She unwittingly left her in the van in the outdoor hospital parking lot on an extremely hot day while she worked. Unfortunately, her daughter was found dead from hyperthermia later that day.

Was Carrie responsible for not remembering? Was she responsible for not paying attention to events that day and for forgetting about her daughter? Initially charged with recklessness and brought to court, the judge ruled that she was not guilty, reasoning that forgetting is an involuntary process. But suppose that she had been charged with negligence or recklessness and was convicted for failing to exercise her capacity to remember. The hippocampus, which is part of the limbic system, is essential for the retrieval of episodic memory. This involves the ability to recall events we have experienced and is distinct from semantic memory of facts and procedural memory of motor functions such as riding a bicycle or driving a car. Functional MRI scans can show that a particular region of the hippocampus, the parahippocampal gyrus, is activated when people are asked to recall certain events. Damage to this region could impair one's ability to recall having done certain things, such as leaving a child in a car. In principle, damage to Carrie Engholm's parahippocampal gyrus, displayed in an fMRI image showing significantly reduced metabolic activity in and

blood flow to this part of the brain, could excuse her from any charge of responsibility or liability for her daughter's death. On the basis of this brain scan, one could argue that she lacked the capacity to recall the crucial event of leaving her daughter in the car.

In all of these cases, structural and functional abnormalities in the frontal lobe or limbic system, or immature development of these brain regions, can impair or even undermine the capacity for reasoning and decision-making. If this capacity is essential to control one's thought and behavior, and if the brain abnormalities I have described impair or undermine this capacity, then it appears that the individuals in the cases I have presented lack this control. Furthermore, if control of one's thought and behavior is necessary for one to have free will and be responsible for what one does or fails to do, then presumably neuroimaging showing these abnormalities suggests that these individuals lack free will and cannot be responsible for their actions or omissions. The impulsive or immoral actions of a violent offender or psychopath, the compulsive behavior of a person with OCD, and the memory lapse of someone like Carrie Engholm would appear to meet Aristotle's metaphysical and epistemic excusing conditions. CT, PET, MRI, or fMRI scans showing structural and functional brain abnormalities correlating with these disorders would appear to confirm that their lack of control of their mental states, actions, and omissions, and hence their lack of free will, was due to something that had gone awry in their brains.

There are problems with these arguments, though. A structural or functional abnormality in, or immature development of, the prefrontal cortex, amygdala, or hippocampus by itself does not necessarily mean that individuals with these brain features lack or have impaired capacity for cognitive, conative, and affective control of their behavior. Images showing abnormalities in regions of the brain that subserve our desires, beliefs, reasons, intentions, decisions, and actions may serve to mitigate responsibility in some cases. But it is more difficult to defend the claim that brain imaging can show that individuals lack free will altogether and should be excused from responsibility for their behavior. In many cases, brain dysfunction alone will not explain violent or otherwise socially inappropriate behavior.

---

6. Here I closely follow Daniel Schacter's account of the Carrie Engholm case in his testimony before the President's Commission on Bioethics, Seventh Meeting, October 17, 2002, Session 3: *Remembering and Forgetting: Physiological and Pharmacological Aspects.* Transcript: 1–40, at 14–15. From http://www.bioethics.gov/transcripts/oct02/session3.html.

See also Schacter, *Searching for Memory: The Brain, the Mind, and the Past* (New York: Basic Books, 1996), and Endel Tulving and Martin Lepage, "Where in the Brain Is the Awareness of One's Past?" in Daniel Schacter and Elaine Scarry, eds., *Memory, Brain and Belief* (Cambridge, MA: Harvard University Press, 2000): 208–28.

If this is correct, then neuroimaging showing brain abnormalities by itself will not be sufficient to conclude that an individual could not control his motivational states and actions, lacked free will, and therefore could not be responsible for them. Let's now consider the shortcomings of brain imaging with respect to our understanding of free will. This will lead to a more realistic view of how useful brain scans might be in influencing our moral and legal practices of holding people responsible.

THE LIMITS OF NEUROIMAGING

Free will is often not an all-or-nothing capacity. Instead, it is a capacity that comes in degrees along a spectrum of control. At one end of the spectrum, persons are in complete control of their motivational states and actions and are completely responsible for what they do or fail to do. At the other end of the spectrum, persons have no control over their motivational states and actions and should be excused from responsibility for what they do or fail to do. But many cases of criminal or immoral behavior fall in a gray area between the two extremes. Just as there are degrees of the ability to restrain impulses or to respond to reasons when acting, there are degrees of control of behavior and of responsibility for it. Different people may possess the cognitive, affective, and conative capacities that lead to action in varying degrees.

There are no obvious problems in holding people responsible or excusing them at either end of the spectrum. When there are no abnormalities in neural processing, Aristotle's metaphysical and epistemic default conditions of voluntary action can be met, and we can safely assume that one can control one's mental states and behavior. When there are severe neurobiological abnormalities resulting in severely impaired executive functions, they would fail to meet the default conditions and provide strong reasons for saying that one could not control one's behavior. For example, the claim that a schizophrenic with full-blown psychosis and severe impairment of cognitive, affective, and conative capacities lacks control of his or her behavior would be supported when these mental impairments correlate with structural and functional abnormalities in the basal ganglia, prefrontal cortex, and hippocampus—regions of

the brain that ordinarily regulate these mental capacities. A similar claim could be supported in the case of a person with severe OCD. The question of what these two conditions imply about behavior control could be analyzed by comparing brain scans of individuals with these conditions with scans of individuals with no impairment of mental capacity and normal brain structure and function.

Still, the hard cases are those that fall between the two extremes. An adolescent or adult with attention deficit/hyperactivity disorder (ADHD) may have difficulty controlling his impulses and attending to cognitive tasks. These behavioral features may correspond to neuroimaging showing abnormally high levels of the neurotransmitter dopamine in the cerebellum and temporal lobes, which are indicators of the disorder. But there can be considerable variation in the behavior of different people with the same disorder. It is not clear that these differences will be solely a function of subtle differences in the activity of neurons and neurotransmitters in the relevant brain regions. Nor will they alone tell us whether or to what extent someone with the disorder can execute his reasons, intentions, and decisions in the actions he wants to perform, or whether or to what extent he can be responsible for them.

Recall Christopher Simmons. The fact that an MRI scan showed that the frontal lobe regulating his executive functions was incompletely developed by itself could not explain why Simmons committed murder. His immature brain would not be enough to excuse him from moral and legal responsibility for his action. If all adolescents have immature frontal lobes, but not all adolescents commit violent acts, then saying that Simmons' frontal lobe was not fully developed when he committed the crime does not offer a convincing reason to excuse him. If a comparison between Simmons' brain at seventeen and the brains of many others of the same age could be made, then there might be some basis on which to argue that he lacked the capacity to control his impulse to kill and respond to reasons against killing. But the data required for a meaningful comparison could only be derived from longitudinal imaging studies involving a large number of subjects. These studies have not yet been conducted, and thus the data are not yet available. In the light of this, it is unclear to what extent images of Simmons' frontal lobe taken at age seventeen could help the Supreme Court Justices to decide whether or not he had the capacity to control his behavior at the time of his crime. Unless we could conclusively show how much frontal lobe volume and function are necessary for any person to control his behavior, it is unclear to what extent brain imaging could help to answer the legal question of Simmons' culpability.

In psychopaths, a significant reduction in the volume of the amygdala, perhaps due to a congenital malformation, might explain their blunted emotional response to other people or to fear-inducing stimuli. This could lead one to conclude that an individual displaying psychopathic characteristics was unable to empathize with others, conform to social norms, or have any understanding of how others could be harmed by his actions. But some researchers have suggested that psychopaths may have at least some understanding of what it means to harm others. This understanding could be enough to influence their motivational states and provide some restraint on their irrational, immoral, or criminal behavior. So we could distinguish between individuals who cannot empathize with others and act in accord with social norms, and those who have the capacity to do this but have difficulty and fail to exercise it. It is not obvious that brain scans showing subtle differences in the volume of and metabolic activity in the amygdala, OFC, or anterior cingulate gyrus of two people will explain why one person does and the other does not respond appropriately to moral reasons. It will not explain why one person refrains from and the other engages in behavior that harms others. Nor is it obvious that differences in the brain images of two individuals performing the same type of action would justify mitigated responsibility in one case and exoneration in the other.

A person's ability to consciously form desires, beliefs, reasons, and intentions and to execute, or refrain from executing, them in action is influenced by the brain, which generates and sustains these mental states. But this ability can be influenced by factors in the social and natural environment as well. Social expectations can color our perception of the choices and actions that are open to us, and factors in the physical space in which we live can limit the availability of options that we can pursue. In addition, some people may put more mental effort into exercising their capacity to control their behavior.

Just because one displays weakness of will in acting against one's all-things-considered better judgment does not mean that one lacks free will altogether. Also, brain scans cannot account for the phenomenology of free will, or why we *feel* in control (or out of control) of our actions. This feeling too can influence one's perception of the alternative courses of action that are open to one and which actions one performs.

Many people with brain damage or incompletely developed brains are not violent and do not display psychopathic behavior. So it is implausible to claim that structural or functional brain abnormalities detected by brain scans always cause these types of behavior. Except perhaps for cases of severe damage to regions of the brain directly regulating the capacity for rational and moral deliberation and choice, how much control one has of one's behavior, and whether or to what extent one is responsible for it, will not be determined by measuring brain structure or function alone.

Regions other than the OFC may play a role in the cognitive processing that subserves reasoning and decision-making. Focusing on this region alone may be an oversimplified way of explaining the link between the brain and behavior. An abnormality in this region would not necessarily mean that the balance between cognitive and emotional processing had been entirely disrupted. The parietal cortex, which regulates our orientation in space and time, may also play a role in maintaining this balance. Moreover, the cerebellum, which lies below the cortex and ordinarily regulates physical balance and coordination, may also play a role in coordinating thought and behavior. Reasoning and executive functions depend on complex neural systems distributed across multiple regions of the cortex, and these functions may also depend on subcortical regions. There are strong links between the executive center in the prefrontal cortex and the parietal cortex, as well as links between these regions and the cingulate gyrus in the limbic system and the cerebellum and basal ganglia in the motor system.

It is thus misleading to think that the ability or inability to control behavior is always confined to the frontal lobe. Contrary to commonsense intuitions, there is no single locus of free will in the brain. Dysfunction in one brain region that subserves mental processes associated with choice and action does not necessarily imply that other regions are also dysfunctional, or that one regional dysfunction alone will adversely affect these mental processes. There are redundancies in the brain. Some systems can compensate for others that have been damaged or incompletely formed and can perform the same tasks associated with these other systems. This is one example of brain plasticity, the ability of nerve cells to modify their activity in response to changes in the body, brain, or external environment. Indeed, in some cases plasticity occurs to such a degree that a person's capacity to control thought and behavior can remain largely intact despite extensive damage to brain regions that ordinarily underlie that capacity.

Neuropsychiatrist Todd Feinberg describes the case of a patient to illustrate this point.[7] "Sonia" was a thirty-two-year-old secretary who was referred for a neurological exam because of mild paranoia but no significant cognitive deficit. Although her neurological exam was normal, Feinberg noticed that her head was unusually large and ordered a CT scan. Surprisingly, the scan showed that more than three-quarters of her cerebral cortex was missing. All that remained was a band of cortex around the outside of her brain. Her fluid-filled ventricles were abnormally large, a condition known as hydrocephalus. When this condition develops suddenly in an adult and is not surgically corrected, the patient can go into a coma. As Feinberg explains, "Sonia" most likely survived with so many of her mental functions intact because her condition was present from birth and her nervous system was able to accommodate itself to the increased intracranial pressure.[8] Because of its plasticity, this patient's brain was remarkably able to adjust to extensive damage that otherwise would have severely impaired her mental capacities. This example shows that a brain scan indicating extensive damage to regions of the brain underlying many of a person's mental states does not prove that such a person cannot control her behavior.

Let's consider neuroimaging in the context of the epistemic condition of free will and responsibility by returning to the case of Carrie Engholm. Earlier, we asked whether a brain scan of her hippocampus

could have answered the question of whether she was able but failed to retrieve her memory of leaving her daughter in the overheated van. There are several complicating factors that make the question much less straightforward than it might appear at first blush.

One function of the anterior cingulate is to monitor cognitive conflicts. Carrie quite possibly was suffering from information overload when she parked her van, with too many cognitive tasks to plan and execute. This could have affected the hippocampus and led to a temporary retrieval block of her episodic memory of putting her daughter in the van. In fact, this block might have been due to dysfunction in either the anterior cingulate or neocortex, both of which play a critical role together with the hippocampus in the retrieval of episodic memory. Nevertheless, a scan of these regions would not be very helpful after the fact, since most likely they would not show the same degree of metabolic activity as when she had the memory lapse. Moreover, it is unlikely that an imaging device showing increased or decreased activity in these regions would be able to tell us whether she could or could not retrieve the memory, or whether she was not even able to form and store a memory of the event. This is also one reason why brain imaging would not be able to separate "true" from "false" memories in the debate on recovered memories that has figured prominently in cases involving charges of rape and incest. Perhaps most important, data that would allow one to draw these crucial distinctions would only be available from group studies. One would have to average data derived from brain imaging across many people before a particular image, or set of images, for a person could have any statistical significance. As brain imaging techniques become more accurate, and databases of patient populations are formed, neuroimaging may eventually be able to help in ascertaining whether one could have but failed to remember an event, thereby causing harm, and could be responsible for the omission. But presently the technology cannot show definitively whether one can or cannot form and store a memory of an event, or whether one can or cannot retrieve a memory that has been formed and stored in the brain.

To convincingly argue that a person had no control over mental states leading to action because of a brain abnormality, one would have to establish

---

7. *Altered Egos: How the Brain Creates the Self* (New York: Oxford University Press, 2001), 103.

8. Ibid., 104.

a causal relationship between the abnormality and the mental states. Brain scans can show correlations between behavior and its underlying neurobiological basis. But *correlation* falls short of *causation*, which is why neuroimaging is limited in assessing whether people have free will and can be responsible for their thoughts and actions. Another reason for this limitation is that brain-imaging data can measure only the statistical likelihood of violent, psychopathic, or otherwise culpable behavior over a population. It cannot predict how an individual will behave in any given situation. What further complicates this problem is that brain-based measures of mental properties have an illusory accuracy and objectivity. A PET or fMRI scan showing abnormalities in regions of the brain is not necessarily diagnostic of an inability to control behavior. This is because the activity can be modulated by the experimental tasks used by the researcher to mimic actual functions of the scanner. There is also the potential for bias in the design of structural or functional imaging of brain-damaged patients, which can influence how data from these experiments is analyzed.

If this bias could be eliminated from neuroimaging, and real-time imaging techniques could be further refined, then we might have a more accurate picture of how the brain influences behavior. But as cognitive neuroscientist Martha Farah points out, "for now, however, this is not the case, and there is the risk that juries, judges, parole boards, the immigration service and so on will weigh such measures too heavily in their decision-making."[9] There is, then, considerable potential for abuse of information derived from brain scans. This could result in the violation of the privacy and confidentiality of sensitive information about people's brains and considerable harm to those who undergo these scans.

Even if neuroimaging were perfected to accurately measure the neural processes associated with our motivational states and actions, it would not directly translate into simple answers to normative questions such as whether or to what degree people can be responsible for their behavior. These judgments will always be influenced by social norms. This point follows from what may be the strongest reason for questioning the use of neuroimaging to make ethical or legal judgments about people's behavior. It would involve moving from empirical claims about the brain to normative claims about how people ought to behave. Free will and responsibility are not fundamentally empirical but normative notions reflecting social conventions and expectations about how people can or should act. Although our understanding of free will and responsibility will undoubtedly become better informed by brain science, normative claims and judgments cannot be reduced to empirical ones. Ultimately, it is not neuroscientists but society that will decide how empirical information about the brain influences our judgments about what constitutes free will and when people can be held responsible for what they do or fail to do. Morality is not just a function of neurobiology.

CONCLUSION

In the future, more sophisticated, higher-resolution, real-time brain scans may enable researchers to identify the precise features of the brain that regulate executive functions such as reasoning and decision-making. Moreover, they may enable researchers to distinguish between true and false memories, to determine when people can form and retrieve memories, and when people are lying or telling the truth. Ideally, the combination of this technology and established clinical criteria will contribute to a clearer understanding of free will and the difference between full responsibility, mitigation, and excuse. If brain scans could enable us to move from a correlation to a causal connection between the brain and the mind, then

9. "Emerging Ethical Issues in Neuroscience," *Nature Neuroscience* 5 (2002): 1127. See also Martha Farah and Paul Root Wolpe, "Monitoring and Manipulating Brain Function: New Neuroscience Technologies and Their Ethical Implications," *Hastings Center Report* 34 (May–June 2004): 35–45.

Judy Illes points out these and other potential problems with neuroimaging in Brain and Cognition: Ethical Challenges in Advanced Neuroimaging (San Diego: Academic Press, 2003). Also, Illes et al., "From Neuroimaging to Neuroethics," Nature Neuroscience 6 (2003): 250, Illes et al., "Ethical and Practical Considerations in Managing Incidental Neurologic Findings in fMRI," Brain and Cognition 50 (2002): 358–65.

the information derived from functional neuroimaging could be a helpful diagnostic tool indeed. But it should supplement, not supplant, existing moral and legal criteria of responsibility. Because it is still an imprecise science, it will be some time before diagnostic brain imaging becomes feasible for these purposes. In particular, if it does become feasible, then as a society we will have to decide how information about the brain can or should be used as evidence in criminal law, analogous to the way in which DNA evidence is now used.

The brain is the most complex and least understood organ in the human body. It is the source of free will, personal identity, and other dimensions of the self, which is why information about the brain is so sensitive and must be protected. In the light of this, neuroscientist Joseph LeDoux points out that brain imaging studies "force us to confront ethical decisions as a society. How far should we go in using brain images to read minds, and how should we use the information we discover? It is testimony to the progress being made that these questions need to be asked."[10]

---

10. *The Synaptic Self: How Our Brains Become Who We Are* (New York: Viking, 2002), 221.

RECOMMENDED SUPPLEMENTARY READING

EMERGING TECHNOLOGIES

Budinger, Thomas F., and Miriam D. Budinger. *Ethics of Emerging Technologies: Scientific Facts and Moral Challenges*. Hoboken, NJ: Wiley, 2006.

Farah, M. J. "Social, Legal, and Ethical Implications of Cognitive Neuroscience: 'Neuroethics' for Short." *Journal of Cognitive Neuroscience* 19, no. 3 (March 2007): 363–364.

Levitt, M., and N. Manson. "My Genes Made Me Do It? The Implications of Behavioural Genetics for Responsibility and Blame." *Health Care Analysis* 15, no. 1 (March 2007): 33–40.

Racine, E. "Identifying Challenges and Conditions for the Use of Neuroscience in Bioethics." *American Journal of Bioethics* 7, no. 1 (January 2007): 74–76.

ENHANCEMENT

Baird, Patricia A. "Altering Human Genes: Social, Ethical, and Legal Implications." *Perspectives in Biology and Medicine.* 37, no. 4 (Summer 1994): 566–575.

Bostrom, N. "Human Genetic Enhancements: A Transhumanist Perspective." *Journal of Value Inquiry* 37, no. 4 (2003): 493–506.

Gardner, William. "Can Human Genetic Enhancement Be Prohibited?" *Journal of Medicine and Philosophy* 20, no. 1 (1995): 65–84.

Garreau, Joel. *Radical Evolution: The Promise and Peril of Enhancing Our Minds, Our Bodies—and What It Means to Be Human*. New York: Doubleday, 2006.

Holtug, Nils. "Does Justice Require Genetic Enhancements?" *Journal of Medical Ethics* 25 (1999): 137–143.

Kamm, Frances M. "Can Enhancement Be Distinguished from Prevention in Genetic Medicine?" *Journal of Medicine and Philosophy* 22, no. 2 (1997): 125–142.

———. "Is There a Problem With Enhancement?" *American Journal of Bioethics* 5, no. 3 (2005): 5–14.

Mehlman, Maxwell. "The Law of Above Averages: Leveling the New Genetic Enhancement Playing Field." *Iowa Law Review* 85 (2000): 517–593.

Miller, Franklin G., and Howard, Brody. "Enhancement Technologies and Professional Integrity." *American Journal of Bioethics* 5, no. 3 (2005): 15–16.

———, eds. *Enhancing Human Traits: Ethical and Social Implications*. Washington, DC: Georgetown University Press, 1998.

Savulescu, J., M. Hemsley, A. Newson, and B. Foddy. "Behavioural Genetics: Why Eugenic Selection Is Preferable to Enhancement." *Journal of Applied Philosophy* 23, no. 2 (2006): 157–171.

Stock, Gregory, and John Campbell, eds. *Engineering the Human Germline: An Exploration of the Science and Ethics of Altering the Genes We Pass to Our Children*. New York: Oxford University Press, 2000.

FREE WILL AND RESPONSIBILITY

Czerner, F. "The Normative Concept of Guilt in Criminal Law Between Freedom of Will and Neurobiological Determinism." *Archiv für Kriminologie* 218, nos. 5–6 (November–December 2006): 129–157.

Hyman, Steven. "The Neurobiology of Addiction: Implications for Voluntary Control of Behavior." *American Journal of Bioethics* 7, no. 1 (2007): 8–11.

Morris, Stephen G. "Neuroscience and the Free Will Conundrum." *American Journal of Bioethics* 7, no. 5 (2007): 20–22.

Reid, Lynette, and Francoise Baylis. "Brains, Genes, and the Making of the Self." *American Journal of Bioethics* 5, no. 2 (2005): 21–22.